an atlas of

ANATOMY
BASIC TO
RADIOLOGY

ISADORE MESCHAN, M.A., M.D.

Professor and Director of the Department of Radiology
at the Bowman Gray School of Medicine of Wake Forest University,
Winston-Salem, North Carolina; Consultant, Walter Reed Army
Hospital; Chairman, Committee on Radiology, National Research
Council, National Academy of Sciences, 1974–1976

· *W. B. SAUNDERS COMPANY* · *Philadelphia* · *London* · *Toronto*

W. B. Saunders Company: West Washington Square
Philadelphia, PA 19105

1 St. Anne's Road
Eastbourne, East Sussex BN21 3UN, England

1 Goldthorne Avenue
Toronto, Ontario M8Z 5T9, Canada

Library of Congress Cataloging in Publication Data

Meschan, Isadore.

An atlas of anatomy basic to radiology.

Includes indexes.

1. Anatomy, Human—Atlases.   I. Title. [DNLM: 1. Radi-
    ography—Atlases.   2. Technology, Radiologic—Atlases.
    WN17 M578ab]

QM25.M47   611′.0022′2   73–89936

ISBN 0–7216–6310–9

Anatomy Basic to Radiology   ISBN 0-7216-6310-9

Last digit is the print number: 9   8   7   6   5   4

To my wife
Dr. Rachel Farrer-Meschan

PREFACE

Among the basic sciences of medicine fundamental to the practice of radiology, the most important is anatomy. In the past I have addressed myself to the anatomic interpretation of normal radiographs, first in the two editions of the *Atlas of Normal Radiographic Anatomy,* and thereafter in an abbreviated version of this, *Radiographic Positioning and Related Anatomy.* Although no attempt was made to include the innumerable variations of normal anatomy, attention was given to changes with growth and development.

In the present text, I have tried to cover the gross anatomy basic to radiologic interpretation in considerably greater depth and from much wider and broader perspectives, recognizing that the radiograph is a two-dimensional representation of all tissues in the coronal and sagittal planes. Vascular anatomy has been added in considerable detail, as have neuroanatomy, the intricacies of the skull, and correlated sagittal and coronal sections of the chest and abdomen. In essence, this is a new text.

The study of anatomy has unique applications to all branches of medicine. It has been my purpose in this text, however, to extract those basic features from the science of anatomy that are especially pertinent to the practice of radiology. It is my hope that the student or practitioner of radiology will find this text of special advantage, since I have culled not only the conventional textbooks of anatomy for this purpose, but also the wider expanse of scientific literature.

Needless to say, on a subject so broad, decisions must be made as to omissions and inclusions; as the author, I accept the responsibility for these decisions based upon my 35 years in the practice and teaching of radiology.

I. MESCHAN

CREDITS
AND
ACKNOWLEDGMENTS

I have borrowed liberally from the broad resources of the literature and in a few instances have sought the critiques of my colleagues as well. To these innumerable sources of information I have tried to make appropriate reference, either in the bibliographies appended to each chapter or in the legends for each illustration as appropriate. The generous cooperation of the authors and publishers of the major anatomy texts in allowing me to reproduce many illustrations is greatly appreciated. Among these, special thanks go to *Cunningham's Textbook of Anatomy* and Cunningham's *Manual of Practical Anatomy, Gray's Anatomy of the Human Body, Morris' Human Anatomy,* Grant's *Atlas of Anatomy,* and Pernkopf's *Atlas of Topographical and Applied Human Anatomy.*

Because this book is also the product of experience during the past 35 years with preceptors no longer living such as Dr. J. P. Quigley and Dr. Eugene Freedman, as well as with students, colleagues, and referring practitioners of all branches of medicine, it is inevitable that some credits will inadvertently be omitted; to these I extend my apologies and my thanks.

There are many books which become absorbed into one's daily experience, among them those written by Dr. L. R. Sante, Jr., Dr. Artur Schüller, Dr. Leo Rigler, and others no longer published; these have undoubtedly played a part in formulating my own ideas and judgments. These treatises are all part of the background of experience, and credit is due to them no less than to those in active use today, to which reference has been made.

Although I have already indicated in the dedication of this book my indebtedness in these endeavors to my wife and collaborator, Dr. Rachel Farrer-Meschan, special reference is required here also for her outright assistance in the writing of the original *Atlas* which has been partially incorporated in the present book.

As always, the various editors and members of W. B. Saunders Company have been extremely helpful in every detail and unstinting in their support. Mr. George Lynch, Mr. Reuben Hawkins, and Mr. Glen Foy—all artists of this and past endeavors —and also the primary sketches of Dr. B. G. Brogdon, now Professor and Chairman of

Radiology of the University of New Mexico, deserve appreciative mention. Special thanks are due to Dr. Thomas T. Thompson and his photographer Mr. Floyd Willard for their generous help in making logetronic prints from the radiographs we have supplied.

Last but not least, the secretaries, Mrs. Edna Snow especially, and also Mrs. Betty Stimson, Mrs. Bernice McCutcheon, and Mrs. Gloria Ruffin, have, in the course of time, applied themselves assiduously to the typing of the text and index, for which great appreciation is due.

I. MESCHAN

CONTENTS

ix

1

Fundamental Background for Radiologic Anatomy

HISTORICAL REVIEW[1]

Wilhelm Konrad Röntgen, while working with a Hittorf-Crookes type light-proof cathode ray tube in 1895, discovered that a piece of cardboard covered with barium platinocyanide crystals would appear fluorescent whenever a charge of cathode rays passed through the tube.

Röntgen discovered that fluorescence would occur despite the placement of certain materials between the tube and the phosphorescent surface, and he collected a variety of substances to show that these substances varied somewhat in their permeability. Aluminum was moderately permeable but a thin sheet of lead was not. The bones of the fingers were revealed when the hand was interposed. Röntgen called these new rays "x-rays" and noted that they would also affect a photographic plate encased in a light-tight cassette. The rays were unlike the cathode rays of the tube in that they could not be deflected by a magnet.

This discovery was the culmination of efforts of many scientists over a period of 300 years and has become the basis of much further research in medical, dental, biologic, chemical, and industrial fields.

Within several years, the far-reaching biologic effects of x-rays on the skin and blood vessels were well known, but the accumulated information along these lines left a trail of martyrs who had exposed themselves in one way or another to these powerful and penetrating rays. A brief discussion of the biologic effects of these rays will be deferred to a later chapter; here, we shall briefly review the manner in which x-rays are produced for medical diagnostic purposes and describe some of the important ancillary materials which enhance the utilization of x-rays in diagnostic radiology.

In the utilization of x-rays as a "dissecting tool" in living tissues, the physician must constantly bear in mind that these rays do not necessarily leave any immediately, visible objective effects on the tissues of the recipient, but may produce delayed effects, particularly when sizeable doses are employed. Fortunately, the amount of radiation employed in diagnostic radiology is minimal but must be taken into account, particularly when these rays are: (1) utilized repeatedly over a long period of time, or (2) utilized in treatment of genetic or embryonic tissues.

NATURE OF X-RAYS

Spectrum of Electromagnetic Radiations. X-rays resemble visible light rays very closely but have the distinguishing feature that their wave lengths are very short—only about 1/10,000 the wave length of visible light. It is this characteristic that permits x-rays to penetrate materials which otherwise would absorb or reflect light. X-rays form a part of the spectrum of electromagnetic radiations, of which the long electric and radio waves are found at one end; the infrared, visible, and ultraviolet light waves in the middle; and the short wave x-rays, gamma rays, and cosmic rays at the other end (Fig. 1–1). These wave lengths are measured in terms of Ångstrom units, where 1 Å is defined as 10^{-8} cm. or 1/100,000,000 cm. The useful range of wave lengths for medical radiography is approximately 0.50 to 0.125 Å.

Propagation of X-rays. It is probable that radiant energy, such as light waves of all kinds, is propagated by means of both waves and corpuscles, with one or the other form predominating, depending upon the energy level of the propagation.

[1]For greater detail see: Glasser, Otto (ed.): The Science of Radiology, Springfield, Illinois, Charles C Thomas, 1933; Bruwer, A. J. (ed.): Classic Descriptions in Diagnostic Radiology, Springfield, Illinois, Charles C Thomas, 1964; Grigg, E. R. N.: The Trail of the Invisible Light, Springfield, Illinois, Charles C Thomas, 1965; Brecher, R., and Brecher, E.: The Rays: A History of Radiology in the U.S. and Canada, Baltimore, Williams and Wilkins Co., 1969.

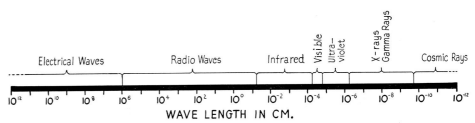

Figure 1–1. Spectrum of electromagnetic radiations.

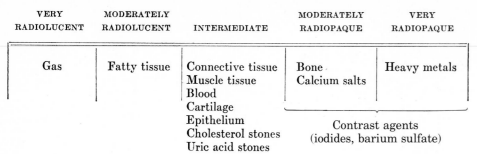

VERY RADIOLUCENT	MODERATELY RADIOLUCENT	INTERMEDIATE	MODERATELY RADIOPAQUE	VERY RADIOPAQUE
Gas	Fatty tissue	Connective tissue Muscle tissue Blood Cartilage Epithelium Cholesterol stones Uric acid stones	Bone Calcium salts	Heavy metals

Contrast agents
(iodides, barium sulfate)

Figure 1–2. Classification of tissues and other substances with medical application in accordance with five general categories of radiopacity and radiolucency.

Radiolucency and Radiopacity. X-rays do not penetrate all matter with similar ease. Some substances such as fats and gases are more readily penetrated than others such as heavy metals, bone, or calcium salts. *Radiolucency* refers to matter which is penetrated by x-rays with relative ease, whereas *radiopacity* is descriptive of matter in which x-rays are absorbed in great measure. Anatomic tissues can be arranged in a scale graduating from the most radiolucent to the most radiopaque (Fig. 1–2), and this difference in opacity when reproduced on photosensitive film makes possible the science of radiography. The x-rays which finally penetrate the anatomic part and produce the x-ray image are spoken of as the "remnant" x-rays (Fig. 1–3).

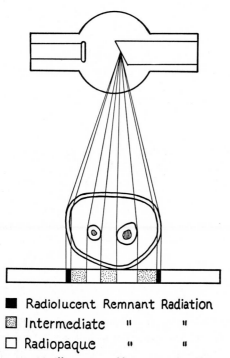

■ Radiolucent Remnant Radiation
▨ Intermediate   "   "
☐ Radiopaque   "   "

Figure 1–3. Diagrammatic illustration of how remnant radiation varies in intensity and radiopacity when x-rays pass through the tissues of the forearm; shown in cross section.

THE PRODUCTION OF X-RAYS

General Principle. In order to produce x-rays, electrons must be obtained and allowed to strike a target with sufficient energy. This is a complex physical process in which most of the electron energy is converted to heat, and a very minute amount (less than 1 per cent) is converted to x-rays.

X-ray Tube. The device in which x-rays are produced is the x-ray tube (Fig. 1–4). This consists of the following essential component parts:

1. An evacuated glass bulb.
2. A negative electrode called the cathode.
3. A positive electrode called the anode.
4. A spiral incandescent filament of tungsten wire, which when heated emits electrons.
5. A means of dissipation of the heat produced when the electrons are made to strike their target, the anode.

Surrounding the filament is a focusing cup (Fig. 1–5) which focuses the electron stream upon the so-called focal spot on the anode. Upon impact with this focal spot, the electrons give rise to a stream of x-rays which are emitted over a 180 degree hemispherical angle surrounding the focal spot. A lead-shielded window (Fig. 1–6) is provided, along with a lead tube casing, so that only a small fraction of these x-rays passes through the portal of the tube.

The actual target is a small rectangular plate of tungsten fused into the beveled end of a large copper bar, causing an angulation of the target of about 20 degrees. This angulation affects the size of the "effective" focal spot. The copper bar acts to dissipate the heat from the target.

The cross-sectional area at the site of origin of the rays (Fig. 1–5) is called the "effective focal spot size" and usually ranges be-

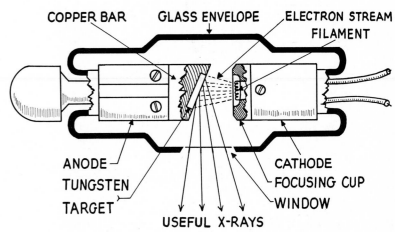

Figure 1–4. Diagram of standard stationary anode x-ray tube.

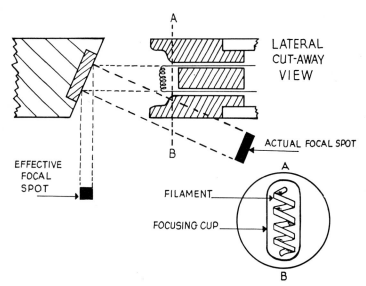

Figure 1–5. Diagram of focusing cup and filament.

tween 0.5 mm. and 2.0 mm., although some special tubes are now made with effective spot sizes of 0.12 mm. which are useful in magnification techniques.

The size of the effective focal spot is responsible for the detail of the roentgen image produced. The smaller the effective focal spot the better the detail, since there is less "shadow effect" (penumbra and umbra) around the image. (See the later section on the geometry of the x-ray image.)

Most x-ray tubes come equipped with two anodes, each of a

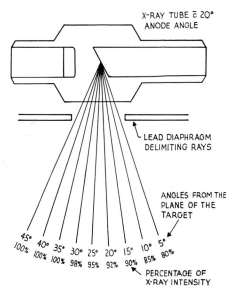

Figure 1–6. Diagram to illustrate stream of x-rays emitted from target through a delimiting lead diaphragm.

different size; since small targets present a greater problem of heat dissipation, the larger target may be necessary when an abundance of x-rays is required to penetrate the large anatomic parts.

The focusing cup helps direct the stream of electrons. Additionally, special grid devices introduced in the x-ray tube facilitate extremely short exposure times when rapid sequential films are necessary.

Electric Circuits

1. *The major electric circuit* (low milliamperage, high voltage) between the anode and the cathode creates a large potential difference, and a stream of electrons known as cathode rays pass from one to the other (see Fig. 1–7).

2. A *filament circuit* provides a means of regulating the number of electrons emitted by a heated filament. This is accomplished by a relatively high amperage (4 to 8 amperes), low voltage circuit from a low voltage step-down transformer.

3. The *rectification circuit* is incorporated to provide a steady stream of electrons in one direction, since the alternating current source of the major x-ray circuit would otherwise cause either an alternation of direction or an intermittent stream of the cathode rays in the x-ray tube.

4. *Timing circuits* are provided to control accurately the duration of the bursts of cathode rays, and thus, x-rays.

5. *Automatic stabilization circuits* supply milliamperage and voltage control for the major x-ray circuit.

6. *External circuitry* is also utilized in relation to image amplification and closed circuit television for fluoroscopy and rapid film sequencing (Fig. 1–7).

The voltage utilized in the major x-ray circuit is measured in terms of thousands of volts (25,000 to 150,000) on most medical diagnostic x-ray machines. This may be regulated at will by various regulatory mechanisms such as the autotransformer.

THE MANNER IN WHICH A BASIC X-RAY MACHINE OPERATES

The Basic Control Panel of an X-ray Machine. There is some variation in control panels of different x-ray machines but there is usually a basic design which can be recognized in all types, if the many automatic features in present day machines are disregarded.

The essential elements of a control panel are shown in Figure 1–7; in the line drawing above the panel, the position of each control is indicated in a schematic diagram. The controls consist of:

1. A main switch to connect the x-ray circuit with the main power supply. This may have a supplemental connection to close the entire x-ray circuit after initially closing only the primary circuit.

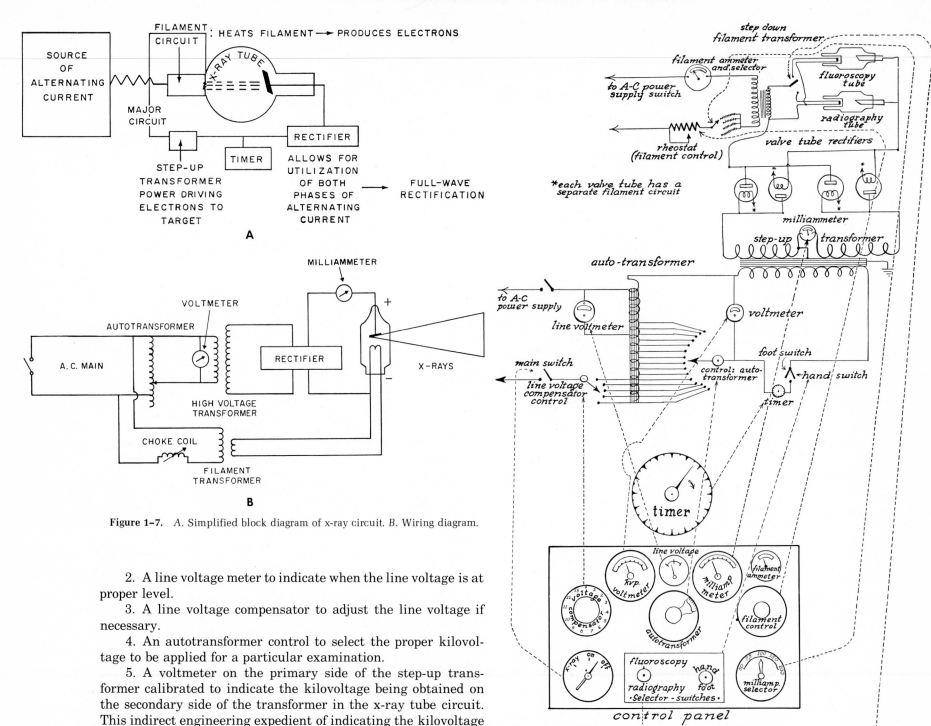

Figure 1–7. *A.* Simplified block diagram of x-ray circuit. *B.* Wiring diagram.

2. A line voltage meter to indicate when the line voltage is at proper level.

3. A line voltage compensator to adjust the line voltage if necessary.

4. An autotransformer control to select the proper kilovoltage to be applied for a particular examination.

5. A voltmeter on the primary side of the step-up transformer calibrated to indicate the kilovoltage being obtained on the secondary side of the transformer in the x-ray tube circuit. This indirect engineering expedient of indicating the kilovoltage in the secondary circuit is necessary because of the difficulty of inserting a suitable high tension voltmeter in a shock-proof manner on the high tension side of the circuit, although this could be done.

6. A timer circuit to cut off automatically the exposure at the preset time.

7. A selector switch to permit selection of either the hand

Figure 1–7 *Continued.* *C.* Diagram illustrating the basic control panel for a universal type x-ray machine, with demonstration of how each item on the panel fits into the basic wiring diagram of a simple x-ray machine.

switch or the foot switch and of either radiography or fluoroscopy. Occasionally, the additional selection of spot-film radiography combined with fluoroscopy is permitted (omitted from the diagram for the sake of clarity).

8. A milliampere selector to indicate automatically the desired milliamperage; this is wired in with an ammeter on the primary side of the filament circuit so that adjustment can be made if necessary by means of the filament control. With age changes in the x-ray tube, slight adjustment may be necessary to obtain the desired milliamperage. In some x-ray machines, this adjustment is automatically obtained. Also, changes in kilovoltage setting require automatic regulation with each change of milliamperage in automatic or monitor controls. In many machines, the filament ammeter does not appear on the control panel, but its equivalent is concealed.

It is possible to trace the action of the operator and the circuit in the following manner:

1. When the operator turns the x-ray switch on, the current passes into the filament circuit and heats the filament, giving rise to an abundance of electrons around the tube filament.

2. Assuming that no further adjustment in line voltage is necessary, the autotransformer is set, the timer is set, the selector switches connected appropriately to either foot switch or hand switch, fluoroscopy or radiography, and the hand or foot switch is turned on.

3. Current passes through the autotransformer and through the primary side of the step-up transformer; then the induced, oppositely directed current passes through the secondary side of the step-up transformer, through the rectifier circuit and then to the x-ray tube.

4. A high potential difference is applied by this means between the tube filament and the target, forcing the electrons derived from the already heated filament to strike the target; thus, x-rays are produced.

Various Methods of Cooling Anode. There are various means of cooling the anode stem (Fig. 1–8):

1. Radial fins outside the glass bulb in continuity with the copper bar (air-cooling).
2. Circulating water within or around the copper bar (water-cooling).
3. Circulating oil around or within the copper bar (oil-cooling).
4. Various combinations of circulating or stationary oil, and circulating water, to cool the oil.

The Rotating Anode. A much more efficient anode is provided if the anode is made to rotate (Fig. 1–9) while the electrons strike the target, so that the electrons never strike a single rectangular area but rather the rim of a wheel which is angled at about 15 degrees. In this type of "rotating anode" tube the effective focal spot can be very small, and yet because the actual

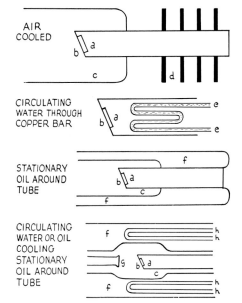

Figure 1–8. Diagram of various types of target-cooling systems. *a*, Copper bar; *b*, tungsten target; *c*, glass envelope—vacuum within; *d*, metal radial fins; *e*, water coils; *f*, oil around tube; *g*, filament; *h*, coils for circulating water or oil within stationary oil.

target is the rim of a wheel it does not heat up as readily as it would in a "stationary anode" type tube.

Advantages and Limitations of Small Focal Spot. As in all instances of light emission, the smaller the light source, the sharper the image produced; just so in radiography, as the focal spot diminishes, the radiographic image becomes sharper. How-

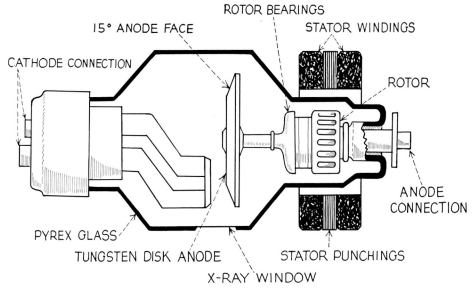

Figure 1–9. Diagram of rotating anode x-ray tube.

ever, the smaller the focal spot, the lower the amount of energy that can be applied without producing damage to the target, so that heat dissipation and mechanical design of the x-ray tube are of fundamental importance in radiography.

Rectification.   The design of the x-ray circuit is also of importance—particularly the mode of rectification—but this is beyond the scope of the present text and can be obtained from many other books devoted to this subject.

SPECIAL PROPERTIES OF X-RAYS IN DIAGNOSTIC RADIOLOGY

The special properties of x-rays which make them so useful in diagnostic radiology are: (1) their *ability to penetrate* organic matter, (2) their ability to produce a *photographic effect* on photosensitive film surfaces, and (3) their ability to produce a *phosphorescence* (fluorescence) in certain crystalline materials.

Penetrability of Tissues and Other Substances by X-rays. Tissues and other substances with medical applications may be classified as indicated in Figure 1–2 on the basis of their density and atomic structure. At one end of the spectrum are the *radiolucent* materials, through which the x-rays pass readily; at the other end are the *radiopaque* substances in which the x-rays are absorbed to a considerable degree in their passage so that little radiation escapes.

The x-rays penetrating an anatomic part may be called the "remnant rays." These are the rays that ultimately affect the x-ray film or fluorescent screen and are responsible for the gradations of black and white on the image. Figure 1–3 is a diagram of x-rays traversing the cross-section of a forearm. The gradations of black, gray, and white as shown on the film beneath the forearm are caused by the remnant radiation after the rays have been absorbed by the interposed tissues such as subcutaneous fat, muscles, and bone. Unfortunately, in the process of passage through an anatomic structure the x-rays (and the secondary electrons produced within the anatomic part) are scattered in all directions, depending upon the energy of the primary x-ray beam. Such *scattered radiation* causes a loss of detail. Special devices must be interposed between the x-ray source and the film to eliminate the scattered rays from the final image. *Coning devices and stationary and moving grids (Potter-Bucky diaphragm),* which help to eliminate such scattered radiation, will be described later.

Photographic Effect of X-rays.   Just as visible or ultraviolet rays alter light-sensitive photographic emulsion, so do roentgen rays, so that when appropriately "developed," "fixed," and "washed," a permanent image is produced. The film employed for this purpose is ordinarily made with a thicker emulsion, although this is not absolutely necessary. The utilization of intensifying fluorescent screens (to be described below) has largely replaced such direct radiography, since less x-irradiation is necessary for

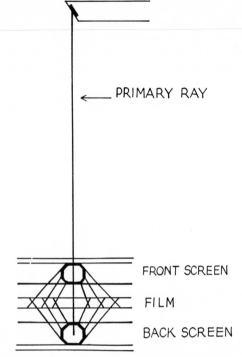

Figure 1–10.   Diagram illustrating fluorescence from intensifying screen.

radiography by intensification techniques. However, when the body part under study (such as an extremity) is not large, and when optimum detail is required, direct radiography may be preferable. Direct radiography is also preferable when it is necessary to be certain that no dust or other similar artefacts may be interposed or projected on the x-ray image.

Fluorescent Effects of X-rays (Fig. 1–10).   When roentgen rays strike certain crystalline materials, phosphorescence results. The spectrum of light so produced will vary with the crystalline substance; at times, it is mostly ultraviolet, at other times, mostly visible, light. Ultraviolet light has proved to be most advantageous in respect to x-ray film emulsion. An intensifying screen consists mostly of a thin coating of crystals on a cardboard surface (Fig. 1–11). Its function is to provide a brighter image than would result from the direct photographic effects of the x-rays alone. Intensifying screens are categorized according to brightness (called "speed") and detail, each being inverse to the other and thus requiring some compromise.

Prior to the advent of image amplification, which has re-

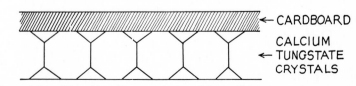

Figure 1–11.   Diagrammatic presentation of intensifying screen in cross section.

placed conventional fluoroscopy, the crystalline substance chosen for its fluorescence produced light in the visible light range. In image amplification requiring electromagnetic enhancement, the "input phosphorescent" and "output phosphorescent" screens are similarly constructed.

Other Fundamental Properties of X-rays. Other fundamental properties of x-rays to be briefly mentioned here are: (1) ionization, (2) chemical effects, (3) heat production, and (4) biologic effects.

Ionization is a primary effect of x-rays whenever these photons strike matter with sufficient energy. It produces various observable phenomena, depending upon the matter affected. Ionization of air by x-rays has been used in the quantitative measurement of radiation.

Chemical effects are produced by x-rays by altering atomic structure. Salt, for example, ordinarily turns yellow from liberation of chlorine.

Heat production is a secondary phenomenon whenever x-rays strike matter. The heat produced in the x-ray tube target is so great that special cooling devices have to be provided. On the other hand, heat production in organic matter may be infinitesimally small—so small that it is difficult to measure.

Biologic effects may be among the most important changes wrought by x-rays, and they are utilized constantly in x-ray therapy. Radiation in diagnostic radiology, however, seldom produces detectable or measureable biologic effects and, hence, further discussion falls outside the scope of this text, except as pertains to radiologic protection (Chapter 2).

ACCESSORIES NECESSARY FOR THE RECORDING OF THE X-RAY IMAGE

The accessories which make radiography and fluoroscopy possible are:

1. The x-ray film.
2. The x-ray cassette, with its enclosed intensifying screens.
3. The x-ray film not requiring an intensifying screen or conventional cassette but placed in a plastic or cardboard folder.
4. The stationary and moving grids, such as the Potter-Bucky diaphragm.
5. Various cones, apertures, and adjustable diaphragms for delimiting the x-ray beam to the body part in question.
6. Body section radiographic equipment.
7. Stereoscopic radiographic accessories.
8. The fluoroscopic screen and the fluoroscope.
9. Image amplifiers used in conjunction with fluoroscopy and radiography.
10. Equipment for television fluoroscopy and radiography with television tape recording.
11. Accessories for spot film radiography.
12. Devices for photographing the output phosphor of an image amplifier; the radiographs may be miniature in size, such as 16 mm., 35 mm., 70 mm., 90 mm., or 100 mm., or cineradiographic sequences.
13. Rapid sequence film changers for either roll film or cut film, or rapid sequence cassette changers for recording rapidly changing x-ray images.
14. Magnification accessories.
15. Contrast media.

Each of these devices will now be briefly illustrated and discussed.

X-ray Film. X-ray film consists of a transparent cellulose acetate or plastic base coated on each side with a photosensitive emulsion such as silver bromide crystals. Rarely, single emulsion films are employed. The emulsion is designed to be most efficiently photosensitized in an ultraviolet radiation range by the light rays emitted by the intensifying screens, when these latter structures are activated by x-rays. X-ray film, with a somewhat different emulsion, is utilized when the film is contained in a light-proof folder without intensifying screens, in which case the film is photosensitized by the x-rays directly. X-ray film is developed in a special developing solution which precipitates the exposed crystals; the unused developing solution clinging to the film is rapidly washed away, and the precipitated silver halide crystals are "fixed" in "hypo" solution. The film is then washed and dried prior to viewing and interpretation. Film processing from start to finish may now be carried out very efficiently in 90 seconds, or even less with appropriate automated equipment.

The X-ray Cassette (Fig. 1–12). The x-ray cassette is a light-proof container for the film, designed to permit easy loading and unloading, while near perfect contact is maintained with the intensifying screens. When the x-ray beam strikes the intensifying screen, ultraviolet and visible light rays are produced and the film is photosensitized. A suitable "x-ray" image is thereby produced, employing fewer x-rays than are necessary when no intensifying screens are used. Unfortunately, any direct particles upon the film or intensifying screen, or defects in either film or screen will also produce an image on the film, so that the x-ray cassette must be cleaned and handled with extreme care.

X-ray Film in a Cardboard or Plastic Holder. When minute foreign bodies are to be detected by x-ray examination, x-ray film in a cardboard or plastic holder is used whenever possible because it eliminates potential artefacts. This film, of course, requires greater radiation exposure for adequate imaging.

The Stationary and Moving Grids (Fig. 1–13) X-rays are scattered in all directions when they strike an object. The grid is a device for collimating the x-rays after transmission through the

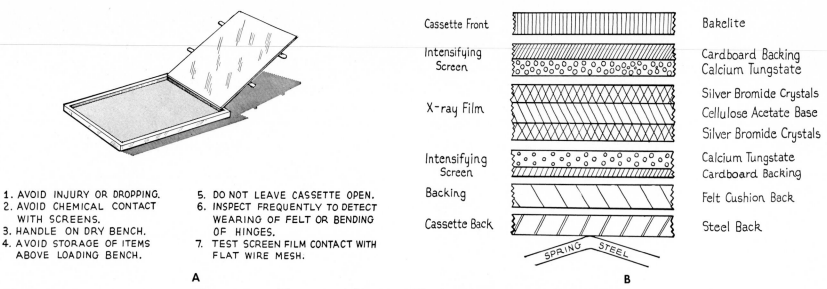

1. AVOID INJURY OR DROPPING.
2. AVOID CHEMICAL CONTACT WITH SCREENS.
3. HANDLE ON DRY BENCH.
4. AVOID STORAGE OF ITEMS ABOVE LOADING BENCH.

5. DO NOT LEAVE CASSETTE OPEN.
6. INSPECT FREQUENTLY TO DETECT WEARING OF FELT OR BENDING OF HINGES.
7. TEST SCREEN FILM CONTACT WITH FLAT WIRE MESH.

A   B

Figure 1-12.   *A.* The cassette and its care. *B.* Diagrammatic cross section of x-ray cassette.

patient so that the image on the film is formed by "orderly" rays which have penetrated the body part. The grid is composed of alternating strips of lead with intervening pieces of wood, bakelite, or plastic. The grid is placed between the part to be radiographed and the film, usually under the table top.

When a focused grid is employed, only the rays in direct radial alignment with the target can pass through the grid, since the scattered rays are absorbed by the lead strips. When the lead strips are parallel with one another, the grid is called unfocused and the target must then be at a distance of at least 40 inches or more from the grid. The diaphragm moves or oscillates during the exposure and thus no lines related to the lead strips are visible on the film. Grids are further characterized by their grid ratio, as shown in the insert, and also by the number of lines per square unit of area. Very fine grids with 140 lines per square inch are available.

Stationary grids usually have very fine lead lines that are barely detectable on the film. Moving grids (the Potter-Bucky diaphragms) are used whenever possible. These are usually oscillating types in modern equipment.

When a stationary grid is incorporated into the cassette front, it is called a grid-cassette. Eight to 10 Kvp. are ordinarily required to compensate for grid absorption.

Cones, Apertures, and Adjustable Diaphragms for Delimiting the X-ray Beam (Figs. 1–14, 1–15).   Cones and aperture dia-

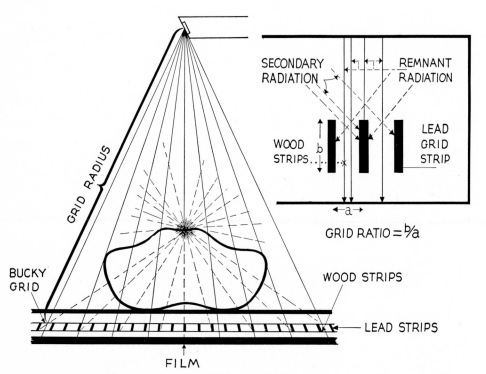

$$\text{GRID RATIO} = b/a$$

Figure 1-13.   Diagram of a Potter-Bucky diaphragm and how it is used.

X-RAY CONING DEVICES

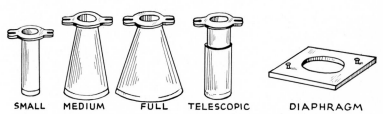

SMALL   MEDIUM   FULL   TELESCOPIC   DIAPHRAGM

Figure 1-14.   Various accessories used to delimit secondary irradiation.

Figure 1–15. *A.* An adjustable cone for various field sizes with a light localizer and centering device. *B.* Diagram illustrating effect of cone in delimiting scattered radiation. *C.* Photograph of another type of adjustable collimator.

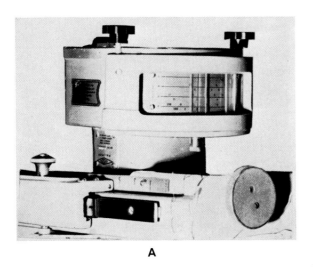

A

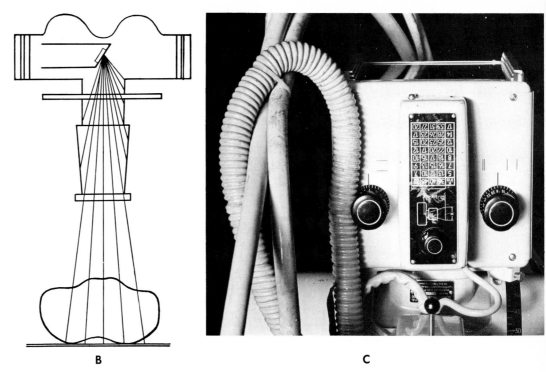

B   **C**

phragms are applied to the x-ray tube window in order to delimit the x-ray beam and reduce the secondary radiation. These coning devices are available in various designs, so it is desirable to choose the cone best suited both to the anatomic part and to the size of the film being exposed. Adjustable cones equipped with light localizers are also available for this purpose; these may be cylindrical in cross section as shown, or rectangular (Fig. 1–15).

Cones have the additional advantage of reducing the stray radiation toward the operator, and thus furnish a very important protective mechanism as well.

Body Section Radiographic Equipment (Fig. 1–16). The body section radiograph is known by various names, depending on slightly different operating principles (i.e., polytome, laminograph, stratograph, tomograph). The main factor in each of these is the movement of the x-ray tube and the x-ray film around a fixed axis or center in either planar or polycycloidal movement. By this means a planar surface or small area of the anatomy is brought into clear perspective while adjoining areas are blurred. In the radiography of the middle ear or larynx the "cuts" are usually no more than 0.5 mm. apart, whereas in larger body volumes such as the chest the usual cuts may be as great as 1 cm. or more apart.

Stereoscopic Radiographic Accessories (Fig. 1–17). To obtain radiographs that can give a true stereoscopic effect, two slightly different views are obtained—first the view as seen by one

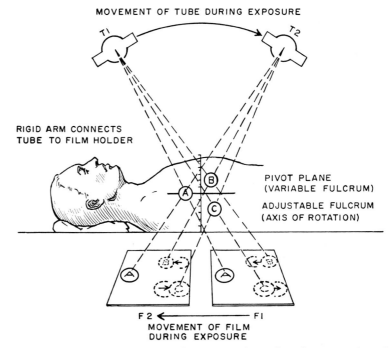

Figure 1–16. The principles of body section radiography. The image of an object such as *A*, located on the pivot plane, remains in focus during movement of tube and film. An object above the pivot plane, *B*, or below, *C*, blurs owing to its realignment between tube and film as they move during exposure.

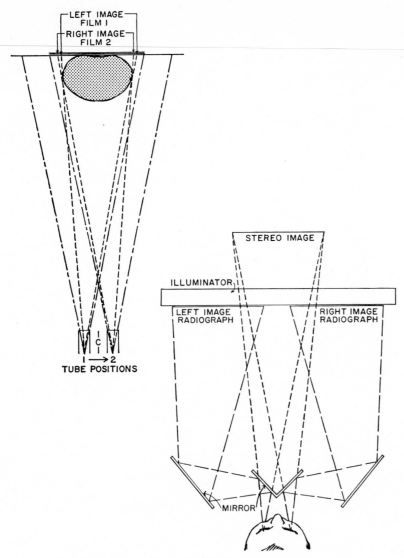

Figure 1–17. The principles of roentgen stereoscopy.

anatomic part in motion. After passing through the patient, the remnant rays strike a special screen composed of fluorescent crystals that transform the x-rays into visible light. Leaded glass protects the observer's head and eyes in the conventional fluoroscope, but electronic amplification of the fluoroscopic image has virtually replaced this older type of equipment.

Electronic Amplification of the Fluoroscopic Image (Fig. 1–19). Instead of the image appearing directly after it strikes the fluoroscopic screen, it is electronically amplified and directed toward an "output phosphor," which may then be viewed through appropriate lens and mirror systems, or by a television camera.

Television Camera. The image may thus be projected by closed circuit television systems to appropriately placed monitors.

Spot Film Radiography. This refers to instantaneous radiography while the patient is being examined by fluoroscopy. Spot film radiography is accomplished by storing a cassette in a lead-protected frame on the fluoroscopic screen, or on the frame support of the image tube. When radiography is desired, a rapid spring release brings the cassette over the patient, and the x-ray technique selector switch rapidly and automatically switches from fluoroscopic exposure values to radiographic factors, and the exposure is made. Often photoelectric ion chambers (or cells) are interposed, so that the exposure is automatically timed to produce an optimum radiographic image.

Radiography with the Image Amplifier. When the image amplifier is used, a movie camera or any other suitable still cam-

eye, and second, that seen by the other eye. This is done by taking two radiographs from two separate tube positions; the amount of tube shift is based on a definite ratio of the normal interpupillary distance. These two radiographs are then placed in a stereoscope or viewed with special prismatic lenses or mirrors so that each eye will see the separate image. The brain fuses the two images into one and the correct spatial, three-dimensional relationship is reconstructed. Unfortunately, not all individuals have this capacity for stereoscopic viewing.

The Fluoroscopic Screen and the Fluoroscope (Fig. 1–18). Fluoroscopy is the study of the x-ray image after its transformation into visible light. By this means the physician may study an

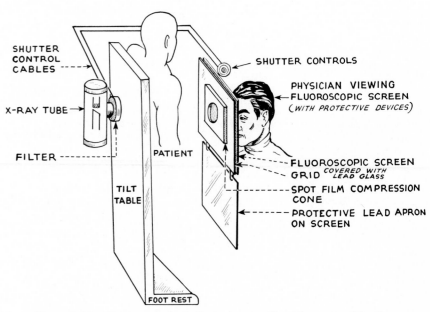

Figure 1–18. Diagram of a basic fluoroscope, without image amplification.

era may be focused on the output phosphor of the image tube, and the image may be totally or in part transmitted to the camera, even while it is being viewed by the television camera system. It is also possible to photograph the television monitor (called *kineradiography*).

Rapid Sequence Film Changers for Roll Film or Cut Film, or Rapid Sequence Cassette Changers. Rapid sequence film changers allow x-ray films to be interposed between two intensifying screens in rapid sequence, and rapid sequence cassette changers allow cassettes to be changed rapidly and mechanically. Films may be changed as rapidly as 12 per second, and cassettes as fast as two per second, simultaneously in each of two planes if desired. Programmers are provided with changers so that appropriate sequences may be chosen. Long films (as long as three 14- by 17-inch films in tandem) may thus be exposed in one apparatus, and may include, for example, the lower aorta and an entire lower extremity simultaneously and in rapid sequence.

Magnification (Fig. 1–20). Magnification of an anatomic part results when the film is placed at a considerable distance from the part. The degree of magnification is directly related to the square of the distance between the film and the focal spot of the x-ray tube, as compared with the distance between the anatomic part and the x-ray tube. When the film-to-focal spot distance is equal to the film-to-anatomic part distance, a magnification of 4 times will result. The limiting factor in this procedure is the size of the focal spot of the x-ray tube, which must be virtually pinpoint in size for optimum detail with magnification. Special high speed fractional focal spot tubes have been manufactured for this purpose, with effective focal spots approaching 0.1 mm. Heat dissipation must be very efficient for x-ray tubes of this design. Magnification of small anatomic parts with films in rapid sequence is becoming available.

Magnification of the x-ray film itself is limited by the grain size of the x-ray film emulsion; usually 6 to 8 times is the maximum magnification possible.

Contrast Media. A body part may be visualized radiographically in the following ways:

1. By its delineation by a naturally occurring fatty envelope or fascia.
2. By its naturally occurring gaseous content, such as lungs and gastrointestinal tract.
3. By its naturally occurring mineral salts, such as the calcium salts of bone.
4. By abnormally occurring gas, fat, or calcium salts in certain pathologic processes.
5. By the introduction of a contrast agent, which may be either *radiolucent* or *radiopaque,* into or around the body part. Such contrast agents should be physiologically inert and harmless. The addition of contrast agents has permitted great strides in anatomic depiction.

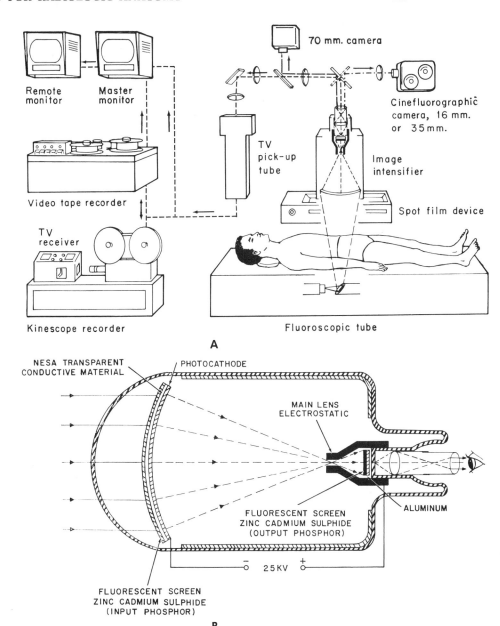

Figure 1–19. *A.* Diagram of presently available fluoroscopic equipment, containing image amplification, cinefluoroscopy, cineradiography, and kineradiography. The amplified image from the output phosphor may be conducted through a lens and mirror system directly to the human eye, directly to a stationary or movie camera device, through a television camera to a television receiver, or through a television camera to a television tape recorder. The image on the television screen may be viewed by the human eye or by an additional camera. *B.* Diagram of image intensifier tube. X-rays which pass through an object form an image on the input phosphor screen emitting visible light proportional to the impinging radiation. The photocathode in contact with this screen is an alkali metal layer that emits electrons proportional to the brightness of the fluorescing screen. This electron image is focused by electrostatic lenses on the output phosphor screen. The electrons are also accelerated by a potential difference of 25,000 volts, and a further increase in brightness results. The proper optical system permits the eye to view the brilliant image. To obtain cineradiography or television fluoroscopy one needs only to substitute a movie or television camera for the eye, or a mirror system, to obtain simultaneous viewing and filming.

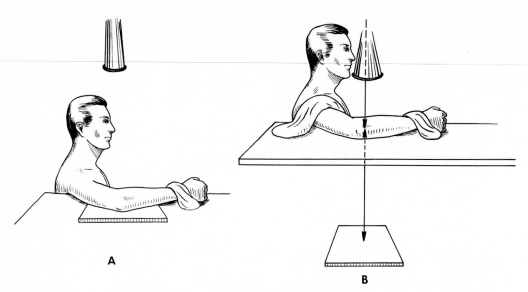

Figure 1–20. *A.* When the film is in close contact with the part being radiographed, and the x-ray tube target is 36 to 40 inches from the film, very little magnification of the part ensues. *B.* When the film is at a considerable distance from the part being radiographed, and the target-to-film distance is 24 to 30 inches, considerable magnification results.

Commonly Used Radiopaque Contrast Media

Barium sulfate is particularly useful in studies of the gastrointestinal tract. It is inert, is not absorbed, and does not alter the normal physiologic function. At times it is used in colloidal suspension to obtain a particular type of mucosa coating, which is most effective for demonstration of small filling defects.

Organic iodides, which are *predominantly excreted by the liver or secreted selectively by the kidneys,* include Hypaque (sodium diatrizoate), Renografin (meglumine diatrizoate), and iothalamates, such as Conray or Angioconray. These compounds are also widely favored for visualization of blood vessels. In low concentrations they may be used for visualization of hepatic and biliary radicles by T-tube and operative cholangiography.

Organic iodides in suspension may be particularly useful in visualization of oviducts (hysterosalpingography) or the urethra (Salpix, Skiodan Acacia, Cystokon, and Thixokon).

Iodized oils, slowly absorbable, are used in myelography (Pantopaque) or bronchography (Dionosil oily).

Radiolucent contrast substances are *gases:* air, oxygen, helium, carbon dioxide, nitrous oxide, and nitrogen. These are commonly used for visualization of the brain (pneumoencephalograms and ventriculograms), joints (arthrograms), and occasionally, the subarachnoid space surrounding the spinal cord (air myelograms). Air may also be used in the pleural space, peritoneal cavity, and pericardial space. Carbon dioxide is of particular value since it is well tolerated and very rapidly absorbed.

OTHER ANCILLARY ITEMS OF X-RAY EQUIPMENT

Shutter Mechanism Over X-ray Tube. Immediately in front of the x-ray tube under the table is a lead shutter mechanism which may be opened and closed in both the vertical and horizontal directions. The shutter is controlled either electrically or by cables connected to knobs on the fluoroscopic screen. The lead is sufficiently thick to prevent any primary radiation from escaping in a forward direction and is so constructed that secondary emanations are also largely absorbed. Thus, the field of vision of the fluoroscopic screen is delimited by these controls beside the screen. This field should always be no larger than is absolutely necessary for visualization of the part in question, and the margins of the shutter itself should always be visible on the screen. The smaller the field, the better the detail—an added inducement for maintaining this standard.

Filtration. Additional filters should always be added in front of the fluoroscopic tube to the extent of 4 mm. of aluminum or more. Only the more highly penetrating rays are effective in radiography and fluoroscopy, and the addition of such filters removes a higher percentage of the less penetrating rays than of the more penetrating. Moreover, the patient's skin has a higher tolerance for the more penetrating rays (this will be more fully described in Chapter 2).

Physical Factors. Ordinarily, 2 milliamperes of current or less are adequate for fluoroscopy. It is common practice to use 85 kilovolts peak for abdominal fluoroscopy, 70 kilovolts for chest, and 60 kilovolts for the extremities. In examining children with the fluoroscope, 0.5 milliamperes and 60 kilovolts need never be exceeded. A small field is imperative for protection of the gonads since a much greater proportion of the entire body of a child is covered by radiation when any single part is radiographed.

Use of X-ray Protective Devices. X-ray protective devices such as lead-lined gloves, lead rubber, or lead glass fiber aprons,

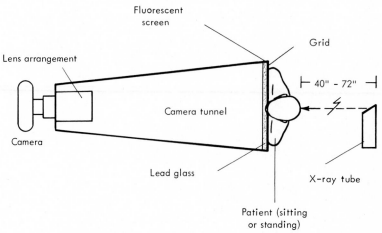

Figure 1–21. Miniature (indirect) radiographs.

and small lead rubber shields dangling beneath the fluoroscopic screen are imperative (see Chapter 2). The operator should never permit his unprotected hands, wrists, or other parts to be exposed to the x-ray beam. Palpation with the hand or other manipulation under the fluoroscope, setting fractures, localizing foreign bodies, or other procedures should be avoided. Intermittent and serial radiography is much to be preferred to such dangerous exposure.

Photoroentgenograms. In photoroentgenography a photograph of the fluoroscopic image is obtained by means of a specially enclosed and constructed camera. Usual film sizes employed for this purpose are 4 × 5 inches, 100 mm., 90 mm., 70 mm., and 35 mm. Photoroentgenography offers an economical method for radiographic survey of large populations. Various optical lens systems and reflex objective systems have been designed to achieve this purpose (Fig. 1–21).

The main disadvantages of this method are (1) loss of accuracy in detail, and (2) increased radiation exposure of the patient. New developments with electronic image amplification and television may overcome these disadvantages, and this method offers great promise for the future.

Roentgen Xeroradiography. In xeroradiography, an x-ray image is produced using a photoconductive surface of selenium on an aluminum plate as a substitute for x-ray film. The plate is contained in a cassette to protect it from casual damage or ambient light (Fig. 1–22). With the cassette open, an electrostatic charge is first placed on the surface of the selenium in darkness. The

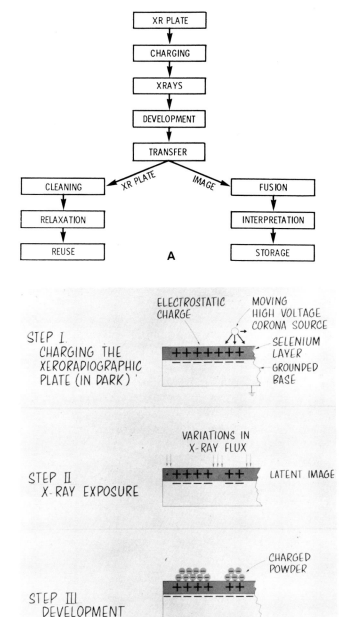

A

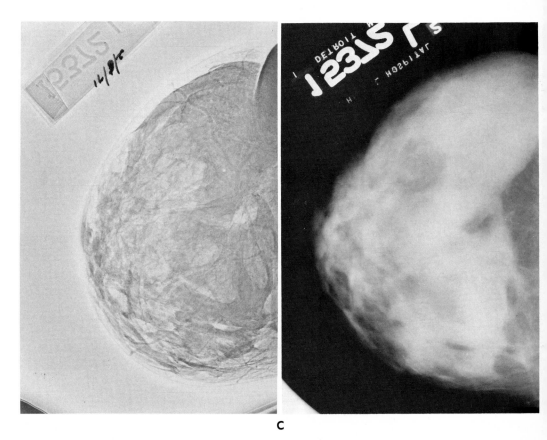

B

C

Figure 1–22. *A.* Schematic view of xeroradiographic process. *B.* Xeroradiographic process. *C.* Comparison of xeroradiographic and film mammograms. The advantages of xeroradiography are shown by these comparison images. All densities are recorded in good detail on the XR (*left*). Note the facility with which the skin, veins, and ducts can be identified as well as the deep structures near the chest wall. The slight thickening of the skin near the inframammary fold is normal. (From Wolfe, J. M.: Xeroradiography of the Breast, 1972. Courtesy of Charles C Thomas, Publisher, Springfield, Illinois.)

plate is then exposed to an x-ray beam in conventional fashion. The selenium photoconductor is discharged thereby in amounts corresponding to the remnant radiation passing through the patient's anatomic part. The remnant radiation produces an electrostatic charge pattern depicting the anatomic part being examined. To make this pattern visible the plate is then developed in a closed chamber into which a blue, finely divided charged plastic powder, called "toner," is sprayed. A powder image on the plate surface is produced in this way (Fig. 1–22 B).

A permanent record of the image may be obtained by transferring the image from the plate to paper or plastic. This may be done by bringing the paper into contact with the toner image and applying pressure, or by charging the back of the paper during the moment of contact. The transferred powder image is then fixed, typically by heating or momentarily softening the plastic layer encapsulating the toner. The residual toner is then removed by brushing the plate appropriately. Actually, the original selenium plate may be reused by heating the photoconductor to about 135 degrees for 30 seconds.

The xeroradiographic image resembles a film image except that (1) there is a greater resolution, (2) small point densities appear to be easier to recognize by virtue of their high contrast, and (3) there is good detail on the image.

This process is gaining application in radiography of the extremities (orthopedic radiology) and in soft tissue roentgenography such as mammography, where it has shown excellent results (Fig. 1–22 C) (Wolfe).

Subtraction Techniques. The principle of subtraction technique has been carefully elucidated by DesPlantes. He demonstrated that in radiographs obtained prior to and after the introduction of a contrast agent, the appearance of the contrast agent can be intensified more clearly by removing interfering bony shadows in the following manner (Fig. 1–23). A negative transparent "diapositive" is obtained from the control radiograph, and this negative is superimposed on the radiograph containing the contrast agent. Since in a negative diapositive the bony structures appear black, this blackness will ordinarily neutralize the bony structures as visualized on the second film when light is transmitted through the two films superimposed over one another. In a third film obtained from the first two, this neutralization process results in virtual obliteration of the bony shadows and a clear demonstration of the contrast agent.

A further modification of this technique has been suggested by Oldendorf and is illustrated in Figure 1–24. In this modification, a second order diapositive is introduced to subtract more of the detail not subtracted by the first. The initial dye-free control film is contact-printed onto a Dupont commercial S film or Eastman commercial film. These two diapositives combined are then superimposed over the succeeding films in an angiographic series to obtain the final subtracted film.

In each instance the control film prior to the introduction of the contrast agent must be obtained in exactly the same position as the later films with the contrast agent in order to get ideal subtraction.

Television subtraction that accomplishes a subtracted image instantaneously is also available.

Rapid Automatic Film Processing. After a latent image is deposited on the film by the x-rays, the cassette or film holder is taken to the darkroom where the film is carefully removed under light conditions that do not allow fogging of the film. The film is loaded directly into automated apparatus (Fig. 1–25 A) and a completely dried and processed film is available for viewing at the

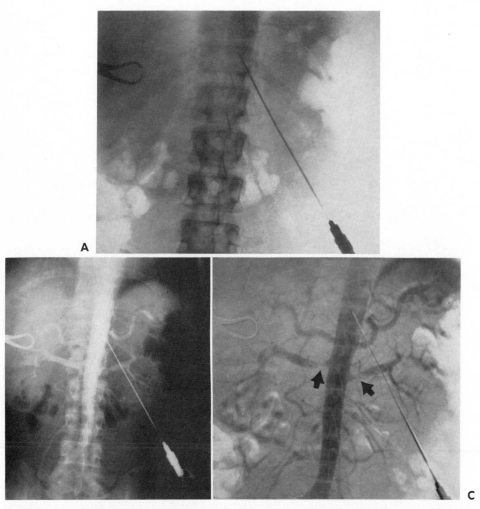

Figure 1–23. Subtraction technique for more accurate delineation of vascular branches. A scout film is first obtained in a position identical to that to be used for delineation of the contrast-filled vascular region. This is reversed so that a negative film (A) is obtained. In this film the bones appear black and the gas shadows appear white. Thereafter, the aortogram (B) is obtained in routine fashion. By superposition of film A over film B, the bone shadows are neutralized and "subtracted out." Film C is thereby obtained. The arrows point to bilateral renal artery stenosis noted more clearly on the postsubtraction film C.

end of 90 seconds. During this process the film is transported through developing, fixing, washing, and drying operations (Fig. 1–25 *B*). Exposure factors must be optimum and control conditions ideal to produce a good radiograph with such automatic film processors.

Wet film processing may still be employed (Fig. 1–25 *B*), and requires that the film be allowed to remain in a developing solution for a definite period of time, depending upon the temperature and degree of exhaustion of the developer. The film is then removed from the developer and inserted into a stop bath, where it is quickly rinsed and transferred to a fixing solution for approximately 10 minutes. It is allowed to fix in hypo solution for at least twice the developing time and then transferred to the "wash" for at least one-half hour, after which it is dried. The rapid processing of film is, however, almost universal now, except with industrial and some thick emulsion films.

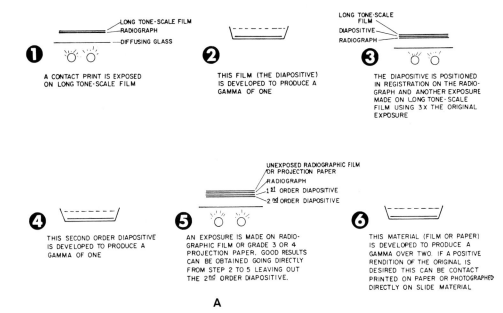

❶ A CONTACT PRINT IS EXPOSED ON LONG TONE-SCALE FILM

❷ THIS FILM (THE DIAPOSITIVE) IS DEVELOPED TO PRODUCE A GAMMA OF ONE

❸ THE DIAPOSITIVE IS POSITIONED IN REGISTRATION ON THE RADIOGRAPH AND ANOTHER EXPOSURE MADE ON LONG TONE-SCALE FILM USING 3X THE ORIGINAL EXPOSURE

❹ THIS SECOND ORDER DIAPOSITIVE IS DEVELOPED TO PRODUCE A GAMMA OF ONE

❺ AN EXPOSURE IS MADE ON RADIOGRAPHIC FILM OR GRADE 3 OR 4 PROJECTION PAPER. GOOD RESULTS CAN BE OBTAINED GOING DIRECTLY FROM STEP 2 TO 5 LEAVING OUT THE 2nd ORDER DIAPOSITIVE.

❻ THIS MATERIAL (FILM OR PAPER) IS DEVELOPED TO PRODUCE A GAMMA OVER TWO. IF A POSITIVE RENDITION OF THE ORIGINAL IS DESIRED THIS CAN BE CONTACT PRINTED ON PAPER OR PHOTOGRAPHED DIRECTLY ON SLIDE MATERIAL

A

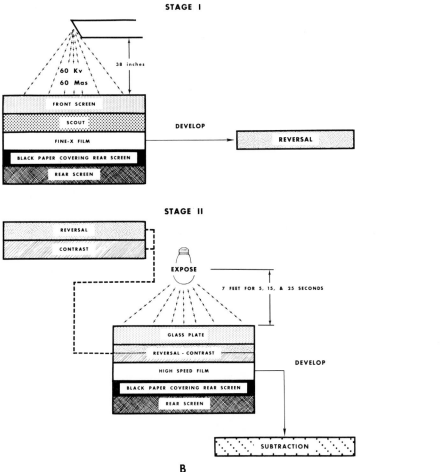

B

Figure 1–24. *A*. Steps in the modified subtraction method as recommended by Oldendorf. With complete subtraction by a good pair of diapositives, greater enhancement will result from using contrast paper in steps 5 or 6. (From Oldendorf, W. H.: Neurology 15:367, 1965.) *B*. Diagrammatic representation of the stages and steps of the subtraction technique. (From Crittenden, J. J., and Stern, C. A.: Amer. J. Roentgenol., 97:523, 1966.)

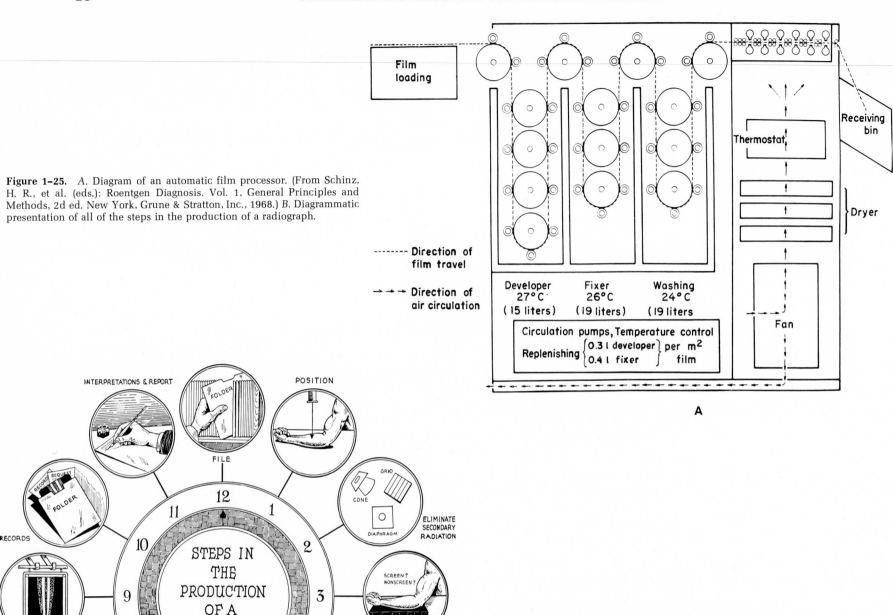

Figure 1–25. *A.* Diagram of an automatic film processor. (From Schinz, H. R., et al. (eds.): Roentgen Diagnosis. Vol. 1, General Principles and Methods, 2d ed. New York, Grune & Stratton, Inc., 1968.) *B.* Diagrammatic presentation of all of the steps in the production of a radiograph.

THE FUNDAMENTAL GEOMETRY OF X-RAY IMAGE FORMATION AND INTERPRETATION

Image Sharpness. X-rays obey the common laws of light. The manner in which any object placed in the path of the x-ray beam is projected depends on: (1) the size of the light source (focal spot), i.e., whether pinpoint or a larger surface, (2) the alignment of the object with respect to the light source (focal spot) and the screen or film, (3) the distance of the object from the light source, (4) the distance of the object from the screen or film, and (5) the plane of the object with respect to the screen or film.

When an image is projected from a pinpoint light source, the borders of the image are sharp, but if the light source is a larger surface, as in the case of the focal spot of an x-ray tube, the image is ill-defined at its periphery owing to penumbra formation (Fig. 1–26). Measures must be taken to reduce the penumbra as much as possible. To accomplish this the focal spot must be as small as possible, and the object-to-film distance as short as possible. The object-to-focal spot distance should be as long as possible (Fig. 1–27). Also, the film should be perpendicular to the central ray arising from the focal spot.

Image Distortion. When the object is not centrally placed with respect to the central ray its image will be distorted, and this distortion may be considerable (Fig. 1–28). Sometimes this distortion is unavoidable if one is to visualize a part, and in some of the radiographic positions, this distortion brings a part into view which otherwise would be hidden (Fig. 1–29). Thus, the phenomenon of projection may be utilized to good advantage.

Image Magnification. The farther an object is from the light source and the closer it is to the film, the less will be the magnification (Fig. 1–27). The magnification of an object as much as 15 cm. from the film when a relatively usual focal spot-film distance is employed (such as 36 inches) is approximately 20 per cent. Such magnification must be considered in interpreting the size of the heart, the pelvis or any other structure which is to be measured.

These various phenomena of magnification, projection, dis-

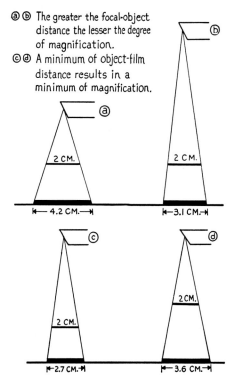

ⓐ ⓑ The greater the focal-object distance the lesser the degree of magnification.

ⓒ ⓓ A minimum of object-film distance results in a minimum of magnification.

Figure 1–27. Diagram illustrating effect of focal-object distance and object-film distance on magnification.

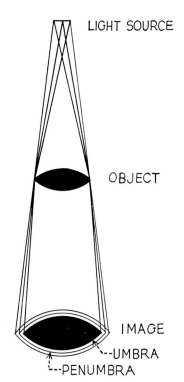

Figure 1–26. Diagram of penumbra formation from surface light source.

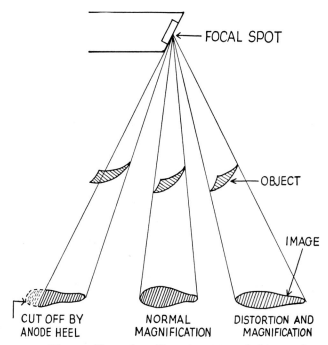

Figure 1–28. Diagram illustrating effect of position of object with respect to central ray on distortion, magnification, and anode-heel effect.

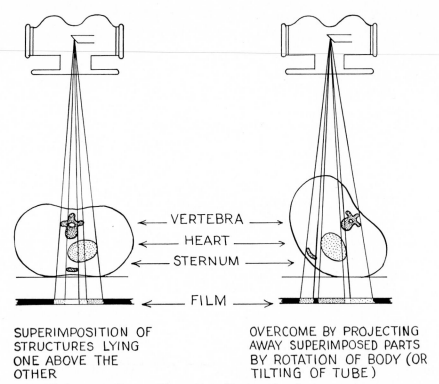

SUPERIMPOSITION OF
STRUCTURES LYING
ONE ABOVE THE
OTHER

OVERCOME BY PROJECTING
AWAY SUPERIMPOSED PARTS
BY ROTATION OF BODY (OR
TILTING OF TUBE)

Figure 1–29. Diagram illustrating utilization of projection to overcome superimposition of anatomic parts.

tortion, and penumbra formation must be constantly borne in mind in viewing radiographic images.

STEPS IN THE PRODUCTION OF A RADIOGRAPH

There are many steps in the production and final interpretation of a radiograph (Fig. 1–25 *B*), and it is well to have some concept of all of them. Given the problem of the radiography of an anatomic part, the following steps are pursued:

1. The patient is placed in a position with respect to the central ray of the x-ray tube in full accordance with our knowledge of the gross anatomy.

2. The most suitable method of eliminating secondary radiation is chosen, whether it be a diaphragm, cone, grid, or all three. In some types of movable grids, a grid movement time must be chosen depending upon the exposure time, and the moving mechanism must be cocked.

3. The proper type of film and the film holder or cassette are placed in position with respect to the central ray, either directly under the anatomic part, or under the grid in a special carriage.

4. Optimum exposure factors are chosen: (*a*) milliamperage; (*b*) kilovoltage; (*c*) time; (*d*) distance; and (*e*) focal spot after the anatomic part has been measured as to its relative size.

5. A latent image is obtained on the film by the x-rays.

6. The cassette or film holder is taken to the darkroom where the film is carefully removed, placed on a film hanger of appropriate size, and allowed to remain in the developing solution for a definite time depending upon the temperature and degree of exhaustion of the developer.

7. The film is removed from the developer and inserted into a stop bath or it is quickly rinsed and transferred to a fixing solution for approximately 10 minutes.

8. The film is then allowed to fix in hypo solution for at least twice the developing time, and then transferred to the "wash" for at least one-half hour.

9. The film is then dried.

10. The finished radiograph is then attached to the original film consultation request, and other pertinent records of the patient in the office, and the entire folder on the patient is brought to the radiologist (physician) for interpretation in the light of all information on the patient.

11. The radiologist writes or dictates his consultation report.

12. The radiologist's report is filed in duplicate in his office, and the original copy is sent to the physician who originally requested the consultation. The patient's films are returned to the central office of the radiologist for filing also.

BASIC PRINCIPLES IN THE INTERPRETATION OF THE ROENTGENOGRAM

1. The radiography must be labeled in respect to laterality—right or left—at the time of exposure; there is no other way in which accuracy can be assured.

2. Sufficient anatomy must be included to allow for specific identification of anatomic characteristics. For example, in a film of bones of the extremities, at least one joint must be included.

3. The basic normal anatomy must be understood well enough to permit the viewer to translate the radiographic anatomy into a three-dimensional perspective, despite the fact that only one or two films may be at hand.

4. Even though a particular substance may have the same density throughout, the image may appear with overlapping detail. Thus, for example, the bones of the pelvis may appear to overlap one another even though they are of a single density, merely because of their spatial relationship. From a single radiograph we are unable to say, unless magnification gives us a clue, which structures lie in front or in back. When reasonably close film-to-target distances are employed we can, however, predict which objects were closest to the film and which farthest (Fig. 1–30).

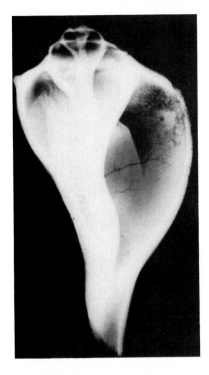
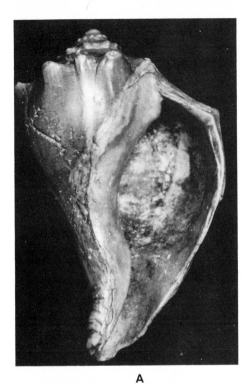
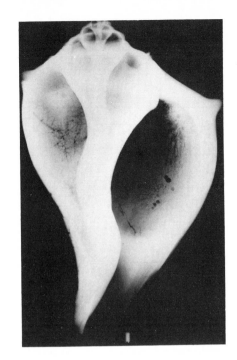

A

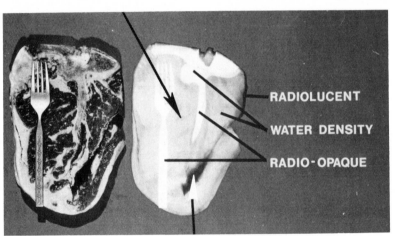

RADIOLUCENT

WATER DENSITY

RADIO-OPAQUE

B

Figure 1–30. A. Radiographs of a conch shell, showing (1) the parts closest to the film have the least magnification and the greatest detail; (2) there is an overlapping of shadows which may produce intensification of the radiograph in certain places. B. Radiograph of a steak showing difference between muscle, bone, and metal.

Actually, a radiograph of an object appears to be a composite of multiple sections of the object superimposed over one another. A good example is a radiograph of a vertebral body. Here the various processes are superimposed over each other in either the lateral or the anteroposterior projection, whichever may be at hand, and it is our knowledge of the three-dimensional anatomy of the vertebral body that allows us to gain a spatial impression of this object (Fig. 1–31).

Lastly, just as the eye must view an anatomic part from two different vantage points to gain a three-dimensional perspective, so must that anatomic part be radiographed from at least two sides. Conventionally, anteroposterior or posteroanterior views and lateral projections of all anatomic parts are obtained. At times, oblique views are also very helpful. This method of obtaining several views of a given anatomic part has the additional advantage of *separating overlying or overlapping structures*—separating the gallbladder, for example, from interfering gas shadows, the stomach from the spine, and so on.

Much of our study in the ensuing chapters will therefore be concentrated upon the interpretation of anatomy as projected in two perpendicular views, and in oblique views that have been standardized for interpretive purposes.

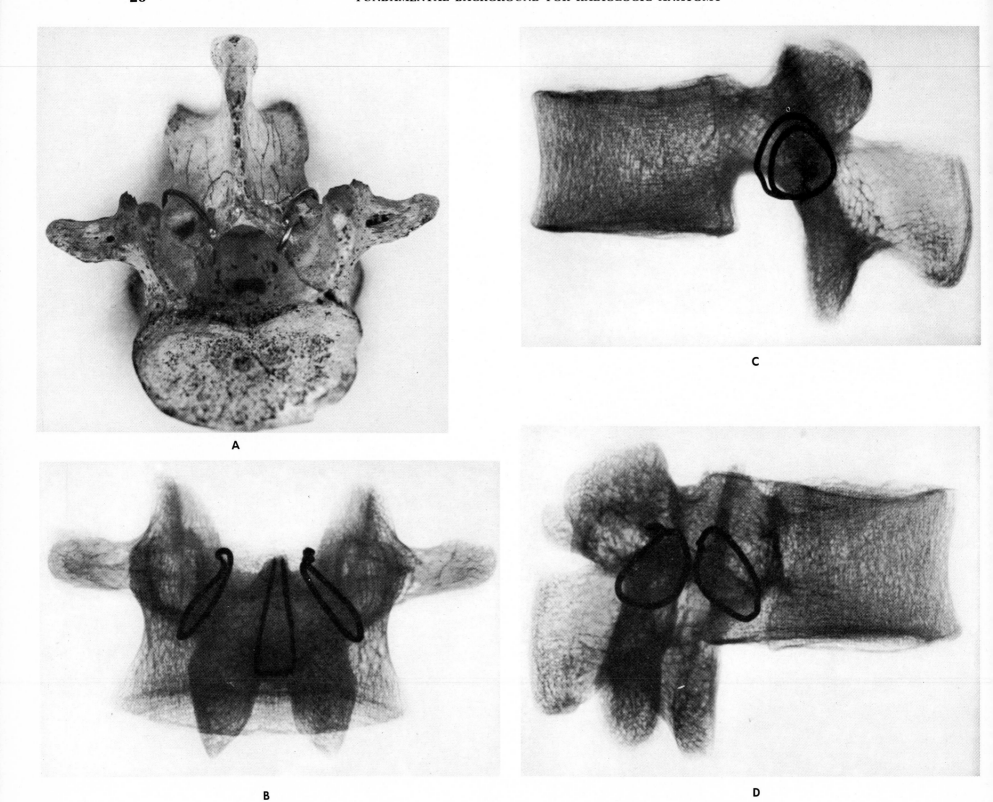

Figure 1–31. Vertebral body with wire delineating the pars interarticularis. *A.* Photograph. *B.* Radiograph in anteroposterior projection. *C.* Radiograph in lateral projection. *D.* Radiograph in oblique projection.

GENERAL TERMS AND CONCEPTS IN DIAGNOSTIC RADIOLOGY

1. *Increased density* denotes a lighter or whiter shadow on the x-ray film or a darker shadow on the fluoroscopic screen, as produced by substances of greater density or thickness.

2. *Decreased density* denotes a darker or blacker shadow on the x-ray film or a lighter one on the fluoroscopic screen. It is produced by substances of low density or slight thickness.

3. *Increased radiolucency (hyperlucency)* implies greater penetrability by the x-rays and has the same connotation as decreased density.

4. *Increased radiopacity* implies diminished penetrability by the x-rays and has the same connotation as increased density.

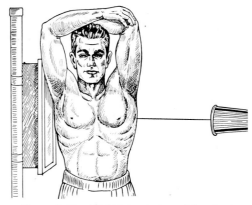

Figure 1–33. Right lateral view of the chest.

5. *Anteroposterior* (Fig. 1–32) indicates that the x-ray beam strikes the anterior aspect of the patient first; *posteroanterior* indicates that the x-ray beam strikes the posterior aspect first.

6. In describing the *laterality* of the patient relative to the x-ray beam, the lateral or oblique projection is always named ac-

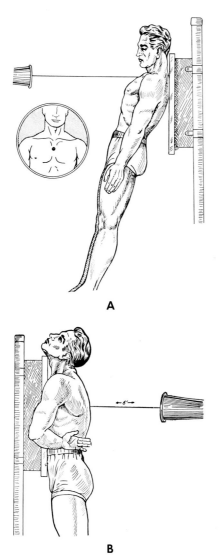

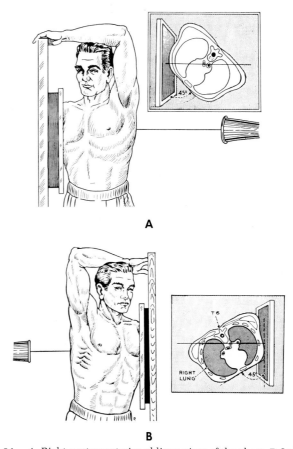

Figure 1–32. *A.* Anteroposterior (apical lordotic) view of the chest. *B.* Posteroanterior view of the chest.

Figure 1–34. *A.* Right posteroanterior oblique view of the chest. *B.* Left posteroanterior oblique view of the chest.

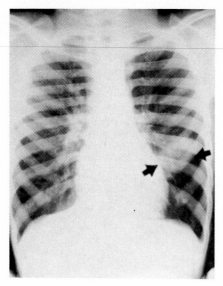

A

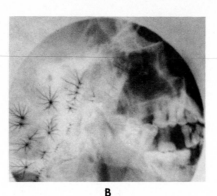

B

Figure 1–35. *A.* "Kissing" artefact caused by two films being in contact with each other during developing process. *B.* Static electricity artefacts.

cording to the *side of the patient closer to the film.* Thus, a *right lateral film* (Fig. 1–33) is taken with the right side of the patient next to the film. A *left lateral* is the reverse.

7. The *oblique* projections are likewise named according to the side of the patient closer to the film. Thus, a *right anterior oblique* radiograph is taken with the right anterior aspect of the patient closer to the film. A *right posterior oblique* (Fig. 1–34 *A*) view is obtained when the right posterior aspect of the patient is nearer to the film. There are also *left anterior* and *left posterior oblique positions* (Fig. 1–34 *B*). The patient or part is usually at

an angle of 45 degrees unless otherwise specified in these oblique views.

8. *Recumbency* indicates that the patient is lying down when the film is taken. He may either be *supine* (on his back) or *prone* (on his abdomen). The beam in these cases is vertical with respect to the patient.

9. The patient is in the *decubitus position* when he is lying on one side while an anteroposterior or posteroanterior film is taken. The beam in these cases is always horizontal. Thus, right lateral decubitus means that the right side of the patient is uppermost. Left lateral decubitus is the reverse. A more accurate terminology is desirable as follows: (1) *horizontal beam study, anteroposterior, with the patient on right (or left) side;* (2) *horizontal beam study, posteroanterior, with the patient on right (or left) side;* (3) *horizontal beam study, with patient supine (or prone) and right (or left) side nearest the film;* (4) *erect position* — with the patient or the anatomic part upright and the beam horizontal. An erect chest film may be obtained with the patient standing or sitting; (5) *semirecumbent, also called semi-erect* — this term implies that the vertical axis of the part being radiographed is at an angle of approximately 45 degrees to the horizontal.

10. *Artefacts* (Fig. 1–35 *A, B*) are changes on the film which do not have an anatomic basis directly related to the part being radiographed but are introduced by some technical fault, such as dirt in the cassette or static electrical charge. Occasionally, artefacts are produced by items of clothing, immobilization devices, or even hair braids projected over the film.

11. *Comparison films* are taken of the opposite side for comparison with a suspected abnormal side. These are very useful, particularly in children, and should be taken whenever possible.

12. *Serial films* are films taken in sequence either during a single study or after longer intervals of time (days or weeks).

REFERENCES

Altschule, M. D.: The use of urographic agents to measure renal clearance and blood flow. Medical Science, *15*:50, 1964.

Barnhard, H. J., and Barnhard, F. M.: The emergency treatment of reactions to contrast media. Radiol. Clin. N. Amer., *3*:51–64, 1965.

Brecher, R., and Brecher, E.: The Rays: A History of Radiology in the U.S. and Canada. Baltimore, Williams and Wilkins Co., 1969.

Bruwer, A. J.: Classic Descriptions in Diagnostic Roentgenology. Springfield, Ill., Charles C Thomas, 1964.

Cahoon, J. B.: Formulating X-ray Techniques. Fifth edition. Durham, N.C., Duke University Press, 1961.

Des Plantes, B. G. Z.: Subtraktion Technique. Stuttgart, Georg Thieme Verlag, 1961.

Etter, L.: Glossary of Words and Phrases Used in Radiology. The Fundamentals of Radiography. Medical Division, Eastman Kodak Co., Rochester, New York. Springfield, Ill., Charles C Thomas, 1960.

Glasser, O.: The Science of Radiology. Springfield, Ill., Charles C Thomas, 1933.

Glasser, O., Quimby, E., Taylor, L., and Weatherwax, J.: Physical Foundations of Radiology. New York, Paul B. Hoeber, 1952.

Grigg, E. R. N.: The Trail of the Invisible Light. Springfield, Ill., Charles C Thomas, 1965.

Hildreth, E. A., Pendergrass, H. P., Tondreau, R. L., and Ritchie, I.: Reactions associated with intravenous urography; discussion of mechanisms of therapy. Radiology, *74*:246–254, 1960 (36 references).

Marshall, T. R., and Ling, J. T.: Clinical evaluation of two new contrast media: Conray and Angioconray. Amer. J. Roentgenol., *89*:423–431, 1963.

Meschan, I., Deyton, W. N., Schmid, H. E., and Watts, F. C.: The utilization of ^{131}I-labeled Renografin as an inulin substitue for renal clearance rate determination. Radiology, *81*:974–979, 1963.

Meschan, I., Hosick, T. A., Schmid, H. E., and Watts, F. C.: Variability in renal clearance rate studies using fresh O[131]IHA, purified product and stored product. J. Nucl. Med., *4*:70–77, 1963.

Meschan, I., Schmid, H. E., Watts, F. C., and Witcofski, R. L.: The utilization of radioactive iodinated Hippuran for determination of renal clearance rates. Radiology, *81*:438–446, 1963.

Oldendorf, W. H.: A modified subtraction technique for extreme enhancement of angiographic detail. Neurology, *15*:336, 1965.

Peterson, H. O.: The radiologist and the special procedures. Amer. J. Roentgenol., *88*:4–20, 1962.

Potsaid, M. S.: Iodinated organic contrast agents. Medical Science, *15*:40–49, 1964.

Roach, J. F., and Hillebae, H. E.: Xeroradiography. J.A.M.A., *157*:899–901, 1955.

Röntgen, W. C.: Über eine neue Art von Strahlen. Sitzungsber. physikalisch. med Ges. Würzburg, *9*:132–141, 1895.

Schinz, H. R., Baensch, W. E., Frommhold, W., Glauner, R., Uehlinger, E., and Wellauer, J. (eds.): Roentgen Diagnosis, Vol. 1., General Principles and Methods. Second Amer. ed. Arr. and ed. by Rigler, L. G. New York and London, Grune and Stratton, 1968.

Schmorl, G., and Junghanns, H.: Die Gesunde und Kranke Wirbelsäule in Roentgenbild und Klinik. Stuttgart, Germany, Georg Thieme, 1951.

Weigen, J. F., and Thomas, S. F.: Reactions to intravenous organic iodine compounds and their immediate treatment. Radiology, *71*:21–27, 1958.

Wolfe, J. N.: Xeroradiography of the Breast. Springfield, Ill., Charles C Thomas, 1972.

2

Protective Measures in X-Ray Diagnosis

INTRODUCTION

Great benefits have resulted from the proper utilization of ionizing radiation, both in the diagnosis and in the treatment of disease. Those who would utilize ionizing radiation for its benefits, however, must be thoroughly cognizant of its hazards.

An understanding of the balance of benefit versus hazard requires the following considerations:

1. Definitions of quantities and qualities of ionizing radiation.
2. The systemic effects of ionizing radiation on the body, as well as the organ-specific effects and their dose relationships.
3. Concepts of "safe," "acceptable," and "tolerance" doses. The differentiation of those occupationally exposed from those in an "uncontrolled" population.
4. Protection of the patient from excessive exposure to ionizing radiation.
5. Representative radiation doses to patients in the various diagnostic examinations.
6. Protection of the radiologist and technician (radiographer).
7. Electrical hazards in relation to handling of equipment.

DEFINITION OF PHYSICAL TERMS

Quality of Ionizing Radiation. The quality of ionizing radiation depends in great part on the *kilovoltage* applied and the so-called *"filters"* inserted in the beam.

X-rays produced by low voltage cathode ray tubes are ordinarily referred to as *"soft"* and do not penetrate the body part for great distances. X-rays produced by high voltage (*"hard"*) cathode rays penetrate more deeply.

24

The term "filters" with respect to radiation refers to a layer of absorbing medium, usually a metal such as aluminum, copper, tin, or lead. This absorbing medium *diminishes* the soft rays relative to the hard ones, but, unlike chemical filters, does not eliminate all soft rays.

Generally, radiation produced by kilovoltages below 60 is considered soft, whereas 120 to 150 kilovolts are moderately penetrating. Hard radiation derived from kilovoltages higher than 150 Kv. are not utilized in conventional diagnostic radiology.

In diagnostic radiology, at least 2 to 4 mm. of aluminum are ordinarily added as filtration at the open diaphragm of the tube to produce an optimum quality of radiation.

Quantification of Ionizing Radiation. Ionizing radiations are radiations consisting of alpha, beta, gamma, neutron rays (or particles) and x-rays which produce biological effects because they ionize, or separate, electrons from their parent atoms in compounds in the body. The *roentgen* (Fig. 2–1) is the internationally accepted unit for quantity of ionizing radiation. It is defined as *"The quantity of x- or gamma radiation such that the associated*

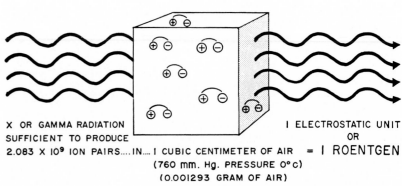

X OR GAMMA RADIATION SUFFICIENT TO PRODUCE 2.083 × 10⁹ ION PAIRS....IN.... I CUBIC CENTIMETER OF AIR = I ROENTGEN (760 mm. Hg. PRESSURE 0°C) (0.001293 GRAM OF AIR) — I ELECTROSTATIC UNIT OR

Figure 2–1. Definition of the roentgen in diagrammatic form.

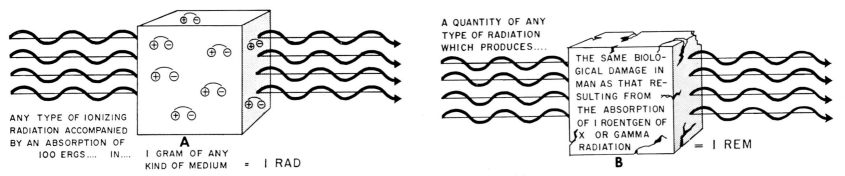

Figure 2–2. *A.* Diagram of the rad. *B.* Diagram of the rem.

TABLE 2–1 RADIATION DOSE RECEIVED BY THE SKIN AND GONADS IN RADIOGRAPHIC EXAMINATIONS (per film)*

Examination	Ku.	mAs.	Focus-Film Distance	Added Filtration	Skin Dose (mr)	Male Gonad Dose (mr)	Female Gonad Dose (mr)
Sinuses	80	40	27 in.	3 mm. Al	1040	0.1	0.05
Hand and wrist, postero-anterior	46	50	27 in.	3 mm. Al	100	0.04	0.01
Chest, postero-anterior	90	3	27 in.	3 mm. Al	8	0.01	0.02
Chest, tomogram (apices) antero-posterior	85	12B	100 cm.	3 mm. Al	110	0.01	0.02
Dorsal spine, antero-posterior	75	80B	110 cm.	3 mm. Al	480	1.0	1.3
Lumbar spine, antero-posterior	75	80B	110 cm.	3 mm. Al	480	0.5[a]	95.0
Lumbar spine, lateral	85	300B	110 cm.	3 mm. Al	2000	2.25	270.0
Lumbar sacral joint, lateral	90	400B	110 cm.	3 mm. Al	3000	2.0	350.0
Pelvis, antero-posterior	75	80B	110 cm.	3 mm. Al	480	20.0[a]	80.0
Abdomen, antero-posterior	75	60B	110 cm.	3 mm. Al	360	0.5[a]	75.0
Abdomen, B meal, prone (H.V.)	90	20B	110 cm.	3 mm. Al	130	1.5	20.0
I.V.P. renal, antero-posterior	75	80B	110 cm.	3 mm. Al	480	0.5[a]	95.0
I.V.P. bladder, antero-posterior	75	80B	110 cm.	3 mm. Al	480	10.0[a]	80.0
Knee, antero-posterior	82	25B	110 cm.	3 mm. Al	180	1.25	0.4
Ankle, antero-posterior	70	30B	36 cm.	1 mm. Al	200	0.1	0.025
Duodenal cap series, postero-anterior (H.V.)	90	15G	18 in.	5 mm. Al + TT	130	0.05	0.05
Fluoroscopy chest (I.I.)	75	90G (3 min.)	18 in.	5 mm. Al + TT	900	3.0	3.0
Fluoroscopy B meal (I.I.)	75	150G (5 min.)	18 in.	5 mm. Al + TT	1500	5.0	5.0

*From Adran, G. M., and Crooks, H. E.: Gonad radiation dose from diagnostic procedures. Brit. J. Radiol., *30*:295–297, 1957.

[a] Lead rubber protection

B – Bucky

G – Stationary grid

H.V. – High voltage screen – Ilford Red Seal film. Other examinations Par Speed screens and Red Seal film extremities.

Ilfex film.

I.I. – Image intensifier, tube current, 0.5 to 1.0 Ma.

corpuscular emission per 0.001293 grams of air produces, in air, ions carrying one electrostatic unit of quantity of electricity of either sign." In everyday radiologic practice it requires approximately 200 to 300 roentgens of x-radiation in the diagnostic quality range to produce a skin erythema. This occurs usually after a latent period of several days. Although the long-term hazards of repeated exposures of this order are great for the technician and the physician, exposures of this order are seldom necessary for patients; hence, an erythema resulting from a diagnostic roentgenologic procedure is almost never observed in a patient.

The *rad* (a word derived from "*r*oentgen *a*bsorbed *d*ose") (Fig. 2–2 A) *is the dose of any type of ionizing radiation accompanied by an absorption of 100 ergs of energy per gram of absorbing material.* In contrast to the roentgen, which is a measure of "ionization in air," the rad is a measure of absorbed dose in terms of ergs of energy. Wherever feasible the *rad* is a more meaningful unit of quantification of ionizing radiation, since it is the absorbed dose which is most significant in the ultimate analysis of biological effect.

The *rem* (derived from "*r*oentgen *e*quivalent *m*an") (Fig. 2–2 B) *is that quantity of any type of ionizing radiation which produces the same biological damage in man as that resulting from the absorption of 1 roentgen of medium energy x-rays.* This, too, is a measure of biological dose, and *is obtained by multiplying the dose in rads by the relative biological effectiveness (RBE) of the irradiation.*

The *RBE is a measure of absorbed radiation, but is the ratio of the absorbed dose in rads of x-rays or gamma rays to the number of rads of a particular radiation producing the same biological effect.* Thus, the RBE for cobalt-60 radiation as compared with 250 Kvp. x-ray radiation is ordinarily given as approximately 0.8 to 0.9.

Radiation Dose Received by the Skin and Gonads in Radiographic Examinations. Table 2–1 summarizes interesting dose data in relation to commonly employed diagnostic radiologic procedures, with usual exposure times and numbers of films. The estimated dose to the ovaries ranges between 0.1 and 0.3 roentgens for the examination of the upper gastrointestinal tract, and 0.1 to 0.8 roentgen for barium enema study of the colon. It is important to know the physical factors employed; thus, in comparing a technique with a target-to-tabletop distance of 30 inches without added filtration and one with a distance of 46 inches and 3 mm. added filtration, it becomes evident that a dosage ratio of almost 10 to 1 exists at the surface. At 10 cm. depth, however, this difference is minimized.

The dose range for single abdominal films to the midpelvis was found to fluctuate between 0.05 and 0.1 R for each exposure.

It is apparent from study of the accompanying table that the exposure most important for consideration is that related to the lumbar spine, pelvis, abdomen, excretory urography, and fluoroscopy.

EFFECTS OF IRRADIATION ON THE BODY

Systemic Effects

Although the biological effects of whole body irradiation must be understood, it is important to realize that in diagnostic radiology relatively small dose levels are utilized, and the whole body effects to be described are usually of academic interest only. *There is little chance for the occurrence of observable deleterious effects with the small doses employed in diagnostic roentgenology.* Effects from whole body irradiation begin to be observable at approximately the 100 rad level. These whole body levels are not obtained in diagnostic radiology. Whole body radiation which exceeds 125 rads may produce severe illness; 250 rads may produce severe illness with loss of hair temporarily, nausea, and even a persistent skin erythema after an initial delay. The person exposed to 250 rads will usually regain his hair and recover fully in a matter of a few months with no *observable* consequences. Very much later in life he may become susceptible to some secondary illness or perhaps even cancer in one form or another. If whole body irradiation of 500 rads occurs, approximately one-half of those exposed will not survive beyond 21 days. The major effects of doses of this order are related to alterations in the bone marrow and reticuloendothelial apparatus. As the whole body exposure level increases to 1500 or 2000 rads, additional effects occur in the gastrointestinal tract, where glandular functions are suppressed, mucosa eroded, and hemorrhage encountered. In doses exceeding 3000 or 4000 rads, additional deleterious effects upon the central nervous system occur.

Fortunately, *dramatic protection is afforded the body by shielding even a part of it from ionizing radiation.* For example, if only one leg is thoroughly shielded, the chance of survival is markedly increased; and of course, irradiation of only a small part of the body has far less dramatic effects. In therapeutic radiology, it is not uncommon to administer 5000 to 6000 rads over a period of 5 to 6 weeks to a given small area of the body in treatment of a malignant tumor, with only moderate or negligible systemic effects.

Organ, Tissue, and Cellular Effects

Radiation Effects on Cells. These effects may be summarized for present purposes as follows:

1. *Radiation suppresses the ability of cells to multiply and reproduce themselves.*

2. *Cells are most sensitive to radiation just before DNA synthesis is well established in their reproductive cycle.* This cycle consists of a resting state, a synthesis period during which DNA is

synthesized rapidly, and a third phase when growth continues but DNA synthesis has largely stopped. Division takes place after this third phase.

3. There is a measure of recovery in irradiated cell populations which is not purely physical. Recovery is enhanced by reducing the temperature.

4. Hypoxic tissues are less subject to the damaging effects of radiation as compared with normally oxygenated tissues. This difference in sensitivity is called the *"oxygen effect."*

5. Generally speaking, *at elevated temperatures* nearly unbearable in the living system, *radiation sensitivity is high.*

6. If the body or the cells being irradiated contain a high concentration of *sulfhydryl (−SH) radicals,* there is a sharp *reduction in radiation sensitivity.* Substances like cysteine and glutathione fall into this category of protective substances.

Superficial Injuries from Ionizing Radiation. Superficial injuries include: (1) epilation, (2) skin damage, (3) brittleness of nails with ultimate destruction of nail bed, (4) lenticular cataracts of the eye, and (5) mucous membrane ulceration of the lips, mouth, and oropharynx. In practically no instance is an immediate effect noted. Depending upon the dose, however, the effects may be seen in days or weeks. If the initial delay period is approximately 1 week, complete repair usually does not ensue for a period of 4 to 6 weeks. Skin carcinomas may result from superficial injury by ionizing radiation after several years.

Hematopoietic Injury. Injury to the reticuloendothelial system results not only in a deprivation of the primordial cells but in thrombocytopenia, lymphopenia, leukopenia, anemia, and loss of specific immune response. Repeated exposure over a prolonged period of time in certain susceptible persons may result in malignant transformation, such as leukemia.

Variability of Tissue or Organ Radiosensitivity. The different tissues, organs, or organ systems throughout the body vary in their *radiation sensitivity.* To a great extent, this *depends upon the relative numbers of undifferentiated, immature, and unspecialized cells as against the number of cells which are highly differentiated.* This relationship was noted very early in the history of radiation biology and has been called the "law of Bergionér and Tribondeau," which states: "... that radiosensitivity of tissues depends upon the number of undifferentiated cells which the tissue contains, the degree of mitotic activity in the tissue, and the length of time that the cells of the tissue stay in active proliferation. . . ."[1] Ordinarily there is a continuous equilibrium between the rate of production of new cells and the disappearance of older, more highly differentiated cells. Radiation interferes with cell division by suppression of DNA synthesis, chromosome breaks, recombinations, and bridging. A tissue with a high rate of mitotic activity may be expected to be radiosensitive. *The hematopoietic*

system is the most radiosensitive, and the central nervous system the most radioresistant; the respiratory and gastrointestinal systems occupy intermediate positions.

A detailed description of the various effects of radiation on the several systems is not included in this text since the *dose levels in diagnostic radiology would not, if properly carried out, induce any detectable change in any of the organ systems of the body.*

Genetic Aberrations and Sterility. Radiation may produce *chromosome breaks, recombinations, bridging, and other alterations in chromosomal constitution.* Radiation *interferes with mitosis* through its effects on the centromeres, resulting in an unequal distribution of chromosomes on the spindle at anaphase. There is also a *high probability of direct gene mutation.*

Apart from the genetic aberrations, the embryo itself is probably in a most sensitive stage in respect to radiation and will be profoundly affected by radiation at any stage of its development. If the embryo is irradiated the reactions induced will depend upon those organ systems which happen to be in a high stage of differentiation at the time. This in turn will determine the kind of abnormality which ultimately could be manifest. In mammals, irradiation of a developing embryo before it becomes implanted in the uterus often results in the death of the embryo. It is here that *exposures in diagnostic radiology can be highly significant,* since it has been shown that "even with doses as low as 200 R, up to 80 per cent of early preimplantation embryos of mice are killed."[1] In the mouse, neonatal death may result from irradiation 7 to 12 days after fertilization; in humans this is probably equivalent to the second through the sixth week of pregnancy. Even doses as low as 25 roentgens in the $7\frac{1}{2}$ day mouse will greatly increase the incidence of skeletal anomalies.

In general, *it is during the first trimester of pregnancy that the embryo is most vulnerable,* and exposure of the embryo during this period should be avoided if at all possible. Irradiation of women of child-bearing age after the first 10 days following the onset of menstruation or during the first trimester of pregnancy should also be avoided if at all possible. Exposure of the pelvis under these circumstances should be limited to emergency procedures. *However, whether or not abnormalities are produced in human embryos during any roentgenologic diagnostic procedure is as yet uncertain.*

Inferences regarding the induction of sterility in man are largely made from comparable data in experimental animals, with full knowledge that this data cannot always be extrapolated. Exposure to radiation in males does not appear to affect sexual capacity or libido, but with sufficient exposure *fertility* may be at least temporarily impaired. Permanent sterility can be produced if sufficiently high doses of radiation are given to the gonads in

---

[1]Pizzarello, D. J., and Witcofski, R. L.: Basic Radiation Biology. Philadelphia, Lea & Febiger, 1967, p. 226.

[1]Pizzarello and Witcofski, p. 260.

isolated fashion. *Sterility would not be likely to result from whole body exposure* since doses required to produce this result would be so high as to bring about one or another of the death-producing radiation syndromes. Sterility may be produced if the number of sperm is sufficiently reduced so that the probability of fertilization of an egg is reduced to unlikely levels. *It is probable that at doses in the diagnostic range of roentgenology there is no clear-cut period of complete sterility or even of functional sterility since doses below 200 or 300 rads would have been administered.* It is possible that "a single dose of about 250 rads" might "bring about sterility for about one year."[1]

In females, a similar situation obtains. Permanent sterilization varies with the age of the individual because older females require smaller doses to be made sterile than do younger ones. Again, the radiation would have to be given directly to the ovaries to bring about sterility—otherwise the dose required for whole body radiation for sterility would cause one or another of the death-producing radiation syndromes. "Induced menopause" may result in individuals nearing the menopause with doses as little as 1000 to 1500 rads. In females 30 years of age or younger, a permanent induced menopause may not result even with doses of 3000 rads.

Reduction in Life Span. Exposure of the entire body to radiation of significant degree shortens the life span. This is true whether the exposures are given over short or long periods of time. Irradiated animals also develop malignant tumors more frequently than do nonirradiated ones. However, even if all deaths due to malignant disease are excluded, the life of an irradiated animal is shorter by statistically significant amounts than that of a nonirradiated one. There are some experiments in rodents, however, in which very small doses of irradiation, accumulated over periods of time, actually produced a life-lengthening effect.

In general, it may be concluded that the amount of shortening of life of small animals after total body irradiation appears to be dependent upon dose, but it is not known whether or not a threshold dose response in respect to this does exist. *Hence, it is doubtful that a life-shortening effect at the usual dose ranges employed in diagnostic roentgenology can ever be demonstrated.*

COMMON SENSE APPROACH TO THE PROBLEM OF HAZARDS DUE TO DIAGNOSTIC RADIOLOGY

The dose levels administered to the skin and gonads in radiographic examinations are usually so low that general effects of irradiation such as superficial injuries, hematopoietic injury,

[1] Pizzarello and Witcofski, p. 250.

induction of malignant tumors, reduction in life span, or other effects such as lenticular cataract and sterility, are not observed. This is true, assuming that appropriate precautions are employed. However, the genetic aspects of roentgen exposure are important (Meschan; Norwood).

If one accepts the age of 30 to 35 years as the age by which most people have produced the majority of their children, we need take into account only this younger population when considering the genetic aspects. Presumably, if the entire population is at risk, the average individual dose must be reduced to 4.8 rads for the total span prior to the 30 to 35 year age limit.

A higher dose (10 times this amount) is permitted for people whose occupation requires a risk exposure to radiation. This is permitted because of the great genetic dilution afforded by the unirradiated public.

Although diagnostic procedures have increased in frequency (Gitlin and Lawrence; Stein), technical improvements have correspondingly diminished exposure.

By present standards, it is estimated that, even if the individual dose is limited to 4.8 rads during the first 30 to 35 years of life, it is probable that a dose of approximately 14 rads to the gonads from *all* sources during the first 30 years of life would not upset the genetic milieu of mankind.

Webster has calculated that the saving of lives by discovery of tuberculosis and cancer by routine chest radiology far exceeds the hazards of the irradiation encountered when good technique is employed. *So long as physicians have proper indication for the examinations chosen for a given patient, and so long as physicians who handle radiation use this valuable tool with the greatest of precision and precaution to themselves and their patients and personnel, the medical usage of radiation in the future is not likely to be deleterious to mankind.*

PROTECTION OF THE PATIENT IN DIAGNOSTIC RADIOLOGY

Exposure of the patient in diagnostic radiology may be considered from the standpoint of protection against both the acute and chronic effects of overexposure, each being discussed in relation to fluoroscopy on the one hand, and radiography on the other.

Safety Recommendations for Fluoroscopy
(Fig. 2–3)

1. *The target-to-tabletop distance, minimum 18 inches.*
2. *Added filtration, 2.5 to 4 mm. of aluminum.*

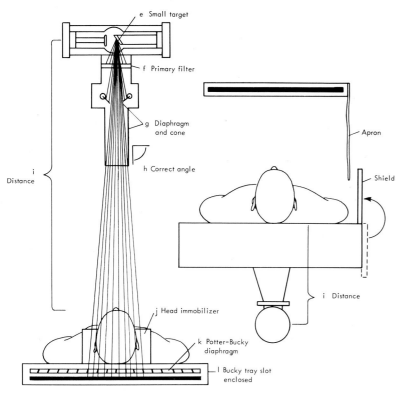

Figure 2–3. Further radiation protection factors diagrammatically illustrated.

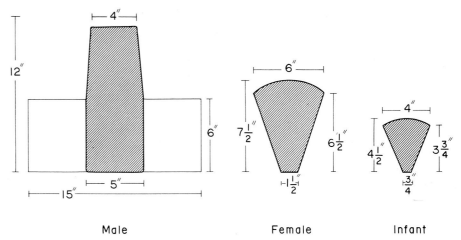

Figure 2–4. Designs of lead gonad shields useful in radiography. These should be ⅛ inch thick lead (or equivalent). They should be placed over the patient's gonads whenever such exposure is not required as part of the diagnostic test.

3. *Whenever possible, protective equipment such as lead rubber should be utilized over the gonads* (Fig. 2–4).

4. *The dosage rate measured in air at the tabletop should be measured frequently, and if possible, kept at a minimum of 5 roentgens per minute (or less).*

5. *The field size should be as small as possible* to cover the anatomic part being studied. In patients under 40 years of age, the gonads should be covered with leaded shielding as protection against scattered radiation (Fig. 2–5).

6. A *self-limiting fluoroscopic timer* should be placed in the circuit and this will automatically shut off the fluoroscope after an appropriate time interval. In general, the timer may be set anywhere between 3 and 5 minutes (Fig. 2–6).

7. *High kilovoltage techniques* with milliamperage settings as low as possible, not to exceed 5 milliamperes, and dial setting appropriately modified to deal with different body thicknesses of infants, children, and adults should be employed. The examination should be conducted as rapidly as warranted.

8. *To diminish exposure, films rather than fluoroscopy should be used whenever feasible.*

9. *Image intensifiers should be employed in fluoroscopy* (Fig. 2–7).

10. *Hand fluoroscopes should never be employed.*

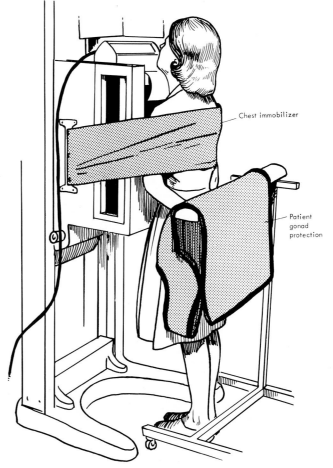

Figure 2–5. Other radiation protection factors.

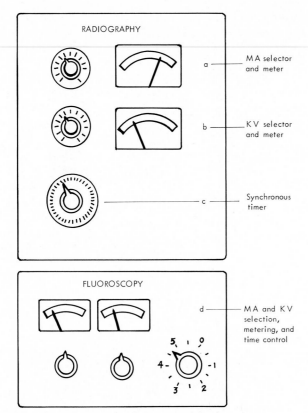

Figure 2–6. Diagram of x-ray control panel to emphasize control of physical factors in radiation protection.

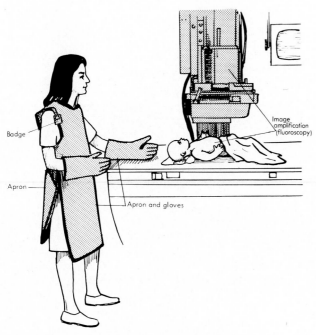

Figure 2–7. Other radiation protection factors.

Safety Recommendations for Radiography

1. Whenever possible, *fast film-screen combinations* should be used if they are suitable for a given purpose *without sacrifice of detail.*

2. *Added filtration,* up to 3 or 4 mm. of aluminum, should almost invariably be used. A minimum of 0.5 mm. of aluminum must be added for beryllium window x-ray tubes for mammography.

3. An adequate range of *adjustable or fixed cones* and *diaphragms* for limiting the useful beam to the smallest dimension necessary in any given examination ought to be available and used.

4. Tests should be made to *insure that leakage of radiation from the tube housing to cones is limited to the degree recommended* by the National Bureau of Standards Handbook 60.

5. For diagnostic examinations in general: (a) *Gonadal exposure must be minimized.* With suitable cones and diaphragms and special lead protective devices, the gonads can be kept out of the direct beam in most cases. In particular, shielding of the testes can be practiced without much difficulty or inconvenience. (b) *Expert assistance and calibration should be sought for every x-ray machine installation.* Dosage factors should be established at tabletop, and the maximum permissible fluoroscopic time posted; tests must ascertain that there is no radiation leakage from the x-ray tube housing. The equipment should be designed to afford a maximum of shielding for the operator.

6. There are *three basic factors* to consider always: (a) *time of exposure,* (b) *distance from the radiation source,* and (c) *shielding provided.*

7. It is recommended that, prior to the examination of all females *under 45 years of age* who could conceivably be pregnant, a brief *menstrual history be obtained.* Rapid immunologic type tests are now available which may, if desired, be performed in minutes prior to radiation exposure. Where impregnation is a possibility, radiation exposure of the embryo should be avoided except in dire emergencies. If pregnancy is known to exist, radiation should be avoided in the first trimester and as much as possible in pregnancy thereafter. When feasible, diagnostic x-ray examinations should be scheduled during the first 10 days following the onset of menstruation.

8. Patients should be immobilized as much as is comfortably possible to avoid movement during the radiographic exposure. (For chest immobilizer in children see Figure 2–8.)

PROTECTION OF PERSONS OCCUPATIONALLY EXPOSED TO RADIATION

In this discussion special emphasis is placed on the protection of physicians and radiologic technicians.

The International Commission on Radiological Protection (ICRP) has made separate regulations for three types of personnel: (1) those occupationally exposed, (2) those near controlled areas or atomic energy establishments, and (3) the population at large. The ICRP has also made separate regulations for different tissues of the body (Johns).

Persons Occupationally Exposed

1. THE BLOOD-FORMING ORGANS, GONADS, AND LENSES OF THE EYES:

The maximum permissible total dose (D) accumulated in these tissues shall be governed by the formula:

$$D = 5 \ (N-18) \text{ rems}$$
$$N = \text{age in years}$$

This formula implies a constant dose rate not exceeding 5 rems per year or 0.1 rems per week. In any period of 13 weeks, a dose rate of 3 rems must not be exceeded.

The ICRP allows for an accidental exposure of 25 rems once in a lifetime, and this accidental dose may be added to that allowed by the above formula.

2. FOR SINGLE ORGANS OTHER THAN THE GONADS, BLOOD-FORMING ORGANS, AND EYES:

A higher dose for these other organs is permitted as follows: skin and thyroid: 8 rems every 13 weeks; hand, forearms, feet and ankles: 20 rems every 13 weeks; other internal organs not mentioned above: 4 rems every 13 weeks.

3. FOR WHOLE BODY EXPOSURE FROM THE UPTAKE OF SEVERAL ISOTOPES:

The same limitations are applied as for blood-forming organs, gonads, and lenses of the eyes.

Persons Near Controlled Areas of Atomic Energy Establishments

The yearly adult dose to the gonads, the blood-forming organs and the lenses of the eyes must be limited to 1.5 rems or less and 3 rems to the skin and thyroid.

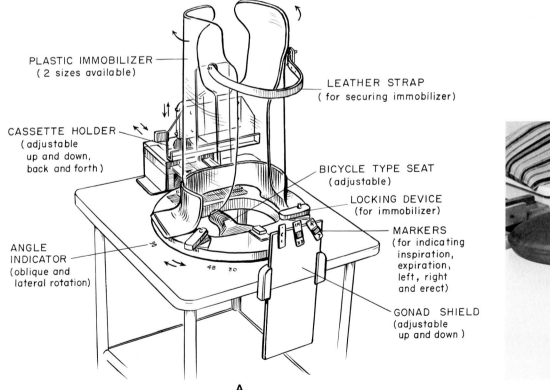

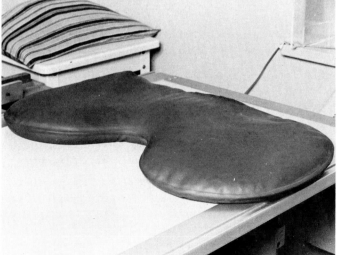

PLASTIC IMMOBILIZER
(2 sizes available)

LEATHER STRAP
(for securing immobilizer)

CASSETTE HOLDER
(adjustable
up and down,
back and forth)

BICYCLE TYPE SEAT
(adjustable)

LOCKING DEVICE
(for immobilizer)

ANGLE
INDICATOR
(oblique and
lateral rotation)

MARKERS
(for indicating
inspiration,
expiration,
left, right
and erect)

GONAD SHIELD
(adjustable
up and down)

A

B

Figure 2–8. A. Pigg-O-Stat infant immobilization device for erect radiography (made by Modern Way Immobilizers, Memphis, Tenn.). B. Photograph of immobilization apparatus useful in pediatric radiology.

For children who live near controlled areas, the yearly dose is limited to 0.5 rems per year (one-tenth of the value for those occupationally exposed).

Public at Large

Here the main concern is the genetic hazard. The dose for those below age 30 must not exceed 5 rems plus the lowest possible contribution from medical procedures. Since the background varies in different parts of the country, this is excluded from consideration. Also, the dose of 5 rems is actually an average figure which includes those who are occupationally exposed—and thus the average for the rest of the population is less. It is estimated that the general population is exposed to about 3 rems from background radiation and about 3 rems from diagnostic procedures.

In order to comply with these rules, physicians and technicians are advised as follows:

1. Personnel must never allow themselves to be exposed to a direct beam of radiation. Immobilization devices must be devised and used. Anesthesia must be employed if immobilization is not feasible.

2. Lead protective gloves and aprons must be worn at all times when the possibility of exposure to scattered radiation exists. These leaded flexible materials must have a lead equivalency of 0.5 mm. (Fig. 2–7). Roentgenoscopic screens with lead rubber drapes also diminish radiation exposure.

3. The physician's unprotected hands, wrists, arms, or other parts should never be exposed to the x-ray beam (Fig. 2–9).

4. Avoid fluoroscopy if films can suffice.

5. Suitable kilovoltage and milliamperage settings in fluoroscopy should be adopted as follows (with image amplifier):

Abdomen	95 Kvp.	2–3 Ma. or less
Chest	70 Kvp.	2 Ma. or less
Thick extremities	60 Kvp.	2 Ma. or less
Thin extremities	50 Kvp.	½–1 Ma.
Children	50–60 Kvp.	½–1 Ma.

6. *General principles of fluoroscopic use:*

(*a*) Shutters must be closed down to no more than 30 to 40 square centimeters.

(*b*) The fluoroscope should be used intermittently, and should be avoided when the patient is not intercepting the beam.

(*c*) The examination should be concluded as quickly as possible, usually within 5 minutes. It is well to have a special timing device in the circuit to turn off the machine automatically when this time is exceeded.

(*d*) When setting fractures or locating foreign bodies, alternation of radiography with manipulation should be used, if possible, rather than fluoroscopy.

(*e*) All x-ray machines should be thoroughly checked before

using for (1) electrical shock properties, (2) radiation leakage around tube housing, (3) roentgen output at the tabletop, (4) scattered irradiation dose pattern around the table with a phantom in place, (5) safe operating voltages and times, and (6) safe continuous fluoroscopic times from the standpoint of the x-ray tube and thermal capacity.

(*f*) All lead protective equipment (aprons and gloves) should be checked frequently for possible leakage.

7. It is well for the physician and his personnel to have frequent blood counts (at least at 6 month intervals), and if there is any opportunity for absorption of internal emitters, frequent urinary assays should also be performed. *A radiation monitoring device should be worn at all times and frequent assays noted in a permanent record.* The film badge or pocket chamber measurement device is ordinarily considered adequate for this purpose, unless there is a single opportunity for excessive exposure, in which case an accurately calibrated milliroentgen pocket chamber would be more accurate and should be employed (Fig. 2–

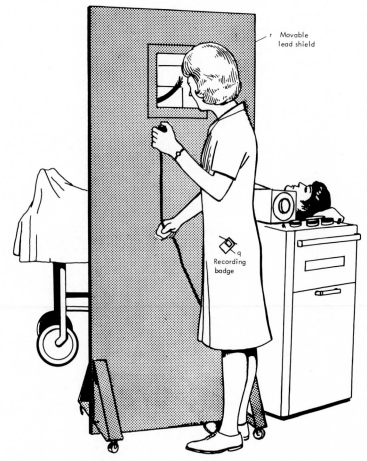

Figure 2–9. Further radiation protection factors diagrammatically illustrated.

9). Metabolic changes are perhaps incurred by physicians even though sufficient protection is worn. The high incidence of leukemia in radiologists, and even among nonradiologists, has already been alluded to; it is possible that when certain susceptible individuals receive even the minimal exposure allowed for in the above methods, they may ultimately develop this form of malignancy.

8. When the mobile x-ray unit is employed, a movable lead shield should also be used to protect the technician or radiologist during the x-ray exposure.

PROTECTION AGAINST ELECTRICAL HAZARDS

A potential electrical hazard may exist within any Radiology Department due to: the high energy side of the x-ray equipment, the presence of explosive anesthetic gases, and hazards caused by sources of low voltages and low currents which may induce ventricular fibrillation in the patient.

1. All exposed cables should be protected against mechanical damage and these should be periodically inspected for defects or abrasions to prevent high energy electrical shock.

2. Explosive anesthetic gases should not be used in the presence of x-ray equipment, if possible. If these are absolutely essential, however, it is well to employ only explosion-proof procedures and apparatus. No switch devices should be permitted below 5 feet from the floor and all switches should be explosion-proof.

All exposed noncurrent-carrying parts of the apparatus should be permanently grounded in acceptable fashion with excellent ground leads.

3. Low voltages and low currents, with their potential of inducing ventricular fibrillation, have become a more frequent hazard in radiology. It has been demonstrated that currents as low as 20 microamperes with voltages as low as 60 millivolts can induce ventricular fibrillation in dogs (Starmer et al.; Weinberg et al.).

When electrodes are applied directly to the human heart, currents as low as 180 microamperes with voltages as low as 100 millivolts will produce ventricular fibrillation (Whalen et al.).

An intracardiac catheter filled with blood or a conducting solution offers an excellent current path directly to the heart, making ventricular fibrillation feasible. A similar hazard exists when there are electrodes from an electrocardiographic monitor in contact with the patient. Grids, when they are dampened, are likewise potentially hazardous. Power injectors connected to catheters are particularly hazardous if they do not have a good separate grounding system, or if they are incorrectly plugged into the wall socket and inadequately grounded (Barry et al.).

In general, the majority of problems associated with electric shock hazards of this type can be solved by providing adequate grounding systems in the angiographic room and connecting them to each item of apparatus that has contact with either the x-ray machine or the patient.

First aid practices such as artificial respiration and emergency treatment for burns should be thoroughly familiar to personnel in case they are needed.

Although the dangers of electric shock are not as extreme in the darkroom, they do exist. Lighting fixtures are the greatest potential hazard in this regard and they must be carefully installed with every attention to proper insulation and grounding.

REFERENCES

Addendum: Maximum permissible radiation exposures to man. Radiology, *71*:263–266, 1958.

Archer, V. W., Cooper, G., Jr., Kroll, J. G., and Cunningham, D. A.: Protection against x-ray and beta radiation; lead glass fabric. J.A.M.A., *148*:106–108, 1952.

Ardran, G. M., and Crooks, H. E.: Gonad radiation dose from diagnostic procedures. Brit. J. Radiol., *30*:295–297, 1957.

Ardran, G. M.: Hazards from increasing use of ionizing radiations: Symposium; The dose to operator and patient in x-ray diagnostic procedures. Brit. J. Radiol., *29*:266–269, 1956.

Aub, J. C., Evans, R. D., and Hempelmann, L. H.: Late effects of internally-deposited radioactive materials in man. Medicine, *31*:221–239, 1952.

Bacon, J. F., and Leddy, E. T.: Protection in roentgenoscopy. Med. Clin. N. Amer., *29*:1036–1041, 1945.

Barry, W. F., Jr., Starmer, C. F., Whalen, R. E., and McIntosh, H. D.: Electric shock hazards in radiology departments. Amer. J. Roentgenol., *95*:976–980, 1965.

Blair, N. A.: Data pertaining to shortening of life span by ionizing radiation. A.E.C. Documents U.R.-442, April, 1956.

Braestrup, C. B.: Past and present radiation exposure to radiologists from the point of view of life expectancy. Amer. J. Roentgenol., *78*:988–992, 1957.

Brucer, M.: The clinical story of radiation damage and definition of radiation complex. Conn. Med., *28*:167–202, 1964.

Brues, A. M., and Sacher, G. A.: Analysis of mammalian radiation injury and lethality. *In* Nickson, J. J. (ed.): Symposium on Radiobiology: The Basic Aspects of Radiation Effects on Living Systems. New York, John Wiley and Sons, 1952, pp. 441–465.

Chamberlain, R. H.: The medical use of ionizing radiation: Benefits and hazards. Mod. Med., *26*:67–73, 1958.

Clark, D. E.: The association of irradiation with cancer of the thyroid in children. J.A.M.A., *159*:1007–1009, 1955.

Crow, J. F.: Genetic considerations in establishing maximum radiation doses. Radiology, *69*:18–22, 1957.

Dahlgren, S.: Thorotrast tumors: A review of the literature and report of two cases. Acta Path. Microbiol. Scand., *53*:147–161, 1961.

Dobzhansky, T.: Genetic loads in natural populations. Science, *126*:191–194, 1957.

Dunn, L. C.: Radiation and genetics. Scientific Monthly, *84*:6–10, 1957.

Failla, G., and McClement, P.: The shortening of life by chronic whole-body irradiation. Amer. J. Roentgenol., *78*:946–954, 1957.

Gitlin, J. N., and Lawrence, P. S.: Population Exposure to X-rays U.S. 1964. U.S. Department of Health, Education and Welfare. Public Health Service Publication, No. 1519. (Excellent bibliography)

Hatano, H.: III. Short term and long term effect: A. Some aspects of radiation biochemistry. Conn. Med., *28*:203–206, 1964.

Henshaw, P. S., and Hawkins, J. W.: Incidence of leukemia in physicians. J. Nat. Cancer Inst., *4*:339–346, 1944.

International Commission on Radiological Protection: Recommendations of the ICRP, 1958. New York, Pergamon Press, 1959.

Johns, H. E.: The Physics of Radiology. Second edition. Springfield, Ill., Charles C Thomas, 1964.

Jones, H. B.: Factors in longevity. Kaiser Found. Med. Bull., *4*:329–341, 1956.

Laughlin, J. S., Meurk, M. L., Pullman, I., and Sherman, R. S.: Bone, skin, and gonadal doses in routine diagnostic procedures. Amer. J. Roentgenol., *78*:961–982, 1957.

Lewis, E. B.: Leukemia and ionizing radiation. Science, *125*:965–972, 1957.

Lincoln, T. A., and Gupton, E. D.: Radiation dose to gonads from diagnostic x-ray exposure. J.A.M.A., *166*:233–239, 1958.

Macht, S. H., and Kutz, E. R.: Detection of faulty roentgenoscopic technique by direct radiation measurements. Amer. J. Roentgenol., *68*:809–814, 1952.

Macht, S. H., and Lawrence, P. S.: National survey of congenital malformations resulting from exposure to roentgen radiation. Amer. J. Roentgenol., *73*:442–446, 1955.

MacKenzie, K. G., Preston, C. D., Stewart, W., and Haggith, J. H.: Thorotrast retention following angiography: A case with postmortem studies. Clin. Radiol., *13*:157–162, 1962.

March, H. C.: Leukemia in radiologists in a twenty year period. Amer. J. Med. Sci., *220*:282–286, 1950.

March, H. C.: Leukemia in radiologists, ten years later. Amer. J. Med. Sci., *242*:137–149, 1961.

Medical Research Council: Hazards to man of nuclear and allied radiation. Command Paper 9780. London, Her Majesty's Stationery Office, 1956.

Meschan, I.: A common sense approach to the problem of the hazards of radiation fall-out and diagnostic radiology. J. Ark. Med. Soc., *57*:488–498, 1961.

Moloney, W. C., and Kastenbaum, M. A.: Leukemogenic effects of ionizing radiation on atomic bomb survivors in Hiroshima City. Science, *121*:308–309, 1955.

Muller, H. I.: Genetic damage produced by radiation. Science, *121*:837–840, 1955.

Myrden, J. A., and Hiltz, J. E.: Breast cancer following multiple fluoroscopies during artificial pneumothorax treatment of pulmonary tuberculosis. Canad. Med. Ass. J., *100*:1032–1034, 1969.

National Council on Radiation Protection and Measurements: Medical X-Ray and Gamma-Ray Protection for Energies up to 10 MeV. NCRP Report No. 33. Washington, D.C., 1968.

National Council on Radiation Protection and Measurements: Medical X-ray and Gamma-Ray Protection for Energies Up to 10 MeV. NCRP Report No. 34. Washington, D.C., 1970.

National Research Council: The biological effects of atomic radiation: Summary reports from the Study by National Academy of Sciences. Washington, D.C., 1956.

Neel, J. Van G., and Schull, W. J.: The effect of exposure to the atomic bomb on pregnancy termination in Hiroshima and Nagasaki. Publication No. 461. Washington, D.C., National Academy of Sciences, National Research Council, 1956.

Norwood, W. D.: Common sense approach to the problem of genetic hazard due to diagnostic radiology. Report based in part on study of exposures in a small American industrial city. J.A.M.A., *167*:1928–1935, 1958.

Pizzarello, D. J., and Witcofski, R. L.: Basic Radiation Biology. Philadelphia, Lea & Febiger, 1967.

Proceedings of Health Physics Society, 114–126. New York, Pergamon Press, 1956.

Ritter, V. W., Warren, S. R., Jr., and Pendergrass, E. P.: Roentgen doses during diagnostic procedures. Radiology, *59*:238–251, 1952.

Russell, L. B., and Russell, W. L.: Radiation hazards to the embryo and fetus. Radiology, *58*:369–376, 1952.

Russell, W. L.: Genetic effects of radiation in mice and their bearing on the estimation of human hazards. Proc. International Conference on Peaceful Uses of Atomic Energy. Vol. 2, Geneva, pp. 382–383, 401–402, 1955.

Sanders, A. P., Sharpe, K., Cahoon, J. B., Reeves, R. J., Isley, J. K., and Baylin, G. J.: Radiation dose to the skin in roentgen diagnostic procedures: Optimum KVP and tissue measurement techniques. Amer. J. Roentgenol., *84*:359–368, 1960.

Seltser, R., and Sartwell, P. E.: Ionizing radiation and longevity of physicians. J.A.M.A., *166*:585–587, 1958.

Seltser, R., and Sartwell, P. E.: The effect of occupational exposure to radiation on the mortality of physicians. J.A.M.A., *190*:1046–1048, 1964.

Simon, N., Muller, H. J., Tessmer, C. F., and Henry, H. F.: Side effects of radiation: Genetics, carcinogenesis, aging, and leukemogenesis. Lippincott's Medical Science, *15*:69–77, 1964.

Simpson, C. L., Hempelmann, L. H., and Fuller, L. M.: Neoplasia in children treated with x-rays in infancy for thymic enlargement. Radiology, *64*:840–845, 1955.

Sonnenblick, B. P.: Aspects of genetic and somatic risk in diagnostic roentgenology. J. Newark Beth Israel Hosp., *8*:81–95, 1957.

Sonnenblick, B. P. (ed.): Protection in Diagnostic Radiology. New Brunswick, N.J., Rutgers University Press, 1959.

Sonnenblick, B. P.: X-rays and leukemia. Lancet, *1*:1197–1198, 1957.

Sorrentino, J., and Yalow, R.: A nomogram for dose determinations in diagnostic roentgenology. Radiology, *55*:748–753, 1950.

Stanford, R. S., and Vance, J.: The quantity of radiation received by the reproductive organs of patients during routine diagnostic x-ray examinations. Brit. J. Radiol., *28*:266–273, 1955.

Starmer, C. F., Whalen, R. E., and McIntosh, H. D.: Hazards of electric shock in cardiology. Amer. J. Cardiol., *14*:537–546, 1964.

Stein, J. J.: The carcinogenic hazards of ionizing radiation in diagnostic and therapeutic radiology. Ca: A Cancer Journal for Clinicians, *17*:278–287, 1967. (Excellent compilation of references)

Stern, C.: Genetics in the atomic age. Eugen. Quart., *3*:131–138, 1956.

Stewart, A., Webb, J., Giles, D., and Hewitt, D.: Malignant disease in childhood and diagnostic irradiation in utero; Preliminary communication. Lancet, *2*:447, 1956.

Stone, R. S.: The concept of a maximum permissible exposure. Radiology, *58*:639–660, 1952.

Ulrich, H.: The incidence of leukemia in radiologists. With a review of the pertinent evidence for radiation leukemia. New Eng. J. Med., *234*:45–46, 1946.

Upton, A. C., Furth, J., and Chirstenberry, K. W.: The late effects of thermal neutron irradiation in mice. Cancer Res., *14*:682–690, 1954.

U.S. National Bureau of Standards: Protection Against Radiations From Radium, Co-60 and Cesium-137 (issue Sept. 1). Handbook 54. Washington, D.C., Supt. of Documents, 1954.

U.S. National Bureau of Standards: X-ray Protection (issue Dec. 1). Handbook 60. Washington, D.C., Supt. of Doc., 1955.

U.S. National Bureau of Standards: Safe Handling of Bodies Containing Radioactive Isotopes. Handbook 65. Washington, D.C., Supt. of Documents, 1958.

U.S. National Bureau of Standards: Maximum Permissible Body Burdens and Maximum Permissible Concentrations of Radionuclides in Air and in Water for Occupational Exposure. Handbook 69. Washington, D.C., Supt. of Documents, 1959.

U.S. National Bureau of Standards: Medical X-ray Protection up to Three Million Volts. Handbook 76. Washington, D.C., Supt. of Documents, 1964.

Van Swaay, H.: Aplastic anaemia and myeloid leukaemia after irradiation of the vertebral column. Lancet, *2*:225–227, 1955.

Warren, S.: Longevity and causes of death from irradiation in physicians. J.A.M.A., *162*:464–468, 1956.

Webster, E. W.: Hazards of diagnostic radiology: A physicist's point of view. Radiology, *12*:493–507, 1959.

Weens, H. S., Clements, J. L., and Tolan, J. H.: Radiation dosage to the female genital tract during fluoroscopic procedures. Radiology, *62*:745–749, 1954.

Weinberg, D. I., Artley, J. L., Whalen, R. E., and McIntosh, H. D.: Electric shock hazards in cardiac catheterization. Circ. Res., *11*:1004–1009, 1964.

Whalen, R. E., Starmer, C. F., and McIntosh, H. D.: Electrical hazards associated with cardiac pacemaking. Ann. N.Y. Acad. Sci., *111*:922–931, 1964.

3

The Development of Bone

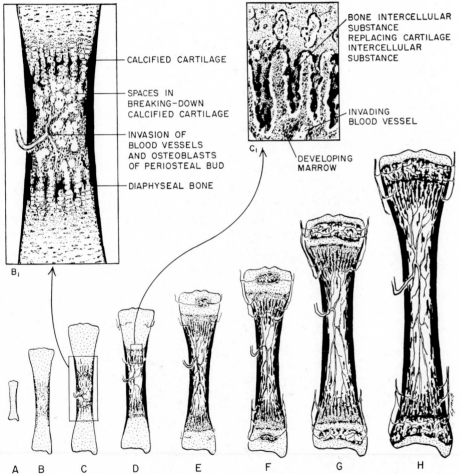

CALCIFIED CARTILAGE

SPACES IN
BREAKING-DOWN
CALCIFIED CARTILAGE

INVASION OF
BLOOD VESSELS
AND OSTEOBLASTS
OF PERIOSTEAL BUD

DIAPHYSEAL BONE

B₁

BONE INTERCELLULAR
SUBSTANCE
REPLACING CARTILAGE
INTERCELLULAR
SUBSTANCE

INVADING
BLOOD VESSEL

C₁

DEVELOPING
MARROW

A   B   C   D   E   F   G   H

Figure 3–1. Diagram to illustrate the growth and ossification of a typical long bone: *A*, Primary cartilaginous anlage. *B*, Primary center of ossification in shaft with early conversion of perichondrium to periosteum. *C*, Further progression of the perichondrial ossification and extension of the partially calcified cartilage upward toward the metaphysis. *D*, Continued absorption of the inner compact bony wall and new bone deposition beneath the periosteum. Note the bone intercellular substance replacing the cartilage intercellular substance and the invasion of the blood vessels from the region of the marrow. *E, F,* and *G,* Commencement and continued ossification of the epiphyses. Note the demarcation between the metaphysis and epiphyseal plate. *H,* The ossification of the epiphyseal plate and cessation of growth. Note the covering of articular cartilage which remains unossified.

36

Osteoblasts, the cells responsible for the deposition of bone, are normally differentiated from mesenchyme in two kinds of environment:

In the first, exemplified by the skull, they form within fibroblastic and collagenous membranes—and bone formed in such an environment is called *intramembranous ossification.*

In the second type of ossification (*endochondral*), osteoblasts develop in a cartilaginous environment. Their source is thought to be perichondrial cells, or fibrous connective tissue cells, and the means by which these penetrate the cartilage cells is described below.

INTRAMEMBRANOUS OSSIFICATION

Intramembranous ossification begins when certain mesenchymal cells differentiate into osteoblasts. These appear in clusters called *centers of ossification.*

Osteoblasts secrete or form the intercellular organic matrix of bone called *osteoid,* and ultimately this matrix surrounds the osteoblasts in a chamber called a *lacuna,* which is then said to contain the *osteocyte,* or bone cell.

Simultaneously, phosphatase is secreted, causing calcification of the osteoid.

Near the margin of the bony anlage the osteoblasts proliferate, producing growth by spiderlike processes or "spicules." These spicules join one another in a lattice-work called *bony trabeculae.* When the lattice spaces predominate, the bone is called *cancellous.* When the trabeculae are compactly arranged and the lattice spaces are sparse, the bone is called *compact* (Fig. 3–2).

The lattice spaces in both cases contain the main blood supply and marrow tissues.

ENDOCHONDRAL OSSIFICATION

Most of the skeleton forms as a result of endochondral ossification (Fig. 3–1).

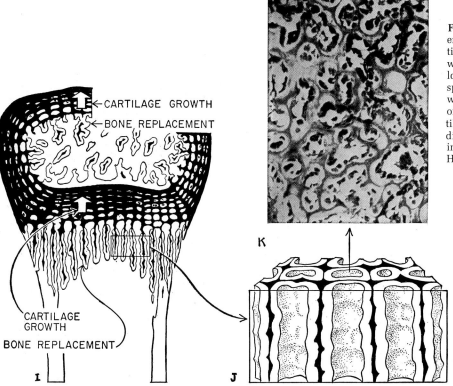

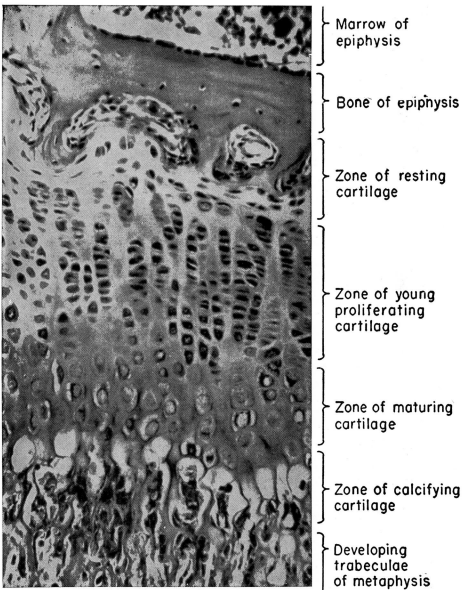

Figure 3-1. *Continued.* I, Diagram which illustrates in longitudinal section an end of a growing long bone. The trabeculae appear stalactite-like in such a preparation. However, if they could be seen in three dimensions, as is illustrated in J, it would be seen that close to the plate the structures that appear as trabeculae in a longitudinal section are slices that have been cut through walls that surround spaces; they are slices cut through walls of tunnels. Photomicrograph K represents what is seen in a cross-section cut through the metaphysis of a growing long bone of a rabbit, close to the epiphyseal disk. In it the trabeculae of bone have cartilaginous cores that surround spaces. These spaces under the periphery of the disk become filled in, forming haversian systems. Such compact bone as is present in the flared extremities of bone is built by such filled-in spaces. (Modified from Ham, A. W.: Histology. 6th ed. Philadelphia, J. B. Lippincott Co., 1969.)

Figure 3-1. *Continued.* L, High-power photomicrograph of a longitudinal section cut through the upper end of the tibia of a guinea pig. This picture illustrates the different zones of cells in the epiphyseal plate. (Modified from Ham, A. W.: Histology. 6th ed. Philadelphia, J. B. Lippincott Co., 1969.)

Figure 3-1 continued on following page.

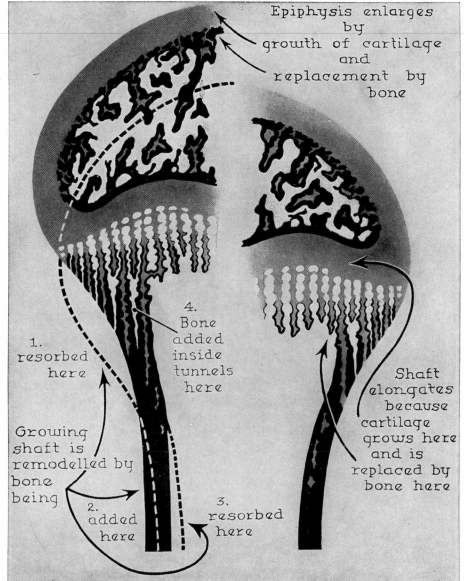

Epiphysis enlarges
by
growth of cartilage
and
replacement by
bone

1.
resorbed
here

Growing
shaft is
remodelled by
bone
being

2.
added
here

4.
Bone
added
inside
tunnels
here

3.
resorbed
here

Shaft
elongates
because
cartilage
grows here
and is
replaced by
bone here

M

Figure 3–1 *Continued.* M, Diagram showing the manner in which bone is deposited and resorbed to account for the remodeling that takes place at the ends of growing long bones that have flared extremities. (From Ham, A. W.: J. Bone Joint Surg., *34A:*701–728, 1952.)

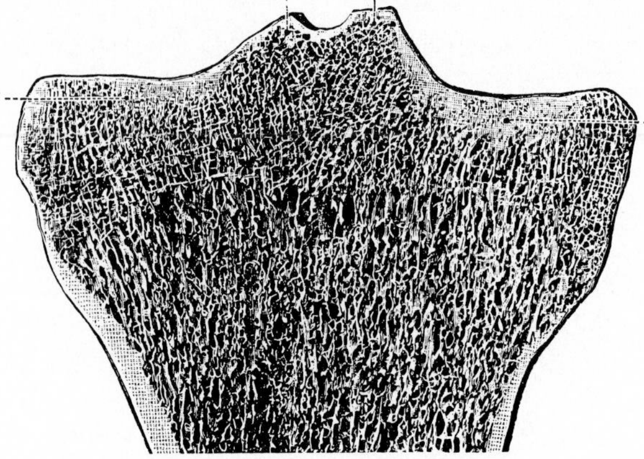

Figure 3–2. Macroscopic longitudinal section through a typical long bone (tibia) to show cancellous and compact bone. (From Toldt, C.: An Atlas of Human Anatomy for Students and Physicians. New York, The Macmillan Co., 1926.)

External tubercle of the spine of the tibia
Tuberculum intercondyloideum laterale

Internal tubercle of the spine of the tibia
Tuberculum intercondyloideum mediale

External tuberosity
Condylus lateralis

Internal tuberosity
Condylus medialis

In the various sites where bones are to form, the mesenchyme of that area begins to differentiate into cartilage with a surrounding membrane called the *perichondrium*.

Cartilage grows by one of two methods:

1. *Interstitial* growth, in which the cartilage cells themselves retain their capacity to divide. This capacity is retained by young cartilage cells only. These cells are responsible for the addition of intercellular substance, which enables the cartilage to expand from within.

2. *Appositional* growth is defined as the adding of new cartilage to a preexisting surface, and is caused by differentiation of the deep perichondrial cells into chondroblasts and later to chondrocytes.

The cartilaginous anlage increases in length by interstitial growth. This growth is greater near the ends than the midsection. The chondrocytes go through a definite cycle of maturation which is characteristic wherever cartilage is undergoing transformation into bone. The areas of such transformation are: (1) the primary center of ossification in the center of the shaft, (2) in linear fashion in the epiphyseal plate, and (3) in the subarticular region of the growing end, where the epiphysis is formed.

This cycle develops as follows:

1. Cartilaginous interstitial growth.

2. Swelling, vacuolation, and maturation of these cells, with the secretion of phosphatase.

3. Intercellular calcification of cartilaginous matrix.

4. Death of the cartilage cells and fragmentation of the calcified intercellular substance.

5. Invasion of the disintegrating calcific zone by blood vessels and osteogenic cells.

6. Elaboration of bony matrix around the calcific foci remaining, forming trabeculae of bone.

With the progressive development of the vascular system, the perichondrium is invaded by blood vessels. The cells which were chondroblasts and chondrocytes within the perichondrium become osteoblasts, and a thin layer or shell of bone is laid down around the cartilaginous anlage. The perichondrium has thus become the periosteum (Fig. 3–1, *B*).

Thereafter, osteogenic cells together with capillaries grow from the inner layer of the periosteum into the breaking down midsection of the cartilage. These vessels provide the osteoblastic source for the primary center of ossification and epiphyseal plate, the latter by extension along the shaft. Ossification gradually extends toward the ends of the anlage (Fig. 3–1, *C*). Periosteum also continues to add bone to the sides of the anlage, and as this becomes more compact, the central area becomes more cancellous, ultimately forming the marrow cavity (Fig. 3–1, *C*).

However, ossification stops short of replacing all the cartilage near the end of the anlage. The cartilage cells on the shaft side of the articular cartilage go through the maturation cycle which is responsible for the ossification of the shaft. Ossification also stops short of "a plate" between the epiphyseal and diaphyseal centers of ossification (*epiphyseal disk or plate*).

In the epiphyseal disk, there are two processes occurring continuously: (1) Proliferation of cartilage cells which tends to thicken the epiphyseal disk and make it grow, and (2) Calcification, death, and replacement of cartilage on its diaphyseal side, which tend to thin it out.

These processes allow the bone to grow, and are identical with the maturation cycle described above. Any interference with any of these processes is quickly reflected in an aberration of bone growth.

Thus, the epiphyseal disk is composed of four different zones passing from the diaphysis to the epiphysis (Fig. 3–1, *L*):

1. Zone of calcified cartilage.

2. Zone of maturing cartilage.

3. Zone of proliferating young cartilage.

4. Zone of "resting" cartilage which binds the plate to the bone of the epiphysis.

The zones of maturing and proliferating cartilage are arranged in columns, and any deviation from regularity is an indication of an abnormal process at work.

The zone of calcified cartilage is thin and intermingles with the bone of the diaphysis arranged in longitudinally disposed trabeculae. This zone of calcified cartilage is seen in the x-ray as the provisional zone of calcification (Fig. 3–3). As rapidly as bone is added to the epiphyseal plate side of the metaphysis, it is resorbed by osteoblasts on the marrow side.

The growth in diameter of the shaft of the bone as well as the normal flaring is accomplished by continuous resorption at the outer periphery of the epiphyseal plate, and by adding to the shaft below this level (Fig. 3–1, *M*). The shaft of the bone grows in width by apposition of new bone under the periosteum while at the same time bone is dissolved away from the inside of the shaft.

These added layers of bone are called circumferential lamellae and tend to surround the entire shaft (Fig. 3–4). Some of these are converted to haversian systems as more and more lamellae are added. The persistent blood supply to these lamellae and haversian systems from the periosteum are contained within canals called Volkmann's canals.

The bone marrow contained in the medullary spaces consists of connective tissue, fat, blood vessels, nerve fibers, and all of the hematogenic elements of the blood and osteogenic elements as well. Yellow marrow differs from red in that it consists mainly of fat.

The periosteum of bone is not normally detected in the radiograph because it is not calcified and offers no contrast to overlying structures. When it is seen, it is an indication of abnormality.

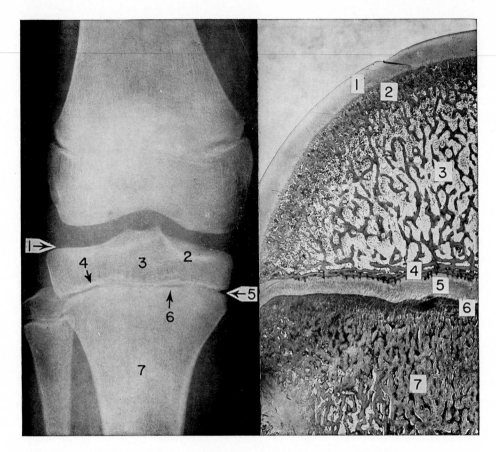

Figure 3–3. Anteroposterior radiograph of the knee and low power photomicrograph of the end of a long bone with related areas labeled. (From Pyle, S. I., and Hoerr, N. I.: Radiographic Atlas of Skeletal Development of the Knee, Springfield, Ill., Charles C Thomas, 1955.)

Radiologic Terms	Histologic Terms
1. Articular cartilage does not show in a film.	1. Articular cartilage.
2. White outline of subarticular margin of epiphysis.	2. Compact bone of subarticular margin.
3. Epiphysis.	3. Epiphysis; spongy bone.
4. Increased density of terminal plate; inner bone margin of epiphysis.	4. Terminal plate.
5. Epiphyseal line; strip of lesser density; epiphyseal plate; diaphyseal-epiphyseal gap. Radiographically, these terms exclude the recently calcified cartilage, which appears as part of the metaphysis.	5. Epiphyseal disk; growth cartilage. Histologically, these terms include the calcified cartilage.
6. Metaphysis; includes both calcified cartilage and newly formed bone (zone of provisional calcification).	6. Metaphysis; includes only newly formed bone of primary ossification.
7. Diaphysis or shaft.	7. Spongy bone of diaphysis.

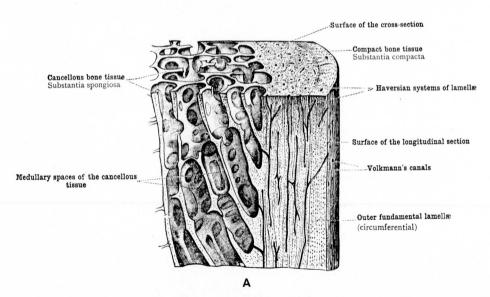

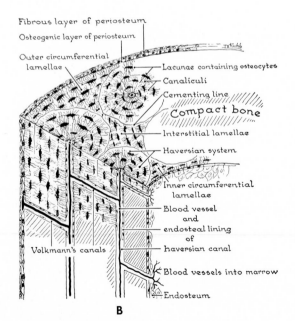

Figure 3–4. *A.* Diagram to illustrate the structure of bone. (From Toldt, C.: An Atlas of Human Anatomy for Students and Physicians. New York, The Macmillan Co., 1926.) *B.* A three-dimensional diagram showing the appearance of both a cross and a longitudinal section of the various components that enter into the structure of the cortex of the shaft of a long bone. The diagram shows the different kinds of lamellae that are present and the relation between the blood vessels of the periosteum, Volkmann's canals, haversian canals, and the marrow cavity. (From Ham, A. W.: Histology. 6th ed. Philadelphia, J. B. Lippincott Co., 1969.)

THE BLOOD SUPPLY OF A LONG BONE

There are three sets of vessels supplying a long bone (Figs. 3–5, 3–6):

1. *The nutrient artery* (or arteries), derived from the original periosteal bud to the primary ossification center.

2. *The metaphyseal and epiphyseal vessels,* entering these regions directly. Epiphyseal vessels are of two types: (a) in epiphyses completely surrounded by articular cartilage (like the head of the femur), the epiphyseal vessel centers between the articular and epiphyseal plate cartilages; (b) in other epiphyses, the vessel may enter the epiphyses directly.

After growth in length ceases, the cartilage of the epiphyseal plate is resorbed and replaced by bony trabeculae (Fig. 3–1, *H*). Anastomoses between the epiphyseal and metaphyseal vessels thus occur and these are called metaphyseal-epiphyseal vessels.

3. *The periosteal vessels* contribute to the arterioles in the haversian systems and Volkmann's canals.

The blood supply of the *bone marrow* is very rich. The nutrient or medullary artery penetrates obliquely through the nutrient foramen where it divides into an ascending and descending branch and supplies an abundance of small arteries to all portions of the medullary portion of the bone.

The terminal arteries end in broad capillaries which simulate sinusoids. Certain of the terminal arteries anastomose with those of the cancellous epiphyses and with the arteries which enter the haversian system of the compact bone from the periosteum, which have already been described. Afferent veins return the blood as companion veins to the arterial system described above.

The nerves accompany the blood vessels throughout.

The *veins* emerge from the long bones in three places: (1) accompanying the nutrient artery, (2) at the articular extremities, and (3) passing out of the compact substance of the bone.

In the flat bones there are tortuous canals in the diploic tissue or veins with occasional perforating canals.

In cancellous tissue, the veins have thin walls supported by a thin, osseous structure.

FACTORS AFFECTING BONE FORMATION

Bone may be laid down in accordance with predetermined congenital pathways (Barnhard and Geyer). It is probable that trabeculae usually develop according to prevailing stress (Feist). Systemic factors which play an essential role in bone formation are shown in Table 3–1 and Figure 3–7.

Phosphatase is found consistently at sites of new bone formation as well as in bone osteolysis. In an acid medium, phosphatase splits bone salts and returns the salt into the solution; in an alkaline medium, phosphatase activity promotes osteogenesis by liberating phosphate ions and precipitating calcium salts. Acid

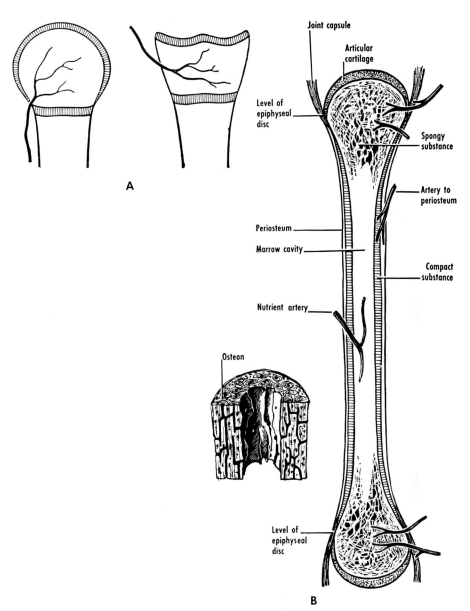

Figure 3–5. A. Drawings to show the two types of epiphyseal blood supply. When separation of the epiphyseal plate occurs (*left*), the blood vessels are torn and the bone of the epiphysis dies. (Preparation by G. Dale and W. R. Harris.) (From Ham, A. W.: Histology. 6th ed. Philadelphia, J. B. Lippincott Co., 1969.) B, Schematic diagram of a long bone and its blood supply. The inset diagram shows the lamellae of the compact bone arranged into osteons. The blood vessels of long bones are: (1) nutrient artery or arteries; (2) periosteal vessels supplying the compact bone; (3) metaphyseal and epiphyseal vessels arising from arteries supplying the joint. These latter pierce the compact bone and supply the spongy bone and marrow. When the epiphyseal plate fuses and becomes ossified the epiphyseal and metaphyseal vessels anastomose. (From Gardner, E., Gray, D. J., and O'Rahilly, R.: Anatomy: A Regional Study of Human Structure. 3rd ed. Philadelphia, W. B. Saunders Co., 1969.)

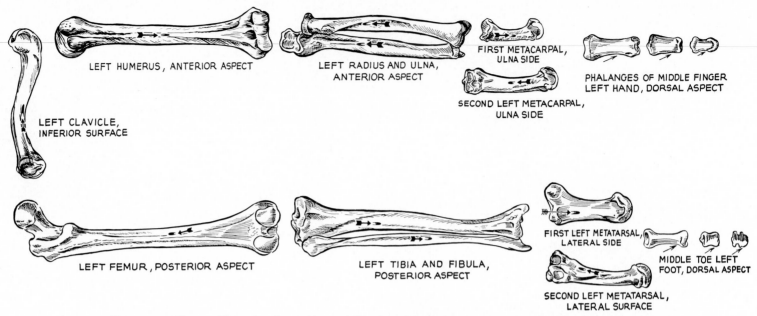

Figure 3–6. Diagram illustrating the position and direction of the various important nutrient foramina of the appendicular skeleton. (Modified from Anson, B. J. (ed.): Morris' Human Anatomy. 12th ed. New York, McGraw Hill Book Co., 1966.)

phosphatase is otherwise confined within the intact prostate gland, from which it may be released by invasive carcinoma.

Calcitonin is secreted in response to hypercalcemia in the thyroid gland (possibly the parathyroid gland as well), and its function seems to be depression of serum calcium levels by inhibition of bone resorption (Aliapoulios, Bernstein, and Balodimos; Foster).

Parathyroid hormone functions principally in the maintenance of a proper level of calcium in the blood by mobilization of calcium. A decrease in the level of serum calcium causes an increase in parathyroid hormone secretion. Parathormone exerts its effects at three distinct levels:

1. Inhibition of phosphate resorption at the renal tubular level, thus leaving a relative excess of calcium ions in the circulation.

2. Promotion of absorption of calcium and phosphorus at the intestinal mucosa level.

3. Direct stimulation of osteoclasts in bones to mobilize calcium.

Vitamin D has three essential roles: absorption of calcium from the ileum, promotion of tubular phosphate excretion much like parathormone in the kidneys, and direct action on bone by potentiating the osteoclastic activity stimulated by parathormone. In addition, it may tend to catalyze bone calcification.

THE CORRELATION OF THE BONE RADIOGRAPH WITH THE PHOTOMICROGRAPH OF BONE

In the normal healthy state, bone is a constantly changing organ and bone formation and resorption are in equilibrium with one another except as required by growth and repair. The accompanying radiograph (Fig. 3–3) and its low power photomicrograph show the following:

The dense white zones immediately adjoining the epiphyseal plate (shown in *4* and *6*) represent zones of compact bone in the former and calcified cartilage and osteoid in the latter. These are called the *zones of provisional calcification.* The compact bone (*2*) is readily differentiated from the spongy bone of the diaphysis (*7*).

TABLE 3–1   FACTORS AFFECTING BONE FORMATION

Exogenous	Gastrointestinal Tract		Blood Serum Levels	Bone	Kidneys
Dietary calcium Phosphorus Vitamins A, C, D[a] Proteins	Acid chyme } Adequate vitamin D }	Favor absorption	Calcium Phosphorus Phosphatase[a] Vitamins Hormones	Storehouse for calcium and phosphorus	Glomerular function Tubular function
	Alkaline chyme } Excessive phos- phates, fatty acids, soaps and carbo- nates Fluoride }	Impair absorption	Pituitary (growth) Calcitonin[a] Adrenal corticosteroids (anabolic and catabolic) Estrogens Androgens Parathormone[a]		

[a]See accompanying text.

The articular cartilage is of an intermediate radiolucency and blends with the surrounding soft tissues which are of intermediate density. It cannot be seen distinctly on the radiograph unless a contrast agent is introduced into the joint. The examination using this procedure is described as *arthrography*. Positive contrast agents such as sodium or meglumine diatrizoate (Renografin or Hypaque) may be used, or gases such as air or oxygen, or double contrast techniques involving a combination of both. The epiphyseal plate (5) is similarly of intermediate density.

Method of Roentgen Analysis of Bones (Fig. 3–8)

Always make at least two perpendicular views of the bone in question and one of the joint.
Study the bone in the following sequence:
1. Soft tissues.
2. Periosteal region.
3. Cortex.
4. Medulla.
5. Joint capsule and joint.
6. Subarticular bone.
7. Epiphysis, epiphyseal plate, and metaphysis.
Make comparison studies of the two comparable sides of the body when appropriate.

BONE AGE VERSUS CHRONOLOGICAL AGE: MATURATION OF THE SKELETON

Introduction. Chronological age refers to the actual age of the patient in days, weeks, or months since birth.

Bone age, on the other hand, refers to the development of the bones as assayed against growth charts which have been constructed after the study of many so-called "normal populations" in different parts of this country—and indeed, in the case of other charts, in many parts of the world.

As a general rule, in any given long bone, the epiphysis which appears first is usually the last to fuse. The fibula, femur, and tibia are frequently exceptions to this rule.

The nutrient canal of a long bone is directed away from the epiphysis, which fuses last.

Some epiphyseal centers, such as those of the innominate bone, scapula, ribs, and vertebrae, do not appear until puberty or thereafter.

Major Factors in Skeletal Maturation

1. Ossification of the long and short bones (usually complete in utero).
2. *Onset of ossification of the epiphyses* (Figs. 3–9, 3–10).
(*Text continued on page 51.*)

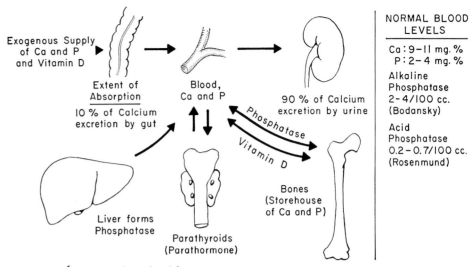

NORMAL BLOOD LEVELS

Ca: 9–11 mg. %
P: 2–4 mg. %
Alkaline Phosphatase 2–4/100 cc. (Bodansky)
Acid Phosphatase 0.2–0.7/100 cc. (Rosenmund)

Exogenous Supply of Ca and P and Vitamin D

Extent of Absorption

10 % of Calcium excretion by gut

Blood, Ca and P

90 % of Calcium excretion by urine

Phosphatase

Vitamin D

Liver forms Phosphatase

Parathyroids (Parathormone)

Bones (Storehouse of Ca and P)

Vitamin D { 1. Absorption of calcium
2. Promotes calcification of osteoid
3. When excessive — osteoporosis

Parathormone: When calcium is deficient in blood, this hormone helps mobilization of Ca from bones.

Figure 3–7. Factors governing calcium metabolism.

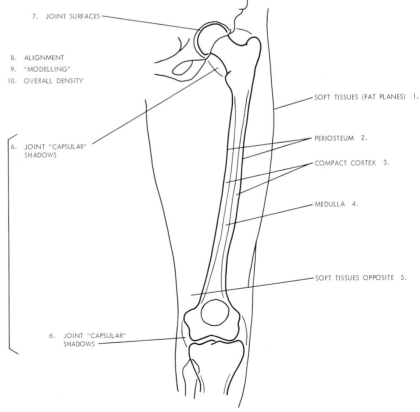

7. JOINT SURFACES

8. ALIGNMENT
9. "MODELLING"
10. OVERALL DENSITY

6. JOINT "CAPSULAR" SHADOWS

SOFT TISSUES (FAT PLANES) 1.

PERIOSTEUM 2.

COMPACT CORTEX 3.

MEDULLA 4.

SOFT TISSUES OPPOSITE 5.

6. JOINT "CAPSULAR" SHADOWS

Figure 3–8. Method of roentgen analysis of bones.

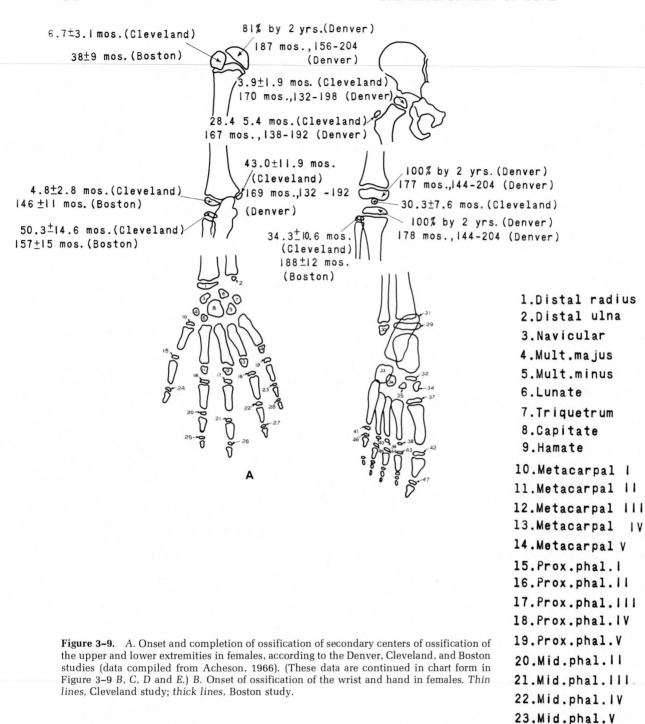

6.7±3.1 mos.(Cleveland)
38±9 mos. (Boston)

81% by 2 yrs.(Denver)
187 mos.,156-204 (Denver)

3.9±1.9 mos. (Cleveland)
170 mos.,132-198 (Denver)

28.4 5.4 mos.(Cleveland)
167 mos.,138-192 (Denver)

43.0±11.9 mos. (Cleveland)
169 mos.,132 -192 (Denver)

4.8±2.8 mos.(Cleveland)
146 ±11 mos. (Boston)

50.3±14.6 mos.(Cleveland)
157±15 mos. (Boston)

34.3±10.6 mos. (Cleveland)
188±12 mos. (Boston)

100% by 2 yrs.(Denver)
177 mos.,144-204 (Denver)

30.3±7.6 mos.(Cleveland)
100% by 2 yrs.(Denver)
178 mos.,144-204 (Denver)

A

MONTHS
10 20 30 40 50 60 70 80 90 100 110

1.Distal radius
2.Distal ulna
3.Navicular
4.Mult.majus
5.Mult.minus
6.Lunate
7.Triquetrum
8.Capitate
9.Hamate
10.Metacarpal I
11.Metacarpal II
12.Metacarpal III
13.Metacarpal IV
14.Metacarpal V
15.Prox.phal.I
16.Prox.phal.II
17.Prox.phal.III
18.Prox.phal.IV
19.Prox.phal.V
20.Mid.phal.II
21.Mid.phal.III
22.Mid.phal.IV
23.Mid.phal.V
24.Dist.phal.I
25.Dist.phal.II
26.Dist.phal.III
27.Dist.phal.IV
28.Dist.phal.V

B

Figure 3–9.   *A.* Onset and completion of ossification of secondary centers of ossification of the upper and lower extremities in females, according to the Denver, Cleveland, and Boston studies (data compiled from Acheson, 1966). (These data are continued in chart form in Figure 3–9 *B, C, D* and *E.*) *B.* Onset of ossification of the wrist and hand in females. *Thin lines,* Cleveland study; *thick lines,* Boston study.

Figure 3–9 *Continued.   C.* Onset of ossification of secondary centers of the ankle and foot in females, according to the Cleveland and Boston studies. (Data compiled from Acheson, 1966.) *Thin lines.* Cleveland study; *thick lines.* Boston study. *D.* Completion of ossification of the wrist and hands in females, according to the Cleveland and Boston studies. (Data compiled from Acheson, 1966.) *Thin lines,* Cleveland study; *thick lines,* Boston study.

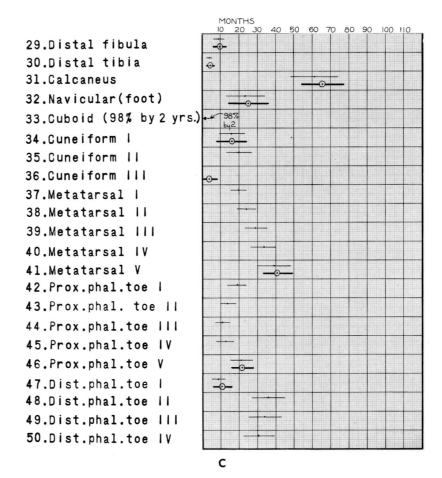

29.Distal fibula
30.Distal tibia
31.Calcaneus
32.Navicular(foot)
33.Cuboid (98% by 2 yrs.)
34.Cuneiform I
35.Cuneiform II
36.Cuneiform III
37.Metatarsal I
38.Metatarsal II
39.Metatarsal III
40.Metatarsal IV
41.Metatarsal V
42.Prox.phal.toe I
43.Prox.phal. toe II
44.Prox.phal.toe III
45.Prox.phal.toe IV
46.Prox.phal.toe V
47.Dist.phal.toe I
48.Dist.phal.toe II
49.Dist.phal.toe III
50.Dist.phal.toe IV

C

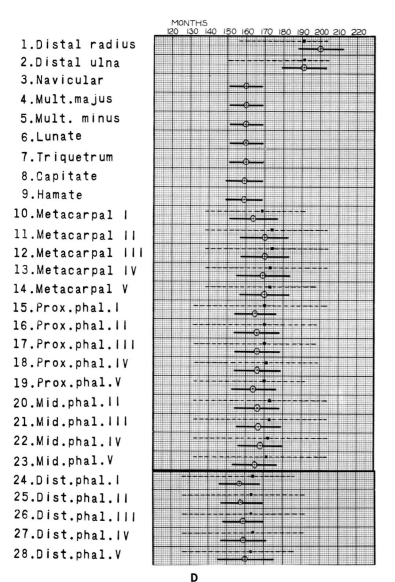

1.Distal radius
2.Distal ulna
3.Navicular
4.Mult.majus
5.Mult. minus
6.Lunate
7.Triquetrum
8.Capitate
9.Hamate
10.Metacarpal I
11.Metacarpal II
12.Metacarpal III
13.Metacarpal IV
14.Metacarpal V
15.Prox.phal.I
16.Prox.phal.II
17.Prox.phal.III
18.Prox.phal.IV
19.Prox.phal.V
20.Mid.phal.II
21.Mid.phal.III
22.Mid.phal.IV
23.Mid.phal.V
24.Dist.phal.I
25.Dist.phal.II
26.Dist.phal.III
27.Dist.phal.IV
28.Dist.phal.V

D

Figure 3–9 continued on following page.

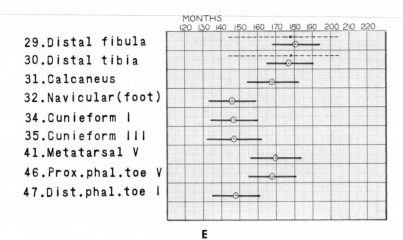

MONTHS
120 130 140 150 160 170 180 190 200 210 220

29. Distal fibula
30. Distal tibia
31. Calcaneus
32. Navicular(foot)
34. Cunieform I
35. Cunieform III
41. Metatarsal V
46. Prox.phal.toe V
47. Dist.phal.toe I

E

Figure 3–9 *Continued.* E. Completion of ossification of the ankle and foot in females, according to the Cleveland and Boston studies. (Data compiled from Acheson, 1966.) *Thin lines,* Cleveland study; *thick lines,* Boston study. F. Onset and completion of ossification of secondary centers of the shoulder and elbow in males according to the Denver, Cleveland, and Boston studies. (Data compiled from Acheson, 1966.)

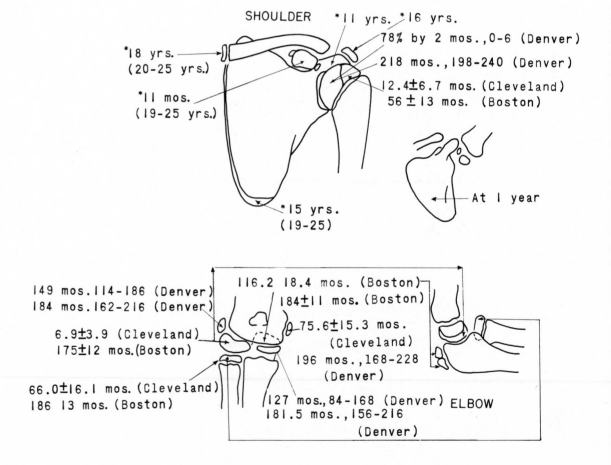

SHOULDER   *11 yrs. *16 yrs.
78% by 2 mos.,0-6 (Denver)
*18 yrs.
(20-25 yrs.)   218 mos.,198-240 (Denver)
12.4±6.7 mos. (Cleveland)
*11 mos.   56±13 mos. (Boston)
(19-25 yrs.)

*15 yrs.
(19-25)

At 1 year

149 mos.114-186 (Denver)   116.2 18.4 mos. (Boston)
184 mos.162-216 (Denver)   184±11 mos. (Boston)

6.9±3.9 (Cleveland)   75.6±15.3 mos.
175±12 mos.(Boston)   (Cleveland)
196 mos.,168-228
(Denver)

66.0±16.1 mos. (Cleveland)
186 13 mos. (Boston)   127 mos.,84-168 (Denver) ELBOW
181.5 mos.,156-216
(Denver)

F   *Schinz-Baensch-Friedl-Uehlinger

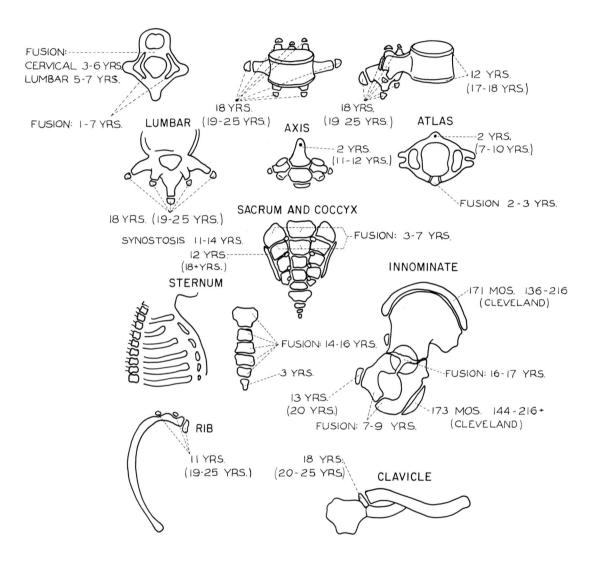

Figure 3–9 *Continued.* G. Ossification onset or fusion of vertebrae, sternum, innominate bone, ribs, and clavicle. (Data modified from Girdany and Golden, 1952.)

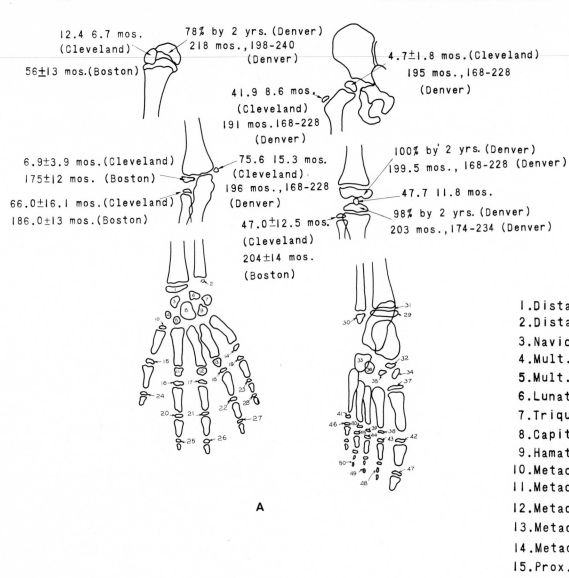

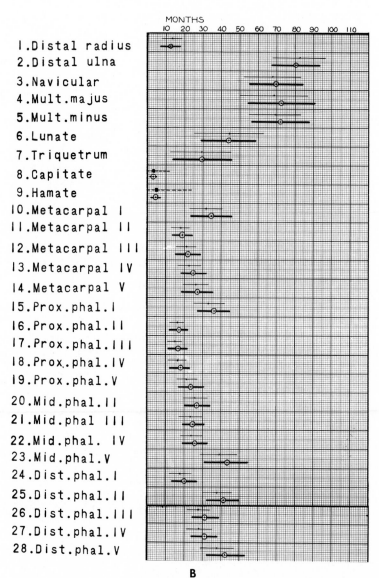

Figure 3–10. *A.* Onset and completion of ossification of secondary centers of ossification of the upper and lower extremities in males, according to the Denver, Cleveland, and Boston studies. (Data compiled from Acheson, 1966.) (These data are contained in chart form in Figure 3–10 *B, C, D,* and *E.*) *B.* Onset of ossification of secondary centers of the wrist and hands in males according to the Cleveland and Boston studies. (Data compiled from Acheson, 1966.) *Thin lines,* Cleveland study; *thick lines,* Boston study.

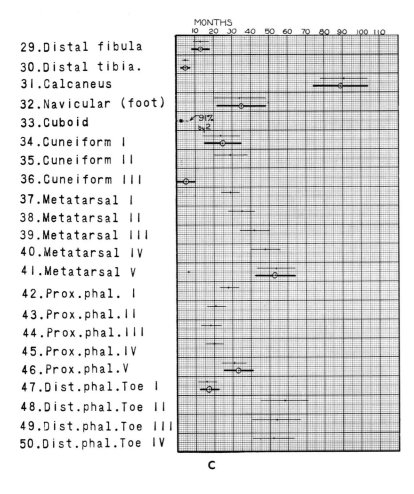

C

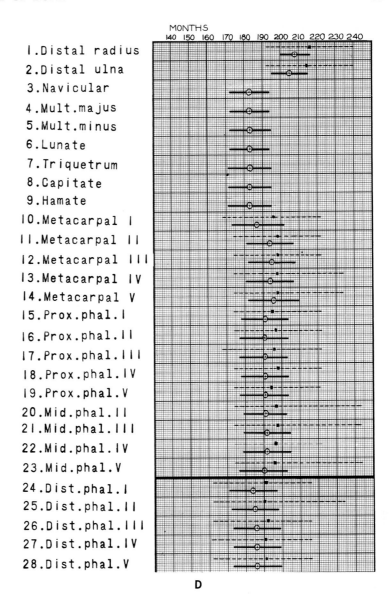

D

Figure 3–10 Continued. C. Onset of ossification of secondary centers of the ankle and foot in males, according to the Cleveland and Boston studies. (Data compiled from Acheson, 1966.) *Thin lines*, Cleveland study; *thick lines*, Boston study. D. Completion of ossification of the wrist and hands in males, according to the Cleveland and Boston studies. (Data compiled from Acheson, 1966.) *Thin lines*, Cleveland study; *thick lines*, Boston study.

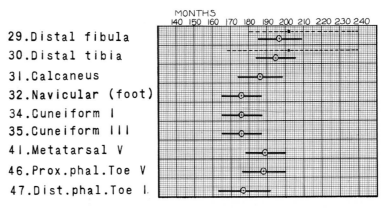

E

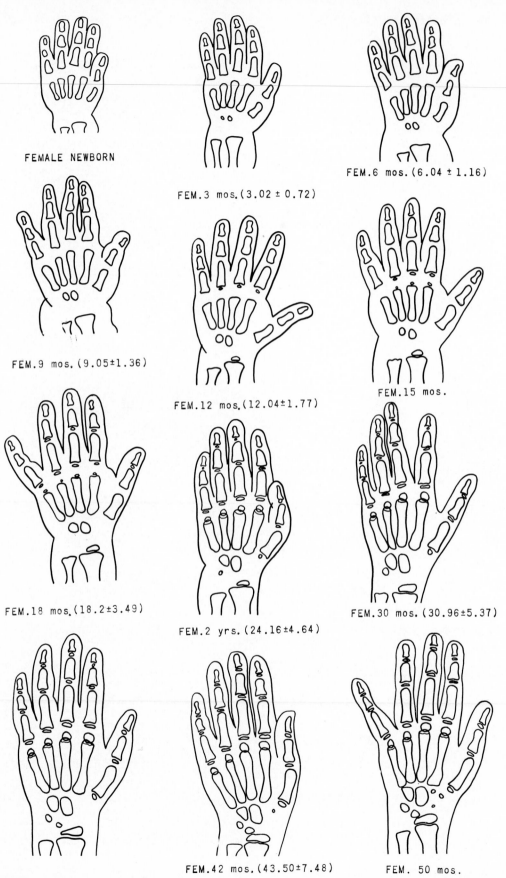

FEMALE NEWBORN

FEM.3 mos.(3.02 ± 0.72)

FEM.6 mos.(6.04 ± 1.16)

FEM.9 mos.(9.05±1.36)

FEM.12 mos.(12.04±1.77)

FEM.15 mos.

FEM.18 mos.(18.2±3.49)

FEM.2 yrs.(24.16±4.64)

FEM.30 mos.(30.96±5.37)

FEM.42 mos.(43.50±7.48)

FEM. 50 mos.

Figure 3–11. A. See opposite page for legend.

Figure 3–11 continued on opposite page.

50

A

3. *Completion of ossification* (Figs. 3–9, 3–10), with fusion of the epiphyses and metaphyses (Todd; Rotch).

4. *Maturation indicators* in the wrist, hand, tarsus, foot, and knee (patella) (Figs. 3–11, 3–12, 3–13).

Generally, the center of the distal end of the femur appears during the 9 months of intrauterine life; the center of the prox-imal end of the tibia and of the head of the humerus also appear toward the end of intrauterine life, often but not invariably. Most of the other centers of long bones appear during infancy and childhood with the exception of the clavicle. This has an epiphysis at its medial end only and this does not appear until the 18th or 20th year. It is one of the last epiphyses to unite.

(*Text continued on page 57.*)

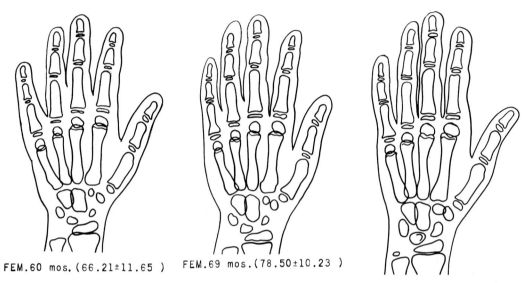

FEM.60 mos.(66.21±11.65)   FEM.69 mos.(78.50±10.23)

FEM.82 mos. (if 84 mos.:89.30±9.64

Figure 3–11 *Continued.* Osseous changes in the wrist and hand and foot in the male and female. A. Female hand and wrist, birth to 18 years. (Modified from Greulich, W. W., and Pyle, S. I.: Radiographic Atlas of Skeletal Development of the Hand and Wrist. 2nd ed. Stanford, Calif., Stanford University Press, 1959.)

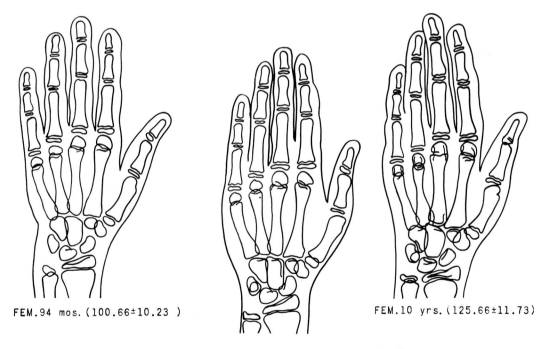

FEM.94 mos. (100.66±10.23)   FEM.10 yrs. (125.66±11.73)

A   FEM.106 mos.(if 9 yrs.:113.86±10.74)

Figure 3–11 continued on following page.

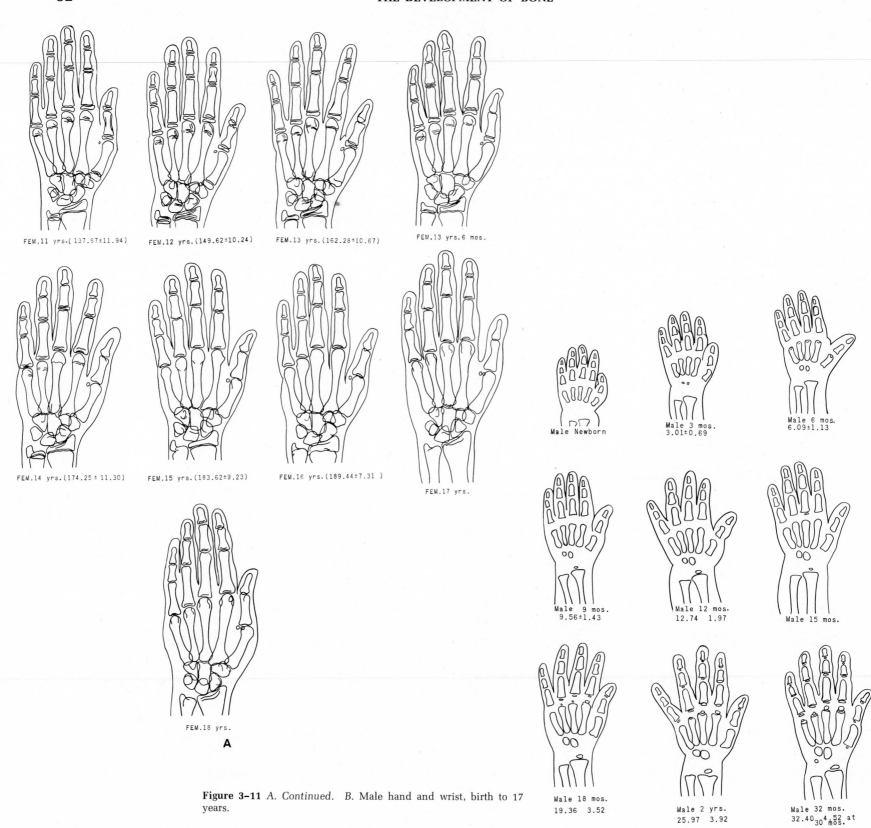

FEM.11 yrs.(137.87±11.94)   FEM.12 yrs.(149.62±10.24)   FEM.13 yrs.(162.28±10.67)   FEM.13 yrs.6 mos.

FEM.14 yrs.(174.25 ± 11.30)   FEM.15 yrs.(183.62±9.23)   FEM.16 yrs.(189.44±7.31)

FEM.17 yrs.

FEM.18 yrs.

A

Male Newborn   Male 3 mos. 3.01±0.69   Male 6 mos. 6.09±1.13

Male 9 mos. 9.56±1.43   Male 12 mos. 12.74 1.97   Male 15 mos.

Male 18 mos. 19.36 3.52   Male 2 yrs. 25.97 3.92   Male 32 mos. 32.40 30±4.52 at mos.

B

Figure 3–11 *A. Continued. B.* Male hand and wrist, birth to 17 years.

Figure 3–11 continued on opposite page.

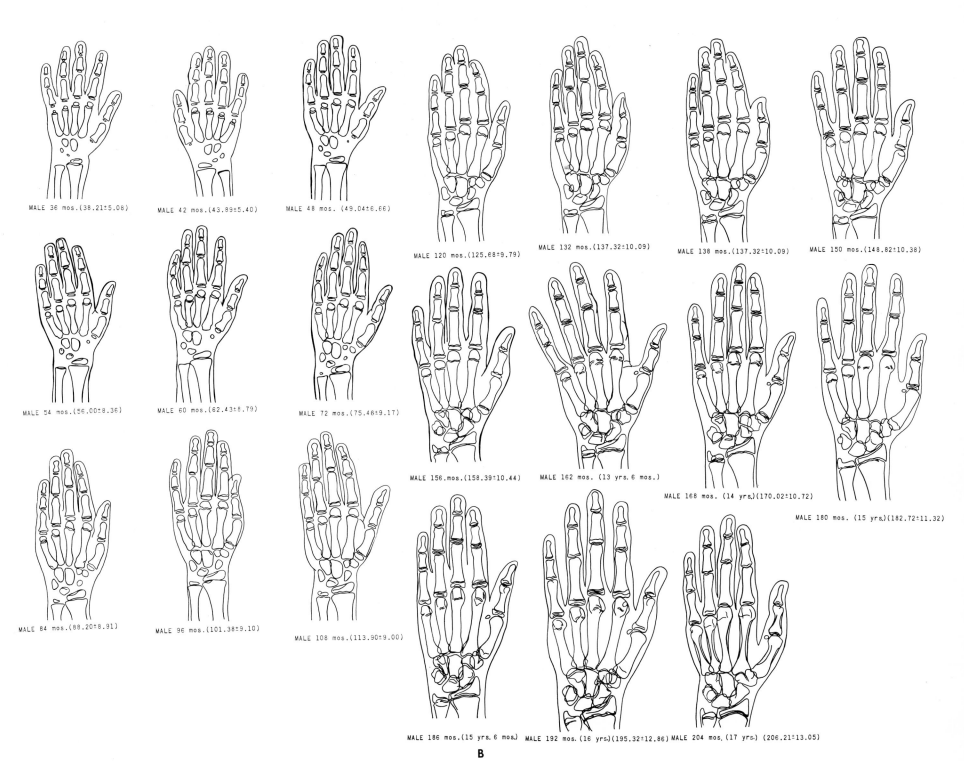

MALE 36 mos.(38.21±5.08)

MALE 42 mos.(43.89±5.40)

MALE 48 mos. (49.04±6.66)

MALE 120 mos.(125.68±9.79)

MALE 132 mos.(137.32±10.09)

MALE 138 mos.(137.32±10.09)

MALE 150 mos.(148.82±10.38)

MALE 54 mos.(56.00±8.36)

MALE 60 mos.(62.43±8.79)

MALE 72 mos.(75.46±9.17)

MALE 156.mos.(158.39±10.44)

MALE 162 mos. (13 yrs. 6 mos.)

MALE 168 mos. (14 yrs.)(170.02±10.72)

MALE 180 mos. (15 yrs.)(182.72±11.32)

MALE 84 mos.(88.20±8.91)

MALE 96 mos.(101.38±9.10)

MALE 108 mos.(113.90±9.00)

MALE 186 mos.(15 yrs. 6 mos.)   MALE 192 mos. (16 yrs.)(195.32±12.86) MALE 204 mos. (17 yrs.) (206.21±13.05)

B

Figure 3–11. *B. Continued.*

Figure 3–11 continued on following page.

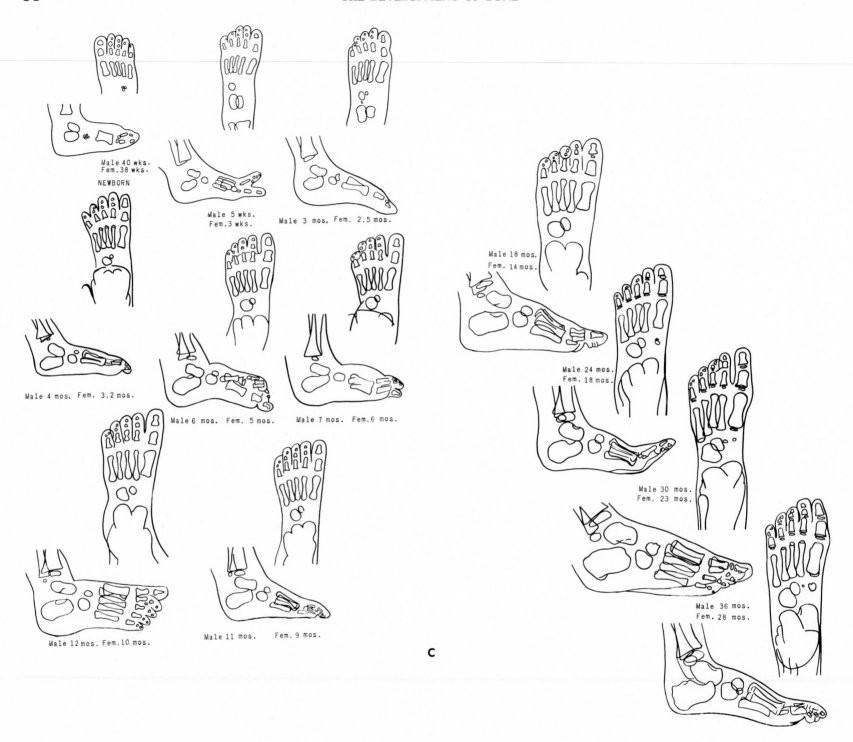

Figure 3–11 *Continued.*   C. Foot and ankle, birth to 17.5 years (male and female).

Figure 3–11 continued on opposite page.

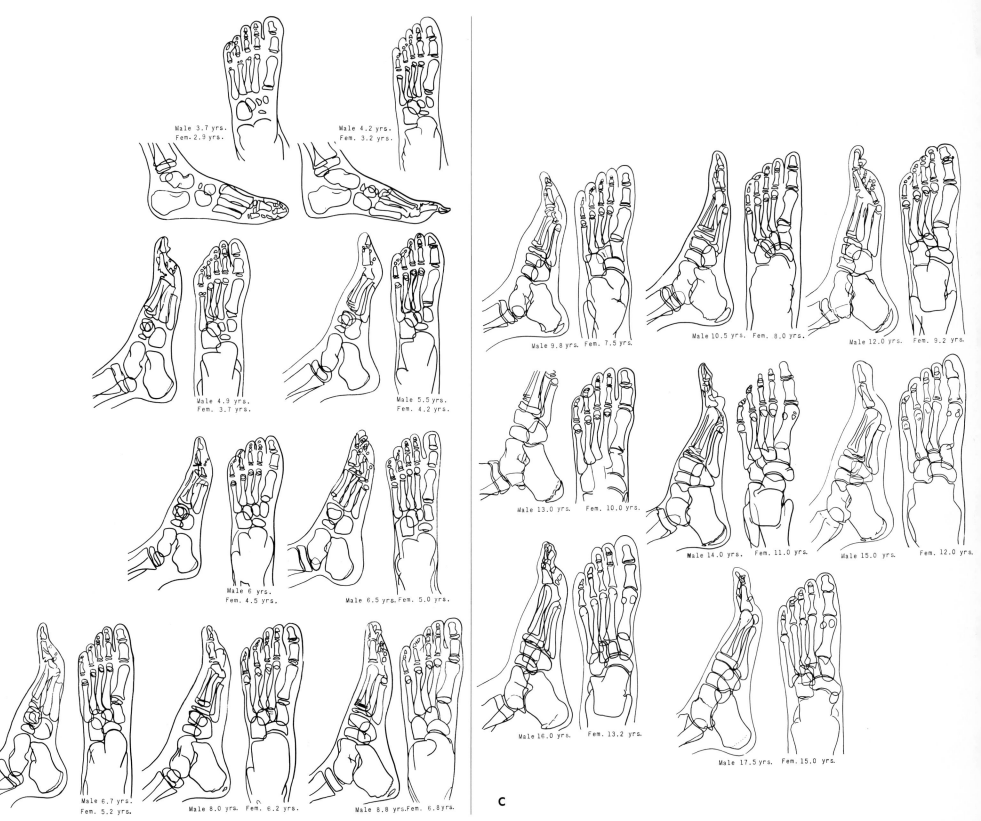

Male 3.7 yrs. Fem. 2.9 yrs.

Male 4.2 yrs. Fem. 3.2 yrs.

Male 4.9 yrs. Fem. 3.7 yrs.

Male 5.5 yrs. Fem. 4.2 yrs.

Male 6 yrs. Fem. 4.5 yrs.

Male 6.5 yrs. Fem. 5.0 yrs.

Male 6.7 yrs. Fem. 5.2 yrs.

Male 8.0 yrs. Fem. 6.2 yrs.

Male 8.8 yrs. Fem. 6.8 yrs.

Male 9.8 yrs. Fem. 7.5 yrs.

Male 10.5 yrs. Fem. 8.0 yrs.

Male 12.0 yrs. Fem. 9.2 yrs.

Male 13.0 yrs. Fem. 10.0 yrs.

Male 14.0 yrs. Fem. 11.0 yrs.

Male 15.0 yrs. Fem. 12.0 yrs.

Male 16.0 yrs. Fem. 13.2 yrs.

Male 17.5 yrs. Fem. 15.0 yrs.

C

Figure 3–11 C. Continued.

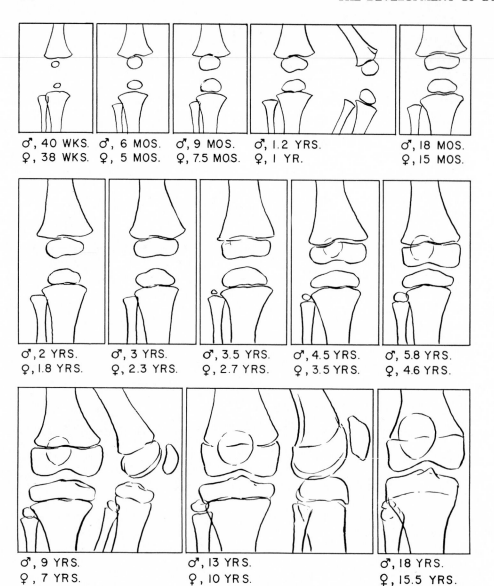

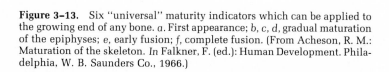

♂, 9 YRS.   ♂, 13 YRS.   ♂, 18 YRS.
♀, 7 YRS.   ♀, 10 YRS.   ♀, 15.5 YRS.

Figure 3–12. Osseous changes in the knee with age in the male and female (after Pyle and Hoerr).

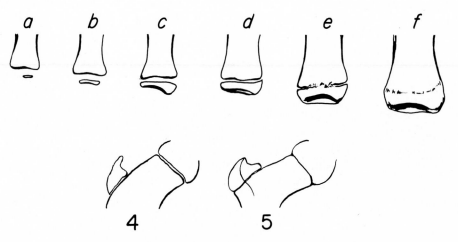

Figure 3–13. Six "universal" maturity indicators which can be applied to the growing end of any bone. *a.* First appearance; *b, c, d,* gradual maturation of the epiphyses; *e,* early fusion; *f,* complete fusion. (From Acheson, R. M.: Maturation of the skeleton. *In* Falkner, F. (ed.): Human Development. Philadelphia, W. B. Saunders Co., 1966.)

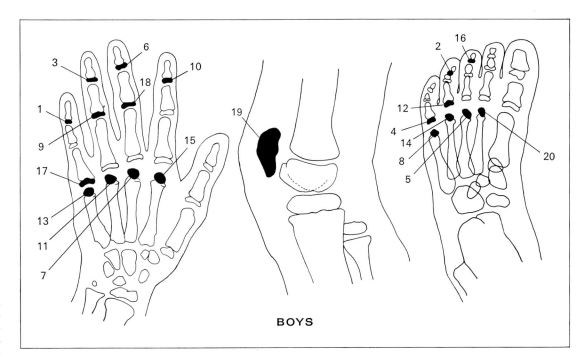

BOYS

Figure 3–14. The 20 centers of maximum predictive value in boys and in girls. The postnatal ossification centers that have the highest statistical "communality" and hence the greatest predictive value in skeletal assessment are located in the hand, foot, and knee. Thus, three radiographs can actually provide more diagnostically useful information than the larger number often made. (From Garn, S. G., Rohmann, C. G., and Silverman, F. N.: Medical Radiography and Photography, 43(2), 1967.)

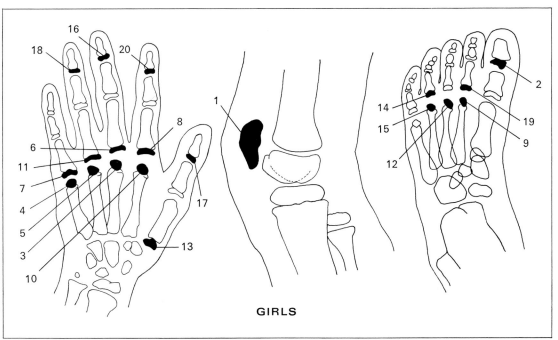

GIRLS

Author's recommendations for assessment of bone age:

1. Radiographs are obtained of the regions indicated in Figure 3–15, depending upon the chronological age of the child.

2. In these regions, onset and completion of ossification (fusion) are studied (Figs. 3–9, 3–10). The "age-at-appearance" percentiles for major postnatal ossification centers can be determined (Tables 3–2, 3–3, 3–4).

3. Maturation indicators are studied in the hand, wrist,

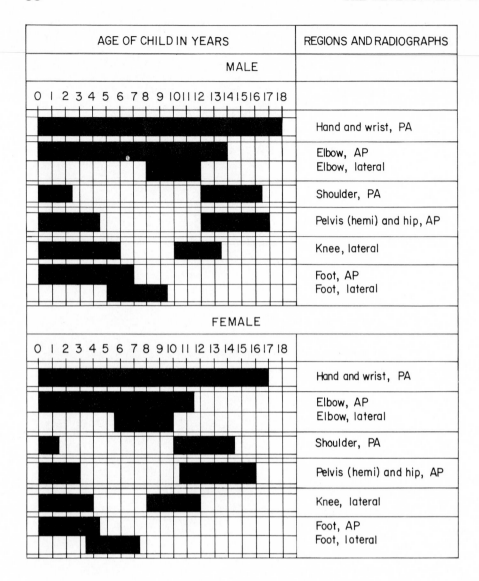

Figure 3-15. Bone age sampling method—suggested filming. (Fels Institute data from Graham, C. B.: Instruction Course. Miami Beach, Amer. Roentgen Ray Soc., 1970.)

tarsus, foot, and knee as indicated by the age of the child. These are tabulated in relation to the given mean age plus the standard deviation (Figs. 3-9, 3-10, 3-11, 3-14).

4. All of these data are interrelated to give the most probable age. The 20 centers of ossification which are most valuable from the standpoint of evaluating postnatal ossification are shown in Figure 3-14. Three radiographs usually suffice. At puberty, however, more attention must be given to the centers of the hip, iliac bones, and the sesamoids of the thumb and other fingers.

There have, of course, been many methods of estimating skeletal maturation and a few of these are reviewed in a companion text, *Analysis of Roentgen Signs.*

Limitations of Skeletal Assessment

1. Skeletal assessment has the greatest validity for normal children.

2. In some cases of endocrinopathy, chromosomal aberration, Morquio's syndrome, or dyschondroplasia, whole groups of ossification centers may fail to appear (Garn et al., 1964).

3. Skeletal assessments have value in distinguishing between small size and retardation, in measuring the effects of thyroid therapy in hypothyroidism, and in steroid therapy in those requiring this form of treatment.

4. Assessment of one bone or joint is not necessarily a guide to the development of other bones or joints.

TABLE 3–2 AGE-AT-APPEARANCE (YEARS-MONTHS) PERCENTILES FOR SELECTED OSSIFICATION CENTERS*

Centers	Boys 5th	50th	95th	Girls 5th	50th	95th
1. Humerus, head	—	0– 0	0– 4	—	0– 0	0– 4
2. Tibia, proximal	—	0– 0	0– 1	—	0– 0	0– 0
3. Coracoid process of scapula	—	0– 0	0– 4	—	0– 0	0– 5
4. Cuboid	—	0– 1	0– 4	—	0– 1	0– 2
5. Capitate	—	0– 3	0– 7	—	0– 2	0– 7
6. Hamate	0– 0	0– 4	0–10	—	0– 2	0– 7
7. Capitellum of humerus	0– 1	0– 4	1– 1	0– 1	0– 3	0– 9
8. Femur, head	0– 1	0– 4	0– 8	0– 0	0– 4	0– 7
9. Cuneiform 3	0– 1	0– 6	1– 7	—	0– 3	1– 3
10. Humerus, greater tuberosity	0– 3	0–10	2– 4	0– 2	0– 6	1– 2
11. Toe phalanx 5M	—	1– 0	3–10	—	0– 9	2– 1
12. Radius, distal	0– 6	1– 1	2– 4	0– 5	0–10	1– 8
13. Toe phalanx 1D	0– 9	1– 3	2– 1	0– 5	0– 9	1– 8
14. Toe phalanx 4M	0– 5	1– 3	2–11	0– 5	0–11	3– 0
15. Finger phalanx 3P	0– 9	1– 4	2– 2	0– 5	0–10	1– 7
16. Toe phalanx 3M	0– 5	1– 5	4– 3	0– 3	1– 0	2– 6
17. Finger phalanx 2P	0– 9	1– 5	2– 2	0– 5	0–10	1– 8
18. Finger phalanx 4P	0–10	1– 6	2– 5	0– 5	0–11	1– 8
19. Finger phalanx 1D	0– 9	1– 6	2– 8	0– 5	1– 0	1– 9
20. Toe phalanx 3P	0–11	1– 7	2– 6	0– 6	1– 1	1–11
21. Metacarpal 2	0–11	1– 7	2–10	0– 8	1– 1	1– 8
22. Toe phalanx 4P	0–11	1– 8	2– 8	0– 7	1– 3	2– 1
23. Toe phalanx 2P	1– 0	1– 9	2– 8	0– 8	1– 2	2– 1
24. Metacarpal 3	0–11	1– 9	3– 0	0– 8	1– 2	1–11
25. Finger phalanx 5P	1– 0	1–10	2–10	0– 8	1– 2	2– 1
26. Finger phalanx 3M	1– 0	2– 0	3– 4	0– 8	1– 3	2– 4
27. Metacarpal 4	1– 1	2– 0	3– 7	0– 9	1– 3	2– 2
28. Toe phalanx 2M	0–11	2– 0	4– 1	0– 6	1– 2	2– 3
29. Finger phalanx 4M	1– 0	2– 1	3– 3	0– 8	1– 3	2– 5
30. Metacarpal 5	1– 3	2– 2	3–10	0–10	1– 4	2– 4
31. Cuneiform 1	0–11	2– 2	3– 9	0– 6	1– 5	2–10
32. Metatarsal 1	1– 5	2– 2	3– 1	1– 0	1– 7	2– 3
33. Finger phalanx 2M	1– 4	2– 2	3– 4	0– 8	1– 4	2– 6
34. Toe phalanx 1P	1– 5	2– 4	3– 4	0–11	1– 7	2– 6
35. Finger phalanx 3D	1– 4	2– 5	3– 9	0– 9	1– 6	2– 8
36. Triquetrum	0– 6	2– 5	5– 6	0– 3	1– 8	3– 9
37. Finger phalanx 4D	1– 4	2– 5	3– 9	0– 9	1– 6	2–10

TABLE 3–2 AGE-AT-APPEARANCE (YEARS-MONTHS) PERCENTILES FOR SELECTED OSSIFICATION CENTERS *(Continued)*

Centers	Boys 5th	50th	95th	Girls 5th	50th	95th
38. Toe phalanx 5P	1– 6	2– 5	3– 8	1– 0	1– 9	2– 8
39. Metacarpal 1	1– 5	2– 7	4– 4	0–11	1– 7	2– 8
40. Cuneiform 2	1– 2	2– 8	4– 3	0–10	1–10	3– 0
41. Metatarsal 2	1–11	2–10	4– 4	1– 3	2– 2	3– 5
42. Femur, greater trochanter	1–11	3– 0	4– 4	1– 0	1–10	3– 0
43. Finger phalanx 1P	1–10	3– 0	4– 7	0–11	1– 9	2–10
44. Navicular of foot	1– 1	3– 0	5– 5	0– 9	1–11	3– 7
45. Finger phalanx 2D	1–10	3– 2	5– 0	1– 1	2– 6	3– 3
46. Finger phalanx 5D	2– 1	3– 3	5– 0	1– 0	2– 0	3– 5
47. Finger phalanx 5M	1–11	3– 5	5–10	0–11	2– 0	3– 6
48. Fibula, proximal	1–10	3– 6	5– 3	1– 4	2– 7	3–11
49. Metatarsal 3	2– 4	3– 6	5– 0	1– 5	2– 6	3– 8
50. Toe phalanx 5D	2– 4	3–11	6– 4	1– 2	2– 4	4– 1
51. Patella	2– 7	4– 0	6– 0	1– 6	2– 6	4– 0
52. Metatarsal 4	2–11	4– 0	5– 9	1– 9	2–10	4– 1
53. Lunate	1– 6	4– 1	6– 9	1– 1	2– 7	5– 8
54. Toe phalanx 3D	3– 0	4– 4	6– 2	1– 4	2– 9	4– 1
55. Metatarsal 5	3– 1	4– 4	6– 4	2– 1	3– 3	4–11
56. Toe phalanx 4D	2–11	4– 5	6– 5	1– 4	2– 7	4– 1
57. Toe phalanx 2D	3– 3	4– 8	6– 9	1– 6	2–11	4– 6
58. Capitulum of radius	3– 0	5– 3	8– 0	2– 3	3–10	6– 3
59. Navicular of wrist	3– 7	5– 8	7–10	2– 4	4– 1	6– 0
60. Greater multangular	3– 6	5–10	9– 0	1–11	4– 1	6– 4
61. Lesser multangular	3– 1	6– 3	8– 6	2– 5	4– 2	6– 0
62. Medial epicondyle of humerus	4– 3	6– 3	8– 5	2– 1	3– 5	5– 1
63. Ulna, distal	5– 3	7– 1	9– 1	3– 3	5– 4	7– 8
64. Calcaneal apophysis	5– 2	7– 7	9– 7	3– 6	5– 4	7– 4
65. Olecranon of ulna	7– 9	9– 8	11–11	5– 7	8– 0	9–11
66. Lateral epicondyle of humerus	9– 3	11– 3	13– 8	7– 2	9– 3	11– 3
67. Tibial tubercle	9–11	11–10	13– 5	7–11	10– 3	11–10
68. Adductor sesamoid of thumb	11– 0	12– 9	14– 7	8– 8	10– 9	12– 8
69. Os acetabulum	11–11	13– 6	15– 4	9– 7	11– 6	13– 5
70. Acromion	12– 2	13– 9	15– 6	10– 4	11–11	13– 9
71. Iliac crest	12– 0	14– 0	15–11	10–10	12– 9	15– 4
72. Coracoid apophysis	12– 9	14– 4	16– 4	10– 4	12– 3	14– 4
73. Ischial tuberosity	13– 7	15– 3	17– 1	11– 9	13–11	16– 0

*Modified by Graham from Garn, S. M., Silverman, F. N., and Rohmann, C. G.: A rational approach to the assessment of skeletal maturation. Ann. Radiol. (Paris), 7:297–307, 1964.

P, proximal; M, middle; D, distal.

5. Irrespective of the "bone age assessment," the genetic pattern of the individual must be taken into consideration. For example, in populations in which axillary and pubic hair are normally scarce, radiographic appraisal of the skeleton has particular value (Garn et al., 1963).

6. If the assessment is based upon developmental data compiled from a population not applicable to the individual being evaluated, allowances must be made for moderate deviations (Graham).

7. Caution must be exercised in "over-requesting" too many osseous centers, which will result in inordinate exposure of the patient to radiation, and in "overinterpreting" with a pictorial age-standard one specific body region such as the hand and wrist, since the specific region may not reflect skeletal maturation as a whole (Table 3–3). Moreover, there are long periods during which little bony change is occurring either in the hand and wrist or in the foot, and a single standard plate is virtually impossible (Graham, 1972).

TABLE 3–3 NUMBER OF OSSIFICATION CENTERS AT DIFFERENT MONTHS OF AGE*

Boys

Age, Mo.	Av. No. Centers =M	Dev. =σ	Range of Variation					
			M−3σ	M−2½σ	M−σ	M+σ	M+2½σ	M+3σ
1	4.8	1.9	0	0	2.9	6.7	9.6	10.5
2	5.7	2.0	0	0.7	3.7	7.7	10.7	11.7
3	6.5	2.0	0.5	1.5	4.5	8.5	11.5	12.5
4	8.9	2.8	0.5	1.9	6.1	11.7	15.9	17.3
5	9.8	2.4	2.6	3.8	7.4	12.2	15.8	17.0
6	11.2	2.4	4.0	5.2	8.8	13.6	17.2	18.4
7	12.5	2.9	3.8	5.2	9.6	15.4	19.8	21.2
8	13.0	1.7	7.9	8.7	11.3	14.7	17.3	18.1
9	13.6	2.7	5.5	6.8	10.9	16.3	20.4	21.7
10	15.2	3.5	4.7	6.4	11.7	18.7	24.0	25.7
11	15.8	3.2	6.2	7.8	12.6	19.0	23.8	25.4
12	16.5	4.9	1.8	4.2	11.6	21.4	28.8	31.2
13–15	19.9	6.3	1.0	4.1	13.6	26.2	35.7	38.8
16–18	23.5	8.4	0	2.5	15.1	31.9	44.5	48.7
19–21	25.5	8.4	0.3	4.5	17.1	33.9	46.5	50.7
22–24	32.3	9.2	4.7	9.3	23.1	41.5	55.3	59.9
25–27	36.8	5.5	20.3	23.0	31.3	42.3	50.6	52.3
28–30	39.8	8.4	14.6	18.8	31.4	48.2	60.8	65.0
31–33	44.1	4.8	29.7	32.1	39.3	48.9	56.1	58.5
34–36	48.5	5.8	31.1	34.0	42.7	54.3	63.0	65.9
37–42	49.5	6.9	28.8	32.2	42.6	56.4	66.8	70.2
43–48	56.6	4.9	41.9	44.3	51.7	61.5	68.9	71.3
49–54	59.3	5.5	42.8	45.5	53.8	64.8	73.1	75.8
55–60	61.8	3.5	51.3	53.0	58.3	65.3	70.6	72.3

Girls

Age, Mo.	Av. No. Centers =M	Dev. =σ	Range of Variation					
			M−3σ	M−2½σ	M−σ	M+σ	M+2½σ	M+3σ
1	4.7	1.9	0	0	2.8	6.6	9.5	10.4
2	6.2	2.3	0	0.4	3.9	8.5	12.0	13.1
3	7.6	2.5	0.1	1.3	5.1	10.1	13.9	15.1
4	8.5	2.8	0.1	1.5	5.7	11.3	15.5	16.9
5	10.4	2.0	4.4	5.4	8.4	12.4	15.4	16.4
6	11.5	1.7	6.4	7.2	9.8	13.2	15.8	16.6
7	12.9	1.4	8.7	9.4	11.5	14.3	16.4	17.1
8	14.6	3.5	4.1	5.8	11.1	18.1	23.4	25.1
9	16.3	2.4	9.1	10.3	13.9	18.7	22.3	23.5
10	18.1	4.4	4.9	7.1	13.7	22.5	29.1	31.3
11	22.7	6.9	2.0	5.4	15.8	29.6	40.0	43.4
12	25.1	8.7	0	3.3	16.4	33.8	46.9	51.2
13–15	28.6	9.2	1.0	5.6	19.4	37.8	51.6	56.2
16–18	32.9	8.8	6.5	10.9	24.1	41.7	54.9	59.3
19–21	41.3	8.6	15.5	19.8	32.7	49.9	62.8	67.1
22–24	47.2	7.1	25.9	29.4	40.1	54.3	65.0	68.5
25–27	50.8	4.8	36.4	38.8	46.0	55.6	62.8	65.2
28–30	53.2	6.5	33.7	36.9	46.7	59.7	69.5	72.7
31–33	55.8	4.8	41.4	43.8	51.0	60.6	67.8	70.2
34–36	60.5	3.0	51.5	53.0	57.5	63.5	68.0	69.5
37–42	59.5	4.5	46.0	48.2	55.0	64.0	70.8	73.0
43–48	61.4	6.6	41.6	44.9	54.8	68.0	77.9	81.2
49–54	63.5	2.2	56.9	58.0	61.3	65.7	69.0	70.1
55–60	64.2	2.3	57.3	58.4	61.9	66.5	70.0	71.1

*From Elgenmark, O.: Acta Paediat., *33* (Suppl. 1), 1946.

TABLE 3–4 PERCENTAGE OCCURRENCE OF NEWBORN OSSIFICATION CENTERS, DISTRIBUTED ACCORDING TO SEX, RACE (NEGRO/CAUCASIAN), AND BIRTHWEIGHT (GRAMS)*

Centers	Weight Ranges					
	<2,000	2,000– 2,499	2,500– 2,999	3,000– 3,499	3,500– 3,999	≥4,000
Calcaneus						
females N/C	100 / 100	100 / 100	100 / 100	100 / 100	100 / 100	100 / 100
males N/C	100 / 100	100 / 100	100 / 100	100 / 100	100 / 100	100 / 100
Talus						
females	100 / 83	100 / 100	100 / 100	100 / 100	100 / 100	100 / 100
males	91 / 73	100 / 100	100 / 100	100 / 99	100 / 100	100 / 100
Femur, distal						
females	50 / 50	94 / 92	99 / 98	100 / 100	100 / 100	100 / 100
males	18 / 9	89 / 75	91 / 85	94 / 100	100 / 100	100 / 100
Tibia, proximal						
females	14 / 0	41 / 54	77 / 76	88 / 86	86 / 91	100 / 91
males	0 / 0	39 / 19	63 / 53	76 / 79	80 / 84	93 / 97
Cuboid						
females	21 / 0	38 / 38	68 / 57	78 / 65	82 / 70	75 / 76
males	0 / 0	23 / 6	44 / 15	58 / 40	68 / 44	100 / 60
Humerus, proximal						
females	0 / 0	11 / 6	23 / 26	53 / 42	39 / 69	100 / 87
males	0 / 0	0 / 8	15 / 14	28 / 42	48 / 49	64 / 59
Capitate						
females	0 / 0	13 / 0	20 / 15	42 / 15	41 / 21	100 / 38
males	0 / 0	7 / 0	16 / 0	21 / 8	26 / 16	31 / 18
Hamate						
females	0 / 0	9 / 0	23 / 11	41 / 13	55 / 2	67 / 33
males	0 / 0	16 / 7	16 / 6	18 / 6	44 / 10	28 / 11
Cuneiform, third						
females	0 / 0	6 / 0	14 / 0	17 / 0	18 / 6	25 / 10
males	0 / 0	4 / 0	8 / 0	15 / 3	14 / 2	14 / 3
Femur, proximal						
females	0 / 0	0 / 0	1 / 0	1 / 1	0 / 0	0 / 0
males	0 / 0	0 / 0	0 / 0	0 / 0	0 / 0	0 / 0

*Modified by Graham from Christie, A.: Prevalence and distribution of ossification centers in the newborn infant. Amer. J. Dis. Child., 77:355–361, 1949.

TABLE 3–5 NORMAL RANGES OF AGE-AT-APPEARANCE OF PRINCIPAL CENTERS*

Age of Child		
Male	*Female*	**Range**
0– 1 year	0– 1 year	±3–6 months
3– 4 years	2– 3 years	±1–1.5 years
7–11 years	6–10 years	±2 years
13–14 years	12–13 years	±2 years plus

*Based on Fels Institute data in Graham, C. B.: Instruction Course. Miami, American Roentgen Ray Society, 1970.

General Rules for Use of Bone Age Data
(Watson and Lowrey)

1. *For children from birth to 5 years:* register skeletal age by the time of appearance of centers of ossification.

2. *For children 5 to 14 years of age:* study maturation factors and penetration of cartilaginous areas by reference to standards.

3. *For children 14 to 25 years of age:* register skeletal age by epiphyseal-diaphyseal union and reference to *Completion of Ossification* tables.

Premature Fusion of Epiphyses (Currarino and Erlandson). Premature fusion of one or more epiphyses is uncommon but may occur under the following circumstances: (1) as a complication of infection or trauma involving the epiphyseal cartilage plate, (2) following scurvy, perhaps as a result of pathologic fracture of the epiphyseal plate, (3) as a complication of hypervitaminosis A, (4) as a developmental error of cartilage formation, (5) in Cooley's anemia, or (6) in the congenital adrenogenital syndrome with virilism (Kurlander).

Premature fusion is diagnosed on the basis of bony alteration of the epiphyseal line. There may be associated deformity and shortening of the affected bone.

In those patients with Cooley's anemia over 10 years of age, premature fusion is a relatively common finding if homozygous thalassemia is also present (it occurs in 23 per cent of these patients). The sites of predilection are the proximal end of one or both humeri and the distal end of one or both femora.

Wolff's Law. Wolff's law postulates that the internal architecture and external structure of bone are related to its function and change with altered function. The arrangement of trabeculae in the upper end of the femur is an example of this principle.

CARTILAGE

Hyaline cartilage forms the articular surfaces of joints, the costochondral junctions, the nasal cartilage, the bronchial rings, and parts of the trachea and larynx. Articular cartilage has the following layerlike structure as one proceeds from the epiphysis adjoining the joint surface proper: a zone of calcified cartilage nearest the bone; a zone of transition, consisting of longitudinal columns of large chondrocytes; and a gliding zone, which is the true articular zone and in which the cells tend to be flat and elongated and lie in the plane of the articular surface. The perichondrium is a continuation of the periosteum laterally but does not extend over the gliding zone proper. The actual thickness of articular cartilage is from 0.2 to 0.5 mm. in small joints, 2 to 3 mm. in larger joints, and as much as 4 mm. in the knee joint. The actual joint space on the radiograph in children is considerably wider since a greater portion of cartilaginous epiphysis is included as well. The osseous articular surfaces are smooth and the limiting contour lines of the joints are sharp in the adult, but they may be irregular and blurred in the child.

Fibrocartilage is found normally in such locations as the intervertebral disks, symphysis pubis, sternoclavicular joints, and articular menisci, and it represents a modified fibrous tissue.

Elastic cartilage is hyaline cartilage to which have been added elastic fibers. It is found in the ligamentum nuchae, ligamentum flavum, the external auditory canal, and the external ear.

Hyaline and elastic cartilage may undergo calcification and degeneration following trauma and during senility.

JOINTS

There are three main types of joints: the movable (diarthroses), the slightly movable (amphiarthroses), and the immovable (synarthroses) (Figs. 3–16, 3–17).

The diarthroses (movable joints) are invested by a joint capsule which consists of two layers: an outer fibroelastic layer continuous with the periosteum and an inner cellular layer, the synovial membrane. The synovial membrane is lined by an incomplete layer of mesenchymal cells which lie upon variable thicknesses of fibrous, adipose, or areolar tissue. The loose areolar tissue may form villi, which are highly vascular and which have considerable regenerative powers when destroyed by disease or trauma. Synovial fluid is secreted by the cells lining the synovial membrane and acts as a lubricant by virtue of its mucin content. In hypertrophic arthritis there is increased mucin formation, and in rheumatoid arthritis there is decreased mucin. The following synovial joints contain fibrocartilaginous menisci: temporomandibular, radiocarpal, sternocostal, sternoclavicular, acromioclavicular, knee, and glenohumeral.

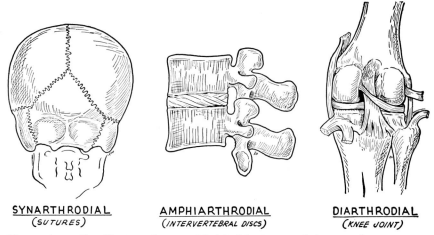

SYNARTHRODIAL
(SUTURES)

AMPHIARTHRODIAL
(INTERVERTEBRAL DISCS)

DIARTHRODIAL
(KNEE JOINT)

Figure 3–16. Classification of joints. (Modified from original drawings by Dr. B. G. Brogdon.)

SCHEMATIC DIAGRAMS SHOWING FOUR STAGES IN THE DEVELOPMENT OF A JOINT

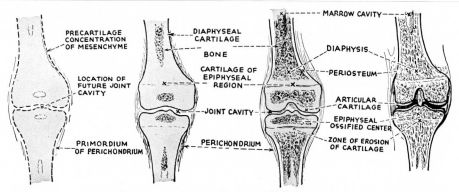

Figure 3–17. (Modified from original drawings by Dr. B. G. Brogdon.)

The amphiarthroses (intervertebral disks) are composed of three parts: the nucleus pulposus, which forms the center of the disk; the annulus fibrosus, which is the fibrocartilaginous substance around the nucleus; and thin hyaline cartilaginous plates which form the upper and lower surfaces of the disk adjacent to the vertebral bodies. The nucleus pulposus absorbs and transmits pressure from one vertebral body to the other and moves about within the annulus fibrosus. Schmorl found that in 38 per cent of autopsied spines there was a protrusion of the nucleus pulposus into the adjoining vertebral bodies (hence called "Schmorl's nodes") and that occasionally such protrusion occurred toward the spinal canal. The disk may be destroyed by pyogenic infection, chronic nonspecific infection, or tuberculosis, but there is considerable resistance to invasion by malignant neoplasm, although the latter may occur also.

The synarthroses (immovable joints) are represented by the sutures in the skull.

GENERAL PRINCIPLES OF IMPORTANCE IN THE RADIOGRAPHIC ANATOMY OF THE SKELETAL SYSTEM

In clinical radiography our emphasis is regional rather than sharply confined to a single anatomic structure. An area is investigated as a whole and it is not unusual, for example, to detect abnormality in the apex of the lung when viewing a shoulder for pain in that region.

The radiographic method for study of a region will vary with the clinical problem at hand. This will become readily apparent when it is evident that numerous views of each anatomic region are possible and only those applicable to the case at hand are utilized. It is, therefore, most important to adapt the radiographic anatomic study to each individual problem.

The epiphyseal development varies somewhat from one individual to another, and in the anatomic study of epiphyses it is most important to compare both sides wherever possible. This is also true for the study of other symmetrical parts of the body such as the two sides of the skull or face. Thus the normal side of a given individual becomes one base line for comparison with the potentially abnormal structure.

In the study of the extremities we always include at least one joint in the radiograph, or one of the joints on either end of that bone, if possible. The main purpose of this is to demonstrate clearly the alignment of the bone with respect to the joints which it serves.

Certain distortions are sometimes inevitable and the observer must become familiar with the normal appearance of such distortion; e.g., when the head of the radius is injured, it is impossible for the patient to extend his elbow fully and a film of the unextended elbow results in considerable distortion (Chapter 4, Figs. 4–23, 4–24).

REFERENCES

Aliapoulios, M. A., Bernstein, D. S., and Balodimos, M. C.: Thyrocalcitonin, its role in calcium homeostasis. Arch. Intern. Med., *123*:88–94, 1969.

Anson, B. J. (ed.): Morris' Human Anatomy. 12th edition. New York, McGraw Hill Book Co., 1966.

Barnhard, H. J., and Geyer, R. W.: Growth and development of bone, normal and abnormal. Radiology, *75*:942–947, 1960.

Caffey, J.: Pediatric X-ray Diagnosis. Fifth edition. Chicago, Year Book Medical Publishers, 1967.

Christie, A.: Prevalence and distribution of ossification centers in the newborn infant. Amer. J. Dis. Child., *77*:355–361, 1949.

Christie, A., Martin, M., Williams, E. L., Hudson, G., and Lanier, J. C., Jr.: Estimation of fetal maturity by roentgen studies of osseous development. Amer. J. Obstet. Gyn., *60*:133–139, 1950.

Copp, D. H.: Parathyroids, calcitonin, and control of plasma calcium. Recent Progress in Hormone Research, *20*:59–88, 1964.

Currarino, G., and Erlandson, M. E.: Premature fusion of epiphyses in Cooley's anemia. Radiology, *83*:656–664, 1964.

Elgenmark, O.: The normal development of the ossific centers during infancy and childhood: clinical, roentgenologic, and statistical study. Acta Paediat., *33* (Suppl. 1):1–79, 1946.

Feist, J. H.: The biological basis of radiological findings in bone disease. Radiol. Clin. N. Amer., 8:182–206, 1970.

Flecker, H.: Time of appearance and fusion of ossification centers as observed by roentgenographic methods. Amer. J. Roentgenol., 47:97–159, 1942.

Foster, G. V.: Calcitonin (thyrocalcitonin). New Eng. J. Med., 279:349–360, 1968.

Garn, S. M., and Rohmann, C. G.: Variability in the order of ossification of the bony centers of the hand and wrist. Amer. J. Phys. Anthropol., 18:219–229, 1960.

Garn, S. M., Rohmann, C. G., and Davis, A. A.: Genetics of hand-wrist ossification. Amer. J. Phys. Anthropol., 21:33–40, 1963.

Garn, S. M., Silverman, F. N., and Rohmann, C. G.: A rational approach to the assessment of skeletal maturation. Ann. Radiol. (Paris), 7:297–307, 1964.

Girdany, B. R., and Golden, R.: Centers of ossification of the skeleton. Amer. J. Roentgenol., 68:922–924, 1952.

Graham, C. B.: Assessment of bone maturation—methods and pitfalls. Radiol. Clin. N. Amer., 10:185–202, 1972.

Graham, C. B.: Roentgenologic evaluation of skeletal development. Instruction course. Miami Beach, American Roentgen Ray Society, 1970.

Graham, C. B.: Skeletal development and assessment of bone age. In Kelley, V. C. (ed.): Brennemann's Practice of Pediatrics. Vol. 4. Hagerstown, Md., Harper and Row, 1972, Pp. 1–14.

Graham, C. B.: Skeletal maturation. In Smith, D., and Marshall, R. (eds.): Introduction to Clinical Pediatrics. Philadelphia, W. B. Saunders Co. (in press).

Greulich, W. W., and Pyle, S. I.: Radiographic Atlas of Skeletal Development of the Hand and Wrist. Second edition. Stanford, Calif., Stanford University Press, 1959.

Ham, A. W.: Histology. Third edition. Philadelphia, J. B. Lippincott Co., 1957.

Ham, A. W.: Some histo-physiological problems peculiar to calcified tissues. J. Bone Joint Surg., 34A:701–728, 1952.

Hoerr, N. L., Pyle, S. I., and Francis, C. C.: Radiographic Atlas of Skeletal Development of the Foot and Ankle. Springfield, Ill., Charles C Thomas, 1962.

Kurlander, G. J.: Roentgenology of the congenital adrenogenital syndrome. Amer. J. Roentgenol., 95:189–199, 1965.

Meschan, I., and Meschan, R.: Analysis of Roentgen Signs. Philadelphia, W. B. Saunders Co., 1973.

Park, E. A.: The imprinting of nutritional disturbances on the growing bone. Pediatrics, 33:815–862, 1964.

Pryor, J. W.: Differences in the time of development of centers of ossification in the male and female skeleton. Anatomical Rec., 25:257–273, 1923.

Pryor, J. W.: The hereditary nature of variation in the ossification of bone. Anatomical Rec., 1:84–88, 1907.

Pyle, S. I., and Hoerr, N. I.: Radiographic Atlas of Skeletal Development of the Knee. Springfield, Ill., Charles C Thomas, 1955.

Pyle, S. I., Waterhouse, A. M., and Greulich, W. W.: A Radiographic Standard of Reference for the Growing Hand and Wrist. Chicago, Year Book Medical Publishers, 1971.

Rotch, T. M.: A study of the development of the bones in childhood by the roentgen method, with a view of establishing a developmental index for the grading and the protection of early life. Trans. Amer. Assoc. Phys., 24:603–630, 1909.

Sontag, L. W., Snell, D., and Anderson, M.: Rate of appearance of ossification centers from birth to the age of five years. Amer. J. Dis. Child., 58:949–956, 1939.

Stein, I., Stein, R. O., and Beller, M. L.: Living Bone in Health and Disease. Philadelphia, J. B. Lippincott Co., 1955.

Stuart, H. C., Pyle, S. I., Cornoni, J., and Reed, R. B.: Onsets, completions and spans of ossification in the twenty-nine bone-growth centers of the hand and wrist. Pediatrics, 29:237–249, 1962.

Tanner, J. M., Whitehouse, R. H., and Healy, M. J. R.: A new system for estimating the maturity of the hand and wrist with standards derived from 2600 healthy British children. Part II. The scoring system. Paris International Children's Center, 1962.

Todd, T. W.: Atlas of Skeletal Maturation, Part I. The Hand. St. Louis, C. V. Mosby Co., 1937.

Watson, E. H., and Lowrey, G. A.: Growth and Development of Children. Fifth edition. Chicago, Year Book Medical Publishers, 1967.

Wilkins, L.: Hormonal influences on skeletal growth. Ann. N.Y. Acad. Sci., 60:763–775, 1955.

4

The Upper Extremity

The primary interest, when reviewing the radiographic anatomy of the extremities without additional contrast agents, lies in the bony structures, since for the most part muscles are blended into a homogeneous mass separated by fat planes. Joint capsular shadows can be distinguished, the fatty subcutaneous layer identified in soft films, and vascular channels may be visualized by special contrast media, but the bones offer the greatest scope to the radiologist and will be the major focus of this chapter.

The main function of the upper extremity is that of a prehensile organ. To perform at maximum efficiency, definite axial relationships between the various parts are maintained. A system of lining has been developed to indicate normal position and alignment, and these will be described in greater detail in subsequent paragraphs.

THE SHOULDER

Related Gross Anatomy. The shoulder girdle consists of the clavicles and scapulas. These structures articulate with one another at the acromioclavicular joint and furnish a suspension type of support for the arm by means of the glenohumeral joint. They are firmly attached to the axial skeleton by the muscles of the vertebral column and the anterolateral thoracic wall.

The *clavicle*, when viewed from above, presents a double curvature (Fig. 4–1). The medial two-thirds of the bone is convex forward and the middle of the shaft is considerably smoother than either of the ends. The posterior border on the medial two-thirds is variably indented and roughened by the "costal tuberosity" for the attachment of the costoclavicular ligament.

The lateral third of the clavicle with an anterior concavity tends to be flattened supero-inferiorly. On its inferior surface is a rough elevation, "the conoid tubercle," which overhangs the coracoid process of the scapula. This may be quite as prominent as the coracoid process in some individuals.

There are three separate centers of ossification for the clavicle—two developing in the fifth to sixth month of fetal life, and the third, the secondary center of ossification, developing between the 16th and the 20th year of life (Fig. 4–1 *E*).

Because of differences in curvature of the clavicle, it must be

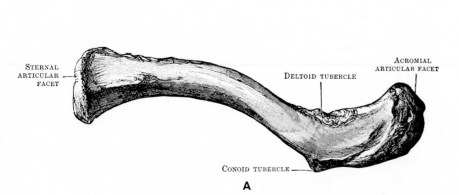

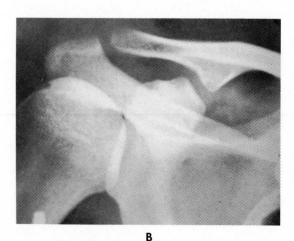

Figure 4–1. *A.* Clavicle viewed from above. (From Cunningham, D. J.: Textbook of Anatomy. 10th ed. London, Oxford University Press, 1964.) *B.* Roentgenogram showing coracoclavicular joint. (From Moore, R. D., and Renner, R. R.: Amer. J. Roentgenol., *78*:86–88, 1957.)

Figure 4–1 continued on opposite page.

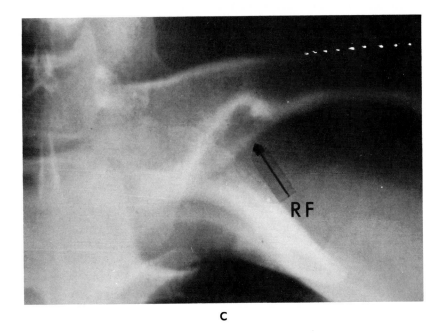

C

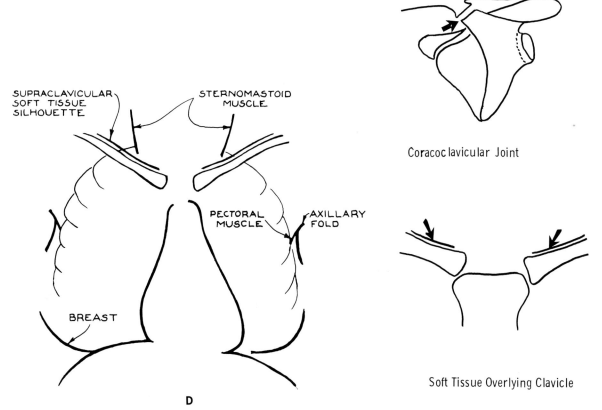

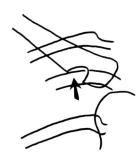

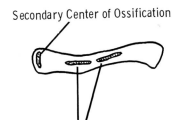

Coracoclavicular Joint

Rhomboid Notch

Soft Tissue Overlying Clavicle

Figure 4–1 *Continued.*   *C.* Radiograph demonstrating the rhomboid notch for a ligament. *D.* Diagram showing the soft tissue overlying the clavicle at the base of the neck. *E.* Diagram illustrating primary and secondary centers of ossification of the clavicle.

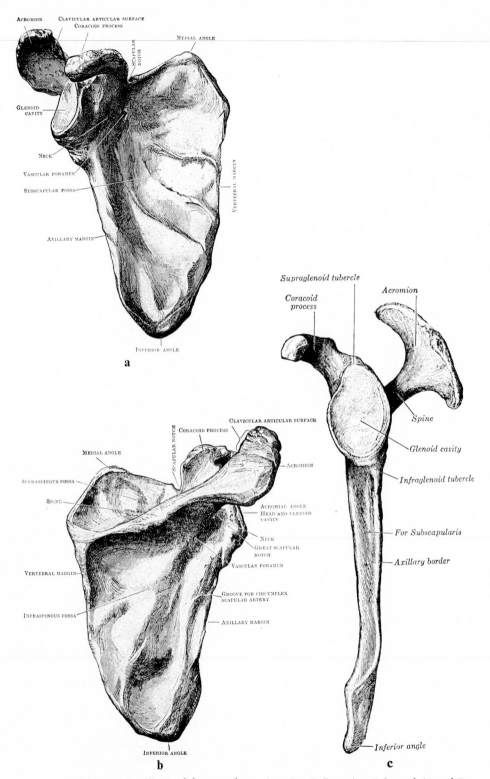

Figure 4-2. Views of the scapula. *A.* Anterior. *B.* Posterior. *C.* Lateral. (*A* and *B* from Cunningham, D. J.: Textbook of Anatomy, 10th ed. London, Oxford University Press, 1964. *C* from Gray, H.: Gray's Anatomy of the Human Body. 24th ed. Philadelphia, Lea & Febiger, 1942.)

visualized from several perspectives, particularly when a greenstick fracture may be suspected in infancy.

A soft tissue shadow parallel to the superior margin of the clavicle, representing the skin and subcutaneous tissues following the clavicle into the supraclavicular fossa, may be identified, (Fig. 4–1 *E*).

Near the outer end of the clavicle there is occasionally a prominence or even a process, the coracoid tubercle, which represents a point of attachment for the coracoclavicular ligament. At times, a true joint forms between the coracoid process of the clavicle and the coracoid process of the scapula (Fig. 4–1 *B*).

Fusion of the secondary center of ossification usually occurs in the middle of the third decade. The shape of the medial end of the clavicle may vary, being rather cup-shaped in early life, and having a more rounded contour in adults.

In some individuals there is a notchlike defect on the inferior medial aspect of the clavicle known as the "rhomboid fossa" or "rhomboid depression" (Fig. 4–1 *C*). This is related to a costoclavicular or rhomboid ligament representing the attachment of the first rib to the clavicle. It is a normal variant.

The *scapula* (Fig. 4–2) is a large flat bone on the dorsal aspect of the thorax between the second and seventh ribs. The body of the scapula is a triangle from which the coracoid process extends anteriorly, and the spine extends posteriorly. The posterior part of the upper surface of the coracoid process is roughened for the attachment of the coracoclavicular ligament. On occasion a small joint may be present between the two bones (Fig. 4–3). The spine continues laterally to form the acromion process which articulates with the clavicle. The anterior surface, or subscapular fossa, is marked by several oblique lines or ridges from which the subscapularis muscle takes origin (in part). The posterior surface is divided by the spine into supraspinatus and infraspinatus fossae. The lateral boundary of the infraspinatus fossa is formed by an oblique ridge of bone which runs from the glenoid cavity downward and backward to the inferior angle of the scapula. This ridge is crossed by an arterial groove and several smaller ridges. These various grooves and ridges are of importance from the standpoint of differentiation from factures.

The various anatomic parts of radiographic significance are the coracoid process, glenoid process, neck, acromion process, spine, inferior angle, axillary border, vertebral border, and supraspinatus fossa.

The scapula is ossified from seven or more centers: one for the body; two for the coracoid process; two for the acromium; one for the vertebral margin; and one for the inferior angle. Ossification of the body begins approximately during the second month of fetal life. At birth, however, much of the scapula is already osseous, but the glenoid cavity, the coracoid process, the acromium, the vertebral border, and the inferior angle are still cartilaginous. Ossification in the center of the coracoid process begins during the 15th to the 18th month after birth, and fusion with the

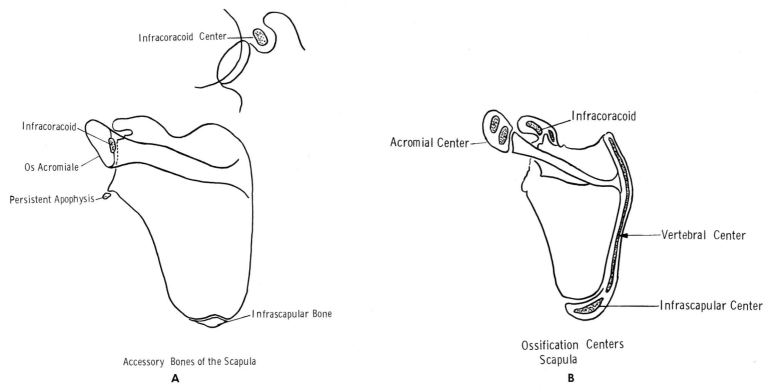

Accessory Bones of the Scapula

A

Ossification Centers
Scapula

B

Figure 4–3.   A. Diagram illustrating accessory bones of a scapula. B. Diagram illustrating the seven ossification centers of the scapula.

rest of the bone does not occur until about the 15th year. Ossification of the remaining parts of the scapula takes place quickly between the 14th and 20th years—first, in the root of the coracoid process; second, near the base of the acromium; third, in the inferior angle and vertebral border; fourth, near the distal portion of the acromium process; and lastly, the vertebral border in its continuation. Further, there are separate ossification centers for the upper third of the glenoid cavity, the lower part of the glenoid cavity, and the tip of the coracoid process. These various centers appear variably between the 10th and 11th years and tend to join with contiguous bony structures between the 16th and 18th years. The various epiphyses, however, do not join with the main bone body until the 25th year (Fig. 4–3 B).

The glenoid process is not yet differentiated in a newborn and seems rippled or irregular even at the age of 8 to 13 years.

A ringlike shadow may be identified closely resembling the end plate of a vertebral body.

There may be a persistent apophysis on the inferior rim of the glenoid process just as a somewhat similar apophysis occurs in the shelving portion of the acetabulum.

When the ossification center fails to fuse at the inferior angle of the scapula with the body of the scapula, an *infrascapular* bone may be identified.

Accessory ossification centers have also been identified in the coracoid process, imparting to the coracoid a shell-like appearance.

Other areas which may persist as separate ossific centers are: the infracoracoid bone and the os acromiale, which represents a persistence of the acromion process ossification center (Fig. 4–3 C).

Radiographic Variation of the Shoulder in Children (Fig. 4–4).   In the scapula at birth, the acromion, the coracoid process, the glenoid cavity, the inferior angle, and the vertebral border are still cartilaginous, and hence are not visualized radiographically. The secondary center of ossification for the coracoid process proper appears about the first year, and fuses with the main body of the scapula around puberty. There is a subcoracoid center of ossification for the lateral part of the coracoid process and upper third of the glenoid cavity which appears at about 10 years of age and fuses at puberty. The other secondary centers of ossification for the margins of the glenoid cavity, the inferior angle, the vertebral border, and two centers for the acromion all appear about puberty and fuse with the main body of the scapula between 20 and 25 years of age. Occasionally, the epiphysis formed from the two acromial centers fails to fuse with the rest of the scapula and remains a separate bone throughout life. When this occurs, the

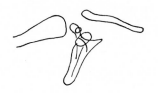

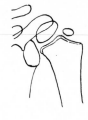

SHOULDER AT BIRTH

SHOULDER, MALE WHITE,
2 YEARS

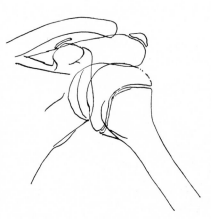

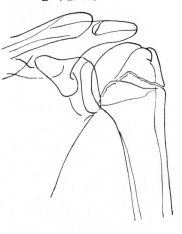

SHOULDER, FEMALE, II YEARS

SHOULDER, FEMALE, 16 YEARS

A

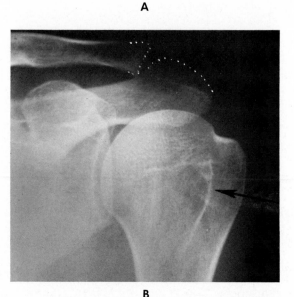

B

Figure 4–4. *A.* Tracings of radiographs to illustrate the osseous changes which occur in the shoulder in different age groups. *B.* Radiograph of adolescent shoulder to show complexity of epiphyseal lines.

condition is usually bilateral and must not be confused with a fracture.

ROUTINE RADIOGRAPHIC STUDIES OF THE SHOULDER REGION

1. **The Shoulder with the Arm in Rotation.** These views are particularly valuable for demonstration of the upper shaft of the humerus and the soft tissue structures in the vicinity of the shoulder joints. Thus, in addition to visualizing the greater and lesser tuberosities and intertubercular sulcus from different anatomic aspects, bursal abnormalities and occasionally distended joint capsules may also be seen.

The views usually obtained are:

(a) Neutral Anteroposterior View of the Shoulder (Fig. 4–5). In this position the patient is rotated approximately 15 degrees so that the shoulder being examined is flat against the table top (or film) and the opposite shoulder is slightly above the table top (or film). The arm is placed along the patient's side in a neutral position with the elbow turned somewhat obliquely. The technical factors will vary depending upon what anatomic parts are to be emphasized.

If the soft tissues happen to be the major interest, and the shoulder is not too muscular, a nonscreen technique would be used with the film in a cardboard or plastic holder. This has the additional advantage of finer detail and less tendency to particulate artefacts. However, if the bony structures are to be investigated primarily, an intensifying screen technique is more desirable.

In this view the greater tuberosity (tubercle) tends to be projected at the upper outer margin of the humerus, and the intertubercular sulcus is seen almost directly "en face." The lesser tuberosity is not seen to best advantage. The junction between the neck and the head of the humerus appears as an angular notch.

The anterior and posterior margins of the epiphyseal line are both seen, and are somewhat irregular. These must not be confused with a fracture.

The glenoid fossa is not seen in complete profile, but its margins can be delineated with considerable clarity. It is particularly important to delineate the inferior margin of the glenoid cavity clearly, since this is the part that becomes roughened or hollowed out in repeated dislocations.

Occasionally, a thin semilunar radiolucent shadow is obtained between the head of the humerus and the glenoid cavity, particularly in children. It is probable that this represents a temporary vacuum in the glenohumeral joint.

The other structures of the scapula are seen in frontal view, but the posterior parts as well as the anterior may be identified. Thus, the coracoid process, spine, subscapular, and infrascapular ridges may be seen. The scapula is projected behind the upper part of the thoracic cage, and thus there is some loss of detail.

The acromion process and its articulation with the clavicle are quite clear. Occasionally, the joint capsule is likewise delineated. The presence of the disk explains the wide separation of the acromioclavicular joint.

The clavicle in most of its length is also seen, and its various anatomic parts clearly delineated.

The bursal structures ordinarily blend with the other soft tissue entities and cannot be delineated. Under abnormal conditions of calcification or calcium deposition in the supraspinatus muscle tendon, these anatomic structures do attain radiographic significance. Special bursal injections with opaque contrast agents will be described later in this chapter. (Fig. 4–15).

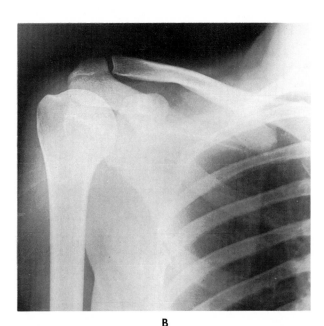

A

B

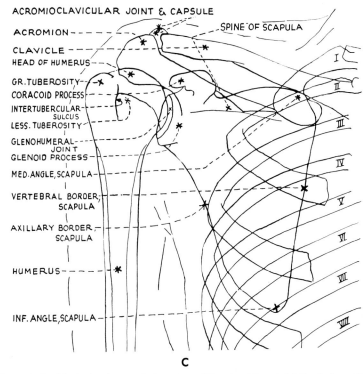

ACROMIOCLAVICULAR JOINT & CAPSULE
SPINE OF SCAPULA
ACROMION
CLAVICLE
HEAD OF HUMERUS
GR. TUBEROSITY
CORACOID PROCESS
INTERTUBERCULAR SULCUS
LESS. TUBEROSITY
GLENOHUMERAL JOINT
GLENOID PROCESS
MED. ANGLE, SCAPULA
VERTEBRAL BORDER, SCAPULA
AXILLARY BORDER, SCAPULA
HUMERUS
INF. ANGLE, SCAPULA

C

Figure 4–5. Neutral anteroposterior view of the shoulder. *A.* Method of positioning patient. *B.* Radiograph. *C.* Labeled tracing of *B.*

Points of Practical Interest with Reference to Figure 4–5

1. The patient may be examined either in the erect position or supine as shown, with the center midway between the summit of the shoulder and lower margin of the anterior axillary fold.
2. To produce better contact of the affected shoulder with the film, rotate the opposite shoulder away from the table top approximately 15 to 20 degrees, supporting the elevated shoulder and hip on sandbags.
3. When looking for faint flecks of calcium in the soft tissues, no-screen film and technique should be employed unless the shoulder is very muscular, in which case the Potter-Bucky apparatus may be employed in addition. When using the Potter-Bucky diaphragm (or grid cassette) it is best to position the cassette so that the central ray will pass through the center of the cassette and the coracoid process.

(b) Anteroposterior View of the Shoulder with Internal Rotation of the Humerus (Fig. 4–6).   The position of the patient is the same except that the entire arm (not just the forearm) is rotated inward. The greater tuberosity is projected along the medial margin of the upper shaft, and the lesser tuberosity is seen, but poorly. The intertubercular sulcus is likewise seen in profile and hence is difficult to identify clearly.

The other structures of the shoulder are essentially the same as previously described.

The bursal structures move with the head of the humerus, and if there is any abnormal calcium within them, the rotation is apt to project it away from the bony structures.

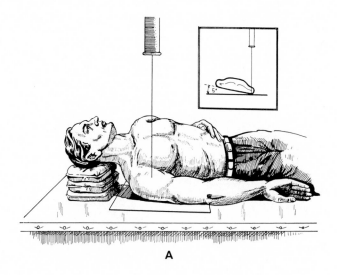

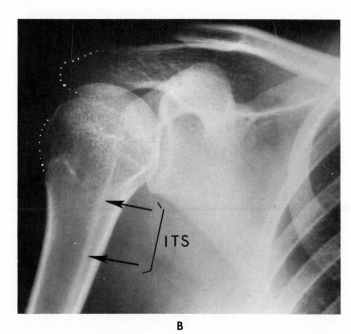

B

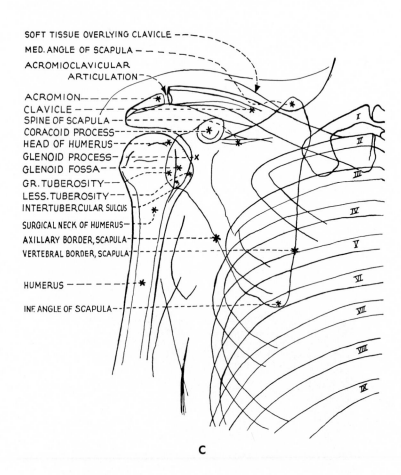

C

Figure 4–6. Anteroposterior view of the shoulder with internal rotation of the humerus. *A.* Method of positioning patient. *B.* Radiograph. *C.* Labeled tracing of *B.*

Points of Practical Interest with Reference to Figure 4–6

1. One must make certain in this position that the entire humerus is rotated inward, not just the forearm and hand.
2. The central ray may pass through the region of the coracoid process.
3. The angle of rotation of the body may be increased to 15 to 20 degrees instead of the 5 degrees as shown. This will produce a slightly better profile view of the glenoid process.
4. It is most important that sandbags be used on the hand and forearm to immobilize the patient. (These have been omitted for clarity in Fig. 4–6 *A.*)

(c) Anteroposterior View of the Shoulder with External Rotation of the Humerus (Fig. 4–7). Again the position of the patient is the same except that the entire arm is rotated externally. Here the lesser tuberosity is projected into silhouette along the upper outer margin of the shaft of the humerus. The other structures of the upper shaft of the humerus are not so clearly shown as in the neutral position.

This additional rotation affords another opportunity to demonstrate abnormal calcium in a bursa without interference by the adjoining bones.

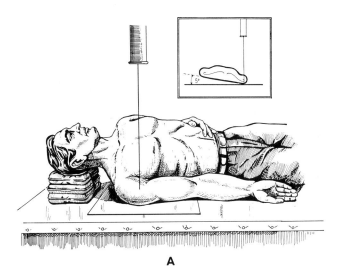

A

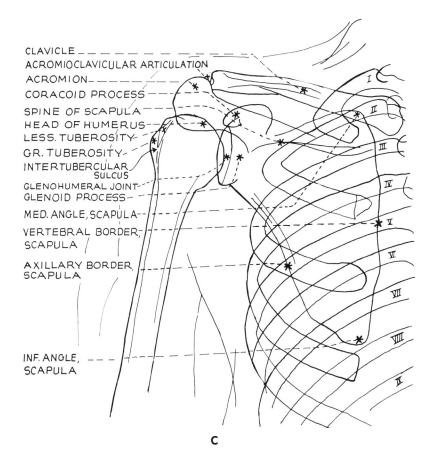

C

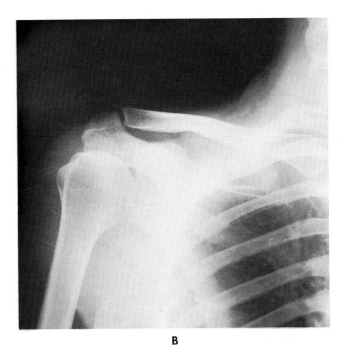

B

Figure 4–7. Anteroposterior view of the shoulder with external rotation of the humerus. *A.* Method of positioning patient. *B.* Radiograph. *C.* Labeled tracing of *B.*

Points of Practical Interest with Reference to Figure 4–7

1. One must make certain to rotate the entire arm externally, not just the forearm and hand. (Sandbags as indicated for Fig. 4–6.)
2. In order to obtain a slightly better profile view of the glenoid process of the scapula, the angle of rotation may be increased from 5 degrees as shown to 15 or 20 degrees.
3. When looking particularly for small flakes of calcium deposit in the soft tissues of the shoulder, one must use a no-screen technique with or without the Potter-Bucky diaphragm. The central ray may be directed through the coracoid process rather than centering as shown.

2. **View of the Shoulder for Greater Detail in Reference to the Glenoid Process** (Fig. 4–8).　In order to see the glenoid process of the scapula in profile, the opposite shoulder must be rotated upward at least 45 degrees. This view is particularly important in cases of chronic dislocation of the shoulder, since in such abnormalities there is frequently erosion of the inferior margin of the glenoid process, seen only in profile in this projection.

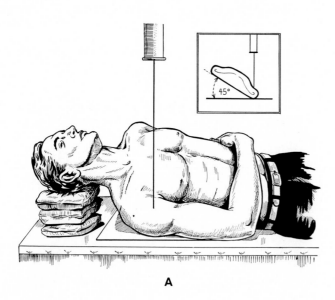

A

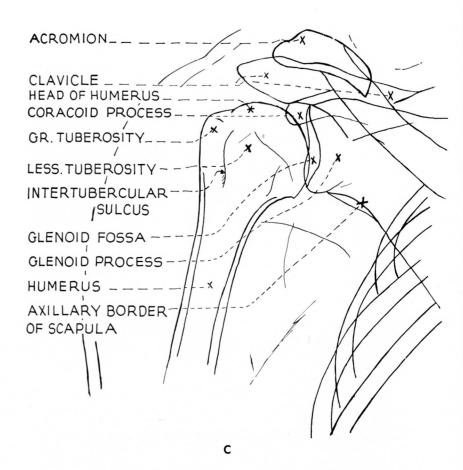

ACROMION

CLAVICLE
HEAD OF HUMERUS
CORACOID PROCESS
GR. TUBEROSITY

LESS. TUBEROSITY
INTERTUBERCULAR
／SULCUS

GLENOID FOSSA

GLENOID PROCESS

HUMERUS

AXILLARY BORDER
OF SCAPULA

C

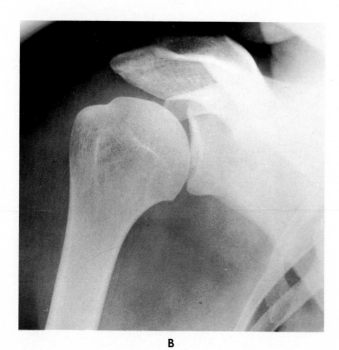

B

Figure 4–8.　View of shoulder for greater detail with reference to the glenoid process. *A.* Method of positioning patient. *B.* Radiograph. *C.* Labeled tracing of *B.*

Points of Practical Interest with Reference to Figure 4–8

1. Adjust the degree of rotation to place the scapula parallel with the plane of the film, and the head of the humerus in contact with it. This will usually come to an angle of 45 degrees as shown.
2. The arm is very slightly abducted and internally rotated, and the forearm is rested against the side of the body.
3. For a more uniform density, respiration is suspended in the expiratory phase.
4. The central ray is directed to a point 2 inches medial and 2 inches distal to the upper-outer border of the shoulder.
5. This view is particularly valuable in cases suspected of chronic dislocation of the shoulder, since in the latter instance the inferior margin of the glenoid process is frequently eroded or contains spurs in contrast to the smooth contour shown.

3. **View of the Shoulder for Testing the Integrity and Degree of Separation of the Acromioclavicular Joint.** In order to demonstrate possible tear of the joint capsule of the acromioclavicular joint a special view must be obtained with the arm in traction (Fig. 4–9). This is done by taking an erect anteroposterior view of the shoulder with a heavy weight in the hand pulling down on the arm. Any latent separation of this joint thus becomes manifest when compared with the width of the joint space of the opposite side.

The comparison with the opposite side is most readily accomplished if both shoulders are filmed simultaneously as shown in Figure 4–9.

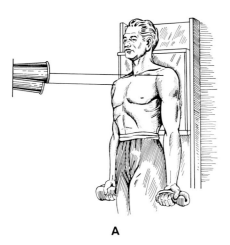

A

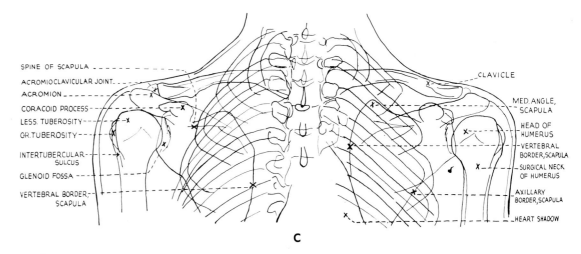

C

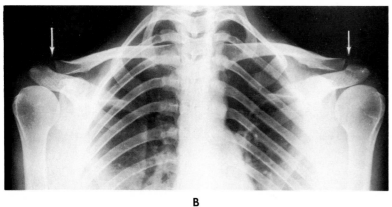

B

Figure 4–9. Detection of integrity of the acromioclavicular joint. A. Method of positioning patient. (In small individuals a single exposure may be obtained as indicated in the illustrations below; in larger patients two separate exposures may be required with the cone centering over each joint separately without moving the patient.) B. Radiograph. C. Labeled tracing of B.

Points of Practical Interest with Reference to Figure 4–9

1. When there is a tear in the acromioclavicular joint capsule, there is a tendency for the distal end of the clavicle to rise above the level of the adjoining acromion process. The two films must be so equivalent in the projection as to make it possible to measure not only the joint space between the clavicle and the acromion process, but also the difference in relation to a horizontal line which would connect the superior margins of the acromion processes.
2. The technique employed should demonstrate the acromioclavicular joint capsule on each side by soft tissue contrast. Hemorrhage and swelling of the joint capsule may thereby be detected as well.

4. **Lateral View of the Shoulder through the Axilla** (Fig. 4–10). In this view, the film is placed perpendicular to the table top and the central ray is directed horizontally into the axilla. The coracoid process is ordinarily projected anteriorly, and the acromion process posteriorly. The other structures are readily identified.

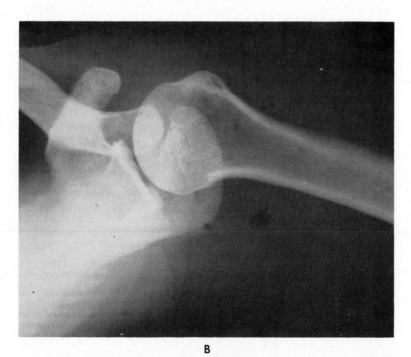

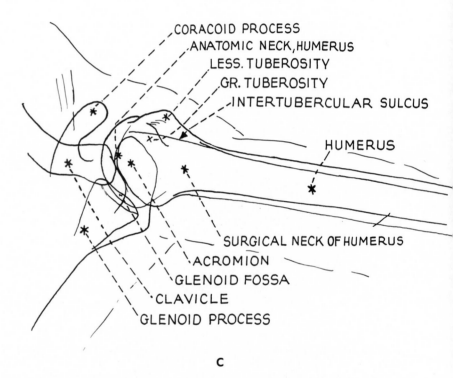

Figure 4–10. Lateral view of shoulder with the central horizontal ray projected through the axilla. *A.* Method of positioning patient. *B.* Radiograph. *C.* Labeled tracing of *B.*

Points of Practical Interest with Reference to Figure 4–10

1. The arm is kept in external rotation, while the forearm and hand are adjusted and supported in a comfortable position.
2. The central ray is directed through the axilla to the region of the acromioclavicular joint.
3. The arm should be abducted as near as possible to a right angle with respect to the long axis of the body.
4. It is important to push the cassette against the patient's neck as far as possible to obtain maximal visualization of the scapula.

5. Lateral View of the Shoulder Projected through the Body

(Fig. 4–11). It is frequently impossible to raise the arm when a shoulder has suffered injury. In order to obtain a lateral projection of the bones of this region, the arm on the affected side is placed against the film. The Bucky apparatus must be utilized to improve detail. The central ray is directed through the body at an upward angle of about 5 degrees. This view does not give the most accurate detail, but demonstrates the relative positions of the gross structures and the alignment of fragments.

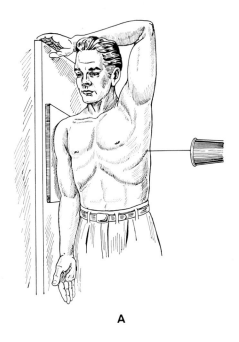

A

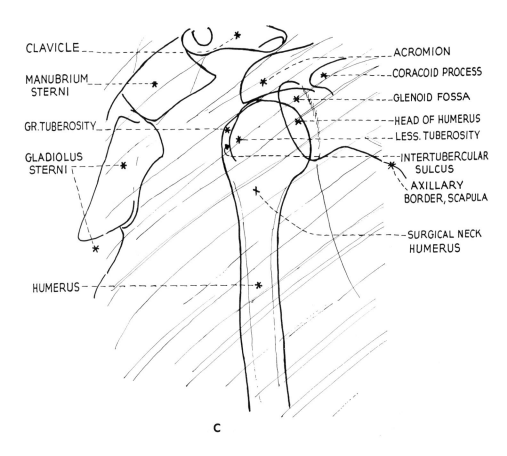

C

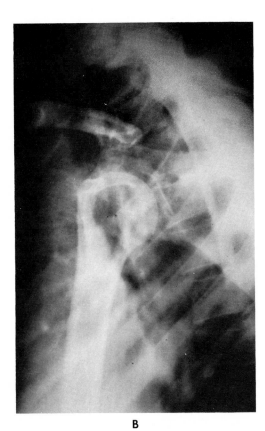

B

Figure 4–11. Lateral view of shoulder with the central horizontal ray projected through the entire body. A. Method of positioning patient. B. Radiograph. C. Labeled tracing of B.

Points of Practical Interest with Reference to Figure 4–11

1. For best results one must employ a screen film, with a vertical Potter-Bucky diaphragm, or grid-front cassette.
2. The cassette is centered to the region of the surgical neck of the affected humerus, as is the central ray. The central ray may be angled cephalad 5 to 15 degrees.
3. The patient stands perfectly perpendicular to the film as shown, raising the opposite shoulder out of the way by resting his forearm upon his head and elevating the opposite scapula.
4. It is best to suspend respiration in full inspiration in this instance so that the lungs, being full of air, will improve the contrast of the bone and decrease the exposure necessary to penetrate the body.
5. This view may be the only method of obtaining a lateral view of the upper humerus if there is a fracture in this location and the patient is unable to abduct the arm.
6. The erect position is shown, but the recumbent position may also be employed, although it is less desirable.

6. **Lateral View of the Scapula** (Fig. 4–12). In this view, the scapula is placed perpendicular to the film, and the central ray strikes it in tangential fashion. The vertebral and axillary margins are projected over one another. Any disturbance in the main body of the scapula or its processes is readily detected in this manner.

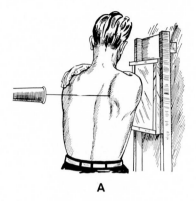

A

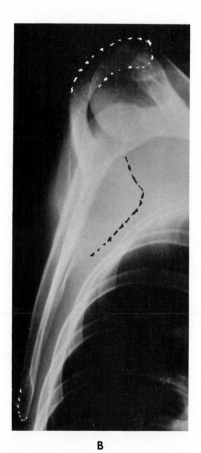

B

Figure 4–12. Lateral view of scapula. *A.* Method of positioning patient. *B.* Radiograph. *C.* Labeled tracing of *B.*

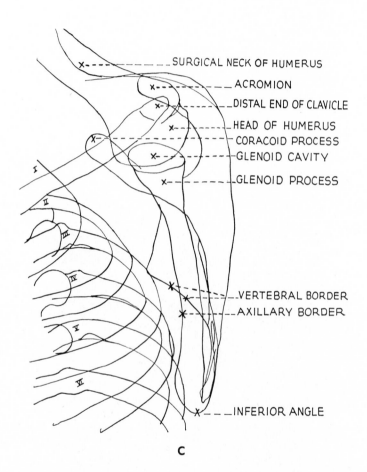

SURGICAL NECK OF HUMERUS
ACROMION
DISTAL END OF CLAVICLE
HEAD OF HUMERUS
CORACOID PROCESS
GLENOID CAVITY
GLENOID PROCESS

VERTEBRAL BORDER
AXILLARY BORDER

INFERIOR ANGLE

C

Points of Practical Interest with Reference to Figure 4–12

1. The Potter-Bucky diaphragm is necessary to obtain best results with this view.
2. The scapula is placed perpendicular to the film after rotating the opposite shoulder out of view, and the central beam is directed over the position of the spine of the scapula after palpation of this part.
3. To rotate the wing of the scapula to its maximum outward limit it is best to rest the forearm of the affected side on the opposite shoulder, bringing the arm of the affected side as close to the anterior chest wall as possible. Although the erect position is preferable, the recumbent position may also be employed in this instance.

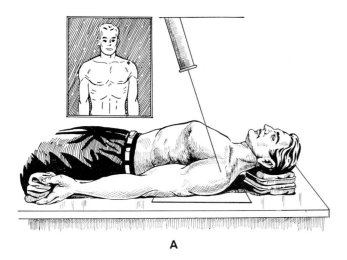

A

7. **Special View of the Clavicle** (Figs. 4–13, 4–14). This is ordinarily an anteroposterior view of the clavicle with the central ray tilted about 5 degrees toward the head to project the clavicle away from the chest and throw it into profile. Occasionally there is an anomalous articulation between the coracoid process and the conoid tubercle of the clavicle; the sternoclavicular joint is not well shown in this view and will be further discussed under the thoracic cage.

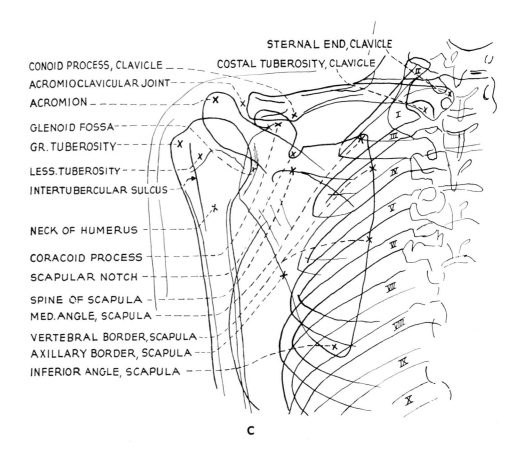

STERNAL END, CLAVICLE
COSTAL TUBEROSITY, CLAVICLE
CONOID PROCESS, CLAVICLE
ACROMIOCLAVICULAR JOINT
ACROMION
GLENOID FOSSA
GR. TUBEROSITY
LESS. TUBEROSITY
INTERTUBERCULAR SULCUS
NECK OF HUMERUS
CORACOID PROCESS
SCAPULAR NOTCH
SPINE OF SCAPULA
MED. ANGLE, SCAPULA
VERTEBRAL BORDER, SCAPULA
AXILLARY BORDER, SCAPULA
INFERIOR ANGLE, SCAPULA

C

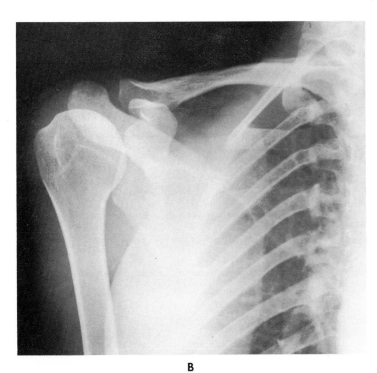

B

Figure 4–13. Special anteroposterior view of clavicle and coracoid process of scapula. *A.* Method of positioning patient. *B.* Radiograph. *C.* Labeled tracing of *B.*

Points of Practical Interest with Reference to Figure 4–13

1. A 5 degree angulation of the tube is usually adequate to project the clavicle away from the rest of the thoracic cage in this view.
2. When interpreting this film, the physician must take into account a considerable element of projection and distortion, since the clavicle is a fair distance from the film.
3. The central ray should pass through the middle of the clavicle in this projection, or through the acromioclavicular articulation as shown.

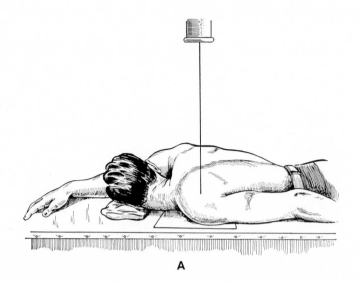

A

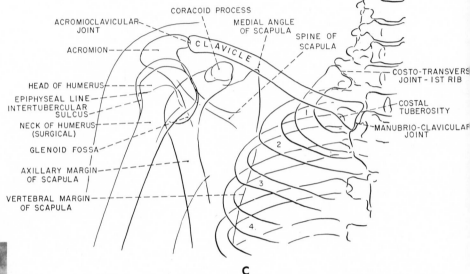

C

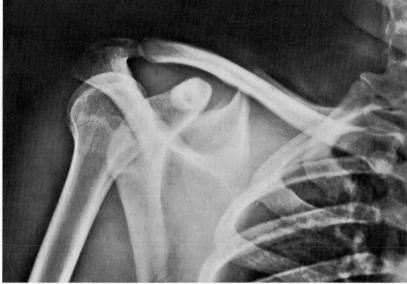

B

Figure 4–14. Special posteroanterior view of clavicle. *A.* Method of positioning patient. *B.* Radiograph. *C.* Labeled tracing of *B.*

Points of Practical Interest with Reference to Figure 4–14

1. This view may be employed with either the erect or the prone position as shown. The erect position is probably more readily obtained if the clavicle is injured.
2. The central ray passes through the center of the clavicle in this instance; an angulation of 10 degrees toward the feet may be employed.
3. Approximately one-half of the clavicle is projected over the bony thorax as shown, but there is less distortion and magnification in this view than in Figure 4–13, and hence it is more desirable in some instances.

8. **Special Views of the Bursae of the Shoulder Joint** (Fig. 4–15). Sodium or methylglucamine diatrizoate may be injected percutaneously directly into the shoulder bursae, placing the injection beneath the coracoid process. On occasion, somewhat similar anatomic presentation may be obtained by injecting the agent directly beneath the acromion process. Ordinarily, 6 to 10 ml. of the contrast agent may be employed until distention is obtained under direct fluoroscopic visualization.

It will be noted that the capsule cannot extend on the lesser and greater tubercles of the humerus because the four short muscles (subscapularis, supraspinatus, infraspinatus, and teres minor) are inserted there, but it can and does extend inferiorly onto the surgical neck *via* the synovial sheath of the biceps (Grant).

It will be noted also that the bursae have two extensions—one that extends along the synovial sheath of the biceps and a subscapular bursa extending beneath the coracoid process.

In some patients the subcoracoid (subscapular) bursa does not communicate with the rest of the shoulder joint and when injected merely distends in and by itself.

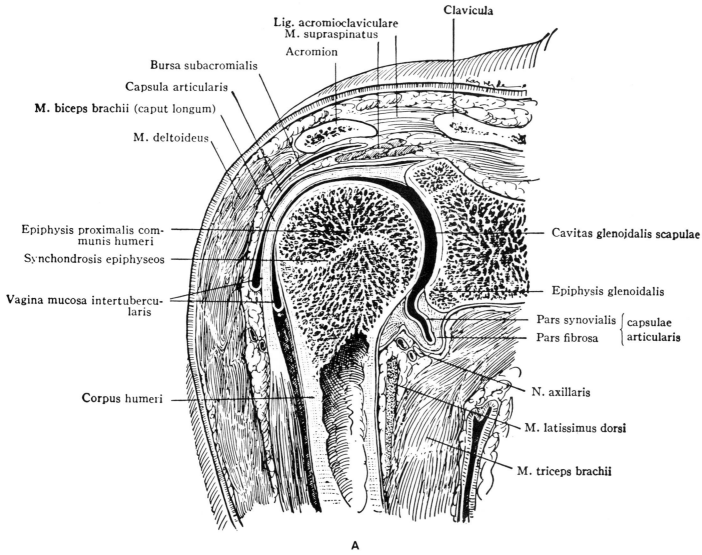

Figure 4–15. A. Subdeltoid bursa and its anatomic relationships. (From Anson, B. J., and Maddock, G. J.: Callander's Surgical Anatomy. 4th ed. Philadelphia, W. B. Saunders Co., 1958.)

Figure 4–15 continued on following page.

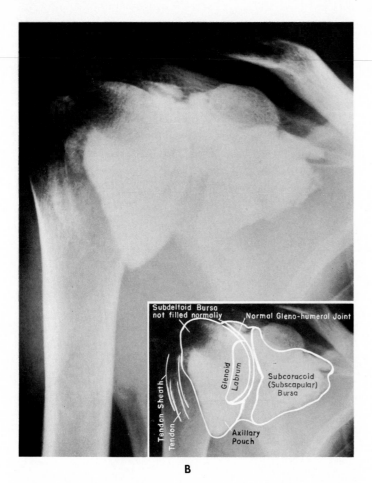

B

Subdeltoid Bursa not filled normally

Normal Gleno-humeral Joint

Tendon Sheath

Tendon

Glenoid Labrum

Subcoracoid (Subscapular) Bursa

Axillary Pouch

Figure 4–15 *Continued. B.* Normal Hypaque arthrogram of an adult's shoulder, demonstrating the normal joint, subscapularis bursa, and dependent axillary pouch. (From Kernwein, G. A., Roseberg, B., and Sneed, W. R., Jr.: J. Bone Joint Surg., 39A:1267–1279, 1957.) *C.* Capsule of shoulder joint (distended), anterior aspect. (From Gray, H.: Gray's Anatomy of the Human Body. 29th ed. Philadelphia, Lea & Febiger, 1973.)

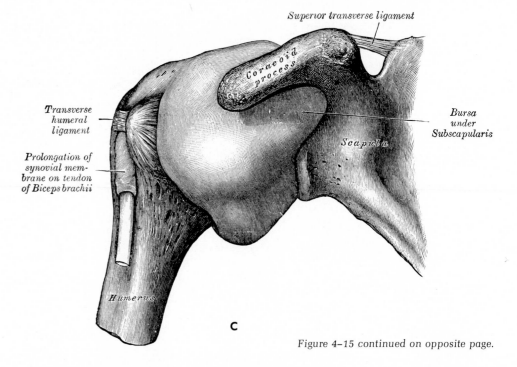

Superior transverse ligament

Coracoid process

Transverse humeral ligament

Scapula

Bursa under Subscapularis

Prolongation of synovial membrane on tendon of Biceps brachii

Humerus

C

Figure 4–15 continued on opposite page.

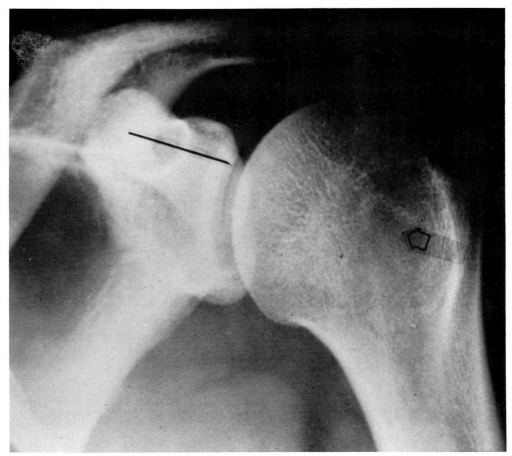

D

Figure 4–15 *Continued.* *D.* The "in vacuo stripe" in the shoulder joint upon first stretching the shoulder joint.

THE ARM

Related Gross Anatomy of the Humerus (Fig. 4–16). The humerus forms the bony support for the arm and articulates with the glenoid process of the scapula; its head is a hemispherical structure mounted obliquely on the upper metaphysis of the humerus. The anatomic neck, greater and lesser tuberosities, and intertubercular groove are readily seen. The epiphyseal line at the base of the head of the humerus is very irregular in its contour and must be differentiated from a fracture, since it is visualized radiographically in its entire circumference.

Immediately below the two tuberosities, the bone contracts and forms the surgical neck.

The shaft or body of the humerus is spiral in contour, being

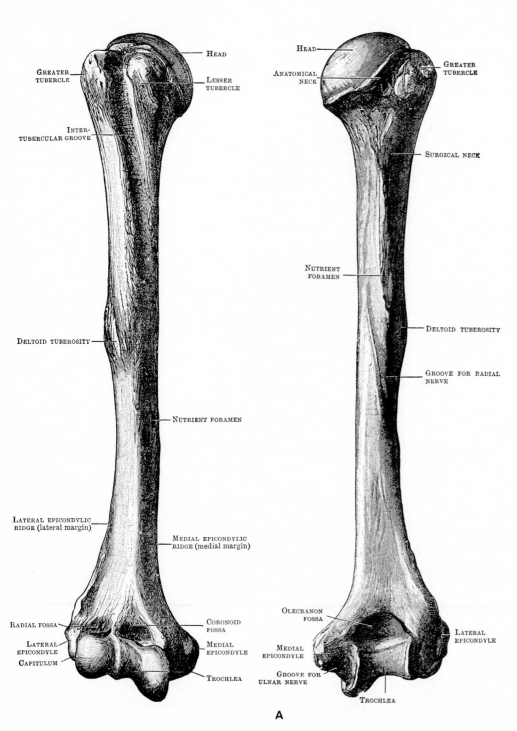

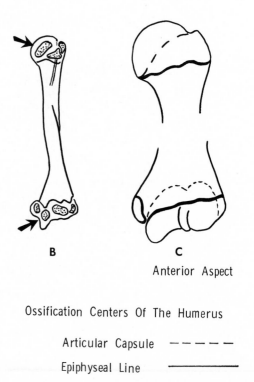

Anterior Aspect

Ossification Centers Of The Humerus

Articular Capsule   – – – – –

Epiphyseal Line   ─────────

Figure 4–16. *A.* Anterior and posterior views of the humerus. (From Cunningham, D. J.: *Textbook of Anatomy.* 10th ed. London, Oxford University Press, 1964.) *B.* Ossification centers of the humerus. At birth the main shaft of the humerus is ossified. The secondary centers of ossification are found in the head, greater tuberosity, lesser tuberosity, capitulum, and lateral part of the trochlea, medial part of the trochlea, medial epicondyle, and lateral epicondyle.

Only the secondary center in the head appears at birth or soon thereafter. Secondary centers in the greater and lesser tuberosities appear between 3 and 5 years of age. The centers for the head and tuberosities coalesce at about the sixth year to form one epiphysis, but the center for the greater tuberosity may remain separate in about half of the cases until union with the shaft occurs. In all individuals with epiphyses comparison films of the opposite side should be obtained, since it may be very difficult at times to assess normality. *C.* Line diagram demonstrating the appearance of the epiphyseal lines in the proximal and distal humerus.

Figure 4–16 continued on opposite page.

rather cylindrical superiorly and flattened inferiorly. Accentuating this spiral appearance is the groove for the radial nerve. The deltoid tubercle forms a prominence near the middle of the shaft laterally and anteriorly.

The flattened distal portion of the humerus tends to be thinner in the central region above the epiphysis. Anteriorly this forms the coronoid fossa, posteriorly the olecranon fossa. The medial and lateral margins or borders form the medial and lateral supracondylar ridges respectively.

The distal end of the humerus resembles a spool in outline, forming the capitulum, the trochlea, and the medial and lateral epicondyles.

The medial epicondyle is smooth posteriorly where a shallow groove for the ulnar nerve is present.

Proximal to the trochlea there are two fossae: anteriorly the coronoid fossa, which receives the coronoid process of the ulna when the forearm is flexed; and posteriorly the olecranon fossa, which receives the olecranon process when the forearm is extended. These fossae are usually separated by a thin plate of bone but sometimes merely by a fibrous tissue so that a supratrochlear foramen or septal aperture may exist.

Immediately proximal to the capitulum there is a third fossa—the *radial fossa*—a small depression receiving the anterior edge of the head of the radius when the forearm is completely flexed. There is also a shallow groove between the capitulum and the trochlea which is occupied by the rim of the head of the radius.

The chief nutrient artery of the shaft of the humerus runs a course of over 2 inches. It is situated on the anteromedial surface or border below the insertion of the coracobrachialis muscle and is directed distally toward the elbow. This must not be confused with a fracture.

The humerus is ossified from eight centers (Fig. 4–16 *B*): the body, the head, the greater tuberosity, the lesser tuberosity, the capitulum, the trochlea, the medial epicondyle, and the lateral epicondyle.

The center for the shaft of the humerus appears about the 42nd day of intrauterine life. A single additional center of ossification appears for the head of the humerus about the time of birth. At 7 months in girls, and at 12 months in boys, the greater tuberosity appears; the lesser tuberosity may actually appear somewhat earlier by an extension from the greater. These three nuclei coalesce between the third and seventh year of age to form a single epiphysis. This epiphysis then joins the main shaft of the humerus between the 17th and 21st year. The distal portion of the humerus ossifies from four centers: the capitulum, which appears during the fifth month in girls and the seventh in boys; the medial epicondyle, which appears in the fourth year in girls and the seventh in boys; the trochlea, which appears during the first year; and the lateral epicondyle, which appears between the eighth and the sixteenth year of age. The nuclei for the lateral epicondyle, capitulum, and trochlea coalesce to form a single epiphysis which joins the main shaft of the humerus between the ages of 10 and 16. The epiphysis of the medial epicondyle joins the shaft independently at about the same time or perhaps a little later.

Occasionally a bony spine of variable size projects distally from the anteromedial surface about 5 cm. proximal to the medial epicondyle. This is the *supracondylar process* and is found in about 1 per cent of Caucasian subjects, and perhaps somewhat less often in Negro races (Terry).

A band of fibrous tissue projecting from the supracondylar process to the distal shaft may contain the median nerve and brachial artery or a large branch thereof. In some cases this "foramen" is occupied by the median nerve alone. This process is the origin of part of the pronator teres muscle, and may also afford an insertion to a persistent inferior part of the coracobrachialis muscle.

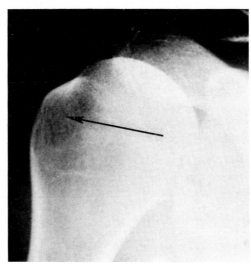

D

Figure 4–16 *Continued.* D. Lucency in the head of the humerus, a normal variant.

Figure 4–16 continued on following page.

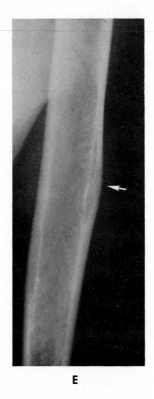

E

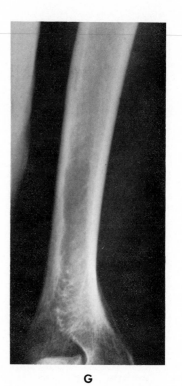

G

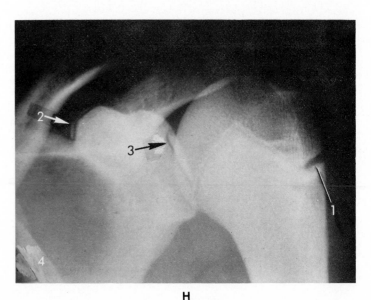

F

H

Figure 4-16 *Continued.* *E.* Close-up radiograph of the deltoid tubercle of the humerus. *F.* Lucency in the distal humerus, a normal variant. *G.* Detailed view of the trabecular pattern of the distal shaft of the humerus. *H.* Radiograph showing the epiphyses of the shoulder region and the epiphyses of the humerus in an adolescent child.

Figure 4-16 continued on the opposite page.

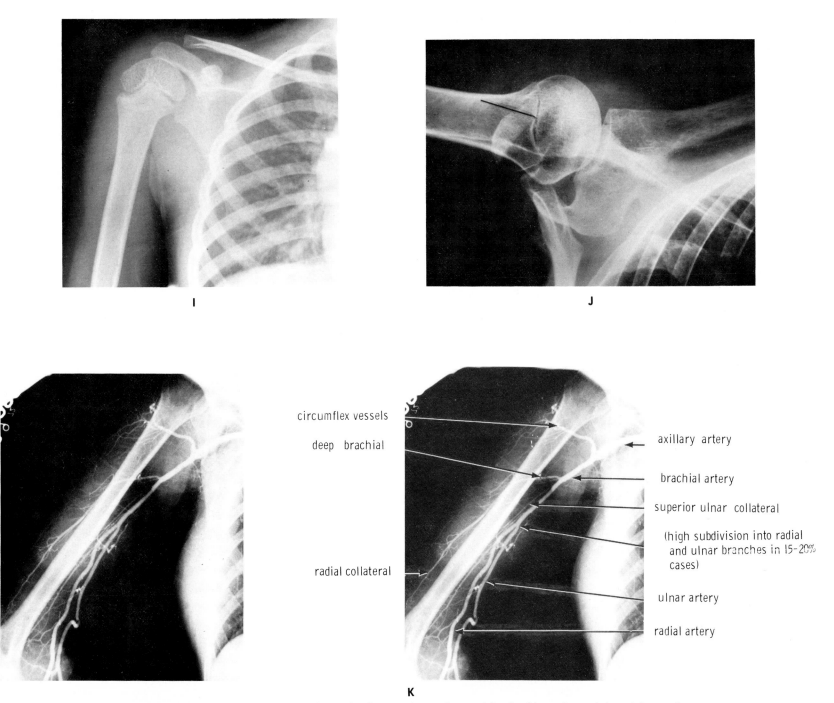

Figure 4–16 *Continued.* *I* and *J*. Radiographs showing the epiphyses of the shoulder region and the epiphyses of the humerus in an adolescent child. *K*. Axillary and brachial arteriogram. Radiograph and labeled rendition of same.

Axial Relationships at the Upper Part of the Humerus. The axial relationships at the head of the humerus to the anatomic neck and shaft are illustrated in Figure 4–17. The original axes as defined by Toldt have been reinvestigated by Keats et al., who showed that the values in males range from 52 to 70 degrees in the angle shown and in females from 50 to 70 degrees. The average for the entire group was 60 degrees with no significant sex variation in the axial relationships (Keats et al.).

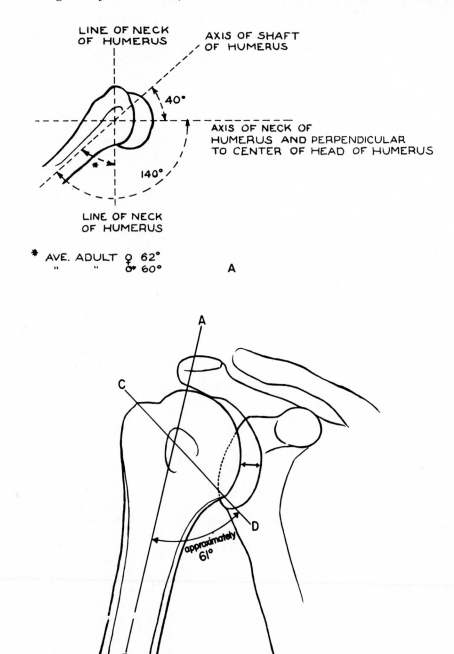

Figure 4–17. A. Axial relationships at the upper part of the humerus. (Modified from Toldt, C.: An Atlas of Anatomy for Students and Physicians. New York, Macmillan Co., © 1926; and Keats, T. E., et al.: Radiology, 87: 904–907, 1966.) B. Axial relationships of the shoulder and measurement of the joint space. The width of the joint space in adults is 0 to 6.0 mm., depending on the degree of rotation of the humerus. More than 6 mm. is significant and is particularly useful in the diagnosis of dislocation of the humeral head. (From Atlas of Roentgenographic Measurement, 3rd ed. by Lusted, L. B., and Keats, T. E. Copyright © 1972 by Year Book Medical Publishers, Inc., Chicago. Used by permission.)

ROUTINE RADIOGRAPHIC STUDIES OF THE ARM

1. **Anteroposterior View of the Arm** (Fig. 4–18). The patient's arm is placed flat upon the film so that the anterior aspect of the humerus points directly upward. The central ray is allowed to pass through the center of the arm, and either the shoulder or the elbow joint or both are included in the film. Most of the anatomic parts of the humerus are readily identified: the head, anatomic neck, surgical neck, greater and lesser tubercles, the intertubercular groove or sulcus, the deltoid tubercle, the medial and lateral epicondyles, the olecranon fossa, the capitulum, and the trochlea articulating with the radius and ulna respectively. Although no great effort is made to identify the soft tissue structures, the position of the radial nerve must always be borne in mind when viewing fractures of the arm.

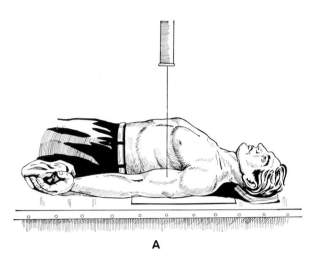

A

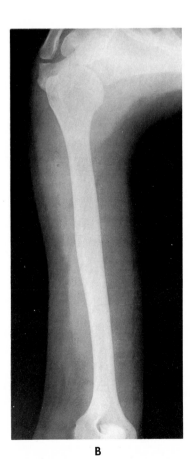

B

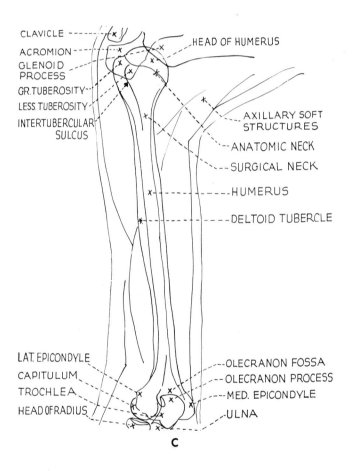

C

Points of Practical Interest with Reference to Figure 4–18

1. The entire humerus from head to epicondyle should be included if at all possible.
2. One must make certain to supinate the hand sufficiently so that both the epicondyles lie flat on the film.
3. The central ray is directed through the midshaft of the humerus.
4. The opposite shoulder may be rotated upward and supported by sandbags in order to place the humerus in better contact with the film.

Figure 4–18. Anteroposterior view of the arm. *A.* Method of positioning patient. *B.* Radiograph. *C.* Labeled tracing of *B.*

2. **Lateral View of the Arm** (Fig. 4–19). In this view, the medial border of the humerus is placed against the film, and the central ray is directed through the midshaft of the humerus on its lateral margin. The medial and lateral epicondyles are projected over one another, and the cubital fossa is seen in profile. The capitulum and the trochlea of the humerus are projected over one

another also. There is a gentle concavity of the distal shaft of the humerus on its anterior aspect.

When the patient is unable to abduct his arm so that a lateral view of the upper shaft of the humerus can be obtained in no other way, the previously described view of the upper arm taken through the body is obtained (Fig. 4–11).

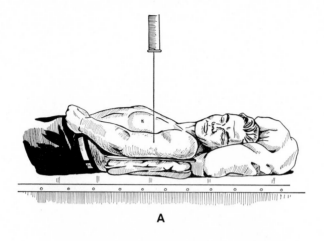

A

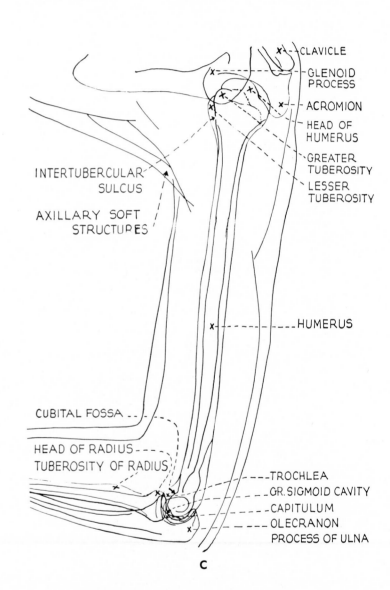

C

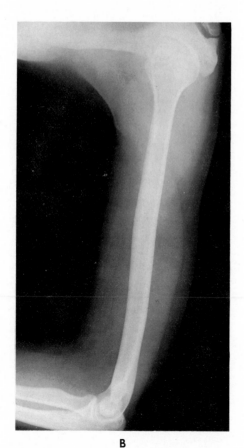

B

Figure 4–19. Lateral view of the arm. *A.* Method of positioning patient. *B.* Radiograph. *C.* Labeled tracing of *B.*

Points of Practical Interest with Reference to Figure 4–19

1. The chosen film size must be adequate to include the entire shaft of the humerus from head to elbow joint.
2. The two epicondyles must be perfectly superimposed over one another and perpendicular to the film surface. To accomplish this, the physician may have to elevate the film on a sandbag, as shown, and flex the forearm, resting the forearm upon the abdomen.
3. An alternative technique allows the patient to sit in a chair and extend the arm across the table, with the arm in perfect contact with the film, particularly in its lower two-thirds.

Variations of Normal. Periosteal thickenings are frequently encountered in the region of the deltoid tubercle.

At times, a double contoured appearance of the lateral border of the upper metaphysis of the humerus may resemble a periosteal proliferation, but it is generally regarded as a normal finding in young persons.

The epiphyseal suture line in the junction of the head and anatomic neck of the humerus does not follow a simple transverse course but assumes an undulatory form. The radiographic appearance may be bizarre, and care must be exercised in interpretation of abnormalities.

Radiolucencies may also appear in: (1) the greater tuberosity of the humerus; (2) the midhumeral shaft, occasionally caused by the projection of soft tissues and the muscular grooves; and (c) the distal shaft in the region of the superimposed olecranon and coranoid fossae.

THE ELBOW

Related Anatomy of the Elbow Joint. The elbow joint is a hinge joint, with the trochlea of the humerus articulating with the greater sigmoid cavity of the ulna, the capitulum of the humerus with the head of the radius, and the head of the radius with the radial notch of the coronoid process of the ulna. The joint capsule is thickened medially and laterally by the ulnar and radial collateral ligaments.

Between the dense outer capsule and the inner synovial membrane are three masses of fat: (1) over the olecranon fossa, (2) over the coronoid fossa, and (3) over the radial fossa.

There are projections of the synovial membrane which tend to subdivide the joint into three communicating parts: (1) humeroradial, (2) humeroulnar, and (3) proximal radioulnar joints.

The annular ligament binds the head of the radius to the radial notch of the ulna; the integrity of this ligament prevents the constant subluxation of the head of the radius by flexion of the biceps brachii muscle.

Because of the obliquity of the trochlea with respect to the shaft of the radius, the forearm in flexion tends to move into a position lateral to the axis of the shaft of the humerus; in extension the "carrying angle" (Fig. 4–21 C) is maintained.

An accessory bone has been described over the anterior aspect of the joint (Simril and Trotter).

The Bursae of the Elbow. Two bursae of the elbow (and sometimes three) are of clinical importance in that they are subject to inflammation: (1) the olecranon bursa, (2) the radiohumeral bursa, and (3) the bursa over the medial epicondyle of the humerus.

The olecranon bursa is subcutaneous and lies over the olecranon process. It ordinarily facilitates the movement of the triceps tendon over the bone at this point. (The inflammation of this bursa gives rise to a condition known as "miners' elbow" or "students' elbow.")

The radiohumeral bursa is situated between the conjoined tendon of the extensor muscles and the radiohumeral joint. Inflammation of this bursa gives rise to a condition known as "tennis elbow."

An inconstant bursa may be found over the medial epicondyle of the humerus.

Axial Relationships at the Elbow (Fig. 4–20, C). The axial relationships of the shaft of the humerus with respect to the forearm are such that an angle is formed measuring an average of 168 degrees (Keats et al.), with the apex of the angle directed medially. This is called the "carrying angle." This axis of the trochlea forms an angle of 84 degrees (average) with the axis of the shaft of the humerus. The axis of the trochlea is parallel with that of the elbow joint, and both are almost perpendicular to the axis of the forearm (average angle, 84 degrees (72 to 99 degrees)).

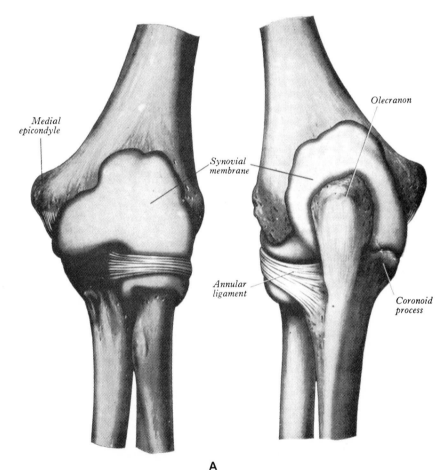

Medial epicondyle

Synovial membrane

Annular ligament

Olecranon

Coronoid process

A

Figure 4–20. *A.* The synovial cavity of the left elbow joint (*left*), partially distended. Anterior aspect. The fibrous capsule of the elbow joint has been removed but the annular ligament has been left *in situ*. Note that the synovial membrane descends below the lower border of the annular ligament.

The synovial cavity of the left elbow (*right*), partially distended. Posterior aspect of the specimen represented at left.

Figure 4–20 continued on following page.

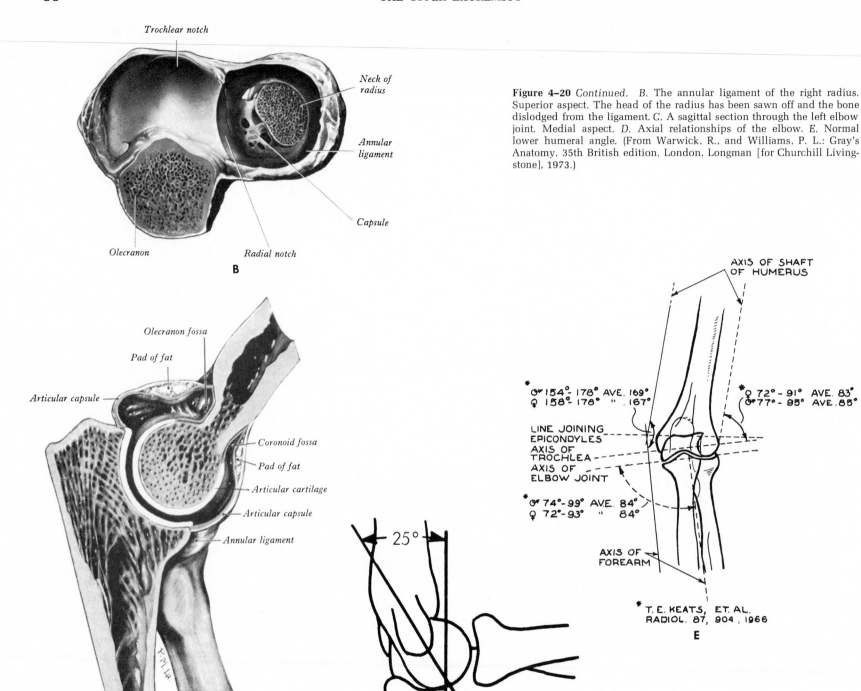

Trochlear notch

Neck of radius

Annular ligament

Capsule

Olecranon

Radial notch

B

Figure 4–20 Continued. B. The annular ligament of the right radius. Superior aspect. The head of the radius has been sawn off and the bone dislodged from the ligament. C. A sagittal section through the left elbow joint. Medial aspect. D. Axial relationships of the elbow. E. Normal lower humeral angle. (From Warwick, R., and Williams, P. L.: Gray's Anatomy. 35th British edition. London, Longman [for Churchill Livingstone], 1973.)

Olecranon fossa

Pad of fat

Articular capsule

Coronoid fossa

Pad of fat

Articular cartilage

Articular capsule

Annular ligament

C

25°

NORMAL LOWER HUMERAL
EPIPHYSIS - 25° ANGLE

D

AXIS OF SHAFT
OF HUMERUS

* ♂ 154°- 178° AVE. 169°
♀ 158°- 178° " 167°

* ♀ 72° - 91° AVE. 83°
♂ 77° - 95° AVE. 85°

LINE JOINING
EPICONDYLES
AXIS OF
TROCHLEA
AXIS OF
ELBOW JOINT

* ♂ 74°- 99° AVE. 84°
♀ 72°- 93° " 84°

AXIS OF
FOREARM

* T. E. KEATS, ET. AL.
RADIOL. 87, 904, 1966

E

Structural Variations of the Elbow with Age (Fig. 4–21). There are usually seven secondary centers of ossification in the elbow: (1) the capitulum and lateral part of the trochlea which appear at 1 to 1½ years of age, (2) the medial part of the trochlea which appears at 10 years of age, (3) the lateral epicondyle which appears at 14 years, (4) the medial epicondyle which appears in females between 5 and 6, and in males between 8 and 9 years, (5) the proximal end of the olecranon which appears at 11 years, (6) the head of the radius which appears between 5 and 6 years in females, and between 5 and 7 in males, and (7) occasionally the radial tuberosity which appears at puberty.

These for the most part fuse around 14 to 15 years of age in the female and between 18 and 21 years in the male, with the exception of the radial tuberosity which fuses very rapidly after it once appears (when it appears separately).

The centers for the capitulum and the trochlea coalesce to

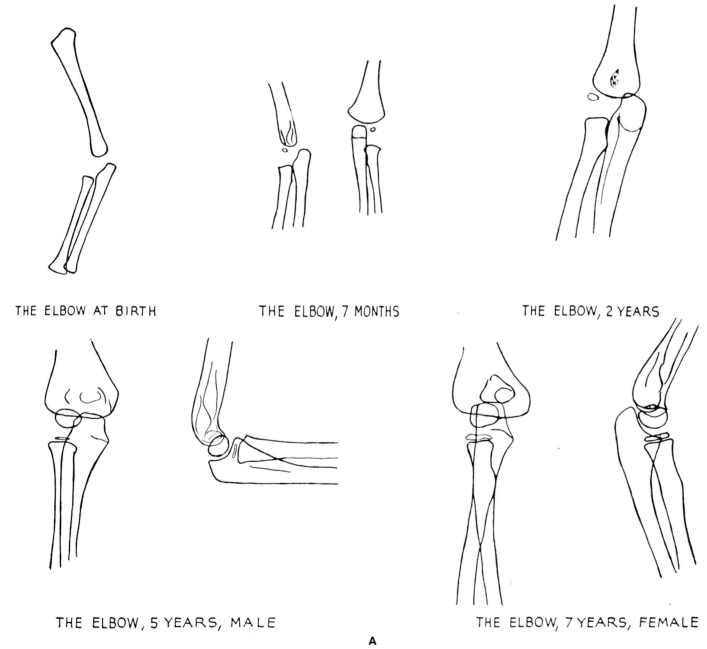

THE ELBOW AT BIRTH   THE ELBOW, 7 MONTHS   THE ELBOW, 2 YEARS

THE ELBOW, 5 YEARS, MALE   THE ELBOW, 7 YEARS, FEMALE

A

Figure 4–21. A. Tracings of radiographs to illustrate the osseous changes which occur in the elbow region in different age groups.

Figure 4–21 continued on following page.

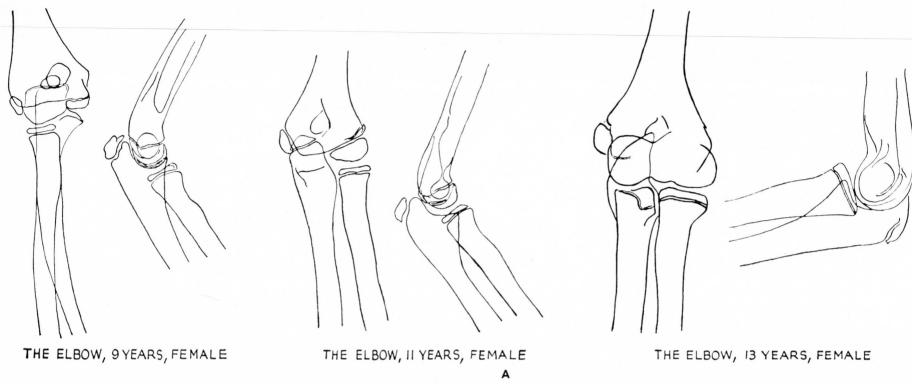

THE ELBOW, 9 YEARS, FEMALE   THE ELBOW, 11 YEARS, FEMALE   THE ELBOW, 13 YEARS, FEMALE

A

Figure 4–21. *A. Continued. B.* Elbow, showing the semilunar notch and olecranon spur. *C.* Cross section of elbow, showing nerve relationships to the joint capsule.

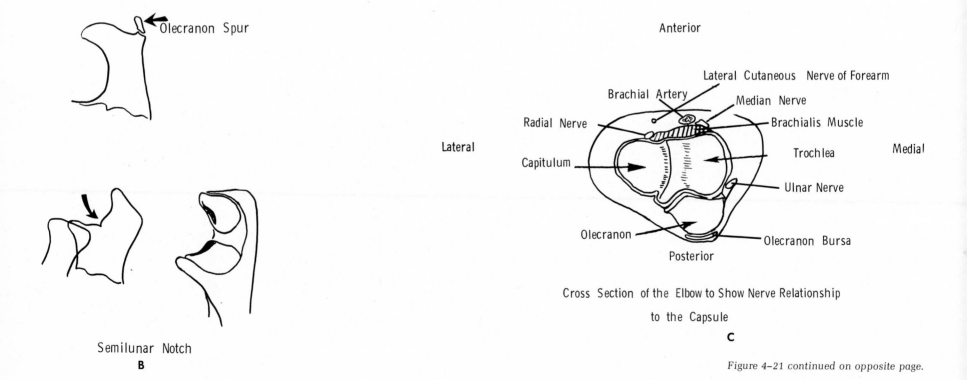

Olecranon Spur

Semilunar Notch

B

Cross Section of the Elbow to Show Nerve Relationship to the Capsule

C

Figure 4–21 continued on opposite page.

form one epiphysis at about 15 years in boys and 13 years in girls, and the lateral epicondyle usually joins the shaft independently. In about one-third of the cases the latter does not appear as a separate center but appears to be ossified by extension from the capitulum.

The ossification center for the olecranon process may be bipartite or multipartite. Fusion of the olecranon epiphysis takes place first in its volar (anterior) portions, and a deep groove may remain for a considerable period of time before this entire epiphysis fuses (Fig. 4–21, 13 year old female). Persistent epiphyses of the olecranon may also occur.

It can thus be seen that the elbow furnishes good opportunity to help establish the so-called bone age of the growing individual, particularly between the ages of 5 and 14. The head of the radius appears after the capitulum and lateral part of the trochlea, which appear very early. The medial epicondyle, the trochlea, the olecranon, and the lateral epicondyle appear sequentially in that order at the ages indicated. *In general, when determining bone age, it is advisable to take views of several areas rather than to rely completely on one.* (See Chapter 3.)

Other Variations of Normal. The olecranon process in profile may exhibit other variations of normal as follows: (1) an olecranon spur which represents the point of attachment of the triceps tendon to the ulna; and (2) a small notch within the semilunar notch caused by a slight irregularity of the articular cartilage in this immediate vicinity (Fig. 4–21, *B*).

Important Nerve Relationships at the Elbow Joint. The radial nerve is in direct contact with the elbow joint capsule on the anterior aspect of the capitulum, and the ulnar nerve is in contact with the ulnar collateral ligament. The median nerve is close to the joint capsule but separated from it by a very thin layer of the brachialis muscle; it is situated near the lateral aspect of the trochlea on its anterior side.

Normal Fat Planes Surrounding the Elbow Joint (Fig. 4–21, *D*). Normally, the major fat plane surrounding the elbow joint runs distally in a gentle ventral curve parallel to the proximal third of the radius. Also, the synovial and adjoining fat planes on the distal aspect of the humerus and the anterior and posterior aspects of the elbow joint are smoothly and relatively closely applied to the distal humerus and the elbow joint. In traumatic bursitis or accompanying fractures there is a widening of the fat planes, ventral or posterior displacement, and blurring. These become important indicators of pathologic processes.

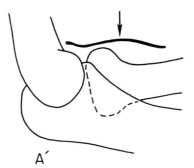

A'

NORMAL ARM. SUPINATOR FAT PLANE ARISES FROM ELBOW JOINT AND RUNS DISTALLY IN GENTLE VENTRAL CURVE PARALLEL TO PROXIMAL THIRD OF THE RADIUS (ARROWS).

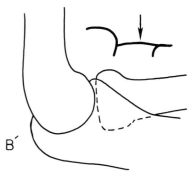

B'

ARM WITH FRACTURE. FAT PLANE WIDENED, BLURRED, AND VENTRALLY DISPLACED.

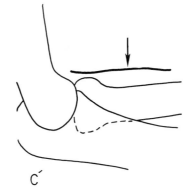

C'

SUPINATOR FAT PLANE IN NORMAL ARM.

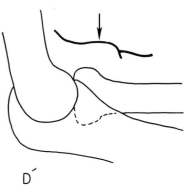

D'

GROSS DISTORTION OF FAT PLANE IN INFECTED ARM.

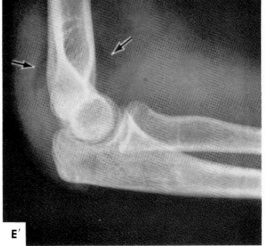

E'

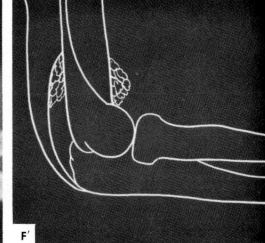

F'

D

Figure 4–21 *Continued.* D. Supinator muscle fat plane on anterior aspect of elbow.

ROUTINE RADIOGRAPHIC STUDIES OF THE ELBOW
REGION

1. **Routine Anteroposterior View of the Elbow** (Fig. 4–22). The patient is immobilized with the volar aspect of the forearm pointing directly upward and the central ray of the x-ray tube projected into the cubital fossa. The anatomic parts are indicated in Figure 4–22.

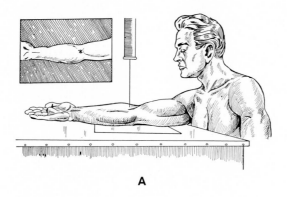

A

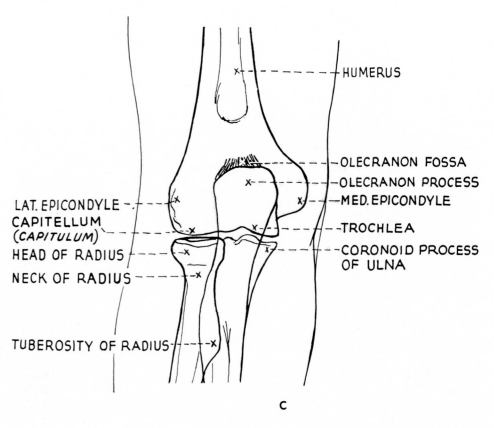

C

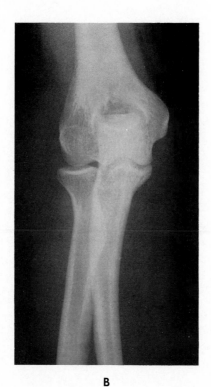

B

Figure 4–22. Anteroposterior view of elbow. *A.* Method of positioning patient. *B.* Radiograph. *C.* Labeled tracing of *B.*

Points of Practical Interest with Reference to Figure 4–22

1. Note that the patient is seated low enough to place the shoulder joint and the elbow in approximately the same plane. This assures a good contact between the distal humerus and the film.
2. The anterior surface of the elbow and the plane passing through the epicondyles must be perfectly parallel with the film. To accomplish this the hand must be completely supinated and usually supported in this position by means of a sandbag. Occasionally also the patient must lean somewhat laterally.
3. The olecranon and coronoid fossae of the humerus, because it is superimposed and is a very thin plate of bone, will frequently appear as a foramen rather than as a bony plate, which may be misleading. A foramen in lieu of this bony plate does occur very rarely in anomalous conditions.

2. **Anteroposterior Views of Distal Humerus and Proximal Forearm.** *When the patient is unable to extend the forearm fully,* an anteroposterior view is first obtained of the distal humerus, and then another of the proximal forearm, each in proper turn being flat on the film cassette or cardboard film holder (Figs. 4–23, 4–24). Another means of overcoming this difficulty is to take the anteroposterior view, gauging an equal angle between the forearm and table top and arm and table top respectively.

Under such circumstances it may also be advisable to obtain a special view of the olecranon process by placing the olecranon process tangentially in the central x-ray beam (Fig. 4–25).

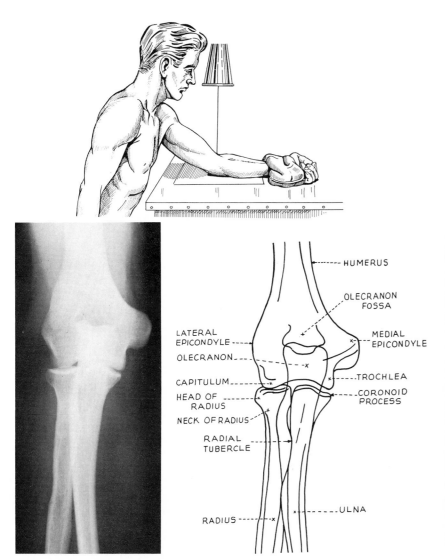

Figure 4–23. Views of the elbow region when the elbow cannot be fully extended. View of the proximal forearm, with a distorted view of the distal humerus. Method of positioning patient, radiograph, and labeled tracing.

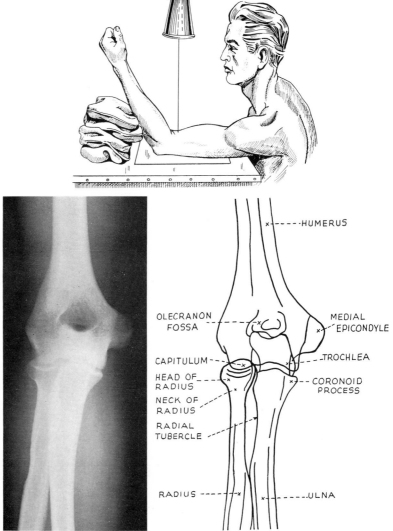

Figure 4–24. Views of the elbow region when the elbow cannot be fully extended. View of distal humerus, with a distorted view of the proximal forearm. Method of positioning patient, radiograph, and labeled tracing.

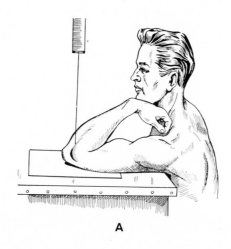

A

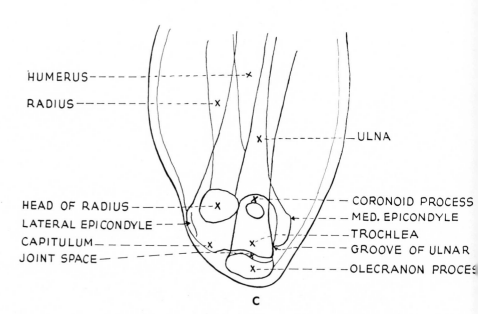

HUMERUS ------------------- x

RADIUS ------------------ x

                                    x ------- ULNA

HEAD OF RADIUS ------ x   x ------- CORONOID PROCESS
LATERAL EPICONDYLE -- ←   ← ------- MED. EPICONDYLE
CAPITULUM _____ x   x ------- TROCHLEA
JOINT SPACE ---- ---   x ------- GROOVE OF ULNAR
                                    x ------- OLECRANON PROCES

C

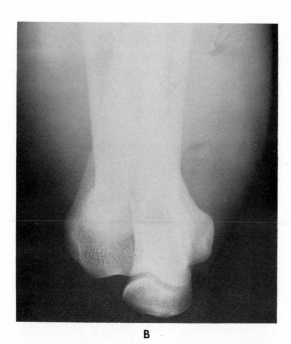

B

Figure 4–25. Views of the elbow region when elbow cannot be fully extended. Special view of the olecranon process. *A.* Method of positioning patient. *B.* Radiograph. *C.* Labeled tracing of *B.*

Points of Practical Interest with Reference to Figure 4–25

1. The patient must be seated in such a way that the entire humerus is in good contact with the table top and film.
2. The elbow is flexed as acutely as possible and the hand pronated.
3. It is important in this instance also to obtain a visualization of the soft tissues immediately outside the olecranon process in view of their frequent involvement by inflammatory process and calcium deposit.

3. **Routine Lateral View of the Elbow** (Fig. 4–26). The elbow is partially flexed, and the forearm is so placed that the thumb points directly upward. The distal portion of the humerus as well as the proximal forearm are seen in lateral profile. The capitulum and trochlea overlap one another completely, and the head of the radius overlaps the coronoid process partially. The radial tubercle points anteriorly. The portion of the forearm adjoining the interosseous crest is also seen.

The student's attention is particularly directed to the practical points of interest in relation to Figures 4–22 to 4–26. Unless the technical details of positioning are accurately followed, considerable distortion and possible inaccuracy in interpretation of the anatomy may result.

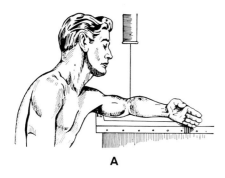

A

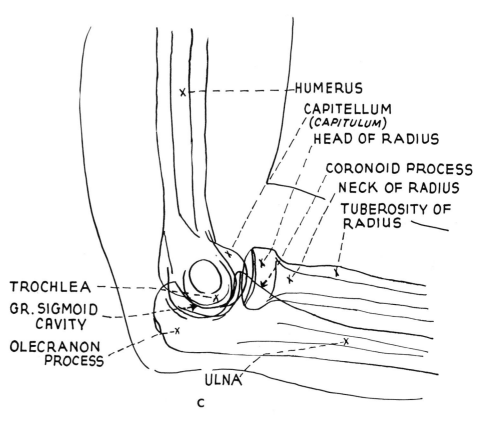

HUMERUS
CAPITELLUM
/ (CAPITULUM)
HEAD OF RADIUS
CORONOID PROCESS
NECK OF RADIUS
TUBEROSITY OF RADIUS
TROCHLEA
GR. SIGMOID CAVITY
OLECRANON PROCESS
ULNA

C

Points of Practical Interest with Reference to Figure 4–26

1. The patient is so placed with respect to the table that the arm is at the same level as the shoulder. Unless this is done the elbow joint proper will not be visualized clearly, and a rather oblique view of the head and neck of the radius will be obtained.
2. The elbow is ordinarily flexed approximately 90 degrees. The center of the film is placed immediately beneath the elbow joint and the central ray passes through the joint and center of the film, the epicondyles of the humerus being superimposed and perpendicular to the film. The forearm is placed so that the thumb points directly upward and the palm of the hand is perpendicular to the table top surface. The fist may be clenched to facilitate maintenance of position. It is best to immobilize the forearm in this position by means of sandbags.
3. Since fractures of the head and neck of the radius are frequently missed by radiographic diagnosis, the contour and structure of these regions must be examined with great care to avoid such an oversight.

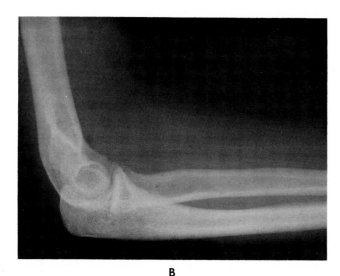

B

Figure 4–26. Lateral view of elbow. *A.* Method of positioning patient. *B.* Radiograph. *C.* Labeled tracing of *B.*

THE FOREARM

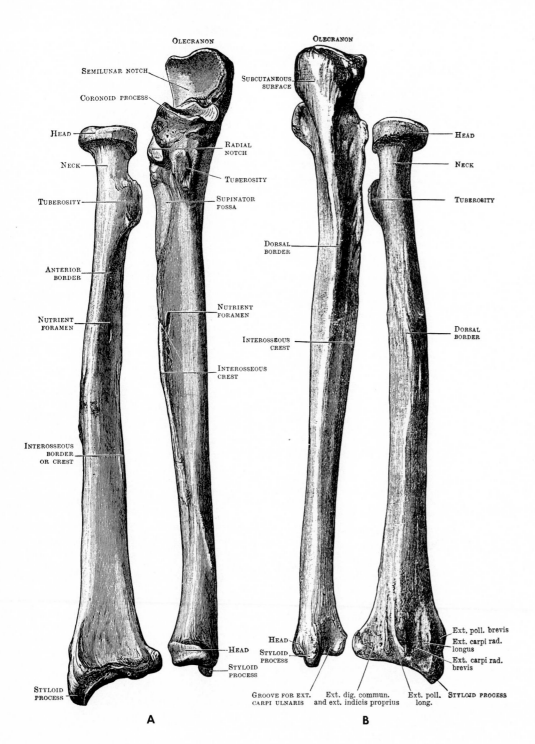

Related Gross Anatomy of the Radius (Fig. 4–27).   The head of the radius is a circular disk whose flat upper surface articulates with the capitulum of the humerus and whose medial edge articulates with the radial notch of the ulna. The head is completely surrounded by a capsular or annular ligament. The neck is the constricted portion below the head. The radial tuberosity is situated anteromedially below the neck. The body gradually increases in size distally and is concave toward the ulna. The sharp medial edge below the radial tuberosity is known as the interosseous crest.

The distal portion of the dorsal surface of the shaft contains numerous grooves for the tendons of muscles and for the attachment of ligaments. These grooves and irregularities must be recognized as normal.

The styloid process is the pointed distal extremity of the shaft of the radius. The distal articular surface articulates with both the navicular and lunate carpal bones and medially with the head of the ulna.

Related Gross Anatomy of the Ulna.   The proximal portion of the ulna contains an articular surface which is concave in the long axis of the bone and convex from side to side. The proximal part is the olecranon and the anterior projection is the coronoid process. The concave portion is the greater sigmoid cavity or semilunar notch. This articulates with the trochlea of the humerus. The radial notch is the articular surface for the head of the radius and is situated on the lateral aspect of the coronoid process. There are several bony ridges for muscular attachment below the coronoid process. The interosseous crest is the sharp lateral edge which gives attachment to the interosseous membrane.

The lower portion of the ulna is small and consists of the head and styloid process, separated by a groove.

The head articulates with the ulnar notch of the radius, *but not with the carpus*, since it is separated from it by a triangular cartilaginous disk.

Figure 4–27.   *A.* Volar aspect of the radius and ulna. *B.* Dorsal aspect of the radius and ulna. (From Cunningham, D. J.: Textbook of Anatomy. 10th ed. London, Oxford University Press, 1964.)

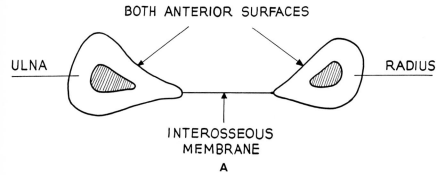

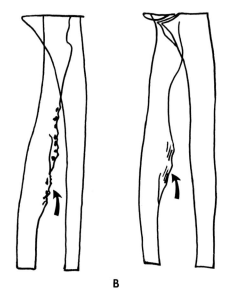

Figure 4–28. *A.* Relationship of the interosseous membrane to the radius and ulna in cross section. (Modified from Toldt, C.: An Atlas of Human Anatomy for Students and Physicians. New York, Macmillan Co., © 1926.) *B.* Irregularities of the interosseal ridge of the radius and ulna. *C.* Cross section through the middle of the forearm, showing relationships of the nerves and arteries to the bones and interosseous membrane.

There is a very slight bowing of the distal half of the ulna medially. In the act of supination, the interosseous borders of the radius and ulna are posterior in position. In cross section, the anterior surfaces of the radius and ulna form almost a perfect semicircle with the interosseous membrane (Fig. 4–28), while the posterior surfaces form a flat surface. This configuration assists materially in the supination and pronation functions of the forearm, and every effort is made to preserve this configuration in the event of fracture.

The functions of supination and pronation are carried out exclusively by the radius with the ulna remaining in relatively constant position unless the humerus is also moved.

The Distal Radioulnar Articulation. The distal radioulnar articulation is separated from the radiocarpal or wrist joint by an articular disk or triangular fibrocartilage. The upper surface of this disk articulates with the head of the ulna, and its lower surface with the lunate and triangular carpal bones. The disk is attached at its apex to the junction of the styloid process and the head of the ulna, and at its base to the lower ridge of the ulnar notch of the radius.

In addition there are volar and dorsal radioulnar ligaments which maintain the capsular integrity of this joint.

The Interosseous Membrane. The interosseous membrane is a broad thin fibrous sheet of tissue which extends between the interosseous crests of the radius and ulna (Fig. 4–28). It commences about 2.5 cm. beneath the tuberosity of the radius. Its purpose is to increase the extent of surface for attachment of the deep muscles of the forearm, and it aids in holding the radius and ulna together.

Its integrity is important from the standpoint of the supination and pronation movements of the forearm.

The interosseous crest at times appears somewhat irregular

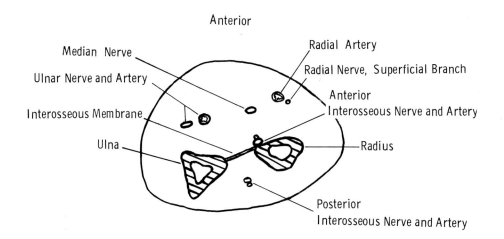

Figure 4–28 continued on following page.

in its margination along the middle of the shaft of the forearm, affecting either the radius or the ulna or both. This slight irregularity may simulate a localized periosteal thickening (Fig. 4–28, E).

General Anatomic Features of the Interosseous Membrane and Its Relationships to Nerves, Arteries, and Bones (Fig. 4–28). The interosseous membrane extends from the proximal to the distal radioulnar joint, and the course of its fibers is from the ulna below to the radius above. Note the strong supinator muscles—the biceps and supinator brevis—which insert into the proximal third of the radius, and the pronator teres muscle which inserts into the middle of the radius. The pronator quadratus muscle inserts into the distal third of the radius. These relationships of supinator and pronator muscles become important in the event of injury, since they function together with the interosseous membrane.

Additionally, the brachioradialis muscle inserts into the lateral aspect of the distal end of the radius, extending from the distal shaft of the humerus.

When injuries of the proximal, middle, or distal third of the shafts of the radius and ulna are sustained, these interrelationships must be carefully defined.

Among the nerves and arteries in the middle of the forearm at the level of the insertion of the pronator teres are: the ulnar nerve and artery, which lie deep in a fibrous septum between the superficial and deep digital flexors.

The anterior interosseous branch of the median nerve is situated on the skeletal plane.

The radial artery is overlapped and considerably protected by the brachioradialis muscle. This artery lies at a significant distance from the radius but at a relatively superficial level. The superficial branch of the radial nerve follows along the anterior border of the extensor carpi radialis brevis muscle.

The posterior interosseous nerve lies between the superficial and deep layers of the digital extensor. Thus, the important nerves and arteries tend to lie in relatively protected sheaths and compartments in the forearm, with the exception of the anterior interosseous nerve and arteries which are closely approximated to the medial anterior aspect of the midshaft of the radius as it adjoins the interosseous membrane.

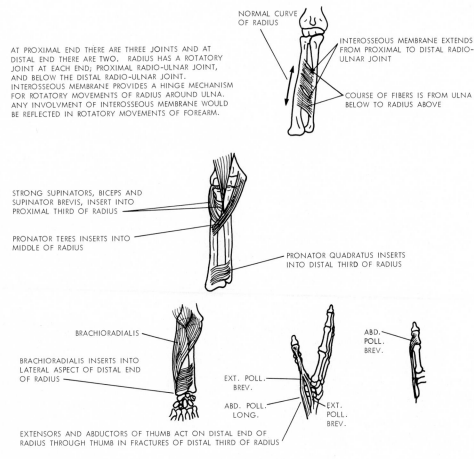

AT PROXIMAL END THERE ARE THREE JOINTS AND AT DISTAL END THERE ARE TWO. RADIUS HAS A ROTATORY JOINT AT EACH END; PROXIMAL RADIO-ULNAR JOINT, AND BELOW THE DISTAL RADIO-ULNAR JOINT. INTEROSSEOUS MEMBRANE PROVIDES A HINGE MECHANISM FOR ROTATORY MOVEMENTS OF RADIUS AROUND ULNA. ANY INVOLVMENT OF INTEROSSEOUS MEMBRANE WOULD BE REFLECTED IN ROTATORY MOVEMENTS OF FOREARM.

NORMAL CURVE OF RADIUS

INTEROSSEOUS MEMBRANE EXTENDS FROM PROXIMAL TO DISTAL RADIO-ULNAR JOINT

COURSE OF FIBERS IS FROM ULNA BELOW TO RADIUS ABOVE

STRONG SUPINATORS, BICEPS AND SUPINATOR BREVIS, INSERT INTO PROXIMAL THIRD OF RADIUS

PRONATOR TERES INSERTS INTO MIDDLE OF RADIUS

PRONATOR QUADRATUS INSERTS INTO DISTAL THIRD OF RADIUS

BRACHIORADIALIS

BRACHIORADIALIS INSERTS INTO LATERAL ASPECT OF DISTAL END OF RADIUS

EXT. POLL. BREV.

ABD. POLL. LONG.

EXT. POLL. BREV.

ABD. POLL. BREV.

EXTENSORS AND ABDUCTORS OF THUMB ACT ON DISTAL END OF RADIUS THROUGH THUMB IN FRACTURES OF DISTAL THIRD OF RADIUS

D

Figure 4–28 *Continued. D. Upper,* General anatomy of the interosseous membrane. *Middle,* Anatomy of the supinator and pronator muscles of the forearm. *Lower,* Anatomy of the brachioradialis and thumb muscles in respect to the bones of the forearm.

ROUTINE RADIOGRAPHIC STUDIES OF THE FOREARM

1. **Routine Anteroposterior View of the Forearm** (Fig. 4–29). The forearm is supinated so that the volar aspect is turned upward, and the central ray passes through the central portion of the forearm. It is important that the palm be turned upward perfectly to obtain the proper perspective.

The various anatomic parts are illustrated in Figure 4–29.

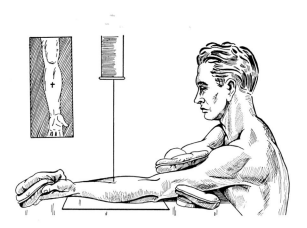

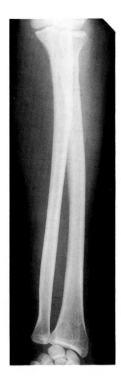
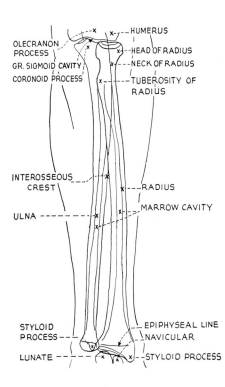

Figure 4–29. Anteroposterior view of forearm. Method of positioning patient, radiograph, and labeled tracing.

2. **Routine Lateral View of the Forearm** (Fig. 4–30). It is helpful in this view to raise the elbow on a small platform into a horizontal position with respect to the shoulder. The elbow is flexed sufficiently to permit a perfect superposition of the proximal portions of the radius and ulna. This is best obtained by making certain that the thumb points straight upward, and the hand and wrist are perfectly perpendicular to the film and table top. The central ray passes through the center of the forearm. The anatomic parts are well illustrated in Figure 4–30.

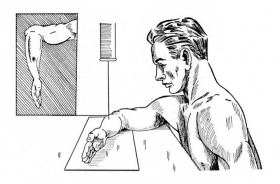

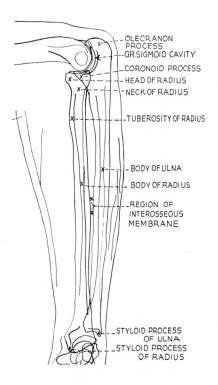

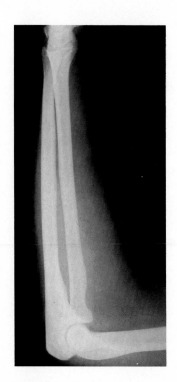

Figure 4–30. Lateral view of forearm. Method of positioning patient, radiograph, and labeled tracing.

Points of Practical Interest with Reference to Figures 4–29 and 4–30

1. When the proximal two-thirds of the forearm are of greatest anatomic interest, the elbow joint is always included. The wrist joint is always included when the major anatomic interest is in the distal one-third of the forearm. Thus, the important technical adjuncts which apply to the elbow joint and wrist also apply here, with the exception that the forearm is always in a supinated position with the volar aspect uppermost in these views.

   In any case, it is well to seat the patient low enough to place the shoulder and the elbow in approximately the same plane, to assure good contact between the distal humerus and the film. A platform on the table top, with the patient's arm and the film on the platform, can achieve the same purpose.

2. In both of these views, it is important to obtain an accurate concept of the integrity of the interosseous membrane. The ability of the patient to pronate and supinate his forearm depends in greatest measure upon the adequacy of this membrane and the space between the two bones of the forearm throughout their lengths. When the bones of the forearm are injured, there is a tendency for the fragments of the radius and ulna to contact one another, forming a bony bridge between them across the interosseous membrane. This tendency must be recognized early and prevented.

THE WRIST

Related Gross Anatomy of the Carpus or Wrist (Fig. 4–31). The carpus consists of eight bones, arranged in two rows. The proximal row is formed by the navicular, lunate, triquetral, and pisiform; the distal row by the greater multangular, lesser multangular, capitate, and hamate. A line joining the superior surfaces and margins of the bones is convex, whereas the volar aspect is concave. The margins of this concavity are formed by the tuberosity of the navicular and the ridge of the greater multangular laterally, and the pisiform and the hook of the hamate medially. The pisiform bone is attached to the volar surface of the triquetrum, and stands out clearly in a lateral profile view of the wrist.

The proximal articulation with the radius is formed by the navicular and lunate bones only. The distal articular surfaces of the wrist bones which articulate with the metacarpals are very irregular.

The articular surface between the two rows of carpal bones is concavoconvex from side to side.

Each carpal bone except the pisiform (which is virtually a sesamoid bone) has six surfaces—with two to four articular surfaces depending upon whether the bone is an outer or inner one, and the remaining surfaces rough for the attachment of ligaments. These multiple surfaces are important since their numerous margins are all visualized radiographically; all radiographs should be viewed with a three-dimensional concept in mind to aid in the interpretation of these lines.

The carpal bones articulate with one another by diarthrodial synovial joints; a similar joint exists between the pisiform and the triquetral bones. Each of the two rows of carpal bones moves as a unit so there are but three functional joints in the wrist: the radiocarpal, the intercarpal, and the carpometacarpal (Fig. 4–31, C).

The important anatomic features of the so-called "carpal tunnel" are indicated in Figure 4–31, D. The position of the median

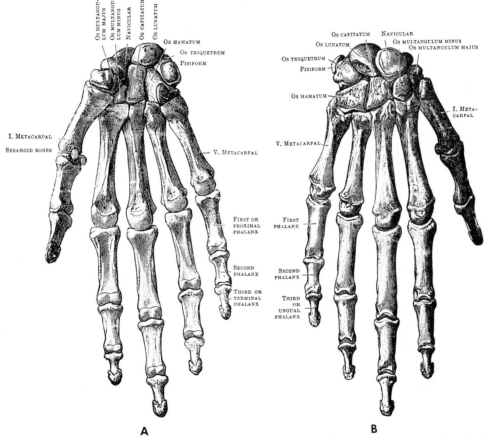

Figure 4–31. *A.* Volar aspect of the bones of the right hand and wrist. *B.* Dorsal aspect of the right hand and wrist.
(From Cunningham, D. J.: Textbook of Anatomy. 10th ed. London, Oxford University Press, 1964.)

Figure 4–31 continued on following page.

nerve in close proximity to the volar carpal ligament becomes significant if the median nerve is "pinched" or impressed upon by the adjoining structures. This gives rise to a so-called "carpal tunnel syndrome" that is basic to median nerve involvement.

The basic blood supply of the carpal navicular (scaphoid) bone is also important because healing of the fractures of this bone depends on the integrity of the blood supply. The arteries of the scaphoid enter on its dorsal aspect in the region of the

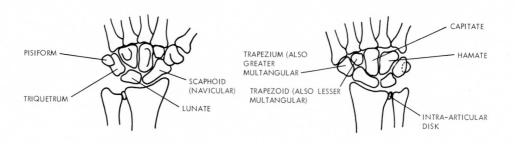

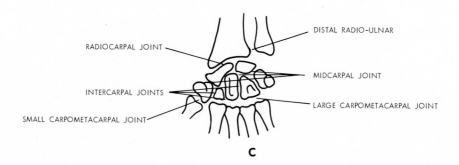

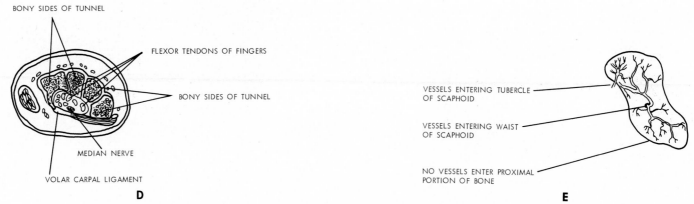

Figure 4–31 *Continued.* C. Joint cavities of the wrist. D. Anatomy of the carpal tunnel. E. Blood supply of the scaphoid (navicular carpal) bone.

tubercle; in the waist of the bone or in midposition avascular necrosis may result if a fragment becomes separated from its blood suppy (Fig. 4–31, *E*).

Axial Relationships at the Wrist (Fig. 4–32). The axis of flexion of the hand is perpendicular to the axis of the forearm, and forms an angle of 10 to 15 degrees with the line connecting the styloid processes of the radius and ulna. Keats et al. measured 25 normal males and 25 normal females in the posteroanterior projection with the results shown in Figure 4–32. The average measurement of the angle formed on the ulnar side between the shaft of the radius and the line drawn between the styloid processes of the radius and ulna was 83 degrees. In the lateral perspective the angle shown measured an average of 85.5 degrees, with ranges as indicated between 79 and 94 degrees in the two groups.

In the straight lateral view of the wrist, the midplane of the carpus is perpendicular to the plane of the radiocarpal joint.

ROUTINE RADIOGRAPHIC STUDIES OF THE WRIST

There are several special views in the case of the wrist which are employed for demonstration of certain anatomic features. In view of the curvature of the navicular carpal bone, a fracture through its midsection may escape detection unless this portion of the bone is brought into relief, and because of the great frequency of distressing symptoms in fracture of the navicular these special views assume considerable importance. It is also helpful to learn to recognize the navicular carpal bone on the straight lateral projection.

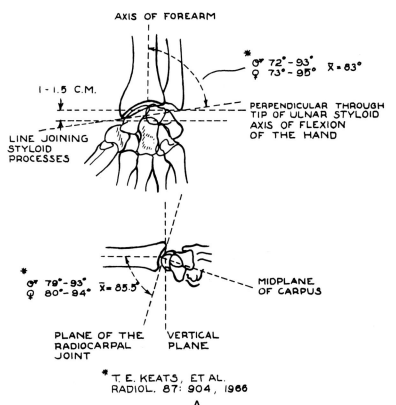

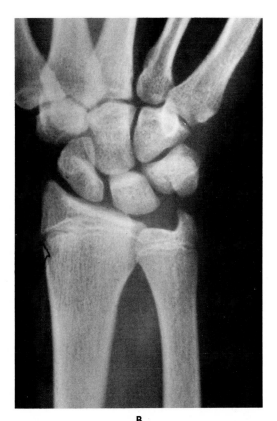

A   B

Figure 4–32. *A.* Axial relationships of the wrist. *B.* Radiographs of the epiphyseal plate of the distal radius in children.

1. **Routine Posteroanterior View of the Wrist** (Fig. 4–33). In this view, the forearm is pronated and the hand placed palm downward on the film. The palm may be spread out or the fist clenched. In the latter case, there is somewhat less overlapping of articular margins in the carpometacarpal joints. The central ray is directed over the middle of the carpus.

The anatomic parts are illustrated in Figure 4–33.

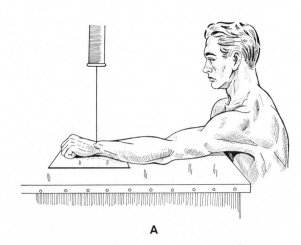

A

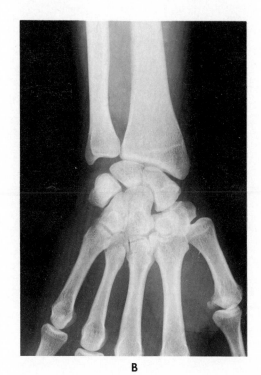

B

ULNA — RADIUS

STYLOID PROCESS — — — — — — — — — — — STYLOID PROCESS

— — — — LUNATE

PISIFORM — — — — — — — — — — — — NAVICULAR

TRIANGULAR — — — —

HAMATE — — — — — — — — — — — GR. MULTANGULAR

CAPITATE — — — — — — — — — — — LESS. MULTANGULAR

METACARPALS — — — — — — — — — — — SESAMOID BONES

— — — THENAR EMINENCE

C

Figure 4–33. Posteroanterior view of wrist. *A.* Method of positioning patient. *B.* Radiograph. *C.* Labeled tracing of *B.*

Points of Practical Interest with Reference to Figure 4–33

1. The posteroanterior projection of the wrist is usually preferable to permit better contact between the carpus and the film than is obtained in the reverse projection. In contrast, however, the anteroposterior view of the forearm is the more desirable since pronation of the hand would cause the two bones of the forearm to cross one another.
2. The central ray is projected immediately over the navicular carpal bone, midway between the styloid processes.
3. The clenched fist as shown places the wrist at a very slight angulation, but because the navicular carpal bone is at right angles to the central ray, it is usually projected without any superimposition, by itself or by adjoining structures.

2. **Routine Lateral View of the Wrist** (Fig. 4–34).   The wrist is placed in the same position as was the case in the lateral view of the forearm, with the thumb upward and the hand and wrist perfectly perpendicular to the film. The central ray is directed over the carpus. The relationship of the carpus to the distal articular margin of the radius is of particular importance here.

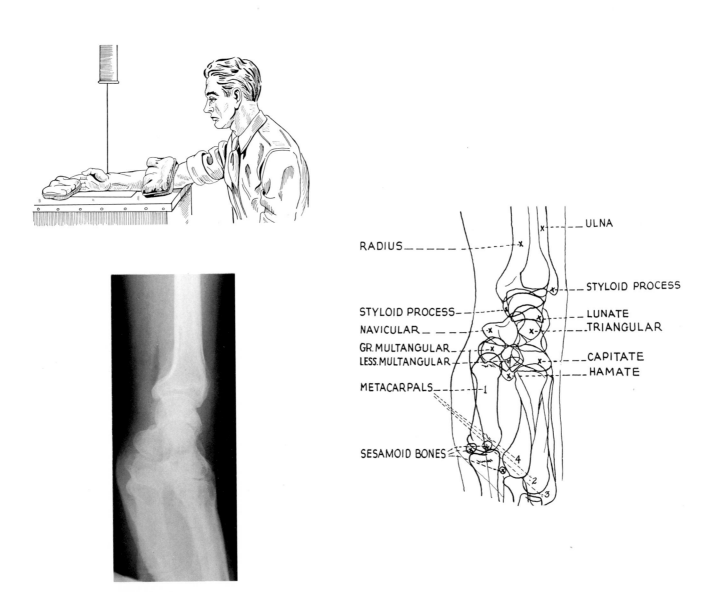

Figure 4–34.   Lateral view of the wrist. Method of positioning patient, radiograph, and labeled tracing.

3. **Special View for Demonstration of the Midsection of the Navicular Carpal Bone** (Fig. 4–35).   The palm is outstretched and placed on the film, spreading the thumb and the index finger. The axis of the central ray bisects the angle between the thumb and the index finger, at an angle of 45 degrees with the horizontal. The central ray is directed over the region of the navicular. A markedly distorted but good view of the midsection of the navicular is thus obtained.

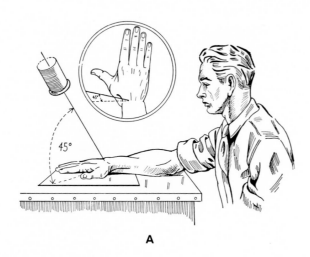

A

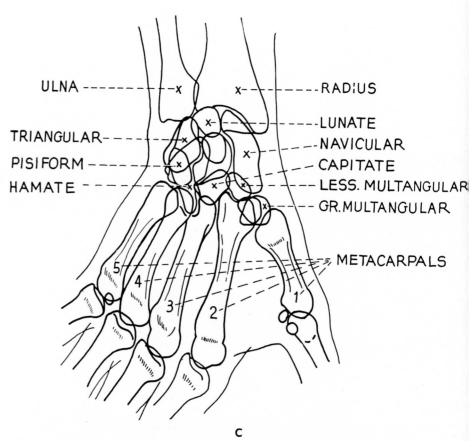

C

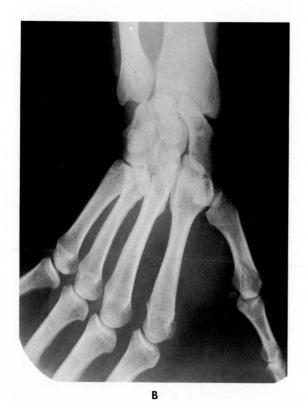

B

Figure 4–35.   Special view for demonstrating navicular carpal bone. *A.* Method of positioning patient. *B.* Radiograph. *C.* Labeled tracing of *B.*

Points of Practical Interest with Reference to Figure 4–35

1. This view is an application of the principle of distortion in order to provide increased clarity of a pathologic process within a bony structure. Actually, a rather distorted and elongated view of the navicular carpal bone is obtained, but for the most part it is completely clear of the adjoining structures, particularly in the area that is most prone to be fractured, namely its midsection. Also its own structure is not superimposed upon itself.
2. This view is also of some value with reference to the base of the first metacarpal, but not to the rest of the carpus.

4. **Oblique View of the Carpus** (Fig. 4–36). In this projection, the wrist is placed to form an angle of 45 degrees with the horizontal, the palm downward, and the radial border of the wrist farthest from the film. The central ray is directed over the middle of the carpus. This view is of value also in obtaining a better perspective of the midsection of the navicular, and less distortion of the other carpal bones than in the markedly distorted view previously described.

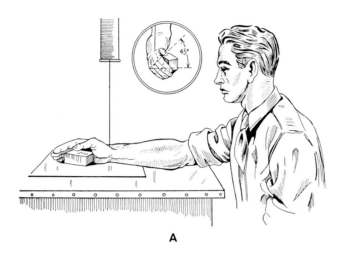

A

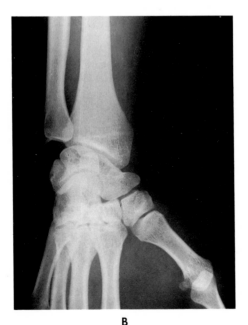

B

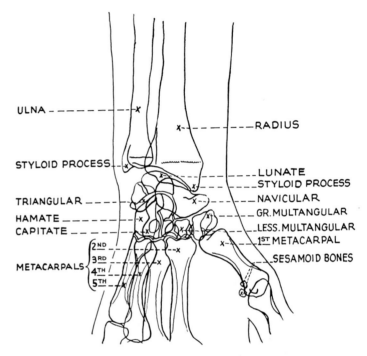

NOTE: IT IS NECESSARY FOR THE STUDENT TO DEVELOP A THREE-DIMENSIONAL CONCEPT, IN THAT ONE VISUALIZES BOTH THE ANTERIOR AND THE POSTERIOR MARGIN OF A SURFACE RIGHT THROUGH ANY INTERVENING STRUCTURE.

C

Figure 4–36. Oblique view of wrist. *A.* Method of positioning patient. *B.* Radiograph. *C.* Labeled tracing of *B.*

Points of Practical Interest with Reference to Figure 4–36

1. The film is placed under the wrist so that the center of the film is approximately 3 to 4 cm. anterior to the carpal bones. This will place the film immediately under the navicular carpal bone when the wrist is slightly pronated to about 45 degrees from the lateral position. The hand is supported on a balsa wood block or sandbag as shown, and the forearm may be immobilized by an additional sandbag.
2. The central ray is directed immediately over the navicular carpal bone.
3. This view is also particularly valuable in obtaining a clear perspective of the joint between the greater multangular and the first metacarpal.

5. **Special Carpal Tunnel View of the Wrist.** (Fig. 4–37). The special carpal tunnel view of the wrist, a modification of the Gaynor-Hart position and the Templeton and Zim carpal tunnel view, is shown in Figure 4–37. If hyperextension of the wrist cannot be maintained as shown, a special ray is directed at an angle of 20 to 30 degrees to the long axis of the hand. The view is particularly designed to show the relationship of the soft tissue structures in the carpal tunnel for definition of any pressure phenomena which may exist in relation to the median nerve.

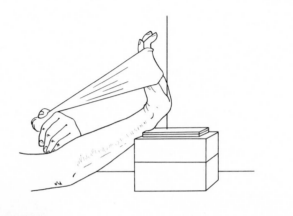

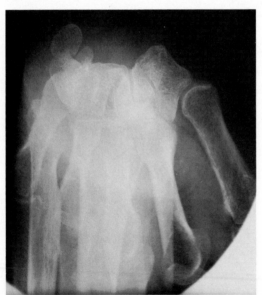
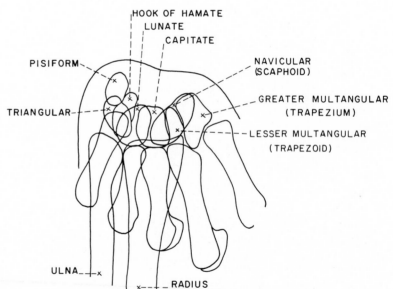

Figure 4–37.   The carpal tunnel view of the wrist (modification of Gaynor-Hart position, and Templeton and Zim carpal tunnel view). Method of positioning patient, radiograph, and labeled tracing.

THE HAND

Related Gross Anatomy of the Metacarpals (Fig. 4–31). These consist of five "long bones in miniature" articulating with the carpus proximally and the phalanges distally. When considered as a group, they form a concavity deep in the palm of the hand. With the exception of the first metacarpal, they are usually triangular in cross section, the apex of the triangle being a palmar ridge. The nutrient canal (Fig. 3–6) is usually in the middle of the shaft and is directed away from the wrist, with the exception of the thumb which runs proximally. The head is a rounded articular surface distally, on each side of which is a prominent tubercle. The second metacarpal is usually the longest, whereas the first is the shortest and widest. The first metacarpal also differs in other respects—its epiphysis is at its base instead of its head and its concavity and ridge are medial rather than palmar.

The other metacarpals differ from one another largely at their bases, which have angular and irregular articular margins and facets. A three-dimensional concept in the mind's eye is of the utmost importance here also.

Related Gross Anatomy of the Phalanges (Fig. 4–31). The thumb has two phalanges, and each of the other four fingers has three, distinguished as proximal, middle, and distal, respectively.

The proximal phalanges are semicylindrical in cross section, the flat aspect being on the palmar side. The base is a concave articular surface, whereas the distal articular surface is "half dumbbell-shaped," with a central groove and two condylelike structures on either side.

The middle phalanx is lacking in the thumb and in the case of the other fingers is distinguished from the first phalanx by having a ridge on its proximal articular surface to correspond with the groove in the adjoining distal articular surface of the first phalanx. The distal end of the second phalanx resembles that of the proximal phalanx. The palmar surface contains a tendinous impression.

The distal phalanges differ by having a club-shaped end known as the ungual *tuberosity* or *tuft.*

The nutrient canals tend to be in the midshaft on the radial side and they are directed distally.

With advancing age there is a tendency for the margins of the shafts to become more and more irregular, particularly in the areas of muscular attachment. These irregularities must not be misinterpreted as periostitis.

Sesamoid Bones (Fig. 4–38). The sesamoid bones are small rounded bones that are embedded in certain tendons. The most frequent of these according to occurrence by percentage (Degen) are shown in Figure 4–38 A. These are: (1) two over the left carpal phalangeal joints of the thumb, occurring in 100 per cent of cases (flexor pollicis brevis muscle), (2) one over the interphalangeal joint of the thumb, occurring in 72.9 per cent of cases, and (3) one over the metacarpal phalangeal joint of the fifth finger, occurring

in 82.5 per cent of cases. Other infrequent sesamoids are also shown.

The sesamoid index has been proposed as an aid in the diagnosis of acromegaly (Kleinberg et al.). The greatest diameter of the medial sesamoid bone at the metacarpal phalangeal joint of the first digit, measured in millimeters with a caliper, is multiplied by the greatest diameter of the same sesamoid image perpendicular to the first diameter. This product is representative of the size of the sesamoid bone and is called the "sesamoid index." When measurements are made bilaterally they are comparable, although not necessarily equal, on both sides. In control individuals of both sexes, the median sesamoid index is 20, with a range of 12 to 29 for both men and women. Among acromegalics, the median for men is 40 (range 30 to 63) and for women, 33 (range 31 to 35). Even among acromegalics, the smaller indices were obtained from persons under 37 years of age, although these were still in the abnormal range. The maximum normal sesamoid index may therefore be assumed to be 29 sq. mm.

The osseous structure of the sesamoid bones may be either spongy or compact.

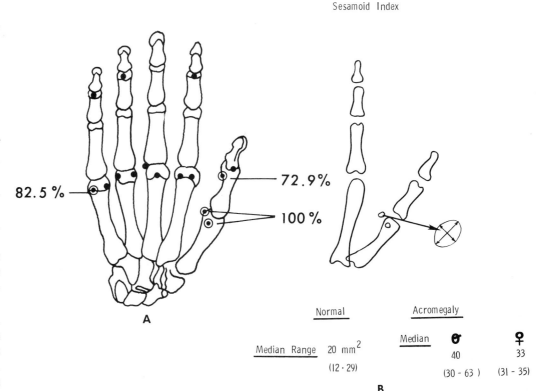

Figure 4–38. A. Schematic drawing (after Degen) of the sesamoids of the adult human hand. The most common are indicated by percentage occurrence. (Degen, St.: Med. Klin., 46:1330, 1959.) B. Diagram of the sesamoid index.

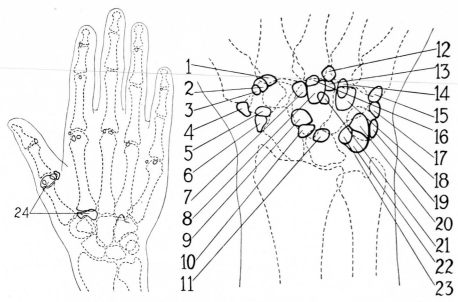

Figure 4–39. Supernumerary bones of the hand. 1, Os trapezoides secundarium; 2, trapezium secundarium; 3, praetrapezium; 4, paratrapezium; 5, epitrapezium; 6, radiale externum; 7, styloid; 8, subcapitatum; 9, os centrale; 10, hypolunatum; 11, epilunatum; 12, ossiculum gruberi; 13, os capitatum secondarium; 14, os hamuli proprium; 15, os vesalianum; 16, parastyloid; 17, ulnare externum; 18, hamular basale; 19, pisiforme proprium; 20, triquetrum ulnare; 21, metastyloid; 22, triquetrum radiale; 23, epipyramis; 24, epiphyses of the head of the first metacarpal and base of the second metacarpal, respectively. (From McNeill, C.: Roentgen Technique. Springfield, Ill., Charles C Thomas.)

Other supernumerary bones that may occur are shown in Figure 4–39.

Cystlike Defects in Carpal Bones. Small cystlike defects varying in size from 2 to 3 mm. are often identified in the carpal bones. They are surrounded by a thin sclerotic border. Histopathologically, these usually represent a circumscribed medullary fibrosis. They are considered to be of no pathologic significance, and may be found in metacarpal bones and phalanges as well. Some investigators believe that in the majority of cases these defects represent vascular canals seen on end; they must not be confused, however, with similar but larger shadows which represent such pathologic entities as ununited fractures, aseptic necrosis, and hemorrhagic cysts (Scholder; Bugnion; Radelli—quoted in Kohler and Zimmer).

The Carpal, Metacarpal, and Phalangeal Signs of Gonadal Dysgenesis (Kosowicz) (Fig. 4–40). Kosowicz noted that a line drawn tangent to the head of the fourth and fifth metacarpals would not traverse the head of the third metacarpal in 90 per cent of normal people, whereas in persons with gonadal dysgenesis, this line transected the head of the fourth metacarpal. This he called the "metacarpal sign."

Similarly, he noted that in normal persons the length of the fourth metacarpal could be compared to the summated length of the proximal and distal phalanges of the fourth finger or three times the length of the distal phalanx of the fourth finger, as shown in Figure 4–40. In patients with gonadal dysgenesis the phalanges were disproprotionately longer than the metacarpals, as shown.

In the carpus, a line drawn as shown tangent to the proximal edges of the navicular and lunate (scaphoid and lunate) normally forms a carpal angle of 134 degrees. A similar line in patients with gonadal dysgenesis forms a much smaller angle of 108 degrees. This Kosowicz called the "carpal angle."

In the normal adult, the carpal angles measure 135 degrees plus or minus 7.2 degrees.

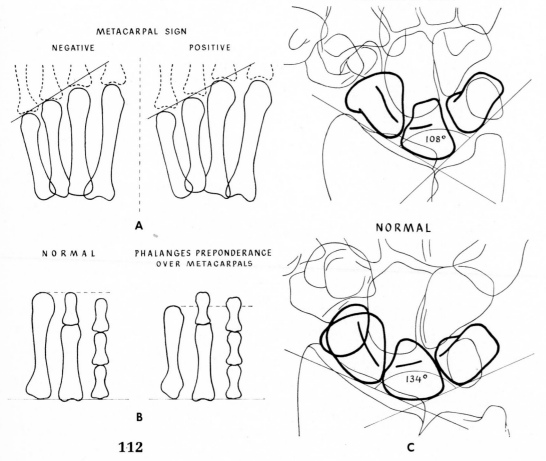

Figure 4–40. A. Line drawing illustrating the metacarpal sign. In the majority of patients with gonadal dysgenesis, a tangent touching the outlines of the fifth and fourth metacarpal heads runs through or touches the head of the third metacarpal. In nearly 90 per cent of normal subjects, this tangent runs above the head of the third metacarpal. B. Line drawing showing the disproportionate length of the phalanges over the metacarpals. The usual proportions of these bones in a normal subject are shown for comparison. C. (Upper) Line drawing of the wrist illustrating the positive carpal sign in a patient with gonadal dysgenesis. The bones of the proximal carpal row are angularly arranged, the carpal angle being 108 degrees. (Lower) In normal subjects the bones of the proximal carpal row form a slight arch. Two lines drawn tangentially to the contours of these bones form a normal carpal angle of 134 degrees. (From Kosowicz, J.: Amer. J. Roentgenol., 93:358, 1965.)

ROUTINE RADIOGRAPHIC STUDIES OF THE HAND

1. **Routine Posteroanterior View of the Hand** (Fig. 4–41). The hand is placed palm downward on the film and the central ray passes through the head of the third metacarpal. In view of the fact that there may be considerable variation in density between the metacarpal and phalangeal areas of the hand, special views are frequently employed to obtain better detail of the fingers. If a single finger is in question, multiple views of the one finger are usually in order.

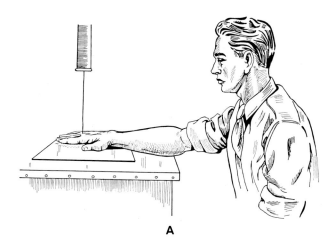

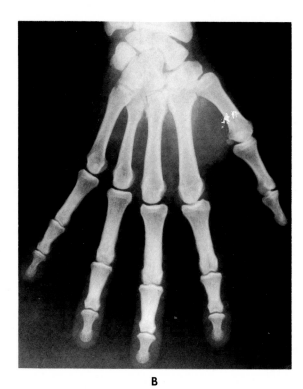

B

Figure 4–41. Posteroanterior view of hand. *A.* Method of positioning patient. *B.* Radiograph. *C.* Labeled tracing of *B.*

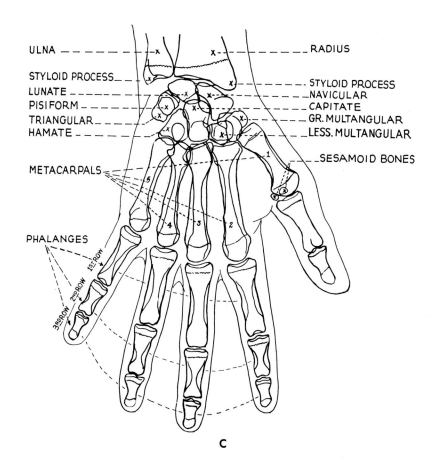

C

Points of Practical Interest with Reference to Figure 4–41

1. The fingers should be spread slightly, completely extended and in good contact with the film.
2. The central ray should pass through the third metacarpophalangeal joint.
3. It is well to immobilize the forearm just above the wrist by means of a sandbag.
4. The greatest care must be exercised to obtain a clear view, particularly of the tufted ends of the distal phalanges as well as the shafts of the phalanges, since many of the pathologic processes of a systemic type will produce minute and very important changes in these structures. The student should obtain a very clear concept of the normal appearance of the phalanges and metacarpals.
5. If a single finger is in question a lighter exposure technique is employed and usually four views of that finger from all perspectives are taken.
6. All the structures are shown in straight posteroanterior projection except the thumb, of which an oblique view is obtained.

2. **Routine Oblique View of the Hand** (Fig. 4–42).   The hand is placed palm downward on the film, with the thumb and thenar portion of the hand raised about 45 degrees from the film and the hypothenar portion of the hand in contact with it. The central ray is once again made to pass through the head of the third metacarpal. This view has the advantage over the direct lateral in that the various anatomic parts do not overlap so much, but exact degree of displacement is impossible to describe except in the straight lateral.

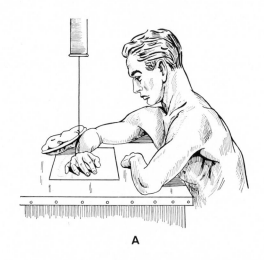

A

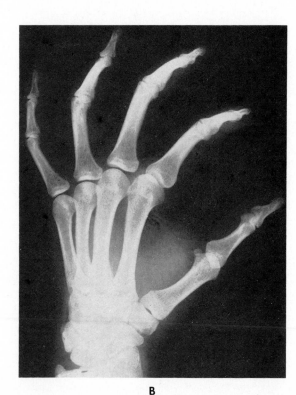

B

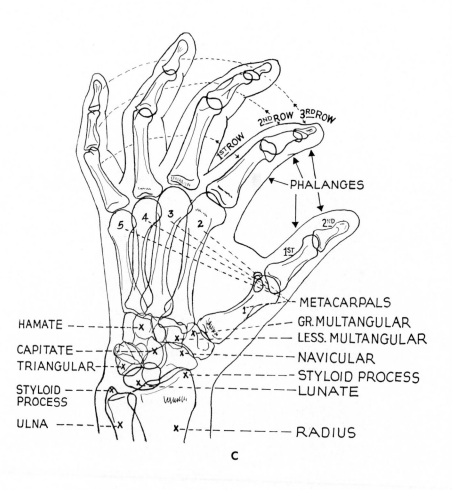

C

Figure 4–42.   Oblique view of hand. *A.* Method of positioning patient. *B.* Radiograph. *C.* Labeled tracing of *B.*

Practical Points of Interest with Reference to Figure 4–42

1. One should adjust the obliquity of the hands so that the metacarpophalangeal joints form an angle of approximately 45 degrees with the film.
2. The central ray is directed vertically through the third metacarpophalangeal joint.
3. Cotton pledgets may be employed to spread the fingers. A 2 inch square of balsa wood placed under the thumb makes an excellent immobilization device.

3. **Straight Lateral View of the Hand** (Fig. 4–43). The hand is placed perpendicular to the film with the thumb pointing upward. The central ray is made to pass through the line of the heads of the metacarpals. It is important to note the normal curvature of the metacarpals in this projection with their concavity on the palmar aspect of the hand. Various sesamoid bones, particularly at the metacarpophalangeal junctions, will be demonstrated clearly.

4. **Various Positions for Views of Fingers and Thumb** (Fig. 4–44). The individual digits are filmed in anteroposterior or posteroanterior perspectives, along with oblique and lateral views with various supporting mechanisms as shown in the accompanying illustration.

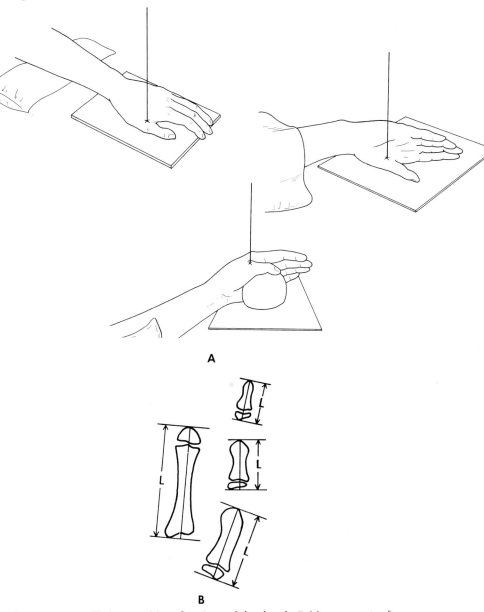

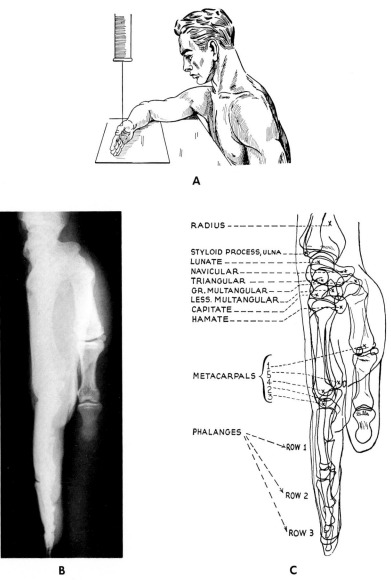

Figure 4–43. Straight lateral view of the hand. Method of positioning patient, radiograph, and labeled tracing.

Figure 4–44. A. Various positions for views of the thumb. B. Measurements of the bones were taken along the longitudinal axis of each bone. The length was defined as the maximal distance between perpendiculars drawn to each end of the bone. For the adult, the nine-year, or the four-year standards, the entire bone, including the epiphysis, was measured. On the one-year standards, only the diaphysis was measured. B. Measurements of the bones were taken along the longitudinal axis of each bone. The length was defined as the maximal distance between perpendiculars drawn to each end of the bone. For the adult, the nine-year, or the four-year standards, the entire bone, including the epiphysis, was measured. On the one-year standards, only the diaphysis was measured. (From Poznanski, A. K., Garn, S. M., and Holt, J. F.: Radiology, *100*:115–129, 1971.)

Points of Practical Importance. The overlapping articulations of the distal row of carpal bones with the bases of the metacarpals are of particular importance. These overlapping surfaces frequently give rise to the impression of fracture unless they are carefully delineated.

The tufted ends (ungual tufts) of the distal phalanges alter their appearance both from injury and metabolic disease. They must be studied carefully from this aspect.

In view of the fact that in the straight lateral view of the hand many of the bones are projected over one another, the oblique view of the hand is more frequently employed. The lateral view is used particularly if a knowledge of the exact degree of anteroposterior displacement is of importance.

VASCULAR ANATOMY OF THE UPPER EXTREMITIES

A diagram of the named arteries of the upper limb is shown in Figure 4–45.

Both extremities are identical, with the exception of the right

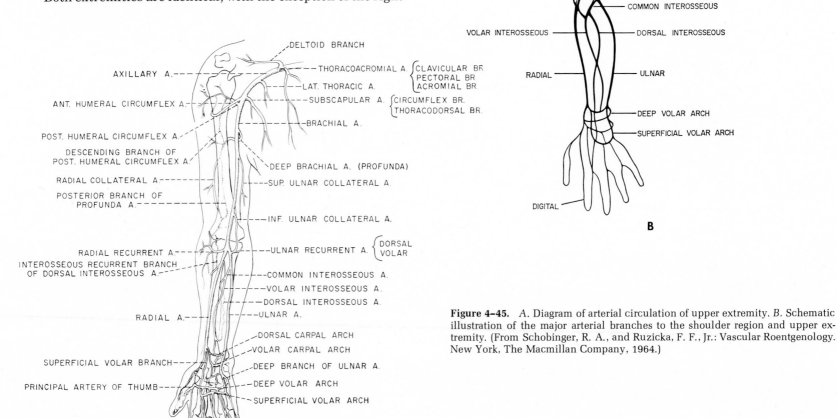

Figure 4–45. *A.* Diagram of arterial circulation of upper extremity. *B.* Schematic illustration of the major arterial branches to the shoulder region and upper extremity. (From Schobinger, R. A., and Ruzicka, F. F., Jr.: Vascular Roentgenology. New York, The Macmillan Company, 1964.)

Figure 4–45 continued on opposite page.

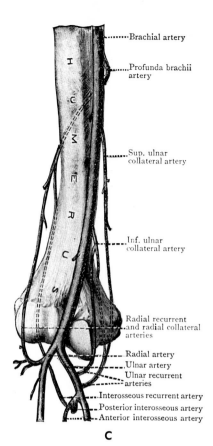

C

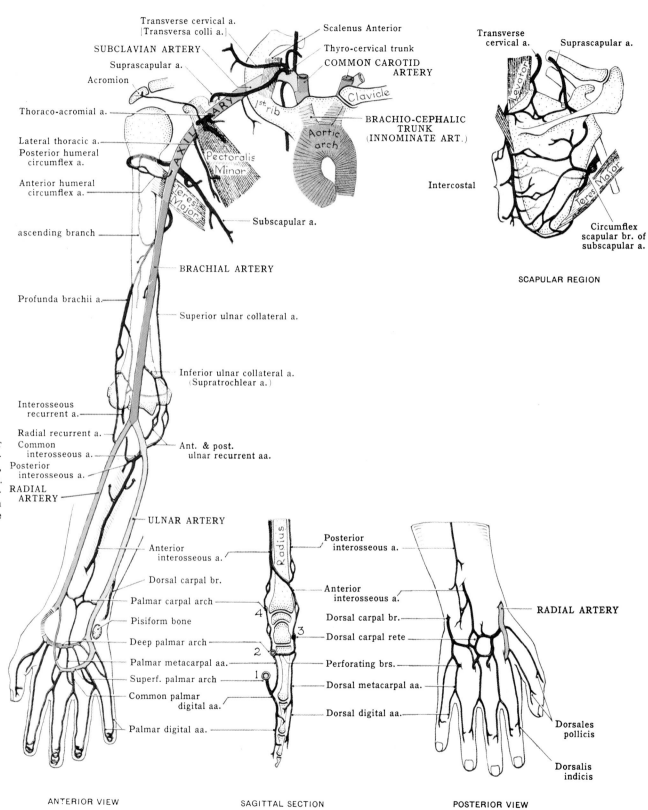

Figure 4–45 *Continued. C.* Diagram of major anastomoses around the elbow joint. (From Cunningham, D. J.: Manual of Practical Anatomy. Vol. 1, 12th ed. London, Oxford University Press, 1959.) *D.* Diagram of named arteries of the upper limb. (Reproduced by permission from J. C. B. Grant: An Atlas of Anatomy, 5th ed. Copyright © 1962. The Williams & Wilkins Co.)

Figure 4–45 continued on following page.

subclavian artery, which arises from the brachiocephalic trunk or innominate artery, whereas the left subclavian artery branches directly from the aortic arch.

The important relationships of the major vessels may be summarized as follows:

1. The *subclavian artery* lies above the level of the clavicle (2 to 3 cm.) and crosses cephalad to the first rib to enter the axilla as the *axillary artery*.

2. The *axillary artery* arises from a small segment between the first rib and the pectoralis minor muscle, crosses beneath the

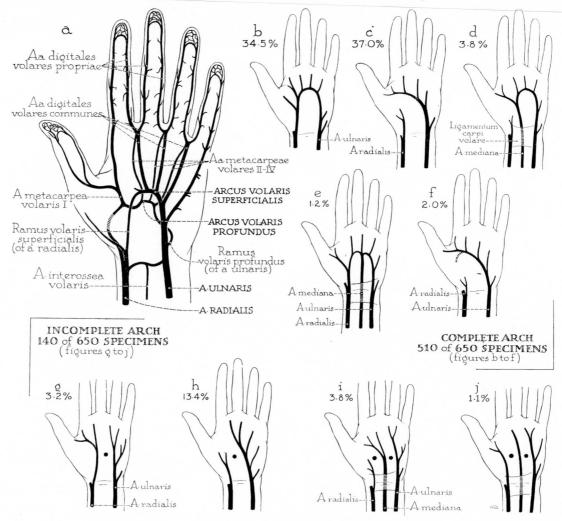

ARCUS VOLARIS SUPERFICIALIS, 650 SPECIMENS

E

Figure 4–45 *Continued.* E. Types of superficial volar arterial arch (b to j) encountered in 650 dissections of the hand, together with the "textbook normal" (a). Shown schematically, with the percentage occurrence of each of the nine types. Variations (b to f) encountered in 510 specimens in which the arch was complete; patterns (g to j) found in the 140 hands in which the arch was incomplete—in the areas indicated by marker. a, The standard, and regularly pictured, pattern of superficial arterial arch with its branches at metacarpal and phalangeal levels— the common and the proper volar digital arteries, respectively. b, The schematized form of the complete radioulnar communication present in slightly more than one-third of the total number of extremities studied. c, A transpalmar arciform continuation of the ulnar artery with a full complement of common volar digital branches. This type occurs more frequently, 37 per cent of cases, than the traditional or "standard" type. d, An arciform arrangement to which the contributors are ulnar and median arteries—the median artery replacing the radial of the type shown in a and b. The ulnomedian type initiates the series of patterns whose frequencies of occurrence show a sharp decline from the commonest varieties, namely, those depicted in b and c. e, An arch to which the 3 arteries contribute. Here a median communication is sent to the center of the arch formed by anastomosis of the radial and ulnar arteries. f, In this type a transpalmar continuation of

the ulnar artery (compare with c) receives a midpalmar contribution from the deep palmar arterial arch, not from the radial artery itself. In the remaining specimens, 140 out of a total of 650 (21.5 per cent), the superficial arterial arch is incomplete, the area of interruption indicated in each diagram by a black dot. g, In specimens of this type, the proper volar arteries are derived equally from the radial and ulnar arteries, without communication across the middle line of the hand. h, Here the ulnar artery is the chief contributor to the set of digital vessels, supplying 3½ digits, that is, toward the thumb, to include the ulnar aspect of the index finger. i, In specimens of this type the median artery reaches the hand to furnish digital arteries (compare with d and e), but without anastomosing the radial and ulnar arteries. Inclining toward the radial side of the hand, the median artery gives off a branch to the thumb. j, In this variety of palmar arterial supply, the deviation of the three source-vessels toward the radial side of the hand is of lesser degree than in the preceding type; the branches of the common volar digital artery derived from the median artery pass only to the facing aspects of the index and middle fingers, the radial and ulnar arteries caring for the areas marginal thereto. (From Coleman, S. S., and Anson, B. J.: Surg., Gynec., Obstet., *113*(4):412, 1961. Used by permission of Surgery, Gynecology and Obstetrics.)

Figure 4–45 continued on opposite page.

pectoralis minor, and thereafter crosses anterior to the teres major muscle to become the *brachial artery.*

3. The *brachial artery* lies on the medial aspect of the humerus at first and descends the arm to the anterior aspect, where it bifurcates into *radial and ulnar arteries* about 1 inch below the crease of the elbow.

The relationships of the radial nerve to the adjoining arteries and humerus are shown in Figure 4–46.

The radial nerve is behind the proximal 2 cm. of the brachial artery, but it then passes down and laterally into the radial groove of the humerus, adjoining the profunda branch (deep brachial artery).

4. The *ulnar artery* descends on the medial side of the forearm, whereas the radial artery is on the lateral. The two ultimately communicate by several arches as shown in sagittal section (Fig. 4–45 *C*).

5. Many of the branches of the arteries are purely muscular and nameless. The major named arteries are shown.

6. Anastomoses are rather common in relation to the brachial artery and its branches. These anastomoses are of some importance in the event that ligation of a major vessel becomes necessary. Those around the elbow are shown in Figure 4–45 *C*.

7. There are four main arches in the vicinity of the wrist and hand and these are formed as shown (Fig. 4–45 *A, D, E, F*). These tend to unite the radial and ulnar arteries of their branches with the interosseous arteries of the forearm, of the dorsum of the hand, and of the digits.

8. The subclavian artery is said to be divided into three un-

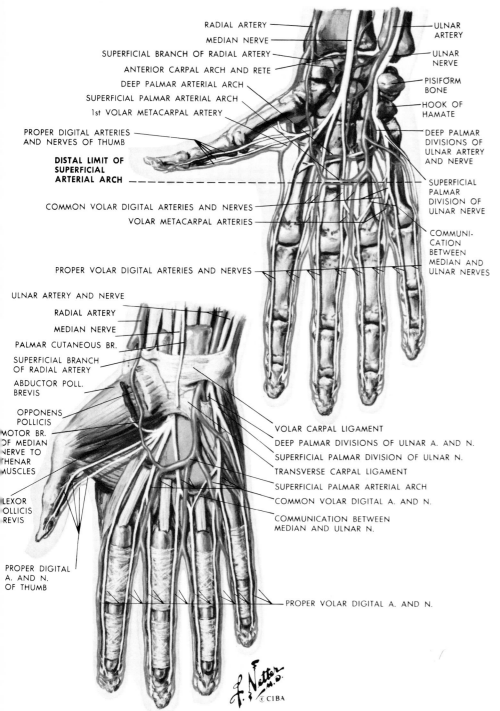

Figure 4–45 *Continued. F.* (Copyright 1969 Ciba Pharmaceutical Company, Division of Ciba-Geigy Corporation. Reproduced with permission from *Clinical Symposia*, illustrated by Frank H. Netter, M.D. All rights reserved.)

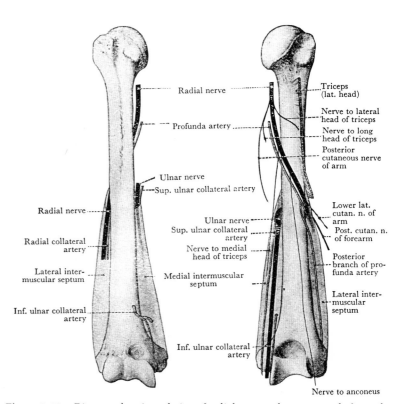

Figure 4–46. Diagram showing relation of radial nerve to humerus, and of vessels and nerves to the intermuscular septa. (From Cunningham, D. J.: Manual of Practical Anatomy. Vol. 1, 12th ed. London, Oxford University Press, 1959.)

equal parts by the scalenus anterior muscle. One portion of the artery is just proximal to this muscle, a second portion lies beneath it, and a third is distal to it over the first rib.

9. The axillary artery passes within 1 cm. of the tip of the coracoid process. The brachial artery lies medial to the humerus proximally and anterior to it distally, where it may be reached for percutaneous catheterization.

10. The deep veins of the upper extremity tend to follow closely the arterial pattern. The superficial veins of the upper limbs are shown (Fig. 4–47). The most important named veins are shown and represent those veins most frequently entered for intravenous puncture. At times, more peripheral veins, particularly on the dorsum of the hand, may also permit entry for percutaneous puncture.

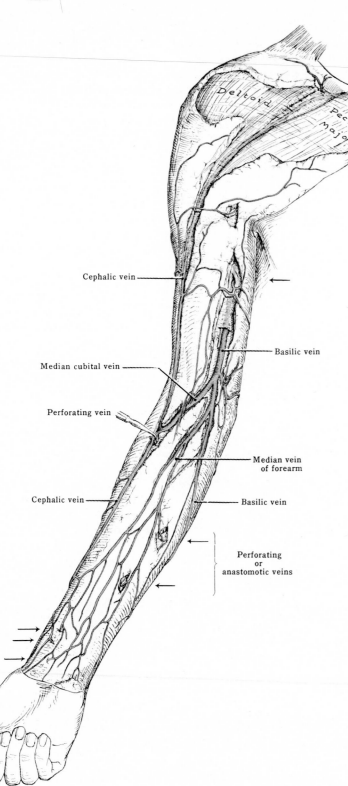

Cephalic vein

Median cubital vein

Perforating vein

Median vein of forearm

Basilic vein

Cephalic vein

Basilic vein

Perforating or anastomotic veins

Figure 4–47.   Superficial veins of the upper limb (dissected and drawn by Miss Nancy Joy). The arrows indicate where perforating veins pierce the deep fascia and bring the superficial and deep veins of the limb into communication with each other. For obvious mechanical reasons the palmar veins are few and small, and the dorsal veins are large. (Reproduced by permission from J. C. B. Grant: An Atlas of Anatomy, 5th ed. Copyright © 1962, The Williams & Wilkins Co.)

LYMPH VESSELS AND LYMPH NODES OF THE UPPER EXTREMITIES

Lymph vessels and nodes are categorized as superficial or deep. Generally, the deep lymph nodes lie along the course of the main blood vessels. The nodes are grouped chiefly in the axilla with a few along the medial side of the brachial artery and at its bifurcation deep in the cubital fossa. Other nodes may be found in relation to the radial, ulnar, and interosseous arteries. The deep lymphatics are much less numerous than the superficial vessels and generally accompany the main blood vessels. The superficial vessels as shown in Figure 4–48 are straight yet sinuous channels with a system of valves that take the main trend of a stream from the hand upward toward the lymph nodes of the axilla.

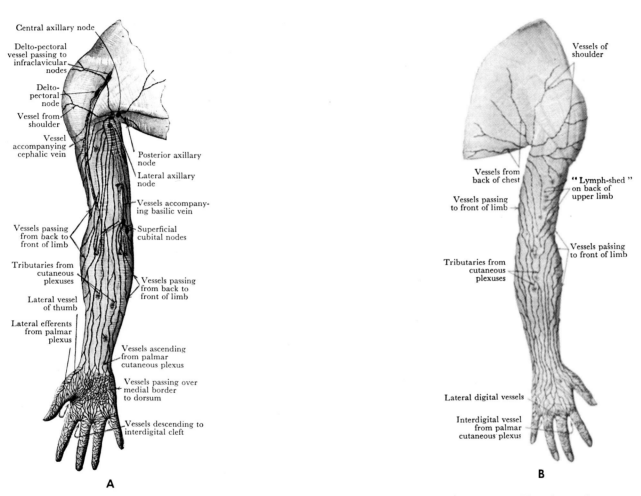

Figure 4–48. *A.* Superficial lymph vessels and lymph nodes of front of upper limb. *B.* Superficial lymph vessels of back of upper limb. (From Cunningham's Manual of Practical Anatomy, Vol. 1. 12th ed. London, Oxford University Press, 1959.)

REFERENCES

Calenoff, L.: Angiography of the hand: guidelines for interpretation. Radiology, *102*:331–335, 1972.

Cunningham, D. J.: Manual of Practical Anatomy. 12th edition. London, Oxford University Press, 1959.

Degen, St.: Über das Auftreten der Knochenkerne am Handskelett von der Geburt bis zur Reife. Mit einem Hinweis auf die Sesambeine der hand. [Appearance of bone rudiments in the hand skeleton from birth to maturity.] Med. Klin. *46/50*:1330–1332, 1951.

DePalma, A. F.: The Management of Fractures and Dislocations. Philadelphia, W. B. Saunders Co., 1959.

Grant, J. C. B.: Atlas of Anatomy. Fifth edition. Baltimore, Williams and Wilkins Co., 1962.

Gray, H.: Anatomy of the Human Body. 29th edition. Goss, C. M., ed. Philadelphia, Lea and Febiger, 1973.

Keats, T. E., and Burns, T. W.: The radiographic manifestations of gonadal dysgenesis. Radiol. Clin. N. Amer., *2*:297–313, 1964.

Keats, T. E., Teeslink, R., Diamond, A. E., and Williams, J. H.: Normal axial relationships of the major joints. Radiology, *87*:904–907, 1966.

Kernwein, G. A., Roseberg, B., and Sneed, W. R. J.: Arthrographic studies of the shoulder joint. J. Bone Joint Surg., *39A*:1267–1279, 1957.

Kleinberg, D. L., Young, I. S., and Kupperman, H. S.: The sesamoid index: an aid in the diagnosis of acromegaly. Ann. Intern. Med., *64*:1075–1078, 1966.

Köhler, A., and Zimmer, E. A.: Borderlands of the Normal and Early Pathologic and Skeletal Roentgenology. Third edition. Translated and edited by S. P. Wilks, New York and London, Grune and Stratton, 1968.

Kosowicz, J.: Gonadal dysgenesis. Amer. J. Roentgenol., *93*:354–361, 1965.

Lusted, L. B., and Keats, T. E.: Atlas of Roentgenographic Measurement. Second edition. Year Book Medical Publishers, 1967.

Moore, R. D., and Renner, R. R.: The coraco-clavicular joint. Amer. J. Roentgenol., *78*:86–88, 1957.

Poznanski, A. K., Garn, S. M., and Holt, J. F.: The thumb in the congenital malformation syndrome. Radiology, *100*:115–129, 1971.

Schobinger, R. A., and Ruzicka, F. F., Jr.: Vascular Roentgenology. New York, Macmillan, 1964.

Simril, W., and Trotter, M.: An accessory bone and other skeletal anomalies of the elbow. Radiology, *53*:97–100, 1949.

Terry, R. J.: New data on the incidence of the supracondyloid variation. Amer. J. Phys. Anthropol., *9*:265–270, 1926.

Wagner, A., and Schaaf, J.: Size and frequency of sesamoid bones in acromegaly. Fortschr. Röntgenstr., *99*:215–219, 1963.

5

The Pelvis and Lower Extremity

The anatomic groups that are considered radiographically in the examination of pelvis and lower extremity are pelvis, hip, thigh, knee, leg, ankle, and foot. Considered also are special examinations for some of the component parts of these regions such as the patella and the calcaneus.

THE PELVIS

Gross Anatomy with Radiographic Significance. The os coxae, innominate, or hip bone (Figs. 5–1, 5–2), together with its fellow of the opposite side, forms the anterior and lateral walls of the bony pelvis. It articulates posteriorly with the sacrum, and the two hip bones articulate anteriorly to form the pubic symphysis.

The hip bone is formed by three separate bones which are firmly united at the acetabulum in the adult: the ilium, ischium, and pubis, each contributing two-fifths, two-fifths, and one-fifth respectively to the deep hemispherical socket which articulates with the head of the femur.

The trabecular pattern of the ilium suggests a moderately cancellous type of bone, with the major direction toward the acetabulum, except at the iliac crest, where the trabeculae tend to run parallel with the crest. There is a roughness visualized on the surfaces of the ilium related to the areas of attachment of the heavy gluteal muscles and the iliacus muscle. The following anatomic parts of the ilium can be identified radiographically: the anterior superior iliac spine; the anterior inferior iliac spine; the posterior superior iliac spine; the posterior inferior iliac spine; the iliac crest; the iliopectineal eminence, which indicates the point of union of the ilium and pubis; the iliac fossa; the auricular surface, for articulation with the sacrum; and the auricular tuberosity or tuberosity of the ilium. There are two notches in the contour of the ilium just above the acetabulum: the posterior notch below the articular auricular surface is the greater sciatic notch;

Figure 5–1. Os coxae, or hip bone, from the lateral aspect. (From Cunningham's Textbook of Anatomy, 6th ed. London, Oxford University Press, 1931.)

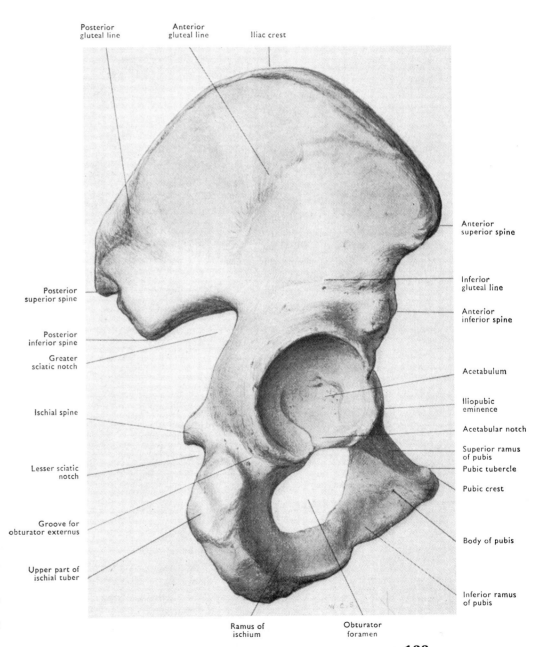

Posterior gluteal line

Anterior gluteal line

Iliac crest

Anterior superior spine

Inferior gluteal line

Anterior inferior spine

Posterior superior spine

Posterior inferior spine

Greater sciatic notch

Acetabulum

Iliopubic eminence

Acetabular notch

Ischial spine

Superior ramus of pubis

Pubic tubercle

Pubic crest

Lesser sciatic notch

Groove for obturator externus

Body of pubis

Upper part of ischial tuber

Inferior ramus of pubis

Ramus of ischium

Obturator foramen

123

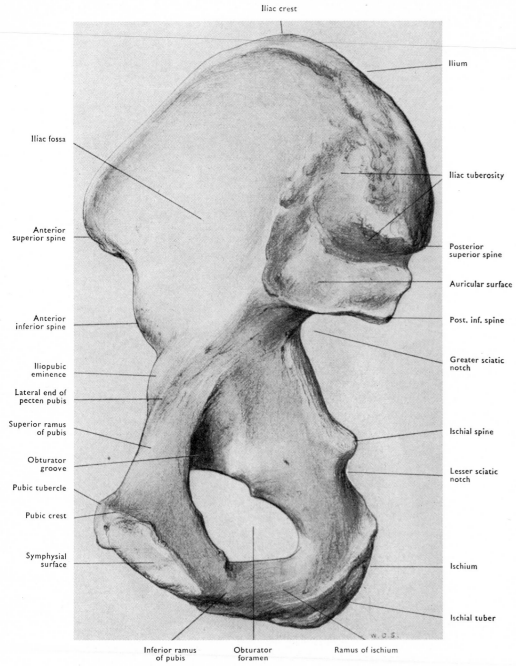

Iliac crest

Ilium

Iliac fossa

Iliac tuberosity

Anterior
superior spine

Posterior
superior spine

Auricular surface

Anterior
inferior spine

Post. inf. spine

Greater sciatic
notch

Iliopubic
eminence

Lateral end of
pecten pubis

Superior ramus
of pubis

Ischial spine

Obturator
groove

Lesser sciatic
notch

Pubic tubercle

Pubic crest

Symphysial
surface

Ischium

Ischial tuber

Inferior ramus   Obturator   Ramus of ischium
of pubis   foramen

Figure 5–2. Os coxae from the medial aspect. (From Cunningham's Textbook of Anatomy, 6th ed. London, Oxford University Press, 1931.)

and the anterior is situated between the anterior inferior iliac spine and the acetabulum and is known as the inferior iliac notch.

The important anatomic landmarks with regard to the ischium are the following: the body of the ischium; the ischial spine, below the greater sciatic notch; the lesser sciatic notch, below the ischial spine; the ischial tuberosity; the superior ramus, which ultimately fuses with the superior ramus of the pubis; and the inferior ramus, which fuses with the inferior ramus of the pubis. The ischial and pubic rami and the bodies of the ischium and pubis enclose an opening called the obturator foramen. Anterosuperiorly it is deeply grooved for passage of the obturator vessels and nerves.

The pubis consists of a body and two rami, and is united with its fellow of the opposite side at the pubic symphysis. The lines of union of the pubis and ischium (ischiopubic synchondrosis) are frequently readily evident on the radiograph, and care must be exercised to differentiate these from fracture.

The acetabulum contains both an articular and a nonarticular portion, the acetabular fossa and lunate surface respectively. The nonarticular portion is formed mainly by the ischium and is continuous with the margin of the obturator foramen. The margins of this socket, although thick, are subject to fracture. In order to visualize the posterior margin of the acetabulum, this structure must be viewed through the head of the femur. The shelving portion of the acetabulum is also of considerable importance, and when defective in development, congenital dislocation of the hip may result. The articular portion resembles a semilunar-shaped cartilage with its concavity directed toward the obturator foramen; it extends in irregular fashion around the ligamentum teres, excluding the latter structure from the synovial cavity. The outer edge of the articular portion is rough and uneven and gives attachment to the glenoidal labrum which deepens the socket. There is a ligament, the transverse ligament, which connects the opposite extremities of this lunate cartilage, forming the acetabular foramen. A nerve and vessels enter the joint through this foramen.

The Bony Pelvis (Figs. 5–3, 5–4).   The bony pelvis is formed by the two hip bones together with the sacrum and coccyx. The iliopectineal line divides the pelvis into two areas, the one above being known as the greater or false pelvis and the one below as the true pelvis. These bony structures are very firmly bound together, and it ordinarily requires considerable trauma to injure this bony cage. The most vulnerable portion is the region of the pubis and its rami. An injury in this location will frequently be accompanied by a "contrecoup" fracture of the opposite wing of the sacrum. Urinary bladder or urethral injury is not infrequently found when the bony pelvis is injured.

The female bony pelvis is of particular importance because of its obstetric implications. The true pelvis is described as having an inlet, a cavity, and an outlet. The contour and dimensions of these are carefully studied in relation to the fetal head (see Chapter 17), and although other factors such as uterine tone are of great importance in this regard, the simpler anatomic details of pelvic struture must also be considered. Apart from actual measurements, the concavity of the sacrum, the pubic angle, the size of the ischial spines, and the mobility and position of the coccyx

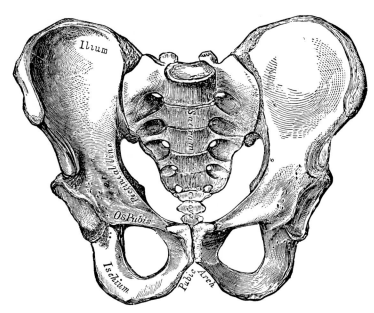

Figure 5–3. The bony pelvis (male). (From Gray's Anatomy of the Human Body, 29th ed. Goss, C. M. (ed.) Philadelphia, Lea & Febiger, 1973.)

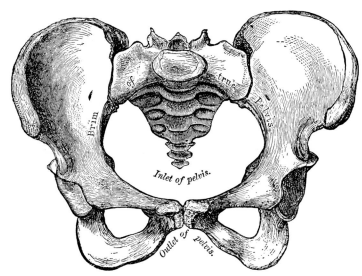

Figure 5–4. The bony pelvis (female). (See Chapter 17 for significance in relation to obstetric radiology.) (From Gray's Anatomy of the Human Body, 29th ed. Goss, C. M. (ed.) Philadelphia, Lea & Febiger, 1973.)

iliac joints are perpendicular to the plane of the intervertebral or apophyseal joints, and thus constitute structural supports for one another. An irregular anteroposterior appearance of the sacroiliac joints is produced by the obliquity of the angle, and for proper interpretation these joints must be visualized in three dimensions. For that reason the oblique projection of the sacroiliac joints has considerable value.

Changes with Growth and Development. The hip bone is ossified from eight centers as shown in Figure 5–5 *A*: one each for the ilium, ischium, and pubis; and five secondary ossification centers—the crest of the ilium, the anterior inferior spine, the tuberosity of the ischium, the pubic symphysis (more frequently in the female than in the male), and an additional epiphysis contained within the Y-shaped sector in the acetabulum. At birth, although the larger part of the bony pelvis is ossified, the three primary centers are separate. However, by age 7 or 8 the inferior rami of the pubis and ischium are almost completely united at their synchondroses. By the age of 13 or 14 the primary centers have grown toward one another within the acetabulum and are separated from each other by a Y-shaped portion of cartilage which may contain traces of secondary ossification centers (Fig. 5–5 *B*). One of the ossification centers contained within the acetabulum, called the os acetabuli, appears at about age 12 and fuses at approximately age 18 on the pubic aspect of the acetabulum. At about puberty, ossification takes place in each of the remaining parts of the innominate bone, and the secondary ossification centers join the primary between the ages of 20 and 25. It is thought that the secondary ossification centers of the crest are particularly helpful in bone age estimation at the time of puberty. At birth, in both sexes, the pelvis is relatively small, but as the lower limbs grow, the pelvis keeps pace with its growth.

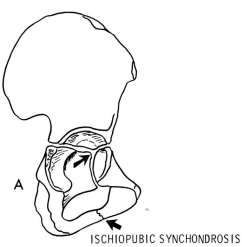

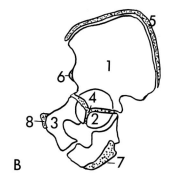

ISCHIOPUBIC SYNCHONDROSIS

OSSIFICATION CENTERS OF HIP BONE

Figure 5–5. *A.* Ossification centers of the hip bone. *B.* Tri-radiate synchondrosis of the hip bone. *1, 4, 5,* and *6* are parts of the ilium; *3* and *8,* the pubis; *2* and *7,* the ischium.

all play an essential part in conversion of the pelvis to a birth canal. A classification for the female bony pelvis as well as differences between the male and female will be detailed in Chapter 17.

The sacroiliac articulations are synovial (diarthrodial) joints and are normally obliquely situated at an angle of approximately 45 degrees to the sagittal plane. It is significant that the sacro-

The pelvic organs gradually descend into the pelvis minor by the sixth year. Growth is similar in both boys and girls until puberty, when it is modified according to the sex of the child (Fig. 5–6).

There is also a change at this time in the lumbosacral angle, and the sacrum tends to sink in between the two innominate bones. The acetabula become deeper and thus tend to stabilize the hip joints.

The pelvis of a woman differs from that of a man in preparation for the child-bearing function in the woman, unless there is an aberration in the female pelvis. This will be discussed more fully in Chapter 17. In women, the pelvis minor is larger in all diameters, and the cavity tends to be less funnel-shaped and is shorter. The female pubic arch is wide and the angle blunt. Mid-

pelvic measurements approach the shape of a sphere and the pelvic inlet in the so-called gynecoid pelvis is circular. Abnormalities in this contour assume considerable importance during parturition.

Some Variations of Normal in the Iliac Bone. These are shown in Figure 5–7. Ordinarily the trabecular arrangement of the hip bone is quite characteristic. Occasionally, however, a vascular channel becomes accentuated as shown in Figure 5–7 A. At times a notch, called the paraglenoidal sulcus of the ilium, appears just lateral to the sacroiliac joint. Apophyses sometimes appear, particularly in the region of the shelving portion of the acetabulum (Fig. 5–7 C).

Other variations of normal in the immediate vicinity of the

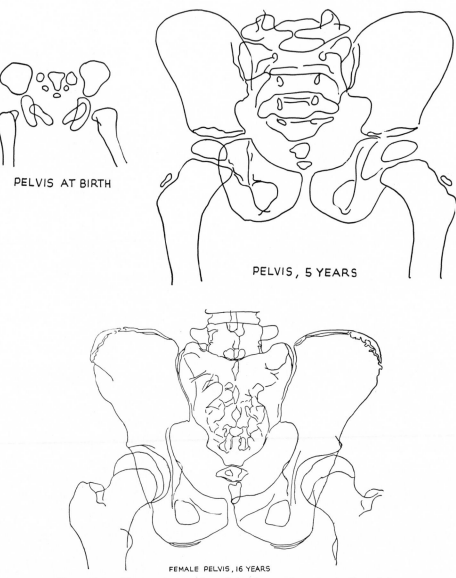

PELVIS AT BIRTH

PELVIS, 5 YEARS

FEMALE PELVIS, 16 YEARS

Figure 5–6. Changes in growth and development as seen in the pelvis.

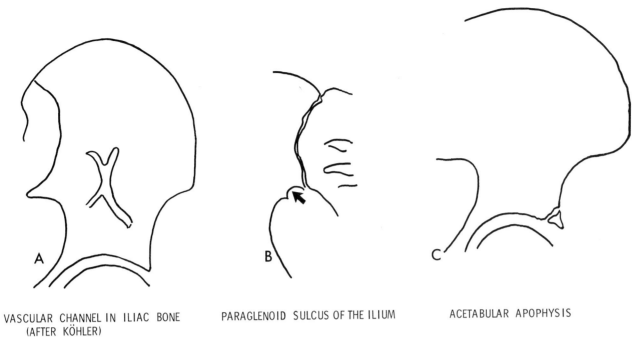

VASCULAR CHANNEL IN ILIAC BONE
(AFTER KÖHLER)

PARAGLENOID SULCUS OF THE ILIUM

ACETABULAR APOPHYSIS

Figure 5–7. Variations of the normal iliac bone.

pubis or pubic symphysis are shown in Figure 5–8. These include: (a) comma-shaped ossification centers and "inferior apophyseal centers" of the pubic symphysis, (b) symmetrical exostoses of the pubic bones which would appear to encroach upon the obturator foramina symmetrically, and (c) very prominent ischial pubic synchondroses.

The relationships of the acetabulum to the hip joint proper will be described more fully in connection with that joint.

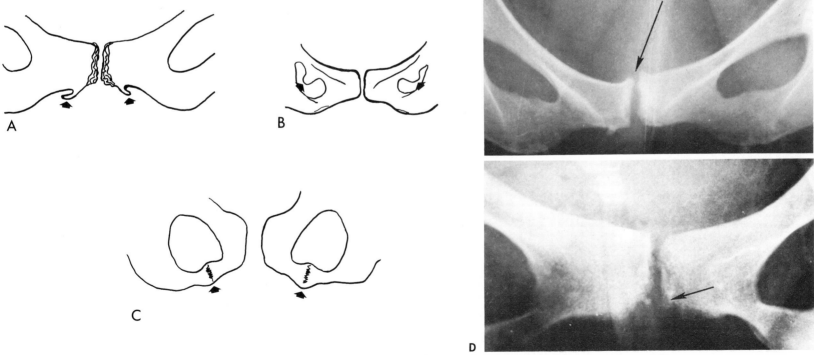

Figure 5–8. Variation of the normal pubis and pubic symphysis. A. Comma-shaped ossification centers and "inferior apophyseal centers" (pubic symphysis) (after Köhler). B. Symmetrical exostoses of the pubic bone (after Köhler). C. Ischial pubic synchondrosis. D. Irregularity of the pubic symphysis.

ROUTINE VIEWS OF THE PELVIS

1. **Anteroposterior View of the Pelvis** (Fig. 5–9).　A 14 × 17 inch cassette is placed crosswise to the table, and the central ray is directed perpendicular to a point about 1 inch superior to the pubic symphysis.

2. **Lateral View of the Pelvis** (Fig. 5–10).　The patient is turned on one side, and the central ray is directed over the highest part of the convexity at about the level of the second sacral segment. The thighs and knees are usually slightly flexed. The lumbar spine is supported with towels or any radiolucent material so that it is horizontal and parallel with respect to the table top. One tries to visualize the pubic symphysis, ischial spines, and tuberosities, as well as the entire sacrum and coccyx in this projection.

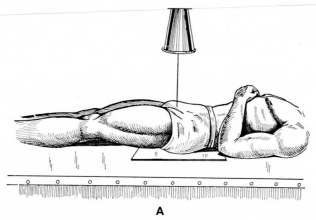

A

Figure 5–9.　Anteroposterior view of the pelvis. *A.* Method of positioning patient. *B.* Radiograph. *C.* Labeled tracing of *B.*

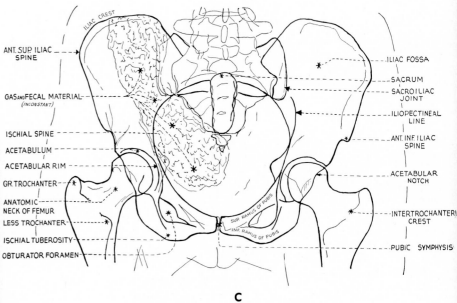

C

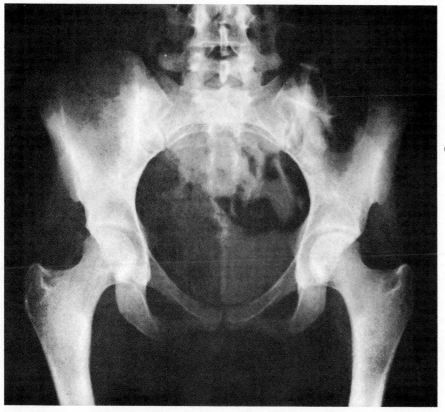

B

Points of Practical Interest with Reference to Figure 5–9

1. Center the patient to the median line of the table with the center of a 14 × 17 inch cassette placed crosswise 1½ inches above the superior margin of the pubic symphysis. This will place the upper border of the film above the iliac crest and the lower border of the film well below the lesser trochanters of the femurs.

2. In order to project the necks of the femurs in their full lengths it is well to invert the feet about 15 degrees and immobilize them with sandbags in this position.

3. The entire pelvis must be symmetrical. This may necessitate placing a folded sheet or balsa wood block under one side.

4. There are various special views for the ilium, the acetabulum, the anterior pelvic bones and the pubes which have not been included in this text. These special views need be employed only on rare occasions.

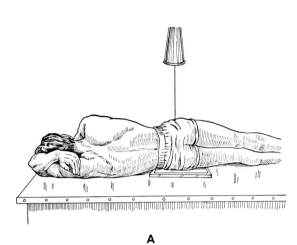

A

Figure 5–10. Lateral view of pelvis and lower lumbosacral spine. *A.* Method of positioning patient. *B.* Radiograph. *C.* Labeled tracing of *B.*

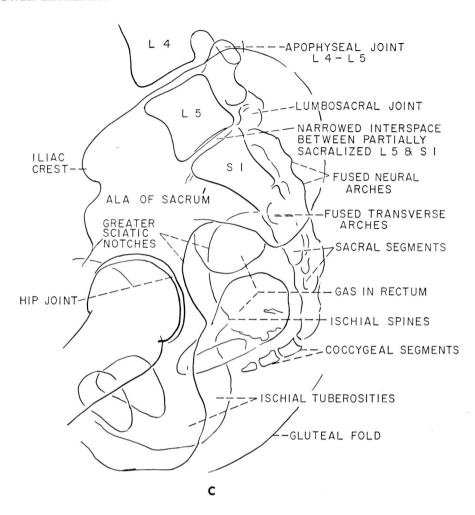

C

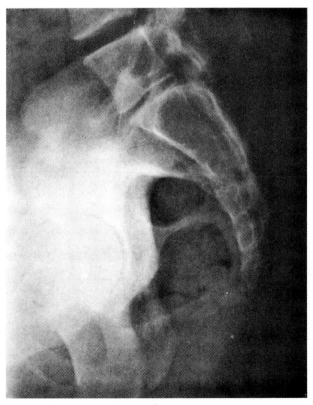

B

Points of Practical Interest with Reference to Figure 5–10

1. The patient is placed in the lateral position, either erect or recumbent, and the film is placed in the Potter-Bucky diaphragm. The knees and hips are slightly flexed to facilitate maintenance of position.
2. The gluteal cleft is placed parallel with the film.
3. Immobilization with a compression band is frequently very helpful. This is applied across the trochanteric region of the pelvis.
4. Center in the midaxillary plane over the depression between the iliac crest and the greater trochanter of the femur.
5. There should be almost perfect superposition of the ischial spines as well as the acetabula in this projection.

3. **Oblique View of the Sacroiliac Joints** (Fig. 5–11). The patient lies on his back with the side in question turned obliquely away from the table top at an angle of about 45 degrees, and the central ray is made to pass through the sacroiliac joint farthest from the film. The apophyseal joints which are closest to the film are shown in best relief, but the sacroiliac joint farthest from the film is the one shown in profile when the pelvis is placed obliquely with respect to the film.

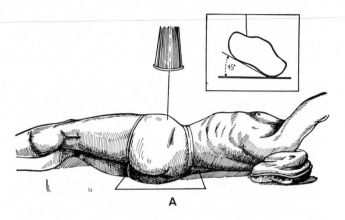

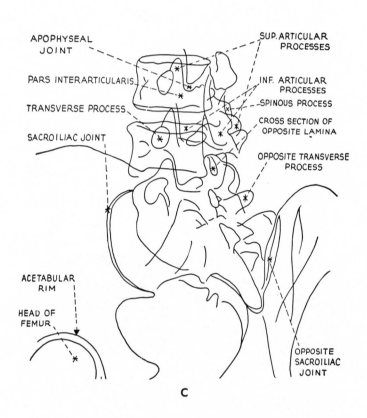

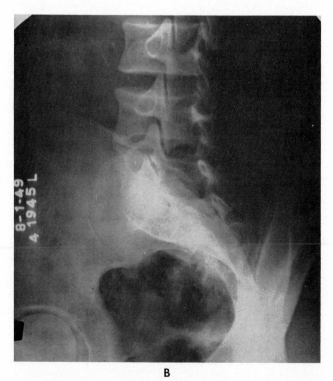

Figure 5–11. Oblique view of the sacroiliac joints and lower lumbar spine. *A.* Method of positioning patient. *B.* Radiograph. *C.* Labeled tracing of *B.*

Points of Practical Interest with Reference to Figure 5–11

1. Elevate the side being examined approximately 45 degrees and support the shoulder and the upper thigh on sandbags, making certain that the sandbags do not appear on the radiograph.
2. The sacroiliac joint that is farthest from the film will appear most clearly and it is this joint that is being examined. The two articular surfaces of the sacroiliac joint closest to the film are superimposed over one another, and hence this joint is not shown to best advantage.
3. A somewhat similar oblique view of the sacroiliac joints may be obtained in the posteroanterior projection by placing the patient obliquely prone instead of supine as noted above.
4. Oblique views of both sacroiliac joints are always obtained because one joint offers some comparison for analysis of the other.
5. The central ray may be angled 5 degrees cephalad. In some patients this improves visualization of the sacroiliac and lumbar apophyseal joints.

4. **Distorted View of the Sacrum** (Fig. 5–12).   In the straight anteroposterior projection of the pelvis, the lower segments of the sacrum and the coccyx are seen to underlie the pubic symphysis and thus are partially obscured. By tilting the tube about 15 degrees toward the head and flexing the thighs so that the sacrum is flat against the table, a somewhat distorted view of the sacrum is obtained, but it is completely visualized. The sacroiliac joints are also distorted, but are shown to good advantage in this projection. This view will also reveal to better advantage a possible articulation of the transverse process of the last lumbar vertebra with the superior surface of the wing of the sacrum or medial portion of the iliac crest. The special view of the pelvic inlet and views for pelvic mensuration are described in Chapter 17.

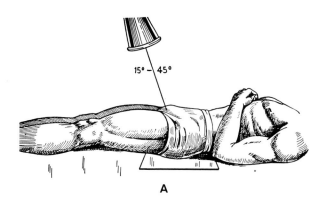

A

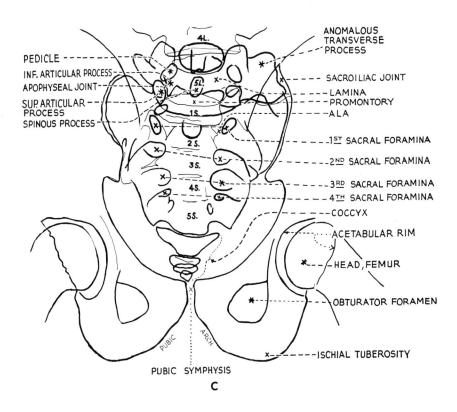

C

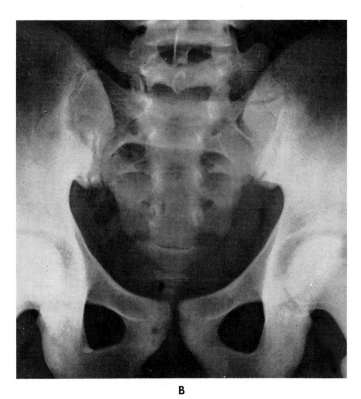

B

Figure 5–12.   Distorted view of sacrum. *A.* Method of positioning patient. *B.* Radiograph. *C.* Labeled tracing of *B.*

Points of Practical Interest with Reference to Figure 5–12

1. For more marked distortion, angulation of the tube up to 45 degrees cephalad may be employed.
2. The central ray is adjusted so that it enters the body just above the pubic symphysis and leaves the body at approximately the upper margin of the sacrum or at the level of the fifth lumbar segment. Care is exercised to center the x-ray film to the central ray of the x-ray tube, otherwise the anatomic structures depicted here will not appear on the film.
3. This view is particularly valuable for demonstrating sacralization of the last lumbar transverse processes as shown in the accompanying diagram. Defects in the neural arch of the fifth lumbar vertebra also appear to advantage in this view.

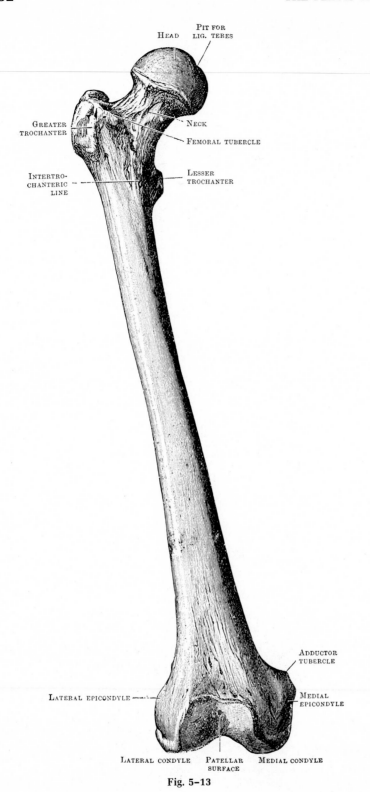

Fig. 5-13

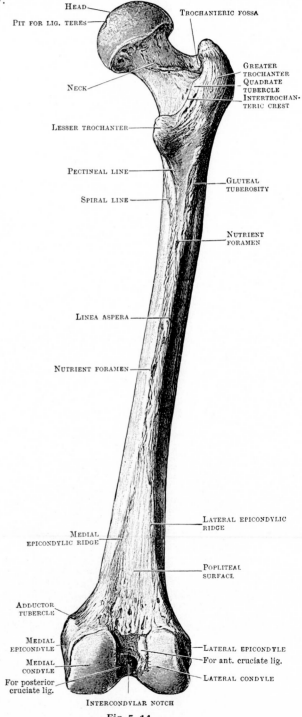

THE THIGH

Correlated Gross Anatomy.   As in the case of the upper extremity, our main radiographic interest concerns the bony structure, although the supportive soft tissues are always studied with equal thoroughness. The femur (Figs. 5–13, 5–14), or thigh bone, is the largest and longest bone in the skeleton, and supports the entire weight of the skeleton between the legs (the locomotor organs) and the pelvis. It curves somewhat medially and posteriorly.

Figure 5–13.   Femur, anterior aspect. (From Cunningham's Textbook of Anatomy, 6th ed. London, Oxford University Press, 1931.)

Figure 5–14.   Femur, posterior aspect. (From Cunningham's Textbook of Anatomy, 6th ed. London, Oxford University Press, 1931.)

Fig. 5-14

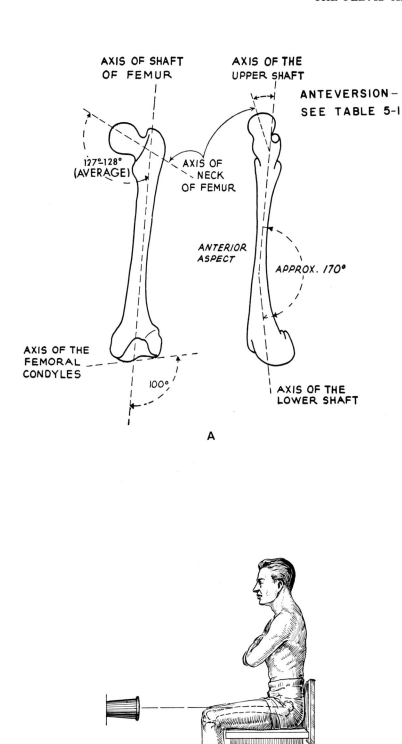

A

B

The head of the femur is a smooth, hemispherical structure which articulates with the acetabulum and contains a small depression a little behind and below its center called the fovea centralis, for the ligamentum teres. The neck of the femur is mounted at an angle with respect to its shaft in two planes (Fig. 5–15):

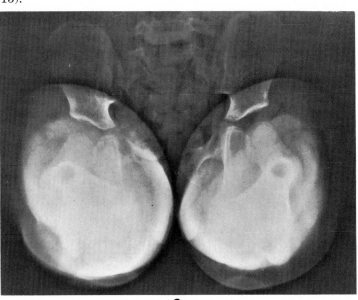

C

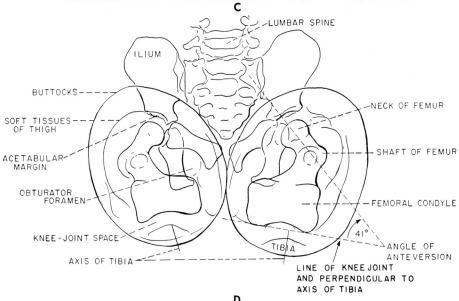

D

Figure 5–15. *A.* Axial relationships of the shaft of the femur (angles are approximations and are not invariable. See text). *B.* Position of patient in a special view designed to measure the degree of anteversion of the neck of the femur with respect to the shaft. Note that the central ray strikes the middle of the shaft of the femur and not the knee joint proper. As noted in *A,* the shaft of the femur arches posteriorly. It is the *proximal* half of the femoral shaft that is horizontal; actually, the distal half of the femur dips downward toward the floor slightly. It is this expedient that permits a diagnostic film to be obtained using lumbosacral spine technical factors. Otherwise, detail procured will be inadequate for measurement. *C.* The film so obtained (intensified). The detail is poor, but adequate to draw the angle of anteversion as indicated in *D. D.* Tracing of *C.* One line is drawn along the inferior margins of the femoral condyles; the other is drawn through the axis of the neck of the femur. The angle between may then be measured.

(a) The mediolateral angle which the neck forms with the shaft of the femur measures about 160 degrees at birth; in the adult, it varies between 110 and 140 degrees (127 degrees on the average).

(b) The neck is anteverted with respect to the shaft, which likewise varies with the age of the individual as indicated in Table 5–1. This angle may measure as much as 50 degrees at birth, and diminishes to about 8 degrees in the adult. A method of measuring this angle for clinical application is important, and is shown in Figure 5–15 *B, C, D*. The diagnosis of anteversion of the hip in the growing child must be made with considerable caution and parallels the diagnosis of congenital dislocation of the hip on the basis of the angle for measuring the shelving portion of the acetabulum (alpha angle for acetabular dysplasia, Fig. 5–26).

The neck of the femur is demarcated from the shaft by a ridge called the intertrochanteric line. This line furnishes the attachment anteriorly for the capsule of the hip joint (Fig. 5–23). The posterior surface of the neck of the femur tends to be concave, and only its medial two-thirds is enclosed within the joint cavity. The superior border of the neck is perforated by large nutrient foramina, although much of the bony nutrition also comes from the capsular attachment. The greater and lesser trochanters form the projections at the extremities of the intertrochanteric line.

The anteversion and the usual elements in radiography causing distortion and magnification (see Chapter 1) make it difficult for the orthopedic surgeon to anticipate the true length of the neck of the femur for purposes of choosing an appropriate nailing and fixation device for repair of a fracture of the neck of the femur. A method of measurement of the neck of the femur to overcome this difficulty has been devised (van Brunt), but is considered outside the scope of this text.

The shaft of the femur is rather cylindrical but a rough longitudinal ridge in its middle third posteriorly spreads out distally to enclose the popliteal surface of the bone. The lateral ridge terminates in the lateral epicondyle, whereas the medial ridge ends in

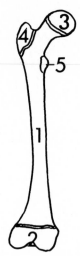

Figure 5–16. Ossification centers of the femur. *1*, Diaphysis; *2*, distal epiphysis; *3*, head; *4*, greater trochanter; *5*, lesser trochanter.

the adductor tubercle just above the medial epicondyle. The nutrient foramen is situated on the posteromedial aspect of the shaft of the femur at the junction of its middle and distal one-thirds, and is directed toward the hip.

The intercondyloid fossa separates the two articular condyles posteriorly, but they are continuous in front, forming a smooth trochlear surface for articulation with the patella. In the lateral projection, each condyle appears to consist of a fusion of the segments of two spheres, giving the condyles a "figure 3" appearance (or reverse "3" for the left femur). The medial condyle is more prominent, thinner, and longer than its lateral fellow, which compensates for the obliquity of the femur.

Changes with Growth and Development. The femur is ossified from five centers (Fig. 5–16): one for the body, one for the head, one for each trochanter, and one for the entire lower condylar portion. At birth, the main body of the femur is ossified, and usually the epiphysis of the distal end is also just beginning to ossify; this is one of the most reliable indicators that the fetus is full term (see Chapter 17). Ossification extends into the neck of the femur after birth. The epiphysis of the head of the femur begins to ossify between 6 months and 1 year of age approximately (see Chapter 3). The epiphysis of the greater trochanter appears later, at 4 or 5 years of age, and that of the lesser trochanter at 9 or 11. All of these secondary epiphyses fuse late in adolescence, earlier in the female than in the male (Fig. 5–17). See also Chapter 3.

TABLE 5–1   NORMAL DEGREES OF ANTEVERSION OF THE FEMORAL NECK*

Age (years)	Anteversion (in degrees)
Birth to 1	30–50
2	30
3–5	25
6–12	20
12–15	17
16–20	11
Over 20	8

*Adapted from Billing, L.: Roentgen examination of proximal femur end in children and adolescents. Acta Radiol. (Suppl.), *110*:1–80, 1954; and Budin, E., and Chandler, E.: Measurement of femoral neck anteversion by a direct method. Radiology, *69*:209–213, 1951.

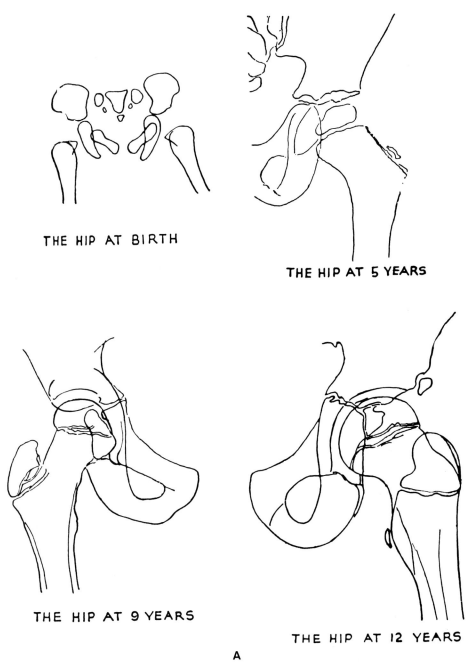

THE HIP AT BIRTH

THE HIP AT 5 YEARS

THE HIP AT 9 YEARS

THE HIP AT 12 YEARS

A

Figure 5–17. A. Changes in growth and development as seen in the hip.

Figure 5–17 continued on following page.

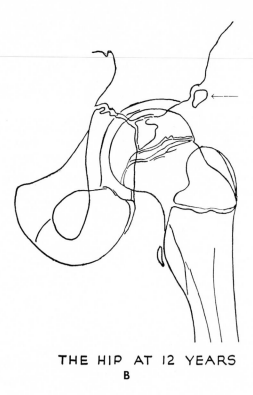

THE HIP AT 12 YEARS
B

Figure 5–17 *Continued.* B. Tracing of radiograph showing the numerous superimposed lines caused by un-united ossification centers. C. Lucencies often found in the neck of the femur. These must be interpreted with great care since they may represent variations of normal. D. Soft tissue structures around the hip joint actually represent the fatty encasement of the gluteal muscles but are often interpreted as the "hip joint capsule." The arrow points to the ilial pectineal line on the inner aspect of the acetabulum. This is often called the obturator fascia. The secondary epiphysis of the ischial tuberosity is also shown (*straight line*). E. Epiphysis of the iliac crest not yet fused to the remainder of the body of the iliac crest.

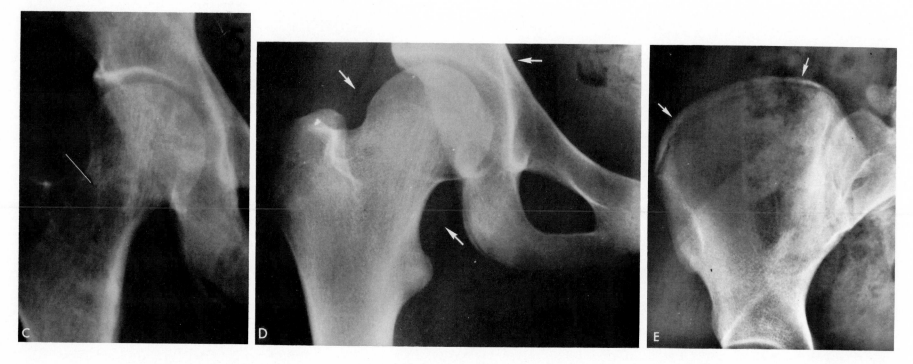

Figure 5–17 continued on opposite page.

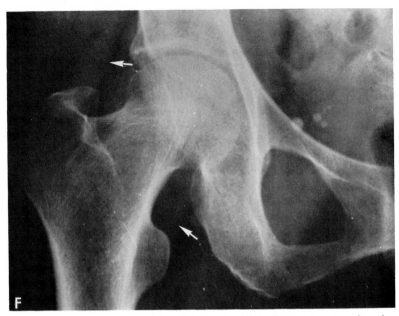

Figure 5–17 *Continued.*   F. Further illustration of the soft tissues surrounding the hip, often referred to as the hip joint capsule.

Axial Relationships of the Shaft of the Femur (Figs. 5–15, 5–18)

1. The axis of the shaft of the femur forms an angle with the axis of the neck of the femur which ranges from 110 to 140 degrees, with an average of 127 degrees for both sexes (Keats et al.).

2. A line drawn along the upper margin of the neck of the femur, as indicated in Figure 5–18, transects the ossified femoral head in both the anteroposterior and lateral projections. This alignment becomes significant in detecting a slipped epiphysis of the head of the femur.

3. A line drawn tangent to the external surfaces of the condyles of the femur and tibia (lines EF and GH, Fig. 5–19) is per-

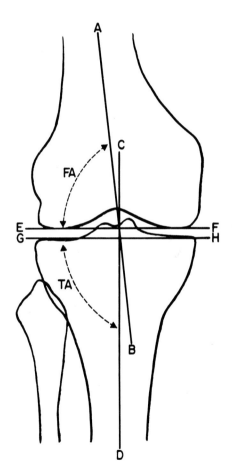

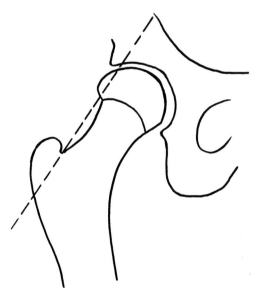

Figure 5–18.   Line along the outer margin of the neck of the femur demonstrating the proper relationship of the head of the femur to the neck. This line should intersect the head in both the anteroposterior and lateral views.

	FA	*TA*
Male	75° — 85°	85° — 100°
Female	75° — 85°	87° — 98°
Average	81°	93°

Figure 5–19.   Axial relationships of the knee joint. (From Atlas of Roentgenographic Measurement, 3d ed., by Lusted, L. B., and Keats, T. E. Copyright © 1972 by Year Book Medical Publishers, Inc., Chicago. Used by permission.)

BLOOD SUPPLY OF THE FEMORAL CAPITAL EPIPHYSIS AND NECK OF THE FEMUR IN CHILDHOOD

BLOOD SUPPLY OF THE FEMORAL HEAD

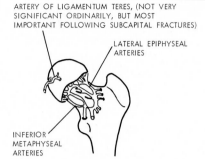

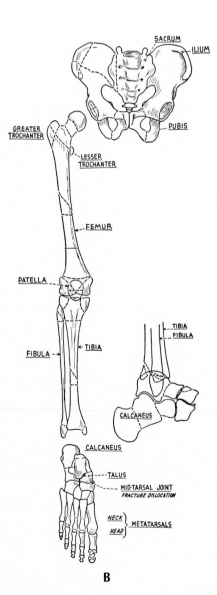

Figure 5–20. *A.* Blood supply of the head and neck of the femur. *B.* The most common sites of fractures of the pelvis and lower extremity.

pendicular to the axis of the shaft of the tibia (line CD) but forms an angle with the axis of the shaft of the femur (line AB). This angulation of the femur with the knee joint produces a slight genu valgum deformity, which is normal. The angle FA averages 81 degrees and is similar in both male and female, whereas the angle for the axis of the shaft of the tibia with the knee joint approximates the perpendicular and averages 93 degrees, ranging from 85 to 100 degrees in the male and 87 to 98 degrees in the female.

4. There is a slight anterior bowing of the shaft of the femur, the axis of the upper two-thirds forming an angle of approximately 170 degrees with the axis of the lower one-third; this latter axis is continuous with that of the leg in the extended position.

5. The axis of the neck of the femur in the true lateral perspective forms an angle with the axis of the upper shaft of the femur ranging from 8 to 50 degrees. Table 5–1 lists the degrees of anteversion showing regression with age.

Blood Supply to the Head of the Femur and Acetabulum. The head of the femur receives *three sets* of arteries: (a) arteries which ascend on the *synovium* on the posterosuperior and posteroinferior parts of the neck to perforate just distal to the head, (b) terminal branches of the *medullary artery* of the shaft, and (c) the *artery of the ligament of the head.* This latter artery enters the head when the center of ossification has extended to the small pit, or ligament, of the head at about the twelfth to the fourteenth year (Grant).

The *acetabular blood vessels,* consisting of an artery and veins, represent branches of the posterior division of the obturator artery and vein and pass through the acetabular foramen, entering the acetabular fossa and ramifying in the fatty areolar tissue therein. A branch from this passes through the ligament of the head of the femur to the head proper. This is partially represented in Figure 5–20. It is thus apparent that the head and neck of the femur have a blood supply highly dependent upon the synovial retinacula, the terminal branches of the medullary artery of the shaft, and a relatively filamentous artery passing through the ligamentum teres. This arrangement presents potential difficulty in the event of injury to this weight-supporting structure.

The Fabella.   The fabella is a frequent sesamoid bone situated in the lateral head of the gastrocnemius muscle, and is projected on the posterior aspect of the lateral femoral condyle (Fig. 5–39). Its usual measurement is about 8 mm. in diameter, and it tends to be spherical in shape.

RADIOGRAPHIC EXAMINATION OF THE THIGH

1. **Routine Anteroposterior View of the Femur** (Fig. 5–21). The patient lies flat on his back, with the film beneath his thigh. The central ray passes through a point just below the midsection of the thigh, and the knee joint (or hip joint) is always included.

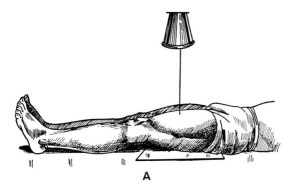

A

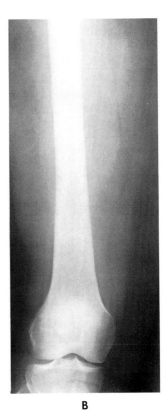

B

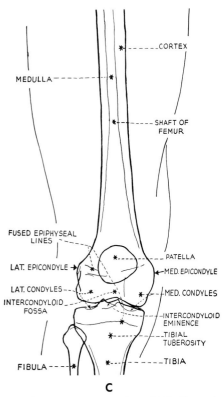

C

Figure 5–21. Routine anteroposterior view of the femur. *A.* Method of positioning patient. *B.* Radiograph. *C.* Labeled tracing of *B.*

2. **Routine Lateral View of the Thigh** (Fig. 5–22). The patient lies on the affected side and the knee is slightly flexed. The opposite thigh is placed so that it will not interfere with the projection. The thigh is placed perpendicular to the film and the central ray passes through a point just distal to the midsection of the thigh. The knee joint is included in this view.

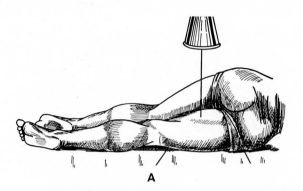

A

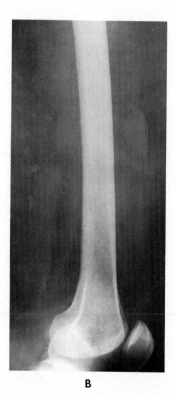

B

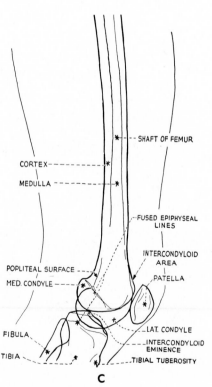

C

Figure 5–22. Routine lateral view of the thigh. *A.* Method of positioning patient. *B.* Radiograph. *C.* Labeled tracing of *B.*

THE HIP JOINT

Correlated Gross Anatomy. The *hip joint capsule* is composed largely of the ileofemoral ligament, which is shaped like an inverted Y attached to the intertrochanteric line anteriorly and deep to the rectus femoris superiorly, and the ischial femoral ligament directed spirally on the posterior aspect of the hip joint. The muscles surrounding the hip joint capsule assist materially in support of this important weight-bearing joint. The radiographic depiction of the "joint capsule" is largely related to the fatty and bursal sheath which encompasses and adjoins these muscles.

The line of attachment of the hip joint capsule is illustrated in Figure 5–23, the capsule being attached anteriorly at the intertrochanteric line and posteriorly at the junction of the middle and distal thirds of the neck of the femur. The joint capsule and surrounding muscles are usually readily identified in radiographs (Fig. 5–17 *D* and *E*) and are of considerable importance because they may be the only manifestation of early hip joint disease.

The bursal structures surrounding the hip joint are also important. As in the case of the shoulder, these are subject to deposits of calcium and inflammation. There may be four or more bursae adjoining the greater trochanter and one adjoining the ischial tuberosity, and some may be larger than others.

There is frequently a small extra ossicle adjoining the superior lip of the acetabulum called an *apophysis* (Fig. 5–17 *B*). This may not be symmetrical on the two sides and must be carefully differentiated from a fracture. This ossicle forms part of the shelving portion of the acetabulum.

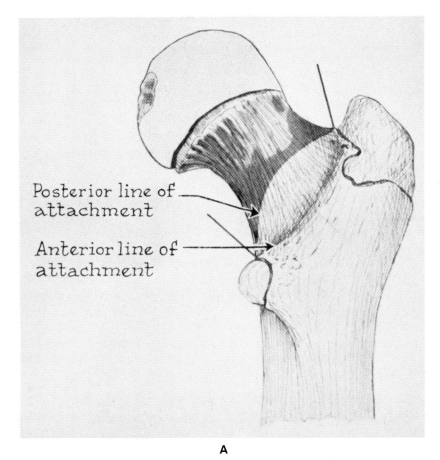

Posterior line of attachment

Anterior line of attachment

A

Figure 5–23. A. The line of attachment of the capsule of the hip joint. (Modified from Perry, in Morris *Human Anatomy*, The Blakiston Co., Publishers.)

Figure 5–23 continued on following page.

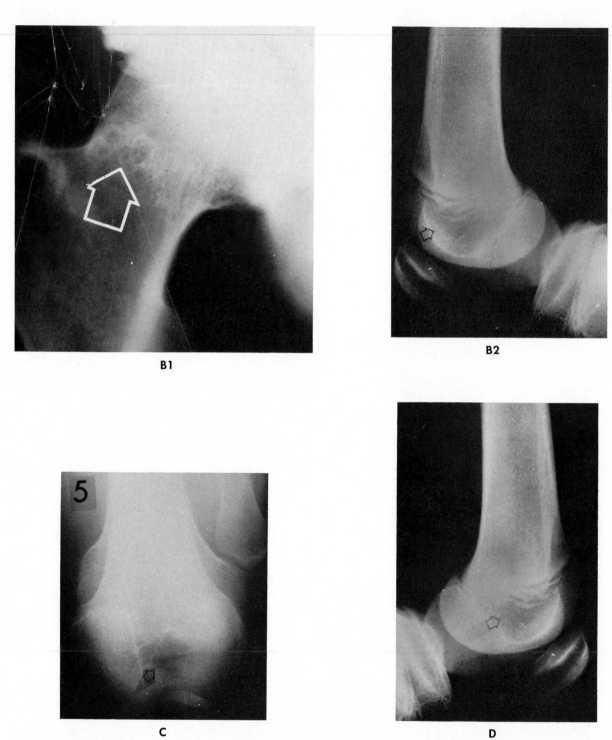

Figure 5–23 *Continued.*   *B* and *C.* Intertubercular lucency often visualized in the proximal (B1) and distal femur in the anteroposterior and lateral views. *D.* Further illustration of the kind of lucency normally seen in the distal femoral condyles, particularly before the distal epiphysis fuses with the main shaft of the femur.

Figure 5–23 continued on opposite page.

Axial Relationships of the Hip (Fig. 5–24). Some of the more useful axial and angular relationships of the hip joint region which assist in the evaluation of the hip joint from a functional point of view are as follows:

1. The angle formed by the axis of the neck of the femur with the axis of the shaft of the femur averages 127 degrees.

2. A horizontal line drawn perpendicular to the axis of the shaft of the femur through the uppermost margin of the greater trochanter should pass through or below the fovea centralis of the head of the femur (Skinner's line).

3. The inferior margin of the neck of the femur forms a continuous arc with the superior and medial margin of the obturator foramen (Shenton's line).

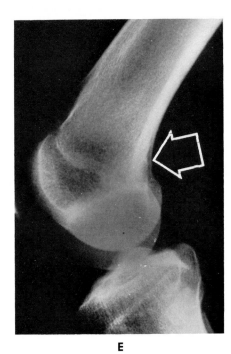

E

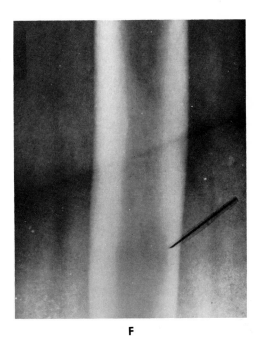

F

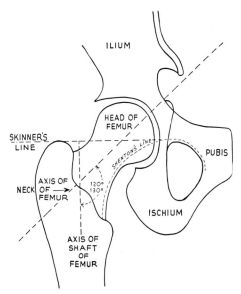

Figure 5–24. Axial relationships of the hip joint.

Figure 5–23 *Continued.*   E. Irregularity and sclerosis of the distal diaphysis of the femur on its posterior aspect, a normal variant. F. The endosteal trabecular pattern of the distal femoral shaft and midfemoral shaft. Notice the tendency for endosteal thickening in the midshaft region and the slight irregularity of the thickness of the sclerotic portion of the bone.

4. Lines indicating the slope of the iliac portions of the innominate bone as well as the shelving portion of the acetabulum are shown in Figure 5–25. These are the acetabular angle and the iliac angle respectively. The range of normal values for these angles is indicated for infants who are less than 3 months of age, and those 3 to 12 months of age. The acetabular angles have a wide range of normal in infants in the former category, but in those 3 to 12 months of age the acetabular angle should not exceed 34 degrees. Likewise, the iliac angle in these infants should not exceed 101 degrees.

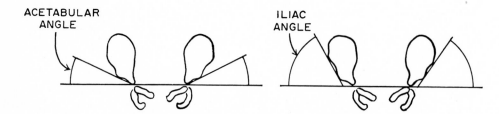

Category	Mean Acetabular Angle	SD	± 2 SD	Actual Range
Young normal infants less than 3 months of age	28°	4.7	37–18	44–12
Normal infants 3–12 months of age	22°	4.2	30–14	34–8
	Mean Iliac Angle			
Less than 3 months	81°	8.0	97–65	97–68
3–12 months	79°	9.0	96–60	101–62

A

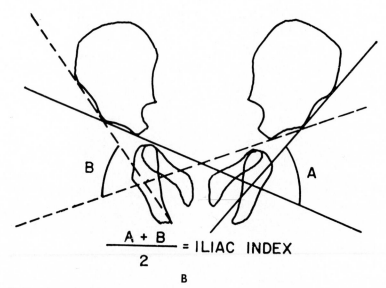

$$\frac{A + B}{2} = \text{ILIAC INDEX}$$

B

Figure 5–25. A. Acetabular and iliac angles. B. Tong's method for measuring the iliac index.

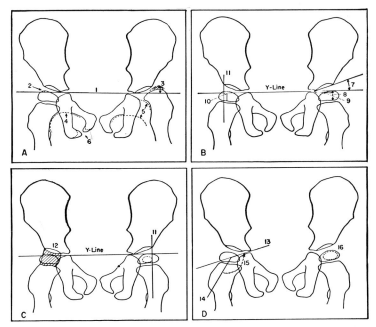

Figure 5-26. Criteria for congenital dislocation of hip. *1*, Y-symphyseal line. *2* and *3.* Normally are equal. *4,* Shenton's line unbroken—normal. *5,* Shenton's line broken—indicates dislocation or fracture. *6,* Fusion delayed, with dislocation. *7,* Not greater than 34 degrees in newborn normally; not greater than 25 degrees after 1 year. *8,* Not less than 6 mm. normally. *9,* Less than 16 mm. normally. *10,* Less than one-half of epiphyseal width normally. *11,* Should cross epiphysis lateral to center normally. *12,* Right angled cylinder normally. *13,* Line: center of acetabulum to center of head. *14,* Axis of neck of femur. *15,* Angle 120 degrees normally. (Modified from Köhler, A., and Zimmer, E. A.: Borderlands of the Normal and Early Pathologic in Skeletal Roentgenology. New York, Grune and Stratton, 1956.)

Other criteria for congenital dislocation of the hip are indicated in Figure 5-26.

5. Since the various measurements given in Figure 5-26 are fraught with some latitude and uncertainty, Andren and von Rosen have worked out a simple method for demonstrating congenital dislocation of the hip in newborns, by keeping the hips dislocated during the x-ray exposure. This is accomplished by forcible abduction, *to at least 45 degrees, with appreciable inward rotation of the femora* (Fig. 5-27). If the hip is normal, the line of femoral shaft will be directed toward the upper edge of the bony acetabular wall, but in the presence of congenital dislocation of the hip, it will point to the anterior superior iliac spine. It should be stressed that the abduction must be at least 45 degrees, or the results will be misleading. Also, owing to the marked anteversion of the femoral necks of the newborn (Table 5-1), a fair degree of inward rotation of the femora is necessary.

6. Klein et al. have described the roentgenographic features of a slipped capital femoral epiphysis in some detail and have proposed the lining technique illustrated in Figure 5-28. The technique consists of the following: the anteroposterior and lateral views of both hips are obtained simultaneously on one film for each view using the straight AP view and frog-leg AP views as illustrated in Figure 5-9 and Figure 5-33. The centering point is about 1½ inches above the pubic symphysis. A line is drawn along the superior margin of the neck of the femur on each hip region. Normally this line transects the head of the femur on both views. When this is not present slipping may be diagnosed and measured, particularly if there is one normal hip on the opposite side.

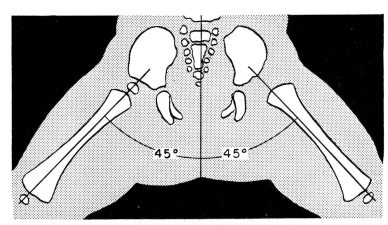

Figure 5-27. Tracing of roentgenograms (postmortem) of newborn with femur abducted and rotated inwards. *Right side,* Normal hip, femoral shaft directed toward edge of acetabular wall. *Left side.* Dislocation, femoral shaft directed toward anterior superior iliac spine. (Ortolani's "clock" could be elicited on this side but not on the right.) (Modified from Andren, L., and Von Rosen, S.: Acta Radiol., 49(2):89-95, 1958.)

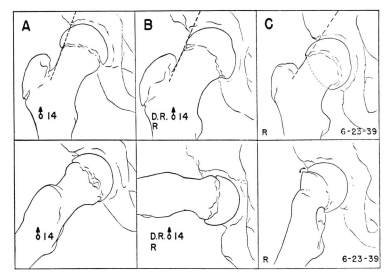

Figure 5-28. Medial and posterior slipping. *A.* Normal hip for comparison. *B.* Medial slipping. In this case slipping is detectable only in the anteroposterior view where the head is not transected by the prolongation of the superior neck line. *C.* Posterior slipping. In the anteroposterior view the posteriorly displaced head is projected through the proximal portion of the neck. In the lateral view the amount of posterior slipping is denoted by the curved arrow. (From Klein, A., et al.: Amer. J. Roentgenol., 66, 1951.)

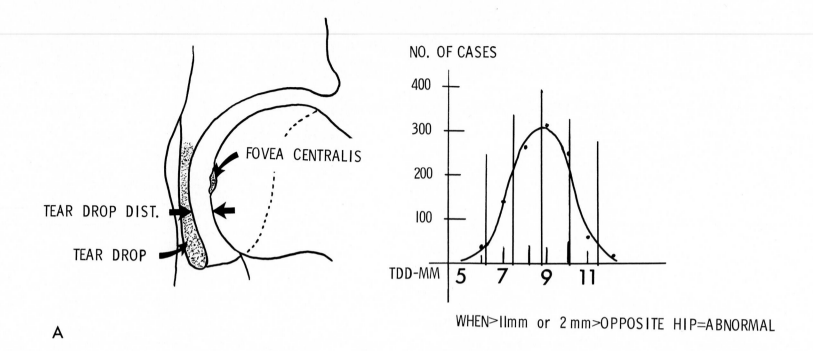

A

NO. OF CASES

WHEN>11mm or 2mm>OPPOSITE HIP=ABNORMAL

ANGLE OF ANTEVERSION

ANGLE OF INCLINATION

B

Figure 5–29. A. Line diagram showing the tear drop distance and the distribution of normal tear drop distances as measured in a large series of normal hips. Note that when the tear drop distance is greater than 11 mm. or when it is 2 mm. greater on one side than on the opposite side, the hip joint may be considered abnormal. This sign is one of the early indicators of osteochondrosis of the hip. (After Eyring, E. J., Bjornson, D. R., and Peterson, C. A.: Amer. J. Roentgenol., *104*:851, 1968.) *B.* Diagrams illustrating methods of measurement of "angle of inclination" and "angle of anteversion" of head and neck of femur.

7. The axial relationships of the neck of the femur to the shaft in regard to anteversion have already been described and do not deserve further attention here (Fig. 5–15, *B, C, D*).

8. The pelvic tear drop distance, when measured in over 1000 normal hips of persons from 1 to 11 years of age, is distributed as shown in Figure 5–29. It may therefore be postulated, when this distance is greater than 11 mm., or when one side differs by more than 2 mm. in comparison with the other side, that the hip joint is abnormal. In the original investigation of Eyring, this method was utilized for detection of early Calvé-Legg-Perthes' disease.

9. Another indicator of joint disease in the growing hip is shown in Figure 5–30. The posterior lip of the acetabulum ordinarily overlaps the shadow of the head of the femur on both sides. In well-exposed and symmetrically positioned film studies of the hips the two sides should appear symmetrical. Likewise, the tear drop appearances should be symmetrical and the tear drop distance should not vary by more than 2 mm. on the two sides.

The triangle A, B, and C may be compared on each of the two sides and these likewise must appear symmetrical.

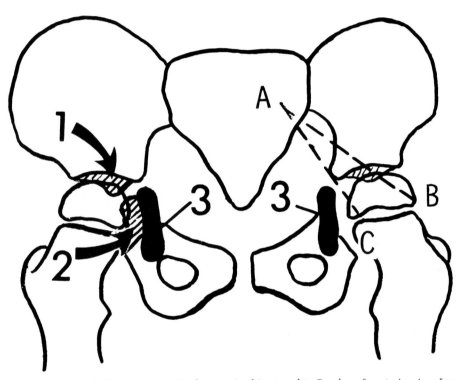

Figure 5–30. Areas to study for asymmetry in the growing hip. *1* and *2*, Overlap of posterior rim of acetabulum; *3*, Tear drops are symmetrical. *A* to *C*, The heads of the femurs appear symmetrical when a triangle is drawn as shown. (After Martin, H. E.: Radiology, 56:842, 1951.)

RADIOGRAPHIC METHODS OF EXAMINATION OF THE HIP JOINT

1. **Routine Anteroposterior View of the Hip** (Fig. 5–31). The patient is placed flat on his back with the *toe of his foot pointing somewhat to the median plane.* This latter measure is necessary so that the neck of the femur is not foreshortened. The central ray passes through a point 1 inch below the center of the inguinal ligament.

2. **Routine Lateral View of the Hip Employing a Horizontal X-ray Beam** (Fig. 5–32). This view may be obtained in either of two ways: the central ray may be directed from the medial aspect of the thigh, or from the lateral aspect of the hip. It is usually ad-

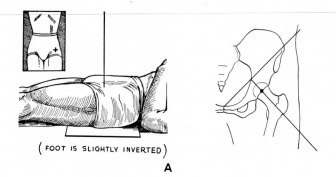

(FOOT IS SLIGHTLY INVERTED)

A

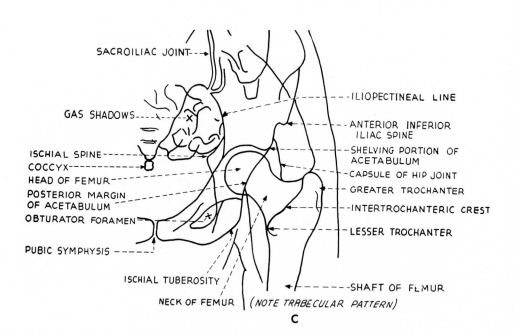

C

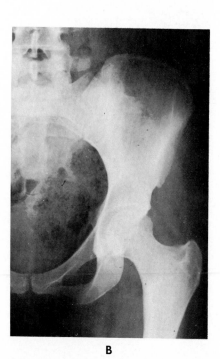

B

Figure 5–31. Routine anteroposterior view of hip. *A.* Method of positioning patient. *B.* Radiograph. *C.* Labeled tracing of *B.*

Points of Practical Interest with Reference to Figure 5–31

1. The patient is placed in a perfectly supine position. The entire pelvis must be symmetrical even when only one side is to be considered.
2. For maximum elongation and detail with regard to the femoral neck the foot is inverted approximately 15 degrees and immobilized by means of a small sandbag in that position.
3. A line is drawn between the anterior-superior iliac spine and the superior margin of the pubic symphysis. The centering point is a point 1 inch distal to the midpoint of this line. This point will ordinarily fall immediately over the hip joint proper.
4. If the foot is everted instead of inverted the lesser trochanter will be shown in maximum detail and the neck of the femur will be completely foreshortened.
5. For maximum detail with regard to both the greater and the lesser trochanter the foot should point directly upward and remain perpendicular to the table top at time the film is obtained.

visable to mark the probable position of the neck of the femur on the patient before proceeding. The central ray is made to pass as nearly perpendicular to this line and central to it as possible. If the medial position of the tube is employed, the film is placed perpendicular to the table top and parallel with the neck of the femur, if possible. A close film-target distance must usually be employed in view of the fact that this part of the body is so thick. Actually, a longer film-target distance in this instance would be more desirable from the standpoint of eliminating as much distortion and magnification as possible. If the central ray is directed from the lateral aspect of the thigh, usually a curved cassette is required in the groin. In this projection, it is important to visualize the entire acetabulum along with the ischial tuberosity and neck of the femur. The pubic symphysis is frequently seen also.

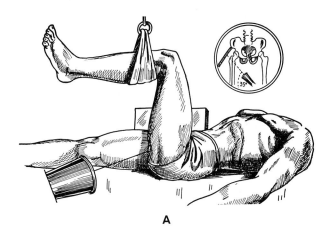

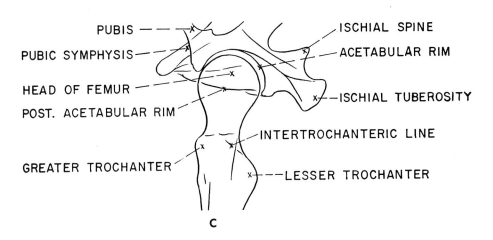

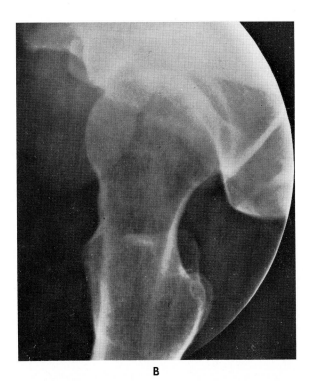

Figure 5–32. Routine lateral view of the hip, employing a horizontal x-ray beam. *A.* Method of positioning patient. *B.* Radiograph. *C.* Labeled tracing of *B.*

Points of Practical Interest with Reference to Figure 5–32

1. The patient is placed in a supine position and the pelvis is elevated sufficiently on a firm pillow or folded sheets to raise the ischial tuberosity approximately 3 cm. from the table top. This support of the gluteus must not extend beyond the lateral margin of the body so that it will not interfere with the placement of the cassette directly on the table top.
2. To localize the long axis of the femoral neck: (a) Draw a line between the anterior-superior iliac spine and the upper border of the pubic symphysis and mark its center point. (b) Next draw a line approximately 4 inches long perpendicular to this midpoint, extending down to the anterior surface of the thigh. This latter line represents the long axis of the femoral neck.
3. Adjust the central ray so that it is perpendicular to the midpoint of this long axis; adjust the film perpendicular to the table top so that the projection of this long axis will fall entirely upon the film.
4. If the foot is maintained in a vertical position the anteversion of the neck of the femur with respect to the shaft will be demonstrated. If the foot of the affected side is inverted approximately 15 degrees the plane of the neck will be parallel with the film and will form a straight line with the axis of the shaft of the femur.
5. The unaffected side may be supported over the x-ray tube or by a sling from above as shown.
6. The thickness of the part traversed by the central ray is comparable to that of a lateral lumbar spine, and the same technical factors used in a lateral lumbar spine film should ordinarily be employed.
7. A grid cassette is a very desirable adjunct for this projection.

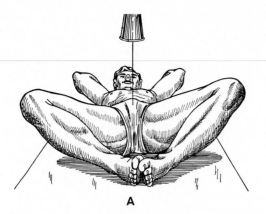

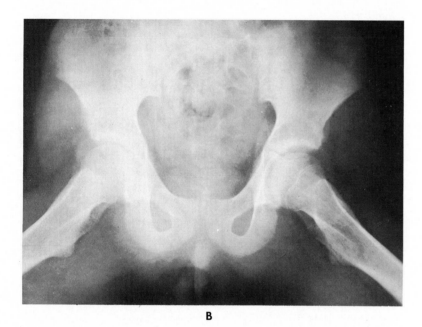

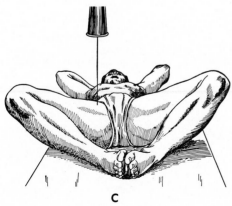

Figure 5–33. Lateral view of both hips, employing the "frog-leg" position. *A.* Method of positioning patient. *B.* Radiograph. *C.* Lateral view of one hip, employing the "frog-leg" position. Method of positioning patient. *D.* Radiograph.

3. **Lateral View of the Hip Employing the Frog-leg Position** (Fig. 5–33). The patient lies flat on his back and places the heel of the affected side on the opposite knee, everting the thigh so that it lies as nearly flat on the table top as possible. Alternatively, he may place both thighs in this position and allow the soles of both feet to touch one another. The central ray passes through a point about 1 inch below the center of the inguinal ligament. When views of both hips are obtained simultaneously in this projection, the central ray passes through the pubic symphysis.

4. **Hip Arthrography with Opaque Contrast Media** (Barnett and Arcomano; Laage et al.). Methylglucamine diatrizoate in 20 per cent solution has been employed for definition of the following anatomic detail: the limbus of the joint; the thickness of the ligamentum teres; the fixation of the capsule to the ilium; the relationship of the uncalcified femoral head to the uncalcified limbus in children; the presence or absence of complete or partial dislocation, especially in children; and the degree of "hour-glassing" of the capsule.

This procedure is performed in selected cases, particularly prior to surgery. A needle is inserted anteriorly into the hip joint, usually just beneath the head of the femur, and 5 to 10 ml. of the methylglucamine diatrizoate solution are injected under fluoroscopic control. Appropriate films are obtained after moving the hip about for approximately 1 minute. Ideally, the films should be obtained with a 0.6 mm. focal spot, either by spot-film fluoroscopic techniques or by vertical x-ray beam and Bucky grid.

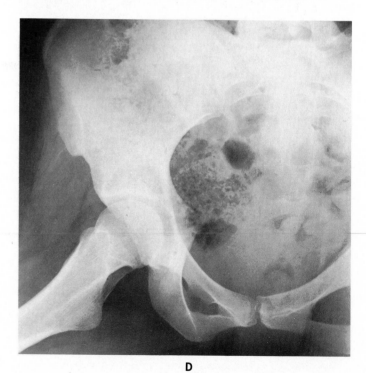

Figure 5–33 continued on opposite page.

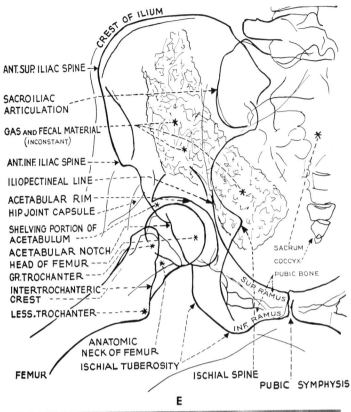

CREST OF ILIUM

ANT. SUP. ILIAC SPINE

SACRO ILIAC
ARTICULATION

GAS AND FECAL MATERIAL
(INCONSTANT)

ANT. INF. ILIAC SPINE

ILIOPECTINEAL LINE

ACETABULAR RIM
HIP JOINT CAPSULE

SHELVING PORTION OF
ACETABULUM

ACETABULAR NOTCH
HEAD OF FEMUR
GR. TROCHANTER
INTERTROCHANTERIC
CREST

LESS. TROCHANTER

ANATOMIC
NECK OF FEMUR
ISCHIAL TUBEROSITY

FEMUR

ISCHIAL SPINE

PUBIC SYMPHYSIS

SACRUM
COCCYX
PUBIC BONE
SUP. RAMUS
INF. RAMUS

E

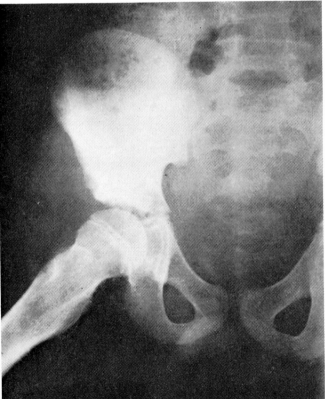

F

Points of Practical Interest with Reference to Figure 5–33

1. The "frog-leg" lateral view of the hip is actually a useful but imperfect lateral perspective of the head, neck, and upper shaft of the femur. The acetabulum remains in an anteroposterior relationship, and the normal anteversion of the neck of the femur with respect to the shaft is not shown. Moreover, this technique cannot be employed after most injuries when the hip joint motion is very limited and painful. Nevertheless, it is particularly useful in analysis of suspected hip abnormalities in children, and in other circumstances when acetabular lateral perspectives are unnecessary. Technically, this view is easier to obtain than the true lateral shown in Figure 5–32.

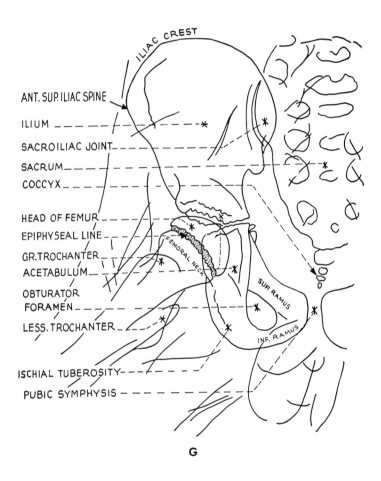

ILIAC CREST

ANT. SUP. ILIAC SPINE

ILIUM

SACROILIAC JOINT

SACRUM

COCCYX

HEAD OF FEMUR

EPIPHYSEAL LINE

GR. TROCHANTER

ACETABULUM

OBTURATOR
FORAMEN

LESS. TROCHANTER

ISCHIAL TUBEROSITY

PUBIC SYMPHYSIS

FEMORAL NECK

SUP. RAMUS

INF. RAMUS

C

G

Figure 5–33 *Continued.* *E.* Labeled tracing of *D.* *F.* Radiograph showing epiphyseal relationship of head of femur. *G.* Labeled tracing of *F.*

THE KNEE JOINT

Correlated Gross Anatomy (Fig. 5–34). The knee joint is composed of the articular margins of the condyles and trochlear surface of the femur, the condyles of the tibia, the patella, and several bursal structures encased by numerous external and internal ligaments, joined by an articular capsule. The internal ligaments extend obliquely between the middle of the articular surface of the tibia to that of the femur, and are known as the anterior and posterior crucial (or cruciate) ligaments.

There are two semilunar cartilages resting upon the upper surface of the tibial plateau which are known as the medial and lateral menisci respectively; these deepen the upper surface of the tibia for articulation with the femur. The peripheral border of each is thick and convex, and is attached to the edge of the tibial condyles by the coronary ligaments, which are actually thickened areas in the joint capsule, and to the tibial plateau as indicated in Figure 5–34.

The medial meniscus is intimately connected with the tibial collateral ligament but the lateral is separated from the fibular collateral ligament by synovial tissue. Their inner borders are concave, thin, and free, their cross sections triangular, and they are composed of fibrocartilage. The lateral meniscus has a smaller diameter and is thicker than the medial (Fig. 5–34). The extremities of both are known as the cornua. The anterior cornu of the medial meniscus is reflected down toward the tibial tuberosity.

The synovial membrane of the knee bulges upward from the patella to form the suprapatellar bursa, situated beneath the tendon of the extensor muscles on the front of the distal femur. This bursa frequently contains folds of synovia producing communicating compartments. There are two additional pouches at the back of the knee joint posterior to the femoral condyles and beneath the origin of the gastrocnemius muscle (Fig. 5–35). The

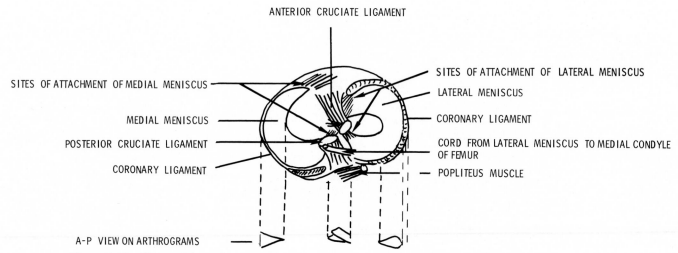

Figure 5–34. The condyles and menisci of the knee joint seen from above. The correlated view on arthrograms is also shown.

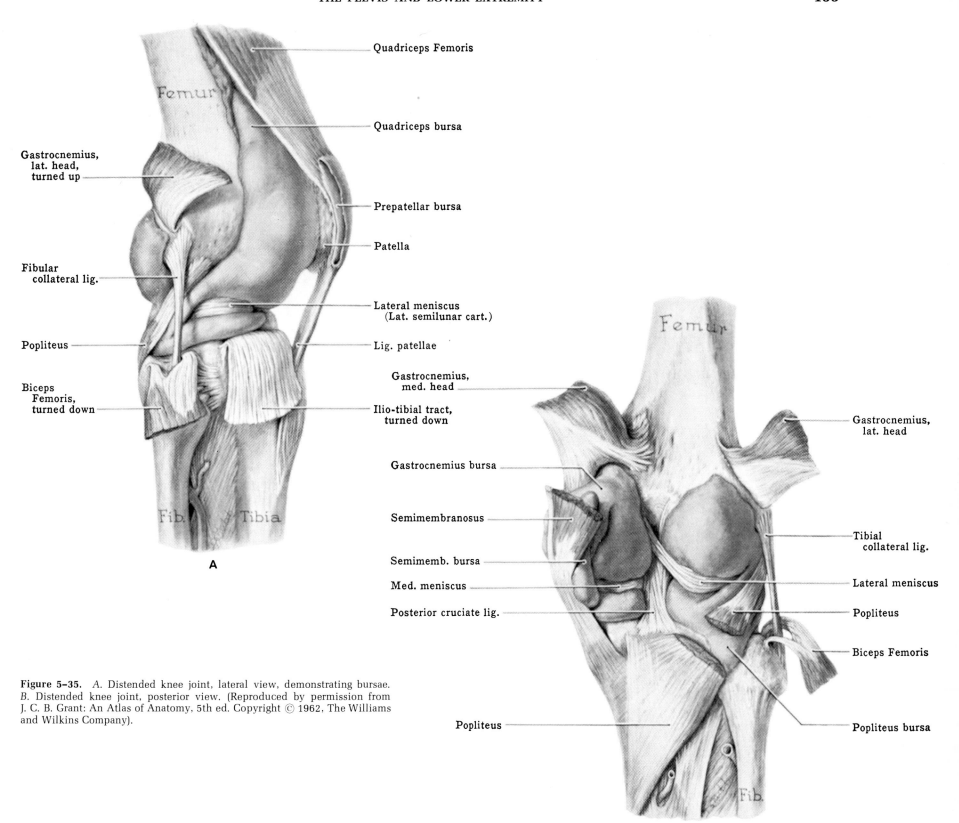

Figure 5–35. *A.* Distended knee joint, lateral view, demonstrating bursae. *B.* Distended knee joint, posterior view. (Reproduced by permission from J. C. B. Grant: An Atlas of Anatomy, 5th ed. Copyright © 1962, The Williams and Wilkins Company).

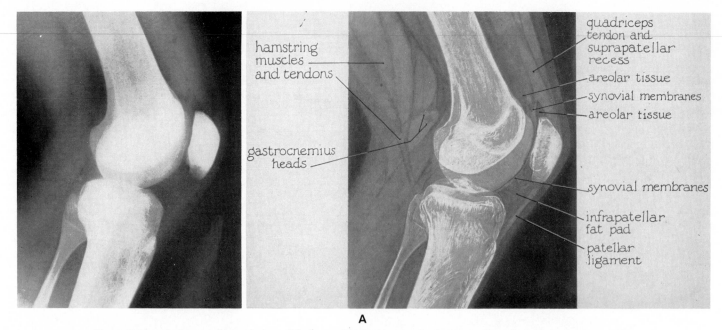

A

Figure 5–36. *A.* A normal lateral view of the knee with the associated soft tissue anatomy which can sometimes be identified either by routine views or by viewing the film with a bright light. (From Lewis, R. W.: Amer. J. Roentgenol., 65, 1951.) *B.* Lines of attachment of the articular capsules of the hip and knee joints, viewed from anterior and posterior aspects.

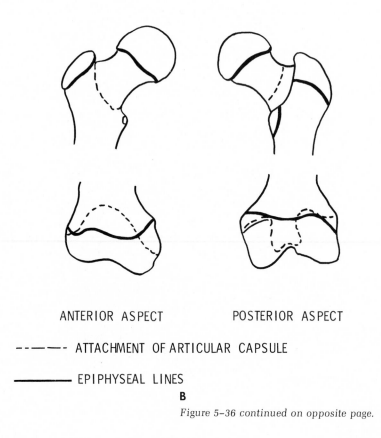

ANTERIOR ASPECT   POSTERIOR ASPECT

– – – – – ATTACHMENT OF ARTICULAR CAPSULE

———— EPIPHYSEAL LINES

B

Figure 5–36 continued on opposite page.

reader is referred to Figure 5–36 *A* and *B*, which demonstrates soft tissue structures around the knee joint (Köhler and Zimmer).

An inconstant posterior pouch extends into the popliteal space in about 13 per cent of knees. When the stalklike communication of this pouch with the knee is obstructed, or when this bursa becomes inflamed, this popliteal bursa is called a "Baker's cyst."

There is a large process of synovial membrane containing a layer of fat within it that projects into the knee on the anteroinferior aspect of the patella known as the patellar synovial fold (ligamentum mucosum) and infrapatellar fat pad, respectively. This process extends upward and posteriorly to the intercondyloid notch of the femur where it is attached in front of the anterior crucial ligament and lateral to the posterior crucial ligament.

Since the cartilaginous structures of the knee are of the same order of radiolucency as the surrounding soft tissue structures, special contrast media must be introduced into the knee joint to demonstrate them. Some appearances of the epiphyseal lines in the proximal and distal femur and the lines of attachment of the articular capsule are demonstrated in Figure 5–36 *B.*

In Figure 5–36 *C variations of normal* in the distal femur and proximal tibia are shown. For example, the distal epiphysis of the femur in a young or growing child may appear irregular and ragged at times, before it is completely ossified. In the adolescent a lucency in the distal femur often may be projected over the condyles. Also in the lateral view there is an irregularity on the posterior aspect of the shaft of the femur just proximal to the condyles which may suggest a periostitis. Note also the indentation in the femoral condyles bilaterally.

In the proximal epiphysis of the tibia the anterior tibial tubercle may appear fragmented when it is incompletely ossified. In the proximal shaft of the tibia on its lateral aspect there may be an irregularity of contour strongly suggestive of a periostitis. This is a normal variant and should not be misinterpreted. It is valuable in demonstrating the bursae, menisci, crucial liga-

ments, reflection of synovia over the popliteus muscle, the infra-patellar fat pad and the cartilage covering the articular margins of the femur, tibia, and patella.

Without special contrast, the infrapatellar fat pad can usually be demonstrated since its fatty tissue produces a triangular radiolucent area. The bursae are not ordinarily identified without contrast media unless they are distended abnormally by fluid.

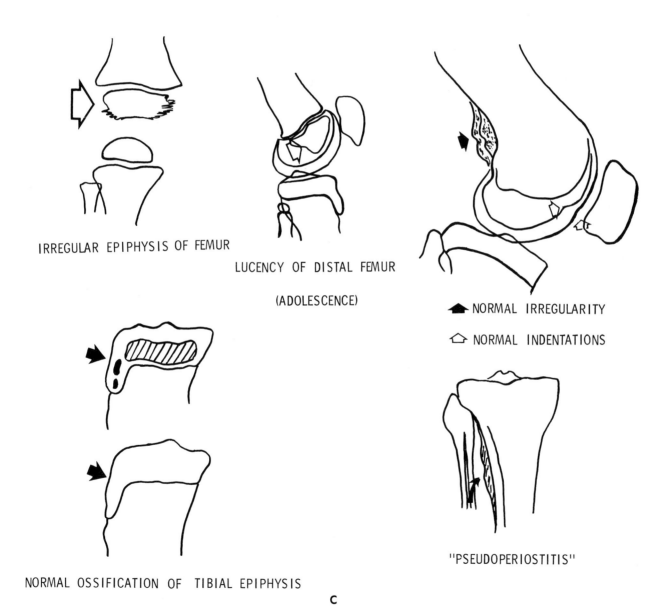

IRREGULAR EPIPHYSIS OF FEMUR

LUCENCY OF DISTAL FEMUR

(ADOLESCENCE)

▲ NORMAL IRREGULARITY

⬠ NORMAL INDENTATIONS

NORMAL OSSIFICATION OF TIBIAL EPIPHYSIS

"PSEUDOPERIOSTITIS"

C

Figure 5-36 *Continued.* C. Variations of normal bony structure in the immediate vicinity of the knee joint.

Axial Relationships of the Knee (Fig. 5–37). 1. In the anteroposterior projection the axis of the femoral shaft forms an angle of 81 degrees, on the average, with the parallel lines representing the knee joint space (range 75 to 85 degrees). The angle formed between the parallel lines of the knee joint space and the axis of the tibial shaft averages 93 degrees, with a range of 85 to 100 degrees. There are minimal differences between male and female in this latter angle (Keats et al.).

2. In the lateral projection when the knee is fully extended, the axis of the lower one-third of the shaft of the femur forms a continuous line with the axis of the shaft of the tibia.

3. The line through the lowermost margins of the femoral condyles is parallel to the line drawn through the upper articular margins of the tibia.

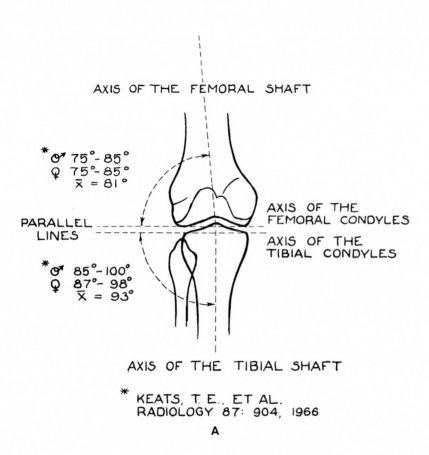

A

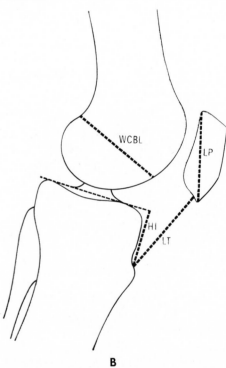

B

Figure 5–37. *A.* Axial relationships of the knee joint. *B.* Tracing of a radiograph of a normal knee showing the relationship of the patella to the femur and the tibia. Four measurements are obtained: LT (length of tendon), length of patellar tendon on its deep or posterior surface; LP (length of patella), greatest diagonal length of patella; WCBL (width of the femoral condyle at Blumensaat's line), both condyles measured at the level of Blumensaat's line and an average obtained; and HI (height of insertion), perpendicular distance from level of tibial condylar surface to the point of insertion of the patellar tendon. The point of insertion is represented on the radiograph by a clearly defined notch.

$$\frac{LT}{LP} = 1.02 \pm 0.13$$

$$\frac{LP}{WCBL} = 0.95 \pm 0.07 \text{ (in each instance, one standard deviation)}$$

$$\frac{LT}{HI} = 1.85 \pm 0.24$$

The length of the patellar tendon does not differ from that of the patella by more than 20 per cent.

TABLE I: DISTANCE FROM THE LOWER POLE OF THE PATELLA TO BLUMENSAAT'S LINE IN 44 KNEES

Distance (cm)	No. of Knees
0.0	0
0.5	3
1.0	15
1.5	12
2.0	9
2.5	3
3.0	2
TOTAL	44

RADIOGRAPHIC METHODS OF EXAMINATION

1. **Routine Anteroposterior View of the Knee** (Fig. 5–38). The patient lies flat on his back and the film is placed under his knee. The central ray passes through a point about ½ inch below the tip of the patella, directly through the knee joint space.

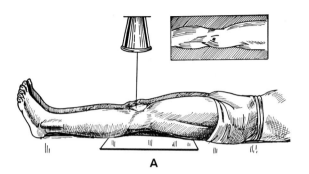

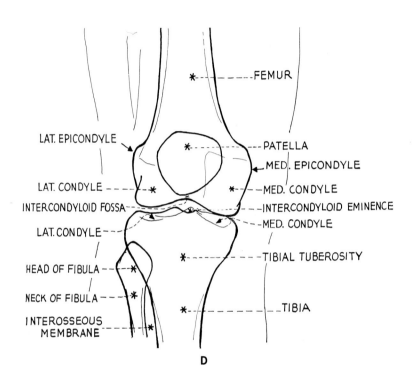

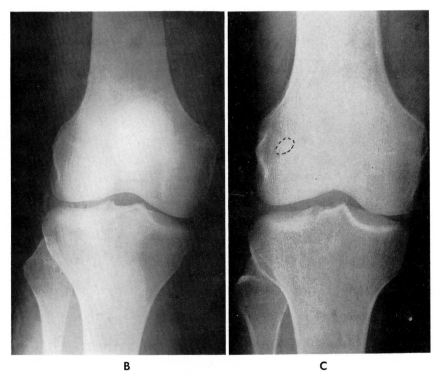

Figure 5–38.   Routine anteroposterior view of the knee. *A*. Method of positioning patient. *B*. Radiograph. *C*. Radiograph showing fabella. *D*. Labeled tracing of *B*.

Points of Practical Interest with Reference to Figure 5–38

1. The knee should be completely extended with the patient in the supine position. If the patient is unable to extend the knee completely, the posteroanterior projection is preferable.
2. Alternatively, if the knee cannot be fully extended the cassette may be elevated on sandbags to bring it into closer contact with the popliteal space. If the degree of flexion of the knee is great, a curved cassette or curved film holder should be employed.
3. The leg is adjusted in the true anteroposterior position and the distal apex of the patella is noted.
4. Center the cassette and the central ray of the x-ray tube approximately 1 cm. below the patellar apex.
5. When radiographing the joint space it may be helpful to tilt the tube approximately 5 degrees cephalad. This will help to give a clear view of the knee joint space because the superimposition of the anterior and posterior margins of the tibial plateau is somewhat more satisfactory.

2. **Routine Lateral View of the Knee** (Fig. 5–39).   The knee is partially flexed, and its lateral aspect placed next to the film. The central ray passes through the knee joint space approximately in the midcondylar plane. In order to superimpose the two tibial condyles, a 5 degree tube angulation of the shaft of the femur may be employed.

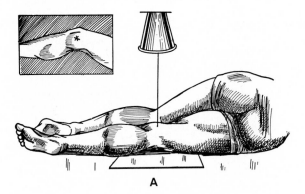

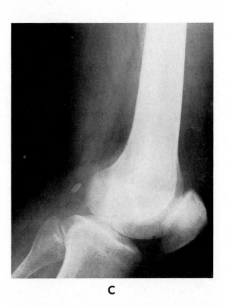

C

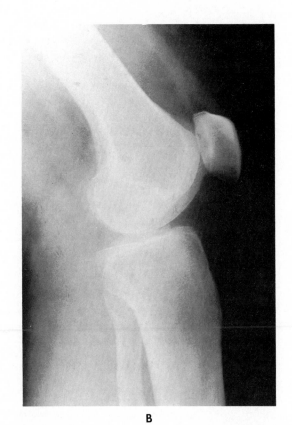

B

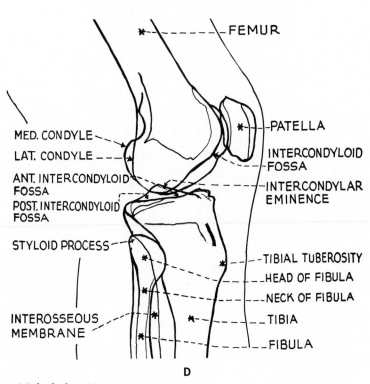

D

Figure 5–39.   Routine lateral view of the knee. *A.* Method of positioning patient. *B.* Radiograph. *C.* Radiograph demonstrating fabella. *D.* Labeled tracing of *B.*

3. **Special View of the Intercondyloid Fossa of the Femur**
(Fig. 5–40).   This projection is employed to obtain a clear visualization of the knee joint space. The knee is bent over a curved cardboard film holder or curved cassette and the central ray is directed into the intercondyloid fossa of the femur as shown. This view may reveal a loose opaque body in the knee when other views fail to show it clearly because of overlying bone.

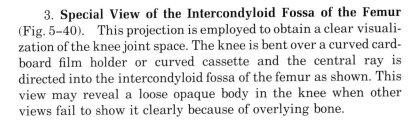

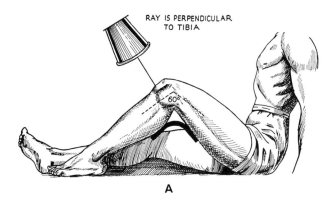

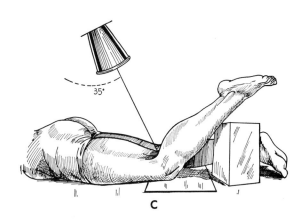

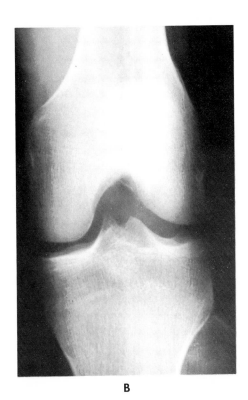

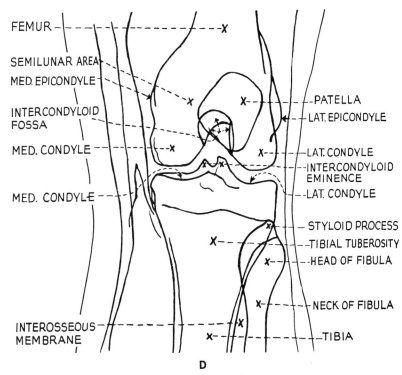

FEMUR

SEMILUNAR AREA
MED. EPICONDYLE

INTERCONDYLOID
FOSSA

MED. CONDYLE

MED. CONDYLE

INTEROSSEOUS
MEMBRANE

PATELLA
LAT. EPICONDYLE

LAT. CONDYLE
INTERCONDYLOID
EMINENCE
LAT. CONDYLE

STYLOID PROCESS
TIBIAL TUBEROSITY
HEAD OF FIBULA

NECK OF FIBULA

TIBIA

Figure 5–40.   Special view of the intercondyloid fossa of the femur. *A.* Method of positioning patient. *B.* Radiograph. *C.* Alternate method of positioning patient. A very similar radiograph is obtained. *D.* Labeled tracing of *B.*

4. **Routine Views in Arthrography of the Knee** (Fig. 5–41). In arthrography of the knee three basic contrast methods are available: (1) absorbable gases only, (2) water soluble positive contrast media, or (3) a combination of gas and water soluble positive contrast media to provide a double contrast technique. (For review see Freiberger et al.; Meschan and McGaw; Somerville; Haveson and Rein).

A suitable sterile tray and a procedure for insertion of the needle into the suprapatellar bursa are shown in Figure 5–41. The sterile tray contains the appropriate skin preparation apparatus, drapes, syringes, and solutions of 1 per cent xylocaine and 60 per cent Renografin with an oxygen tank adjoining, if oxygen or air is to be employed for double contrast.

A spreading device such as that shown in Figure 5–44 may be employed, or a pillow may be placed under the distal femur and a sandbag over the ankle to open the part of the joint being examined.

When the needle is properly placed, air can be injected with only gentle pressure on the plunger of the syringe. A small amount of air or oxygen is injected prior to the further instillation of 5 to 10 cc. of methylglucamine diatrizoate 60 per cent (up to 15 cc. may be utilized). The knee is actively flexed several times and the patient may be allowed to walk about for about 1 minute.

Thereafter, with the patient in a prone or oblique position, a pillow is placed under the lower end of the femur and the x-ray beam is arranged to fall tangential to the posterior aspect of the medial meniscus, which will be uppermost. The beam is centered at the level of the tibial plateau. A sandbag is placed over the ankles to widen the joint space and allow a maximum amount of air to surround the contrast-coated meniscus. Usually six exposures are made, and the patient is rotated 30 degrees toward the supine position after each exposure. Always the central beam is adjusted to the level of the tibial plateau. As the more anterior portions of the meniscus are examined, the legs may be flexed at the knee and the sandbag may be placed under the heel to allow moderate flexion.

The lateral meniscus is filmed in the same way.

The examination is completed by obtaining anteroposterior and lateral Bucky roentgenograms with a vertical x-ray beam.

Generally, spot-film fluoroscopic control is best if a small focal spot (0.6 mm.) is available. Otherwise, an overhead tube must be employed in conjunction with fluoroscopy to obtain the best detail.

Normal air (pneumo-) arthrograms are illustrated in Figure 5–42, accompanied by labeled tracings. Figure 5–43 demon-

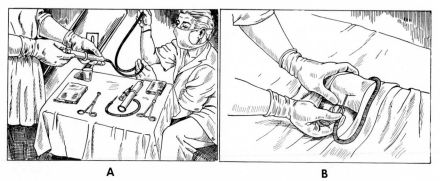

A   B

Figure 5–41. Technique of arthrography of the knee. A. The syringe is loaded with contrast agent (and possibly a small amount of air—usually 10 to 15 cc. of 50 per cent methylglucamine diatrizoate—is adequate). B. The needle is inserted under the superior margin of the patella into the suprapatellar bursa as shown.

If a small focus x-ray tube is available (0.6 mm. or less) radiography can be performed under spot-film fluoroscopic control. Otherwise, the patient may be positioned afterward under fluoroscopic control, but in such a case films are obtained with an overhead small focal spot tube.

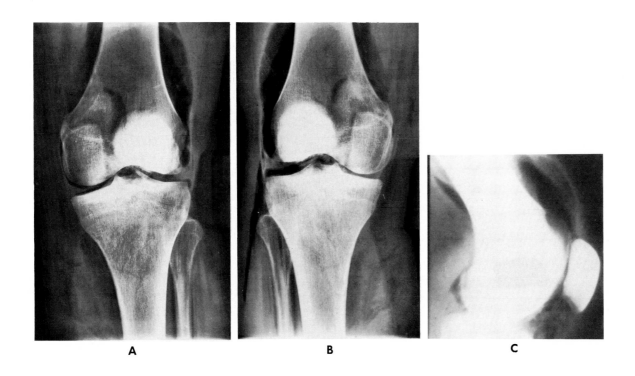

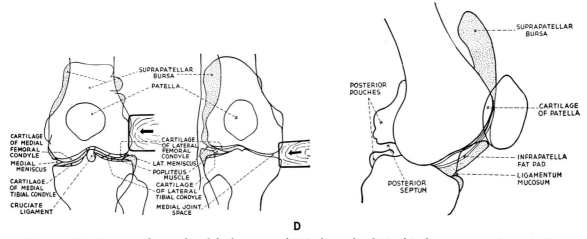

Figure 5–42. Pneumoarthrography of the knee. *A* and *B*. Radiographs obtained in the posteroanterior projection, first with the medial knee joint spread, and next with the lateral knee joint spread. *C*. Radiograph of the knee in a straight lateral projection. *D*. Labeled tracings of radiographs.

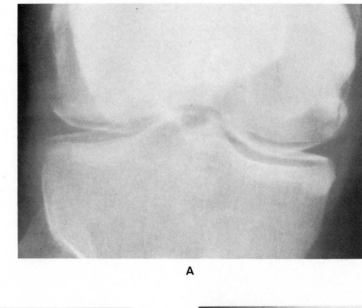

A

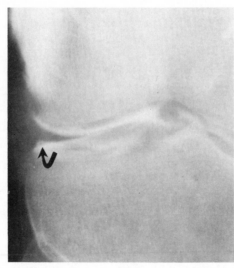

B

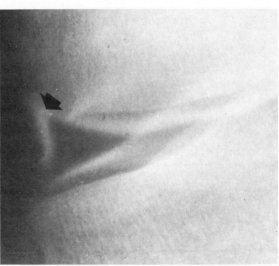

C

Figure 5–43. Opaque contrast arthrograms of the knee. *A* and *B* represent normal or variations of normal. The arrow in *B* points toward a normal undulation often found in the lateral meniscus. *C* shows a fracture through the medial meniscus and its appearance with opaque media.

strates normal arthrograms obtained with water soluble positive contrast media and a very small additional amount of air.

As will be noted, the *medial meniscus* is a crescentic triangular structure in cross section. The superior and inferior surfaces are well defined and free within the joint space. The base of the triangle is wedged against the coronary ligament. Low contrast substance is ordinarily present between the meniscus and the coronary ligament.

The *lateral meniscus* is usually somewhat more variable in its cross-sectional pattern and more loosely attached to its lateral collateral ligament. A small amount of contrast agent may occasionally be seen between the base of the triangle and the coronary ligament. The margins of the meniscus are smooth and the apex of the triangle does not normally extend beyond the middle of the appropriate condyle. An elongated meniscus extending far into the joint space suggests an abnormality called a *discoid*

meniscus, whereas a meniscus which is short or irregular in its contour suggests a tear or abnormality.

THE PATELLA

The patella is a triangular sesamoid bone developed in the tendon of the quadriceps femoris muscle (Fig. 5–45). Its anterior surface is perforated by many small openings which transmit nutrient vessels, and this roughened appearance must be recognized as a normal condition. Its anterior surface is covered by one or more bursae, and its posterior surface is articular, articulating with the anterior aspects of both femoral condyles.

Ossification of the patella begins about the third year of life and is usually completed about the age of puberty.

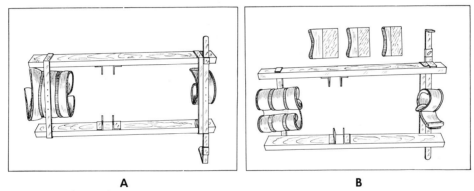

Figure 5–44. Special device for spreading the knee for pneumoarthrography. *A.* Top view. *B.* Bottom side up. The blocks of wood are adjusted in the slots and act as a fulcrum against the knee while the ankle in its brace is moved in one direction or the other, depending on which side of the knee joint is being spread.

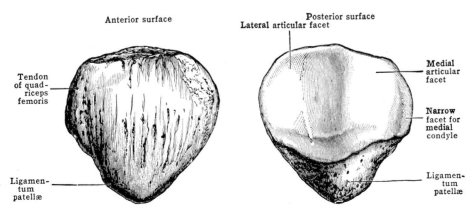

Figure 5–45. The patella, anterior, posterior and superior views. (From Anson, B. J. (ed.): Morris' Human Anatomy, 12th ed. Copyright © 1966 by McGraw-Hill, Inc. Used by permission of McGraw-Hill Book Company.)

Occasionally a segmentation of the patella persists throughout life, separating the upper outer quadrant on the articular aspect of the bone from the rest of the patella. This is called a bipartite patella (Fig. 5–46). More rarely, there may be a third segment; this constitutes a tripartite patella (Fig. 5–46 B). These entities are important from the standpoint of differentiation from fracture.

In view of the distance of the patella from the film in the anteroposterior projection, a certain amount of distortion of the patella is obtained in this view. Also, projection may produce some confusion as to the exact position of the patella with relation to the distal femur. This is overcome by obtaining the posteroanterior view of the patella which furnishes considerably greater detail regarding patellar structure and position.

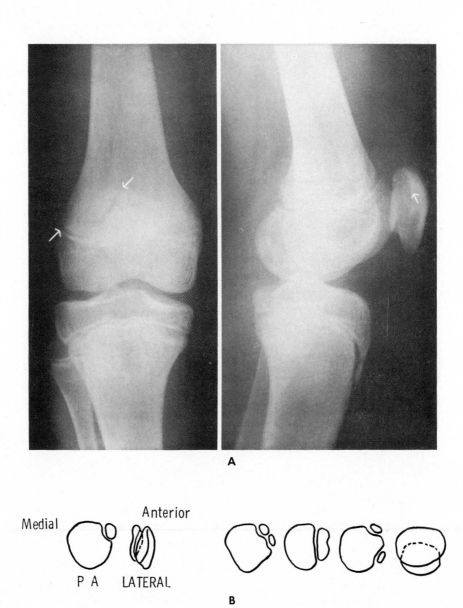

A

B

Figure 5–46.   A. Bipartite patella. B. Various shapes of patella partita.

RADIOGRAPHIC METHODS OF EXAMINATION OF THE PATELLA

1. **Posteroanterior View of the Patella** (Fig. 5–47). The patient lies prone with the film beneath the patella. *A relatively short film-target distance is employed* so that most of the knee will be distorted, and the patella will be more clearly defined because it is close to the film. The central ray in this instance can pass either through the knee joint proper, as illustrated, or through the patella.

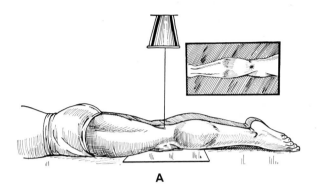

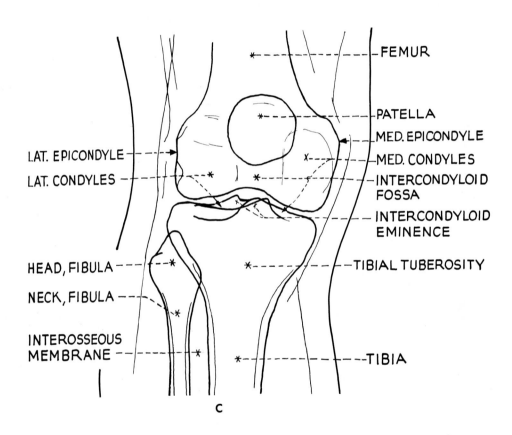

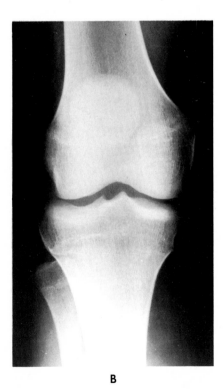

B

Figure 5–47. Posteroanterior view of the patella. *A.* Method of positioning patient. *B*, Radiograph. *C.* Labeled tracing of *B*.

Points of Practical Interest with Reference to Figure 5–47

1. The patient is placed in the prone position with the ankles and the feet ordinarily supported by sandbags.
2. The film is centered to the patella and the central ray adjusted so as to pass through the center of the patella. The heel may have to be rotated outward slightly to accomplish this.
3. Ordinarily, it is desirable to use a telescopic cone, bringing the cone fairly close to the knee in order to produce a distortion of the superimposed femoral condyles and a clearer concept of the patella, which lies next to the film.
4. This view definitely gives better detail of the patella than that obtained with the anteroposterior projection.

2. **Special Tangential View of the Patella** (Fig. 5–48). The two views usually employed in this connection are illustrated in the accompanying diagrams. Frequently, the anterior margin of the patella is found to be irregular owing to the fact that it is penetrated by several nutrient vessels from its anterior aspect. This imparts a serrated appearance to the patella.

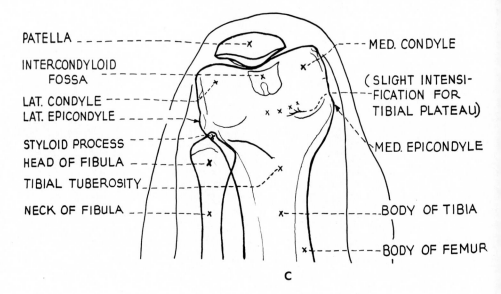

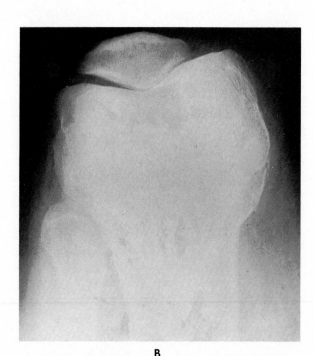

Figure 5–48. Special tangential view of the patella. *A.* Method of positioning patient. *B.* Radiograph. *C.* Labeled tracing of *B.*

Points of Practical Interest with Reference to Figure 5–48

1. This view may be obtained with the patient either prone or supine. If the patient is in the prone position, the thigh is placed flat against the table and the leg flexed by means of a band wrapped around the ankle, the ends of which are held by the patient's hand. If the patient is supine, the film is placed along the distal aspect of the thigh as shown.
2. The central ray is directed at right angles to the joint space between the patella and the femoral condyles, and the degree of central ray angulation will depend upon the degree of flexion of the knee. Ordinarily the central ray should be parallel with the articular margin of the patella.
3. The outer margin of the patella as projected in this view frequently has a rather serrated and irregular appearance which must not be interpreted as abnormal. This serrated appearance is caused by points of tendinous attachments to the bony substance of the patella, as well as by penetration by nutrient vessels.

THE LEG

Correlated Anatomy of the Tibia.   The upper end of the tibia (Figs. 5–49, 5–50) contains the medial and lateral condyles which articulate with the corresponding condyles of the femur. Anteriorly, the condyles meet to form the tuberosity of the tibia,

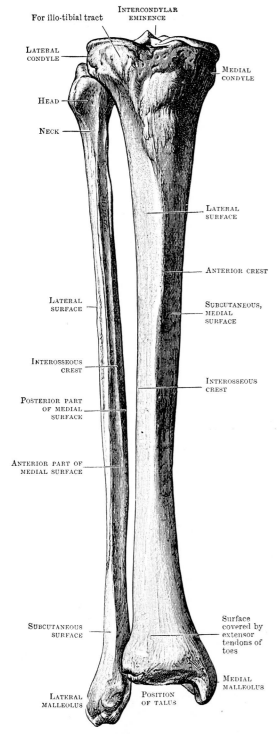

Fig. 5–49

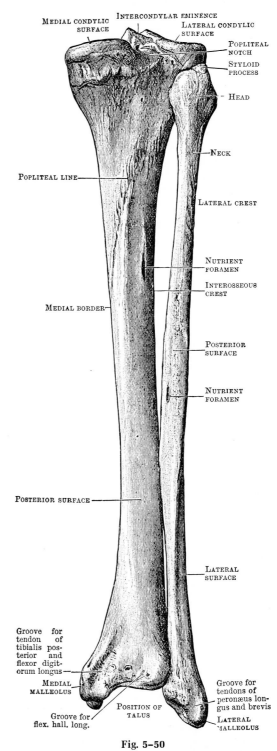

Fig. 5–50

Figure 5–49.   Tibia and fibula, anterior aspect. (From Cunningham's Textbook of Anatomy, 6th ed. London, Oxford University Press, 1931.)

Figure 5–50.   Tibia and fibula, posterior aspect. (From Cunningham's Textbook of Anatomy, 6th ed. London, Oxford University Press, 1931.)

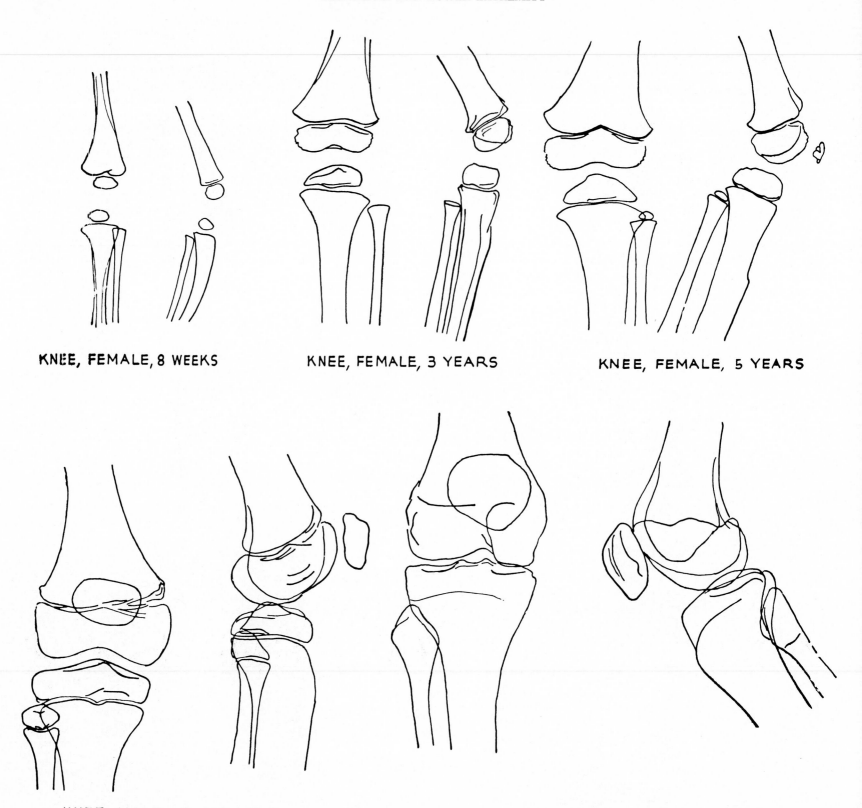

KNEE, FEMALE, 8 WEEKS

KNEE, FEMALE, 3 YEARS

KNEE, FEMALE, 5 YEARS

KNEE, MALE, 9 YEARS

KNEE, FEMALE, 17 YEARS

Figure 5-51. Changes in growth and development as seen in the knee.

which receives an attachment of the ligamentum patellae. Between the ligament and the anterior upper aspect of the tuberosity, there is a prominent, more superficial bursa. (This bursa is subject to inflammation in persons who must rest their weight upon this structure for one reason or another, such as frequent kneeling or scrubbing floors.)

The shaft of the tibia has a prominent crest (the anterior crest) anteriorly in its upper two-thirds, which gradually extends medially toward the medial malleolus. The lateral border of the tibia forms the interosseous crest, to which the interosseous membrane is attached.

The lower end of the tibia presents the medial malleolus on the medial aspect, a smooth anterior aspect, and a roughened posterior aspect. The posterior surface contains two grooves—the medial receiving the tendons of the tibialis posterior and flexor digitorum longus muscle, and the lateral the flexor hallucis longus muscle. The lateral aspect is indented for its articulation with the fibula. The distal articular surface extends along the lateral aspect of the medial malleolus, and the entire surface articulates with the talus tarsal bone.

There are several items of particular radiographic interest in this bone (Fig. 5–36 C). The tibial tuberosity is a rather variable structure in its appearance and is subject to degenerative changes during the growth period. Not infrequently, the tuberosity will appear different on the two sides.

The upper margin of the interosseal crest is frequently of a lesser density than the remainder of this ridge, and simulates a periosteal elevation or thickening. This appearance is normal, however, and should not be interpreted as a periostitis.

There is a slight normal curvature of the tibia, both laterally and anteriorly. On the other hand, the fibula tends to curve somewhat posteriorly, producing an ovoid aperture in the interosseal region in the lateral view. These slight curvatures must be considered in studying the lines of weight bearing in the leg.

Correlated Anatomy of the Fibula. The fibula (Figs. 5–49, 5–50) in man bears none of the weight of the trunk, and is important only from the standpoint of its muscular attachments and its participation in the formation of the ankle joint. The head of the fibula is a rather bulbous structure which rises to a pointed apex known as the styloid process that is considerably roughened for attachment of muscles and ligaments. Medially, it articulates with the lateral condyle of the tibia. The shaft of the fibula contains numerous longitudinal and oblique grooves which furnish muscular attachment; the interosseous crest on the medial aspect gives attachment to the interosseous membrane. The lateral malleolus is particularly important because of its frequent participation in injuries to the ankle area. The upper medial surface articulates with the talus tarsal bone and is smooth, but the rest of the malleolus is very roughened and grooved. It gives attachment to numerous ligaments around the ankle and is grooved posteriorly for the peroneal tendons. The tip of the lateral malleolus

affords attachment to the calcaneofibular ligament of the ankle, which is particularly subject to tear and strain in inversion injuries.

In view of the great importance of the malleoli, special views of these structures from several perspectives should be obtained, and minute abnormalities require the closest inspection. The irregularities which may occur normally must be understood; only then can abnormal irregularities be recognized.

Changes with Growth and Development (Fig. 5–52). The tibia and fibula are each ossified from three centers of ossification—one for the body and one for each extremity. The center for the upper epiphysis of the *tibia* appears before or shortly after birth. It has a thin, tongue-shaped process anteriorly which forms the tuberosity. The center of ossification for the tibia's lower epiphysis appears considerably later, usually around the second year. The lower epiphysis joins the body of the tibia somewhat

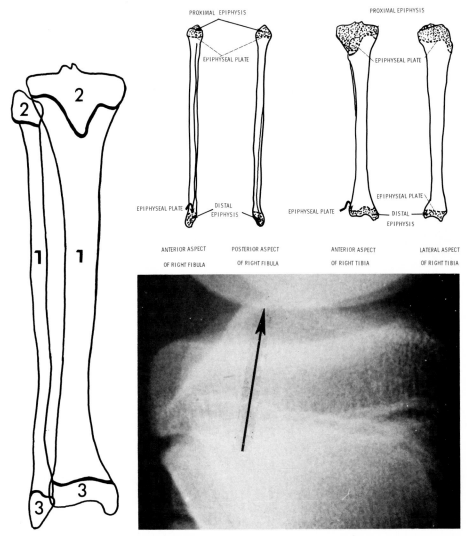

Figure 5–52. Ossification centers of the tibia and fibula.

earlier than the upper epiphysis—approximately 18 years for the lower epiphysis and 20 for the upper (see Chapter 3). Occasionally there are additional centers of ossification for the medial malleolus or the tongue-shaped process of the upper epiphysis.

Ossification in the *fibula* begins in its lower end in the second year approximately and in the upper epiphysis about the fourth year. In this instance, the lower epiphysis is also the first to ossify, uniting with the body of the fibula during the 20th year, whereas the upper epiphysis unites somewhat later—usually about the 25th year.

The epiphyseal line is somewhat wavy and irregular, especially in the upper epiphysis (Fig. 5–51).

The fibula is thicker in the child than in the adult when compared with the tibia, and once it begins to ossify it grows distally more rapidly than the medial malleolus. This rapid growth ultimately accounts for the fact that it is slightly more distal than the medial malleolus.

Compartments of the Leg in Cross Section (Fig. 5–53). In cross section of the middle of the leg several compartments can be identified: first is a compartment anterior to the interosseous membrane and extending between the tibia and fibula; this contains the extensor muscles. Resting upon the interosseous membrane within the anterior compartment are the anterior tibial vessels. Immediately posterior to the interosseous membrane is the tibialis posterior muscle. Between this muscle and the intermuscular septum on the posterior aspect of the tibia, but separated from the tibia by the flexors of the toes, are the posterior tibial vessels and the tibial nerve.

The peroneal vessels lie just lateral to these on the posterior aspect of the tibialis posterior muscle just medial to the fibula. The anterior and posterior crural septa surround the peroneal muscles on the lateral aspect of the fibula, forming a lateral compartment. The intermuscular septum extends transversely across the leg as shown, separating the flexors of the toes from the calf muscles, which consist of the soleus, the gastrocnemius, and the plantaris.

Farther down the leg in its lower third, the anterior tibial artery moves in front of the tibia.

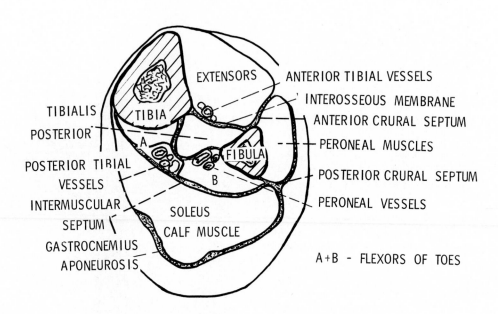

Figure 5–53. Cross section of compartments of the leg in its midsection.

RADIOGRAPHIC METHODS OF EXAMINING THE LEG

1. **Routine Anteroposterior View.**

2. **Lateral View** (Figs. 5–54, 5–55). The diagrams are self-explanatory. It is important to emphasize only that in the anteroposterior projection the toes point slightly medially. If possible, both the knee joint and the joint between the tibia and talus should be included so that the line of weight bearing can be accurately drawn. In any event, one of these joints should always be shown.

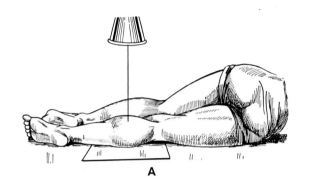

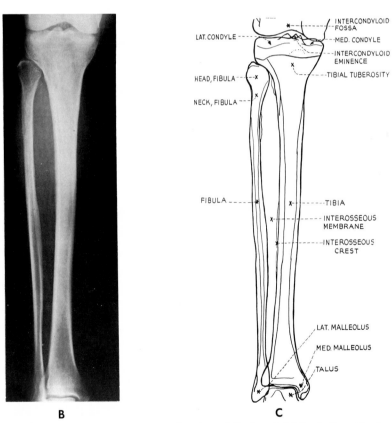

Figure 5–54. Routine anteroposterior view of the leg. *A.* Method of positioning patient. *B.* Radiograph. *C.* Labeled tracing of *B.*

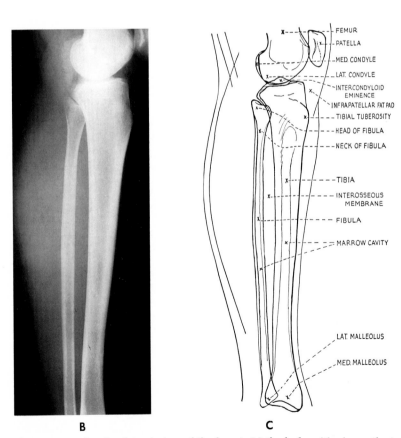

Figure 5–55. Routine lateral view of the leg. *A.* Method of positioning patient. *B.* Radiograph. *C.* Labeled tracing of *B.*

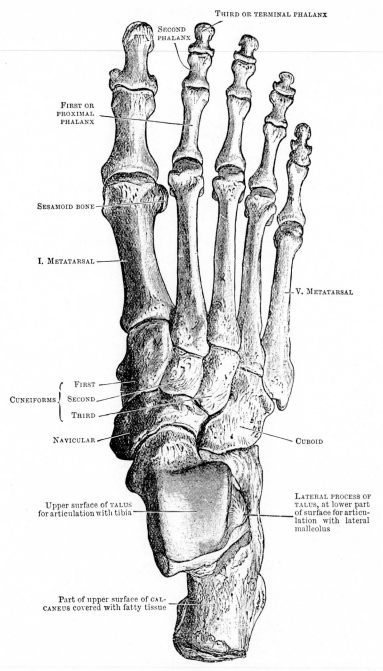

SECOND PHALANX

THIRD OR TERMINAL PHALANX

FIRST OR PROXIMAL PHALANX

SESAMOID BONE

I. METATARSAL

V. METATARSAL

CUNEIFORMS { FIRST SECOND THIRD }

NAVICULAR

CUBOID

Upper surface of TALUS for articulation with tibia

LATERAL PROCESS OF TALUS, at lower part of surface for articulation with lateral malleolus

Part of upper surface of CALCANEUS covered with fatty tissue

Fig. 5–56

THE TARSUS

Correlated Gross Anatomy (Figs. 5–56, 5–57). There are seven tarsal bones—the calcaneus, talus, navicular, cuboid, and three cuneiform bones. Each has approximately six surfaces, some surfaces being articular and others roughened by ligamentous attachments.

The talus supports the tibia, articulating with the malleolus

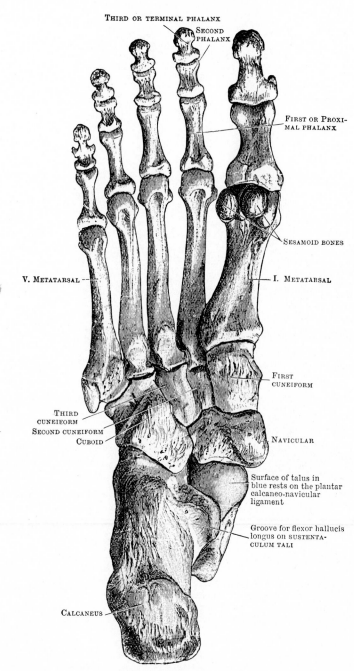

THIRD OR TERMINAL PHALANX

SECOND PHALANX

FIRST OR PROXIMAL PHALANX

SESAMOID BONES

V. METATARSAL

I. METATARSAL

FIRST CUNEIFORM

THIRD CUNEIFORM

SECOND CUNEIFORM

CUBOID

NAVICULAR

Surface of talus in blue rests on the plantar calcaneo-navicular ligament

Groove for flexor hallucis longus on SUSTENTACULUM TALI

CALCANEUS

Fig. 5–57

Figure 5–56. Dorsal view of foot. (From Cunningham's Textbook of Anatomy, 6th ed. London, Oxford University Press, 1931.)

Figure 5–57. Plantar view of foot. (From Cunningham's Textbook of Anatomy, 6th ed. London, Oxford University Press, 1931.)

on each side, the calcaneus below, and the navicular in front. Anteriorly, the head of the talus articulates with the navicular. Inferiorly, there are two separate articular surfaces for the calcaneus—one which articulates with the sustentaculum tali, and another larger one which articulates with the calcaneus proper. Occasionally, there is a separate ossicle along the posterior margin of the larger calcaneal articular surface known as the *os trigonum.* It is important radiographically when it is necessary to differentiate it from a fracture.

The calcaneus is the largest tarsal bone and forms the heel of the foot. Superiorly and anteromedially it articulates with the talus. Anteromedially where it supports the talus there is a well-marked process known as the sustentaculum tali. Anteriorly, it articulates with the cuboid. Unlike the other tarsal and carpal bones, there is a secondary epiphysis situated on the heel aspect of the calcaneus which begins to ossify in the sixth to the tenth year, uniting with the body of the bone between the thirteenth and the twentieth year. This ossification varies considerably in different people, and even on the two feet of a single person. *The bone of this epiphysis tends to be somewhat more compact than that of most epiphyses, and any interpretations of abnormality in this epiphysis, with regard either to its irregularity or its density, must be considered cautiously.*

Boehler's angle for the normal calcaneus (Fig. 5–58) is a line drawn from the posterior superior margin of the talocalcaneal joint through the posterior superior margin of the calcaneus, making an angle of approximately 30 to 35 degrees with a second line drawn from the posterior superior margin of the talocalcaneal joint to the superior articular margin of the calcaneocuboid joint. Less than 28 degrees is quite definitely abnormal and poor position from the functional standpoint.

The navicular bone is situated between the talus behind and the three cuneiforms in front. Its tuberosity is a prominent eminence on its medial aspect, its superior surface is somewhat irregular and variable in appearance. There is not infrequently a small extra ossicle adjoining the tuberosity known as the *accessory navicular* which, like the os trigonum, owes its importance to the fact that it must not be confused with a fracture in this region.

The three cuneiform bones are wedge-shaped bones situated between the navicular behind and the first three metatarsals in front. Although they are in the same line posteriorly, the first and third project farther anteriorly than does the second. This forms a recess into which the base of the second metatarsal fits.

The cuboid, as its name indicates, is an irregular cube in shape and is situated between the calcaneus behind and the fourth and fifth metatarsals in front. In addition, it also articulates with the third cuneiform, and occasionally also with the navicular and talus.

One of the most frequent sesamoid bones of this region is the *peroneal sesamoid,* which is situated between the cuboid and the base of the fifth metatarsal, in the tendon of the peroneus longus

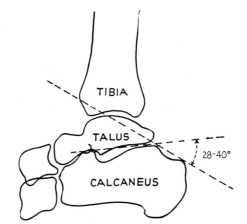

Figure 5–58. The criteria for a normal calcaneus. (Boehler.)

muscle. An accessory first cuneiform is another frequent extra ossicle arising from the separate ossification of the plantar and dorsal aspects of the first cuneiform, and is situated in the tendon of the tibialis anterior muscle.

The most frequent sesamoid bone of the ankle area is the os trigonum, situated over the medial surface of the head of the talus in the tendon of the tibialis posterior muscle (see Fig. 5–59).

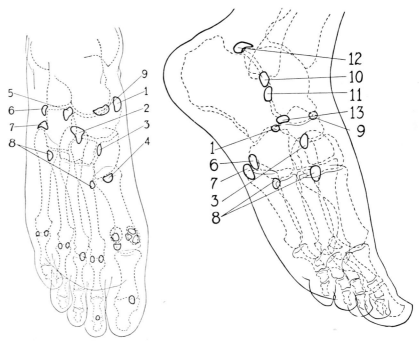

Figure 5–59. Schematic diagram showing sesamoid bones and supernumerary bones of the foot. 1 Os tibiale externum; 2, processus uncinatus; 3, intercuneiforme; 4, pars peronea metatarsalia I; 5, cuboides secundarium; 6, os peroneum; 7, os vesalianum; 8, intermetatarseum; 9, accessory navicular; 10, talus accessorius; 11, os sustentaculum; 12, os trigonum; 13, calcaneus secundarius. The most common of these are: 1, 6, 7, 9 and 12. (From McNeill, C.: Roentgen Technique. Courtesy of Charles C Thomas, Publisher, Springfield, Illinois.)

The Ankle Joint (Fig. 5–60). The ankle joint is formed by the lower ends of the tibia and fibula and the upper surface of the talus, apart from ligamentous structures. The synovial membrane of this joint is extensive, being very loose and extending beyond the actual articulation. Because the medial and lateral malleoli are subject to frequent injury, this joint is of considerable importance in traumatic medicine. Since a portion of the lateral malleolus is obscured by the talus, oblique views are necessary to show the lateral malleolus clearly in its entirety. The so-called trimalleolar fracture is actually a clinical misnomer since there are not three malleoli in this region; the term, however, refers to a combined fracture of the posterior articular margin of the tibia and medial malleolus which may or may not be continuous, as well as a coexisting fracture of the lateral malleolus. The ankle joint space is a regular structure, with a parallelism of the articular margins that is demonstrated in Figure 5–61 *A*.

Axial Relationships of the Ankle. The axial relationships of the ankle were measured in 50 normal adult subjects and are illustrated in Figure 5–61 *B* (Keats et al.). In this diagram several relationships may be noted.

First, the axis of the shaft of the tibia is perpendicular to the horizontal plane of the ankle joint and is continuous with the vertical axis of the talus. The line tangent to the articular surface of the medial malleolus, CD, forms an angle which averages 53 degrees (ranging from 45 to 65 degrees, as indicated) with the horizontal plane of the ankle joint. The line tangent to the articular surface of the lateral malleolus forms an average angle of 52 degrees (range, 45 to 63 degrees) with the horizontal plane of the ankle joint.

Generally, in a straight anteroposterior view of the ankle the lateral tibial tubercle overlaps the distal fibula just above the lateral malleolus. The absence of such an overlap indicates tibiofibular diastasis from a torn tibial fibular ligament. This, in turn, suggests that a search be made for a fracture of the fibular shaft about 6 cm. above the lateral malleolus.

The Tarsal Joints. The tarsal joints, together with the tar-

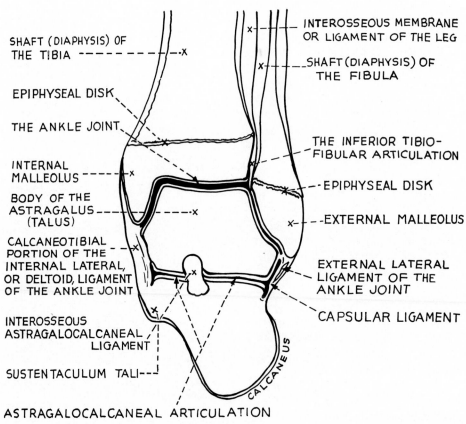

Figure 5–60. Coronal section through the ankle joint. (After Toldt, C.: An Atlas of Anatomy for Students and Physicians. New York, Macmillan Co., © 1926.)

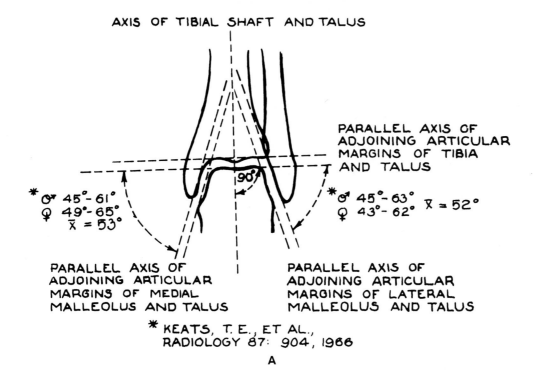

AXIS OF TIBIAL SHAFT AND TALUS

PARALLEL AXIS OF
ADJOINING ARTICULAR
MARGINS OF TIBIA
AND TALUS

90°

* ♂ 45°- 61°
♀ 49°- 65°
x̄ = 53°

* ♂ 45°- 63°
♀ 43°- 62° x̄ = 52°

PARALLEL AXIS OF
ADJOINING ARTICULAR
MARGINS OF MEDIAL
MALLEOLUS AND TALUS

PARALLEL AXIS OF
ADJOINING ARTICULAR
MARGINS OF LATERAL
MALLEOLUS AND TALUS

* KEATS, T. E., ET AL.,
RADIOLOGY 87: 904, 1966

A

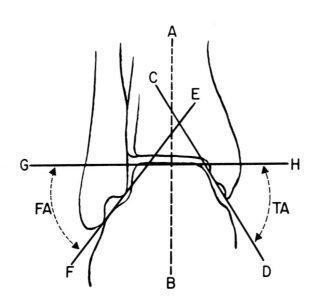

	Males	Females	Av.
FA	45° - 63°	43° - 62°	52°
TA	45° - 61°	49° - 65°	53°

B

Figure 5–61. *A.* Diagram illustrating parallelism of articular surfaces of the ankle joint. *B.* Measurement of axial angles of the ankle. (From Atlas of Roentgenographic Measurement, 3d ed., by Lusted, L. B., and Keats, T. E. Copyright © 1972 by Year Book Medical Publishers, Inc., Chicago. Used by permission.)

sometatarsal, metatarsophalangeal, and interphalangeal joints, constitute the joints of the foot.

Changes with Growth and Development (Fig. 5–62). Ossification of the tarsus begins at birth in the following tarsal bones: the calcaneus, the talus, and occasionally the cuboid. Thereafter, the third cuneiform begins to ossify by the first year, the navicular by the third year, and rapidly thereafter, the second cuneiform and first cuneiform by the third and fourth years, respectively (for greater detail see Chapter 3). The centers of ossification for the navicular tarsal bone may be multiple originally but rapidly fuse into one. The calcaneus is the only tarsal bone with a secondary center of ossification. That part of this bone that ultimately forms the medial and lateral tubercles ossifies at 8 years in girls and 10 years, approximately, in boys, uniting at 15 years and 18 years respectively. Otherwise, ossification of all the tarsal bones is complete by puberty or shortly thereafter. The posterior tubercle of the talus may develop as a separate bone called the os trigonum.

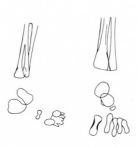

THE ANKLE AT BIRTH

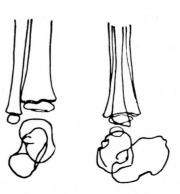

THE ANKLE AT 3 YEARS

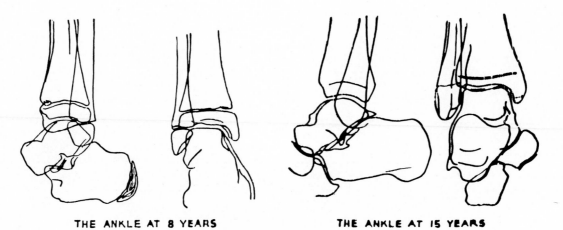

THE ANKLE AT 8 YEARS   THE ANKLE AT 15 YEARS

Figure 5–62. Changes in growth and development as seen in the ankle.

RADIOGRAPHIC METHODS OF EXAMINATION OF THE ANKLE

1. **Routine Anteroposterior View of the Ankle** (Fig. 5-63). The patient lies flat, with the toe pointing slightly medially. The central ray passes through the center of the talotibial joint. The lateral malleolus is partially obscured on this view, and the tarsal bones distal to the talus are not shown to good advantage.

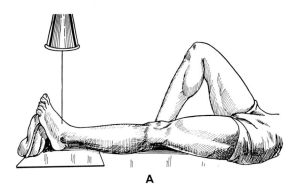

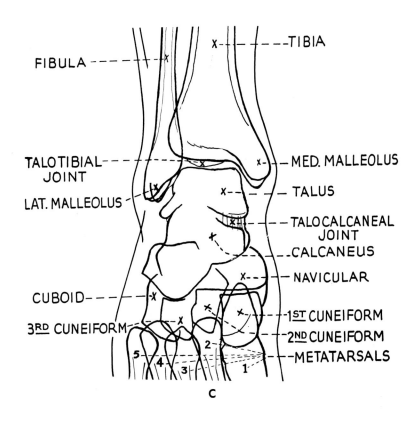

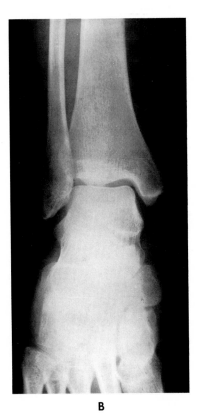

Figure 5-63. Routine anteroposterior view of the ankle. A. Method of positioning patient. B. Radiograph. C. Labeled tracing of B.

Points of Practical Interest with Reference to Figure 5-63

1. If less overlapping of the distal tibia and fibula is desired, the foot should be inverted slightly. This expedient will increase the clarity of the lateral malleolus particularly, but will interfere with the measurement of the distance between the talal articular margin and the malleoli.

2. In young individuals, in whom the distal epiphyses of the tibia and fibula are not yet united to their respective shafts, it is particularly important to obtain comparison films of the opposite normal side. Otherwise it may be very difficult to be certain about the absence of a slight fracture through the epiphyseal disk.

3. Although the ligaments around the ankle are not visualized radiographically, it is important to have an accurate knowledge of their relationships. Often the more important aspects of trauma and injury to the ankle concern abnormalities in the ligaments rather than in the bones.

2. **Routine Lateral View of the Ankle** (Fig. 5–64). The ankle is placed against the film so that the lateral malleolus is in the central ray. The foot is perpendicular to the film, and the two malleoli should be projected directly over one another. This view shows the lateral relation of the talotibial joint, the anterior and posterior lips of the medial malleolus, and the lateral malleolus through the medial.

3. **Oblique View of the Ankle** (Fig. 5–65). This view is illustrated in the accompanying diagram. Its main purpose is to show the lateral malleolus and tibiofibular joint to better advantage.

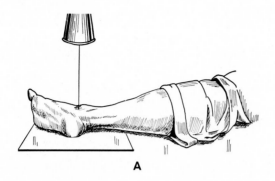

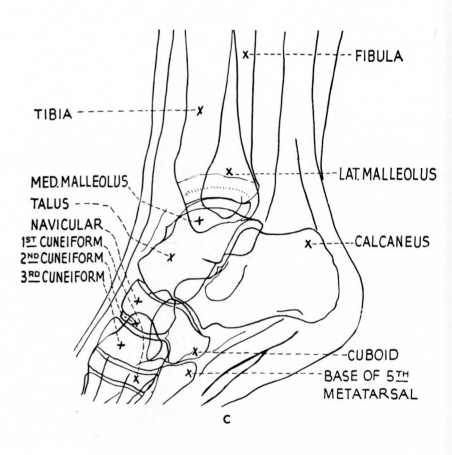

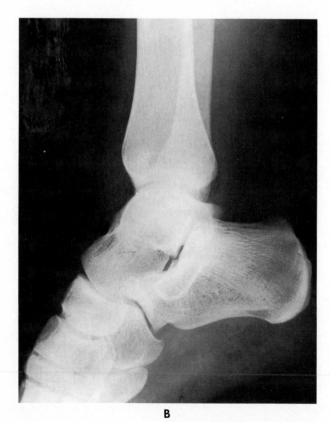

Figure 5–64. Routine lateral view of ankle. *A.* Method of positioning patient. *B.* Radiograph. *C.* Labeled tracing of *B.*

Points of Practical Interest with Reference to Figure 5–64

1. The affected leg and ankle are so placed that the sagittal plane of the leg is perfectly parallel with the table top and film. The film holder and central ray are centered to a point approximately 2 cm. proximal to the tip of the lateral malleolus. A sandbag or balsa wood block placed under the distal one-third of the foot facilitates true alignment.
2. The unaffected side is sharply flexed and placed in a comfortable position forward so that no movement will occur during the exposure of the film.

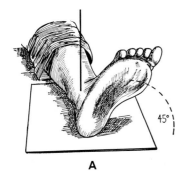

A

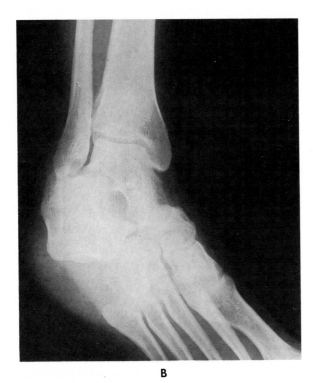

B

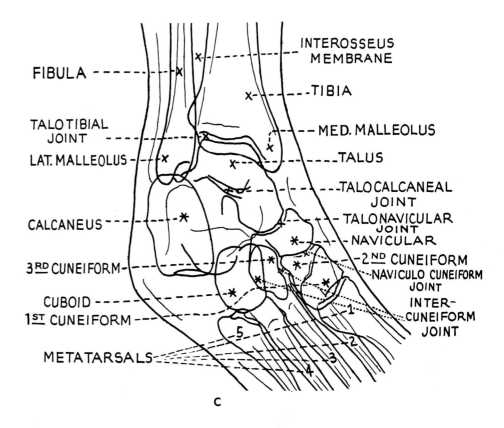

C

Figure 5–65. Oblique view of ankle. *A.* Method of positioning patient. *B.* Radiograph. *C.* Labeled tracing of *B.*

Points of Practical Interest with Reference to Figure 5–65

1. As much as possible, the leg should be kept in the anteroposterior position while the foot is inverted approximately 45 degrees. Immobilize the leg with sandbags placed across it and against the plantar surface of the foot.
2. The central ray is directed to the middle of the talotibial joint.
3. This view permits an unobstructed projection of the lateral malleolus and of the space between the talus and malleolus where so frequently injury may be manifest.

4. **Special Tangential View of the Calcaneus** (Fig. 5–66). This view demonstrates the posterior two-thirds of the calcaneus in excellent, though distorted, profile. Fracture of the body of the calcaneus and of its posterior aspect will be shown in this projection.

THE METATARSALS

Correlated Gross Anatomy. There are five metatarsal bones articulating with the tarsus behind and the phalanges in front. They are slightly convex on their dorsal and concave on their ventral aspects. The bases are wedge-shaped, and the heads semicircular. One each side of the head, there is a depression surmounted by a tubercle. The inferior surfaces of the heads are grooved to allow passage of the flexor tendons.

The first metatarsal is the shortest and thickest of the series, and the second metatarsal is the longest.

The fifth metatarsal articulates with the cuboid by means of a long triangular facet, which may on occasion be separate from the rest of the base as an ununited extra ossicle. Also, in younger people in whom this basilar epiphysis has not united with the shaft of the fifth metatarsal, differentiation from fracture may be difficult. A fracture line in this location is usually transverse, but the epiphyseal line is oblique.

A normal slight medial angulation of the first metatarsophalangeal joint may on occasion become excessive, in which case the abnormality of hallux valgus results. There is a bursa adjoining the head of the first metatarsal which is prone to become inflamed in this condition.

The Phalanges of the Foot. Except for the great toe, the three phalanges of each digit tend to be considerably smaller than

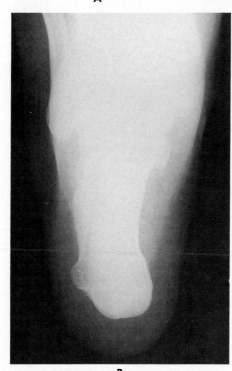

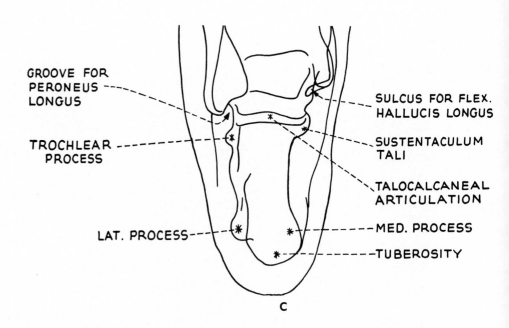

Figure 5–66. Special tangential view of calcaneus. *A.* Method of positioning patient. *B.* Radiograph. *C.* Labeled tracing of *B.*

Points of Practical Interest with Reference to Figure 5–66

1. The ankle is placed over the film so that the talotibial joint falls over the central portion of the film.
2. The plantar surface of the foot should be as near to right angles with the table top and film as possible in acute flexion.
3. The central ray should be centered to the midpoint of the film. It will usually enter the plantar surface at the level of the bases of the fifth metatarsals and emerge in the region of the upper tarsus.
4. Ordinarily all portions of the calcaneus between the tuberosity and the sustentaculum tali are included.
5. An alternate view may be obtained by placing the patient prone, the film perpendicular to the table top and in contact with the sole of the foot, and directing the central ray through the heel at an angle of 45 degrees caudad.

the phalanges of the hand. The great toe, like the thumb, has two phalanges which are usually moderately stout bones.

Since the toes tend to have a plantar curvature and concavity, the phalanges may be foreshortened and partially projected over one another in the radiographs. If one wishes to obtain accurate detail regarding the phalanges of the third, fourth, and fifth toes particularly, it is necessary to straighten the toes manually to obtain an undistorted, full-length view.

The phalanges of the foot are very small replicas of the phalanges of the hand, the structures of the two bearing close resemblance.

Sesamoid Bones of the Foot (Fig. 5–59). A pair of sesamoid bones which begin to ossify about the fifth year is constant under the metatarsophalangeal joint of the great toe in the tendons of the flexor hallucis brevis. Occasionally there are three sesamoid bones in this location, or one of them may be bivalved and appear fractured (bipartite sesamoids). Additional sesamoids occur over the interphalangeal joint of the great toe, the metatarsophalangeal joints of the second and fifth toes, and, less frequently, of the third and fourth.

The sesamoid and supernumerary bones of the foot are actually very numerous and the most common of these are illustrated in Figure 5–59.

Variations from the Normal

1. *Variations in the Sesamoid Bones.* Considerable variation may occur in size and shape of sesamoids, but always on the plantar aspect. The following sesamoids are seen regularly: two at the head of the first metatarsal; one at the head of the second; and one at the head of the fifth. Rarely, there are two at the head of the fifth metatarsal and one at the fourth. More rarely, a sesamoid is seen on the medial side of the head of the third metatarsal.

Bipartite and multipartite sesamoids occur, especially at the first metatarsal but elsewhere as well. A bipartite sesamoid is usually much larger than a normal or fractured one. A fractured sesamoid looks only slightly bigger than its counterpart on the opposite foot (Fig. 5–67).

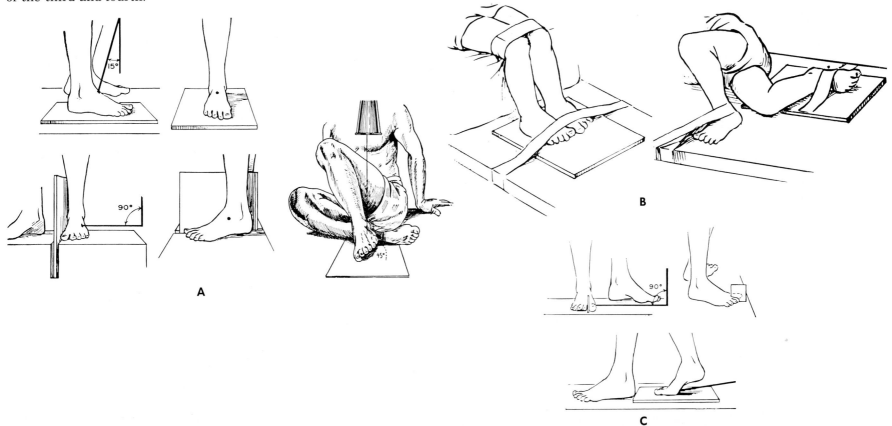

Figure 5–67. *A.* Standard projections of the foot. 1, Weight-supporting dorsoplantar view; 2, weight-supporting lateral view (film support as devised by Gamble and Yale); 3, recumbent oblique (dorsoplantar) projection. *B.* Special technique for dorsoplantar and lateral views of the feet in children (modified from Davis and Hatt). *C.* Special projections of the foot. *Upper,* Special lateral view of the great toe; *lower,* special axial projection for the ball of the foot and for the sesamoids (modified from Gamble and Yale). (*A, B,* and *C* from Meschan, I.: Sem. Roentgenol., 5:327–340, 1970. Reprinted by permission of Grune & Stratton, Inc.)

2. *Variations in the Shape of the Phalanges.* The proximal phalanx tends to be more regular in outline than the middle and terminal phalanges. Marked underdevelopment of the terminal phalanges is common except for the great toe, although it too may vary in shape. A conical or bell-shaped epiphysis, which may occur in the proximal phalanges of the second to the fourth toes, is illustrated in Figure 5–68 (Laurent and Brombart, quoted from Köhler and Zimmer).

3. *Variations of Individual Bones* (Köhler and Zimmer; Pirie; Willis). Many of these variations are illustrated in Figure 5–69. (1) Single or multiple synostoses between adjacent margins of the calcaneus, cuboid, talus, navicular, and metatarsals are common. (2) Periostitis along the diaphysis of the fifth metatarsal will at times be simulated by overlapping of the plantar and dorsal edges at the lateral wall of the first metatarsal bone, which in this region arches moderately inward. (3) The sustentaculum tali may be unduly prominent on the medial border of the os calcis. (4) The trochlear process of the os calcis may appear as a separate ossicle or apophysis. (5) The "secondary calcaneus" may be fused with the anterior articular surface of the calcaneus, producing a

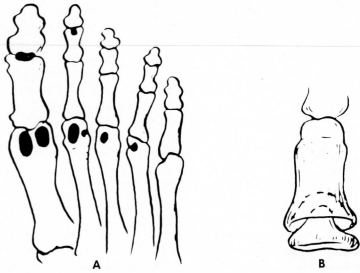

Figure 5–68. *A.* The most frequent sesamoids of the foot (modified from Köhler and Zimmer). *B.* Conical or bell-shaped epiphysis. According to Laurent and Brombart, they occur in the proximal phalanges of the second to the fourth toes. (From Meschan, I.: Sem. Roentgenol., 5:327–340, 1970. Reprinted by permission of Grune & Stratton, Inc.)

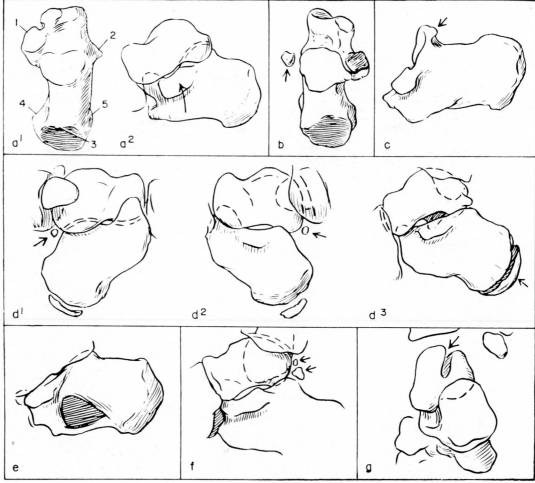

Figure 5–69 continued on opposite page.

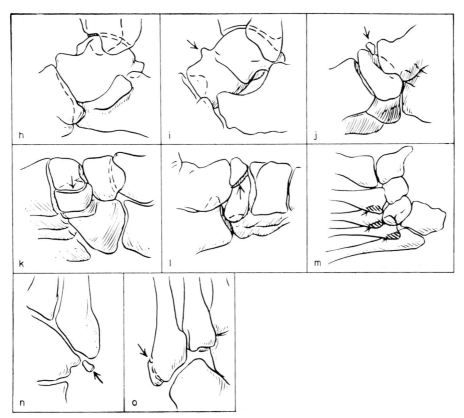

Figure 5–69 *Continued.* Variations of individual bones of the foot. a¹. Normal os calcis: (1) sustentaculum tali; (2) trochlear process; (3) tuberosity; (4) medial process; and (5) lateral process, a². Unduly prominent sustentaculum tali on the medial border of the os calcis (arrow). b. The trochlear process of the os calcis as a separate ossicle or apophysis. c. Secondary calcaneus fused with the anterior articular surface of the calcaneus and having a swallow tail prominence. This usually articulates with the talus and the cuboid. d, Variations in the appearance of the calcaneal epiphysis (arrow in d³). The arrows in d¹ and d² point to a small os trigonum. e. Cystlike appearance within the trabecular pattern of the os calcis due to locally increased spongy architecture. f. Bipartite os trigonum (arrows). g. Cleft talus (from DeCuveland). h. Spur on the anterior superior aspect of the talus near its anterior articular margin, producing a "turned-up" appearance. i. The talar beak (arrow), an irregular spur on the upper margin of the talus, reported especially in athletes. j. Os supranaviculare. Generally, this small bone coalesces with the navicular. k. Bipartite first cuneiform bone (arrow). l. Bipartite navicular bone (arrow). m. Normal radiolucencies at the base of the third, fourth, and fifth metatarsal bones (arrows) due to indentation and overlap. n. The os vesalianum, located in the angle between the cuboid and the tuberosity of the fifth metatarsal (arrow), may be mistaken for a fracture. o. An apophysis at the base of the fifth metatarsal (arrow) may simulate a fracture. (Modified from Kohler and Zimmer. Reprinted from Meschan, I.: Sem. Roentgenol. 5:327–340, 1970. Reprinted by permission of Grune & Stratton, Inc.)

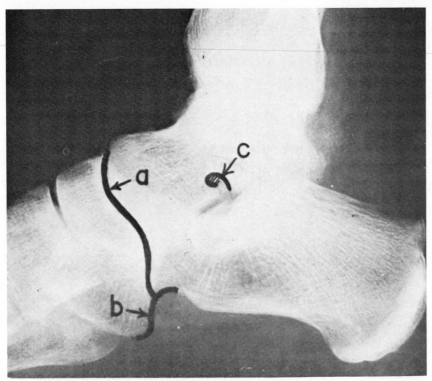

Figure 5-70. Normal design of the medial and lateral forefoot. The midtarsal joint line (*a*). Continuous line relationship between os calcis and cuboid (*b*). Sinus tarsi (*c*). (From Meschan, I.: Sem. Roentgenol., 5:327–340, 1970. Reprinted by permission of Grune & Stratton, Inc.)

swallowtail prominence on the superior aspect of this bone. Usually, however, it articulates with the talus and the cuboid. (6) There may be a cystlike appearance within the trabecular pattern of the os calcis caused by locally increased spongy architecture. (7) The os trigonum may appear bipartite. (8) The talus may have a cleft within it. (9) There may be a spur on the anterosuperior aspect of the talus near its anterior articular margin, producing a "turned up" appearance. (10) There may be a tailor beak, an irregular spur on the upper margin of the talus, especially in athletes. (11) The navicular tarsal bone may appear bipartite. (12) There are often radiolucencies at the bases of the third, fourth, and fifth metatarsal due to indentation and overlap. (13) There may be an apophysis at the base of the fifth metatarsal which may simulate a fracture (Fig. 5–69).

Important Anatomic Angles and Interrelationships of the Bones of the Foot (Figs. 5–70 to 5–76). It has been common practice to refer to the foot arches as longitudinal and transverse. It is probably best, however, to be much more specific in defining configuration and alterations of the foot. The longitudinal arch extends between the calcaneus and the heads of the metatarsals, while the transverse arch is situated under the metatarsals and is supported medially and laterally by the first and fifth metatar-

sals, respectively. Weight-bearing films are necessary to demonstrate these arches.

Figure 5–70 demonstrates the normal structure of the medial and lateral forefoot in a properly positioned lateral view of the foot. The midtarsal joint line A forms a continuous line on the anterior aspect of the talus and the posterior aspect of the cuboid. The *sinus tarsi* normally represents an important functional component in the interrelationships of foot stress, and radiographically, it is an index of a normal position for the calcaneus and talus (Gamble and Yale).

Likewise, on a satisfactory lateral projection of the foot the *sustentaculum tali,* the *lateral tuberosity of the calcaneus,* and the *groove on the cuboid for the perineus longus* muscle should be readily identifiable (Fig. 5–71).

The *calcaneal pitch* (Fig. 5–72) is an index of the height of the foot framework. It is considered low when it is between 10 and 20 degrees; medium, between 20 and 30 degrees; and high, greater than 30 degrees. The calcaneal pitch is obviously a better reference measurement than the so-called longitudinal arch.

The *diagonal axis of the talus* as shown in Figure 5–72 *B* is also a fair indicator of the proper relationship of the talus to the os calcis. Normally it is horizontal or nearly so.

The *length patterns of the metatarsal bones* have specific ratios to each other. The first metatarsal is usually shorter than the second, which is the longest. The third metatarsal is also shorter than the second. The fourth is shorter than the third, and the fifth is shorter than the fourth. Ordinarily, the second, third and fourth metatarsal shafts are approximately the same width in the dorsoplantar view. A *metatarsal distal joint angle* drawn as shown in Figure 5–73 measures approximately 135 degrees.

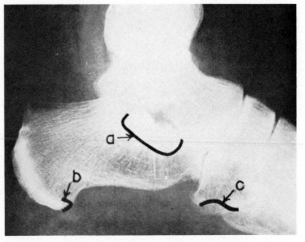

Figure 5-71. The sustentaculum tali (*a*), lateral tuberosity of the calcaneus (*b*), and the groove on the cuboid (*c*) for the peroneus longus muscle. These elements should be identifiable when relationships are normal. (From Meschan, I.: Sem. Roentgenol., 5:327–340, 1970. Reprinted by permission of Grune & Stratton, Inc.)

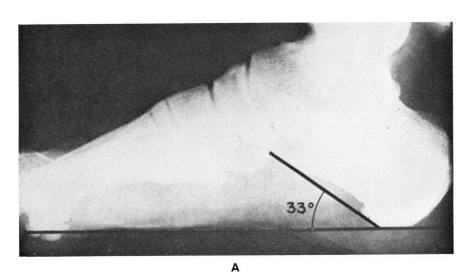
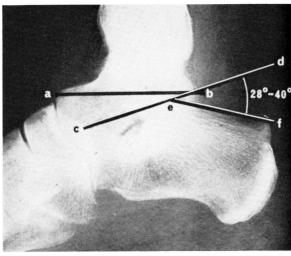

A   B

Figure 5–72. *A.* The calcaneal pitch is an index of the height of the foot framework. In this instance, the pitch is high since it exceeds 30 degrees. *B.* Boehler's critical angle of the os calcis; *cd* is drawn from the most superior anterior aspect of the os calcis to the joint space between the talus and the os calcis; *ef* is drawn from this joint to the most superior posterior point on the tuberosity of the os calcis. The diagonal axis of the talus (*ab*) is nearly horizontal. (From Meschan, I.: Sem. Roentgenol., 5:327–430, 1970. Reprinted by permission of Grune & Stratton, Inc.)

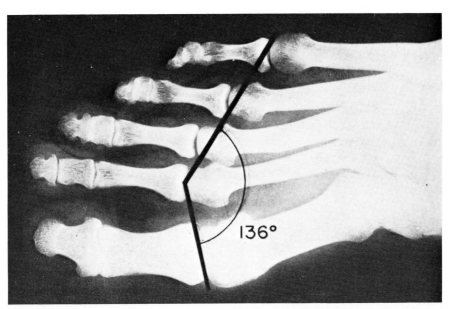

Figure 5–73. Length pattern of metatarsal bones. The first metatarsal is shorter than the second, which is the longest; the third metatarsal is shorter than the second; the fourth is shorter than the third; and the fifth is shorter than the fourth. Ordinarily, the second, third, and fourth metatarsal shafts are approximately the same width in the dorsoplantar view. (From Meschan, I.: Sem. Roentgenol., 5:327–340, 1970. Reprinted by permission of Grune & Stratton, Inc.)

In the dorsoplantar view (Fig. 5–74) there are other interesting relationships: note the line drawn from the center of the calcaneus to the medial aspect of the head of the third metatarsal. This may be considered the *midline of the foot*. The *midaxis of the talus* forms an angle with this line of approximately 15 degrees. Note also the "*sine wave*" formed by the midtarsal joint line AB. It ordinarily is bisected by the midline of the foot. When the midline is drawn as in Figure 5–74 B, there is a relatively perpendicular relationship to the transverse axis of the navicular (CD), and an angle of approximately 15 degrees is formed with the longitudinal axis of the first metatarsal.

In the lateral projection the usual tarsometatarsal relationships are indicated in Figure 5–75. The superior surfaces of the talus, navicular, and first cuneiform tend to form a fairly straight line (line AB). The inferior surfaces of the navicular and first cuneiform also tend to form a straight line (line CD), parallel to AB. The cuneiform-metatarsal joint (lines EF and GH) is almost perpendicular to lines AB and CD. The degree of its obliquity from the horizontal depends on the angular relationship of the long axis of the talus to the calcaneal pitch.

The *talocalcaneal angle* in the dorsoplantar view in children usually measures 20 to 40 degrees (Fig. 5–76). The line through the axis of the talus points to the head of the first metatarsal, while the axial line of the os calcis points to the fourth metatarsal. When these two lines are extended they generally pass through the midshafts of these metatarsals. The longitudinal axes of the second, third, and fourth metatarsals are nearly parallel.

The *midtalar and midcalcaneal lines* in the lateral view meet near the anterior margin of the cuboid, forming an acute angle. The midtalar line, when extended, coincides with the midaxis of the shaft of the first metatarsal.

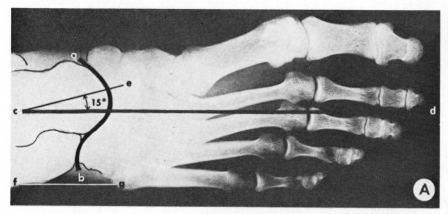 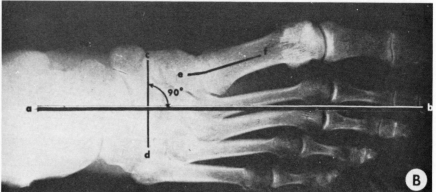

Figure 5–74. Relationships of the midline of the foot in the dorsoplantar view. *A.* The midline of the foot is represented by *cd* (see text); *dce* indicates a normal angle of approximately 15 degrees with the midaxis of the talus. The lateral border of the foot (*fg*) is parallel to *cd*. The partial sine wave curve formed by the midtarsal joint line (*ab*) is bisected by *cd*. *B.* The midline is represented by *ab*. There is a perpendicular relationship to the transverse axis of the navicular (*cd*), and an angle of approximately 15 degrees with the longitudinal axis of the first metatarsal (*ef*). (From Meschan, I.: Sem. Roentgenol., 5:327–340, 1970. Reprinted by permission of Grune & Stratton, Inc.)

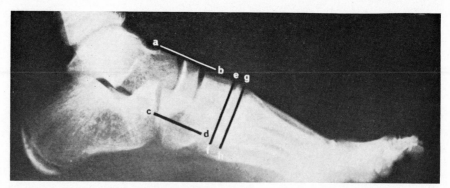

Figure 5–75. Tarsometatarsal relationships in the lateral projection. The superior surfaces of the talus, navicular, and first cuneiform tend to form a fairly straight line (*ab*). The inferior surfaces of the navicular and first cuneiform also tend to form a straight line, *cd*, parallel to *ab*. The cuneiform-metatarsal joints (*ef* and *gh*) are almost perpendicular to *ab* and *cd*. The degree of their obliquity with respect to the horizontal depends on the angular relationship of the long axis of the talus to the calcaneal pitch. (From Meschan, I.: Sem. Roentgenol., 5:327–340, 1970. Reprinted by permission of Grune & Stratton, Inc.)

The *longitudinal arch* is an obtuse angle, apex cephalad, formed by lines along the inferior margin of the os calcis and the inferior cortex of the fifth metatarsal.

The *talocalcaneal angle* in the dorsoplantar projection varies in normal children from 15 to 50 degrees and is age-dependent (Templeton et al.). In infants and young children, the talocalcaneal angle ranges from 30 to 50 degrees. There is a progressive decrease in this angle up to the age of 5, after which the angle seems to level off with respect to age. In children over 5, the talocalcaneal angle varies from 15 to 30 degrees. In the lateral view, the midtalar, midcalcaneal angle varies normally from 25 to 50 degrees. The obtuse angle on the plantar aspect of the foot ranges between 150 and 175 degrees and is not age-dependent as is the talocalcaneal angle.

A line drawn through the central long axis of the talus passes longitudinally through the shaft of the first metatarsal on the lateral weight-bearing roentgenogram in children over 5 years; but in infants and young children, the talus is positioned more vertically, and the midtalar line passes inferior to the shafts of the first metatarsals.

Growth and Development Changes in the Foot. The main shafts of the metatarsals are ossified at birth, and the epiphysis for the base of the first and the heads of the others appear at approximately 2 years in females and 3 years in males, fusing at approximately 15 to 18 years respectively (see Chapter 3). The base of each of the phalanges ossifies from separate centers of ossification which appear at 2 years in females and approximately 3 years in males, fusing at about 15 and 18 years respectively (Fig. 5–77) (see Chapter 3 for accurate tabular details).

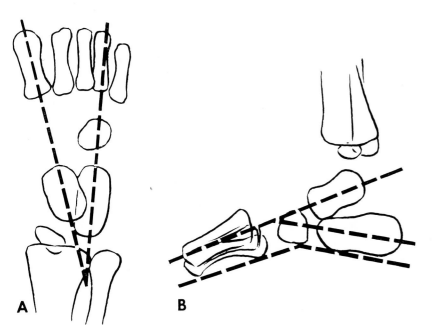

A   **B**

Figure 5–76. Talocalcaneal angle in the dorsoplantar (*A*) and lateral (*B*) views in children. (From Davis, L. A., and Hatt, W. S.: Radiology, 64:818, 1955.)

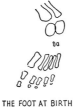

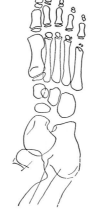

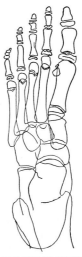

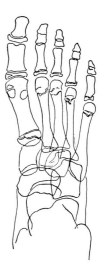

Figure 5–77. Changes in growth and development as seen in the foot.

THE FOOT AT BIRTH

THE FOOT AT 5 YEARS

THE FOOT AT 8 YEARS   THE FOOT AT 16 YEARS

RADIOGRAPHIC METHODS OF EXAMINATION OF THE
TARSUS AND FOOT

1. **Anteroposterior View of the Foot** (Fig. 5–78).
2. **Lateral View of the Foot** (Fig. 5–79).
3. **Oblique View of the Foot** (Fig. 5–80). These projections
are designed to show the tarsus as well as the metatarsals and

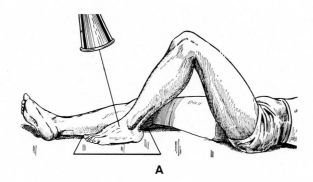

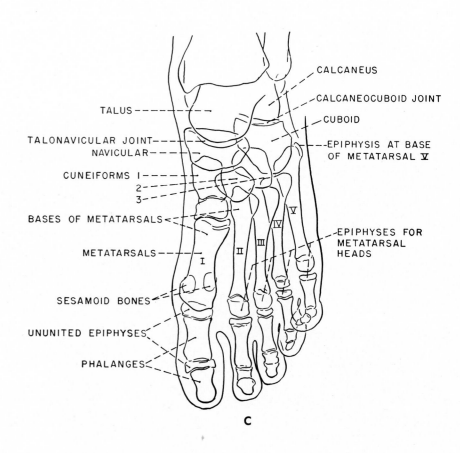

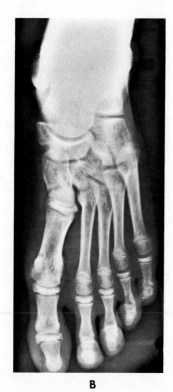

Figure 5–78. Anteroposterior view of the foot. A, Method of positioning patient.
B, Radiograph. C, Labeled tracing of B.

Points of Practical Interest with Reference to Figure 5–78

1. It will be noted that for visualization of the entire tarsus, both this view and
   the anteroposterior view of the ankle (Fig. 5–63) are necessary. The talus is
   not shown to good advantage in this projection, whereas the more distal tarsal
   bones are not presented clearly in the anteroposterior view of the ankle.
2. This view may also be required if the patient is unable to stand and bear his
   weight.

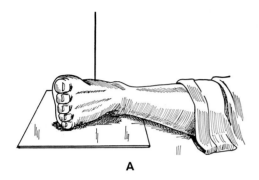

A

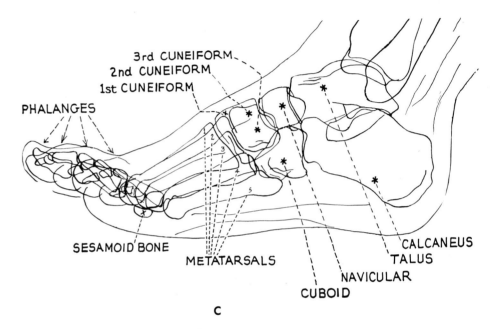

C

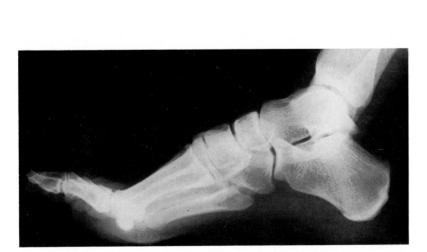

B

Figure 5–79. Lateral view of the foot. *A*, Method of positioning patient. *B*, Radiograph. *C*, Labeled tracing of *B*.

Points of Practical Interest with Reference to Figure 5–79

1. The knee may be elevated slightly on a sandbag so that the sagittal plane of the foot is perfectly parallel with the table top and film. The center of the tarsus is placed over the center of the film.

2. The ankle is immobilized by means of a sandbag.

3. The recumbent position is especially useful for showing the bony structure. If a view of the longitudinal arch under weight-bearing conditions is desired, an erect film with the patient standing is obtained using a similar technique.

4. If it is desired to obtain a coned-down lateral view of the body of the calcaneus, the foot is positioned similarly, but the central ray passes through the central portion of the calcaneus rather than through the center of the tarsus. This view of the calcaneus is particularly valuable for demonstration of Boehler's critical angle (see text).

phalanges of the foot. The exposure factors will vary slightly, depending upon whether it is desired to show the phalanges or the tarsus to best advantage. The accompanying diagrams show the positions in which these views are obtained. The lateral view is frequently obtained in the standing position, particularly if one is interested in demonstrating the integrity of the longitudinal arch. Occasionally coned-down films of the great toe may be obtained, since it is so frequently the area of major interest. The oblique view of the foot is of more value than the lateral, since the configuration of the metatarsal bones and phalanges is obscured in the latter, owing to the fact that they are projected over one another.

ANGIOLOGY OF THE LOWER EXTREMITY—BASIC ANATOMY

Arteries

Introduction. The abdominal aorta terminates by dividing into two *common iliac arteries*. These arteries arise opposite the left aspect of the fourth lumbar vertebra, and each of them terminates opposite the lumbosacral articulation by bifurcating into (a) an *external iliac artery* which continues to the lower extremity, and (b) an *internal iliac artery* which descends into the minor

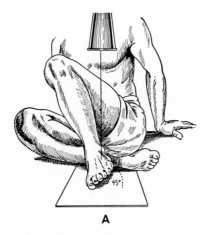

A

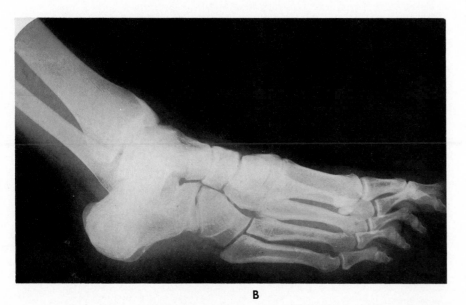

B

Figure 5–80. Oblique view of the foot. *A,* Method of positioning patient. *B,* Radiograph. *C,* Labeled tracing of B.

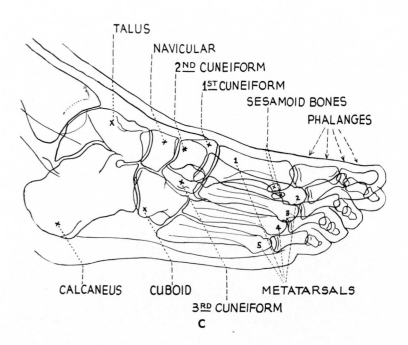

C

Points of Practical Interest with Reference to Figure 5–80

1. This view is particularly valuable (a) to demonstrate the intertarsal joints; (b) to outline the various tarsal bones more clearly; and (c) to demonstrate the joint between the tarsus and the fourth and fifth metatarsals as well as the structural detail of the base of the fifth metatarsal.
2. This oblique projection is employed when structural detail of the bones of the foot is of paramount interest. It is ordinarily obtained in combination with the anteroposterior projection of the foot. When, however, a foreign body must be localized accurately, the true lateral projection of the foot is employed instead of this oblique projection.

pelvis. Since the external iliac artery is the branch primarily involved with the lower extremity it may be considered at this point in the text. The other branches will be discussed in relation to the abdomen and its viscera.

At the inferior margin of the inguinal ligament, midway between the anterior superior iliac spine and the pubic symphysis,

the external iliac artery passes into the thigh and thereafter is called the femoral artery (Fig. 5–81).

The branches of the *external iliac artery* are: the *inferior epigastric*, the *deep circumflex iliac*, and several *small and variable branches to the psoas muscle* and adjoining lymph nodes.

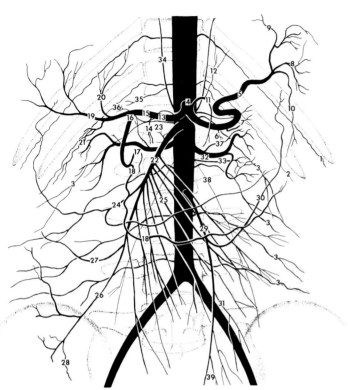

Figure 5–81. Legend:*

1. Intercostal
2. Subcostal
3. Lumbar
4. Celiac trunk
5. Splenic
6. Dorsal pancreatic
7. Pancreatica magna
8. Terminal branches of splenic
9. Short gastric
10. Left gastroepiploic
11. Left gastric
12. Esophageal branches of left gastric
13. Common hepatic
14. Right gastric
15. Hepatic proper
16. Gastroduodenal
17. Superior pancreaticoduodenal
18. Right gastroepiploic
19. Right branch of hepatic proper (Right hepatic)
20. Left branch of hepatic proper (Left hepatic)
21. Cystic
22. Superior mesenteric
23. Inferior pancreaticoduodenal

24. Middle colic
25. Intestinal
26. Ileocolic
27. Right colic
28. Appendicular
29. Inferior mesenteric
30. Left colic
31. Sigmoid
32. Renal
33. Accessory renal
34. Phrenic (Inferior phrenic)
35. Superior suprarenal
36. Middle suprarenal
37. Inferior suprarenal
38. Testicular (Internal spermatic) or Ovarian
39. Superior rectal (Superior hemorrhoidal)
40. Superior sacral
41. Common iliac
42. External iliac
43. Inferior epigastric
44. Deep iliac circumflex (Deep circumflex iliac)
45. Internal iliac (Hypogastric)
46. Iliolumbar

47. Lateral sacral
48. Superior gluteal
49. Inferior gluteal
50. Internal pudendal
51. Middle rectal (Middle hemorrhoidal)
52. Obturator
53. Uterine
54. Inferior vesical
55. Superficial epigastric
56. Femoral (Common femoral)
57. External pudendal
58. Profunda femoris (Deep femoral)
59. Femoral (Superficial femoral)
60. Perforating
61. Superficial iliac circumflex
    (Superficial circumflex iliac)
62. Medial femoral circumflex
    (Medial circumflex femoral)
63. Lateral femoral circumflex
    (Lateral circumflex femoral)
64. Ascending branch of lateral femoral circumflex
65. Descending branch of lateral femoral circumflex

*Anatomic terms are based on Nomina Anatomica (N.A.) with two exceptions: *intestinal* (no. 25) is employed as a combining form for the jejunal and iliac arteries. *Accessory renal* (no. 33) occurs with sufficient frequency to warrant its inclusion. Commonly used synonyms are indicated parenthetically.

(From Muller, R. F., Figley, M. M., Rogoff, S. M., and DeWeese, V. A.: Arteries of the lower extremity. Used by permission of Eastman Kodak Company, Radiography Markets Division, Rochester, New York.)

The collateral circulation for the external iliac artery (in case of thrombosis or obstruction) is illustrated by Figure 5–82.

The *femoral artery* is the continuation of the external iliac artery and represents the main blood supply to the extremities.

Femoral Artery.   The course and main branches of the femoral artery are indicated in Figure 5–83. At its termination it lies close to the medial side of the femur. Its major branches lie in the proximal one-third of the thigh, where it is rather superficially placed.

The *adductor canal* extends distally from the middle third of the thigh. The canal terminates at the adductor hiatus and transmits the femoral artery from the middle third of the thigh, containing, in addition, the femoral vein, the saphenous nerve, and the nerve to the vastus medialis muscle.

The branches of the femoral artery assume special importance in the event of thrombosis or obstruction of the femoral artery in any of its sectors. The largest branch of the femoral artery is the *deep femoral.* It finally perforates the great adductor muscle and terminates in branches to the lower portion of the hamstring muscles.

The branches of the *deep femoral* are: the *medial femoral circumflex,* the *lateral femoral circumflex,* and the *perforating and muscular branches.*

Popliteal Artery.   The *popliteal artery* is the continuation of the femoral artery through the popliteal fossa. It extends from the adductor hiatus at the junction of the middle and distal thirds of the thigh to the lower border of the popliteal muscle, where it terminates by dividing into *anterior and posterior tibial arteries.* The tibial nerve and popliteal vein accompany the popliteal artery, the tibial nerve being the most superficial of the structures found in the popliteal fossa.

Various arterial anastomoses around the right knee joint are shown in Figure 5–84.

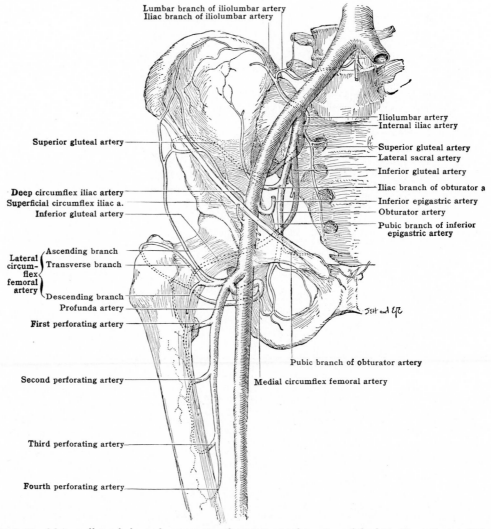

Figure 5–82.   Major collateral channels connecting the arteries in the region of the hip. (From Anson, B. J. (ed.): Morris' Human Anatomy, 12th ed. Copyright © 1966 by McGraw-Hill, Inc. Used by permission of McGraw-Hill Book Company.)

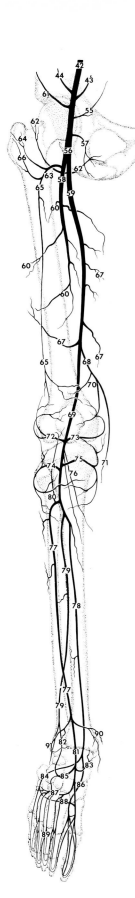

Figure 5–83.   Legend:*

42. External iliac
43. Inferior epigastric
44. Deep iliac circumflex (Deep circumflex iliac)
45. Internal iliac (Hypogastric)
46. Iliolumbar
47. Lateral sacral
48. Superior gluteal
49. Inferior gluteal
50. Internal pudendal
51. Middle rectal (Middle hemorrhoidal)
52. Obturator
53. Uterine
54. Inferior vesical
55. Superficial epigastric
56. Femoral (Common femoral)
57. External pudendal
58. Profunda femoris (Deep femoral)
59. Femoral (Superficial femoral)
60. Perforating
61. Superficial iliac circumflex
    (Superficial circumflex iliac)

62. Medial femoral circumflex
    (Medial circumflex femoral)
63. Lateral femoral circumflex
    (Lateral circumflex femoral)
64. Ascending branch of lateral femoral
    circumflex
65. Descending branch of lateral femoral
    circumflex
66. Transverse branch of lateral femoral
    circumflex
67. Muscular branches of femoral and
    profunda femoris
68. Descending genicular (Supreme genicular)
69. Popliteal
70. Articular branch of descending genicular
71. Saphenous branch of descending genicular
72. Superior lateral genicular
73. Superior medial genicular
74. Inferior lateral genicular
75. Inferior medial genicular
76. Sural

77. Anterior tibial
78. Posterior tibial
79. Peroneal (Fibular)
80. Anterior tibial recurrent
    (Recurrent anterior tibial)
81. Dorsalis pedis
82. Perforating branch of peroneal
83. Medial tarsal
84. Lateral plantar
85. Lateral tarsal
86. Medial plantar
87. Arcuate
88. Deep plantar branch of dorsalis pedis
89. Dorsal metatarsal, plantar metatarsal,
    dorsal digital, and plantar digital
90. Medial anterior malleolar
91. Lateral anterior malleolar

*Anatomic terms are based on Nomina Anatomica (N.A.) with one exception. The term *muscular branches of femoral and profunda femoris* (no. 67) has been included because these branches are often observed in arteriograms of the lower extremities. Commonly used synonyms are indicated parenthetically, and the N.A. term *fibular*, accepted by the Sixth International Congress of Anatomists as an alternative for *peroneal* (no. 79), is shown in brackets.

(From Muller, R. F., Figley, M. M., Rogoff, S. M., and DeWeese, V. A.: Arteries of the lower extremity. Used by permission of Eastman Kodak Company, Radiography Markets Division, Rochester, New York.)

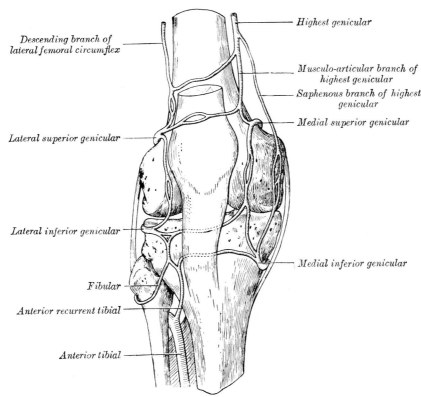

Highest genicular

Descending branch of lateral femoral circumflex

Musculo-articular branch of highest genicular

Saphenous branch of highest genicular

Medial superior genicular

Lateral superior genicular

Lateral inferior genicular

Medial inferior genicular

Fibular

Anterior recurrent tibial

Anterior tibial

Figure 5–84.   Circumpatellar anastomosis. (From Gray's Anatomy of the Human Body, 29th ed., Goss, C. M. (ed.) Philadelphia, Lea & Febiger, 1973.)

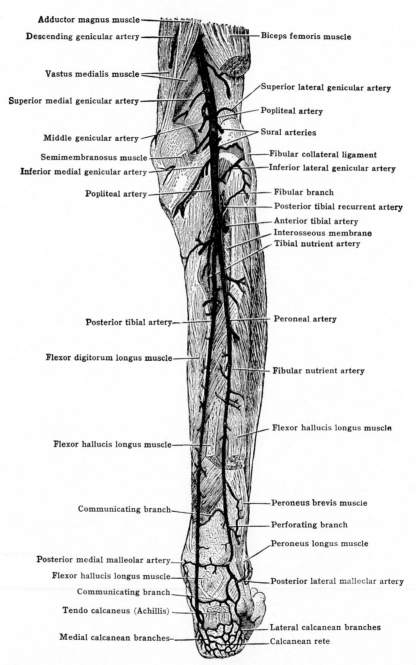

Adductor magnus muscle

Descending genicular artery

Biceps femoris muscle

Vastus medialis muscle

Superior lateral genicular artery

Superior medial genicular artery

Popliteal artery

Middle genicular artery

Sural arteries

Semimembranosus muscle

Fibular collateral ligament

Inferior medial genicular artery

Inferior lateral genicular artery

Popliteal artery

Fibular branch

Posterior tibial recurrent artery

Anterior tibial artery

Interosseous membrane

Tibial nutrient artery

Posterior tibial artery

Peroneal artery

Flexor digitorum longus muscle

Fibular nutrient artery

Flexor hallucis longus muscle

Flexor hallucis longus muscle

Peroneus brevis muscle

Communicating branch

Perforating branch

Peroneus longus muscle

Posterior medial malleolar artery

Flexor hallucis longus muscle

Posterior lateral malleolar artery

Communicating branch

Tendo calcaneus (Achillis)

Lateral calcanean branches

Medial calcanean branches

Calcanean rete

Figure 5–85.   The posterior tibial, popliteal, and peroneal arteries and their major branches (after Toldt). (From Anson, B. J. (ed.): Morris' Human Anatomy, 12th ed. Copyright © 1966 by McGraw-Hill, Inc. Used by permission of McGraw-Hill Book Company.)

The branches of the popliteal artery are: the *sural*, the *genicular*, and the *muscular*. As previously indicated, the popliteal artery continues into the leg as the anterior and posterior tibial artery.

Posterior Tibial Artery. The posterior tibial artery is usually the larger of the two terminating branches of the popliteal artery, extending distally into the leg between the superficial and deep muscles in the posterior compartment of the leg. As it passes distally it inclines to the medial side of the leg. It terminates by dividing into *medial* and *lateral plantar* arteries after traversing a middle path between the medial malleolus and the medial process of the tubercle of the calcaneus. *A line drawn from the center of the popliteal fossa to a spot midway between the medial malleolus and the point of the heel will ordinarily indicate its course.*

The main branches of the *posterior tibial artery* (Fig. 5–85) are the *fibular circumflex*, the *peroneal*, the *tibial nutrient*, the *communicating*, the *posterior medial malleolar*, and the *medial calcaneal*. There are also branches to the muscles of the leg.

Peroneal Artery (Fig. 5–85). The peroneal artery is also situated posteriorly, arising from the posterior tibial artery about 2½ cm. below the distal border of the popliteal muscle. It descends along the medial crest of the fibula and gives rise to a large perforating branch which reaches the anterior compartment of the leg. It also provides *posterior lateral malleolar* branches and terminates on the lateral surface of the calcaneal tubercle by breaking up into *lateral calcaneal branches.*

The branches of the *peroneal* artery are the *fibular nutrient*, the *communicating*, the *perforating*, the *posterior lateral malleolar*, and the *lateral calcaneal*, with numerous muscular and cutaneous branches in its immediate vicinity.

Anterior Tibial Artery (Fig. 5–86). The anterior tibial artery courses anteriorly between the two heads of origin of the posterior tibial muscle, above the proximal part of the interosseous membrane and into the anterior compartment of the leg. It runs distally as far as the anterior side of the ankle joint. Distal to the ankle joint it becomes the *dorsalis pedis artery. The course of the anterior tibial artery may be indicated by a line drawn from the front of the head of the fibula to a point midway between the two malleoli.*

It is accompanied in its course by the deep peroneal nerve and by accompanying veins. The branches of the anterior tibial artery are the *posterior tibial recurrent*, the *anterior tibial recurrent*, the *medial anterior malleolar*, the *lateral anterior malleolar*, and many muscular branches to the extensors of the toes and the anterior tibial muscle.

Plantar Arteries. There are lateral and medial plantar arteries which are formed by the terminal branches of the posterior tibial artery. These give rise to plantar metatarsal arteries and other smaller branches around the digits as shown in Figure 5–87.

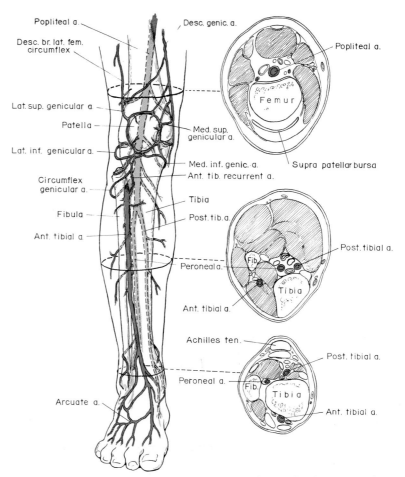

Figure 5–86. Three-dimensional perspective of the popliteal artery and its major branches, around the knee and terminally, as seen in arteriographic study.

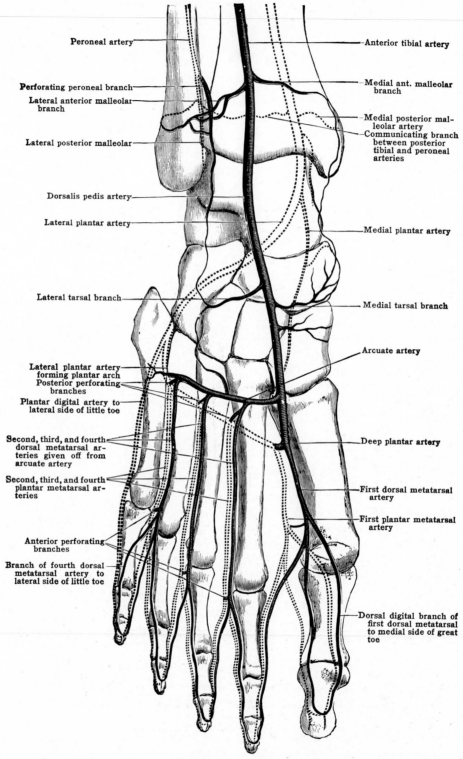

Peroneal artery

Perforating peroneal branch

Lateral anterior malleolar branch

Lateral posterior malleolar

Dorsalis pedis artery

Lateral plantar artery

Lateral tarsal branch

Lateral plantar artery forming plantar arch
Posterior perforating branches
Plantar digital artery to lateral side of little toe

Second, third, and fourth dorsal metatarsal arteries given off from arcuate artery

Second, third, and fourth plantar metatarsal arteries

Anterior perforating branches

Branch of fourth dorsal metatarsal artery to lateral side of little toe

Anterior tibial **artery**

Medial ant. malleolar branch

Medial posterior malleolar artery
Communicating branch between posterior tibial and peroneal arteries

Medial plantar **artery**

Medial tarsal **branch**

Arcuate artery

Deep plantar **artery**

First dorsal metatarsal artery

First plantar metatarsal artery

Dorsal digital branch of first dorsal metatarsal to medial side of **great** toe

Figure 5–87. Scheme of the distribution and anastomoses of the arteries of the right foot. *Dotted lines,* plantar arteries; *solid lines,* dorsal arteries. (After Walsham. Reprinted from Anson, B. J. (ed.): Morris' Human Anatomy, 12th ed. Copyright © 1966 by McGraw-Hill, Inc. Used by permission of McGraw-Hill Book Company.)

Dorsalis Pedis Artery (Fig. 5–87). This is the continuation of the anterior tibial artery. It extends from the ankle joint to the proximal end of the first interosseous space, where it divides into the *first dorsal metatarsal artery* and the *deep plantar artery*. The *deep plantar* joins the *lateral plantar* artery to complete the *plantar arch*.

The branches of the dorsalis pedis extend to the anterior aspect of the foot and the digits involving metatarsal and arcuate branches in this region.

Veins

Lower Extremity. There are two groups of veins of the inferior extremity (Fig. 5–88): superficial, and deep. Superficial veins merge chiefly into two main trunks: (1) the *great saphenous*, lying anteromedially, and (2) the *small saphenous*, lying posterolaterally. The great saphenous joins the *femoral vein;* the small saphenous joins either the *popliteal*, the *deep femoral*, or the *great saphenous vein.*

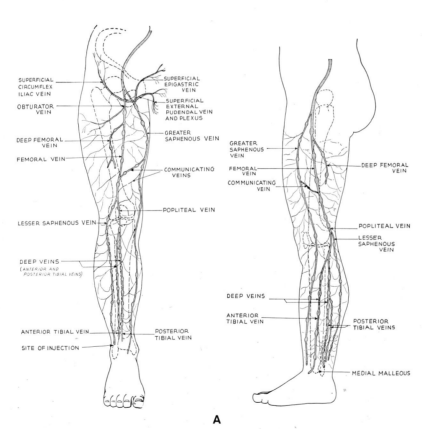

Figure 5–88. *A.* Diagram of the anatomy of conventional venograms of the leg. *Left,* Anteroposterior projection. *Right,* Lateral projection.

Figure 5–88 continued on opposite page.

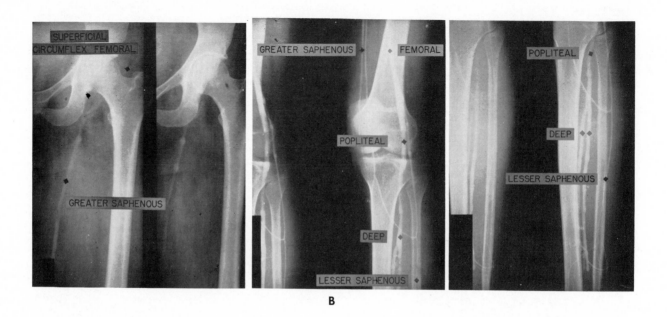

B

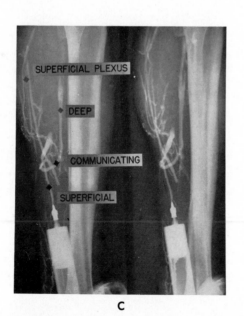

C

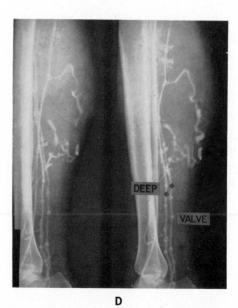

D

Figure 5–88 *Continued.* *B,* Representative conventional venograms of the lower extremity demonstrating primarily the lesser and greater saphenous veins and several deeper veins of leg and thigh. (Courtesy of Dr. E. C. Baker, Youngstown, Ohio.)
    C. Venograms of leg demonstrating the communicating veins joining superficial and deep veins. *D.* Venograms of deep veins of leg, showing their paired nature. (Courtesy of Dr. E. C. Baker, Youngstown, Ohio.)

Figure 5–88 continued on opposite page.

The deep veins accompany their corresponding arteries. There are numerous valves in all of the veins of the lower extremity—more numerous in the deep veins than in the superficial.

Pelvis. The major veins of the pelvis (Fig. 5–89) empty into either the *internal iliac (hypogastric) vein* (with the exception of the median sacral and the iliolumbar veins, which are tributaries of the common iliac veins) or the *testicular* or *ovarian veins*, which terminate in the *inferior vena cava* and the *left renal vein.*

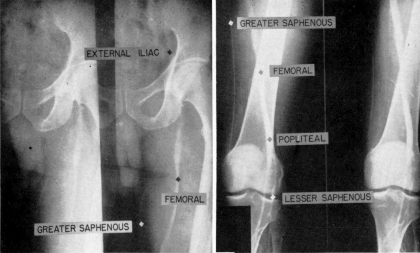

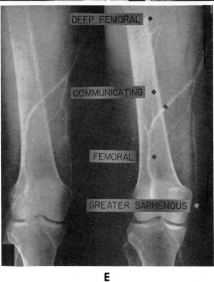

E

Figure 5–88 *Continued.* E. Venograms demonstrating the external iliac vein, and the femoral vein and its major tributaries. (Courtesy of Dr. E. C. Baker, Youngstown, Ohio.)

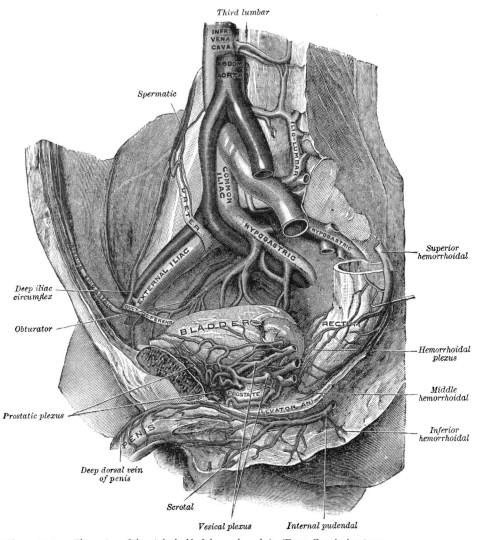

Figure 5–89. The veins of the right half of the male pelvis. (From Gray's Anatomy of the Human Body, 29th ed., Goss, C. M. (ed.) Philadelphia, Lea & Febiger, 1973.)

Lymphatic System

Introduction. Lymphatic capillaries are drained by thin, delicate lymphatic vessels which are richly distributed throughout the body (Fig. 5–90). The lymphatic vessels converge upon and unite into larger trunks (Fig. 5–91), emptying ultimately into the thoracic duct or directly into the great veins at the base of the neck. Intermittently, lymphatic vessels are interrupted by lymph nodes. These act as filtration stations where the lymph comes into intimate contact with the reticuloendothelial lymphoid and lymphocytic elements of the hematopoietic system. It would appear that it is the function of the lymphatic system to absorb interstitial fluid derived from blood plasma and to return it along with lymphocytes to the general circulation. There are abundant valves distributed throughout the lymphatic channels imparting to the lymphatics a rather beaded appearance. They tend to prevent the backward flow of lymph toward the capillaries

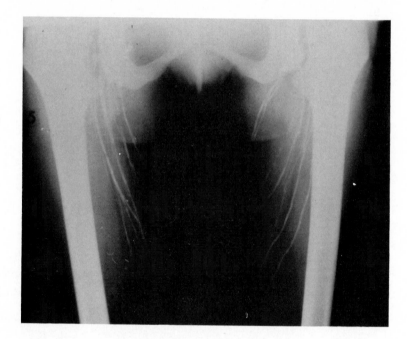

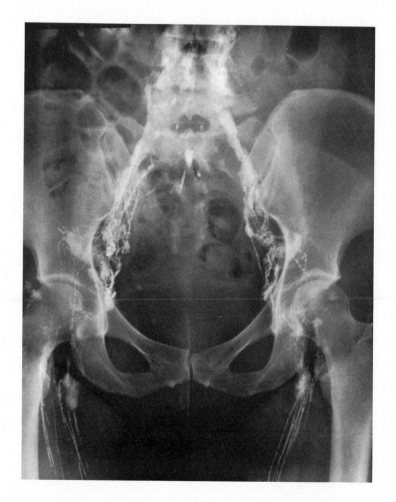

Figure 5–90. Radiograph demonstrating the superficial lymphatics of the thigh.

Figure 5–91. Lymphangiogram of groins and pelvis.

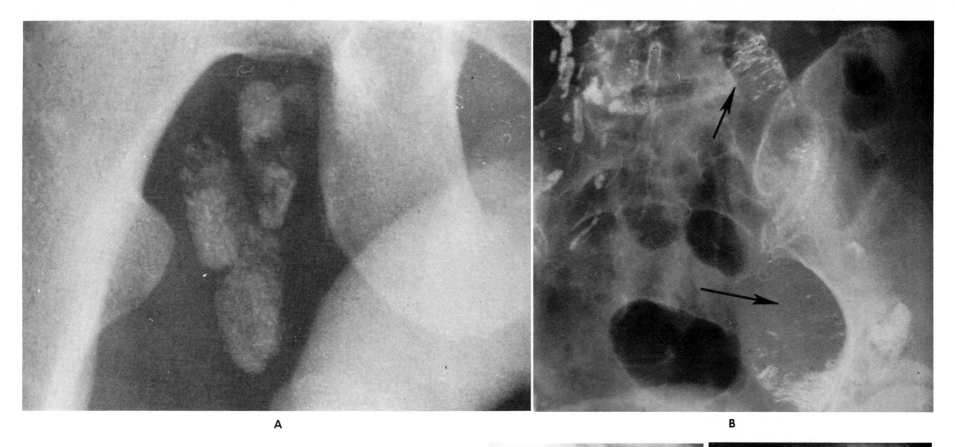

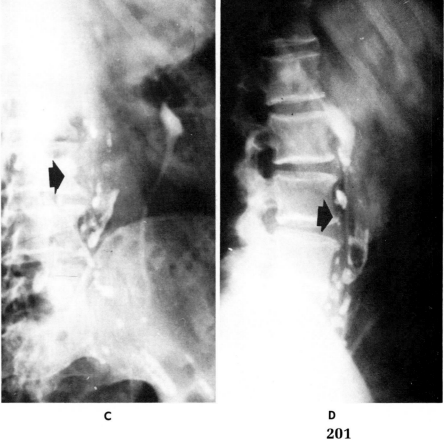

Figure 5–92. *A.* Magnified radiograph of a normal lymph node obtained after a lymph-angiogram. *B.* Lymph node in lymphadenitis from focal nephritis. *C* and *D.* Lymph nodes in lymphosarcoma for comparison with the normal.

and thus aid in directing the movement of the lymph toward the venous system.

Lymph nodes are generally ovoid structures varying considerably in size but not exceeding 3 cm. in any dimension (Fig. 5–92). They may be spherical or flattened on one or more sides in relation to some organs. Each node has a hilus where the arteries

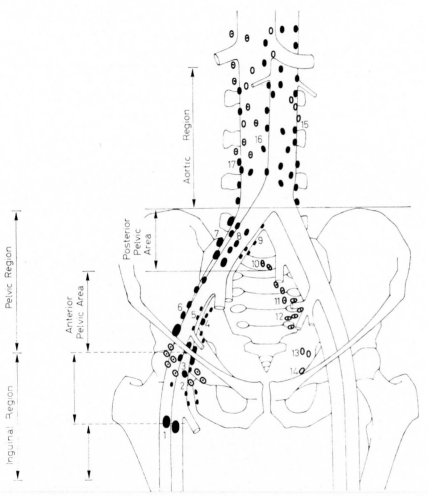

Figure 5–93. Topographic roentgen anatomy of the inguinal, iliac, and aortic lymph nodes (anteroposterior). *Inguinal lymph nodes:* 1, inferior superficial inguinal (subinguinal) lymph nodes; 2, superior superficial (crural group) and deep inguinal lymph node group; 3, superior superficial inguinal lymph nodes (perineal and genital group). *Pelvic lymph nodes:* 4, medial external iliac lymph nodes; 5, intermediate external iliac lymph nodes; 6, lateral external iliac lymph nodes; 7, lateral common iliac lymph nodes; 8, intermediate common iliac lymph nodes; 9, medial common iliac lymph nodes; 10, promontorial (subaortic) lymph nodes; 11, lateral sacral lymph nodes; 12, superior gluteal lymph nodes; 13, inferior gluteal lymph nodes; 14, obturator lymph nodes. *Aortic lymph nodes:* 15, left aortic lymph nodes; 16, preretroaortic lymph nodes; 17, right aortic lymph nodes. ●, Routinely demonstrated by lymphangiography; ⊙, facultatively demonstrated by lymphangiography. (From Fuchs, W. A. et. al.: Lymphography in Cancer. New York, Springer Verlag, 1969.)

enter and the veins and efferent lymphatics emerge. The radiographic structure of the follicles and cords making up the lymph nodes is characteristic; variations from this general structure are usually significant in respect to inflammatory or neoplastic processes which may be contained therein.

Lymph Nodes of the Lower Extremity (Fig. 5–93). There are three general groups of lymph nodes in the lower extremity: (1) the superficial inguinal, (2) the deep inguinal, and (3) the popliteal. The superficial inguinal are the most numerous – 10 to 20 in number – and they receive the subcutaneous drainage of the gluteal region, the external genitalia, the perineal region, and the anterior and lateral abdominal walls to the level of the umbilicus, as well as the entire superficial drainage of the lower extremity. All the efferent vessels from these nodes pass directly to the deep inguinal nodes, and some pass directly to the lower external iliac nodes.

The deep inguinal nodes number from one to three and lie medial to the femoral vein. They receive lymphatics from the penis, clitoris, and lower extremity and secondary drainage from the superficial inguinal node. Their efferent vessels lead to the external iliac nodes.

The popliteal nodes are deep within the popliteal fossa, receiving the anterior and posterior tibial lymph vessels and vessels coming from the knee joint proper. Efferent vessels from the popliteal nodes terminate in the deep inguinal nodes.

Additionally, there are lymphatics accompanying arteries and veins and occasionally inconstant nodes in the course of some of the vessels.

Lymph Vessels of the Lower Extremity. The collecting lymph vessels of the lower extremity form two main groups: (1) a medial group that follows the great saphenous vein and ends in the superficial inguinal nodes (Fig. 5–94), and (2) a lateral group that curves around to join the medial group partly in the leg and partly in the thigh. In addition, there are deep vessels following the course of the arteries in the lower extremity.

General Techniques of Lymphography. Most methods of lymphography are based on modifications of the classic lymphographic technique of Kinmouth (1952; 1955). First, a vital dye that is absorbed selectively by the lymphatic vessels is injected to identify small capillaries and lymphatics. Patent blue-violet is favored by Fisch. A superficial skin incision is then made in the immediate vicinity of a web space in the foot (or elsewhere on the body, as the case may be), and a lymphatic channel is carefully prepared so that it can be entered with a fine needle or a polyethylene micro tube. Ordinarily, the fine needle is used first to prepare the opening into the vessel for the introduction of the polyethylene tube. The oily contrast medium is then slowly injected with the aid of an electric pump or other device that permits a constant rate of flow.

Generally the pressure of the injection is adapted by the apparatus to the lymphatic vessels. Ethiodol, the contrast agent of

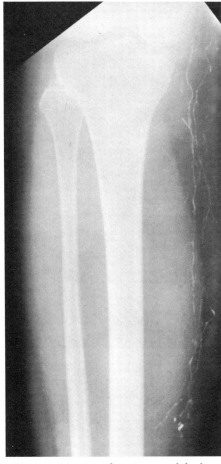

Figure 5–94. Lymphangiogram of the leg.

oblique films of the injected part are obtained. Radiographic examination is repeated 24 hours later (Fig. 5–95 *I, J*), usually in conjunction with an intravenous pyelogram. The emphasis in these later films is on nodal groups only, particularly of the groin, pelvis, and abdomen. The lymphatic vessels themselves are generally empty at that time and the lymph nodes can be seen to best advantage.

Pulmonary embolization may occur after lymphography of the extremities. A slight fever may appear in about 10 per cent of the patients for some hours in the evening of the day of the examination. Other complications include headache, sleeplessness, diarrhea, transitory deterioration of the general condition, abnormal taste sensations, and retrosternal burning.

The iodine released by the metabolism of Ethiodol may interfere with radioisotopic studies of the thyroid gland for years. If thyroid function studies are contemplated they should always be performed before lymphography.

Radiographic Correlation. The roentgenologic picture of a lymph node completely filled by Ethiodol shows a rather typical homogeneous stippling caused by droplets of the contrast agent that are retained in the sinuses (Fig. 5–92). There is ordinarily a sharp marginal outline on the shadow of the lymph node, which is round or bean-shaped. Ethiodol may be demonstrated in lymph nodes up to 3 years following lymphography, and there is a slow

choice,[1] is kept at a temperature of 37 degrees by a warming device built under the syringe holder in the pressure injector. The mean injection rate is .03 to .04 ml. per minute.

Approximately 5 ml. of Ethiodol is sufficient for an extremity, but the amount of contrast medium varies with weight, age, and body build of the patient.

After completing the injection, the microcatheter is removed. Usually, the lymph vessels need not be ligated since lymph fistulas are not apt to occur. The wound, however, is rinsed and closed in two layers. The patient is then transferred to the radiology department where anteroposterior, lateral, and often,

---

[1] Another contrast agent used in Europe is Ultra Fluid Lipiodol (Guerbet and Sons, St. Ouen, Paris). The iodine content of this agent (corresponding to Ethiodol in the United States) is 38 per cent, its density at 15 degrees C. is 1.28, and its viscosity is 0.6 poise. The LD_{50} for this agent injected intravenously is 2 ml. per kg. body weight (Guerbet, quoted in Fisch, p. 16).

	Mean (cm)	Standard Deviation
Size of nodes		
Normal	1.9	0.42
Abnormal	3.1	0.96
Proposed normal range: 2.6 cm or less		
Measurement A		
Normal	2.0	0.61
Abnormal	3.3	1.32
Proposed normal range: 3.0 cm or less		
Measurement B		
Normal	0.9	0.47
Abnormal	1.8	1.24
Proposed normal range: 2.0 cm or less		
Measurement C		
Normal	1.0	0.52
Abnormal	2.2	1.17
Proposed normal range: 2.0 cm or less		

A

Figure 5–95. A. Size and position of nodes in lymphoma. Each group had 60 normal and 60 abnormal cases. (From Abrams, H. L.: Angiography, 2nd ed. Vol. 2. Boston, Little, Brown & Co., 1971.)

Figure 5–95 continued on following page.

Size of nodes

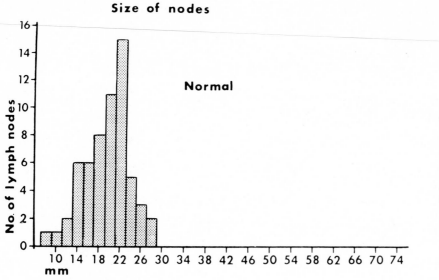

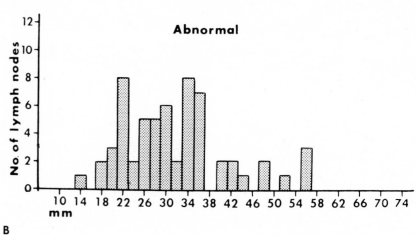

B

Measurement A

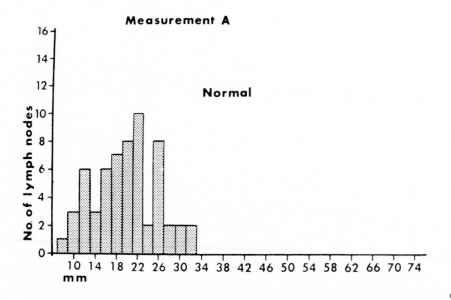

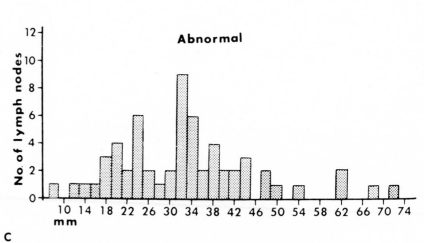

C

Figure 5–95 *Continued.*   B, Size of the lymph nodes in a graphic representation of 60 normal and 60 abnormal lymphangiograms. Mean values were 1.9 and 3.1 cm for the normal and abnormal groups with a standard deviation of 0.42 and 0.96, respectively. The diameters of 58 of 60 nodes were 2.6 cm or below. This is the proposed normal range for node size. C, Graphic representation of the anterior spine-to-node distances (measurement A) in 60 normal and 60 abnormal patients. This distance is the measurement on the cross-table lateral film from the anterior surface of the lumbar vertebral body at its mid-point to the anterior surface of the adjacent node group. The mean values in 60 normal and 60 abnormal studies were 2.0 cm and 3.3 cm with standard deviations of 0.61 and 1.31, respectively. When 3.0 cm was considered as the upper limit of normal, there were only 2 normal cases with a larger measurement. (From Abrams, H. L.: Angiography, vol. 2, 2nd ed. Boston, Little, Brown & Co., 1971.)

Figure 5–95 continued on opposite page.

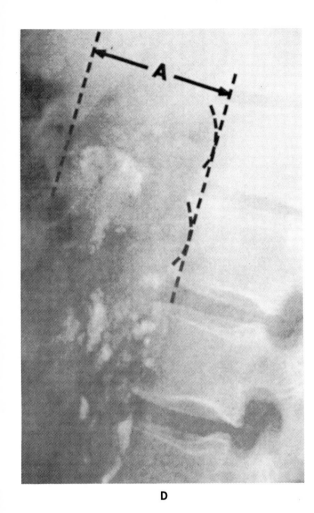

D

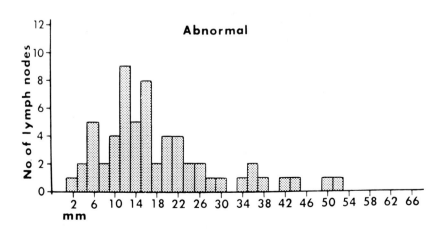

E

Figure 5–95 *Continued.* Distance from anterior spine to node (measurement A) in Hodgkin's disease. *D.* Lateral film demonstrates multiple lymph nodes extending far anteriorly from the twelfth thoracic to second lumbar vertebrae. Measurement A is 5.5 cm. The inferior vena cavogram was normal. If the lateral film had been omitted, correct evaluation of this proved positive case would have been difficult. *E.* Lymphangiographic appearance of Hodgkin's disease. Spine-to-node distances. The right lateral spine-to-node distance (measurement B) is the measurement from the right lateral border of a lumbar vertebral body at its mid-point to the most lateral border of the right juxtacaval node group. In this case it is 2.5 cm beyond the normal limit. The left lateral spine-to-node distance (measurement C) is within the normal range (1.8 cm). *F.* Right lateral spine-to-node distance (measurement B), distribution curves on 60 normal and 60 abnormal cases. This is the measurement from the right lateral border of a lumbar vertebral body at its mid-point to the most lateral border of the right juxtacaval lymph node group. The proposed upper limit of normal is 2.0 cm.

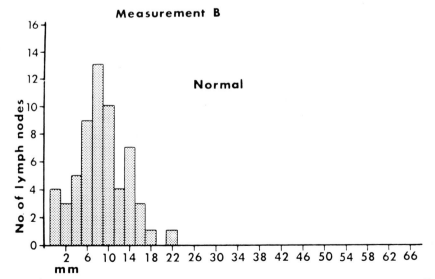

F

Figure 5–95 continued on following page.

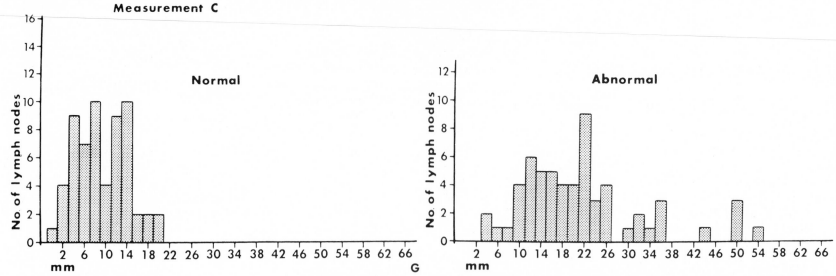

Measurement C

Normal

Abnormal

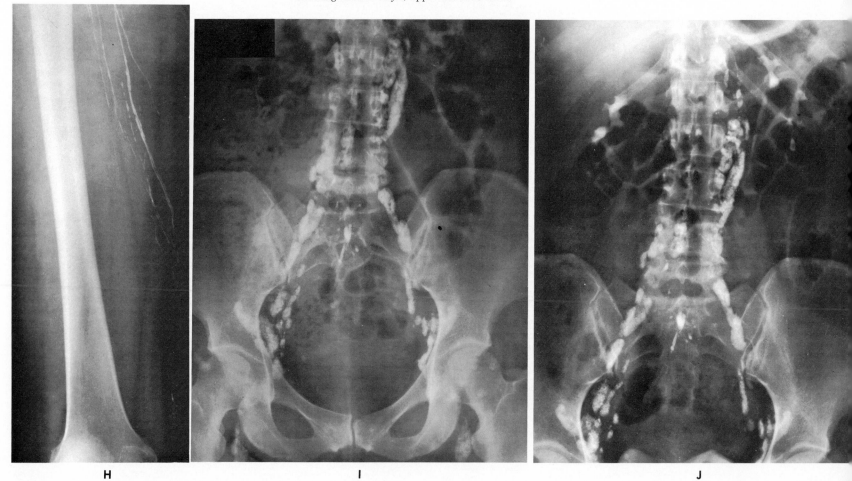

Figure 5–95 *Continued.* *G,* Left lateral spine-to-node distance (measurement C), distribution curves on 60 normal and 60 abnormal lymphangiograms. This is the measurement from the left lateral surface of the mid-point of the vertebral body to the most lateral border of the left para-aortic lymph node groups. The upper normal limit is 2.0 cm. (From Abrams, H. L.: Angiography, Vol. 2, 2nd ed. Boston, Little, Brown & Co., 1971.) *H–J.* Lymphangiograms: *H.* superficial lymphatics of thigh; *I.* 24 hour AP study of pelvis and lower abdomen; *J.* 24 hour study of abdomen showing cisterna chyli, upper left at L2 level.

H   I   J

decrease in the amount stored. The sharpness of outline slowly fades. (At the end of 1 year visualization of lymph nodes is possible in just over 60 per cent of cases; at the end of 2 years, approximately 11 or 12 per cent can be visualized [Abrams].) Lymph nodes tend to form in groups or chains, and at times it may be impossible to delineate clearly a single lymph node.

Radiographs of lymphatic vessels taken immediately after injection—properly called lymphangiograms—show the vessels to best advantage in contrast to later studies—properly called lymphadenograms—which emphasize nodal visualization. Lymphatic channels are long and tortuous, untapered, and measure 2 to 3 mm. in maximum diameter. Typically, these tubular channels are frequently interrupted by the appearance of valves, giving rise to innumerable alternating constrictions every few millimeters.

In early lymphangiograms, lymph nodes may also be seen. In these early films, the lymph node often appears as a ring with a darker central nucleus. Interpretation of lymph nodes, however, should not be undertaken until the later lymphadenograms have been made.

Measurements Useful in Evaluation of Lymphadenograms. Abrams has obtained various measurements of normal and abnormal lymph nodes as well as relationships of nodal groups to the spine. These are tabulated in Figure 5–95 *A*, where the size of nodes with a proposed normal range is given; measurements A, B,

and C as illustrated in Figure 5–95 are further tabulated both graphically and on radiographs.

Since the size of nodes in abnormal groups varies considerably, normality is difficult to describe. Generally, a normal lymph node measures from 3 to 15 mm. in diameter and does not exceed 30 mm. in any dimension. The normal range proposed by Abrams is 2.6 cm. or less.

The anterior spine-to-node distance (measurement A) on a cross-table lateral film from the anterior surface of the lumbar vertebral body at its midpoint to the anterior surface of the adjacent node group is 2.0 cm. plus or minus 0.61 cm.; the adjacent node group measures 2.0 cm. plus or minus 0.61 cm.; and the proposed normal range for this measurement is 3.0 cm. or less.

The right lateral spine-to-node distance (measurement B) distribution curve is also shown. This is the measurement from the right lateral border of a lumbar vertebral body at its midpoint to the most lateral border of the right juxtacaval lymph node group. Here the proposed upper limit of normal is also 2.0 cm. The left lateral spine-to-node distance (measurement C) distribution curve is also shown. This is the measurement from the left lateral surface of the midpoint of the vertebral body to the most lateral border of the left para-aortic lymph node groups. Here the proposed upper limit for normal is also 2.0 cm. or less.

These measurements are based on 60 normal and 60 abnormal cases.

REFERENCES

Andren, L., and von Rosen, S.: The diagnosis of dislocation of the hip in newborns and the primary results of immediate treatment. Acta Radiol., *49*:89–95, 1957.

Angell, F. L.: Fluoroscopic technique of double contrast arthrography of the knee. Radiol. Clin. N. Amer., *9*:85–98, 1971.

Arcomano, J. P., Stunkle, G., Barnett, J. C., and Sackler, J. P.: Muscle group signs and pubic varus as a manifestation of hip disease in children. Amer. J. Roentgenol., *89*:966–969, 1963.

Bardsley, J. L., and Staple, T. W.: Variations in branching of the popliteal artery. Radiology, *94*:581–587, 1970.

Barnett, J. C., and Arcomano, J. P.: Hip arthrography in children with Renografin. Radiology, *73*:245–249, 1959.

Bergvall, U.: Phlebography in acute deep venous thrombosis of the lower extremity. A comparison between centripetal, ascending and descending phlebography. Acta Radiol. (Diag.), *11*:148–166, 1971.

Bierman, H. R.: Selective Arterial Catheterization. Springfield, Ill., Charles C Thomas, 1969.

Billing, L.: Roentgen examination of proximal femur end in children and adolescents. Acta Radiol. (Suppl.), *110*:1–80, 1954.

Boehler, L.: Diagnosis, pathology and treatment of fractures of the os calcis. J. Bone Joint Surg., *13*:75–89, 1931.

Bron, K. M., Baum, S., and Abrams, H. L.: Oil embolism in lymphangiography. Radiology, *80*:194, 1963.

Budin, E., and Chandler, E.: Measurement of femoral neck anteversion by a direct method. Radiology, *69*:209–213, 1951.

Caffey, J., Ames, R., Silverman, W., Ryder, C. T., and Hough, G.: Congenital dislocation of the hip. Pediatrics, *17*:632–641, 1956.

Chait, A., Moltz, A., and Nelson, J. H., Jr.: The collateral arterial circulation in the pelvis. Amer. J. Roentgenol., *102*:392–400, 1968.

Cohen, A. S., McNeill, J. M., Calkins, E., Sharp, J. T., and Schubart, A.: The "normal" sacroiliac joint: analysis of 88 sacroiliac roentgenograms. Amer. J. Roentgenol., *100*:559–563, 1967.

Davis, L. A., and Hatt, W. S.: Congenital abnormalities of the feet. Radiology, *64*:818, 1955.

DeRoo, T.: An improved simple technique for lymphangiography. Amer. J. Roentgenol., *98*:948–951, 1966.

Elliott, G. B., and Elliott, K. A.: Fate of oily contrast media after lymphography. Amer. J. Roentgenol., *104*:851–859, 1968.

Eyring, E. J., Bjornson, D. R., and Peterson, C. A.: Early diagnostic and prognostic signs in Legg-Calvé-Perthes disease. Amer. J. Roentgenol., 93:382–387, 1965.

Fisch, U.: Lymphography of the Cervical Lymphatic System. Philadelphia, W. B. Saunders Co., 1968.

Fischer, H. W.: Lymphangiography and lymphadenography with various contrast agents. Ann. N.Y. Acad. Sci., 78:799, 1959.

Fischer, H. W., and Zimmerman, G. R.: Roentgenographic visualization of lymph nodes and lymphatic channels. Amer. J. Roentgenol., 81:517, 1959.

Freiberger, R. H., Killoran, P. J., and Cardona, G.: Arthrography of the knee by double contrast method. Amer. J. Roentgenol., 97:736–747, 1966.

Fuchs, W. A.: Complications in lymphography with oily contrast media. Acta Radiol., 57:427, 1962.

Gamble, F. O., and Yale, I.: Clinical Foot Roentgenology. Baltimore, The Williams & Wilkins Company, 1966.

Grant, J. C. B.: Atlas of Anatomy. Baltimore, Williams and Wilkins Co., 1962.

Haveson, S. B., and Rein, B. I.: Lateral discoid meniscus of the knee: arthrographic diagnosis. Amer. J. Roentgenol., 109:581–586, 1970.

Insall, J., and Salvati, E.: Patella position in the normal knee joint. Radiology, 101:101–104, 1971.

Jing, B. S.: Improved technique of lymphangiography. Amer. J. Roentgenol., 98:952–956, 1966.

Keats, T. E., Teeslink, R., Diamond, A. E., and Williams, J. H.: Normal axial relationships of the major joints. Radiology, 87:904–907, 1966.

Kim, S. K., and Jones, W. R.: A pelvic phlebogram. A case report and review of the literature. Amer. J. Roentgenol., 93:940–942, 1965.

Kinmonth, J. B.: Lymphangiography in man. Clin. Sci., 11:13, 1952.

Kinmonth, J. B., Harper, R. A. K., and Taylor, G. W.: Lymphangiography by radiological methods. J. Fac. Radiol. (London), 6:217, 1955.

Kinmonth, J. B., Taylor, G. W., and Harper, R. A. K.: Lymphangiography: a technique for its clinical use in the lower limb. Brit. Med. J., 1:940, 1955.

Klein, A., Joplin, R. J., Reidy, J. A., and Haneline, J.: Roentgenologic features of slipped capital femoral epiphysis. Amer. J. Roentgenol., 66:361–374, 1951.

Köhler, A., and Zimmer, E. A.: Borderlands of the Normal and Early Pathologic and Skeletal Roentgenology. Third edition. New York, Grune and Stratton, 1968.

Laage, H., et al.: Horizontal lateral roentgenography of the hip in children. A preliminary report. J. Bone Joint Surg., 35-A:387–398, 1953.

Lewis, R. L.: A roentgen study of soft tissue pathology in and about the knee joints. Amer. J. Roentgenol., 65:200–219, 1951.

Lindblom, K.: Arthrography of knee, roentgenographic and anatomic studies. Acta Radiol. (Suppl.), 74:1–112, 1948.

Martin, H. E.: Geometrical–anatomical factors and their significance in the early x-ray diagnosis of hip-joint disease in children. Radiology, 56:842, 1951.

Meschan, I.: Radiology of the normal foot. Sem. in Roentgenol., 5:327–340, 1970.

Meschan, I., and McGaw, W. H.: Newer methods of pneumoarthrography of the knee with evaluation of procedure in 315 operated cases. Radiology, 49:675–711, 1947.

Pirie, A. H.: Extra bones in the wrist and ankle found by roentgen rays. Amer. J. Roentgenol., 8:569, 1921.

Pugh, D. G., and Winkler, N. T.: Scanography for leg length measurement: an easy satisfactory method. Radiology, 87:130–133, 1966.

Sanders, R. J., and Glaser, J. L.: Clinical uses of venography. Angiology, 20:388–405, 1969.

Schaffer, B., Koehler, P. R., Daniel, C. R., Wohl, G. T., Rivera, E., Meyers, W. A., and Skelley, J. F.: A critical evaluation of lymphangiography. Radiology, 80:917–930, 1963.

Somerville, E. W.: Flexion contractures of the knee. J. Bone Joint Surg., 42-B:730–735, 1960.

Staple, T. W.: Arthrographic demonstration of ileopsoas bursa extension of the hip joint. Radiology, 102:515–516, 1972.

Sutton, D.: Arteriography. Edinburgh and London, E. & S. Livingstone, Ltd., 1962.

Templeton, A. W., McAlister, W. H., and Zim, I. D.: Standardization of terminology and evaluation of osseous relationship in congenitally abnormal feet. Amer. J. Roentgenol., 93:374, 1965.

Tong, E. C.: The iliac index angle—a simplified method for measuring the iliac index. Radiology, 91:376–377. 1968.

Turner, A. F., and Budin, E.: Arthrography of the knee. Radiology, 97:505–508, 1970.

van Brunt, E.: A method of measuring the femoral neck in surgical treatment of fractures. Amer. J. Roentgenol., 76:1163–1165, 1956.

Viamonte, M., Altman, D., Parks, R., Blum, E., Bevilaqua, M., and Recher, L.: Radiographic pathologic correlation in the interpretation of lymphangioadenograms. Radiology, 80:903, 1963.

Vix, V. A., and Ryu, C. Y.: The adult symphysis pubis: normal and abnormal. Amer. J. Roentgenol., 112:517–525, 1971.

Wallace, S., Jackson, L., Dodd, G. D., and Greening, R. R.: Lymphatic dynamics in certain abnormal states. Amer. J. Roentgenol., 91:1187, 1964.

Wallace, S., Jackson, L., Schaffer, B., Gould, J., Greening, R. R., Weiss, A., and Kramer, S.: Lymphangiograms: their diagnostic and therapeutic potential. Radiology, 76:179, 1961.

Willis, T. A.: The function of the long plantar muscles. Surg., Gyn. & Obstet., 60:150, 1935.

6

The Skull

A study of the radiographic anatomy of the skull can be conveniently divided into three parts: (1) a general survey, (2) detailed consideration of certain areas of the skull which are important from a radiographic standpoint, and (3) radiography of the brain by pneumoencephalography, ventriculography, and angiography. Only the first of these will be undertaken in this chapter; the other two subjects will be discussed in Chapters 7 and 8 respectively.

Introduction. There are 22 bones in the skull, including the mandible, firmly bound together at immovable joints called sutures or primary cartilaginous joints (with the exception of the temporomandibular joints).

These are subdivided into the bones of the calvarium (or brain case) and the bones of the face and mandible (Fig. 6–1).

The calvarium or cranium is composed of eight bones: the paired parietal and temporal bones, and the frontal, occipital, sphenoid, and ethmoid bones, which are single. The temporal bones contain the ossicles of the ear.

The cranial cavity lodges the brain and is formed by the frontal, parietal, occipital, temporal, sphenoid, and ethmoid bones. The roof of the cranial cavity is composed of the frontal, parietal, occipital, and squamous portions of the temporal bones, and the greater wings of the sphenoid bone. These bones are largely flat and are composed of a dense outer layer known as the outer table, a less dense middle zone known as the diploë, and another dense inner zone known as the inner table.

In adults with a well-developed brain, the skull is large but relatively thin. The calvarial thickness varies widely among different individuals. The thickest part of a normal vault should not exceed 1 cm.; if it measures more, some degree of cerebral underdevelopment or a systemic disease, whether active or healed, should be suspected (Ethier). The inner table varies very little in thickness except in places where it is eroded by vascular structures and brain markings. It is usually thinner than the outer table (Ethier).

The middle table or diploë is composed of an irregular network of bony trabeculae and vascular spaces that form a mosaic-like pattern.

The outer table varies even less in thickness than does the inner table and appears rather smooth. It tends to be thicker anteriorly when the frontal sinuses are not well developed. Often it is thin along the parietal eminences. It may be perforated by many venous structures.

Temporal enostoses are small bony ridges on the inner table of the squamous portion of the temporal bone, and are frequently seen along the inferior half. Usually they are somewhat triangular in shape. Generally, they tend to project over the sellar region, and must not be misinterpreted as representing parasellar or suprasellar calcification.

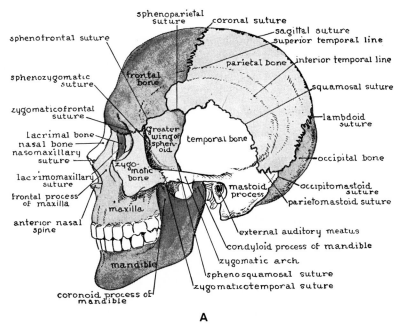

A

Figure 6–1. *A.* Lateral view of the skull, showing the bones of the calvarium, face, and mandible.

Figure 6–1 continued on following page.

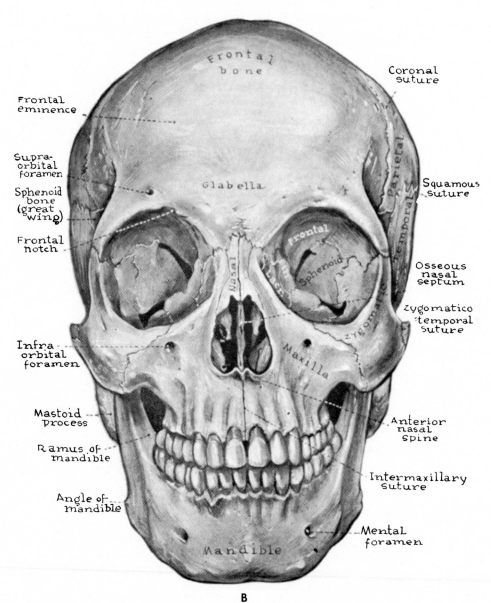

B

Figure 6–1 *Continued.* B. Skull viewed from the front. (*A* and *B* from Pendergrass, E. P. et al.: The Head and Neck in Roentgen Diagnosis, 2nd ed., 1956. Courtesy of Charles C Thomas, Publisher, Springfield, Illinois.)

Figure 6–1 continued on opposite page.

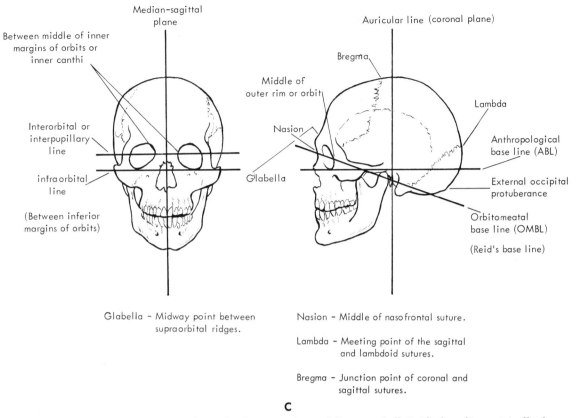

Glabella – Midway point between
supraorbital ridges.

Nasion – Middle of nasofrontal suture.

Lambda – Meeting point of the sagittal
and lambdoid sutures.

Bregma – Junction point of coronal and
sagittal sutures.

C

Figure 6–1 *Continued.* C. Commonly used reference points and lines on skull. Reid's base line, originally described as a line from the infraorbital rim to the external auditory meatus, is seldom used as a reference line because the canthomeatal line, from the outer canthus of the eye to the external auditory meatus, is more clearly defined on the patient.

The *anthropological base line* joins the infraorbital point at the superior border of the external auditory meatus. The *orbitomeatal base line* joins the outer canthus of the eye at the *central* point of the external auditory meatus. These two lines meet at an angle of 10 degrees.

THE BONES OF THE CALVARIUM

The *frontal bone* anteriorly forms the forehead and the anterosuperior portion of the cranial vault, the roof of the orbits, and the greater part of the floor of the anterior cranial fossa. The frontal sinuses are air spaces contained within the frontal bones, and these will be described in detail later.

The *parietal bones* form the greater portion of both sides of the skull. These meet superiorly in the midline to form the sagittal suture, articulating with the frontal bone anteriorly to form the *coronal suture,* and posteriorly with the occipital to form the *lambdoid suture.* Inferiorly they adjoin the temporal bone at its squamous portion to form the *squamous suture.*

The *occipital bone* (Fig. 6–2) is situated at the lower posterior portion of the skull. It forms the posterior part of the roof of the brain, as well as the greater part of the floor of the posterior cranial fossa. It contains a large oval aperture, the foramen magnum, which permits communication between the cranial cavity and the vertebral column. The foramen magnum divides the bone into three sections: (*a*) the squamous portion, which articulates with the parietal and temporal bones at the lambdoid suture, (*b*) the pars lateralis, lateral to the foramen magnum, which contains the condyles for articulation with the first cervical vertebra, and (*c*) the basilar portion anterior to the foramen, which articulates with the basilar portion of the sphenoid bone at the basisphenoid suture. Unlike other sutures at the base of the skull, this basisphenoid suture is open at birth, and remains so for several years.

The *temporal bone* (Fig. 6–3) forms the side of the skull below the parietal bones, and the base of the skull in front of the occipital bone. This bone contains the internal ear, the middle ear, the bony part of the external ear, a small cavity adjoining the middle ear called the tympanic antrum, and numerous air cells throughout. The following major parts of the temporal bone are: squamous, mastoid, tympanic, petrous, styloid process, and temporomandibular fossa. This bone is clinically important because of its

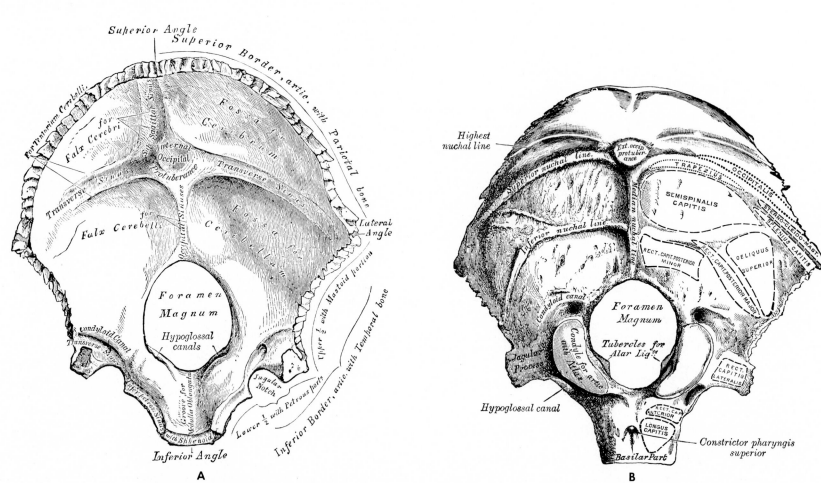

Figure 6–2.   *A.* The occipital bone, inner surface. *B.* Occipital bone, outer surface. (From Gray's Anatomy of the Human Body, 29th ed., Goss, C. M. (ed.) Philadelphia, Lea & Febiger, 1973.)

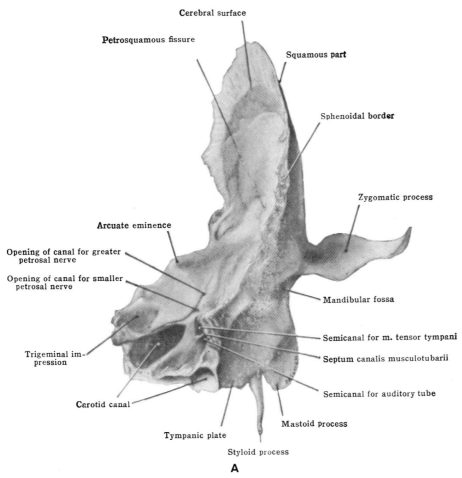

Cerebral surface

Petrosquamous fissure

Squamous part

Sphenoidal border

Zygomatic process

Arcuate eminence

Opening of canal for greater
petrosal nerve

Opening of canal for smaller
petrosal nerve

Mandibular fossa

Semicanal for m. tensor tympani

Septum canalis musculotubarii

Trigeminal im-
pression

Semicanal for auditory tube

Carotid canal

Mastoid process

Tympanic plate

Styloid process

A

Figure 6–3. *A.* The left temporal bone, anteromedial view. (From Anson, B. J. (ed.): Morris' Human Anatomy, 12th ed. Copyright © 1966 by McGraw-Hill, Inc. Used by permission of McGraw-Hill Book Company.)

Figure 6–3 continued on the following page.

association with the auditory and vestibular mechanisms and must be studied exhaustively radiographically. A more detailed consideration will be given in Chapter 7.

The *sphenoid bone* (Fig. 6–4) lies in the floor of the cranial cavity posterior to the orbits. It encloses air spaces beneath the sella turcica called the sphenoid sinuses. It is a bone shaped somewhat like a bird, having a body, greater and lesser wings (both of which form portions of the superior and lateral walls respectively of the orbit), and paired downward projections called the pterygoid processes or plates.

The *ethmoid bone* is situated between the orbits and below the frontal bone (Fig. 6–5). It contains numerous small air cells called the ethmoid sinuses; the superior and middle nasal conchae project from its medial aspect and participate in the formation of the nasal turbinates.

THE FACIAL BONES

The skeleton of the face is composed of 14 bones (including the mandible); the nasal bones, maxillae, lacrimals, zygomata, palatine and inferior nasal conchae are paired, and the vomer and the mandible are single.

The face also contains numerous cavities—namely, the orbits, the nasal cavities, the paranasal sinuses (contained within the maxillary, frontal, ethmoid, and sphenoid bones), as well as the mouth.

The nose and nasal cavity and the paranasal sinuses are anatomic subdivisions that require special radiographic techniques for demonstration; these will be discussed in Chapter 7.

The bones contributing most significantly to the contour of the face are the maxillae, the zygomatic bones, and the mandible.

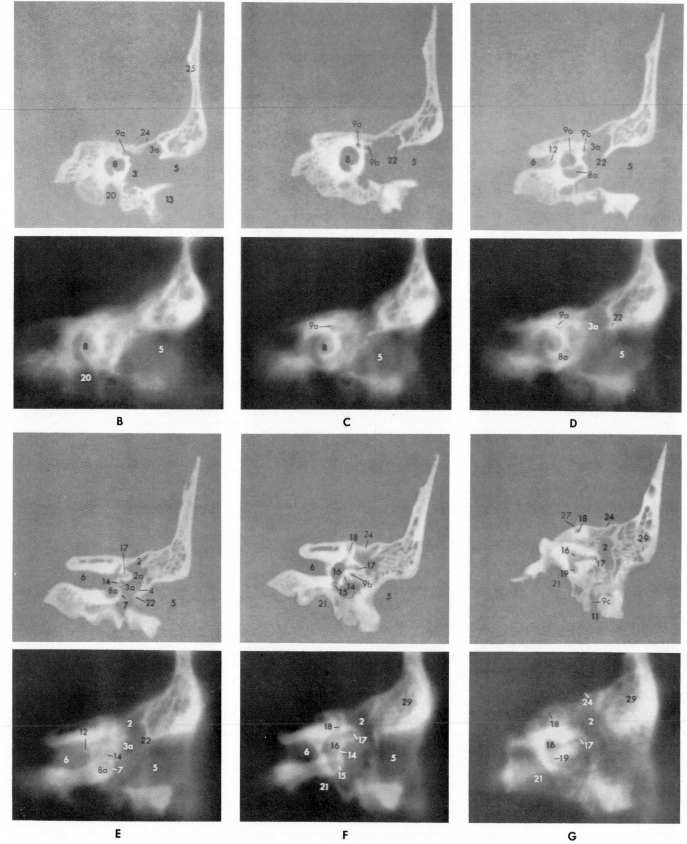

Figure 6–3 Continued.   See opposite page for legend.

Figure 6–3 continued on the opposite page.

Figure 6-3 *Continued.* *B–G.* Anteroposterior (frontal) projection. Six pairs of radiographs (*top*) and tomograms (*bottom*) of a dried left temporal bone. Each pair represents a different level, or plane. The progression of levels from left to right is anterior to posterior, and there is about 1 mm to 1.5 mm between levels. The medial aspect of the bone is on the left; the lateral aspect, on the right. Structures seen particularly well in the anteroposterior projection include the internal auditory canal in its long axis and the epitympanic recess (attic).

Legend:

1 Mastoid process
2 Mastoid antrum
2a Aditus of antrum
3 Middle ear (tympanic cavity)
3a Epitympanic recess (attic)
4 Lateral wall of attic
5 External auditory canal
6 Internal auditory canal
7 Promontory of middle ear
8 Cochlea
8a Basal turn of cochlea
9a Facial nerve canal, petrous segment
9b Facial nerve canal, tympanic segment
9c Facial nerve canal, mastoid (descending) segment
10 Styloid process
11 Stylomastoid foramen
12 Crista transversa (crista falciformis)
13 Mandibular fossa
14 Oval window (fenestra vestibuli)
15 Round window (fenestra cochleae)
16 Vestibule
17 Lateral semicircular canal
18 Superior semicircular canal
19 Posterior semicircular canal
20 Carotid canal
21 Jugular fossa
22 Scutum (spur)
23 Sinus plate
24 Tegmen
25 Squamous portion of temporal bone
26 Crus commune (common limb)
27 Arcuate eminence
28 Petrous apex
29 Mastoid air cells

(From Schaefer, R. E.: Med. Radiography and Photography, *48*:1, 1972. Published by Radiography Markets Division, Eastman Kodak Company.)

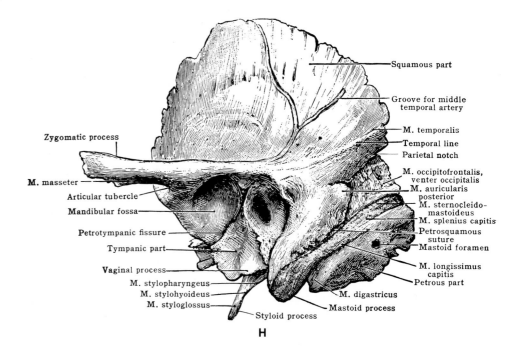

H

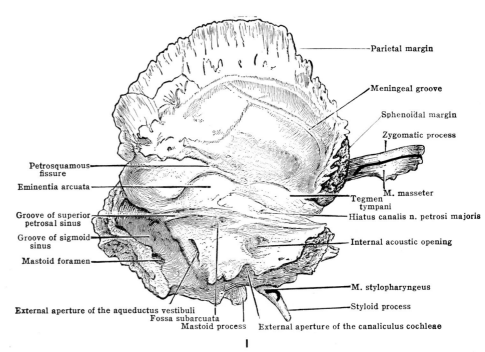

I

Figure 6-3 *Continued.* *H.* The left temporal bone, lateral view. *I.* The left temporal bone, medial view. (From Anson, B. J. (ed.): Morris' Human Anatomy, 12th ed. Copyright © 1966 by McGraw-Hill, Inc. Used by permission of McGraw-Hill Book Company.)

Figure 6-3 continued on the following page.

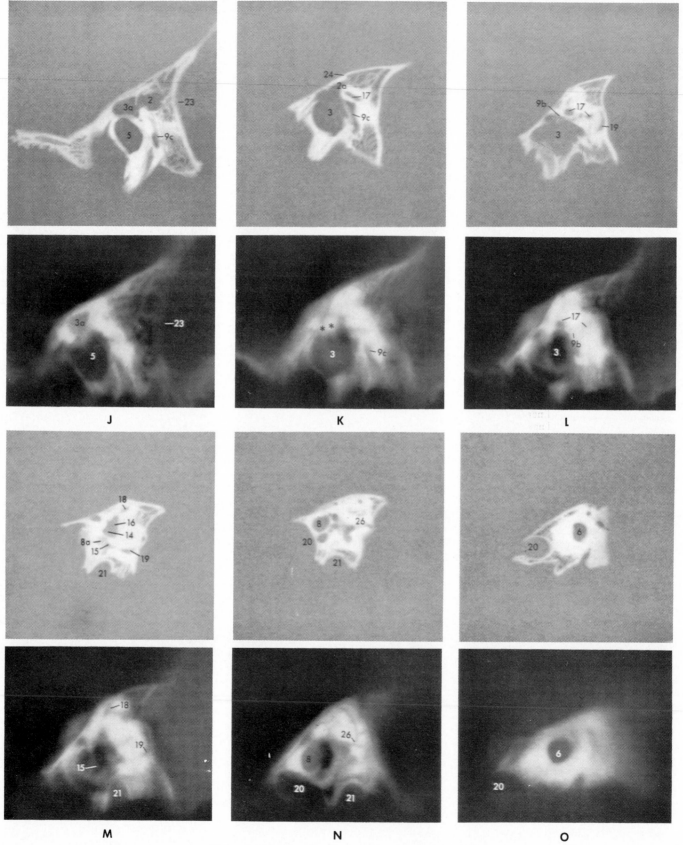

Figure 6-3 Continued.   See opposite page for legend.

Figure 6-3 continued on the opposite page.

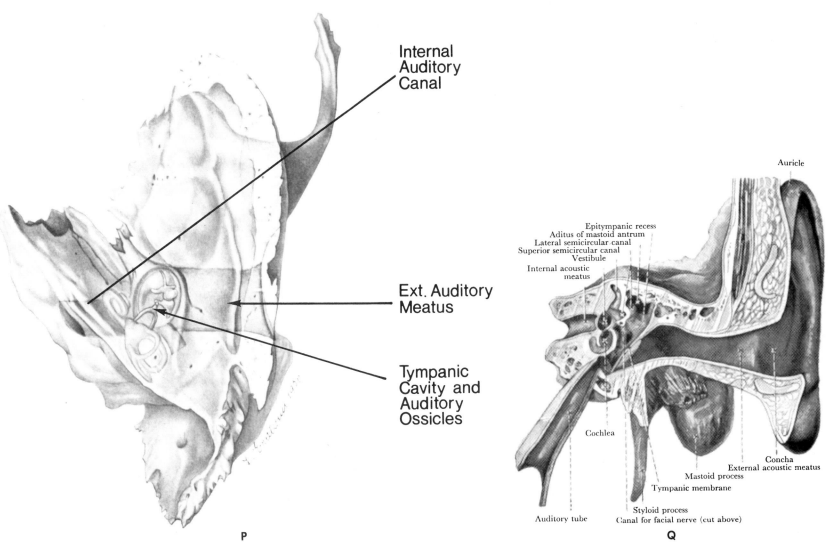

Internal
Auditory
Canal

Ext. Auditory
Meatus

Tympanic
Cavity and
Auditory
Ossicles

Auricle

Epitympanic recess
Aditus of mastoid antrum
Lateral semicircular canal
Superior semicircular canal
Vestibule
Internal acoustic
meatus

Cochlea

Concha
External acoustic meatus
Mastoid process
Tympanic membrane
Styloid process
Auditory tube   Canal for facial nerve (cut above)

P   Q

Figure 6–3 *Continued.*   P. The three subdivisions of the ear projected on the bony framework. (From Pernkopf, E.: Atlas of Topographical and Applied Human Anatomy. Vol. 1. Philadelphia, W. B. Saunders Co., 1963.) Q. The parts of the ear (semi-diagrammatic). (From Cunningham's Manual of Practical Anatomy, 12th ed. London, Oxford University Press, 1958.)

Figure 6–3 *Continued.*   J–O. Lateral projection. Six pairs of radiographs (*top*) and tomograms (*bottom*) of a dried left temporal bone. Each pair represents a different level, or plane. From left to right, the levels progress from the lateral surface of the bone mediad. The posterior aspect of the bone is on the right. The lateral projection reveals the relation between the epitympanic recess and the mastoid antrum and shows the mastoid (descending) segment of the facial nerve canal. In the specimen used for this projection, the malleus and the incus happened to be present in their normal configuration. The tomogram made in the second level (K, *bottom*) clearly shows these ossicles (*asterisks*); the handle of the malleus is anterior, and the long process of the incus is posterior.

Legend:

1 Mastoid process	9b Facial nerve canal, tympanic segment	20 Carotid canal
2 Mastoid antrum	9c Facial nerve canal, mastoid (descending) segment	21 Jugular fossa
2a Aditus of antrum	10 Styloid process	22 Scutum (spur)
3 Middle ear (tympanic cavity)	11 Stylomastoid foramen	23 Sinus plate
3a Epitympanic recess (attic)	12 Crista transversa (crista falciformis)	24 Tegmen
4 Lateral wall of attic	13 Mandibular fossa	25 Squamous portion of temporal bone
5 External auditory canal	14 Oval window (fenestra vestibuli)	26 Crus commune (common limb)
6 Internal auditory canal	15 Round window (fenestra cochleae)	27 Arcuate eminence
7 Promontory of middle ear	16 Vestibule	28 Petrous apex
8 Cochlea	17 Lateral semicircular canal	29 Mastoid air cells
8a Basal turn of cochlea	18 Superior semicircular canal	
9a Facial nerve canal, petrous segment	19 Posterior semicircular canal	

(From Schaefer, R. E.: Med. Radiography and Photography, 48:1, 1972. Published by Radiography Markets Division, Eastman Kodak Company.)

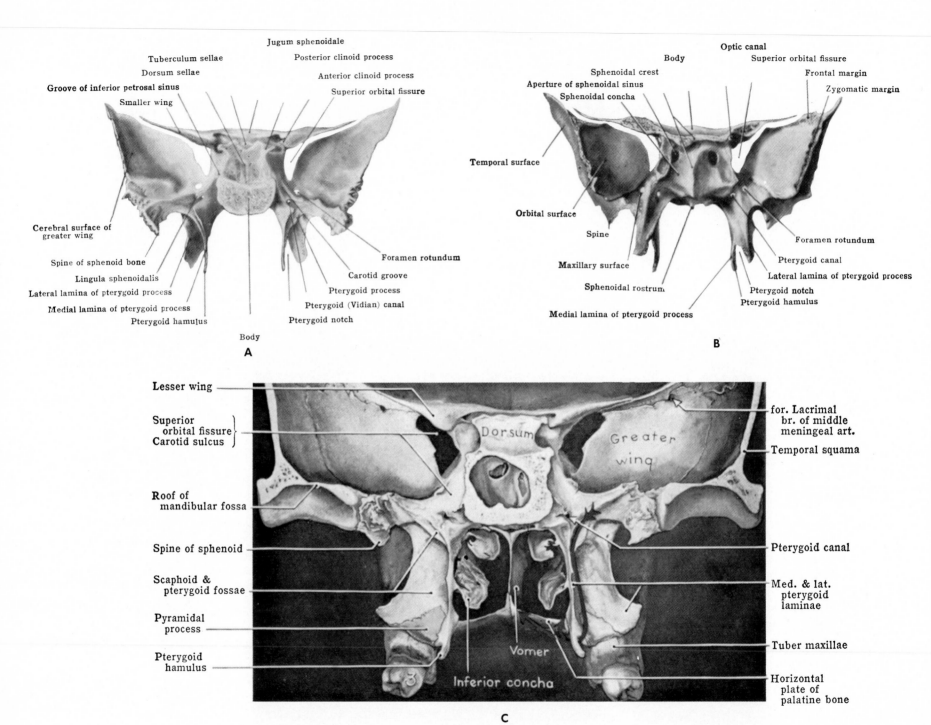

Figure 6–4. The sphenoid bone. A. Posterior view. B. Anterior view. (From Anson, B. J. (ed.): Morris' Human Anatomy, 12th ed. Copyright © 1966 by McGraw-Hill, Inc. Used by permission of McGraw-Hill Book Company.) C. Coronal section of the skull at the sphenoid bone. (Reproduced by permission from J. C. B. Grant: An Atlas of Anatomy, 5th ed. Copyright © 1962, The Williams and Wilkins Co.)

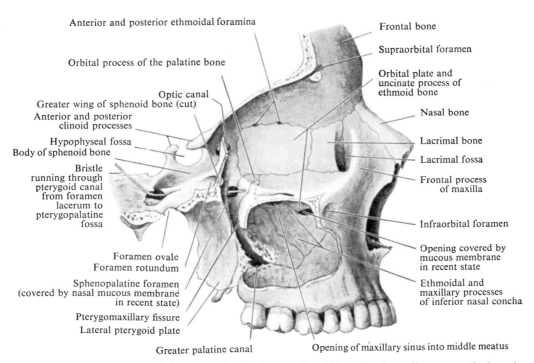

Figure 6–5. Sphenoid bone, medial wall of orbit [including ethmoid bone] and maxillary sinus. The lateral and postero-medial walls of the maxillary sinus have been partly removed to indicate the lateral relations of the palatine bone. Note how the medial wall of the maxillary sinus is completed by the palatine plate, the ethmoidal and maxillary processes of the inferior nasal concha and the uncinate process of the ethmoid. (Reprinted by permission of Faber and Faber Ltd. from Anatomy of the Human Body, by Lockhardt, Hamilton, and Fyfe, Faber and Faber, London; J. B. Lippincott Company, Philadelphia.)

The Maxillae. The two maxillae form the upper jaw (Fig. 6–1B). Each maxilla has a body and four processes. The body encloses a large pyramidal air space called the maxillary sinus. The processes extend upward to the frontal bone and medial wall of the orbit, laterally to the zygoma, downward to form the alveolus and upper dental arch, and medially to form the anterior larger part of the hard palate on its own side.

The maxilla articulates with the frontal bone at the maxillofrontal suture between the frontal process of the maxillary bone and the frontal bone, with the nasal bones at the nasomaxillary suture, with the lacrimal bone at the lacrimomaxillary suture, with the maxilla of the opposite side of the palate at the intermaxillary suture, with the zygoma at the maxillozygomatic suture, and with the ethmoid bone between the orbital processes of the ethmoid and the maxillary bone at the maxillo-ethmoidal suture.

The Zygomatic Bone. The zgyomatic bone (Fig. 6–1B) forms the anterior part of the zygomatic arch and unites with the frontal and sphenoid bones above, and the zygomatic process of the temporal bone behind to form the zygomatic arch. It forms the so-called malar prominence of the face, and is particularly subject to

injury around the orbit. It articulates with the maxilla below at the maxillozygomatic suture.

Radiographically, the maxillae and the zygomatic bones must be demonstrated both from the frontal projection and the supero-inferior projection to determine accurately any displacement of a bony fragment that may be present. Because of the marked local swelling that accompanies injuries of these areas, such displacement is not demonstrable by clinical means.

The zygomatic arches are thin segments of bone formed by the fusion of the zygomatic processes of the zygomatic and temporal bones. Special views are usually required to demonstrate the arch in its entirety in the so-called axial projection. The remainder of the skull must be "under-penetrated" by the x-ray exposure to show the zygomatic arches clearly (Fig. 6–48).

The Lacrimal Bone. The lacrimal bone lies below the inner canthus of the eye in the medial wall of the orbit and helps form the groove in which the lacrimal sac lies. It is the smallest bone of the face and the most fragile. It is surrounded by the following sutures: the lacrimo-ethmoidal, the lacrimofrontal, and the lacrimomaxillary.

The Inferior Nasal Concha. This bone helps form the infe-

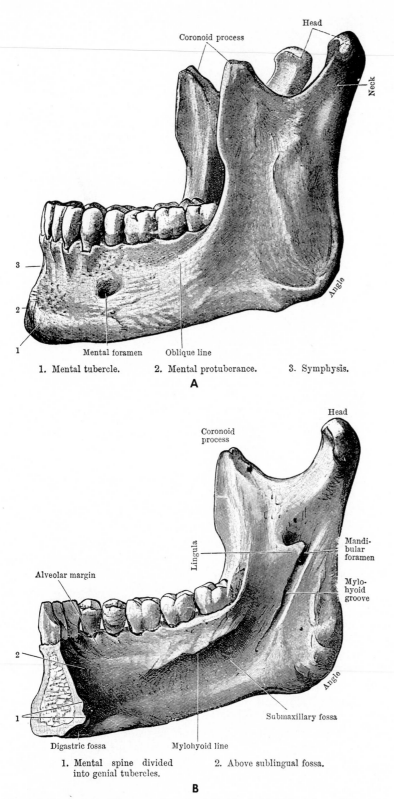

1. Mental tubercle.   2. Mental protuberance.   3. Symphysis.

A

1. Mental spine divided   2. Above sublingual fossa.
**   into genial tubercles.**

B

Figure 6–6. A. Mandible, seen from the left side. B. Medial surface of the right half of the mandible. (From Cunningham's Textbook of Anatomy, 6th ed. London, Oxford University Press, 1931.)

rior nasal turbinate and will be described later in the discussion of the nasal cavity (Chapter 7).

The Vomer. The vomer forms the posterior and postero-inferior part of the nasal septum, and is best seen in the view of the base of the skull (Fig. 6–20).

The Palatine Bones. These bones are likewise best outlined in the view of the base of the skull. They form the posterior quarter or third of the corresponding part of the hard palate (Fig. 6–20) and contribute to the formation of the nasal cavity also.

The Mandible (Fig. 6–6). The mandible is the lower jaw bone and is composed of two bodies united in the midline at the symphysis and two rami at either end of the body. Two processes project upward from each ramus—the coronoid anteriorly, the condyloid posteriorly—and the sigmoid notch lies between. The condyloid process is composed of an articular head and a neck. The mandibular foramen on the medial aspect of the ramus leads to the mandibular canal, the foramen transmitting the inferior alveolar vessels and nerve, and the canal their mylohyoid branches. The mental foramen is anterior on the lateral aspect of the body of the mandible and transmits the mental vessels and nerve.

The mylohyoid groove (which parallels the mandibular canal) and mylohyoid line on the mandible frequently impart a sclerotic appearance to the mandible that is normal. These markings, in contrast to the areas of diminished density produced by the mandibular and mental foramina, may lead to an erroneous impression of bone destruction.

The Teeth (Stafne) (Figs. 6–7, 6–8). We have considered the teeth out of the scope of this text. Ordinarily, for accurate visualization of the teeth, special intraoral films are taken of each region. The integrity of the periodontal membrane is most important in this regard. Moreover, in a young person the normal den-

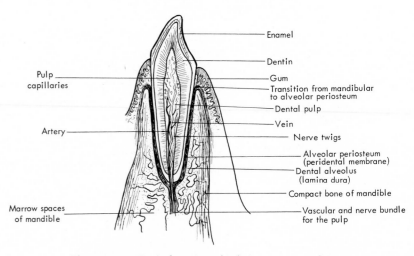

Figure 6–7. Vertical section of inferior canine tooth in situ.

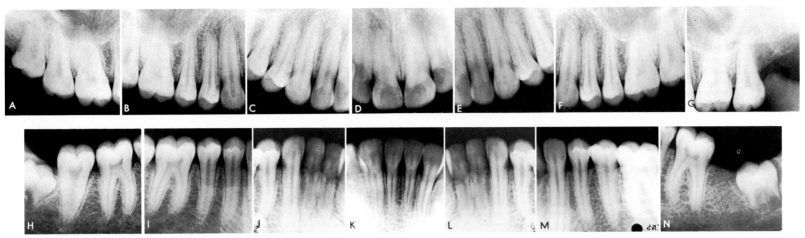

Figure 6–8. Representative intraoral dental films. *A.* Right upper molar area. *B.* Right upper bicuspid area. *C.* Right upper cuspid area. *D.* Upper incisor area. *E.* Left upper cuspid area. *F.* Left upper bicuspid area. *G.* Left upper molar area. *H.* Right lower molar area. *I.* Right lower bicuspid area. *J.* Right lower cuspid area. *K.* Lower incisor area. *L.* Left lower cuspid area. *M.* Left lower bicuspid area. *N.* Left lower molar area.

tal anlage must be differentiated from an abnormality such as a periapical abscess and granuloma.

There are several types of intraoral dental films, each with its own purpose. Small intraoral films are most accurate for visualization of the apex and periapical structures; occlusal films (approximately $2\frac{1}{2} \times 3\frac{1}{2}$ inches) are larger and are placed between the teeth to obtain an inferosuperior perspective of one alveolus or an associated abnormality of the jaw. Bite-wing films are used particularly for demonstration of dental crown abnormalities; they show the relationship of the upper and lower rows of teeth to one another.

The Mandibular Joint (Fig. 6–9). The mandible articulates with the temporal bone at the temporomandibular fossa and is the only freely movable bone of the face. The range of motion is free in all directions. The condyles move forward to the articular tubercles when the mouth is opened, and subluxation must therefore be interpreted with caution.

A plate of fibrocartilage is interposed between each articular margin of the mandible and temporal bone. This cartilage or disk is connected with the articular capsule throughout its circumference. Thus, there are two synovial sacs or spaces in the one joint, and they do not communicate unless the disk is perforated.

No examination of the temporomandibular joints is complete unless an effort is made to demonstrate the extent and character of movement of the condyloid process with relation to its articulating fossa when the mouth is opened. Occasionally we have found the view of the skull in Towne's position (Fig. 6–44) of particular value for demonstration of the articular tubercles and the necks of the condyloid processes.

Body section radiographs of the temporomandibular joint are also of considerable value (Fig. 6–52 *D*).

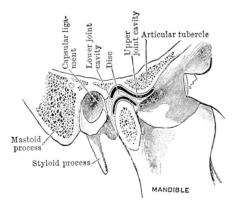

Figure 6–9. Anteroposterior section through the temporomandibular joint. (From Cunningham's Textbook of Anatomy, 6th ed. London, Oxford University Press, 1936.)

LINES, IMPRESSIONS, CHANNELS, AND SUTURES OF THE CRANIAL VAULT

There are various lines and impressions on the cranial vault which are of great radiographic significance.

1. **Granular Pits or Arachnoidal (Pacchionian) Granulation Impressions** (Fig. 6–10). These are small irregular parasagittal impressions that lodge the arachnoidal granulations. They are usually found in the parasagittal region of the vault adjoining the superior sagittal sinus. Occasionally, however, they are found in a more lateral situation along meningeal or diploic

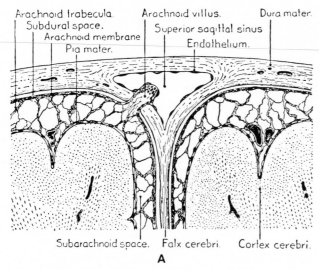

Arachnoid trabecula.   Arachnoid villus.   Dura mater.
Subdural space.   Superior sagittal sinus
Arachnoid membrane   Endothelium.
Pia mater.

Subarachnoid space.   Falx cerebri.   Cortex cerebri.

A

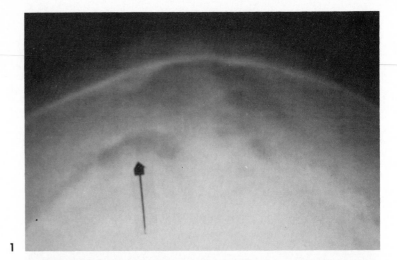

1

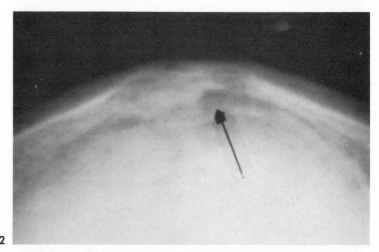

2

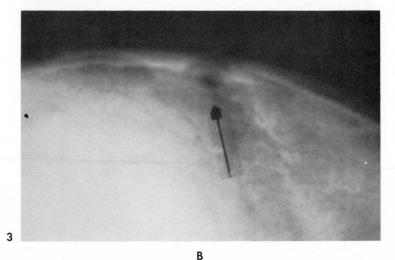

3

B

veins, and not infrequently even the experienced observer has considerable difficulty in distinguishing them from abnormal areas of bone absorption. They are occasionally also found in the occipital bone. Ordinarily, the impressions involve only the inner bony table, into which minute channels radiate.

2. **Arterial and Venous Grooves.** The arterial grooves (Fig. 6–11) are narrow branching grooves for the meningeal vessels— the middle meningeal being the largest. The main groove begins at the foramen spinosum, traverses the squamous temporal bone, and divides into an anterior and a posterior branch which are clearly visible on the parietal bones. These meningeal vessels are so closely applied to the bone that they are likely to be torn when the skull over them is injured (especially the veins, which lie between the arteries and the skull and have thinner walls). The inner table here is very thin and brittle, and may crack even if the outer table remains intact.

The margins of these grooves usually have a slightly denser appearance than the surrounding bone, and the course of the arteries is relatively smooth and undulating, never sharply angled as in a fracture. This characteristic appearance, together with their usual location, is their distinguishing feature.

Arterial grooves in the calvarium may be differentiated from venous grooves in that they tend to taper progressively as they ascend toward the superior aspect of the skull. Venous grooves change very little in caliber throughout their course. The most common venous groove is the bregmatic, which runs along the coronal suture and contains a large meningeal vein that empties into the sphenoparietal or superior longitudinal sinus (Fig. 6–11 *D*).

There are two vascular grooves along the outer table of the cranial vault that have a straight linear appearance and may be confused with fractures. One is supraorbital and is said to be due to the supraorbital artery; the other is located in the outer table of the squamous portion of the temporal bone just above the external auditory meatus and anterior to it. This one is said to be produced by the middle temporal branch of the superficial tem-

Figure 6–10. *A.* Schematic diagram of a coronal section of the meninges and cerebral cortex. (Weed, Amer. J. Anat.: courtesy of Wistar Institute.) *B.* The appearance of arachnoidal granulations in close-up views. (1) Towne's view. (2) A straight posteroanterior film of the skull. (3) Lateral projection.

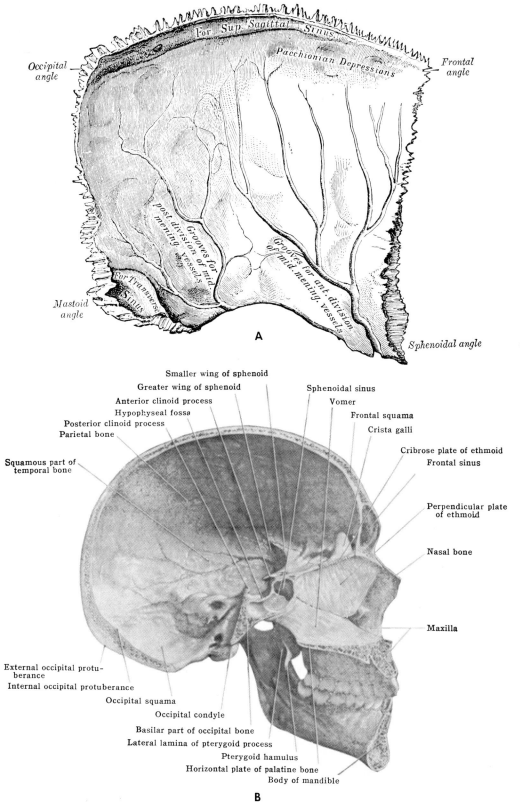

A labels:

Occipital angle

For Sup Sagittal Sinus

Pacchionian Depressions

Frontal angle

Grooves for post. division of mid. mening. vessels

Grooves for ant. division of mid. mening. vessels

For Transverse Sinus

Mastoid angle

A

Sphenoidal angle

B labels:

Smaller wing of sphenoid

Greater wing of sphenoid

Anterior clinoid process

Hypophyseal fossa

Posterior clinoid process

Parietal bone

Squamous part of temporal bone

Sphenoidal sinus

Vomer

Frontal squama

Crista galli

Cribrose plate of ethmoid

Frontal sinus

Perpendicular plate of ethmoid

Nasal bone

Maxilla

External occipital protuberance

Internal occipital protuberance

Occipital squama

Occipital condyle

Basilar part of occipital bone

Lateral lamina of pterygoid process

Pterygoid hamulus

Horizontal plate of palatine bone

Body of mandible

B

Figure 6–11. *A*. The left parietal bone, inner aspect showing vascular grooves. (From Gray's Anatomy of the Human Body, 29th ed. Goss, C. M. (ed.) Philadelphia, Lea & Febiger, 1973.) *B*. The skull, sagittal section. (From Anson, B. J. (ed.): Morris' Human Anatomy, 12th ed. Copyright © 1966 by McGraw-Hill, Inc. Used by permission of the McGraw-Hill Book Company.)

Figure 6–11 continued on the following page.

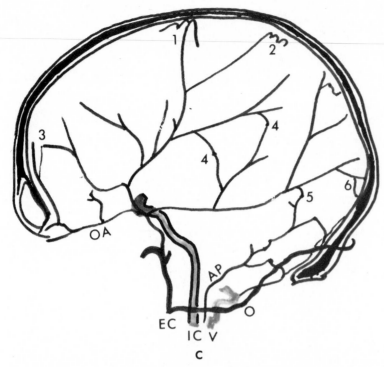

C

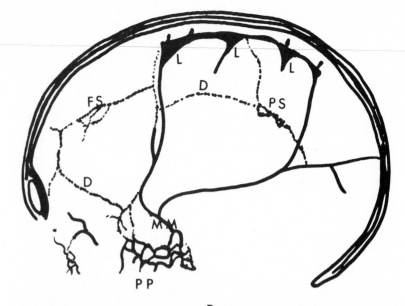

D

Figure 6-11 *Continued.* C. Diagrammatic and radiographic appearance of arterial and venous impressions on the bones of the calvarium. (A) Diagram of meningeal artery circulation. The middle meningeal artery arises from the external carotid (EC), passes through the foramen spinosum of the sphenoid bone and enters the cranium. It runs forward in a groove on the great wing of the sphenoid bone and divides into two branches, the anterior and posterior. The anterior branch crosses the great wing of the sphenoid and then divides into branches that spread out between the dura mater and internal surface of the cranium. Some of its branches pass upward as far as the vertex of the skull, and others backward to the occipital region. The posterior branch curves backward on the squamous portion of the temporal bone and reaches the parietal, where its branches supply the posterior part of the dura mater and cranium. The various anastomoses of the branches of the middle meningeal are numbered. 1 indicates anastomoses with branches of the pericallosal artery; 2 represents anastomoses with branches of the middle cerebral artery that reach the calvarium; 3 is the site of anastomoses with the meningeal branches of the ophthalmic artery (OA), which arises from the internal carotid artery (IC) at the carotid siphon; 4 represents anastomoses between the posterior and anterior branches of the middle meningeal; 5 indicates anastomoses between the meningeal branches of the ascending pharyngeal artery and the posterior branch of the middle meningeal; 6 is the site of anastomoses between the posterior branch of the middle meningeal and the occipital artery and its meningeal branches (O). The vertebral artery (V) sends out meningeal branches that anastomose with those of the ascending pharyngeal and posterior branch of the middle meningeal. (From Meschan, I.: Seminars in Roentgenol., 9:125–136, 1974. Used by permission.)

poral artery. These grooves tend to taper and branch, as do other arterial grooves generally (Ethier; Schunk and Maruyama) (Fig. 6–11 *G*).

A diagram of the arteries supplying the cranium with special reference to their communications is shown in Figure 6–11 *C*. There are three separate intercommunicating systems: (1) the cerebral and cerebellar, (2) the meningeal-osseous, and (3) the vessels to the superficial soft parts and bone. The entire venous

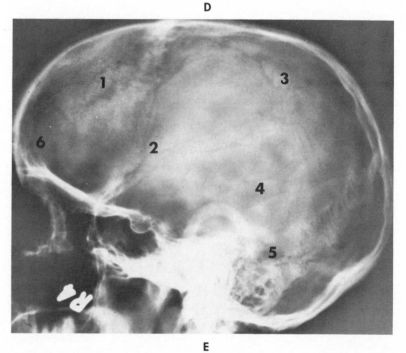

E

Figure 6-11 *Continued.* D. Diagram showing the main middle meningeal veins. Generally, the middle meningeal veins accompany the middle meningeal arteries and thus there is an anterior and a posterior branch complex, as in Fig. 6–11 C. The dotted lines indicate some of the main diploic veins that can be identified on many skull films (D). The "frontal star" (FS) is a cluster of frontal diploic veins that ultimately anastomose with the middle meningeal. The "parietal star" (PS) is a similar collection in the parietal bone that ultimately draws into the middle meningeal, posterior or anterior. The lacunae (L) are venous lakes that communicate with the middle meningeal veins. Arachnoid granulations generally protrude into the lacunae. PP, pharyngeal plexus. E. Lateral view demonstrating vascular impressions: 1, parietal star; 2, middle meningeal artery and vein, anterior division; 3, parietal star; 4, middle meningeal vein, posterior branch; 5, lateral sinus; 6, meningeal communications with the ophthalmic artery and vein. (From Meschan, I.: Seminars in Roentgenol., 9:125–136, 1974. Used by permission.)

Figure 6–11 continued on opposite page.

system is shown in Figure 6–11 *H*. The most important vessels of the meningeal-osseous system are the middle meningeal arteries and their accompanying middle meningeal veins, and the diploic veins. The subcutaneous, muscular, and periosteal arteries and veins, comprising the third system, are especially important at the attachments of muscles and at the *emissary foramina,* to be considered later.

There are numerous intercommunications between the three systems. The main trunks of the cerebral arteries at the base of the skull supply small meningeal and dural communications. There are also parasagittal branches to the dura in the tentorial region. There are similar communications with the ophthalmic arteries and with the arteries of the auditory apparatus. On the venous side, the intercommunications occur at the base, parasagittally, at the tentorium, and at the falx. These communications are particularly significant in pathologic conditions.

The meningeal arteries in bone canals are generally accompanied by two meningeal veins which are disproportionately small when compared with their respective arteries, except in such areas as the parasagittal region where the veins increase in size as they open into the superior sagittal sinus. The anterior branch of the middle meningeal artery, which extends towards the bregma, has an accompanying vein that is usually larger than the artery. In older persons especially it lies in a prominent deep groove. In the parasagittal region, the meningeal veins gradually form lateral lacunae, and the pacchionian granulation impressions in the bone indicate this portion of their course. Normally, there may be a difference of 1 mm. in diameter between the veins on the two sides. When larger differences are found, pathologic processes may be suspected.

Lateral lacunae should be considered widenings of the parasagittal portions of the meningeal veins. They are usually lacking at birth (as are the arachnoidal granulations) and develop later to form large irregular spaces filled with these granulations. The lacunae are widest where the meningeal veins empty into them. They communicate with neighboring cerebral veins and with the

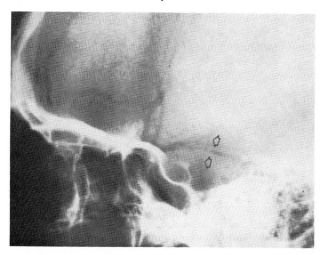

F

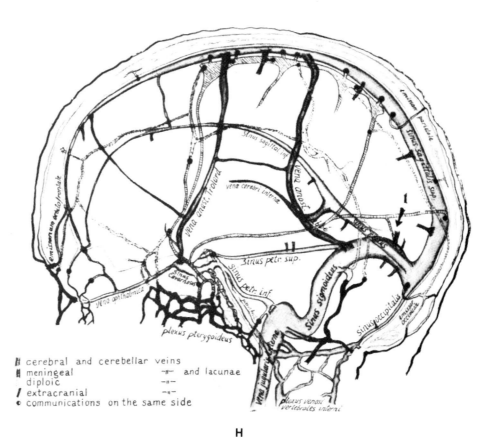

H

Figure 6–11 *Continued.* *F.* PA demonstrating some of the venous impressions. 1, venous lacuna, showing the branching veins communicating with it; 2, arachnoid granulation impression; 3, diploic venous impressions. *G.* The middle temporal branch of the superficial temporal artery (arrows). (*F* and *G* from Meschan, I.: Seminars in Roentgenol., 9:125–136, 1974. Used by permission.) *H.* Diagram of the veins and dural sinuses of the cranium and their communications. (From Lindblom, K.: Acta Radiol. (Stockholm), Suppl. 30, 1936.)

G

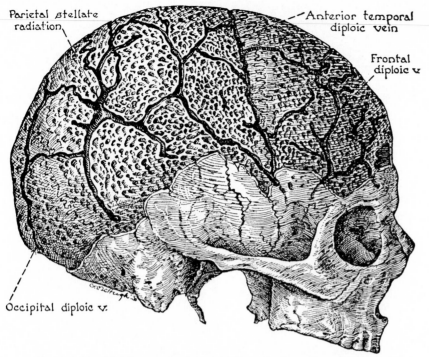

Figure 6–12. Diploic venous plexuses of the calvarium. (From Bailey, P.: Intracranial Tumors. 1957. Courtesy of Charles C Thomas, Publisher, Springfield, Illinois.)

The middle meningeal artery can be followed from its entry into the base of the skull more or less completely out to its third and fourth order branches (Fig. 6–11 C). The artery and its branches become relatively deeper and more visible with increasing age and accompanying deposition of bone on the inner table. The arteries' share of this space in this sulcus relative to that of the veins varies from patient to patient. In the posterior groove, the artery takes up a relatively large portion; the reverse is often true anteriorly. The grooves have irregular outlines, branch dichotomously, and diminish progressively in size as they extend distally.

Lindblom has measured these grooves as follows: a distinct arterial groove at the pterion has an average breadth of 1.5 mm. with a maximum of 2 mm., and the groove for the posterior main trunk measures 1 mm. with a maximum of 2 mm. According to Lindblom, any marked difference in the size of the grooves on the two sides is abnormal.

3. **Venous Plexuses Within the Diploë.** The venous plexuses within the diploë (Fig. 6–12) are impressions within the diploë found in each of the frontal, parietal, and occipital bones, giving the skull a mosaic appearance on the radiograph. In the parietal bones particularly, they have been referred to as the "parietal star" or "spider." At times these appear unusually accentuated. It is usually hazardous, however, to interpret any abnormality on the appearance of the venous diploë alone. Besides diploic veins there are diploic lakes that appear as irregular, grossly oval or round areas of radiolucency and rarely exceed 2 cm. in widest diameter. They are most common in the parietal bones. They are well demarcated and the bone around them is intact.

Diploic veins begin to appear at about 5 years of age. Between

vein of Trollard. The bone depressions for the lacunae are most clearly seen radiographically in an axial projection of the vertex. Somewhat similar lengthened depressions may be produced by sinusoidal cerebral veins, and at times they are difficult to differentiate, particularly on the lateral views alone.

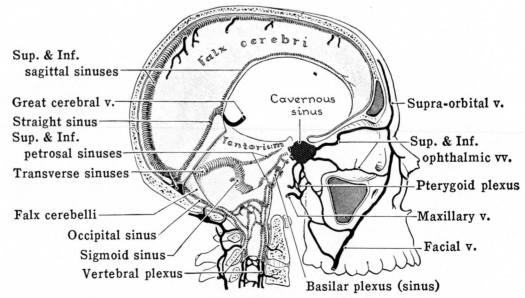

Figure 6–13. Diagram of the venous sinuses of the dura mater. (Reproduced by permission from J. C. B. Grant: An Atlas of Anatomy, 5th ed. Copyright © 1962, The Williams and Wilkins Co.)

5 and 30 years of age one or more diploic veins may reach widths as great as 3 mm. After age 30, this is not at all uncommon in the frontal or parietotemporal regions. A difference in size between corresponding veins on the two sides is found in about 5 per cent of individuals, but usually does not exceed 1 mm. (Lindblom).

4. **Venous Sinuses.** The venous sinuses (Fig. 6–13) produce their impression on the inner table of the skull so that they appear as radiolucent channels bounded by curved bony ridges. The lateral sinus (or transverse sinus) is the largest of these, and has its origin near the internal occipital protuberance, passing forward around the occipital bone with a slight upward convexity to the pneumatic portion of the mastoid bone. Here it curves downward to become the sigmoid sinus.

The sphenoparietal sinus is another commonly prominent venous sinus. It begins in connection with the anterior parietal diploic vein, just posterior to the coronal suture, and then courses along the inferior surface of the lesser wing of the sphenoid to become a tributary of the cavernous sinus.

The point of junction of the lateral sinuses and the superior sagittal sinus is virtually the point of confluence of all the major dural sinuses, and hence is called the *sinus confluens*. It has a variable appearance, resembling a crossroad with or without a bony island contained within it (Fig. 6–14).

5. **Emissary Veins.** In the cranial vault, emissary veins are most frequent in the regions of the occipital protuberance and the parasagittal and posterior aspects of the parietal bone. These represent anastomotic channels between intracranial and extracranial vascular systems. Some of the emissary veins achieve consid-

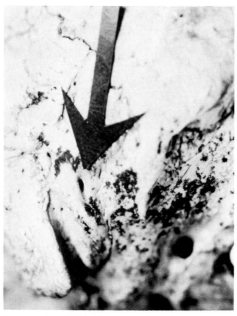

Figure 6–15. Photograph of the mastoid region, demonstrating the site of the mastoid emissary vein.

erable size. One of the most significant of these is the mastoid emissary vein, which is situated near the sigmoid sinus and can be identified posterior to the pneumatized portion of the mastoid (Fig. 6–15). This may contain a small branch of the occipital artery, or it may be in a canal several centimeters in length and 1 to 10 millimeters in width.

An emissary vein up to 2 mm. in diameter may extend from the superior sagittal sinus down to the region of the incisura supra orbitalis.

Also, and quite distinct from the thinning-out of the parietal bones to be described, the parietal bone may contain enlarged *parietal foramina* (Fig. 6–16); this tendency toward enlarged foramina is apparently inherited. Ordinarily extremely small (not greater than 1 mm.), and transmitting an emissary vein, these are situated close to the sagittal suture, about 1 to 1½ inches above the lambdoid suture just medial to the parietal tuberosity.

6. **The Sutures** (Fig. 6–17 *A, B*). A number of important sutures mark the superior portion of the skull: the *sagittal suture* marks the junction of the two parietal bones superiorly, and extends from the bregma, which is its junction with the coronal suture, to the lambda, which is its junction with the lambdoid suture. The *coronal suture* is situated between the parietal bones posteriorly and the frontal bone anteriorly. It ends by joining the sphenoid bone laterally, and this point of union is known as the *pterion* on either side. The *lambdoid suture* is situated between the parietal bone anteriorly and the interparietal portion of the occipital bone posteriorly. Its point of junction with the squamosal suture is known as the *asterion*. When the interparietal portion of the occipital bone exists as an independent element (the

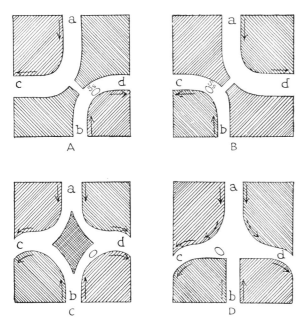

Figure 6–14. Schematic diagram of the sinus confluens, showing variations in its appearance. (From Pendergrass, E. P. et al.: The Head and Neck in Roentgen Diagnosis, 2nd ed., 1956. Courtesy of Charles C Thomas, Publisher, Springfield, Illinois.)

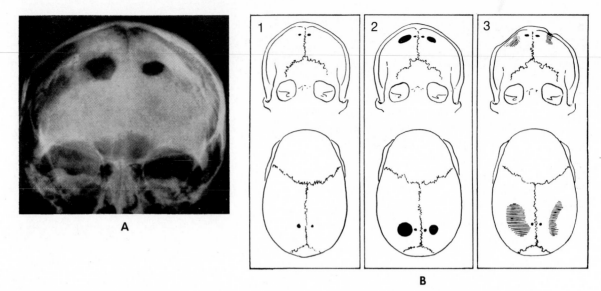

B

Figure 6–16. A. Roentgenograph of a patient with enlarged parietal foramina. (From Pendergrass, E. P. et al.: The Head and Neck in Roentgen Diagnosis, 2nd ed., 1956. Courtesy of Charles C Thomas, Publisher, Springfield, Illinois.) B. Three types of defects in parietal bone. (1) Normal defects in parietal bone containing veins; (2) Emissary foramina and fenestrae (enlarged parietal foramina) shown in same skull; (3) Two forms of thinness shown, quadrangular on left and grooved on right, in association with emissary foramina. (From Nashold, B. S., Jr., and Netsky, M. G.: J. Neuropathol. Exp. Neurol., 18:432, 1959.)

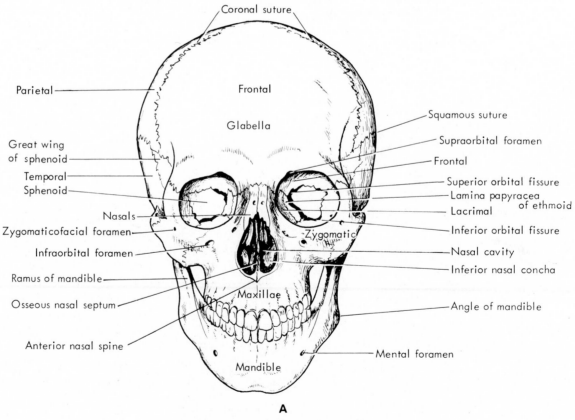

A

Figure 6–17. A. Skull viewed from the front.

Figure 6–17 continued on opposite page.

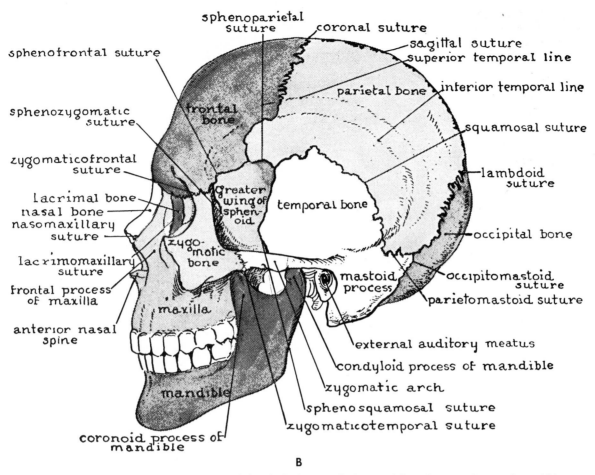

Figure 6–17 *Continued.* B. Lateral view of the skull showing the bones of the calvarium, face, and mandible. (From Pendergrass, E. P., et al.: The Head and Neck in Roentgen Diagnosis, 2nd ed., 1956. Courtesy of Charles C Thomas, Publisher, Springfield, Illinois.)

inca bone), a *transverse occipital suture* is formed between it and the occipital bone proper.

The two halves of the frontal bone normally fuse by the fifth or sixth year of childhood, and this line of fusion disappears; however, in about 10 per cent of cases this suture persists—it is called the *metopic suture* (Fig. 6–18), and extends from the frontonasal suture to the coronal suture. Occasionally this suture may persist incompletely, leading to an erroneous interpretation of skull fracture.

On the lateral aspect of the skull, the *sphenofrontal, sphenoparietal,* and *squamosal sutures* form a continuous irregular line outlining the upper outer margin of the greater wing of the sphenoid and the squamous temporal bone. These extend from the posterior margin of the frontal bone to the occipital bone. There are several important variations in the interrelationship of the frontal, temporal, sphenoid, and parietal bones. Occasionally, the sphenoparietal suture is lacking, and the coronal suture is directly continuous with the suture between the greater wing of the sphenoid and the squamous temporal bone. On other occasions, there is an extra bone at this crossing, known as the *epipteric*

bone (example of sutural or wormian bone). Other variations are shown in Figure 6–19. The *sphenozygomatic suture* is situated between the zygomatic bone and the greater wing of the sphenoid. The *zygomaticofrontal suture* is situated between the frontal process of the zygoma and the inferolateral portion of the frontal bone.

Extending horizontally from the squamosal suture to the lambdoid suture is a small irregular suture that remains rather prominent throughout life, known as the *parietomastoid suture*. It is situated between the mastoid process of the temporal bones and the parietal bone. On the posterior aspect of the mastoid process and between the latter and the occipital bone is the *occipitomastoid* suture. The *zygomaticotemporal suture* joins the zygomatic processes of the zygomatic and temporal bones. This is usually situated at the junction of the anterior and middle thirds of the zygomatic arch.

The superior and inferior temporal lines are muscular and fascial attachment ridges situated 2 to 3 cm. above the squamosal sutures in the parietal bones, and should not be confused with sutures.

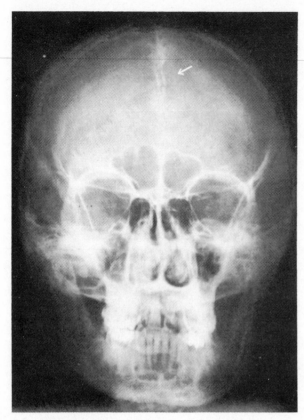

Figure 6–18. Film showing metopic suture.

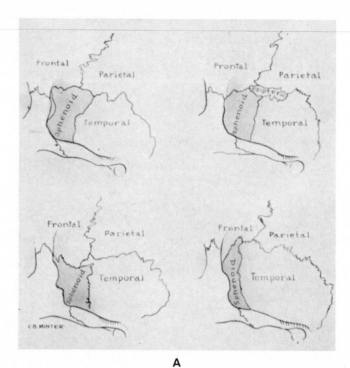

A

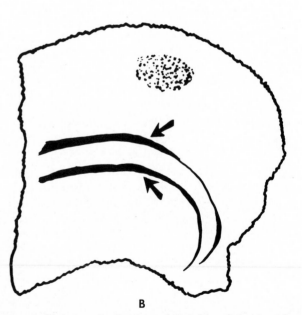

B

On the basilar aspect (Fig. 6–20), the occipital bone articulates with the mastoid process at the occipitomastoid suture, and with the petrous temporal bone at the *occipitopetrosal suture.* The basilar portion of the occipital bone articulates with the body of the sphenoid at the *basisphenoid suture.* The sphenosquamosal suture can be identified once again between the sphenoid and the squamous temporal bone medial to the mandibular fossa for articulation with the mandible; the *sphenopetrosal suture* is situated anteriorly between the sphenoid and the petrous temporal bone. The *median palatine suture* is situated between the two palatine processes of the maxillae, and the *transverse palatine suture* between the palatine processes of the maxilla and the palatine bone. The vomer articulates with six bones: two of the cranium—the sphenoid and the ethmoid; and four of the face—the two maxillae and the two palatine bones. It also joins with the septal cartilage of the nose.

Sutural (or wormian) bones are occasionally found to lie within a suture, particularly at its junction with another suture. This is especially true of the lambdoid suture, and in the region of the pterion (Fig. 6–21).

The sutures ordinarily present a very irregular appearance and follow the rather definite anatomic pattern described here

Figure 6–19. *A.* Variations in the interrelationship of the frontal, temporal, sphenoid, and parietal bones. (From Pendergrass, E. P. et al.: The Head and Neck in Roentgen Diagnosis, 2nd ed., 1956. Courtesy of Charles C Thomas, Publisher, Springfield, Illinois.) *B.* Line diagram showing the superior and inferior ridges of the parietal bones. The dotted areas indicate the parietal fossa. (From Meschan, I.: Seminars in Roentgenol., 9:125–136, 1974. Used by permission.)

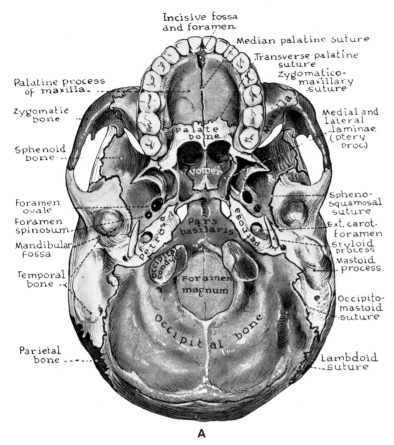

Figure 6-20 labels:
Incisive fossa and foramen
Median palatine suture
Transverse palatine suture
Zygomatico-maxillary suture
Palatine process of maxilla
Zygomatic bone
Sphenoid bone
Maxilla
Palate bone
Vomer
Medial and lateral laminae (ptery. proc.)
Foramen ovale
Foramen spinosum
Pars basilaris
Petrous
Mandibular fossa
Occipital condyle
Temporal bone
Foramen magnum
Spheno-squamosal suture
Ext. carot. foramen
Styloid process
Mastoid process
Occipito-mastoid suture
Parietal bone
Occipital bone
Lambdoid suture

A

The mendosal suture closes first, several weeks after birth. The metopic suture begins to close in the second year and is usually completely obliterated by age 3, but in about 10 per cent of cases it may persist throughout life. The fissure between the exoccipital and supraoccipital portions of the occipital bone—the so-called innominate synchondrosis—disappears between the second and third years of life. The other sutures of the head usually do not close until at least age 30 or somewhat later.

Sometimes a suture produces a double line, owing to the separate appearance of the suture on its inner and outer table aspect; these differences are greatest in the region of the sagittal suture and in the medial portions of the coronal and lambdoid sutures.

Wormian (Sutural) Bones. Sutural bones persisting within a suture and not incorporated into the adjacent bone during mineralization and maturation are called *wormian bones* after the Danish anatomist Olaus Worm. The largest of these is the interparietal bone, which is triangular in shape and represents the interparietal portion of the occipital bone above the mendosal suture. A fetal wormian bone, usually disappearing by birth and

Figure 6-20. *A.* The skull viewed from below. (From Pendergrass, E. P. et al.: The Head and Neck in Roentgen Diagnosis, 2nd ed., 1956. Courtesy of Charles C Thomas, Publisher, Springfield, Illinois.) *B.* Radiograph of the bone of the skull. For details of anatomy see subsequent descriptions and labels.

and illustrated. Under the age of 6, the sutures are considerably wider than they are in the adult, beginning with the relatively widespread appearance in the newborn (Fig. 6-35). The appearance of the normal degree of separation at the various age levels must be clearly recognized so that diastasis of a suture can be diagnosed in the child or the adult following trauma.

The width of neonatal sutures varies greatly between 1½ and 10 or 11 mm. for the coronal and lambdoid sutures. Taveras and Wood (1964) indicated that the most reliable site for measurement is the top of the coronal sutures in the lateral view. In children older than 3 years, the width at the vertex of this suture should be less than 2 mm. Between 2 and 12 months of age it should be no more than 3 mm.

The posterior, anterolateral, anterior, and posterolateral fontanelles are closed by 8 weeks, 3 months, 15 to 18 months, and 2 years, respectively. Closure of the anterior fontanelle marks the disappearance of the last remnant of the membranous calvarium.

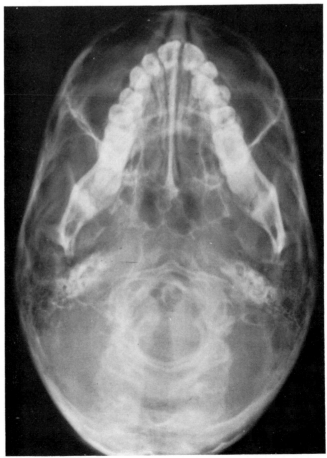

B

fusing with the supraoccipital bone at the posterior margin of the foramen magnum, is the so-called *Kerckring's bone,* described by Caffey in 1953.

Sutural Sclerosis. Often a dense band of sclerosis occurs along sutures owing to a continuous bridging process across the suture. These bands vary in size and may be as large as 15 mm. Sutural sclerosis is a normal physiologic process that becomes more apparent with advancing age.

7. **The Digitate or Convolutional Markings** (Fig. 6–22). These are irregular areas of increased and decreased density throughout the skull that are caused by thinning of the inner table from pressure produced by the convolutions or gyri of the brain. In persons under approximately 16 years of age, these may be readily detectable normally. Beyond this age, or when unduly accentuated in the younger age groups, they may indicate increased intracranial pressure and are of pathologic significance.

8. **Thinning of the Bones of the Calvarium.** The parietal bone superiorly and laterally may on occasion be unusually thin owing to a lack of development of the diploë. There may be a bony dehiscence, the inner table being less affected than the outer. This thinning is usually bilateral, but may be unilateral, a variation that is usually normal but occasionally has pathologic significance (Steinbach and Obota).

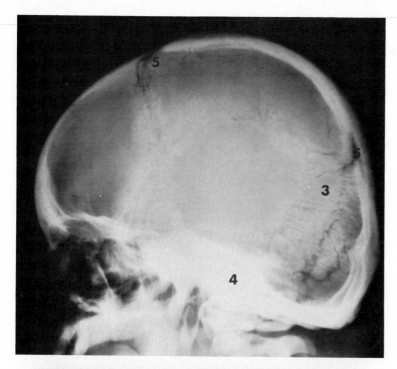

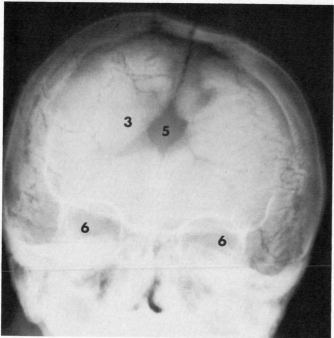

Figure 6–21. Sutural bones in a patient with cleidocranial dysostosis. (3) The numerous wormian bones; (4) the flattened base of the skull; (5) the large open fontanelles; (6) reverse sloping of the petrous ridges associated with flattening of the skull.

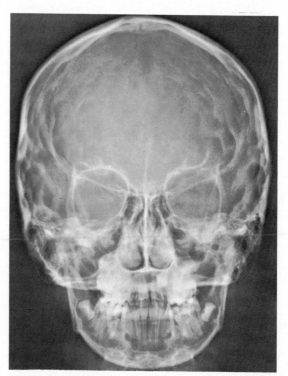

Figure 6–22. Radiograph showing accentuated convolutional markings in a normal young adolescent.

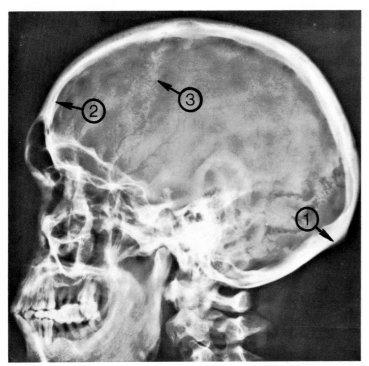

Figure 6-23. Some normal thickened areas of the calvarium. (1) Occipital protuberances; (2) thickening above the frontal sinuses; (3) sclerotic sutural margins.

9. **Thickened Areas of the Calvarium** (Fig. 6-23). The internal and external occipital protuberances ordinarily project inward and outward respectively from the occipital bone, forming thickened areas of bone in these locations. Occasionally, the external protuberance is a considerable process of bone.

There is not infrequently thickened bone immediately above the frontal sinuses, and in the vicinity of the junction of sutures.

There is occasionally also a small exostosis in the external acoustic meatus which may be a minute nodule, or large enough to fill the entire meatus. These are usually bilateral, and when unilateral tend to be more frequent on the left side.

Miscellaneous bone ridges have already been mentioned in connection with the superior and inferior temporal ridges. In the *occipital bone*, the superior and inferior nuchal lines mark the origin of prominent muscles. Detectable ridges may be seen radiographically (Fig. 6-18). In the *frontal bone*, the superciliary arch, located just above the supraorbital foramen or notch and the supraorbital margin, is a readily apparent prominence. The arches of the two sides are separated by the *glabella* (Fig. 6-17). The lateral extremity of the supraorbital margin ends in the zygomatic process, which articulates with the zygomatic bone. The temporal line, which converges upon the zygomatic process, represents the anterior end of the superior and inferior temporal lines of the parietal bone previously described.

In the *sphenoid bone*, the temporal surface of a prominent infratemporal crest is divided into a superior part, which forms part of the wall of the temporal fossa and affords attachment to the temporal muscle, and an inferior part, which forms part of the wall of the infratemporal fossa and to which the lateral pterygoid muscle is attached. The infratemporal crest is usually readily identifiable on the lateral radiograph of the skull.

10. **Depressions in the Contour of the Calvarium.** There may be normal depressions in the contour of the calvarium in the region of the bregma or lambda. When greatly accentuated these may be an indication of developmental deficiency or abnormality, but otherwise may be considered a normal variant.

A Correlated Anatomic and Radiographic Survey of the External Aspect of the Base of the Skull

Viewed from the external aspect, the base of the skull (Fig. 6-20) is divisible into three portions.

1. The anterior portion consists principally of the palatine processes of the maxillary bone, palatine bone, and the upper alveolus bearing the teeth.

2. The middle portion lies between the posterior edge of the hard palate and the anterior margin of the foramen magnum. This contains the basilar portion of the occipital bone, the petrous portions of the temporal bone, the body and greater wings and laminae of the sphenoids, and the vomer. The *foramen lacerum* is an irregular aperture situated at the junction of the petrous apex along with the basilar occipital bone and the sphenoid. Within the petrous ridge posterolateral to the foramen lacerum is the entrance opening for the carotid canal, and still more laterally is the *stylomastoid foramen* from which the facial nerve emerges from the skull. The *jugular foramen* is formed between the apex of the petrous temporal bones and the occipital and is slightly larger on the right than the left. Within the sphenoid bone, just anterior to the petrous portion of the temporal bone, are three major orifices, called (reading from front to back): the *foramen rotundum* (concealed), the *foramen ovale,* and the *foramen spinosum.* The foramen rotundum is somewhat hidden under the pterygoid processes of the sphenoid. The pterygoid processes together with the vomer and the palatine bone form the *choanae,* or posterior nares, which open into the nasal cavity. Lateral to the choanae are the *pterygoid fossae* and the internal auditory or eustachian tubes which connect with the middle ear. The foramen rotundum transmits the maxillary nerve; the foramen ovale, the mandibular nerve; and the foramen spinosum, the middle meningeal vessels.

3. The posterior portion contains the *foramen magnum.* On either side of this area are the occipital condyles, and immediately anterolateral to these condyles are the *jugular* and *hypoglossal foramina.* The jugular foramen transmits the internal jugular vein, the ninth, tenth, and eleventh cranial nerves, and the

lateral and inferior petrosal dural venous sinuses. The hypoglossal foramen transmits the hypoglossal nerve (twelfth cranial nerve) and a small artery. The lateral margin of this portion is formed by the mastoid process of the temporal bone on either side. A line drawn from one external acoustic meatus to the other would pass through the following parts: the stylomastoid foramen, the root of the styloid process, the jugular foramen, the hypoglossal canal, the anterior margin of the occipital condyle, and the anterior margin of the foramen magnum, in that order lateromedially.

In the lateral roentgenogram (Fig. 6–23), the base of the skull appears as a steplike, irregular structure that descends from the frontal sinuses to the upper margin of the cervical spine. Each succeeding step represents a separate subdivision of the inside of the cranium, and these will be described in greater detail when considering the internal aspect of the cranial cavity.

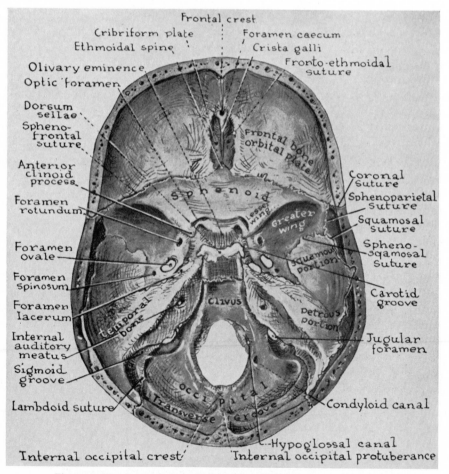

Figure 6–24. Internal aspect of the base of the skull. (From Pendergrass, E. P. et al.: The Head and Neck in Roentgen Diagnosis, 2nd ed., 1956. Courtesy of Charles C Thomas, Publisher, Springfield, Illinois.)

A Correlated Anatomic and Radiographic Consideration of the Internal Aspect of the Cranial Cavity

The floor of the cranial cavity is divided into three fossae (Fig. 6–24) called the anterior, middle, and posterior respectively.

The *anterior cranial fossa* extends between the frontal bone and the sharp posterior margins of the lesser wings of the sphenoid. It is located over the nasal cavity and the orbits, and houses the frontal lobes of the brain. It is formed by the orbital plate of the frontal bone, the cribriform plate of the ethmoid, the lesser wings of the sphenoid, and the ventral part of the body of the sphenoid. The tuberculum sellae and the anterior clinoid processes of the sella turcica form part of the posterior boundary of the fossa centrally. The crista galli rises from the cribriform plate, which ordinarily is depressed. The frontal and ethmoidal air sinuses encroach to a variable extent on the anterior cranial fossa in front and below.

The posterior margin of the lesser wings of the sphenoid marks the location of the anterior part of the lateral cerebral fissure (Sylvian fissure), and hence helps to demarcate the position of the frontal from the temporal lobes of the brain (see Fig. 6–25).

In the lateral view of the skull, the floor of this fossa has a very irregular appearance related to the impressions formed by the convolutions of the brain. A mind's eye impression of this irregularity must be retained by the student if he is to interpret fractures or abnormalities in bony structure such as occur with some brain tumors in this area.

The *middle cranial fossa* is at a slightly lower level than the anterior, and resembles a bird with outstretched wings. The midportion, formed by the body of the sphenoid, is elevated above the lateral parts and contains the sella turcica, the optic foramina united by the chiasmatic groove, and the carotid grooves. The front elevation of the sella turcica is composed of the tuberculum sellae and the anterior clinoid processes, whereas the back of the sella is composed of the dorsum sellae and the posterior clinoid processes. The curved hollow between the two is called the hypophyseal fossa since it houses the pituitary body of the brain. The carotid groove begins at the medial side of the irregular foramen lacerum and ends medial to the anterior clinoid processes. The cavernous venous sinus lies at the side of the carotid groove and the internal carotid artery is virtually embedded in this sinus.

The lateral portions of the middle cranial fossa are largely formed by the temporal bone, and also by the great wing of the sphenoid and a small portion of the parietal bones. The temporal lobes of the brain are housed here. The posterior margin of the fossa is grooved and contains the superior petrosal venous sinus.

The more important foramina of the middle cranial fossa are: (1) the *optic foramen* for the optic nerve and ophthalmic artery; (2) the *superior orbital fissure,* for passage of the ophthalmic nerve, the third, fourth, and sixth cranial nerves, several small arteries, and sympathetic nerves; (3) the *foramen rotundum*, which transmits the maxillary nerve; (4) the *foramen ovale*, which transmits the mandibular nerve, the lesser superficial petrosal nerve, and the accessory meningeal artery; (5) the *foramen spinosum*, which transmits the middle meningeal artery and the recurrent branch of the mandibular nerve; and (6) the *foramen lacerum*, which is crossed by the internal carotid artery and its sympathetic plexus as it emerges from the carotid canal.

In the lateral radiograph of the skull, the superposition of the mastoid and petrous portions of the temporal bone between the middle and posterior cranial fossae may cause some confusion. Various special views are employed to demonstrate these structures clearly; these special anatomic studies will be described later (Chapter 7).

The *posterior cranial fossa* is below the level of the middle fossa and lodges the cerebellum, pons, and medulla oblongata. It is bounded posteriorly by the transverse sulcus of the occipital bone, and is roofed by the tentorium cerebelli. This tentorium is an arched lamina that covers the superior surface of the cerebellum and supports the occipital lobes of the cerebrum. In the median part of the posterior cranial fossa is the foramen magnum, dividing the occipital bone into three parts as already mentioned. The hypoglossal canal is seen on the medial aspect of its thickened anterior margin above the occipital condyle for articulation with the first cervical vertebra. The *internal occipital crest* is the ridge between the foramen magnum and the internal occipital protuberance. The *clivus* or *basiocciput* is the broad extension of the occipital bone forward to its junction with the basisphenoid. The transverse sinus sweeps around the occipital bone to the margin of the sigmoid groove at the lateral margin of the petrous temporal bone and curves forward to the jugular foramen. This latter leads downward to the lower surface of the skull and there is situated opposite the lower margin of the external acoustic meatus, separated from it by the styloid process. The jugular foramen transmits the large venous sinuses (inferior petrosal and lateral) and the ninth, tenth, and eleventh cranial nerves as well as meningeal branches from the occipital and accessory pharyngeal arteries. The *internal acoustic meatus,* which is situated in the anterior wall of the posterior cranial fossa, is a short canal in the petrous portion of the temporal bone and is separated laterally by thin bone from the internal ear. It transmits the auditory and facial nerves.

Towne's position (Fig. 6–44) affords an excellent opportunity to study many structures in the middle and posterior fossae. The posterior two-thirds of the foramen magnum is shown quite clearly, and very frequently the neural arch of the first cervical vertebra is seen through it. The spinous process of the second cervical vertebra may also be seen. The dorsum sellae is frequently seen faintly identified along with the posterior clinoid processes.

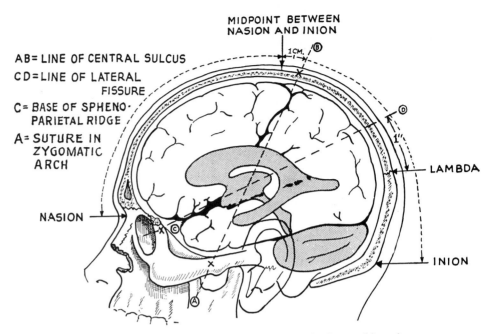

Figure 6–25. Diagram of the brain: relationship of the central sulcus and lateral fissure to the ventricles and skull.

The petrous portion of the temporal bone extends laterally from the foramen magnum. In this structure, the internal acoustic meatus, the arcuate eminence (under which lie the semicircular canals), the tegmen tympani, and the mastoid process can be identified. The occipital bone extends above these ridges on either side. Extending from the region of the tegmen tympani is a rather broad suture, the occipitomastoid suture, which intersects the parietomastoid suture. Extending inward from this intersection is the lambdoid suture. The junction of these three sutures is the *asterion.* In the midline the lambdoid suture meets the sagittal suture at the lambda. The grooves for the venous sinuses in the occipital bone and the increased density in the region of the internal occipital protuberance have already been described.

BASIC ANATOMY OF THE BASAL FORAMINA AND CANALS OF THE SKULL

Greater Palatine Foramen (Fig. 6–26). The greater palatine foramen is situated in the posterior angle of the palate and connects the pterygopalatine canal with the oral cavity. It transmits the greater palatine artery and the greater or anterior palatine branch of the sphenopalatine nerve, which in turn supply the gums and mucous membranes of the hard palate and adjoining soft palate. *Radiologically,* this foramen may be visualized on the

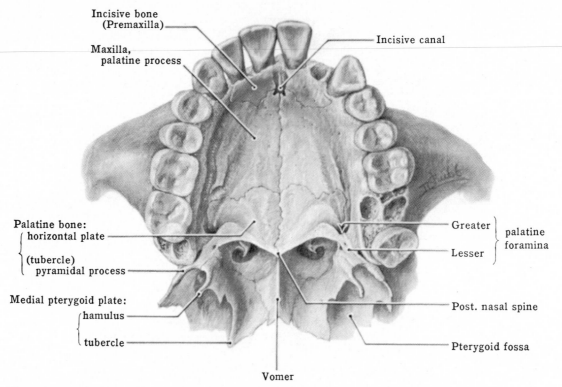

Incisive bone
(Premaxilla)

Maxilla,
palatine process

Incisive canal

Palatine bone:
horizontal plate

(tubercle)
pyramidal process

Medial pterygoid plate:
hamulus

tubercle

Greater
Lesser
} palatine
foramina

Post. nasal spine

Pterygoid fossa

Vomer

Figure 6–26. The bony palate. (Reproduced by permission from J. C. B. Grant: An Atlas of Anatomy, 5th ed. Copyright © 1962, The Williams & Wilkins Company.)

submentovertical projection in the lateral aspect of the palate anterior to the medial pterygoid plate and lesser palatine foramen. It usually measures about 2 mm. in diameter.

Lesser Palatine Foramen (Fig. 6–26). The lesser palatine foramen may be multiple and is situated in the pyramidal process of the palatine bone posterior to the greater palatine foramen. This foramen transmits the lesser palatine nerve and various smaller branches of the greater palatine artery and distributes them to the soft palate, uvula, and tonsils. The lesser palatine foramen is occasionally visualized on standard submentovertical projections just anterior to the medial pterygoid plate. There may be one or two foramina on each side, 1 mm. in diameter, with well-defined margins.

Foramen Rotundum (Fig. 6–27 *E, F*). The medial wall of the foramen rotundum is formed by the lateral wall of the sphenoid sinus, separated only by a few millimeters. The foramen connects the middle cranial fossa with the pterygopalatine fossa. The average length of the canal (or foramen rotundum; the terms are used synonymously) is 3.4 mm., with a range of 2 to 5 mm. (Sondheimer). The other dimensions quoted are 2.9 mm., with a range of 2 to 4 mm., as the average height, and the average width is 3.2 mm., with a range of 1.5 to 4 mm. The left side is slightly wider. The measurements similarly obtained by Lindblom in 1936 were

3×3 mm. to 3.5×4 mm. The foramen rotundum transmits the second division of the trigeminal nerve or maxillary nerve. A few small emissary veins may also traverse this foramen.

The recommended projections for the foramen rotundum are the Caldwell's and Water's, or a slight modification of the latter (Taveras and Wood), decreasing the angle of the orbitomeatal line from 37 to 25 degrees. The foramen is projected into the upper part of the maxillary antrum relatively free of overlying shadows (Fig. 6–47).

Gross congenital asymmetry of the foramina is relatively infrequent but can occur (Shapiro and Robinson).

Pterygospinous and Pterygoalar Bars and Foramina (Fig. 6–27 *A*). The internal and external pterygoid muscles are separated by a thickened fascia cranially, known as the pterygospinous and pterygoalar ligaments. These may occasionally calcify or ossify. When calcified, they are known as bars and may be visualized radiographically, especially on tomography. Tebo (1968) has reported an incidence of 4.3 per cent of these bars. The pterygospinous bar is always medial and the pterygoalar bar always lateral to the foramen ovale. The space enclosed by the pterygoalar bar is called the pterygoalar foramen, and this transmits the major motor branches of the mandibular nerve to the muscles of mastication. This bar may be as wide as 4 mm. and is visible as an

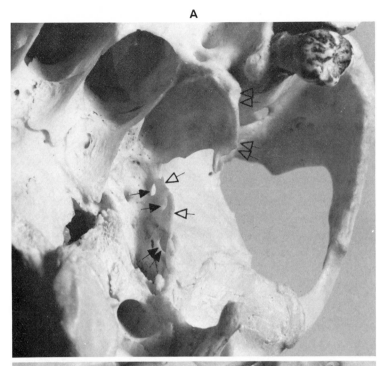

A

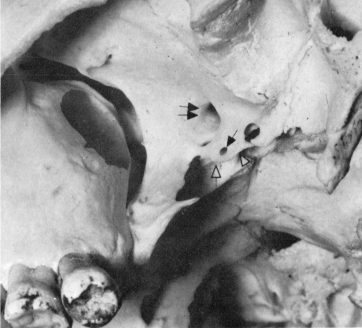

B

Figure 6–27. Photographs (*A* and *B*) and roentgenograms (*C* and *D*) of large pterygospinous bar (open arrows). In *A*, origin from the lateral pterygoid plate (double open arrows) and course of the bar medial to foramen spinosum (double solid arrows) are apparent. Single solid arrows indicate pterygospinous foramina. In oblique view, *B*, foramen ovale is indicated by double solid arrows.

Figure 6–27 continued on the following page.

increased density over the lateral margin of the foramen ovale. The pterygoalar bar is clinically important because of its lateral position, particularly in relation to injections of the mandibular nerve and the gasserian ganglion.

Foramen Spinosum (Fig. 6–20). The foramen spinosum is a small opening in the posteromedial aspect of the greater wing of the sphenoid connecting the infratemporal fossa with the middle cranial fossa. It is usually 2 to 4 mm. long and oval or round in cross section. It varies between 2 and 3 mm. in diameter (Lindblom), the difference between long and short diameters averaging 0.5 mm. It transmits the middle meningeal artery and also the middle meningeal vein or veins emptying into the pterygoid plexus. The recurrent or meningeal branch of the mandibular nerve enters the skull through this foramen and sends a branch to the mucous membrane of the mastoid air cells.

The foramen spinosum is usually well demonstrated in the full axial projection. Lindblom found it to average 2 mm. in width, with a minimum of 1 mm. and a maximum of 3.5 mm. The two foramina are rather symmetric, differing only by 1.5 mm. in 1 per cent and 1 mm. in 2 per cent.

Sondheimer's measurements on 50 basal projections with a focal spot-to-film distance of 40 inches were as follows: average, 2.3 by 3 mm.; smallest, 1 by 1 mm.; largest and longest, 3 by 5 mm.; widest, 3.5 by 2.5 mm. A difference of more than 1 mm. between the foramina on the two sides was found in 12 per cent of the roentgenograms, of exactly 1 mm. in 20 per cent of the films, and the remainder differed by 0.5 mm. or were equal in size.

Foramen of Vesalius (Sphenoid Emissary Foramen). The foramen of Vesalius is a small inconstant opening in the medial aspect of the greater wing of the sphenoid, anteromedial to the foramen ovale, connecting the medial aspect of the middle fossa with the region of the scaphoid fossa in which the tensor veli palatini originates. It is usually 1 mm. in diameter but may be very slightly larger in about 5 per cent of the specimens (Boyd); it is bilateral in 15 per cent of the cases and unilateral in about 22 per cent. An emissary vein connecting the cavernous sinus and the pterygoid plexus is transmitted through this foramen. Sometimes there are two foramina on one side (Schüller).

The Canal of Arnold or Innominate Canaliculus. The innominate canaliculus is a small canal occasionally found a few millimeters posterior to the foramen ovale and medial to the foramen spinosum. The canal transmits the lesser superficial petrosal nerve. Occasionally, this canal carries the preganglionic parasympathetic fibers to the parotid gland via the otic ganglion. The innominate canaliculus is seen in the submentovertical projection (Fig. 6–28) as a slitlike opening extending toward the foramen ovale between the petrosphenoid synchondrosis and the foramen spinosum.

Foramen Lacerum. (Fig. 6–20). This is actually an aperture filled inferiorly with fibrocartilage. It is located at the base of the medial pterygoid plate and bounded anteriorly and laterally by

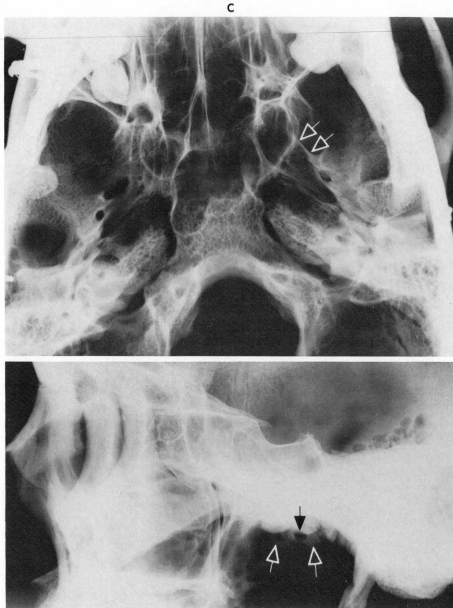

Figure 6–27 *Continued.* C. Submentovertical roentgenogram demonstrates that pterygospinous bar (arrows) partially obscures foramen ovale. *D.* Pterygospinous bar (*open arrows*) and pterygospinous foramen (solid arrow) in lateral projection. (*A* to *D* from Sondheimer, F. H.: Basal foramina and canals. *In* Newton, T. H., and Potts, D. G.: Radiology of the Skull and Brain. The Skull, Vol. 1, Book 1, St. Louis, C. V. Mosby Co., 1971.)

Figure 6–27 continued on the opposite page.

the greater wing of the sphenoid. Posteriorly, it is bounded by the apex of the petrous portion of the temporal bone and medially by the sphenoid and basiocciput. The posterior end of the pterygoid canal opens in front of the foramen, and the rostral opening of the carotid canal ends on its posterior aspect. Its size is quite variable. Although it has been thought that the carotid artery traverses this fissure, this is probably not true—the carotid merely rests on the endocranial aspects of the cartilage that fills the foramen lacerum. The structures actually passing through the foramen lacerum are the meningeal branch of the ascending pharyngeal artery and the nerve of the pterygoid canal. Sometimes a vein that connects the cavernous sinus and the pterygoid plexus also traverses this canal.

The foramen lacerum may be seen on the submentovertical projection as an irregular spiculated structure (Fig. 6–20).

Pterygoid Canal (Vidian Canal). The pterygoid canal is

in the body of the sphenoid that connects the foramen lacerum with the pterygoid palatine fossa. Its posterior opening is below the foramen rotundum, and it flares like a trumpet as it extends forward and opens into the pterygopalatine fossa. Its average length is 14.5 mm., with a range of 6 to 20 mm. (Sondheimer). The width averages 1.5 mm. and ranges from 0.5 to 2.5 mm. The canal transmits the nerve of the pterygoid canal (vidian nerve), an autonomic nerve, which enters the sphenopalatine ganglion. The artery of the pterygoid canal, or vidian artery, arises from the third part of the internal maxillary artery and is distributed to the upper pharynx and eustachian tube. *Radiologically,* the pterygoid canal is visualized on routine Caldwell and Water's views (Figs. 6-42 and 6-47), where it appears as a 1 to 2 mm. round lucency with sclerotic margins. It is better demonstrated by tomography.

Carotid Canal. The carotid canal is situated in the inferior aspect of the petrous portion of the temporal bone, in front of and medial to the tympanic cavity and cochlea. The carotid artery enters the cranial cavity or middle fossa between the lingula and the petrosal process of the body of the sphenoid. The average width of the carotid canal at the bend is 5.5 mm., ranging between 5 and 6.5 mm., and its length is 3 to 4 cm. (Lindblom). It transmits the internal carotid artery; several small veins from the cavernous sinus that surround the carotid artery and drain into the internal jugular vein; and the internal carotid nerve, which is a continuation of the superior cervical ganglion of the sympathetic trunk, dividing into two branches in the canal.

Radiographically, the full axial view (Fig. 6-46) is the best projection for demonstration of the carotid canal. However, the length of the canal may be seen on Stenver's projection (Fig. 7-38). Tomograms are most satisfactory for this purpose (Fig. 6-3).

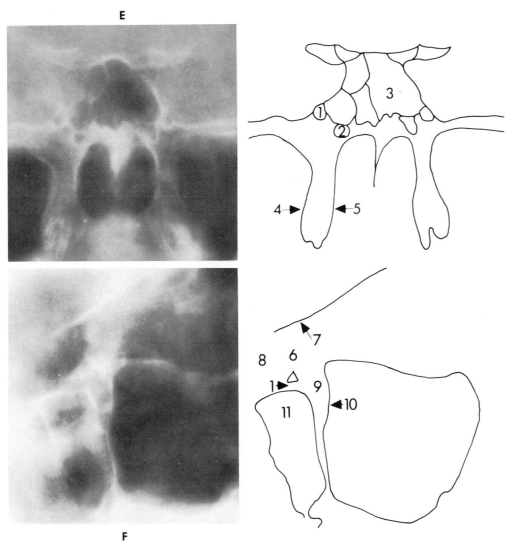

Figure 6-27 *Continued.* E. Coronal tomogram through the foramen rotundum and the pterygoid canal and line drawing of E. *1,* Foramen rotundum; *2,* pterygoid canal; *3,* sphenoid sinus; *4,* lateral pterygoid plate; *5,* medial pterygoid plate. F. Lateral tomogram through the foramen rotundum and line drawing of F, *1,* Foramen rotundum; *6,* superior orbital fissure; *7,* roof of orbit; *8,* middle cranial fossa; *9,* pterygopalatine fossa; *10,* posterior wall of maxillary antrum; *11,* pterygoid process. (From Potter, G. D.: Radiog. Clin. N. Amer., 10:27, April, 1972.)

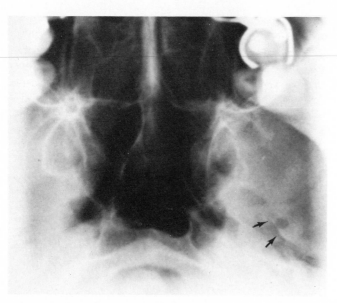

Figure 6–28. Small canaliculus innominatus (arrows) is seen medial to the foramen. (From Sondheimer, F. H.: Basal foramina and canals. *In* Newton, T. H., and Potts, D. G.: Radiology of the Skull and Brain. The Skull, Vol. 1, Book 1. St. Louis, C. V. Mosby Co., 1971.)

Jugular Foramen (Fig. 6–29). The jugular foramen opens into the base of the skull between the lateral edge of the occipital bone and the inferomedial aspect of the petrous pyramid. It connects the posterior fossa with the upper cervical region. The stylomastoid foramen and styloid process are lateral to the foramen. The occipital condyle is medial to it, and the exocranial opening of the carotid canal is anterior to it. It is separated from the carotid canal by a thin bony ridge. A fibrous or bony septum divides the jugular foramen into an anterior *pars nervosa* and a posterior sector, *pars vascularis.*

The size and shape of the jugular foramen vary considerably (DiChiro et al.). There is frequent asymmetry between the foramina on the two sides, with the right side equal to or larger than the left in 70 to 90 per cent of the cases. However, DiChiro et al. considered a difference of more than 20 mm. between the two canals to be pathologic.

The jugular foramen transmits the inferior petrosal sinus, which joins the internal jugular vein within or slightly below the jugular foramen, and the glossopharyngeal or ninth nerve. This nerve branches into the tympanic nerve of Jacobson within the jugular foramen, and this supplies the parotid gland and mucous membrane of the middle ear and continues as the lesser superficial petrosal nerve.

The internal jugular vein originates in the lateral portion of the jugular foramen as a jugular bulb, which represents a continuation of the transverse sinus. It is joined by the inferior petrosal sinus. The vagus nerve or tenth nerve leaves the skull through the posterior portion of the jugular foramen with the accessory nerve but separate from the glossopharyngeal nerve. Within the jugular foramen the vagus nerve gives rise to the nerve of Arnold, its auricular branch. The accessory or eleventh nerve is a motor nerve divided into a cranial portion and a spinal portion. These are usually united within the jugular foramen in a common sheath with the vagus. When the eleventh nerve leaves the foramen its cranial portion joins the vagus and is distributed to the muscles of the pharynx and larynx; the spinal portion enters the skull through the foramen magnum, pierces the dura over the jugular bulb, and joins the cranial portion for a short distance. It then leaves the skull through the jugular foramen and is distributed to the sternocleidomastoid and trapezius muscles.

Meningeal branches of the ascending pharyngeal and occipital arteries also enter the skull through the jugular foramen, ending in the dura of the posterior fossa.

The radiologic depiction of the jugular foramen is not feasible on the standard roentgenograms of the skull, and various special views have been devised, some of which are illustrated (Figs. 6–54, 6–55, 6–56). Polytomography is ideal for this purpose.

Foramen Ovale. The foramen ovale (Fig. 6–20) is visualized best in the submentovertical projections, and an axial view with a 10 to 13 degree caudad angulation of the central ray is best for this purpose (Fig. 6–46). Basal tomography, of course, permits still better definition. The foramen is usually directed somewhat ventrally and laterally. From the axial view, Lindblom found the

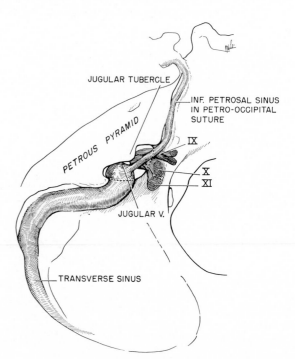

Figure 6–29. Contents of the normal jugular foramen. Glomus jugulare tumors arise most often from the jugular vein adventitia, but can also arise from the sheath of cranial nerves ix, x, or xi. (From Strickler, J. M.: Amer. J. Roentgenol., 97:601–606, 1966.)

following measurements in *adults:* 5 × 8.5 mm. (minimum 3 × 5.5 mm.; maximum 7 × 11 mm.), or 34 sq. mm. in oval cross-sectional area. A magnification of 13 per cent was used in these measurements. Measurements directly on the skeleton without magnification were: 4 × 7 mm., or 22 sq. mm. (minimum 3 × 6 mm.; maximum 4.5 × 10 mm.). In *children* under 5 years of age the average was 30 sq. mm. (magnified value).

Orley's measurements in 1949 were 2 to 7.5 mm. (width) times 5 to 11 mm. (length). Sondheimer's measurements (quoting Radoievitch et al. in 300 specimens) were 3 to 10 mm. (width) times 6 to 14 mm. (length). The smallest foramen measured 3 × 7 mm. and the largest 8 × 14 mm. The foramina on the two sides did not differ by more than 4 mm. in any direction and were otherwise symmetrical, with a difference on the two sides of 2 mm. or less in 80 per cent of the cases.

The foramen ovale transmits the mandibular nerve (third division of the trigeminal nerve) primarily. There is also an ovale emissary sinus—of some significance since injections are made into this area for treatment of trigeminal neuralgia. The accessory meningeal branch of the internal maxillary artery enters the skull through the posterolateral portion of the foramen ovale; middle meningeal veins also occasionally pass through the foramen in its posterior aspect (Henderson).

Foramen Magnum (Fig. 6–30). The foramen magnum is formed within the basal part of the occipital bone. The occipital condyles contribute to the anterior half of the lateral borders of the foramen magnum. Note the occipital condyle and the condy-

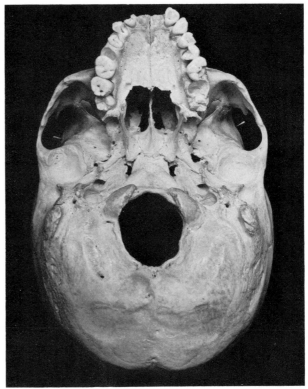

A

NORMAL MEASUREMENTS OF FORAMEN MAGNUM IN
NORMAL AND ARNOLD-CHIARI SKULLS*

	Age in Years	Sex	Width[a]	Length[a]
Normal	1–3	Female	31 ± 3 mm.	39 ± 4.5 mm.
	1–3	Male	31 ± 2.5	40 ± 5.4
	3–7	Female	34 ± 2.4	39 ± 4.8
	3–7	Male	34 ± 2.4	43 ± 3.7
	7 and greater	Female	35 ± 2.8	44 ± 3.5
Arnold-Chiari	1–3	Female	36 ± 4	50 ± 7
	1–3	Male	38 ± 3.8	46 ± 7
	3–7	Female	43 ± 4.6	51 ± 6.4
	3–7	Male	44 ± 3	51 ± 5.3
	7 and greater	Female	46 ± 5	52 ± 4.8
		Male	46 ± 3.4	54 ± 4.8

[a]40 degree half-axial view in supine position for the width measurement. Magnification 25 per cent. For length measurements, focus-object 75 cm. Object-film distance 15 cm. Magnification 20 per cent.

B

Figure 6–30. *A.* Photograph of foramen magnum. *B.* Normal measurements of foramen magnum in normal and Arnold-Chiari skulls. (From Kruyff, E., and Jeffs, R.: Skull abnormalities in the Arnold-Chiari malformation. Acta Radiol. (Diag.), 5:9–24, 1966.)

SPHENOID ANGLE AND FACIAL ANGLE

SPHENOID ANGLE : *ANGLE BETWEEN SPHENOID AND CLIVUS (ALSO CALLED "BASAL ANGLE")*

FACIAL ANGLE : *ANGLE BETWEEN SLOPE OF FACIAL BONES AND LINE DRAWN BETWEEN ALVEOLUS AND FORAMEN MAGNUM AS SHOWN.*

NASO-PINEAL ANGLE : *ROOT OF NOSE TO MIDPOINT OF DIAPHRAGMA SELLAE AND FROM THIS TO PINEAL GLAND (NORMAL: 138.5°-157.5°) SECOND LIMB OF ANGLE: 3.9-53 CM. (± 2 STAND. DEV.) [ISLEY ET AL]*

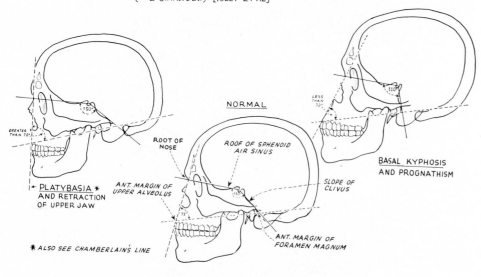

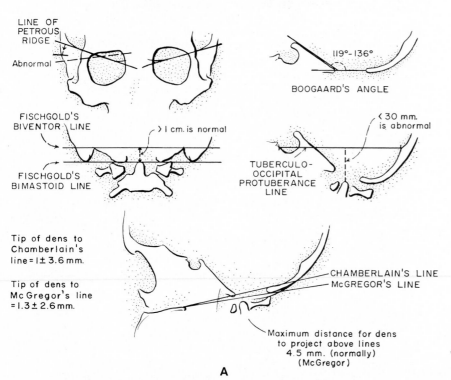

Figure 6–31. A. Measurements at the craniovertebral junction, including the sphenoid and facial angles, as well as the various alignment techniques for the odontoid process with respect to the base of the skull.

Figure 6–31 continued on opposite page.

loid fossa in the accompanying pictures; this fossa articulates with the lateral mass of the atlas when the head is extended.

The supraoccipital segment of the occipital bone is on the posterior aspect of the foramen magnum. From below, the hypoglossal or anterior condyloid canal can be seen; this contains a bony spicule that separates the hypoglossal nerve from the meningeal branch of the ascending pharyngeal artery. The posterior condyloid canal is present on both sides. Also to be identified are the jugular foramen and an emissary vein in the midocciput. The foramen magnum transmits the medulla oblongata and its meninges, the spinal portion of the spinal accessory nerves, the vertebral artery, the anterior and posterior spinal artery, and the veins that communicate with the internal vertebral venous plexus. A cranial attachment of the dentate ligament also occurs at the level of the foramen magnum, situated between the vertebral artery and the hypoglossal nerve. The posterior longitudinal ligament continues through the foramen magnum as the tectorial membrane.

The hypoglossal canal transmits the hypoglossal nerve and the meningeal branch of the ascending pharyngeal artery and its emissary vein.

The average width of the foramen magnum measured in 42 dried adult skulls at the level of the posterior aspect of the occipital condyle was 2.9 cm., with a range of 2.5 to 3.4 cm. The average length of the foramen magnum was 3.4 cm., with a range of 3.2 to 3.6 cm. (Coin and Malkasian).

The occipital veins that are readily demonstrable communicate between the dural sinus and the suboccipital venous plexus and scalp vein, and represent potential routes for spread of infections. They are considered an anatomic site for venous sinus thrombosis.

The foramen magnum is well shown in the Chamberlain-Towne projection (Fig. 6–44). Within the foramen are projected the posterior clinoid processes and the dorsum sellae; or, at times, the posterior arch of the atlas and the jugular tubercles. The structures revealed depend upon the degree of angulation in this projection. Ordinarily there are radiolucent defects on either side of the condyles that are due either to the condyloid canals or to prominent sigmoid grooves, but occasionally the condyloid fossa may be demonstrable.

The anterior configuration of the foramen magnum varies between an angular appearance, small prominent accessory ossicles, or even a keyhole appearance (Kollman).

The foramen magnum measures about 20 mm. from front to back and about 15 mm. from side to side in neonates, but in adults it is usually round and measures about 35 mm. in diameter (see Table with Fig. 6–30).

Measurements at the Craniovertebral Junction. Chamberlain's line, McGregor's line, the *digastric line,* which joins the right and left digastric notches, and the *bimastoid line,* which joins the tips of the right and left mastoid processes, are shown in Figure 6–31. In about 50 per cent of normal persons, the tip of the odontoid is at or below Chamberlain's and McGregor's lines. *If more than half the odontoid process is above one of these lines, basilar invagination is probably present.* In normal patients the digastric line is 11 mm. ± 4 mm. above the middle of the atlanto-occipital joints. *Basilar invagination is almost certainly present when the atlanto-occipital joints are above the digastric line.* Other conditions causing the odontoid process to be high in relation to various lines, such as Chamberlain's, McGregor's, and Fishgold's, include *occipitalization of the atlas, platybasia, a high atlas, a short clivus,* or combinations of these.

The *basal angle* is measured by the angle between the plane of the clivus and the plane of the midline portion of the base of the anterior fossa. Usually, a line is drawn from the *tuberculum sellae to the anterior lip of the foramen magnum* (basion) and to the *nasofrontal suture* on a lateral skull. The angle between these two lines is the basal angle, as the term is used anthropologically. Primates all have basal angles greater than 150 degrees, whereas most mammals below the primates have basal angles measuring close to 180 degrees. In man, the foramen magnum is approximately horizontal and is situated at the bottom of the skull so that the spinal axis is at an angle to the clivus. The average basal angle in man measures 137 degrees, ranging from 123 to 152 degrees.

Clivus

Gross Anatomy (Fig. 6–24). The clivus is situated between the foramen magnum and the dorsum sellae. It includes the basioccipital bone and the body of the sphenoid bone to some extent. Its lateral margins are formed by the petro-occipital fissure superiorly and by the synchondrosis between the basioccipital and the exoccipital bones inferiorly. Anteriorly, it blends with the sphenoid sinus.

The length of the clivus averages about 3.4 cm., with a range of 3.1 to 4 cm. (Coin and Malkasian). The pons and the ventral surface of the medulla oblongata lie in close relationship to the clivus and may contribute to its impressions. These structures are separated from the clivus by the pontine and medullary basal cisterns. The clivus is best depicted radiologically by sagittal tomography laterally, and by frontal tomography, in which the plane of the cut is parallel to the slope of the clivus. The clivus is usually concave posteriorly but may, in rare instances, be either flat or slightly convex posteriorly (DiChiro and Anderson).

From the fourth to the twelfth year, pneumatization from the sphenoid sinus may extend into the clivus for a variable distance and the clivus may become completely pneumatized.

From the embryologic standpoint, the close relationship of the clivus to the origin of the notochord and a notochordal rem-

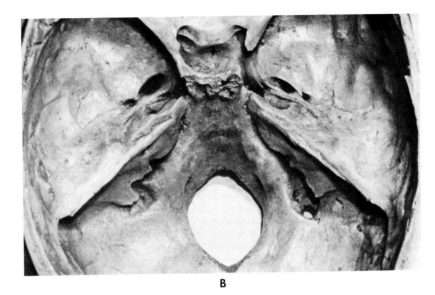

B

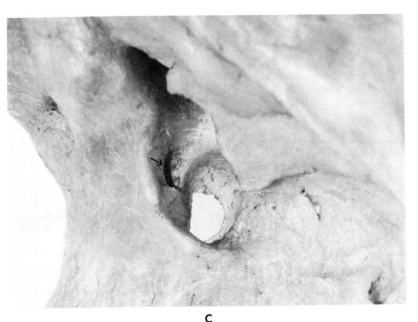

C

Figure 6–31 *Continued.* B. Local deepening at the termination of the sigmoid groove on the right side, with defect of the osseous floor. C. Magnification of B. The intracranial opening of the condyloid canal is indicated with an arrow. (From Gathier, J. C., and Bruyn, G. W.: Amer. J. Roentgenol., *107:*516, 1969.)

nant is highly significant, since a chordoma is the most common tumor of the clivus originating from a notochordal remnant.

Hypoglossal Canal. The hypoglossal canal runs outward and forward through the condyle of the occiput, transmitting the 12th cranial nerve, the meningeal branch of the ascending pharyngeal artery, and a plexus of emissary veins. The canal lies on or very near a line joining the external auditory canals.

This canal may be seen end-on in views designed to show the petrous ridge (Stenver's view, Chapter 7), the mastoid process (Law's or Runström views, Chapter 7), and the optic foramina.

Body section radiography is essential in order to visualize the canal in its three dimensions. Therefore, the radiography of this canal will be discussed in Chapter 7.

On the average the hypoglossal canal is oval, its outer opening measuring 7 × 6 mm. with the long axis horizontal. The longest diameter of the outer opening of the canals measured by Kirdani was 11 mm. and the shortest was 4 mm. The average measurement of the inner opening was 7.5 × 6 mm., the smallest diameter being 4 mm. and the largest 12 mm. In comparing the inner and outer openings of the same canal, Kirdani found a difference of up to 4 mm. between the two openings.

The midcanal tends to be rounded and averages 6 mm. in diameter, ranging between 4 and 11 mm. A variation of up to 3 mm. on the two sides is normal. The average length of the canal is 11 mm. and the difference in length between the two canals of the same subject does not exceed 5 mm. normally. In some canals there is a bony septum and at times this is bilateral (Kirdani).

Condyloid Foramen and Fossa (Gathier and Bruyn). The sigmoid fossa is close to the termination of the sigmoid venous sinus. It is located just dorsal to the jugular incisure where the sigmoid or transverse sinus bends sharply to the jugular fossa. The opening of the condyloid canal is visible in the medial wall of the sigmoid fossa.

The condyloid fossa generally appears behind each condyle as a depression that receives the posterior margin of the superior facet of the atlas, when the head is bent backward. The condyloid foramen itself, which is found in the floor of this fossa, is traversed by an emissary vein passing from the transverse sinus (Fig. 6–2 B).

NORMAL CALCIFICATION WITHIN THE CALVARIUM THAT IS VISIBLE RADIOGRAPHICALLY

Pineal Gland. The pineal gland (or body) is located between the posterior ends of the two thalami in a depression lying between the two superior colliculi. Its stalk is usually separated by a small recess of the cavity of the third ventricle of the brain. The ventral part of this stalk is continuous with the posterior commissure of the cerebrum (see Chapter 7).

The pineal contains a variable amount of gritty, calcareous matter, and in most patients its greatest radiologic value is the possibility of detecting it, on plain radiographs of the skull. Its importance in this regard was first recognized by Schüller in 1912, and its normal range of position has been defined and redefined in extensive studies by many authors since then: Vastine and Kinney (1927), redefined in 1930 by Dyke; Fray (1938); Don (1964); Pawl and Walter (1965); and Murase, et al. (1970).

The incidence of pineal glandular calcification has varied in different studies from 33 per cent to 76 per cent (Kitay and Altschule). Vastine and Kinney reported an incidence of 80 per cent in Caucasian men and of 69 per cent in women over age 60. A considerably lower incidence has been reported in other racial groups—10 per cent in Japan, 8 per cent in India, 5 per cent in Nigeria—usually in somewhat younger age groups (Kieffer and Gold). Dyke reported an incidence of 5 per cent in Caucasian children under age 10, and of 55 per cent in patients over 20. Don's study was made with a group of Chinese, Indian, and Malay patients, both men and women.

There are wide variations in the normal dimensions of the pineal, which normally averages about 5 mm. in length and 3 mm. in height and width. When the calcification is greater than 10 mm. in diameter, a pathologic process may be suspected, *especially in patients in the first two decades of life.*

In the frontal projection, a shift of the pineal of 3 mm. or more from the midline may be regarded as significant, unless the skull is markedly rotated. Slight rotations, even up to 15 per cent, may have no effect because of the remarkably central location in the vertical axis. Displacement of the pineal gland in the lateral view may be determined by a variety of methods which are illustrated in the following section.

Dyke modified the original classic work of Vastine and Kinney (1927) on localization of the pineal gland on lateral roentgenograms of the skull, by suggesting that the range of normal proposed in it be moved forward 4 mm. (Fig. 6–32 C-F). Later, Taveras and Wood, and also Oon, pointed out that even this modification causes a significant number of normal pineal bodies to appear displaced posteriorly, and further modifications were suggested by these authors. Special rulers were devised so that the limits of normal range up to 17 mm., and variations of 2 to 3 mm. outside this range are probably normal. Using these modified ruler methods, pineal gland measurement varies 20 mm. in the anteroposterior dimension and 18 mm. in the superoinferior dimension in the lateral roentgenogram.

Fray proposed two different methods for pineal gland localization. One of these was a proportional method in which an elastic band was constructed and placed upon the lateral roentgenogram, stretching between the predetermined points on the cranial vault originally suggested by Vastine and Kinney and later by Dyke. Fray noted an accuracy of 93 per cent in the anteroposterior dimension and 94 per cent in the superoinferior dimension. Fray's second method was based on angles drawn on a previously constructed overlay. Oon found that Fray's angles generally produced poor results.

The method advocated by Oon is illustrated in Figure 6–32 G. Identification is required of T, the tuberculum sellae, and B, the basion or anterior margin of the foramen magnum. A perfect lateral film of the skull must be obtained, using a target-to-film distance of 70 cm. or 28 inches. This method requires a fixed focal

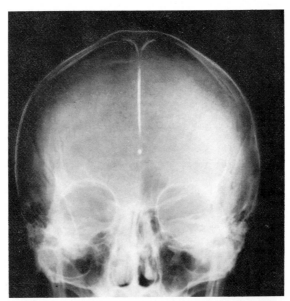

Figure 6-32. *A.* Radiograph demonstrating calcification in the pineal gland and falx cerebri in a posteroanterior view. *B.* Radiograph of the skull (lateral projection) demonstrating calcium deposit in the pineal gland, habenula, and glomera of the choroid plexuses. The habenula is the U-shaped structure immediately anterior to the pineal gland (intensified.)

A

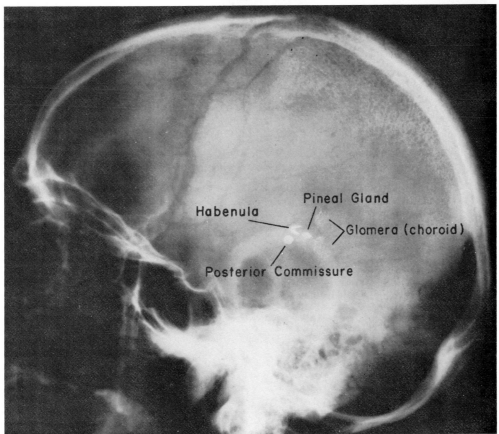

B

Figure 6–32 continued on the following page.

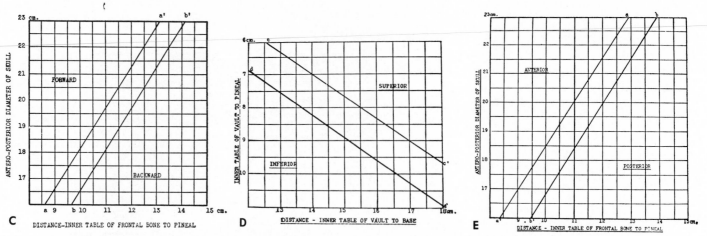

Figure 6–32 *Continued.* *C* and *D.* Determination of the normal position of the pineal gland: method of Vastine-Kinney, as modified by Dyke. Pineals that fall between the lines a-a′ and b-b′ are in the normal zone, while those that fall anterior to this zone are displaced forward and those posterior to it are displaced backward. Likewise, in the vertical plane, the normal zone lies between the lines c-c′ and d-d′. When the pineal falls above it is displaced superiorly, and when it falls below it is displaced inferiorly. *E.* Dyke's modification of the Vastine-Kinney graph in the anteroposterior plane. The normal zone is 4 mm. anterior to the comparable Vastine-Kinney graph. (From Golden, R.: Golden's Diagnostic Roentgenology. Baltimore, The Williams & Wilkins Company, 1936–1963.)

Figure 6–32 continued on the opposite page.

distance because proportional variations are not accounted for, and a perfect roentgenogram is necessary since any movement of the head would nullify the results obtained.

The technique is as follows: line TB is drawn. Point C is located 1 cm. posterior to point T, and a line is erected perpendicular to C. In most instances this perpendicular line will pass through the pineal gland, and the center of the pineal will fall at 5 cm. on this perpendicular.

Oon studied this technique in a group of Chinese, Indian, and Malay individuals, both male and female. Seventy per cent of this group had brachycephalic skulls, 22 per cent had mesocephalic skulls, and 8 per cent had dolichocephalic skulls. In his scattergram of these various studies, Oon achieved an accuracy of 98 per cent if a deviation of 10 mm. from this accepted point P was taken as the upper limit of normal.

To achieve this rate of accuracy Oon pointed out that a true lateral skull position and adequate roentgenographic penetration are essential for the visualization of the basiocciput and the basion. The basion, however, may be indicated by locating a point 5 mm. directly above the apex of the visualized odontoid process. It is also important to utilize a target-to-film distance of 70 cm. or 28 inches—otherwise magnification would also nullify the accuracy of this technique.

A further modification of this technique was proposed by Pawl and Walter in 1965. This is shown in Figure 6–32 *H.* A line is constructed along the base of the skull from the nasion to the lowermost portion of the basiocciput just posterior to the opisthion (line A). From this point a perpendicular line is drawn through the center of the calcified pineal body to the inner table of the vault (line B). A point is then measured on the second line which is one-half the distance from the inner table of the cranial vault to the base line (line A). The pineal should lie 1 cm. below this point. A third line is then constructed parallel to line A and perpendicular to line B, and also passing through the calcified pineal body (line C). A point is measured on this line one-half the distance from the inner table of the frontal bone to the outer table of the occipital bone. The pineal body should lie 1 cm. posterior to this point. In a study of 120 cases utilizing this technique, 100 per cent of the cases were found to lie within 5 mm. above or below the intersection of lines B and C. In the anteroposterior diameter, 98.5 per cent of cases were situated within 5 mm. of this intersection.

With regard to visualization of the calcified pineal gland in the frontal perspective, Schüller pointed out in 1918 that a lateral pineal shift was an extremely important diagnostic aid, and this observation has now become firmly established. Deviations greater than 3 mm. from the midline are highly significant.

It is important to distinguish calcification of the pineal body from calcification in the posterior and habenular commissures, which may at times give the pineal body a multicentric appearance. Localization charts for habenular calcification may also be used (McCrae) (Fig. 6–32 *L, M*).

Slight rotations in the frontal projections may still show the pineal in the midline (Agnos and Wollin).

Alternate methods of localization of the pineal gland have been suggested by a number of authors (Fray; Lilja; Murase et al.). Two of these are shown in accompanying diagrams (Fig. 6–32 *J, K*).

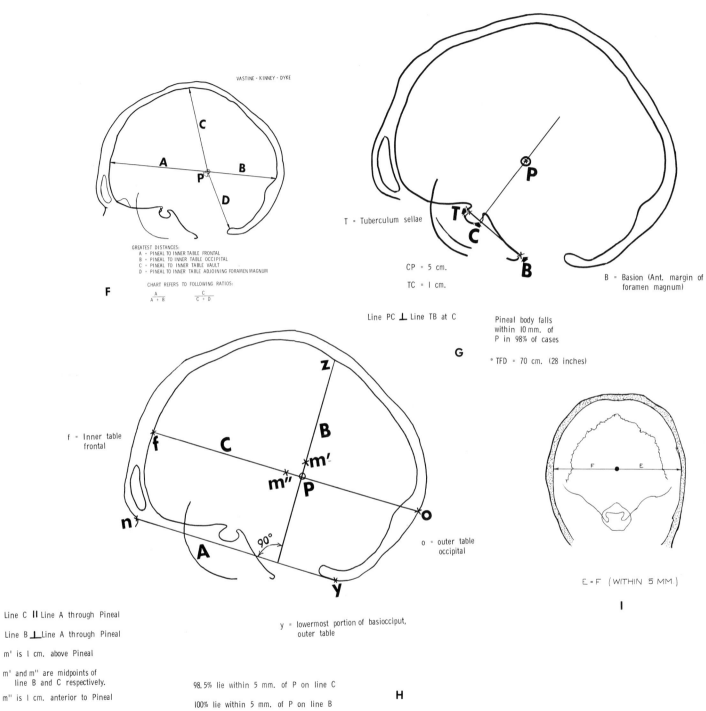

VASTINE - KINNEY - DYKE

GREATEST DISTANCES:
A - PINEAL TO INNER TABLE FRONTAL
B - PINEAL TO INNER TABLE OCCIPITAL
C - PINEAL TO INNER TABLE VAULT
D - PINEAL TO INNER TABLE ADJOINING FORAMEN MAGNUM

CHART REFERS TO FOLLOWING RATIOS:
$\frac{A}{A+B}$ $\frac{C}{C+D}$

F

T = Tuberculum sellae

CP = 5 cm.

TC = 1 cm.

Line PC ⊥ Line TB at C

B = Basion (Ant. margin of
foramen magnum)

Pineal body falls
within 10 mm. of
P in 98% of cases

° TFD = 70 cm. (28 inches)

G

f = Inner table
frontal

o = outer table
occipital

y = lowermost portion of basiocciput,
outer table

Line C ∥ Line A through Pineal

Line B ⊥ Line A through Pineal

m' is 1 cm. above Pineal

m' and m'' are midpoints of
line B and C respectively.

m'' is 1 cm. anterior to Pineal

98.5% lie within 5 mm. of P on line C

100% lie within 5 mm. of P on line B

H

E = F (WITHIN 5 MM.)

I

Figure 6–32 *Continued*   *F.* Lateral view of the skull indicating points from which measurements are made to determine position of the pineal body by the Vastine-Kinney method, as modified by Dyke. Pineals that fall between the lines a-a′ and b-b′ are in the normal range. (C) Inner table of the vault; (D) inner table of the cerebellar fossa at the foramen magnum. (From Golden, R.: Golden's Diagnostic Roentgenology. Baltimore, The Williams & Wilkins Company, 1936–1963.)

   G. Localization of the pineal gland by the method of Oon. (From Oon, C. L.: Amer. J. Roentgenol., *92*:1242– 1248, 1964.) *H.* Localization of the pineal gland by the method of Pawl and Walter. (From Pawl, R. P., and Walter, A. K.: Amer. J. Roentgenol., *105*:287–290, 1969.) *I.* Anteroposterior and lateral views of the skull, showing the pineal gland and the four measurements taken.

Figure 6–32 continued on the following page.

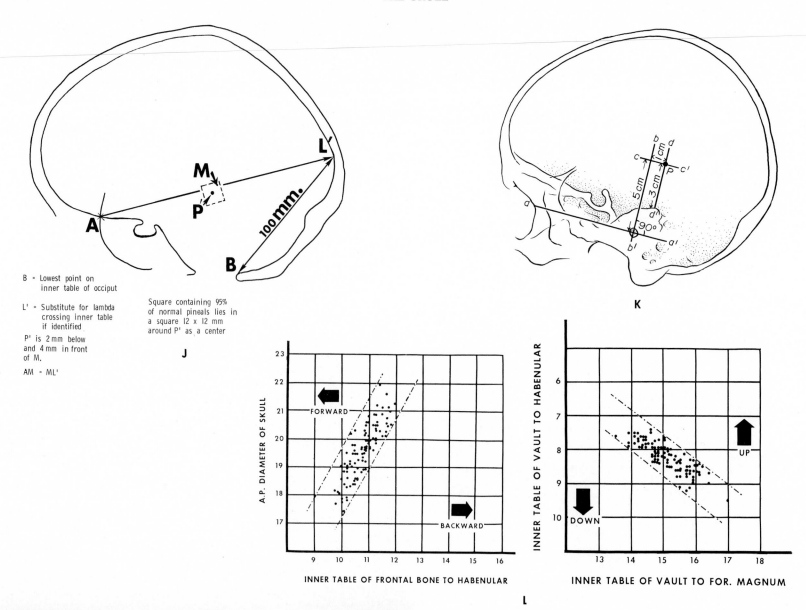

B = Lowest point on
inner table of occiput

L' = Substitute for lambda
crossing inner table
if identified

P' is 2 mm below
and 4 mm in front
of M.

AM = ML'

Square containing 95%
of normal pineals lies in
a square 12 x 12 mm
around P' as a center

J

A.P. DIAMETER OF SKULL

FORWARD

BACKWARD

INNER TABLE OF FRONTAL BONE TO HABENULAR

INNER TABLE OF VAULT TO HABENULAR

UP

DOWN

INNER TABLE OF VAULT TO FOR. MAGNUM

L

K

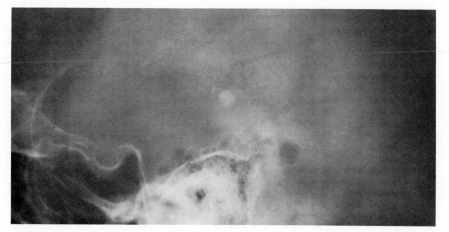

M

Figure 6–32. *Continued.* *J.* Localization of the pineal gland by the method of Murase et al. *K.* Alternate technique for localization of the pineal gland in relation to the orbitomeatal line. (From Murase, Y. et al.: Amer. J. Roentgenol., *110:*92–95, 1970.) *L.* McCrae's graphs for normal localization of habenular calcification. *M.* Inverted "C" appearance of habenular calcification in relation to the pineal gland calcification. (From McRae, D. L.: Amer. J. Roentgenol., *94:*541–546, 1965.)

In the method suggested by Murase et al., a line is drawn as shown between point A and point L′ and a midpoint M is indicated. A is the crossing point of the curved line formed by the anterior border of the middle cranial fossa and the curved line formed by the superior surface of the orbital roof. When both points are identified in the lateral radiograph for both orbits, a point midway between these is taken as point A.

Point L′ is 100 mm. above the lowest point on the inner table of the occiput as identified on the radiograph (point B). As an alternate for L′ the inner table crossing of lambda may be substituted. P′ is a point 2 mm. below and 4 mm. in front of M. A square 12 × 12 mm. containing 95 per cent of normal pineals can be drawn using P′ as a central point.

Apart from the Vastine-Kinney method, the pineal gland may also be located by measuring 5 cm. above the orbitomeatal line and 1 cm. behind on a line drawn perpendicularly both to this line and to a line drawn from the middle of the external auditory meatus. A third alternate diagram is also shown (Fig. 6–32 I).

Other Areas of Calcification. *Habenular calcification* can be recognized in lateral roentgenograms of the skull as a C-shaped area of calcification in the pineal region. It represents calcification in the taenia habenulae (choroid plexus of third ventricle) and is separated from the pineal body by the habenular commissure. This calcification was identified in 89 out of 187 normal skull roentgenograms showing pineal calcification. The localization of habenular calcification may be made on lateral radiographs of the skull (Fig. 6–32 L, M). First, the measurements from the inner table of the frontal bone to the apex of the C-shaped habenular calcification are made. These are compared with the anteroposterior diameter of the skull, using the outer table of the skull for this latter measurement (McRae). McRae considers these charts more accurate than comparable charts for localization of the pineal gland. Habenular calcification is situated about 3 to 5 mm. anterior to the pineal gland in about 30 per cent of a normal North American population, and may be present in about 50 per cent of people in whom the pineal is not detectably calcified (Kieffer and Gold; Stauffer et al.).

The *falx cerebri* (Fig. 6–32 A) is calcified in about 7 per cent of adults and may be seen on the anteroposterior or posteroanterior projection as a thin stripelike shadow. Unless the calcium is very extensive, this cannot be detected with accuracy on the lateral projections of the skull, but may appear as a faint plaquelike structure. It is such a rigid structure that it is not readily displaced by a space-occupying lesion unless a mass lesion has been present many years, and thus has less value than the pineal gland in assisting the radiologist.

The *glomera of the choroid plexuses* (Fig. 6–33) at the junction of the posterior and temporal horns of the lateral ventricles frequently undergo calcification, and are to be found symmetrically 2.5 to 3 cm. on either side of the midline in the anteroposterior projections and behind and superior to the pineal gland in

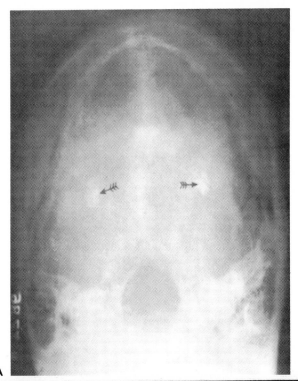

A

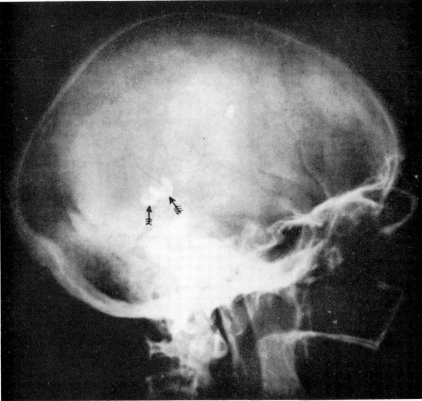

B

Figure 6–33. Roentgenogram showing calcification in the glomera of the choroid plexuses. *A.* Towne's position. *B.* Lateral view.

the lateral projections. Occasionally they will be displaced by a space-occupying lesion, and in that case permit an accurate diagnosis of that condition. Slight asymmetries, however, must be interpreted with caution.

The *petroclinoid ligament* (Fig. 6-34), situated posterior to the sella turcica, may also be calcified in about 12 per cent of adults, and appears as a thin shadow extending from the dorsum sellae to the petrous ridge. It forms the superior border of Dorello's canal through which the sixth cranial nerve passes in its course from the posterior to the middle cranial fossa.

Occasionally there is a *calcific bridge between the anterior and posterior clinoid processes of the sella turcica,* but usually this overbridged appearance of the sella turcica is due to the overlapping shadows of the anterior and posterior clinoids (since the interclinoid distance of the anterior clinoids is considerably greater than that of the posterior) on the lateral roentgenogram of the skull, and not actually to a true bridging of the bone. If a middle clinoid process is present, the interclinoid calcification will be attached to it. This outlines the *caroticoclinoid foramen* through which the internal carotid artery passes at its siphon. Carotid arterial calcification in this location is usually more irregular and curvilinear and can often be detected in frontal perspective as a circular structure lateral to the sella turcica.

There may be *calcium deposit* in the wall of the *superior sagittal venous sinus within the dura* (Fig. 6-34 *B*). It may be

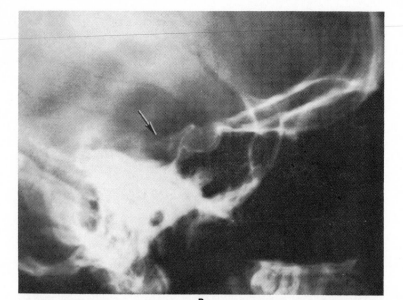

B

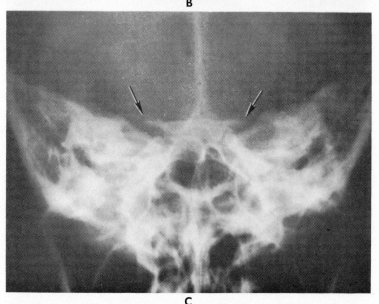

C

Figure 6-34.   A. Radiograph showing calcification in the petroclinoid ligament. B. Slightly oblique radiograph showing the configuration of the petroclinoid ligament when the lateral is not true. C. Radiograph in Towne's projection showing the petroclinoid ligaments extending between the posterior clinoid processes and dorsum sellae and the petrous ridge (intensified).

Figure 6-34 continued on the opposite page.

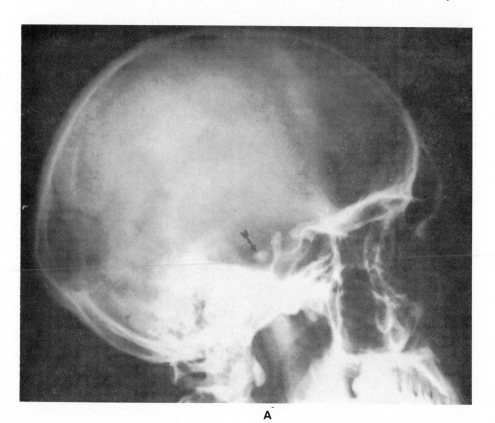

A

located next to the parietal bone, or near its junction with the sinus confluens particularly. This is without pathologic significance. Single or multiple plaques of calcified dura may be scattered almost anywhere over the dura. They are usually flat and sharply marginated. Differentiation from meningioma is usually possible since the latter affects the overlying bone by a mixture of hypervascularity, lucency, and bone sclerosis (except when meningioma occurs in the falx or tentorium at a considerable distance from overlying bone).

Occasionally small *granular calcified areas may appear in the basal ganglia* (Fig. 6–34 C). They are situated on either side of the midline largely within the middle cranial fossa. It is not completely certain that patients may not suffer from this calcium deposit, since the patients in whom this calcification was found had variable abnormalities that might or might not be related to it.

Calcification may occur *in the cerebral arteries,* particularly the internal carotid artery adjoining the sella turcica. This entity, however, does not belong in a discussion of normal calcium deposit.

Calcification in the *tentorium cerebelli* is quite uncommon and can usually be recognized by its plaque-like appearance and location near the margin of the tentorial incisura (duBoulay). If bilateral, it has an inverted V appearance.

Calcifications of arachnoid granulations, when present, appear as round, uniform calcific densities near the appropriate granulation impressions in the calvarium. Microscopically, calcification is not infrequently present in the region of the basal cisterns (Hassler).

THE BLOOD SUPPLY OF THE CALVARIUM AND ITS VENOUS DRAINAGE

The bones of the calvarium do not have single nutrient arteries as do the bones of the extremities, and most of their arterial supply on the deeper surfaces is derived from the meningeal arteries in the depths of the meningeal grooves. A few other small arterioles penetrate the outer surface of the occipital bone and temporal bones, especially near the attachment of the temporal muscles.

Actually most of the circulation of the calvarium is of a venous nature in the diploë, and in general there is one major diploic channel for each cranial bone (Fig. 6–12). This tends to branch in stellate fashion, having a very irregular course. Usually the diploic veins lie closer to the inner table than to the outer.

Thus the following diploic channels can be identified: the frontal diploic veins (which may open exteriorly into the veins in the vicinity of the supraorbital notch); the parietal diploic vein, which seems to be in the shape of a star and hence is referred to as the "parietal star"; the temporal diploic vein, which anastomoses freely with the middle meningeal veins; the occipital diploic veins; and numerous anastomoses with the venous channels in the dura mater.

THE SKULL AT BIRTH AND ITS GROWTH AND DEVELOPMENT

The Skull at Birth. The cranial vault at birth (Fig. 6–35) is quite large in relation to the bones of the face, since the teeth and

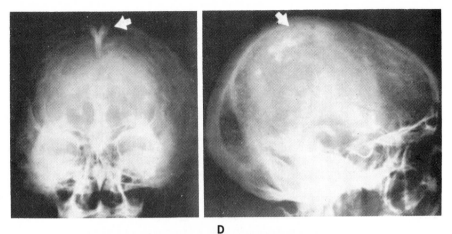

D

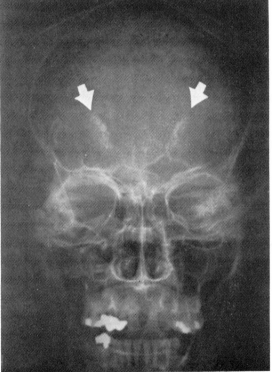

E

Figure 6–34 *Continued.* D. Calcium deposit in the dura mater and falx cerebri. Posteroanterior and lateral projections. (Courtesy of Chalmers S. Pool, M.D.) E. Calcification of the basal ganglia, posteroanterior projection.

air sinuses are so rudimentary. The bones of the cranial vault are also quite widely separated and filled with fibrous tissue. The edges of these are not yet serrated as they are in the adult. Strictly speaking, there are *seven* fontanelles: in addition to the *anterior frontal* and *posterior occipital* fontanelles, there are the *anterior frontal* and *posterior occipital* fontanelles, there are the paired *sphenoid fontanelles,* at the junction of the squamous por-

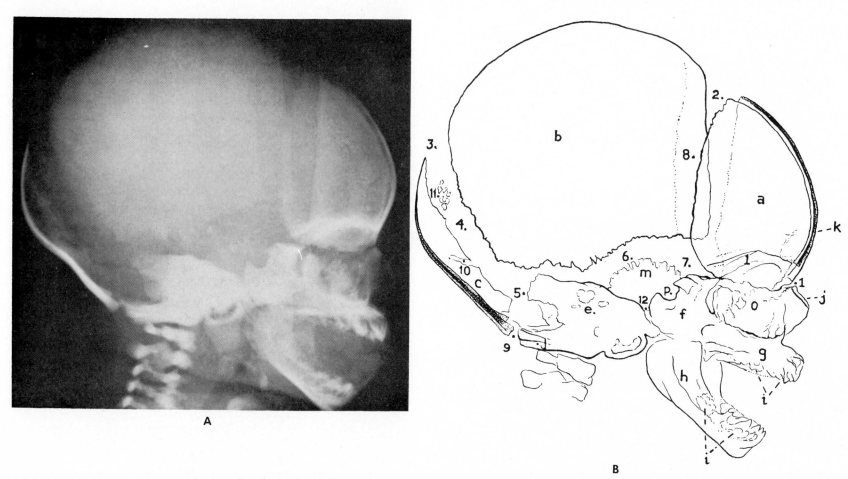

Figure 6–35. Normal neonatal skull. *A.* Roentgenogram, lateral view. *B.* Labeled tracing of *A.* (a) Frontal bone, (b) parietal bone, (c) squamous portion of occipital bone, (d) exoccipital portion of occipital bone, (e) superimposed petrous pyramids of temporal bone, (f) body of sphenoid, (g) upper maxilla, (h) mandible, (i) partially mineralized deciduous teeth, and dental crypts, (j) nasal bone, (k) squamosa of the frontal bone, (l) horizontal plates of the frontal bone, (m) squamosa of the temporal bone, (o) orbit, (p) pituitary fossa; (1) frontonasal suture, (2) anterior fontanelle, (3) posterior fontanelle, (4) lambdoidal suture, (5) posterolateral fontanelle, (6) squamosal suture, (7) anterolateral fontanelle, (8) coronal suture, (9) synchondrosis between exoccipitals and supraoccipital portions of occipital bone, (10) mendosal suture, (11) multiple ossification centers (wormian bones) in lambdoidal suture, (12) occipito-sphenoid synchondrosis. (From Caffey, J.: Pediatric X-ray Diagnosis, 6th ed. Chicago, Year Book Medical Publishers, 1972.)

Figure 6–35 continued on the opposite page.

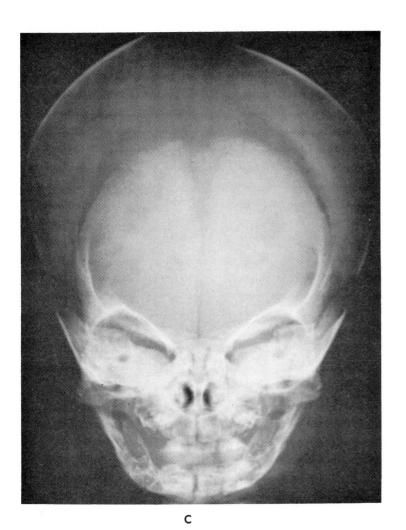

C

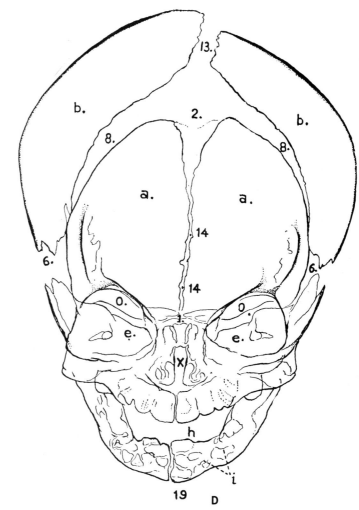

D

Figure 6–35 *Continued.* C. Roentgenogram, posteroanterior view. *D.* Labeled tracing of C. (a) Frontal bone, (b) parietal bone, (e) superimposed petrous pyramids of temporal bone, (h) mandible, (i) partially mineralized deciduous teeth, and dental crypts, (o) orbit, (x) nasal septum, (2) anterior fontanelle, (6) squamosal suture, (8) coronal suture, (13) sagittal suture, (14) metopic suture dividing the frontal bone, (19) symphysis of mandible. (From Caffey, J.: Pediatric X-ray Diagnosis, 6th ed. Chicago, Year Book Medical Publishers, 1972.)

Figure 6–35 continued on the following page.

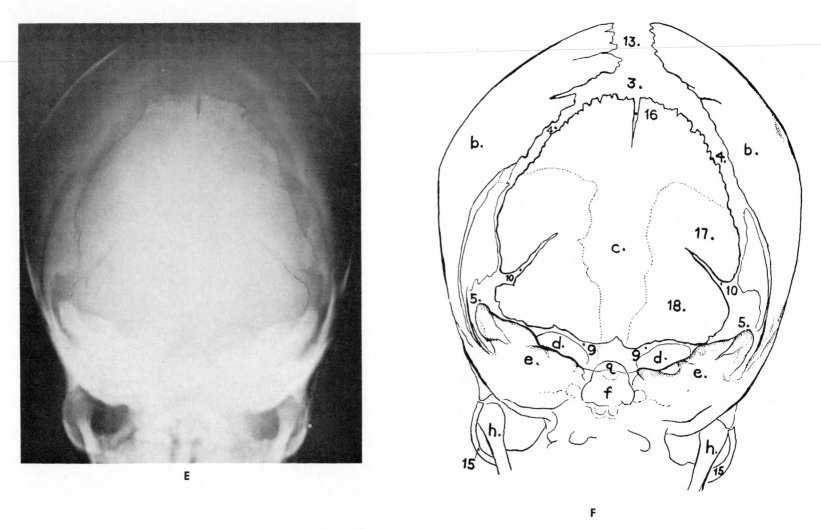

Figure 6–35 *Continued.* E. Roentgenogram, anteroposterior view. Modified Towne's projection. F. Labeled tracing of E. (b) Parietal bone, (c) squamous portion of occipital bone, (d) exoccipital portion of occipital bone, (e) superimposed petrous pyramids of temporal bone, (f) body of sphenoid, (h) mandible, (q) basioccipital portion of occipital bone, (3) posterior fontanelle, (4) lambdoidal suture, (5) posterolateral fontanelle, (9) synchondrosis between exoccipital and supraoccipital portions of occipital bone, (10) mendosal suture, (13) sagittal suture, (15) zygomatic arch, (16) superior median fissure of occipital bone, (17) interparietal portion of occipital bone, (18) supraoccipital portion of occipital bone. (From Caffey, J.: Pediatric X-ray Diagnosis, 6th ed. Chicago, Year Book Medical Publishers, 1972.)

tions of the temporal bones with the coronal suture; the paired *mastoid* fontanelles between squamous portions of the temporal bones and the lambdoid suture on either side; and the *sagittal fontanelle* situated at the obelion just above the lambda. These are usually all closed by the age of 2, the posterior and sphenoid fontanelles closing shortly after birth or at least by 6 months of age, and the mastoid fontanelles closing by the first year. When closure of the fontanelles occurs, irregularities in the bony structure may form the sutural bones already mentioned.

Bones in the anterior fontanelle and its contiguous sutures are normal and relatively common variants that do not interfere with normal growth of the skull (Girdany and Blank). The anterior fontanelle bone is usually single and may or may not develop a diploic space. Fusion between the fontanelle bone and the surrounding bones of the skull occurs usually before the fifth year of life.

At birth the occipital bone is divided into four parts (Fig. 6–36 *D*). There is an incomplete cleft between the interparietal and supraoccipital portions of the bone, which may be misinterpreted as a fracture if one is not familiar with this developmental phenomenon; there are also two lateral parts on either side of the foramen magnum, and the basilar part in the center anteriorly.

The two lateral parts fuse with the supraoccipital portion during the third year, and with the basilar portion during the fourth or fifth year. The basisphenoid suture (suture between the sphenoid and the basilar part of the occipital bone) does not fuse until about the age of 25. A knowledge of these sutural developments is of paramount importance when interpreting skull radiographs.

The *sphenoid* bone is formed in five separate parts: a median and two lateral portions, in addition to the two sphenoidal conchae. The median part consists of the body and the small wings; each lateral part consists of the pterygoid process and a great wing. The dorsum sellae is still mostly cartilaginous at birth and ossifies slowly. It therefore appears considerably elongated and shallow. The sphenoid sinuses are not aerated, but their rudiments are present in the conchae. Extension of the rudimentary sinus by absorption of the spongy bone does not begin until the sixth or seventh year, and fusion of the concha with the sphenoid does not occur until the eighth or ninth year.

There are two synchondroses in the immediate vicinity of the sphenoid bone in infants and children: (1) a *spheno-occipital synchondrosis* (Fig. 6–36 D), and (2) an *intersphenoid synchondrosis* (Fig. 6–36 D). Although the intersphenoid synchondrosis is rather prevalent in younger age groups (64 per cent according to Shopfner et al.), there is a progressive decrease with age and after three years it is absent. Although originally this synchondrosis was thought to represent the cranial pharyngeal canal or Rathke pouch remnant in its migration from the pharynx to the sella, it would appear unlikely under these circumstances.

The spheno-occipital synchondrosis disappears by the 25th year ordinarily when the sphenoid and occipital bones are completely fused.

In newborn children there is a synchondrosis between the squamous portions of the occipital bone and the two condyles that come together near the center of the posterior margin of the foramen magnum. There may be an unoccupied area 6 or 8 mm. wide in this immediate vicinity, which may be filled by an accessory ossification center.

The *temporal* bone is divided into four parts—the petromastoid, the squamous, the tympanic, and the styloid process. The mastoid process has not yet begun to develop at birth, and the osseous portion of the external auditory meatus is lacking. (The tympanic membrane therefore lies near the surface of the head and its obliquity is different from that of the adult.) The mandibular fossa is shallow and large, and looks laterally as well as downward.

The *ethmoid bones* at birth already contain the sinuses in each labyrinth, but the perpendicular plate and the cribriform plate are not yet completely formed or ossified. The ossification of the perpendicular plate is not complete before the fifth or sixth year, and the cribriform plate is ossified usually during the second year. Fusion of the ethmoid and sphenoid does not occur until about 25 years of age.

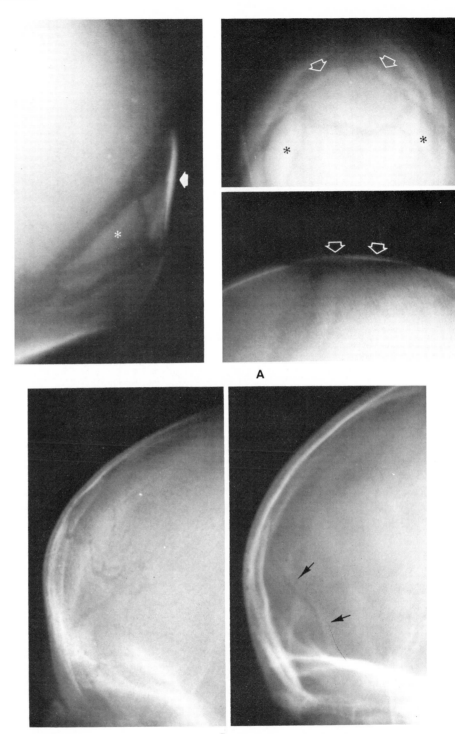

Figure 6–36. *A.* Lateral projection (*left*) and Towne's projection (*upper right*), showing interparietal bone located in the region of the posterior fontanelle (arrows). Additional accessory bones are seen between the lambdoid and mendosal sutures (*). Note concentric skin folds in Towne's projection. *Lower right,* Anterior fontanelle bone, lateral-tangential view (arrows). *B. Left,* Normal frontal vascular grooves in a neonate. *Right,* Normal vascular groove in an older child (arrows). (From Swischuk, L. E.: Radiol. Clin. N. Amer., *10*:277–290, 1972.)

Figure 6–36 continued on the following page.

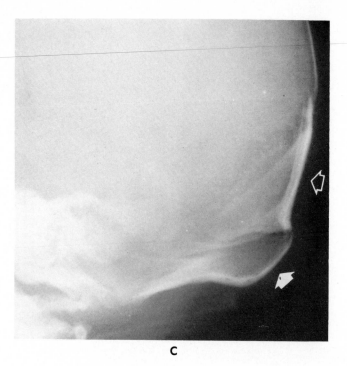

C

The inferior nasal concha is already ossified at birth, and arises as a separate bone.

The *frontal* bone at birth is divided into halves by the frontal suture, which, when it persists into adult life, is called the "metopic" suture. The frontal and parietal eminences or tuberosities are more convex and more prominent in the child than in the adult. Obliteration of the frontal suture usually occurs by the fifth or sixth year of life. The superciliary arch grows more prominent with age. The supraorbital notch is more centrally placed in the newborn child than in the adult.

The *maxillae* are vertical and of small height, accounting for the short distance between the palate and the orbits. The maxillary sinus at this time is a mere groove in the lateral wall of the middle meatus. The alveolar process is also very small and hollowed out for the dental sacs. The maxillary sinus is ordinarily not significantly aerated before 2 or 3 years of age, and its growth (Fig. 6–37) contributes considerably to the growth of the face in general. Sometimes there are septae in the maxillary sinus which persist throughout life.

The vertical plates of the palatine bones are short at birth; the nasal bones are low and flat, and the nasal cavity is situated almost entirely between the orbits. At this time the orbital opening is large and nearly circular with sharp margins; the orbital fissures are wide, and the lacrimal fossa is deep and looks forward instead of laterally.

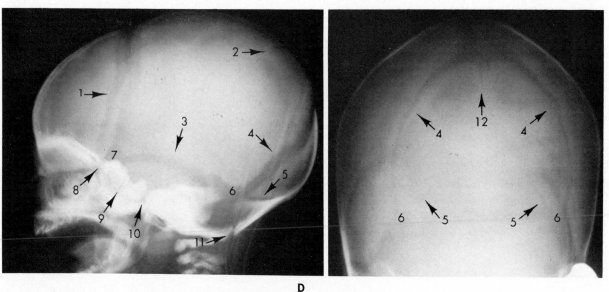

D

Figure 6–36 *Continued.* C. Bathrocephaly. Peculiar bulging of the occipital bone seen in neonates (solid arrow). It usually disappears as the infant grows older and is frequently accompanied by an interparietal bone (upper arrow). D. Normal lateral (*left*) and Towne's (*right*) projections of the neonatal skull. Note that the sutures appear unduly wide and prominent, and that the parietal bone is underossified. (1) Coronal suture, (2) posterior parietal fissure, (3) squamosal suture, (4) lambdoid suture, (5) mendosal suture, (6) posterior lateral fontanelle, (7) anterior lateral fontanelle, (8) frontosphenoid synchondrosis, (9) intersphenoid synchondrosis, (10) spheno-occipital synchondrosis, (11) innominate or posterior occipital synchondrosis, (12) median occipital fissure. (From Swischuk, L. E.: Radiol. Clin. N. Amer., *10*:277–290, 1972.)

Figure 6–36 continued on the opposite page.

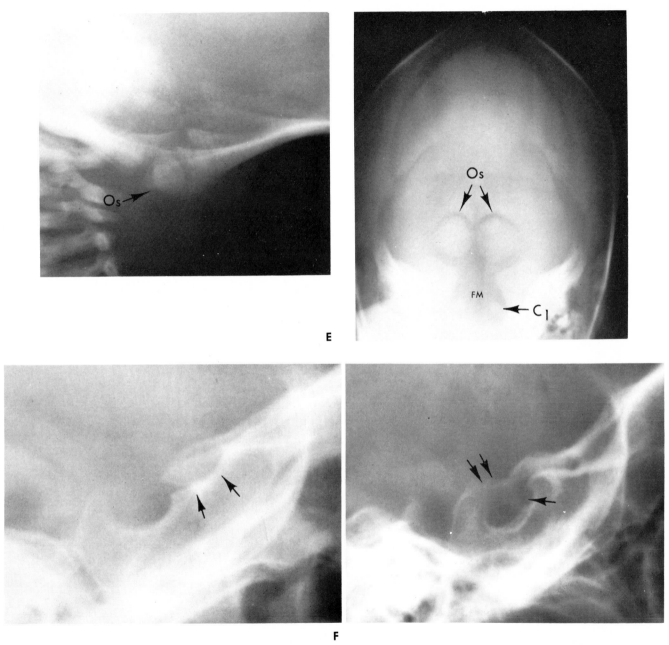

Figure 6–36 *Continued.* E. Lateral (*left*) and Towne's (*right*) projections showing occipital ossicles (Os). Note normal, incompletely fused arch of the first cervical vertebra (C₁), mendosal suture (5), posterior lateral fontanelle (6), and innominate or posterior occipital synchondrosis (11). Foramen magnum (FM). *F. Left,* Normal sella showing exaggerated elongation and scalloping of the chiasmatic groove (arrows). This is a normal variation. *Right,* Bony bridging between the anterior and posterior clinoids (double arrows), and vertical bone strut, the middle clinoid (single arrow). (From Swischuk, L. E.: Radiol. Clin. N. Amer., *10*:277–290, 1972.)

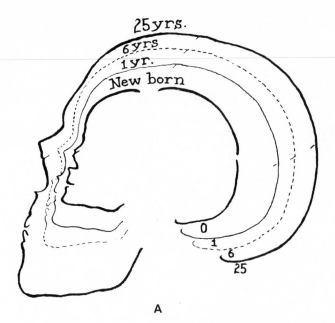

A

Age, Yr.	Cranium of Adult Dimensions				Face of Adult Dimensions			Volume Ratio
	Width	Height	Length	Bizygo-matic Width	Bigonial Width	Height	Length	Cranium Face
0				56		38	40	8 : 1
2	86	92	86	80		68	70	5 : 1
6	92	96	90	83	83	80	80	3 : 1
12	98	99	96	90	93	89	87	2.5 : 1
	max. attained by 15 yr. of age							
18	100	100	100	100	100	100	98	2 : 1

B

Figure 6–37. *A.* Proportionate growth of the facial bones and calvarium during infancy, childhood, and early manhood, shown in medial longitudinal section of the skull. (From Pediatric X-ray Diagnosis, 6th ed., by Caffey, J. Copyright © 1972 by Year Book Medical Publishers, Inc. Used by permission.) *B.* Percentage of adult facial and cranial dimensions achieved at different age levels. (From Growth and Development of Children, 6th ed., by Lowrey, G. H. Copyright © 1973 by Year Book Medical Publishers, Inc., Chicago. Used by permission. [Reprinted from Moyers, R. E., and Hemrend, B.: The Growth of the Craniofacial Skeleton. Toronto, privately printed, 1939.])

Growth and Age Changes of the Skull (Figs. 6–37, 6–39 *C*, 6–41 *A*).   The growth of the facial bones exceeds the growth of the cranial vault. The capacity of the cranium at birth is fully two-thirds that of the adult, and in the adult the volume occupied by the face roughly equals that occupied by the cranium.

At birth the volume of the neural cranium is 8 to 9 times as great as the volume of the face. At 2 years of age this ratio is 5 to 1; at 6 years, 3 to 1; and in the adult it is 2 to 1 (Watson and Lowrey).

A well-positioned lateral roentgenogram of the skull shows clearly the relative areas in the midsagittal plane of the neural cranium and the face. At birth the midsagittal neural cranial area is 4 to 4½ times as large as the facial area when the jaws are closed. In a child of 2 years, this area is 3 to 3½ times as great as the area of the face. At 6 years the ratio is approximately 2½ to 1, and in the adult it ranges from 1½ or 2 to 1.

The accompanying radiographs (Figs. 6–38, 6–39) demonstrate the type of growth that occurs in the face. The mastoid process begins to be well pneumatized by the age of 6, and the frontal sinuses likewise tend to develop air cells. The frontal sinuses are really outgrowths from the ethmoidal labyrinth, and have an origin similar to that of the ethmoid air cells.

The growth of the alveolar processes parallels dental growth, and in old age, owing to the loss of the teeth, there is a diminution in the size of the jaws because of the absorption of the walls of the

alveoli; the chin protrudes and the angle of the mandible becomes more obtuse.

At approximately the age of 7 the orbits, the laminae cribrosae of the ethmoids, the body of the sphenoid, the petrous part of the temporal bones, and the foramen magnum have reached their adult size (Fig. 6–40). The measurement of interorbital distance may be significant in certain pathologic states, and a method for such measurement, separating normal infants from those with mongolism, is proposed and presented in Figure 6–40.

At puberty there is another rapid increase in the rate of growth in all directions, especially in the frontal and facial regions, owing to a further increase in the size of the air sinuses; the skull and face begin to take on a more definitive appearance at this time.

With advancing age the cranial sutures fuse progressively until eventually they are completely united. Apparently the endocranial aspects of the sutures fuse in a more orderly fashion, whereas the ectocranial serrated margin is subject to considerable variation. Closure of sutures correlates less often with age in females than in males. The sutures in females tend to remain open longer or fail to fuse at all. The fundamental model of closure in the vault was described in 1924 and 1925 by Todd and Lyon, who noted that closure in the vault begins in the sagittal suture at age 22, in the coronal at age 24, and in the lambdoid at 26. Complete fusion results by 35, 41, and 47 years respectively.

The sutures bordering the squamous portion of the temporal bone rarely close completely even in old age, but usually begin to close at about the age of 35. The closure pattern in a large series of patients is quite irregular. Radiologically, the sagittal suture often is closed by the age of 35 to 40 and usually after the age of 50. The lambdoid and especially the coronal sutures frequently are closed at least in part after the age of 50, whereas the others are frequently if not uniformly identifiable in some views even into the 90s. Generally, variations in the pattern of suture closure are of no clinical significance except for obvious early closure before adulthood, in which case synostosis of the cranial bones becomes extremely likely. The metopic suture, when present in adults, usually remains open indefinitely.

An interesting radiolucency closely resembling pacchionian depressions is not infrequent in the occipital bone. It is close to the midline just below the transverse sinuses or torcular Herophili and seems to be associated with aging, since it has been found only in adults beyond middle age.

Heinrich, in 1941, produced a table from Lorenz that showed the incidence of pineal calcification to be about 70 per cent at the age of 20, but after the age of 60 it was present in only 79 per cent of skulls, a 9 per cent increase in calcification over a period of 40 years or more.

The nasal septum in the child is also different from that of the adult. It is thick and pale in color compared with that of adults. On each side, the posterior ends of the middle conchae are conspicuous. Just above the soft palate, the posterior ends of the inferior nasal conchae are visible. The superior nasal conchae may be seen high in the nasal cavity adjoining the nasal septum.

The Cronqvist Cranial Index. Cronqvist in 1968 constructed new cranial indices to establish more reliable and objective criteria of assessing the size of the cranial vault. For these measurements only lateral and anteroposterior views are obtained. The measurements include the greatest length from inner table to inner table, the greatest width from inner table to inner table on frontal perspective, and the greatest height between the

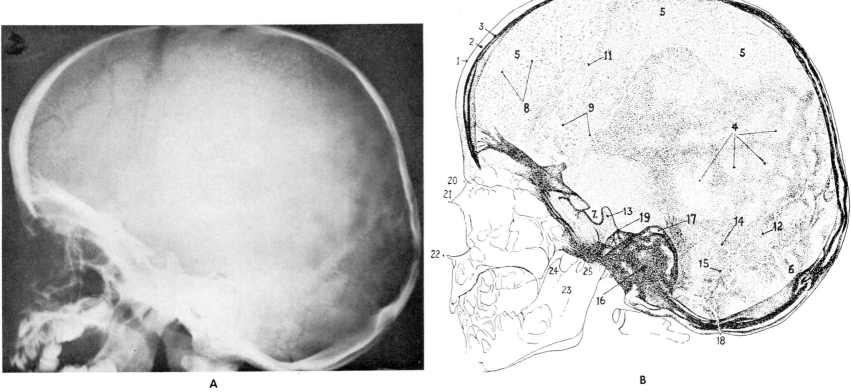

A   B

Figure 6–38. Normal skull at 2 years of age. *A.* Radiograph, lateral view. *B.* Labeled tracing of *A.* (1) Outer table, (2) diploic space, (3) inner table, (4) convolutional markings, (5) fine honeycomb of diploic structure, (6) internal occipital protuberance, (7) pituitary fossa, (8) diploic veins, (9) vascular grooves, (10) anterior fontanelle, (11) coronal suture, (12) lambdoidal suture, (13) dorsum sellae, (14) parietomastoid suture, (15) occipitomastoid suture, (16) petrous pyramids, (17) small temporal pneumatic cell, (18) synchondrosis between exoccipital and supra-occipital areas, (19) spheno-occipital synchondrosis, (20) nasofrontal suture, (21) nasal bone, (22) anterior nasal spine, (23) mandible, (24) coronoid process of mandible, (25) articular process of mandible. (From Caffey, J.: Pediatric X-ray Diagnosis, 6th ed. Chicago, Year Book Medical Publishers, 1972.)

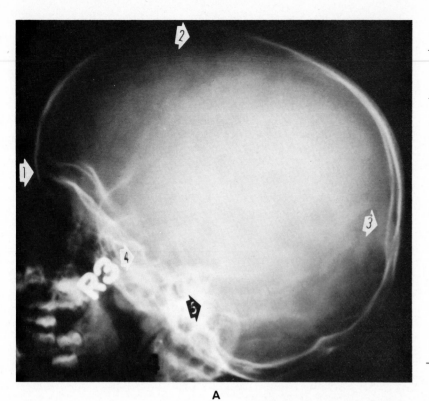

AVERAGE HEAD AND CHEST CIRCUMFERENCE
OF AMERICAN CHILDREN

Age	Mean Head Circumference		Standard Deviation		Chest Circumference		Head-Chest Ratio
	INCHES	CM.	±INCHES	±CM.	INCHES	CM.	
Birth	13.8	35	0.5	1.2	13.7	35	1:1
1 month	14.9	37.6	0.5	1.2			
2 months	15.5	39.7	0.5	1.2			
3 months	15.9	40.4	0.5	1.2	16.2	40	1:1
6 months	17.0	43.4	0.4	1.1	17.3	44	1:1
9 months	17.8	45.0	0.5	1.2			
12 months	18.3	46.5	0.5	1.2	18.3	47	1:1
18 months	19.0	48.4	0.5	1.2	18.9	48	1:1
2 years	19.2	49.0	0.5	1.2	19.5	50	1:1
3 years	19.6	50.0	0.5	1.2	20.4	52	0.96:1
4 years	19.8	50.5	0.5	1.2	21.1	53	0.95:1
5 years	20.0	50.8	0.6	1.4	22.0	55	0.93:1
6 years	20.2	51.2	0.6	1.4	22.5	56	0.91:1
7 years	20.5	51.6	0.6	1.4	23.0	57	0.90:1
8 years	20.6	52.0	0.8	1.8	24.0	59	0.88:1
10 years	20.9	53.0	0.6	1.4	25.1	61	0.87:1
12 years	21.0	53.2	0.8	1.8	27.0	66	0.81:1
14 years	21.5	54.0	0.8	1.8	29.0	72	0.75:1
16 years[a]	21.9	55.0	0.8	1.8	31.0	77	0.71:1
18 years[a]	22.1	55.4	0.8	1.8	33.0	82	0.68:1
20 years[a]	22.2	55.6	0.8	1.8	34.5	86	0.65:1

[a]Chest circumference for males only.

A   **B**

Figure 6–39. *A.* Lateral radiograph of a skull of a 4-year-old with pertinent areas of growth change indicated. (1) Frontal sinus region, (2) coronal sutures, (3) lambdoid sutures, (4) sella turcica, (5) mastoids. The frontal and mastoid areas become pneumatized, the sella becomes more completely ossified, and the sutures become more like those of the adult. *B.* Average head and chest circumference of American children. (Measurements taken from Growth and Development of Children, 6th ed., by Lowrey, G. H. Copyright © 1973 by Year Book Medical Publishers, Inc., Chicago. Used by permission.)

inner table of the parietal bone and the base of the skull. This last measurement is the maximum perpendicular distance between the vault and the skull and a line drawn *from the nasion to the posterior margin of the foramen magnum.* The sum of these measurements is divided by the maximum distance between the inner margin of the two necks of the mandible as measured in the anteroposterior view (M) (Fig. 6–41). The quotient is then multiplied by a factor of 10:

$$\text{Cronqvist cranial index (CCI)} = \frac{H + L + W}{M} \times 10$$

Cronqvist found the normal range ± 2 standard deviations to be 51 to 56. The intermandibular distance reflects growth of the cranial base and yet is not generally affected by intracranial content.

Austin and Gooding in 1971 applied Cronqvist's index to a North American population and found many false-positive measurements, particularly in children under 2 years of age. Austin and Gooding hypothesize that the index may vary with age, and in their analysis of 262 American children they found that the CCI was a function of age, decreasing in value as age increases, as shown in Figure 6–41 *B.* In the newborn (71 cases), this index was

57 ± 5 (2 standard deviations). In 5-year-olds the CCI was 53 ± 5.

One major exception to these indices is found in hypopituitarism. Here, although somatic growth is retarded and the face underdeveloped, the neural growth is normal; hence, an illusion of a large calvarium is produced (Nellhaus).

Microcrania has been defined as "head circumference 2 or more standard deviations below the mean for age and sex," and similarly, "macrocrania is a head circumference greater than 2 standard deviations above the mean" (Pryor and Thelander).

Schechter and Zingesser developed a method of measurement of the supratentorial part of the calvarium, as opposed to the infratentorial, in an effort to differentiate those pathologic states characterized by a disparity between the two. This they called the "perimeter ratio." It may be noted from Figure 6–41 *C* that this ratio normally remains constant. The method of measurement is shown in the graphic illustration.

Sex Differences. Until the age of puberty, there is little difference between the male and female skulls. However, an adult woman's skull is as a rule lighter and smaller than, and its cranial capacity about 10 per cent less, than a man's (Gray).

The walls of the female skull are thinner, and its muscular

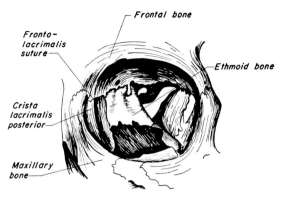

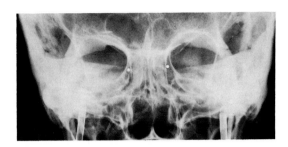

A

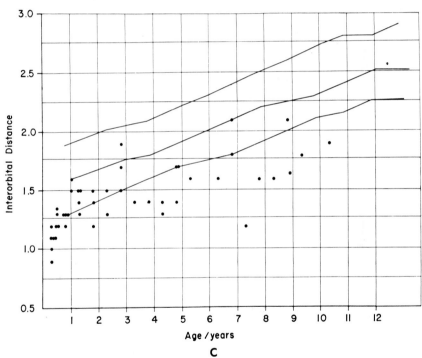

Age (Months)	Critical Level (cm.)
3	1.45
6	1.47
9	1.49
12	1.50
24	1.57
36	1.63
48	1.70
60	1.76
72	1.83
84	1.90
96	1.97
108	2.01
120	2.10
132	2.16
144	2.23

B

C

Figure 6–40. *A. Left,* Anatomy of orbit showing point of reference for measurement of interorbital distance. (Adapted from Sobotta, J.: Descriptive Human Anatomy. New York, Hafner Publishing Company, Inc., 1954.) *Right,* Roentgenogram of skull (anatomic specimen) with metallic markers at the juncture of the crista lacrimalis posterior with the frontolacrimalis suture. Note that the smooth curve is continuous with the medial rim of the orbital margin. The interorbital distance would be measured between the medial edges of the metallic markers. (From Gerald, B. E., and Silverman, F. N.: Amer. J. Roentgenol., 95:154–161, 1965.)

B. Interorbital measurements at various ages, separating patients with mongolism from normal infants and children. These measurements are 78 per cent accurate. C. Unsmoothed curves of normal interorbital distances (in centimeters) and distribution of measurements in mongols. (From Gerald, B. E., and Silverman, F. N.: Amer. J. Roentgenol., 95:145–161, 1965.)

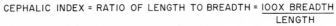

CEPHALIC INDEX = RATIO OF LENGTH TO BREADTH = $\dfrac{100 \times \text{BREADTH}}{\text{LENGTH}}$

MODULUS = $\dfrac{\text{LENGTH} + \text{BREADTH} + \text{HEIGHT}}{3}$

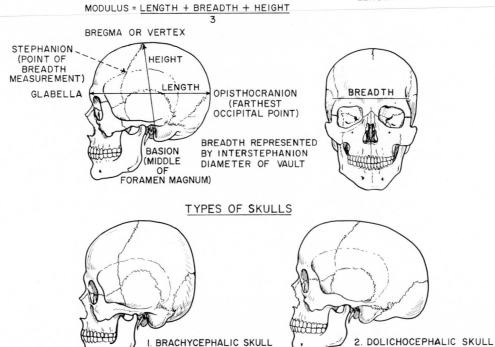

TYPES OF SKULLS

A

Age	(L + H + W) ± 2 S.D. (mm.)	Cranial Index of Cronqvist (± 2 S.D.) $\dfrac{L + H + W}{M} \times 10$
1 mo.	327 ± 26	57 ± 5
2– 3 mo.	355 ± 43	58 ± 4
4– 6 mo.	391 ± 30	57 ± 4
7– 9 mo.	421 ± 42	57 ± 5
10–12 mo.	421 ± 36	56 ± 6
1 yr.	441 ± 45	56 ± 6
2 yr.	456 ± 32	56 ± 7
3 yr.	470 ± 45	55 ± 5
4 yr.	464 ± 34	52 ± 6
5 yr.	465 ± 37	53 ± 5

CRANIAL SIZE IN CHILDREN (Cronqvist)
(after Austin and Gooding)

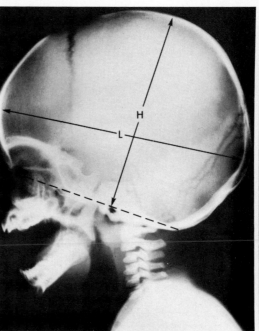
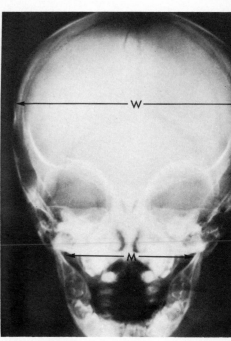

B

Figure 6–41. *A.* Important cranial indices and types of skulls. *B.* Cranial size in children. *Left,* Lateral roentgenogram. L, the greatest length between the inner tables of the skull; H, the greatest height, measured as the maximum perpendicular distance between the vault of the cranial cavity and a line drawn from the nasion to the posterior margin of the foramen magnum. *Right,* Anteroposterior roentgenogram. W, the greatest width between the inner tables of the skull; M, the maximum distance between the inner margins of the two necks of the mandible. (From Austin, J. H. M., and Gooding, C. A.: Radiology, *99*:642, 1971.)

Figure 6–41 continued on the opposite page.

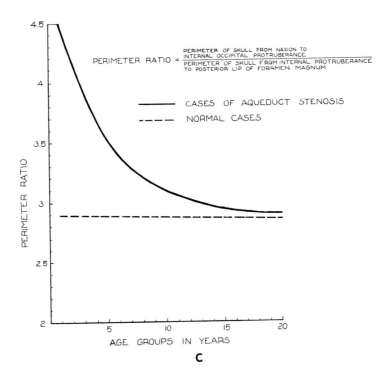

PERIMETER RATIO = PERIMETER OF SKULL FROM NASION TO INTERNAL OCCIPITAL PROTRUBERANCE / PERIMETER OF SKULL FROM INTERNAL PROTRUBERANCE TO POSTERIOR LIP OF FORAMEN MAGNUM

———— CASES OF AQUEDUCT STENOSIS

– – – – NORMAL CASES

C

SPHENOID ANGLE AND FACIAL ANGLE

SPHENOID ANGLE: ANGLE BETWEEN SPHENOID AND CLIVUS (ALSO CALLED "BASAL ANGLE")

FACIAL ANGLE: ANGLE BETWEEN SLOPE OF FACIAL BONES AND LINE DRAWN BETWEEN ALVEOLUS AND FORAMEN MAGNUM AS SHOWN.

NASO-PINEAL ANGLE: ROOT OF NOSE TO MIDPOINT OF DIAPHRAGMA SELLAE AND FROM THIS TO PINEAL GLAND (NORMAL: 138.5° – 157.5°) SECOND LIMB OF ANGLE: 3.9 – 5.3 CM. (± 2 STAND. DEV.) [ISLEY ET AL]

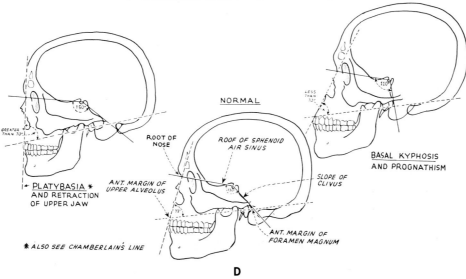

D

Figure 6–41 Continued.   C. The "perimeter ratio" as an indicator of cerebral aqueduct stenosis. (From Schechter, M. M., and Zingesser, L. H.: Radiology, 88:905–916, 1967.) D. The terms sphenoid angle and basal angle as defined in the text are synonymous. According to McGregor, 95 per cent of the population have a basal angle between 122 and 148 degrees.

Figure 6–41 continued on the following page.

NORMAL SIZE OF AVERAGE CAUCASIAN SKULL[a]

Mean	Males (mm.)	Females (mm.)
Length	182	174
Breadth	145	135
Height	132	125

CAPACITY OF ADULT CAUCASIAN SKULL[b]

	Mean (cc.)	Maximum (cc.)	Minimum (cc.)
Males	1450	1790	1220
Females	1300	1550	1090

[a]Broch, quoted by Schwartz, C. W., and Collins, L. C.: The Skull and Brain Roentgenologically Considered. Springfield, Illinois, Charles C Thomas, Publisher, 1951.
[b]Welcker, quoted by Schwartz and Collins.

E

Figure 6–41 *Continued.* E. Normal skull size.

ridges usually less strongly marked; the glabella, superciliary arches, and mastoid processes are less prominent and the air sinuses are smaller. The upper margin of the orbit tends to be sharper, the forehead more vertical, the frontal and parietal eminences more prominent, and the vault somewhat flatter than in men. At times, however, the characteristics are relatively indistinct and sex determination by skull appearance is extremely difficult or impossible.

ROUTINE RADIOGRAPHIC POSITIONS FOR STUDY OF THE SKULL

So many positions have been described for radiographic study of the skull that usually the radiologist must compromise on certain ones, depending on the anatomic part or parts he wishes to demonstrate to best advantage. We have been very arbitrary in choosing these projections, depending on the anatomic indications for each.

Routine Survey of the Bones of the Calvarium

1. *Posteroanterior View with a 15 Degree Tilt of the Tube Caudally (Caldwell's Projection)* (Fig. 6–42). This has the advantage over the straight posteroanterior projection (Fig. 6–43) in that it permits visualization of the orbital structures unobstructed by the petrous ridges. It permits the visualization of the superior orbital fissure with the surrounding lesser and greater wings of the sphenoid to better advantage (Fig. 7–15). On the other hand, the petrous ridge is obscured to a greater extent behind the maxillary antra and ethmoids. The other bones of the cranial vault are well visualized in either case.

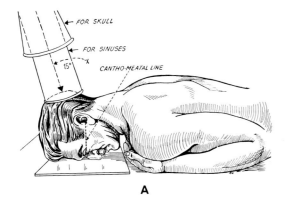

A

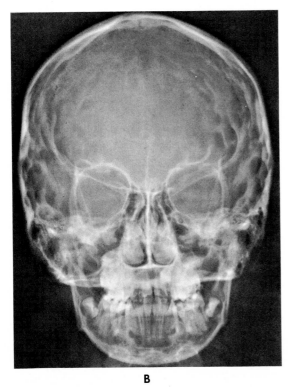

B

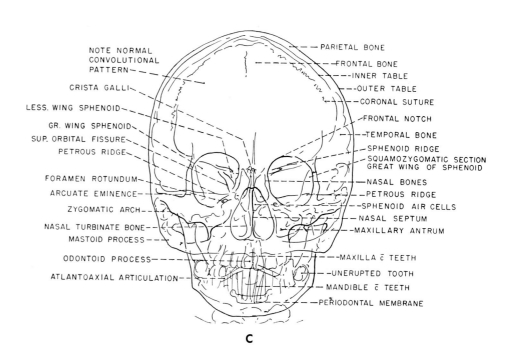

C

Figure 6–42. Caldwell's projection of the skull. A. Position of patient. Note canthomeatal line is perpendicular to the film. (The original Caldwell projection for sinuses was 23 degrees with respect to the glabello-meatal line, which is the same as 15 degrees with respect to the canthomeatal line, but somewhat more variable and hence a less accurate designation.) B. Radiograph. C. Labeled tracing of B.

Points of Practical Interest with Reference to Figure 6–42

1. The patient's head is adjusted so that the sagittal plane is perfectly perpendicular to the table top; the canthomeatal line (outer canthus of the eye to the tragus of the ear or external acoustic meatus) should be perpendicular to the plane of the film also. It may be necessary to support the patient's chin on either his fist or on a folded towel.
2. The central ray is centered to the glabella and angled toward the feet approximately 15 degrees with respect to the canthomeatal line.
3. It will be noted that in this view the petrous ridges are projected near the inferior margins of the orbits, and hence a clearer concept of the orbits is obtained than would be possible without the 15 degree angulation. Also, the lesser and greater wings of the sphenoid bone are projected in the orbits. In the straight posteroanterior view of the skull these are obscured by the petrous ridges which are for the most part projected into the orbits.
4. If the frontal bone in itself is the point of major interest, a straight posteroanterior view of the frontal bone is obtained without angulation of the tube.

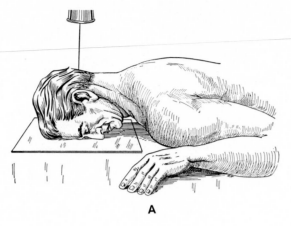

A

2. *Straight Posteroanterior View of the Skull* (Fig. 6–43). In this view the bones of the calvarium are visualized in undistorted frontal projection. The petrous ridges are projected into the orbits.

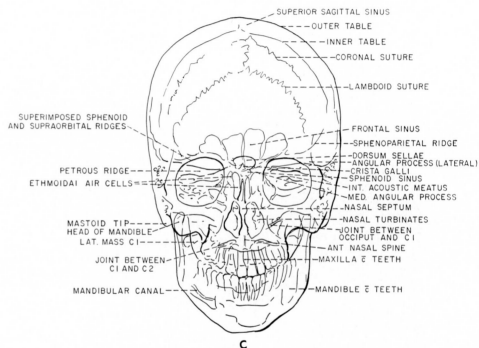

SUPERIOR SAGITTAL SINUS
OUTER TABLE
INNER TABLE
CORONAL SUTURE
LAMBDOID SUTURE
SUPERIMPOSED SPHENOID AND SUPRAORBITAL RIDGES
FRONTAL SINUS
SPHENOPARIETAL RIDGE
DORSUM SELLAE
ANGULAR PROCESS (LATERAL)
PETROUS RIDGE
CRISTA GALLI
SPHENOID SINUS
ETHMOIDAL AIR CELLS
INT. ACOUSTIC MEATUS
MED. ANGULAR PROCESS
NASAL SEPTUM
MASTOID TIP
NASAL TURBINATES
HEAD OF MANDIBLE
JOINT BETWEEN OCCIPUT AND C I
LAT. MASS C I
ANT NASAL SPINE
MAXILLA c̄ TEETH
JOINT BETWEEN C I AND C 2
MANDIBULAR CANAL
MANDIBLE c̄ TEETH

C

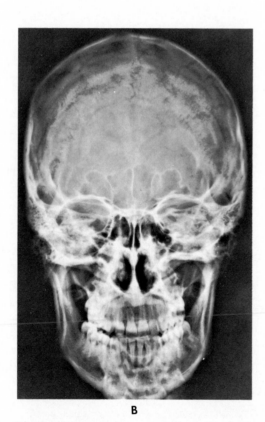

B

Figure 6–43.　Straight posteroanterior view of the skull. *A*. Position of patient. *B*. Radiograph. *C*. Labeled tracing of *B*.

Points of Practical Interest with Reference to Figure 6–43

1. This view differs from the Caldwell position in that the central ray of the x-ray tube is perpendicular to the film and coincides with the canthomeatal line. It will be noted that the petrous ridges are projected into the orbits, completely obscuring the orbital contents; the sphenoid ridges are projected over the petrous ridges and are likewise considerably obscured.
2. The posterior instead of the anterior cells of the ethmoid sinuses are shown, and the dorsum sellae is seen as a curved line extending between the orbits just above the ethmoids.

3. *Anteroposterior View with a 30 Degree Tilt of the Tube Caudally (Towne's Position)* (Fig. 6–44). This view demonstrates the entire occipital bone, foramen magnum, and dorsum sellae, along with a clear view of the petrous ridges. Often these structures are partially or completely obscured.

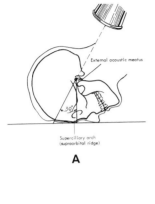

A

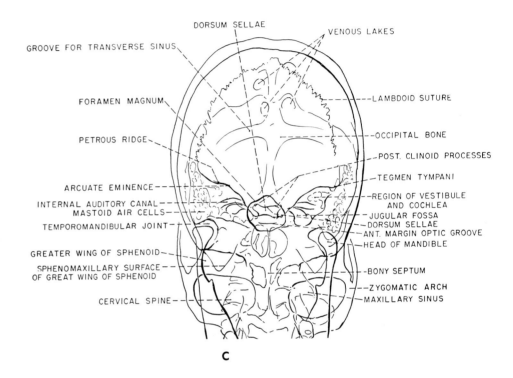

C

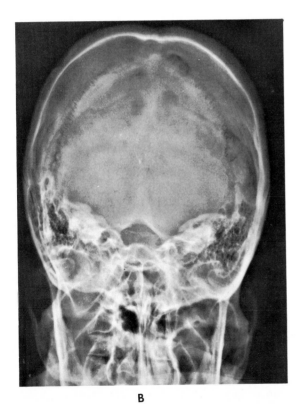

B

Figure 6–44. Towne's projection of the skull. *A.* Position of patient. *B.* Radiograph. *C.* Labeled tracing of *B.*

Points of Practical Interest with Reference to Figure 6–44

1. The sagittal plane of the patient is placed perpendicular to the table top and along the midline of the table.
2. The head is adjusted so that the canthomeatal line is approximately perpendicular to the table top. This will require that the chin be somewhat depressed upon the neck.
3. The central ray is adjusted at an angle of 30 degrees toward the feet so that it enters the forehead ordinarily at the hairline, and leaves the posterior portion of the cranium in the region of the external occipital protuberance.
4. For better projection of the dorsum sellae into the foramen magnum an angle of somewhat more than 30 degrees may be employed (up to 45 degrees).
5. A similar view may be obtained with the patient prone and the tube angled 30 degrees toward the head rather than toward the feet. In this instance the central ray would enter the head in the region of the external occipital protuberance and leave the cranium in the region of the forehead approximately 4 cm. above the superciliary arches. This is called the "reverse Towne's projection."

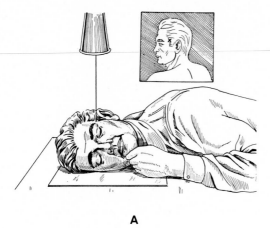

A

4. *Both Lateral Projections of the Skull* (Fig. 6–45), *First with One Side Close to the Film, and Then with the Other Side.* These views demonstrate the bones of the calvarium and base of the skull in the lateral perspective. The best visualization of the sella turcica is also obtained with this projection.

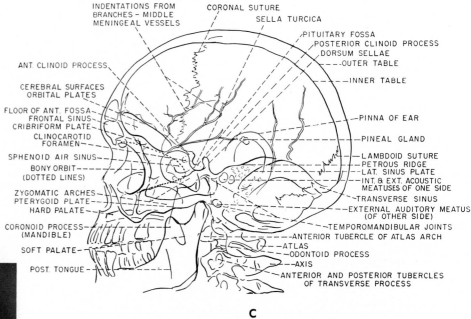

C

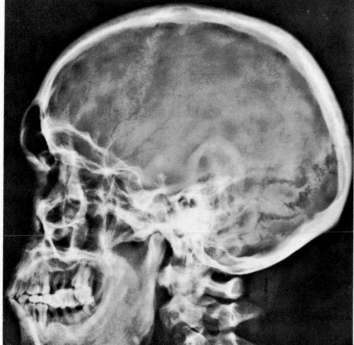

B

Figure 6–45. Lateral view of the skull. *A.* Position of patient. *B.* Radiograph. *C.* Labeled tracing of *B.*

Points of Practical Interest with Reference to Figure 6–45

1. The position of the head is adjusted so that its sagittal plane is parallel with the table top and with the film. Its coronal plane is centered to the longitudinal axis of the table. The film is placed transversely in the Potter-Bucky diaphragm beneath the skull.
2. A support is placed under the chin; usually the clenched fist of the patient is adequate in this regard.
3. The central ray passes through a point 1 inch above the midpoint of the line joining the outer canthus of the eye with the tragus of the ear (canthomeatal line). This will ordinarily fall immediately over the sella turcica.
4. To evaluate a good lateral projection the two halves of the mandible should be almost perfectly superimposed over one another. If the two rami of the mandible are obliquely projected at fair distances from each other, the projection of the skull is too oblique and should be repeated.
5. A rather oblique and distorted view of the upper cervical spine is obtained in this lateral view of the skull. This view must not be used routinely for examination of this segment of cervical spine.
6. A "perfect" position for the lateral skull film may be obtained more easily by placing the patient supine, and directing the beam horizontally. The cassette in a Bucky tray is then vertical.

5. *The Axial View of the Skull (Verticosubmental)* (Fig. 6–46). This projection allows a direct visualization of the base of the skull and the various foramina contained therein. It also provides another view of the petrous ridges, the ethmoid and sphenoid, along with the facial bones and orbit.

Any or all of these projections may be obtained stereoscopically.

In view of the complexity of the base of the skull, supplementary anatomic views are given in the format proposed and presented by Binet (1974), keeping references such as Potter and Newton and Potts well in mind. So many important and overlapping structures appear in the basal view that it is well to see the skull as a series of cuts, as shown in Figure 6–46 *D*. Six cuts are presented in Figure 6–46 *D* (borrowed from Binet and relabeled): these are described in detail in Figures 6–46 *E* through *J*.

The first section (Fig. 6–46 *E*) is at the level of the nasopharynx; it emphasizes particularly the position of the *torus tubarius*, the *eustachian tube*, and the *fossa of Rosemüller*, lateral to the torus, as well as the fact that "the lateral nasopharyngeal walls are not convex outward but instead are concave or sigmoidal in contour" (Rizzuti and Whalen). It is also evident from this cut that "the posterior wall of the nasopharynx does not project behind the anterior arch of the atlas."

In the second section (Fig. 6–46 *F*), traversing the maxillary antrum, the neural arch of C1, and the odontoid process, the air-filled *maxillary antrum* is clearly defined and the *medial and lat-*

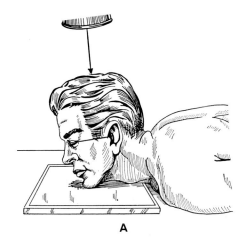

A

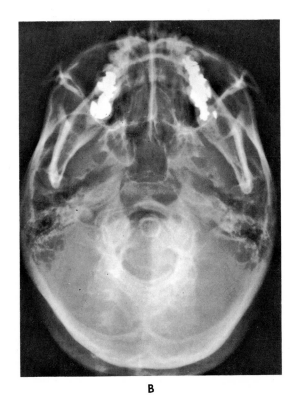

B

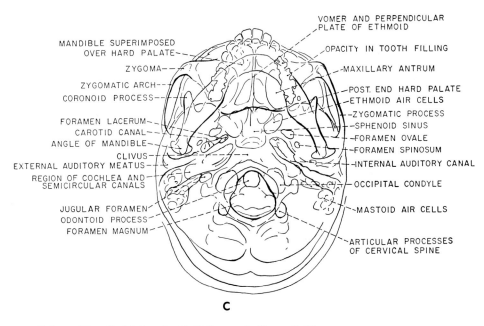

C

Figure 6–46. Axial view of the skull. *A.* Position of patient. *B.* Radiograph. *C.* Labeled tracing of *B.*

Points of Practical Interest with Reference to Figure 6–46

1. The head should be rested on the fully extended chin. The more closely perpendicular the line of the face is to the film the more satisfactory will be this projection.
2. If possible, the canthomeatal line should be parellel with the table top and the film.
3. The central ray should pass through the sagittal plane of the skull perpendicular to the canthomeatal line at its midpoint. It may be necessary to angle the central ray caudally to maintain this relationship if the patient is unable to extend the chin sufficiently.
4. This view is particularly valuable for visualization of the facial bones in tangential projection. It is used in combination with the frontal view of the facial bones in every instance.
5. This view is also valuable for visualization of the posterior ethmoid and sphenoid cells.

Figure 6–46 continued on the following page.

Figure 6–46 *Continued.* *D* to *J.* Common Legend for All Illustrations*

1. Anterior arch atlas 92%	33. Internal carotid artery groove
2. Anterior clinoid process 34%	34. Jugular foramen 1%
3. Anterior condyloid canal	35. Lamina papyracea 92%
4. Anterior margin middle cranial fossa 87%	36. Lateral pterygoid plate 98%
5. Anterior wall maxillary antrum	37. Lateral wall of orbit 87%
6. Clivus 74%	38. Mandibular head 91%
7. Condyloid fossa	39. Mastoid 83%
8. Condyloid process of the mandible	40. Maxillary antrum 90%
9. Cribriform plate	41. Medial pterygoid plate 95%
10. Crista galli 88%	42. Medial wall maxillary antrum
11. Dorsum sellae	43. Nasopharynx 46%
12. Ethmoid sinus 94%	44. Occipital condyle 59%
13. Eustachian tube 10%	45. Odontoid process
14. Exocranial opening, internal carotid artery canal	46. Optic foramen
15. External auditory canal 92%	47. Oropharynx
16. Foramen lacerum 40%	48. Posterior arch C1
17. Foramen magnum 4%	49. Posterior clinoid process 5%
18. Foramen of Vesalius	50. Posterior condyloid canal 1%
19. Foramen ovale 51%	51. Posterior process C2
20. Foramen rotundum 10%	52. Posterior wall maxillary antrum
21. Foramen spinosum 86%	53. Pterygopalatine fossa
22. Foramen transversarium 34%	54. Sella floor
23. Fossa of Rosenmüller 55%	55. Sella side wall 10%
24. Frontal sinus 72%	56. Sella turcica
25. Glenoid fossa 90%	57. Sphenoid sinus 92%
26. Greater palatine foramen 26%	58. Sphenoid sinus septum 94%
27. Horizontal semicircular canal 37%	59. Superior orbital fissure 10%
28. Inferior orbital fissure 13%	60. Styloid process
29. Infraorbital nerve canal 5%	61. Torus tubarius 51%
30. Internal auditory canal 62%	62. Tuberculum sellae 56%
31. Internal carotid artery	63. Turbinate 95%
32. Internal carotid artery canal 60%	64. Vidian canal 3%

*The percentages listed after many of the items indicate how often these items were interpreted as normal on review of 50 unselected base views.

(*D*, *E*, and *J* from Binet, E. F.: *Seminars in Roentgenol.* 9:137, 1974. Used by permission of Grune & Stratton, Inc. Parts *F* to *I* reprinted from Med. Radiography and Photography, courtesy of Radiography Markets Division, Eastman Kodak Company.)

Figure 6–46 continued on the opposite page.

eral walls of the pterygoid plates project posteriorly in the fashion of an inverted C. These structures lie at the posteroinferior *margin of the pterygopalatine fossa,* which is often invaded by neoplasms and juvenile angiofibromas.

The component parts of the nasal cavity and the upper cervical spine are also shown to good advantage.

The third section (6–46 *G*), traversing the clivus and falling just above the foramen magnum, is rather complex: The *clivus* is projected as an X-shaped structure. The *foramen lacerum* and the *canal for the internal carotid artery,* as well as the petrous apex, are readily seen. The sphenoid sinus and nasal structures are easily identified landmarks. The *foramen rotundum,* the *foramen*

spinosum, the *foramen ovale,* the *inferior orbital fissure,* and the *jugular foramen* are clearly seen. The relationship of the latter to a portion of the internal carotid artery canal is shown. The condyloid fossa and the contained process are also readily identified. The foramen magnum has also been cut through at this level, as pointed out earlier. The *posterior condyloid canal* and *condyloid fossa* are shown, but probably are not important clinically. The *anterior condyloid canal* is just anterior to the occipital condyle, and is important to identify on any view because of its frequent involvement in primary and secondary metastatic disease of the base of the skull.

In the fourth section (Fig. 6–46 *H*), through the superior

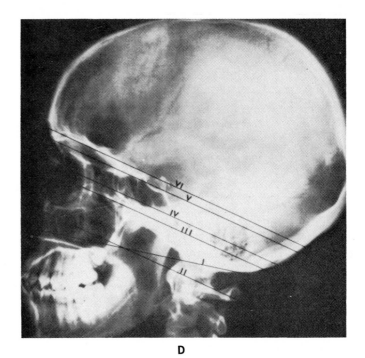

D

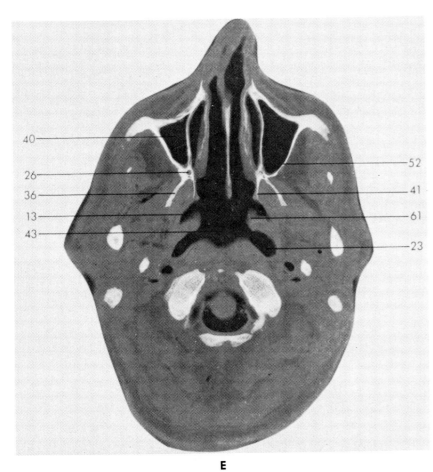

E

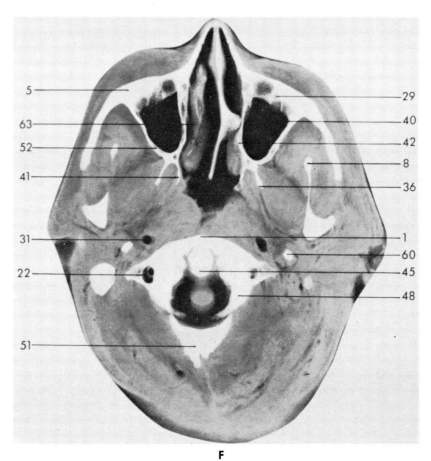

F

Figure 6–46. *Continued.* D. Lateral view, indicating the levels of the base of the skull at which the cadaver heads were sectioned. E. Nasopharynx (Level I). F. Maxillary antrum (Level II).

orbital fissure, the nasal contents, the lateral wall of the orbit, the base of the sphenoid sinus, and the external auditory canal can be identified as clear landmarks. The *internal carotid artery canal* is shown best. The mastoid air cells may be clearly seen.

The fifth section (Fig. 6–46 *I*) extends from the glabella to the base of the sella turcica, traversing the crista galli, and on to the *internal auditory canal.*

In the sixth section (Fig. 6–46 *J*), the line of cut goes through the top of the sella turcica, at the level of the anterior clinoid processes and the top of the orbits. Just medial to the anterior clinoid process is the *optic foramen.* The *dorsum sellae* and *posterior clinoid processes* are also demonstrated here. The anterior margin of the middle cranial fossa is clearly demarcated.

Figure 6–46 continued on the following page.

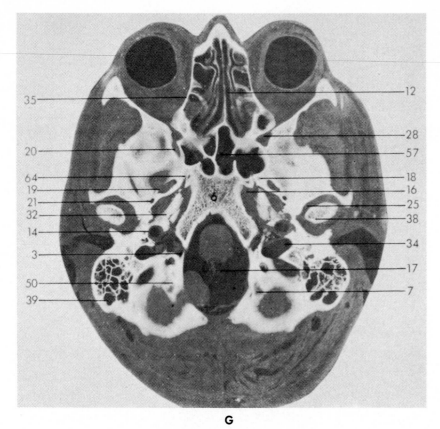

G

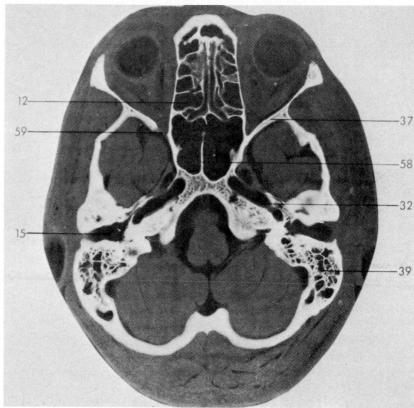

H

Figure 6–46 *Continued.* *G.* Clivus (Level III). *H.* Superior orbital fissure (Level IV).

Figure 6–46 continued on the opposite page.

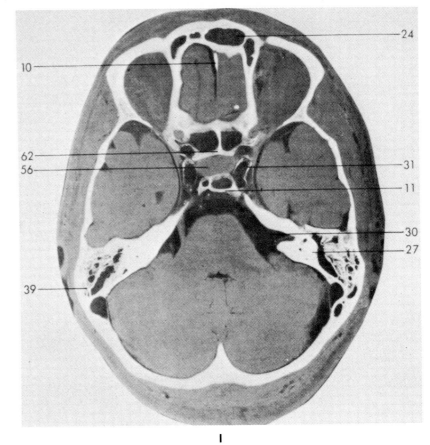

I

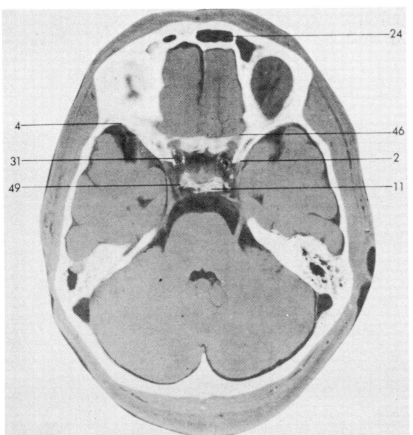

J

Figure 6–46 Continued.   *I.* Internal auditory canal (Level V). *J.* Anterior clinoid process (Level VI).

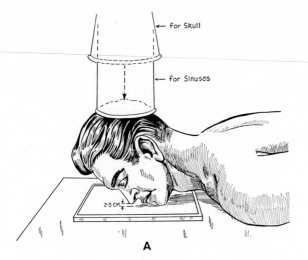

A

Special Study of the Facial Bones Apart from the Nose.

1. *Posteroanterior View of the Face* (Fig. 6–47), *with the Nose Raised Off the Film About 2 to 3 cm., and the Chin on the Film (Water's Projection).* This view affords an excellent opportunity to study the maxillae, zygomata, orbits, and nasal cavity.

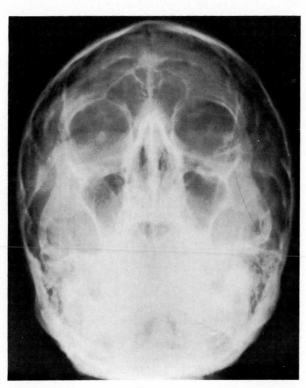

B

NASAL BONES

VENOUS LAKES
(PACCHIONIAN VILLI
IMPRESSIONS)

FRONTAL SINUSES

SUPRAORBITAL NOTCH

CALCIUM IN FALX
CEREBRI

FRONTOZYGOMATIC
SUTURE

MENINGEAL ARTERIES

ETHMOID AIR CELLS AND
NASAL TURBINATES

LAT. WALL LACRIMAL CANAL

NASAL SEPTUM

INFRAORBITAL FORAMEN

INF. MARGIN, ORBIT

UPPER ALVEOLAR RIDGE

FORAMEN ROTUNDUM

ZYGOMA

MAXILLARY ANTRUM

TEMPORAL PROCESS

CORONOID PROCESS

ZYGOMATIC ARCH

HEAD OF MANDIBLE

PETROUS RIDGE

MASTOID AIR CELLS

ANGLE MANDIBLE

ANTERIOR ARCH ATLAS

ODONTOID PROCESS

FORAMEN MAGNUM

ATLAS (POSTERIOR ARCH)

INT. OCCIPITAL PROTUBERANCE

C

Figure 6–47. Posteroanterior view of the face (Water's projection). *A*. Position of patient. *B*. Radiograph. *C*. Labeled tracing of *B*.

2. *Submentovertical View of the Skull (Axial View)* (Fig. 6–48). This view resembles the verticosubmental view closely, in that it permits visualization of the foramina at the base of the skull, the petrous ridges, and the ethmoid and sphenoid bones. It allows a somewhat more satisfactory tangential perspective of the maxillary bones, zygomata, zygomatic arches, orbits, and nasal cavity than does the other.

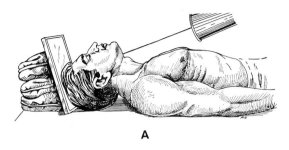

A

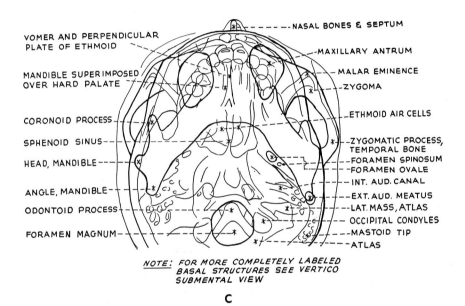

NASAL BONES & SEPTUM

VOMER AND PERPENDICULAR PLATE OF ETHMOID

MAXILLARY ANTRUM

MANDIBLE SUPERIMPOSED OVER HARD PALATE

MALAR EMINENCE

ZYGOMA

ETHMOID AIR CELLS

CORONOID PROCESS

SPHENOID SINUS

ZYGOMATIC PROCESS, TEMPORAL BONE

HEAD, MANDIBLE

FORAMEN SPINOSUM

FORAMEN OVALE

INT. AUD. CANAL

ANGLE, MANDIBLE

EXT. AUD. MEATUS

ODONTOID PROCESS

LAT. MASS, ATLAS

OCCIPITAL CONDYLES

FORAMEN MAGNUM

MASTOID TIP

ATLAS

NOTE: FOR MORE COMPLETELY LABELED BASAL STRUCTURES SEE VERTICO SUBMENTAL VIEW

C

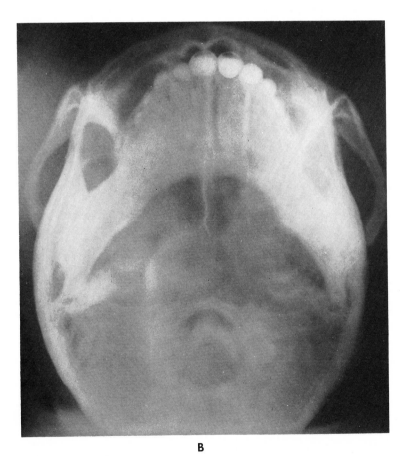

B

Figure 6–48. Axial view of the face (submentovertical view). *A.* Position of patient. This view, using a slightly "lighter" exposure technique, is utilized for visualization of the zygomatic arches in the inferosuperior projection. *B.* Radiograph. *C.* Labeled tracing of *B.*

Points of Practical Interest with Reference to Figure 6–48

1. The film and the patient's head are placed so that the canthomeatal line is parallel with the surface of the film.
2. The central ray is directed perpendicular to the midpoint of the canthomeatal line in the sagittal plane of the patient's skull.
3. A similar view may be obtained with the patient in the sitting position and his head leaning backward against a firm support; or in the supine position by placing a pillow under the upper back. Whenever possible a grid cassette or Potter-Bucky diaphragm should be employed.
4. In this view a clearer concept of the anterior ethmoid cells is obtained, and ordinarily the facial bones and mandible are projected over one another.
5. This view is also valuable for visualization of the zygomatic arches, since they are thrown into bold relief by means of this projection. However, a lighter exposure technique must be employed for this purpose.

3. *Lateral View of the Face* (Fig. 6–49). This is a straight lateral projection of the face, obtained in a fashion similar to the lateral view of the sphenoid, except that the entire face is included. For the anatomic description of this view, the student should also note the lateral sphenoid sinus view (Fig. 7–13).

Routine Study of the Zygomatic Arches (Fig. 6–47). This very frequently is part of a facial bone survey, and actually can be seen on the routine films if a bright light source is employed in viewing the submentovertical film. However, if a special further study is desirable, it is well to obtain a verticosubmental projection (Fig. 6–46), employing soft tissue technique so that the zygomatic arches are not "burned out." Other oblique projections may also be employed.

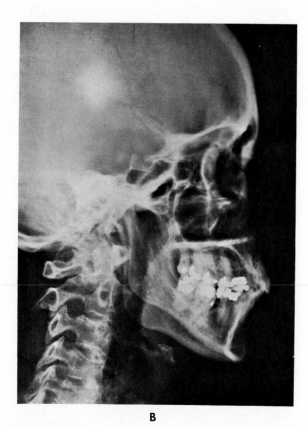

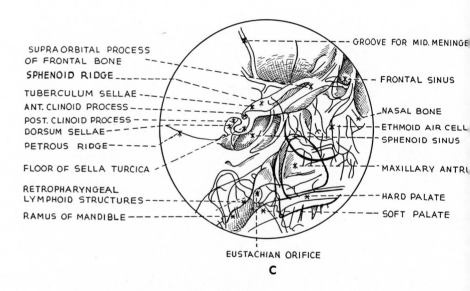

Figure 6–49. Lateral view of the face. *A.* Position of patient. *B.* Radiograph. *C.* Labeled tracing of *B.*

Points of Practical Interest with Reference to Figure 6–49

1. The sagittal plane of the head is adjusted so that it is perfectly parallel with the film and the table top.
2. The cassette may be placed directly under the head without utilizing the Potter-Bucky diaphragm, provided that the extended cone is likewise placed directly in contact with the opposite side of the head.
3. Center to the region of the sella turcica over a point 2.5 cm. anterior to and 2 cm. above the external acoustic meatus. Alternatively, one may center at a point about 2 cm. above the midpoint of the canthomeatal line.

Routine Study of the Mandible. Various obliquities can be obtained, depending upon whether the body of the ramus is to be demonstrated to better advantage.

1. *Straight Posteroanterior View of the Mandible* (Fig. 6–50). The chin is flexed on the neck, and the mandible is placed flat on the film. A short film-target distance is employed so as to avoid loss of detail caused by the cervical spine.

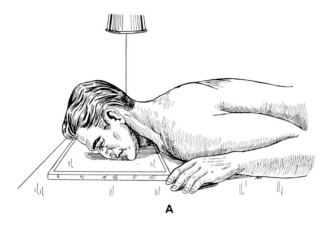

A

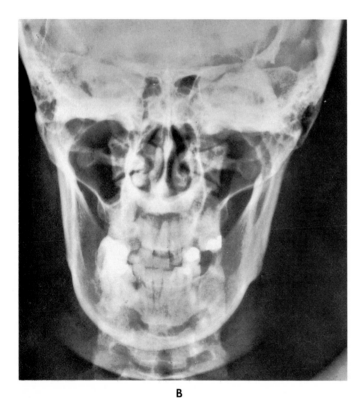

B

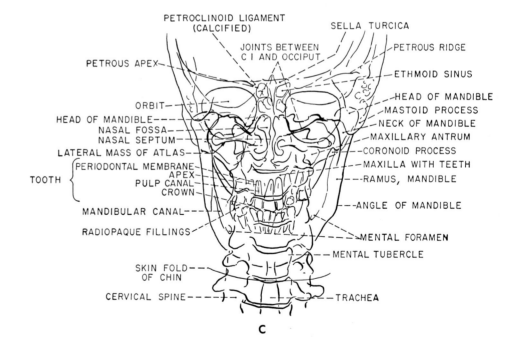

C

Figure 6–50. Posteroanterior view of the mandible. *A.* Position of patient. *B.* Radiograph. *C.* Labeled tracing of *B.*

2. *Oblique Projection of Each Side of the Mandible* (Fig. 6–51). Both the mandible and the tube are placed in the oblique position as shown in order to obtain an unobstructed view.

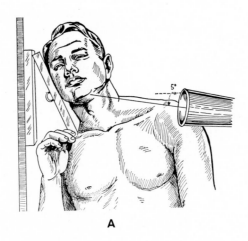

A

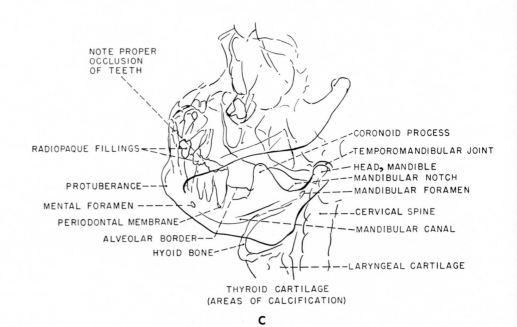

C

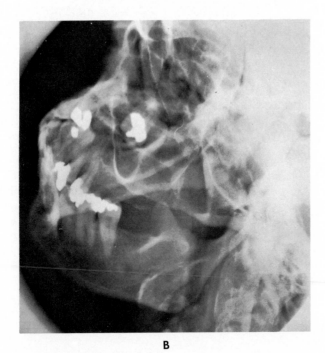

B

Figure 6–51. Oblique view of the mandible. *A.* Position of patient. *B.* Radiograph. *C.* Labeled tracing of *B.*

Points of Practical Interest with Reference to Figure 6–51

1. The film is placed against the patient's cheek at an angle of approximately 15 degrees with the vertical.
2. The broad surface of the mandibular body is placed parallel with the plane of the film.
3. To avoid distortion, a long target-to-film distance may be employed.
4. For better detail with regard to the ramus of the mandible the central ray may be directed inward, centering over the ramus of the mandible, and the ramus of the mandible may be brought into a position more directly parallel with the plane of the film.
5. If more information about the body of the mandible near the symphysis is desired, the head is rotated so that this area is nearer the film.
6. It is ordinarily easier to obtain an erect view of the injured mandible than a recumbent, although the recumbent view may be obtained in somewhat similar fashion.

3. *Special View of the Temporomandibular Articulation* (Fig. 6–52). Law's position is employed as for demonstration of the mastoid process, except that in this instance *two views* are obtained of each temporomandibular joint, with the *mouth open on the one*, and the *mouth closed on the other*. This allows a proper perspective of the apparent normal subluxation that occurs when the mouth is opened, as well as the structural appearance of the joint.

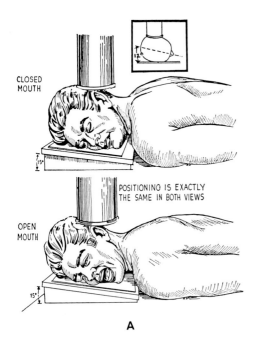

CLOSED MOUTH

15°

POSITIONING IS EXACTLY THE SAME IN BOTH VIEWS

OPEN MOUTH

15°

A

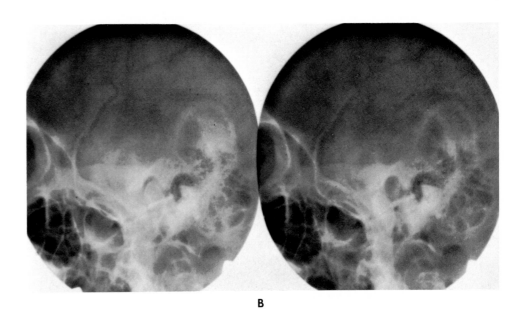

B

Figure 6–52. Views of the temporomandibular joint with the mouth open and closed. *A.* Position of patient. *B.* Radiograph. *C.* Labeled tracings of *B.* *D.* Body section radiograph—mouth closed.

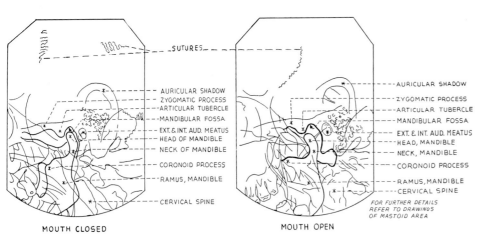

SUTURES

AURICULAR SHADOW
ZYGOMATIC PROCESS
ARTICULAR TUBERCLE
MANDIBULAR FOSSA
EXT. & INT. AUD. MEATUS
HEAD OF MANDIBLE
NECK OF MANDIBLE

CORONOID PROCESS

RAMUS, MANDIBLE

CERVICAL SPINE

MOUTH CLOSED

AURICULAR SHADOW
ZYGOMATIC PROCESS
ARTICULAR TUBERCLE
MANDIBULAR FOSSA
EXT. & INT. AUD. MEATUS
HEAD, MANDIBLE
NECK, MANDIBLE
CORONOID PROCESS
RAMUS, MANDIBLE
CERVICAL SPINE

FOR FURTHER DETAILS REFER TO DRAWINGS OF MASTOID AREA

MOUTH OPEN

C

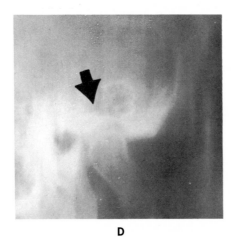

D

4. *Intraoral View of the Body of the Mandible* (Fig. 6–53). This is obtained by placing an occlusal film in the mouth as far back as possible, and directing the central ray through the submental region.

Panoramic views of the mandible may be obtained by several methods. In one technique the centered electron beam hits a pyramid-shaped anticathode, which has been introduced as a focus into the oral cavity. The rays are reflected outward from the oral cavity and pharynx, striking the film which has been placed on the outside of the mandible. A plain panoramic view of the mandibular arch is obtained with this technique.

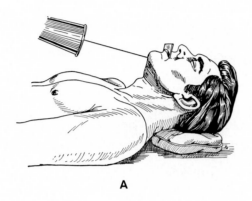

A

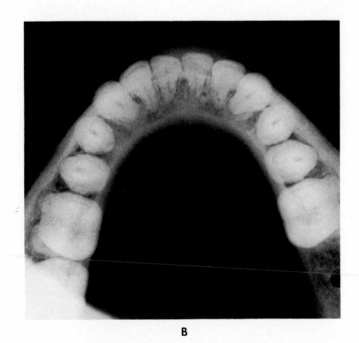

B

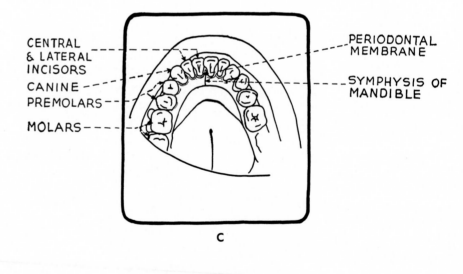

C

Figure 6–53. Occlusal view of the mandible (intraoral). *A.* Position of patient. *B.* Radiograph. *C.* Labeled tracing of *B.*

Figure 6–53 continued on the opposite page.

There are at least three other panoramic x-ray units available, all having the following features in common: (1) the x-ray source rotates around the patient's head, and (2) the x-ray film is held in a cassette with intensifying screens which also rotates around the patient's head.

In Figure 6–53 *D* the specific principles of these units are illustrated. A routine panoramic radiograph of the mandible and maxilla so obtained is illustrated in Figure 6–53 *E*. The position of the patient's head when using an x-ray unit for panoramic radiography such as that shown in Figure 6–53 *D* (1) is shown in Figure 6–53 *F*.

Apart from radiography of the mandible and maxilla, this technique can also be applied in sialography and in clinical pantomography of the jaws (Soila and Paatero; Pappas and Wallace). There is an inherent enlargement factor in these units because of the short distance between the x-ray tube-target and the film, and the great distance between the film and the object being radiographed.

These units are capable of recording curved sections of the body, an advantage which is especially useful in radiography of the dental arch. Actually, in the dental arch three arcs are usually filmed: (a) the left buccal segment, (b) an anterior segment, and (c) a right buccal segment. Centers of rotation of the two sides of the mandible are located behind the third mandibular molar tooth on the side opposite that being radiographed. The anterior segment has a center of rotation just behind the incisors at about the level of the mandibular bicuspids.

The cassette is made of a flexible plastic material with intensifying screens wrapped around a curved metal film holder. Films are ordinarily 6 by 12 inches in size. Grids are usually not employed.

If the system is very slightly eccentric to the mandible, either one of the parotid glands may be brought into focus by rotating the head so that the midsagittal plane is 20 to 25 degrees from the vertical center line.

Pantomography (Soila and Paatero) has been developed to obtain body section radiographs of curved surfaces. Again, the jaws are especially suitable targets for this technique, but it has been used in other areas of the body as well. As described earlier, the method employs a fixed source of radiation while the object and film are rotated on holders having equal radii and moving at equal speeds through a peripheral frictional arrangement.

For concentric pantomography, which is best suited to structures like the jaw, the object is placed concentrically on the holder. In eccentric pantomography, the object is placed eccentrically on the holder. Stereoscopic films may be produced by shifting the tube horizontally or vertically.

Although panography and pantomography have been most applicable to the needs of dental specialists, it is becoming increasingly apparent that the general radiologist would also find benefit in the utilization of these techniques.

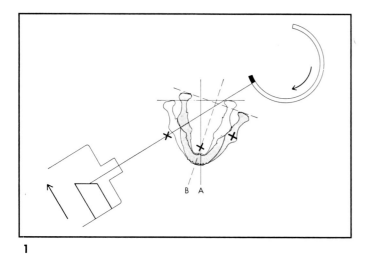

1

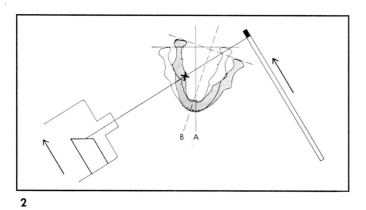

2

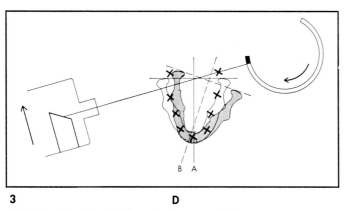

3   **D**

Figure 6–53 *Continued.* *D.* Schematic drawings of three panoramic x-ray units. The *X*'s in drawings 1 and 2 indicate the centers of rotation for the x-ray source. These shift as the x-ray source moves around the face. The *X*'s in drawing 3 indicate the path that the x-ray source follows as it moves around the face. (From Pappas, G. C., and Wallace, W. R.: Dental Radiography and Photography, 43(2):27, 1970.)

Figure 6–53 continued on the following page.

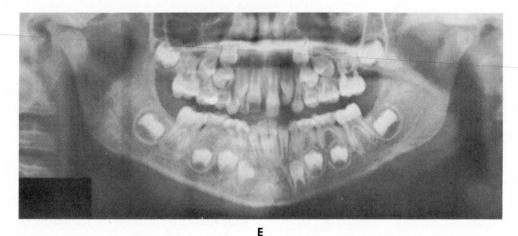

E

Figure 6–53 *Continued.* E. Routine panoramic radiograph. F. Position of the patient's head when using the x-ray unit in Figure 6–53 D for panoramic radiography. *Left*, Conventional position. *Right*, Modified position. (From Pappas, G. C., and Wallace, W. R.: Dental Radiography and Photography, *43*(2):27, 1970.)

5. *Intraoral Views of the Teeth* (Stafne) (Fig. 6–8). Small contact films of the incisor, canine, premolar, and molar areas are obtained of both sides (both upper and lower dental arches). Emphasis in these views is on the apical and periapical structure of the teeth, although a fairly good perspective of the crowns of the teeth is also obtained. For better demonstration of the crowns of the teeth, so-called bite-wing views are obtained.

6. *Methods for Demonstration of the Jugular Foramen* (Figs. 6–29, 6–54, 6–55, 6–56). There are several possible techniques for visualization of the jugular foramen.

(*a*) A modified Water's view may be used, in which the mouth is open as wide as possible and the canthomeatal line and roentgenographic table form an angle of 37 degrees (35 to 37 degrees). The x-ray beam is directed perpendicularly to the table in the posteroanterior (or anteroposterior) projection at the level of the external auditory meatus. A cone is employed to include both the jugular foramina for best detail (Kim and Capp).

(*b*) A modified Law's position may be used for demonstration of the jugular foramen. The left side of the face is against the roentgenographic table when the left jugular foramen is examined (and vice versa for the right jugular foramen). The face is tilted to the side toward the table to make a 5 degree angle between the sagittal suture line and the table. The chin is tilted toward the table to make a 15 degree angle between the nasal axis line and the table. The x-ray tube is tilted 15 degrees caudad, and the central beam is directed to the external auditory meatus of the ear to be examined (Kim and Capp).

(*c*) Transoral projection, open mouth.

(1) Patient is supine with one pillow elevating his ipsilateral shoulder.

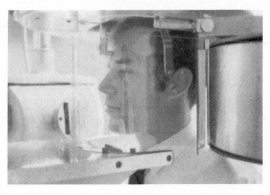
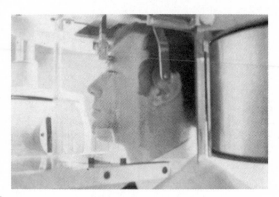

F

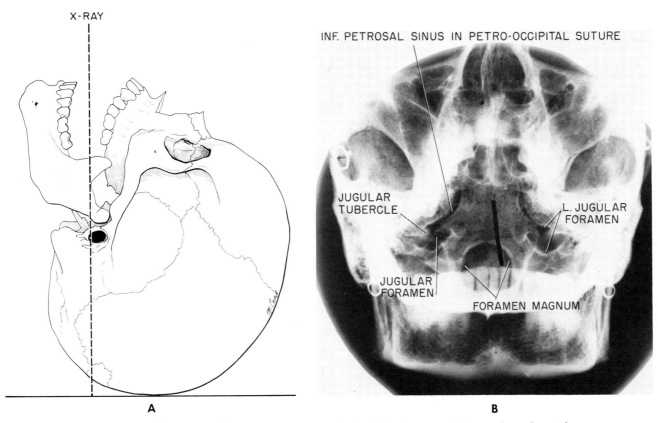

X-RAY

A

INF. PETROSAL SINUS IN PETRO-OCCIPITAL SUTURE

JUGULAR TUBERCLE

L. JUGULAR FORAMEN

JUGULAR FORAMEN

FORAMEN MAGNUM

B

Figure 6–54. A. Transoral projection. The x-ray beam perpendicular to the film passes between the molars and through the plane of the jugular foramina, which lies just caudad to the external auditory meatus at the infratragal notch. B. Transoral view of both jugular foramina in a dry skull. (From Strickler, J. M.: Amer. J. Roentgenol., 97: 601–606, 1966.)

(2) The x-ray beam is perpendicular to the table and midline over the patient.

(3) Patient's mouth is opened wide with a cork or other nonopaque object.

(4) With the patient's nose and chin in the midline, extend or flex his head as necessary to align the central beam through the infratragal notch of the ear and the gap between the upper and lower molars as palpated through the cheek.

(5) Exposure factors are slightly less than those used for the base of the skull (Strickler).

(d) Oblique open mouth view. Follow steps (1) through (4) as for the transoral view of Strickler. Keeping the patient's chin and nose in a straight line parallel to the midplane, roll the patient's head 10 degrees or less to one side. This maneuver centers the x-ray beam over the jugular foramen and along the jugular canal on the side away from which the face is turned. Repeat, turning the face to the opposite side for the other jugular foramen.

(e) In this view the patient is supine with pillows elevating his shoulders. The x-ray beam is perpendicular to the table and midline over the patient. With the patient's mouth closed and his nose and chin in the midline, raise the patient's chin until the central ray is aligned through (a) the infratragal notch of the ear, and (b) the point 2 cm. caudad to the lower edge of the chin as viewed from the lateral position. Edentulous patients are positioned the same way (Fig. 6–29).

Roentgenograms and tracings of them are shown for each of these positions.

Routine Method of Study of Radiographs of the Skull (Fig. 6–57). As indicated in the preceding section, there are numerous variations of normal. These must be understood—there can be no substitute for careful attention to detail and extensive experience. In outline form, the routine method for study of frontal and lateral perspectives of the skull is as follows:

1. Note the shape of the skull as a whole, especially the relationship of the vault to the base in all views.

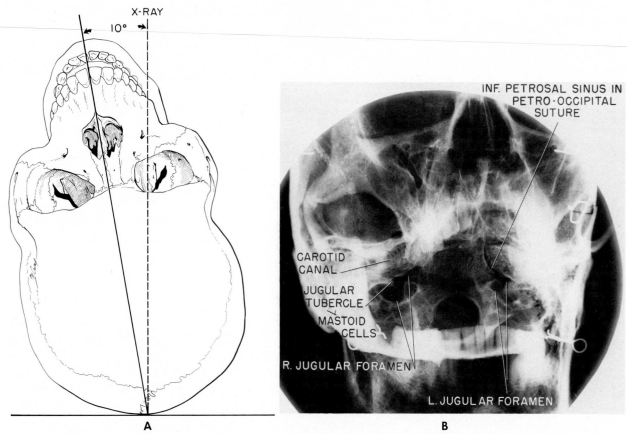

Figure 6–55. *A.* Oblique open-mouth projection. When the face is turned 10 degrees or less to the left from mid-line, the x-ray beam remains perpendicular to the film and becomes centered through the right jugular foramen. *B.* Oblique open-mouth view of right jugular foramen in a dry skull. The walls of the carotid canal are clear and sharp in this "down the hatch" view. (From Strickler, J. M.: Amer. J. Roentgenol., 97:601–606, 1966.)

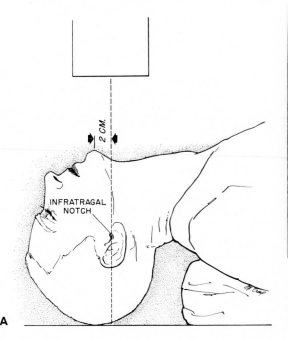

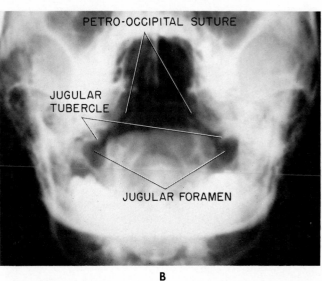

Figure 6–56. *A.* Position for modified base view of both jugular foramina. *B.* Transoral view of the jugular foramina in the same normal patient. (From Strickler, J. M.: Amer. J. Roentgenol., 97:601–606, 1966.)

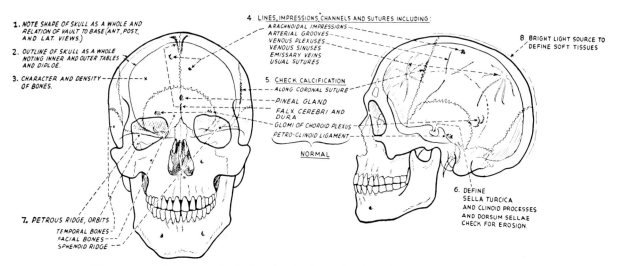

Figure 6–57. Routine method of study of radiographs of skull—frontal and lateral views.

2. Study the outline of the skull as a whole, noting the thickness of the inner and outer tables and diploë and any special characteristics therein.

3. Study the character and density of the bones of the calvarium.

4. Study the lines, impressions, channels, and sutures, including such anatomic detail as the arachnoidal impression, arterial grooves, venous plexuses and sinuses, emissary veins, and the usual sutures.

5. Check all calcification, such as may be found in the dura, the falx cerebri, the pineal gland, the glomi of the choroid plexuses, the petroclinoid ligament, and the habenular commissure.

6. Carefully define the sella turcica, with its anterior and posterior clinoid processes and the tuberculum sellae. The floor must be clearly defined on both sides, if possible in both the frontal and lateral perspectives. The size is measured in the lateral view, and if necessary a volume is computed from lateral and frontal views as well.

7. The petrous ridges, orbits, sphenoid ridges, temporal bones, and facial bones are carefully studied bilaterally. The acoustic canals and foramina are compared and measured. The region of the tegmen tympani and mastoid is carefully observed.

8. A bright light source to define the soft tissues of the scalp is always helpful.

REFERENCES

Agnos, J. W., and Wollin, D. G.: The effect of rotation of the skull on the measured position of the pineal gland. J. Can. Assoc. Radiol., *9*:40–44, 1958.

Anson, B. J. (ed.): Morris' Human Anatomy. 12th edition. New York, McGraw-Hill, 1966.

Austin, J. H. M., and Gooding, C. A.: Roentgenographic measurement of skull size in children.

Binet, E. F.: The base of the adult skull. Sem. in Roentgenol., *9*:137–150, 1974.
    Radiology, *99*:641–646, 1971.

Boyd, G. I.: Emissary foramina of the cranium in anthropoids. J. Anat., *65*:108–121, 1930.

Caffey, J.: Accessory ossicles of the supraoccipital bone. Amer. J. Roentgenol., *70*:401–412, 1953.

Caffey, J.: On the accessory ossicles of the supraoccipital bone. Amer. J. Roentgenol., *70*:401–412, 1953.

Coin, C. G., and Malkasian, D. R.: *In* Newton, T. H., and Potts, D. G.: Radiology of the Skull and Brain. St. Louis, C. V. Mosby Co., 1971.

Cronqvist, S.: Roentgenologic evaluation of cranial size in children. Acta Radiol. (Diag.), 7:97–111, 1968.

Cunningham, D. J.: Manual of Practical Anatomy. Vol. 3, 12th edition. London, Oxford University Press, 1959.

DiChiro, G., and Anderson, W. B.: Clivus. Clin. Radiol., *17*:211–223, 1965.

DiChiro, G., Fisher, R. L., and Nelson, K. B.: The jugular foramen. J. Neurosurg., *21*:447–460, 1964.

Dorst, J. B.: Changes of the skull during childhood. *In* Newton, T. H., and Potts, D. G.: Radiology of the Skull and Brain. St. Louis, C. V. Mosby Co., 1971.

duBoulay, G. H.: *Principles of X-ray Diagnosis of the Skull.* Washington, Butterworth, 1965.

Dyke, C. G.: Indirect signs of brain tumor as noted in routine roentgen examinations: displacement of pineal shadow. Amer. J. Roentgenol., *23*:598–606, 1930.

Ethier, R.: *In* Newton, T. H., and Potts, D. G.: Radiology of the Skull and Brain. St. Louis, C. V. Mosby Co., 1971.

Etter, L.: Atlas of Roentgen Anatomy of the Skull. Springfield, Ill., Charles C Thomas, 1955.

Fischer, E.: Quoted in Newton, T. H., and Potts, D. G.: Radiology of the Skull and Brain. St. Louis, C. V. Mosby Co., 1971.

Fray, W. W.: Roentgenologic study of orientation of pineal body: comparison of proportional and graphic method in absence of tumor of brain. Arch. Neurol. Psychiat., *38*:1199–1207, 1938.

Fray, W. W.: Roentgenological study of pineal orientation. III. Comparison of method used in pineal orientation. Amer. J. Roentgenol., *39*:899–907, 1938.

Gathier, J. C., and Bruyn, G. W.: The so-called condyloid foramen in the half-axial view. Amer. J. Roentgenol., *107*:515–519, 1969.

Girdany, B. R., and Blank, E.: Anterior fontanel bones. Amer. J. Roentgenol., *95*:148–153, 1965.

Graber, T. M.: Panoramic radiography in orthodontic diagnosis. Amer. J. Orthodontics, *53*:799–821, 1967.

Grant, J. C. B.: Atlas of Anatomy. Fifth edition. Baltimore, Williams and Wilkins Co., 1962.

Gray, H.: Gray's Anatomy of the Human Body. 24th and 29th editions. Philadelphia, Lea and Febiger, 1942, 1973.

Hassler, O.: Calcification of the intracranial arachnoid: a microradiological and histological study of the occurrence and appearance of calcification, with special reference to the trigeminal nerve. J. Neurosurg., *27*:336–345, 1967.

Heinrich, A.: Alternsvorgonge in roentgenbild. Leipzig, Georg Thieme, 1941.

Henderson, W. R.: A note on the relationship of the human maxillary nerve to the cavernous sinus and to an emissary sinus passing through the foramen ovale. J. Anat., *100*:905–908, 1966.

Kieffer, S. A., and Gold, L. H. A.: Intracranial physiologic calcifications. Sem. in Roentgenol., *9*:151–162, 1974.

Kim, S. K., and Capp, M. P.: Jugular foramen and early roentgen diagnosis of glomus jugulare tumor. Amer. J. Roentgenol., *97*:597–600, 1966.

Kirdani, M. A.: The normal hypoglossal canal. Amer. J. Roentgenol., *99*:700–704, 1969.

Kitay, J. E., and Altschule, M. D.: The Pineal Gland, Cambridge, Harvard University Press, 1954.

Kollmann, J.: quoted in Newton, T. H., and Potts, D. G.: Radiology of the Skull and Brain. St. Louis, C. V. Mosby Co., 1971, p. 905.

Lilja, B.: On localization of calcified pineal bodies under normal and pathologic conditions. Acta Radiol., *15*:659–667, 1934.

Lindblom, K.: A roentgenographic study of the vascular channels of the skull. Acta Radiol. (Suppl. 30), 1936.

Love, J. G., Camp, J. D., and Eaton, L. M.: Symmetrical cerebral calcification particularly of basal ganglia, demonstrable roentgenologically, associated with cyst of cavum septi pellucidi and cavum vergae. Proc. Staff Meet. Mayo Clin., *13*:225, 1938.

Moreau, M. H.: Radiological localization of the pineal gland. Acta Radiol., *5*:65–67, 1966.

Murase, Y., Tanaka, S., Futamura, A., Ito, T., Imamura, K., and Sakata, K.: A new single measurement of pineal calcification in the lateral craniogram. Amer. J. Roentgenol., *110*:92–95, 1970.

Nellhaus, G.: Head circumference from birth to 18 years: practical composite international and inter-racial graphs. Pediatrics, *41*:106–114, 1968.

Nellhaus, G.: Head circumference in children with idiopathic hypopituitarism. Pediatrics, *42*:210–211, 1968.

Newton, T. H., and Potts, D. G. (eds.): Radiology of the Skull and Brain, Vol. 1. St. Louis, C. V. Mosby Co., 1971.

Oon, C. L.: New method of pineal localization. Amer. J. Roentgenol., *92*:1242–1248, 1964.

Orley, A.: Neuroradiology. Springfield, Ill., Charles C Thomas, 1949.

Pappas, G. C., and Wallace, W. R.: Panoramic sialography. Dental Radiography and Photography, *43*:27–33, 1970.

Pawl, R. P., and Walter, A. K.: Localization of the calcified pineal body on lateral roentgenograms. Amer. J. Roentgenol., *105*:287–290, 1965.

Pendergrass, E. P., Schaeffer, J. P., and Hodes, P. J.: The Head and Neck in Roentgen Diagnosis. Second edition. Springfield, Ill., Charles C Thomas, 1956.

Pernkopf, E.: Atlas of Topographical and Applied Human Anatomy, Vol. 1. Philadelphia, W. B. Saunders Co., 1963.

Phillips, J. E.: Principles and function of the orthopantomograph. Oral Surg., *24*:41–49, 1967.

Potter, G. D.: Sectional Anatomy and Tomography of the Head: An Atlas of Sectional Anatomy of the Head. New York, Grune & Stratton, 1971.

Pryor, H. B., and Thelander, H.: Abnormally small head size and intellect in children. J. Pediat., *73*:593–598, 1968.

Schaefer, R. E.: Roentgen anatomy of the temporal bone. Med. Radiography and Photography, *48*:1, 1972.

Shapiro, R., and Robinson, F.: The foramina of the middle fossa: a phylogenetic, anatomic and pathologic study. Amer. J. Roentgenol., *101*:779–794, 1967.

Schechter, M. M., and Zingesser, L. H.: The radiology of aqueductal stenosis. Radiology, *88*:905–916, 1967.

Schüller, A.: Die roentgenographische Darstellung Einiger Nervenkanale des Schadelbasis. Fortschr. Roentgenstr., *57*:640–641, 1938.

Schüller, A.: Roentgen-Diagnostik der Erkrankungen Des Kopfes. Wien, Holder, 1912.

Schultz, A. H.: quoted in Newton, T. H., and Potts, D. G.: Radiology of the Skull and Brain. St. Louis, C. V. Mosby Co., 1971.

Schunk, H., and Maruyama, Y.: Two vascular grooves of the external table of the skull which simulate fractures. Acta Radiol., *54*:186–194, 1960.

Schwartz, C. W., and Collins, L. C.: The Skull and Brain Roentgenologically Considered. Springfield, Ill., Charles C Thomas, 1951.

Soila, P., and Paatero, Y. V.: Clinical pantomography of the jaws. Radiology, *66*:818–823, 1956.

Sondheimer, F. K.: Basal foramina and canals. *In* Newton, T. H., and Potts, D. G.: Radiology of the Skull and Brain. St. Louis, C. V. Mosby Co., 1971.

Stafne, C. S.: Oral Roentgenographic Diagnosis. Philadelphia, W. B. Saunders Co., 1958.

Stauffer, H., Snow, L., and Adams, A.: Roentgenographic recognition of habenular calcification as distinct from calcification in the pineal body: its applications in cerebral localization. Amer. J. Roentgenol., *70*:83–92, 1953.

Steinbach, H., and Obota, W.: The sign of thinning of the parietal bones. Amer. J. Roentgenol., *78*:39–45, 1957.

Strickler, J. M.: New and simple techniques for demonstration of the jugular foramen. Amer. J. Roentgenol., *97*:601–606, 1966.

Swischuk, L. E.: Radiol. Clin. N. Amer., *10*:277–290, 1972.

Taveras, J. M., and Wood, E. H.: Diagnostic Neuroradiology. Baltimore, Williams and Wilkins Co., 1964.

Tebo, H. G.: The pterygospinous bar in panoramic roentgenography. Oral Surg., *26*:654–657, 1968.

Todd, T. W., and Lyon, D. W.: quoted in Newton, T. H., and Potts, D. G.: Radiology of the Skull and Brain. St. Louis, C. V. Mosby Co., 1971.

Updegrave, W. H.: Panoramic dental radiography. Dental Radiography and Photography, *36*:75–83, 1963.

Vastine, J. H., and Kinney, K. K.: Pineal shadow as aid in localization of brain tumors. Amer. J. Roentgenol., *17*:320–323, 1927.

Watson, E. H., and Lowrey, G. A.: Growth and Development of Children. Fifth edition. Chicago, Year Book Medical Publishers, 1967.

7

Detailed Consideration of Certain Areas of the Skull

There are certain regions of the skull which require special radiographic techniques for demonstration of anatomic detail, in addition to the usual routine examination obtained for a survey of the calvarium or face.

These may be subdivided into the following: (1) the nose and nasal cavities, (2) the paranasal sinuses (which are intimately related to the nasal cavities), (3) the mouth and hard palate (see Chapter 13), (4) the orbits, (5) the temporal bone, its contents, subdivisions and development, and (6) the sella turcica.

THE NOSE

There are two anatomic divisions of the nose: (1) the external skeleton and (2) the nasal cavity.

External Skeleton of the Nose (Fig. 7–1). The lower part of the framework of the nose is formed by cartilages. These cartilages are not individually identifiable radiographically, although with soft tissue technique they can be readily demonstrated. Cartilage also forms part of the anterior portion of the nasal septum, and here too the radiographic examination is not of much value.

The rest of the framework of the nose, however, is osseous, and as such can be demonstrated with considerable accuracy radiographically. The two nasal bones meet in the midline to form the dorsum and the bridge of the nose, and together they form the upper portion of the pyriform aperture. Laterally, this aperture is bounded by the maxillae, which are continued inferiorly and anteriorly to form the nasal spine. The nasal bones articulate superiorly with the frontal bone, laterally with the frontal processes of the maxillae, and internally with the nasal septum (perpendicular plate of the ethmoid). Occasionally, because of extra centers of ossification, vertical or transverse sutures are found that must not be misinterpreted as fractures. The deep surface of each nasal bone is largely covered by mucoperiosteum and is grooved for the anterior ethmoidal nerve (external

nasal branch of the nasociliary nerve). There is also a vascular foramen in the nasal bones that may lead to confusion.

Injuries to the nose are frequently accompanied by injuries to adjoining structures, particularly the nasal septum and lacrimal bones. In the routine examination of this region one should be cognizant of these close relationships.

Since the nasal bones are projected over one another, and since the usual skull exposure overpenetrates the nasal bones, special views to demonstrate the nose are employed, as will be described below.

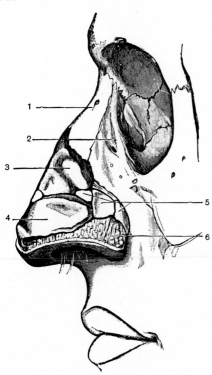

Figure 7–1. Diagram illustrating bones and cartilages of external nose. (1) Nasal bone, (2) frontal process of maxilla, (3) lateral cartilage, (4) greater alar cartilage, (5) lesser alar cartilage, (6) fatty tissue of ala nasi. (From West, C. M., in Cunningham's Textbook of Anatomy, 6th ed. London, Oxford University Press, 1931.)

288

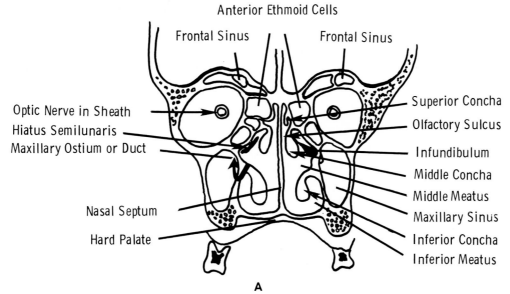

Figure 7–2. A. Coronal section of head showing paranasal sinuses.

Nasal Cavity (Fig. 7–2).   The nasal cavity extends from the nares in front to the choanae behind. It is divided into two halves or nasal fossae by the nasal septum and its base is formed by the roof of the mouth, consisting of the palatine processes of the maxilla anteriorly and the horizontal processes of the palate bone posteriorly. The nasal septum is formed by cartilage anteriorly and by the perpendicular plates of the ethmoid and vomer posteriorly. The lateral wall of each nasal fossa is subdivided into three or four regions called meatuses by the corresponding nasal conchae or turbinate bones. The superior and middle conchae are part of

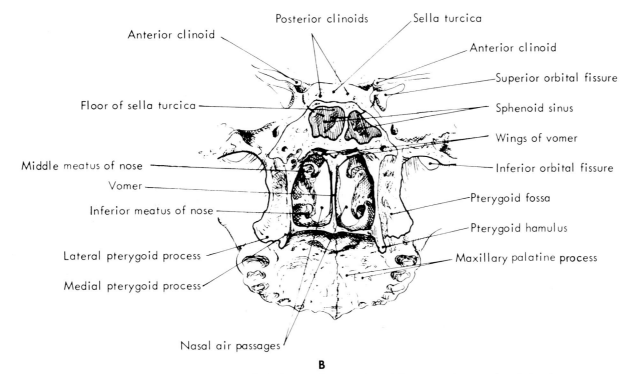

Figure 7–2 *Continued.*   B. Coronal section through nasopharynx, viewed from posterior aspect and showing osseous posterior nasal apertures.

the ethmoid bone, whereas the inferior concha is a separate bone. The superior, middle, and inferior meatuses are those regions which lie under their respective conchae. A fourth and very small meatus may lie above the superior meatus (sphenoethmoidal recess). The following openings are found in the nasal cavity (Fig. 7–3): (1) opening into the *inferior meatus* is the nasolacrimal duct; (2) the *middle meatus* contains openings from the middle ethmoidal air cells, the maxillary sinus, the anterior ethmoidal cells, and the frontal sinus; (3) the *superior meatus* contains the orifice which communicates with the posterior ethmoidal cells; and (4) the sphenoid cells open into the *sphenoethmoidal recess.*

The nasolacrimal passageways are occasionally investigated radiographically.

ROUTINE RADIOGRAPHIC STUDY OF THE NOSE

Much of the nose is cartilaginous; although this can be moderately well visualized using soft tissue technique, most of the radiologist's study in this regard centers on the nasal bones, nasal cavity, and bony nasal septum.

1. **Both Lateral Views of the Nasal Bones** (Fig. 7–4). A small film is placed as close to the side of the nose as possible, perpendicular to the central ray. Soft tissue technique is employed. The anterior nasal spine is also usually included. The various sutures, vascular foramen, and groove for the anterior ethmoidal nerve are carefully differentiated from any anatomic abnormality.

2. **Tangential Superoinferior View of the Nasal Bones** (Fig. 7–5). A film is placed in the mouth between the teeth, and the central ray is directed tangentially to the nasal bones and perpendicular to the film from a superior vantage point. This permits a superoinferior perspective of these bones, provided the glabella does not protrude too far forward.

3. **Posteroanterior View of the Nose with a 15 Degree Tilt of the Tube Caudally (Caldwell's Projection)** (Fig. 7–11). This technique is identical to that employed in paranasal sinus survey, and in this instance is employed to show the bony nasal septum to best advantage. It also demonstrates the nasal cavity moderately well.

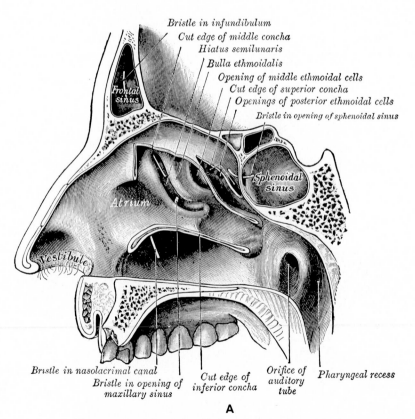

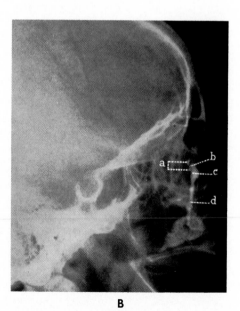

A   **B**

Figure 7–3. A. Lateral wall of nasal cavity demonstrating apertures leading into it. (From Gray's Anatomy of the Human Body, 29th edition, Goss, C. M. (ed.) Philadelphia, Lea & Febiger, 1973.) B. Lateral view of nasolacrimal system. (*a*) Lacrimal puncta, (*b*) canaliculi, (*c*) lacrimal sac, (*d*) lacrimal duct. Contrast medium: 1 to 2 cc. warmed Sinugrafin. (From Pendergrass, E. P. et al.: The Head and Neck in Roentgen Diagnosis, 2nd ed., 1956. Courtesy of Charles C Thomas, publisher, Springfield, Illinois.)

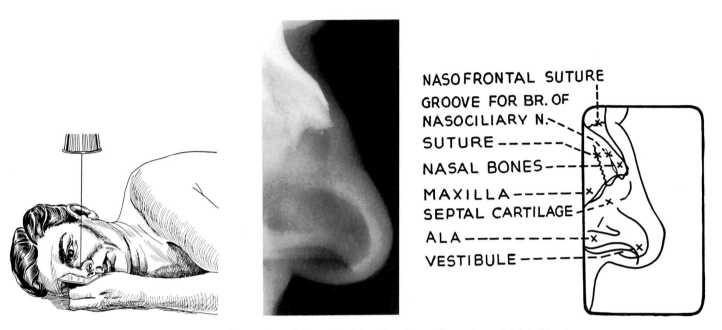

Figure 7–4. Lateral view of nasal bones. Position of patient, radiography and labeled tracing.

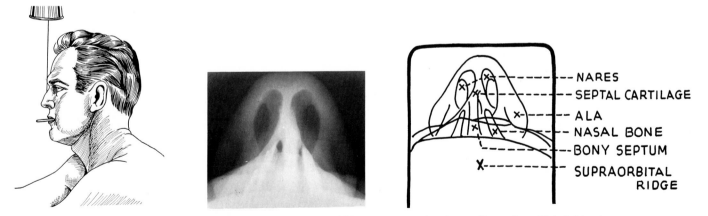

Figure 7–5. Tangential supero-inferior view of nasal bones. Position of patient, radiograph, and labeled tracing.

THE PARANASAL SINUSES

The radiographic anatomy of the paranasal sinuses is particularly complex because of two factors: (1) the sinuses are projected over one another to a great extent and anatomic detail is thus obscured, and (2) there is a great range of normal variants of the sinuses among different individuals in various age groups, as well as in the same age groups.

The paranasal sinuses have already been identified as paired cavities in the frontal, maxillary, ethmoid, and sphenoid bones. They communicate with the nasal cavity and are lined by mucous membrane continuous with that of the nose. In the adult sinuses there are numerous complete and incomplete membranous and bony septa, some of which communicate independently with the nasal cavity.

The frontal sinus communicates with the middle meatus anteriorly through an orifice in the inferior portion of the sinus; the posterior ethmoid cells open into the superior meatus of the nose; the sphenoid sinuses communicate with the nose by means of an orifice in the sphenoethmoidal recess; the maxillary sinuses and the nasal cavity are continuous through an opening which lies in the middle meatus; this orifice is situated high in the wall of the antrum so that emptying of the antrum cannot occur in the erect position except by overflow, or unless the head is inverted. These details are of considerable clinical importance. It has already been indicated that the orifice of the nasolacrimal duct is situated in the inferior meatus.

Maxillary Sinuses (Fig. 7–6 *A*).   The maxillary sinuses are the largest of the sinuses at birth, and each unaerated sinus containing myxomatous tissue measures approximately $8 \times 4 \times 6$ mm. at birth (Pendergrass, Schaeffer, and Hodes). Prior to the fifth year the entire sinus is medial to the intraorbital foramen.

Since pneumatization of the *alveolar process* ordinarily *does not begin before 6 years of age*, and usually is not evident until the 10th or 11th year, the relationship of the teeth to the floor of the maxillary sinuses is not so important in children as in adults. In the adult, usually the roots of the molars and second premolar are embedded just outside the floor of the maxillary antrum, and are important in that any inflammatory process of these teeth may transmit inflammation to the closely adjoining antrum and sinus. When, however, the sinus is small, only the second and third molars may be in close relationship with the maxillary sinuses.

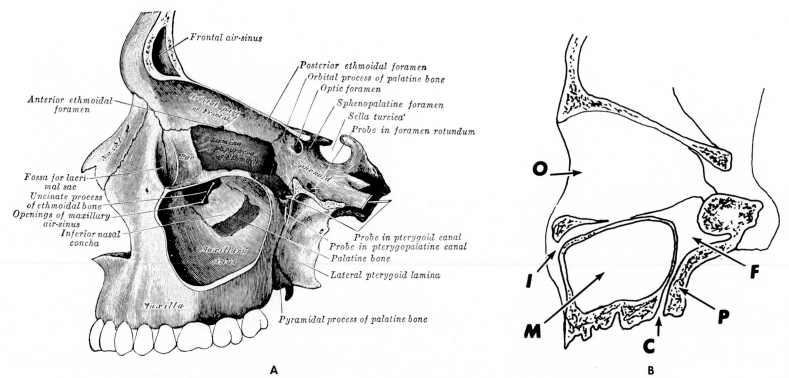

Figure 7–6.   A. Left maxillary sinus opened from lateral side. (From Gray's Anatomy of the Human Body, 29th edition, Goss, C. M. (ed.) Philadelphia, Lea & Febiger, 1973.) B. Diagram of pterygopalatine fossa and canal. (O) orbit, (I) infraorbital canal, (M) maxillary sinus, (C) pterygopalatine canal, (P) pterygoid process, (F) pterygopalatine fossa.

Figure 7–6 continued on the opposite page.

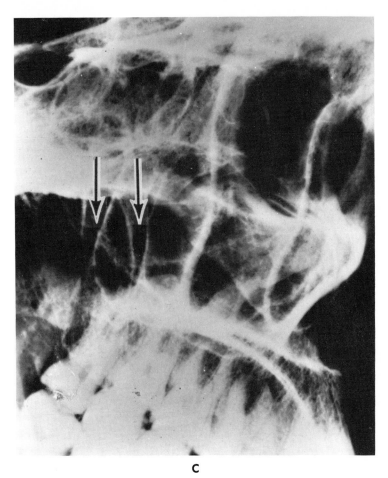

C

Figure 7–6 *Continued.* *C.* Lateral skull roentgenogram rotated 10 degrees away from the true lateral. (*B* and *C* from Potter, G. D.: Amer. J. Roentgenol., *107*:520, 1969.) See text.

The maxillary ostium communicates with the deep aspect of the posterior half of the ethmoidal infundibulum. Since it is located at the highest point in the maxillary antrum, drainage from the maxillary sinus is difficult, except in about one-third of cases where an additional aperture, the accessory maxillary ostium, communicates directly with the middle nasal meatus.

The measurements of the adult maxillary sinus, according to Schaeffer, are as follows: posterosuperior diagonals, 38 mm.; anterosuperior diagonals, 38.5 mm.; superoinferior, 33 mm.; anteroposterior, 34 mm.; medial lateral, 23 mm.

In the frontal projection on the radiograph, the maxillary sinus is rather triangular in outline, with the apex situated medially between the orbit and the nasal aperture. The shape is very variable, and there are numerous irregular septa which are projected over the sinus. Most of these represent folds or incomplete partitions, but not infrequently there are complete divisions of the antra into separate chambers. The base of the maxillary

sinus is formed by the alveolar process and this margin is constant compared with the variability of the antrum as a whole.

The mucoperiosteal lining of the cavity of the sinus is sufficiently dense in outline to be seen and is arbitrarily regarded as normal when it is not over 1 mm. in thickness. Normally no fluid is visible in the sinus in the erect position. The mucous membrane is particularly well demonstrated after the injection of iodized oil (Fig. 7–14) into the maxillary antrum, and any thickened areas are more accurately demonstrated in this manner than in conventional radiographs.

The *pterygopalatine fossa and canal* may be identified on the posterior aspect of the maxillary antrum in the lateral skull roentgenogram. As shown in Figure 7–6 *B*, the pterygopalatine fossa and canal form an inverted triangular radiolucency in this projection. The fossa and canal are approximately 3 cm. in length, bounded superiorly by the body of the sphenoid, anteriorly by the posterior wall of the maxillary antrum, and posteriorly by the pterygoid process of the sphenoid bone. At this point where the pterygopalatine fossa becomes narrower inferiorly, the pterygopalatine canal is formed.

In the true lateral skull or face roentgenogram there is a superimposition of the two canals and hence, for best demonstration of each canal separately, the head is rotated 10 degrees away from the true lateral so that the two triangular radiolucencies can be visualized separately (Fig. 7–6 C).

A study of the configuration of this region is of some significance, particularly in long-standing mass lesions involving the nasopharynx where a *bowing* of the pterygopalatine fossa and canal occurs (Potter).

The projections most valuable for demonstration of the maxillary antra are: (1) Water's projection (Fig. 7–12), with the mouth open or closed, (2) a similar projection obtained in the erect position (Fig. 7–12 C) for demonstration of any fluid levels, and (3) the axial (Figs. 6–46, 6–48) or verticosubmental view, which gives a superoinferior perspective of the antra.

In the Water's projection, the shadows of the upper lips are projected over the antra and may lead to confusion unless their presence is recognized.

Ethmoid Sinuses. The ethmoid sinuses or cells form the medial wall of each orbit on the one hand, and the lateral wall of the upper one-half of the nose on the other. The cells may vary in number and size—there may be 18 or more small ones or a few large cavities.

The ethmoid sinuses are subdivided into three primary groups: (1) anterior, (2) middle, and (3) posterior. The anterior and middle groups communicate with the middle nasal meatus; the posterior group communicates with the superior and supreme nasal meatuses. The anterior ethmoid sinuses are in turn divided into two secondary groups: a frontal anterior group, opening into the frontal recess of the middle nasal meatus, and an infundibular anterior group, opening into the ethmoid infundibulum of the middle nasal meatus.

The middle ethmoid cells drain into the middle nasal meatus opening on the convex surface of the ethmoid bulla or into a prominent suprabullar furrow (Fig. 7–7).

The openings of the posterior ethmoid cells are located superior to the attachment of the middle nasal concha, and the cells communicate with either the superior or supreme nasal meatuses.

In the newborn infant the anterior ethmoid cells measure, on the average, 5 × 2 × 2 mm., and the posterior group measures 5 × 4 × 2 mm. In the adult, the average measurements of the anterior group are 20.6 mm. in height, 22.6 mm. in length, and 11 mm. in width. The corresponding diameters of the superior group are 20.8 mm., 20.5 mm., and 12 mm. respectively (Anson, 1966).

There is a tendency for the ethmoid cells to grow into and encroach upon the surrounding bony structures such as the frontal bone, the maxillary bones, the sphenoid and the ethmoid conchae. In the great majority of cases the frontal sinus is devel-

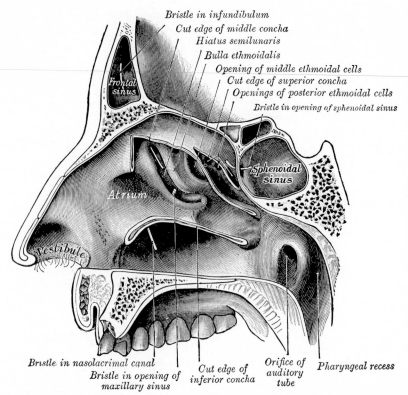

Bristle in infundibulum
Cut edge of middle concha
Hiatus semilunaris
Bulla ethmoidalis
Opening of middle ethmoidal cells
Cut edge of superior concha
Openings of posterior ethmoidal cells
Bristle in opening of sphenoidal sinus

Frontal sinus

Sphenoidal sinus

Atrium

Vestibule

Bristle in nasolacrimal canal
Bristle in opening of maxillary sinus
Cut edge of inferior concha
Orifice of auditory tube
Pharyngeal recess

Figure 7–7. Lateral wall of nasal cavity showing apertures leading into it. (From Gray's Anatomy of the Human Body, 29th ed. Goss, C. M. (ed.) Philadelphia, Lea & Febiger, 1973.)

oped from a frontal anterior ethmoid cell, which gradually grows into the frontal bone.

In infancy, it is extremely difficult to interpret lack of aeration of ethmoid cells on the radiograph, since they are so poorly pneumatized, yet relatively well developed. In the adult, the cells are of variable size and location and overlap one another and the sphenoid sinuses, so that again they are difficult to see clearly.

In the posteroanterior view, the cells of the upper half of the ethmoid area represent the anterior cavities and those of the lower half represent the posterior cells.

The usual radiographs which demonstrate these cells to best advantage are: (1) Caldwell's position (Fig. 7–11), (2) straight lateral view of the face (Fig. 7–13), (3) the special view of the optic foramina, which is best taken stereoscopically (Fig. 7–20), and (4) the axial or verticosubmental view already described in the case of the base of the skull and the maxillary antra (Figs. 6–46, 6–48).

Frontal Sinuses (Fig. 7–8). The frontal sinuses are situated above the bridge of the nose between the inner and outer tables of the frontal bone. They vary greatly in size, but tend to be pyriform in shape. There is usually one sinus on each side, and they are usually asymmetrical (Fig. 7–9). Not infrequently, they extend into the orbital plate of the frontal bone, and fractures of this plate allow free air to escape into the oribital soft tissues, giving rise to an important radiographic sign of this injury. The frontal paranasal sinuses communicate with the middle nasal meatus through a canal called the infundibulum of the frontal sinus, or nasofrontal duct. The nasofrontal duct also communicates with the ethmoid infundibulum, and thence by way of the ostium of the maxillary sinus into the maxillary. Sometimes anterior ethmoid cells may encroach upon the nasofrontal duct, causing it to be constricted, sinuous in its course, and a poor drainage channel. At times, when the sinus itself opens into the frontal recess by a direct single frontal ostium, no duct is present.

The average measurements of the adult frontal sinuses are: height, 27.9 mm.; width, 23.25 mm.; depth, 19.25 mm., with a combined volume of 14 cc. (range 1 to 45 cc.). The frontal sinus by the second year measures approximately $5 \times 3 \times 4$ mm., and by the sixth year $8 \times 4 \times 6$ mm. Embryologically, the frontal sinus is ethmoidal primarily before it is frontal.

Radiographically it may not be possible to identify the frontal sinuses until about 2 years of age. They do not reach the level of the roofs of the orbits until about the eighth year of life. They may be entirely lacking in some people.

Although the frontal sinuses may be demonstrated by any of the sinus views, the most valuable views in this regard are: (1) Caldwell's projection (Fig. 7-11); and (2) straight lateral view of the face (Fig. 7-13).

Sphenoid Sinuses.   The sphenoid sinuses are two cavities situated in the body of the sphenoid bone, frequently extending into the contiguous structures. They are often so closely intermingled with the ethmoid sinuses that they cannot be clearly distinguished. The two cavities are usually asymmetrical and contain incomplete osseous septa, which give the impression of multiple sinuses. The dimensions of the average sphenoid sinus are: height, 22 mm.; width, 18 mm.; length, 12 mm. The capacity ranges from 0.5 to 30 cc., average approximately 7.5 cc. (Anson, 1966).

An aperture, the sphenoid ostium, allows the sphenoid sinus to communicate with the superior nasal fossa. It usually opens into the posterior wall of the sphenoethmoidal recess above the uppermost nasal concha, but occasionally it opens laterally. The sphenoid ostium is, on the average, 14 mm. above the floor of the sphenoid sinus, and thus does not favor good drainage from this sinus. The average sphenoid sinus at term measures 6 to 8 cubic mm. in volume, but by the second year it measures $4 \times 3.5 \times 2$ mm.; at the fifth year, $7 \times 6.5 \times 4.5$ mm., and by the ninth year, $5 \times 12 \times 10$ mm.

The anatomic relationships of the sphenoid sinuses are of the utmost importance. The sella turcica, which houses the pituitary gland and hypophyseal stalk, is situated above them, and not infrequently pneumatization is present in the dorsum sellae or clinoid processes. The optic chiasma is situated immediately anterior to the hypophyseal stalk. Lateral to the sphenoid air cells are the cavernous venous sinuses, through which course the internal carotid artery and the third, fourth, sixth, and ophthalmic and maxillary branches of the fifth cranial nerve. There may actually be an impression upon the sphenoid sinus by the optic nerve. The petrous apex may be in very close association with the sphenoid sinus, and occasionally directly contiguous with it. The vidian nerve, which supplies sympathetic and parasympathetic fibers to the sphenopalatine ganglion, lies close to the floor of the sphenoid sinus. These various relationships become of particular significance in the event of any pathologic process contained within these sinuses.

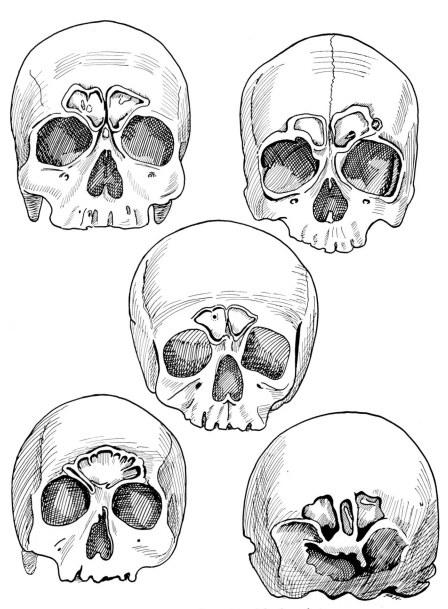

Figure 7-8.   Variations in configuration of the frontal sinuses.

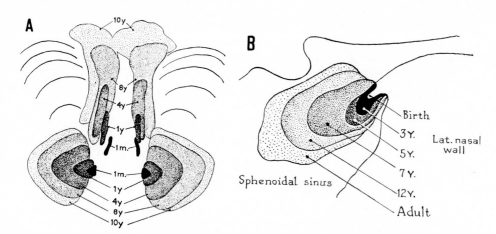

Figure 7-9. Diagrams illustrating growth of frontal and maxillary (*A*) and sphenoid (*B*) sinuses. (From Pediatric X-ray Diagnosis, 6th ed. by Caffey, J. Copyright © 1972 by Year Book Medical Publishers, Inc. Used by permission. Redrawn from Scammon in Abt's Pediatrics.)

The sphenoid sinus does not begin to be pneumatized until the third or fourth year of life, and its gradual growth backward is illustrated in Figure 7–9 *B*.

The radiographic positions that we find most useful for evaluation of the sphenoid sinuses are: (1) Water's position (Fig. 7–12) with the mouth open (both erect and recumbent); (2) lateral view of the face (Fig. 7–13), which projects both sinuses over one another; (3) the axial, or verticosubmental view (Figs. 6–46, 6–48).

Blood Supply of the Nasopharynx (Fig. 7–10). The major arterial supply of the nasal cavity is derived from the *sphenopalatine artery,* a branch of the internal maxillary; the *anterior* and *posterior ethmoidal branches of the ophthalmic portion of the ophthalmic artery;* the *descending palatine artery,* a branch of the internal maxillary; and the *superior labial branch of the external maxillary,* which supplies the nasal vestibule and adjoining parts.

The venous plexuses are drained posteriorly by the sphenopalatine vein to the pterygoid plexus, and also superiorly to the superior ophthalmic vein and anteriorly to join the facial vein.

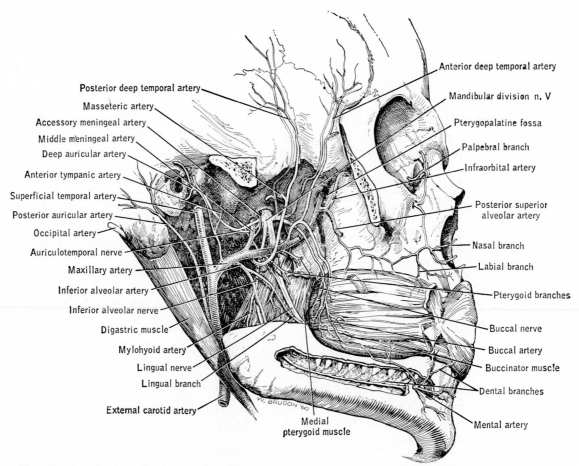

Figure 7-10. Blood supply of nose and middle meningeal artery within the skull (after Spalteholz). (From Anson, B. J. (ed.): Morris' Human Anatomy, 12th ed. Copyright © 1966 by McGraw-Hill, Inc. Used by permission of the McGraw-Hill Book Company.)

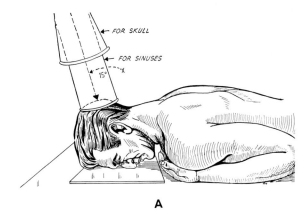

A

ROUTINE PROJECTIONS FOR STUDY OF THE PARANASAL SINUSES

Every effort is made to see the paranasal sinuses as clearly as possible, and certain projections are more valuable for some of the sinuses than for others.

1. **Posteroanterior Nose-Forehead Position with 15 Degree Tilt of the X-ray Tube Caudally (Caldwell's Projection)** (Fig. 7–11). Since we are primarily interested in the paranasal sinuses here, the cone may be placed directly on the head, and it is then unnecessary to utilize the Potter-Bucky diaphragm. This view shows the frontal and ethmoid sinuses to best advantage, while the maxillary sinuses are obscured by the petrous ridges. The sphenoid sinuses are likewise obscured by the ethmoid bones.

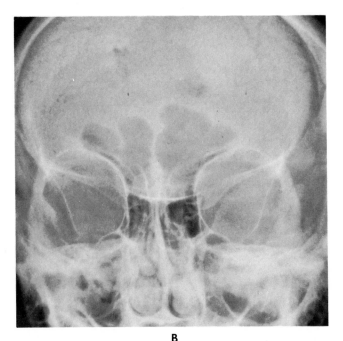

B

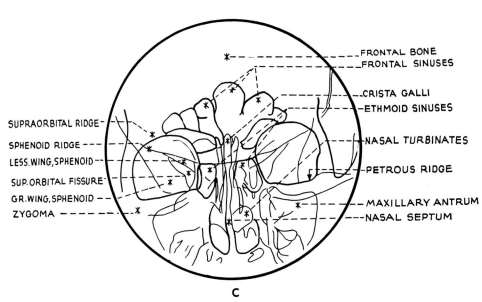

C

Figure 7–11. Caldwell's projection for the paranasal sinuses. *A.* Position of patient. *B.* Radiograph. *C.* Labeled tracing of *B.*

Points of Practical Interest with Reference to Figure 7–11

1. In this view, the petrous ridge is projected along the inferior margin of the orbit. The anatomic structures of major interest here are the frontal sinuses, the ethmoid sinuses, the bony nasal septum, and the orbital contents, not including the optic foramina, however. The superior orbital fissure and the bony structures immediately surrounding it are seen to maximum advantage. These margins must be clearly identified.
2. Although the maxillary antra can be delineated here, they are not seen to good advantage because they are obscured by the projection of the petrous ridges.
3. The degree of aeration of the nasal air passages is also important, and can be evaluated in this projection. The middle and superior nasal turbinates can usually be identified — when they are swollen or hypertrophied, interference with aeration may result.

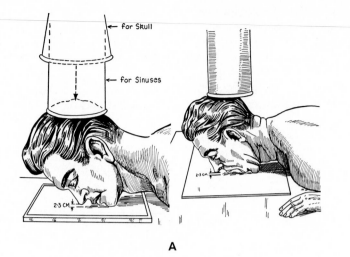

A

2. **Posteroanterior View with the Chin on the Film, and the Nose Raised 2 or 3 cm. from the Film (Water's Projection)** (Fig. 7–12). This view allows the maxillary antra to be clearly seen and projects the petrous ridges beneath them. The frontal and ethmoid sinuses are only moderately visualized. A good view of the sphenoid sinuses is obtained through the open mouth. Also, *it is well to obtain this view in both the recumbent and the erect positions* for demonstration of possible fluid levels within the maxillary antra.

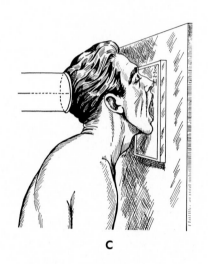

C

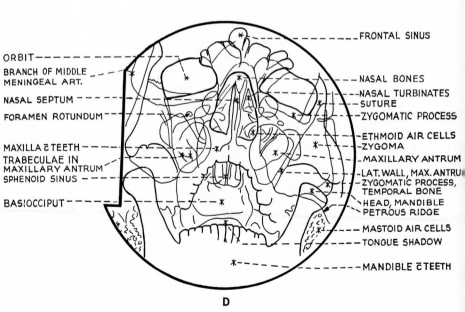

D

ORBIT
BRANCH OF MIDDLE MENINGEAL ART.
NASAL SEPTUM
FORAMEN ROTUNDUM
MAXILLA c̄ TEETH
TRABECULAE IN MAXILLARY ANTRUM
SPHENOID SINUS
BASIOCCIPUT

FRONTAL SINUS
NASAL BONES
NASAL TURBINATES
SUTURE
ZYGOMATIC PROCESS
ETHMOID AIR CELLS
ZYGOMA
MAXILLARY ANTRUM
LAT. WALL, MAX. ANTRUM
ZYGOMATIC PROCESS, TEMPORAL BONE
HEAD, MANDIBLE
PETROUS RIDGE
MASTOID AIR CELLS
TONGUE SHADOW
MANDIBLE c̄ TEETH

B

Figure 7–12. Water's projection for the paranasal sinuses. *A.* Position of patient: *left,* mouth closed; *right,* mouth open. *B.* Radiograph, mouth open. *C.* Position of patient for erect film. *D.* Labeled tracing of *B.*

3. **Lateral Projection of the Paranasal Sinuses** (Fig. 7–13). A straight lateral view of the sinuses shows the sphenoid air cells to best advantage, and also allows another perspective of the frontal sinuses. The maxillary and ethmoid sinuses are not shown clearly in this view because of the considerable bony trabeculae lying in the central ray pathway. Nevertheless some further visualization of these structures is thus obtained.

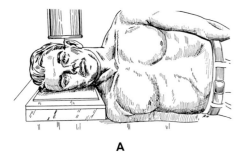

A

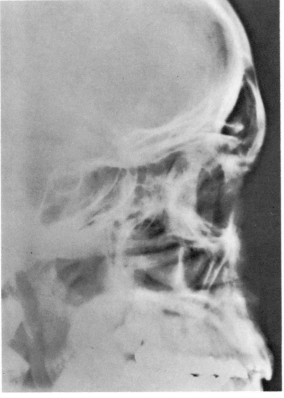

B

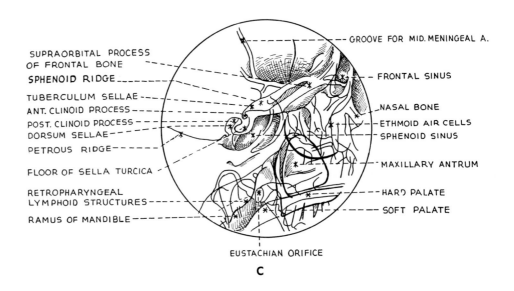

C

GROOVE FOR MID. MENINGEAL A.

SUPRAORBITAL PROCESS OF FRONTAL BONE

SPHENOID RIDGE

TUBERCULUM SELLAE

ANT. CLINOID PROCESS

POST. CLINOID PROCESS

DORSUM SELLAE

PETROUS RIDGE

FLOOR OF SELLA TURCICA

RETROPHARYNGEAL LYMPHOID STRUCTURES

RAMUS OF MANDIBLE

FRONTAL SINUS

NASAL BONE

ETHMOID AIR CELLS

SPHENOID SINUS

MAXILLARY ANTRUM

HARD PALATE

SOFT PALATE

EUSTACHIAN ORIFICE

Figure 7–13. Lateral projection of the paranasal sinuses. *A.* Position of patient. *B.* Radiograph. *C.* Labeled tracing of *B.*

Points of Practical Interest with Reference to Figure 7–13

1. The structures that must be clearly identified in this view are the frontal sinuses, the sphenoid sinuses, the sella turcica, and the retropharyngeal lymphoid structures and adjoining air space.
2. The maxillary antra and ethmoids may have confusing appearances, since so many anatomic structures are projected over one another in these planes. The nasal turbinates especially may simulate the appearance of a tumor within the maxillary antra. The walls of the orbits are considerably obscured, but some effort should be made to delineate these as well as possible.

4. **Use of Iodized Oil in the Maxillary Antra** (Fig. 7–14). Occasionally it is desirable to demonstrate the thickness of the mucous membrane of the antra as accurately as possible. To do so, iodized oil is introduced either through trocar puncture or through the natural ostium into each antrum, and erect and recumbent Water's views are taken, along with oblique views of each antrum. Occasionally a 24 hour study is obtained to test the ciliary function in the removal of this foreign material. The greater part of the iodized oil would be removed in this interval under normal conditions.

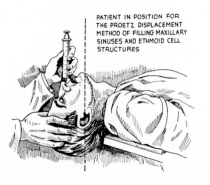

PATIENT IN POSITION FOR THE PROETZ DISPLACEMENT METHOD OF FILLING MAXILLARY SINUSES AND ETHMOID CELL STRUCTURES

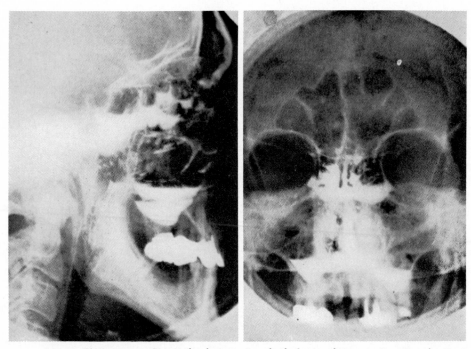

Figure 7–14. Proetz displacement method of sinus diagnosis. Position of patient and radiographs. (From Applicability of Lipiodol in Roentgenography and the Technique of Its Use, E. Fougera & Company, Inc.)

The Proetz technique for the displacement method of sinus diagnosis and treatment is as follows (Proetz):

1. The patient is placed in the supine position, and the head is extended backward so that a line drawn between the chin and the external auditory meatus is perpendicular to the examining table.
2. The iodized oil (such as Dionosil oily) is instilled into the nose through the nostril. Usually 4 to 8 cc. suffices.
3. Negative pressure is applied first to one nostril while the other is closed, and then the other. The pharynx is closed off at the same time by the patient's elevating the soft palate voluntarily.
4. The patient is then placed in the erect position.
5. Posteroanterior and both oblique views are thereafter made of the sinuses in both the erect and recumbent positions. In the recumbent positions, it is usually advisable to obtain these views in both the supine and prone positions.
6. An exposure of the sinuses is made in 72 hours, at which time they should be practically empty under normal conditions.

In this method there is only partial filling of the various sinuses, since the air is never permitted to escape completely; hence if it is desired to demonstrate the structure of an entire sinus, a horizontal x-ray beam must be employed for several views while rotating the patient in various positions.

For best filling and visualization of the maxillary antra, it is probably best to inject the sinuses directly rather than by this indirect means.

Proetz places considerable emphasis on the emptying time of the sinuses in this method of examination also, in that a delay in emptying beyond 72 hours implies impaired ciliary function and probable inflammation.

THE ORBIT

The orbit is shaped like a four-sided pyramid with its base directly toward the face and its apex directed backward and medially. It contains the eyeball and its associated muscles, vessels, and nerves and other structures (Fig. 7–15).

The apex of the orbit corresponds with the optic foramen, which transmits the optic nerve and ophthalmic artery.

The bones entering into the formation of the orbit are as follows:

The roof is formed by the orbital plate of the frontal bone and posteriorly by the lesser wing of the sphenoid. At the lateral angle the fossa for the lacrimal gland is situated.

The floor is formed by the orbital processes of the maxilla, zygomatic and palatine bones. The nasolacrimal canal lies at its medial angle, containing the nasolacrimal duct. There is a groove on its surface which terminates anteriorly in the infraorbital canal through which the infraorbital artery and maxillary nerve emerge on to the face.

The lateral wall is formed by the great wing of the sphenoid and the zygomatic bone. Between the greater and lesser wings of the sphenoid at the posterior portion of this wall is the superior orbital or sphenoidal fissure connecting the orbit and the cranium. The inferior orbital fissure lies between the lateral wall and the floor (Fig. 7–16).

The medial wall is formed by the frontal process of the maxilla, the lacrimal bone, the lamina papyracea of the ethmoid and the body of the sphenoid. Anteriorly lies a hollow which contains the lacrimal sac; posteriorly, at the junction of the medial wall with the roof, lie the anterior and posterior ethmoidal canals. The measurement of interorbital distance for boys and girls is shown in Figure 7–16 *B–E,* and the method of measurement of this distance is illustrated. This measurement is utilized in evaluation of hypertelorism—increased distance between the orbits—and hypotelorism—diminished distance between the orbits.

(Incidentally, Hansman, who is responsible for the graph of interorbital distance, is also to be credited with measurement of the skull thickness on a lateral roentgenogram in the region of lambda.)

Throughout the period from infancy to adulthood the interorbital distance for girls is narrower than it is for boys. Starting at approximately 18 months of age there is a gradual increase in the size of this measurement for both sexes. At about 13 years of age the measurement for girls begins to level off, but the boys' measurement continues to increase until the age of approximately 21 years.

The base of the pyramid, which is seen as the facial boundary, is quadrilateral in shape. It is bounded superiorly by the supraorbital margin of the frontal bone, and above this margin the superciliary arch extends medially to the glabella. The zygomatic and maxillary bones form the sharp infraorbital margin; the frontal process of the maxilla and the inferior angular process of the frontal bone form the medial. The zygomatic bone and the zygomatic process of the frontal bone form the lateral margin.

The axis of each orbit is directed forward and in a lateral direction, but the axes of the eyeballs are anteroposterior and parallel. A detailed anatomic study of the lateral walls of the orbit and the maxillary antrum in the submentovertical view is shown in Figure 7–17. The distinguishing characteristics of the orbital line are: (1) its anterior portion is a bony protuberance that represents the sphenozygomatic suture. The great wing of the sphenoid is thickened at this site. (2) It fuses with the temporal line posteriorly.

Anteriorly and laterally the antral line curves smoothly to join the zygoma; this curve is concave laterally. Medially the antral line curves in its posterior aspect to join the posterior antral wall; this portion of the curve is convex laterally. The antral line,

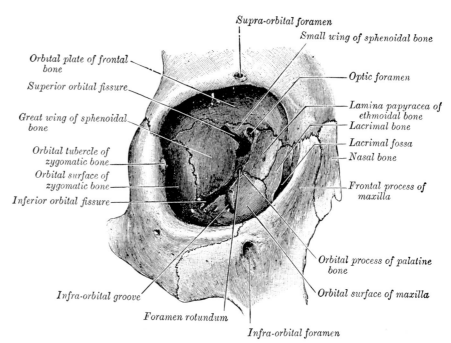

Figure 7–15. The anatomy of the orbit. (From Gray's Anatomy of the Human Body, 24th ed. Lewis, W. H. (ed.) Philadelphia, Lea & Febiger, 1942.)

moreover, has no bony prominence at its anterior extremity and does not join with the temporal line posteriorly (Whalen and Berne).

The sutures seen in the orbit are: the sutures around the lacrimal bone—the lacrimo-ethmoidal, lacrimofrontal, lacrimomaxillary; the sphenofrontal, between the lesser wing of the

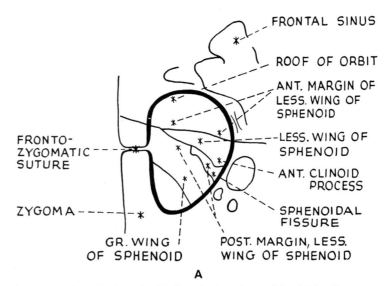

Figure 7–16. A. Tracing of orbital projection obtained by Caldwell's position.

Figure 7–16 continued on the following page.

Age (Months)	Critical Level (cm.)
3	1.45
6	1.47
9	1.49
12	1.50
24	1.57
36	1.63
48	1.70
60	1.76
72	1.83
84	1.90
96	1.97
108	2.01
120	2.10
132	2.16
144	2.23

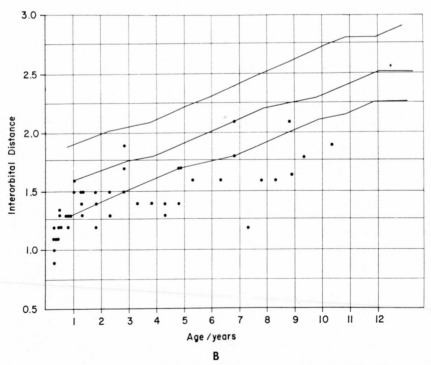

B

Figure 7–16 *Continued.   B. Upper,* Interorbital measurements at various ages, separating patients with mongolism from normal infants and children. These measurements are 78 per cent accurate. *Lower,* Unsmoothed curves of normal interorbital distances (in centimeters) and distribution of measurements in mongols. (From Gerald, B. E., and Silverman, F. N.: Amer. J. Roentgenol., 95:154–161, 1965.)

Figure 7–16 continued on the opposite page.

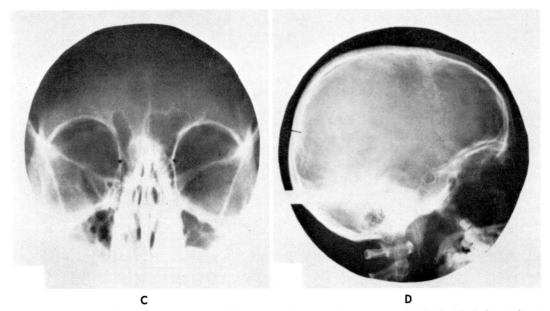

C   **D**

Figure 7–16 *Continued.*   C. Roentgenogram of the paranasal sinuses in a 17 year old girl. The black dots indicate the points at which the interorbital distance is measured. *D.* Lateral roentgenogram of the skull of a boy of 11 years 9 months. The straight line at lambda indicates the measurement of skull thickness. (*C* and *D* from Hansman, C. F.: *Radiology, 86:88,* 1966.)

sphenoid and the frontal bone; the sphenozygomatic, between the greater wing of the sphenoid and the zygomatic; and the maxillo-ethmoidal, between the orbital process of the maxillary bone and the ethmoid.

Superior Orbital Fissure.   This fissure lies between the roof and lateral wall of the orbit and between the lesser and greater wings of the sphenoid bone. It is the largest and most important communication between the middle cranial fossa and the orbit and transmits such structures as the third, fourth, and sixth cranial nerves, the superior ophthalmic vein, and the ophthalmic division of the fifth cranial nerve. A branch of the middle meningeal artery sometimes traverses this aperture, connecting internal and external carotid arteries.

Asymmetry occurs normally between the two orbital fissures in about 9 per cent of specimens (Kornblum and Kennedy). Normally, a sphenoid strut of bone separates the optic canal from the superior orbital fissure. The root of the greater wing of the sphenoid usually separates the inferior aspect of the fissure from the foramen rotundum.

Inferior Orbital Fissure.   This fissure lies between the greater sphenoid wing and the floor of the orbit (maxilla). The following structures pass through this fissure from the orbit to the sphenopalatine and temporal fossa: the inferior ophthalmic vein, the sphenopalatine branches of the internal maxillary artery, and a number of nerves.

Growth, Development, and Measurements.   The orbits attain adult dimensions at the age of about 12 years. Orbital measurements vary considerably but are usually quite symmetrical, and disparities between the two sides of as little as 2 mm. are significant (Potter). The dimensions quoted by Last are: depth of

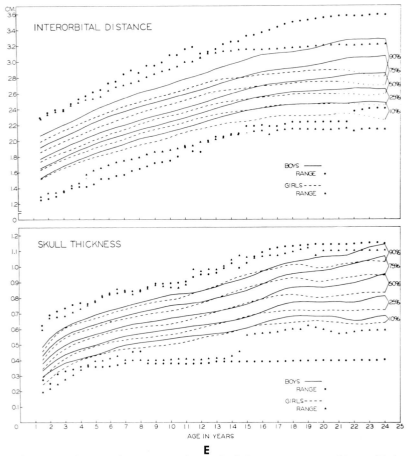

E

Figure 7–16 *Continued.*   *E.* Percentile standards for measurements of interorbital distance (upper graph) and skull thickness (lower graph) for both sexes. The ranges for the two dimensions are indicated. (From Hansman, C. F.: *Radiology, 86:88,* 1966.)

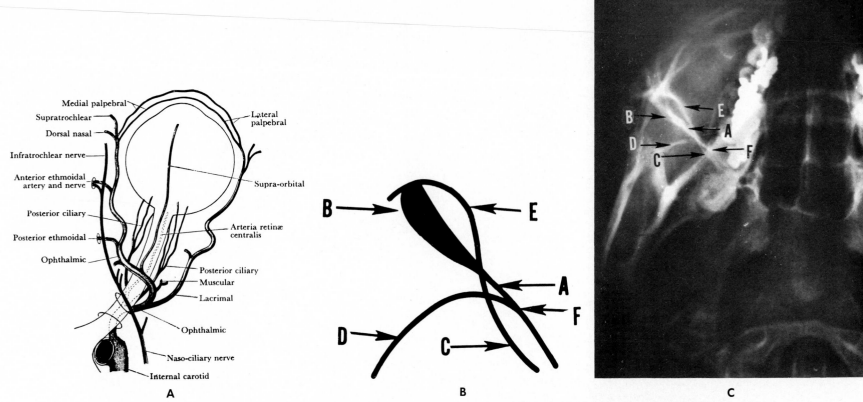

Figure 7–17. *A.* Diagram of the ophthalmic artery and its branches. (From Cunningham's Manual of Practical Anatomy, 12th ed. Vol. 3. London, Oxford University Press, 1959.) *B.* Drawing of the "triple line shadows" as seen in a submentovertical projection. (A) Orbital line, (B) sphenozygomatic suture (protuberance), (C) posterior portion of antral line (convex laterally), (D) temporal line, (E) anterior portion of antral line (concave laterally), and (F) fusion of orbital and temporal lines. *C.* Submentovertical roentgenogram of the right in a normal patient (labels in *B* apply to *C* also). (*B* and *C* from Whalen, J. P., and Berne, A. S.: Amer. J. Roentgenol., 91:1009, 1964.)

Figure 7–17 continued on the opposite page.

orbit, 40 mm.; height of orbital opening, 35 mm.; width of orbital opening, 40 mm.; volume of orbit, 30 cc.

The optic canal, containing the optic nerve, the optic nerve sheath, the ophthalmic artery, and an extension of the subarachnoid space, passes through the sphenoid bone from the middle cranial fossa to the apex of the orbit. The roof of the canal measures 8 to 10 mm., whereas the floor and lateral wall are only 6 to 8 mm. (Potter and Trokel). The optic canals converge posteriorly. The angle of the axis of the canal to the midsagittal plane is ordinarily the same on both sides, although it does, in 16 per cent of adults, vary from one side to the other (Keyes).

The greatest diameter of the adult optic canal may vary from 3 to 6.5 mm. The canals are usually symmetrical, varying less than 1 mm. in 90 per cent of normal adults (Goalwin). In children, the average maximum diameter is 4 mm. in the neonate and 5

mm. at 6 months, enlarging slowly to an average size of 5.5 mm. between 3 and 5 years of age (Evans et al.; Lombardi, 1967).

The optic canal increases from a length of 2 mm. at birth to 4 to 9 mm. at 5 years of age. Some of the asymmetrical appearances of the canal are:

1. A keyhole anomaly that may be unilateral; it is present in about 4 per cent of the general population (Kier, 1966).
2. A figure-of-8 optic canal. In these cases the ophthalmic artery passes between the posterior and the anterior portions, and Kier estimated the incidence of this anomaly to be 1.2 per cent in the general population.
3. A so-called duplicate optic canal.
4. An appearance suggestive of three canals that is produced by the optic canal, paroticoclinoid canal, and the pneumatized anterior clinoid process.

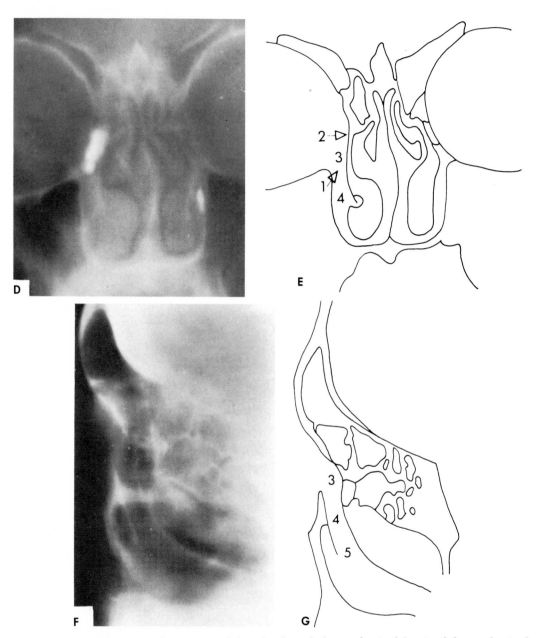

Figure 7–17 *Continued.* F. Coronal tomogram of the orbit through the nasolacrimal fossa and the nasolacrimal canal. There is contrast material in the right nasolacrimal sac. The course of the nasolacrimal canal is vertical. The medial wall of the nasolacrimal fossa produces a medical curvature of the medial wall of the orbit. E. Line drawing of D. 1, Opening of superior end of nasolacrimal canal (dehiscence in floor of orbit); 2, medial wall of nasolacrimal fossa; 3, nasolacrimal fossa, 4, nasolacrimal canal. F. Lateral tomogram of the orbit through the nasolacrimal fossa and the nasolacrimal canal. The course of the nasolacrimal canal is directed posteriorly going from superior to inferior. G. Line drawing of F. 3, nasolacrimal fossa; 4, nasolacrimal canal; 5, inferior opening of nasolacrimal canal in the inferior meatus. (From Potter, G. D.: Radiol. Clin. N. Amer., 10:23, April, 1972.)

Figure 7–17 continued on the following page.

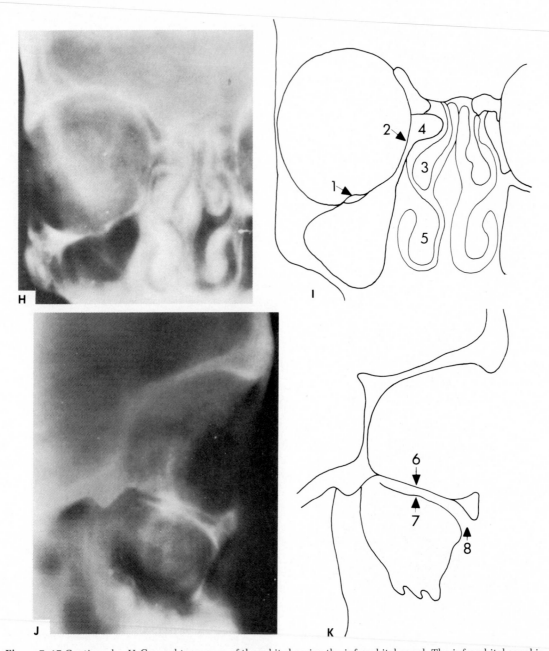

Figure 7–17 *Continued.*   *H.* Coronal tomogram of the orbit showing the infraorbital canal. The infraorbital canal is a faint oval. *I.* Line drawing of *H. 1*, infraorbital canal; *2*, lamina papyracea; *3*, middle turbinate; *4*, ethmoid air cells; *5*, inferior turbinate. *J.* Lateral tomogram of the orbit showing the infraorbital canal. The floor of the infraorbital canal should not be mistaken for a depressed fracture of the floor of the orbit. *K.* Line drawing of *J. 6*, Floor of orbit (roof of infraorbital canal); *7*, floor of infraorbital canal; *8*, infraorbital foramen. (From Potter, G. D.: Radiol. Clin. N. Amer., *10*:23, April, 1972.)

Ophthalmic Arterial and Venous Complex (Wheeler and Baker; Russell and Miller). The main trunk of the ophthalmic artery arises as a branch from the medial aspect of the internal carotid artery at its carotid siphon, at the site where it first exits from the cavernous sinus. The artery courses forward and somewhat upward, accompanying the optic nerve into the optic canal. Artery and nerve separate as they leave the canal, with the artery passing along the medial wall of the orbit and giving off branches to the globe and other orbital structures (Fig. 7–18). It gradually diminishes in size and ends by dividing into the *nasal* and *supratrochlear* (frontal) arteries.

The significant branches of the ophthalmic artery include (1) the *ocular,* and (2) the *orbital,* with other branches as shown in Figure 7–18. The ocular branches supply the central retinal artery and the long and short posterior ciliary arteries to the globe. These are the only arteries of supply to the retina. The largest branch is the *lacrimal,* which accompanies the lacrimal nerve. Additionally, there are supraorbital muscular, posterior ethmoid, nasal, and supratrochlear arteries. An anterior ethmoid artery may also be differentiated. The lacrimal and anterior ethmoid arteries communicate with the recurrent and anterior meningeal arteries (Fig. 7–26).

The major venous drainage of the orbit occurs via the superior ophthalmic vein (Fig. 7–19 *A, B*). This vein originates at the superior medial portion of the orbit at the confluence of the supraorbital frontal and angular veins. Leaving the orbit via the superior orbital fissure, it enters the cavernous sinus. As shown in Figure 7–19, radiologically there are three segments to be considered:

1. The first extends from the inner portion of the orbital roof in the vicinity of the trochlea of the superior oblique muscle to the junction of the anterior and middle thirds of the orbital roof.

2. From there, the second part continues under the superior rectus muscle to produce an outward and backward-facing curve. This second segment at the outer wall of the orbit crosses the underlying optic nerve and the ophthalmic artery.

3. In another change in direction, the vein runs along the outer wall of the orbit, crossing the sphenoid bone to leave the orbit via the inferior portion of the superior orbital fissure. This third segment may be joined by a small, inconstantly visualized inferior ophthalmic vein which arises from the numerous small veins in the inferior anterior portions of the orbit (Russell and Miller; Lombardi and Passerini).

ROUTINE RADIOGRAPHIC STUDY OF THE ORBITS

This study will vary somewhat, depending upon the anatomic relationship one wishes to demonstrate. The consideration for localization of foreign bodies in the eye is out of the scope of this text, and may be obtained from any manual of radiographic technique.

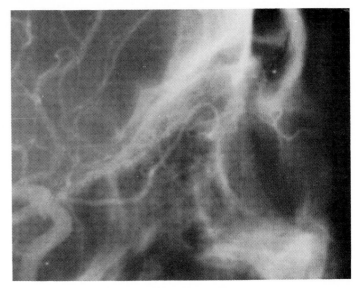

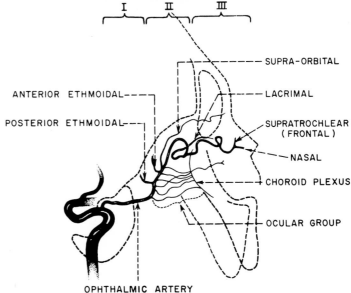

Figure 7–18. Lateral arteriogram and schematic drawing showing normal ophthalmic arterial complex. (Roman numerals indicate division into zones.) (From Wheeler, E. C., and Baker, H. I.: Radiology, *83:*26, 1964.)

1. **Caldwell's Projection.** Ordinarily, Caldwell's projection (Figs. 7–11, 7–16) (posteroanterior view with a caudal 12 to 15 degree tilt of the tube) permits the least interrupted posteroanterior view of the orbit.

2. **Lateral View of Each Orbit Employing a Short Film-target Distance So As to Obscure the More Distant Orbit** (Fig. 7–13). This permits a lateral perspective, although it is not very satisfactory because there is too much interference between the two sides.

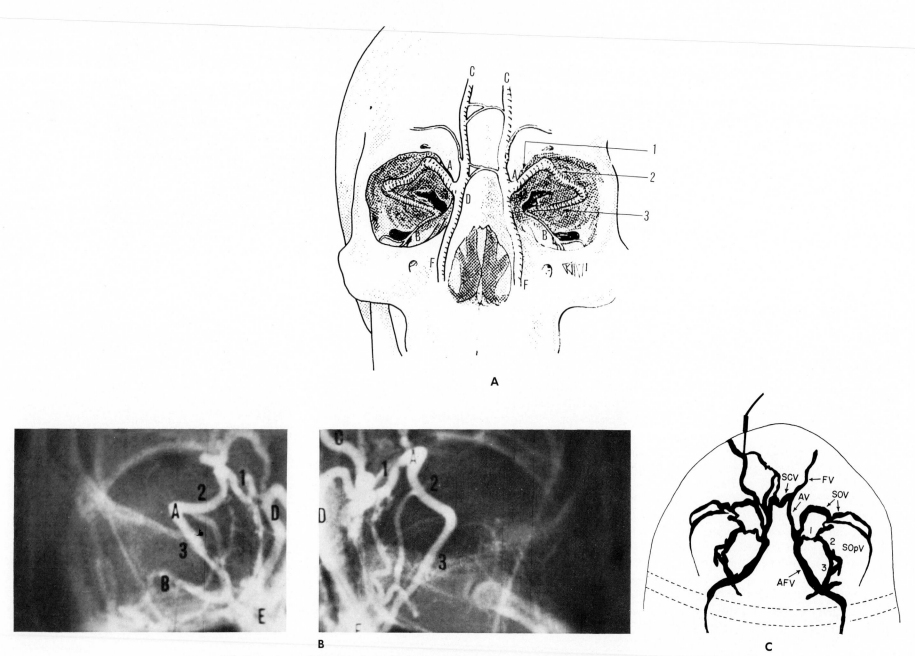

Figure 7–19. *A.* Schematic drawing of normal orbital veins. *B.* Composite of two cases (right and left) taken in the angled anteroposterior direction. Normal studies. (A) Superior ophthalmic veins divided into three portions (*1, 2, 3*), (B) inferior ophthalmic veins (inconstantly visualized), (C) frontal veins, (D) angular veins, (E) cavernous sinus, (F) facial veins. (From Russell, D. B., and Miller, J. D. R.: Radiology, *103:*267, 1972.) *C.* A tracing of the orbital venogram in Water's view. (FV) Frontal vein, (AV) angular vein, (SCV) superficial connecting vein, (SOV) supraorbital vein, (SOpV) superior ophthalmic vein. (AFV) anterior facial vein, (1) first segment, (2) second segment, (3) third segment.

Frontal, angular, superficial connecting, and supraorbital veins in order of decreasing choice of venous puncture. (From Lee, K. F., and Lin, S. R.: Amer. J. Roentgenol., *112:*341, 1971.)

3. **Special View of the Optic Foramen** (Fig. 7–20).   Because of the medial and inferior position of the optic foramen, it is not seen clearly except in the oblique projection demonstrated. An oblique view of the ethmoid air cells is also obtained in the same film study.

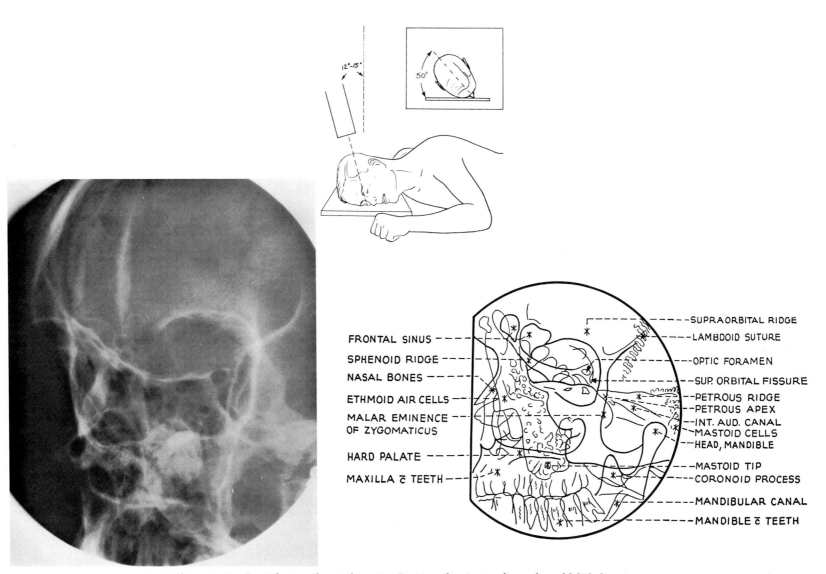

Figure 7–20.   Special view of optic foramina. Position of patient, radiograph, and labeled tracing.

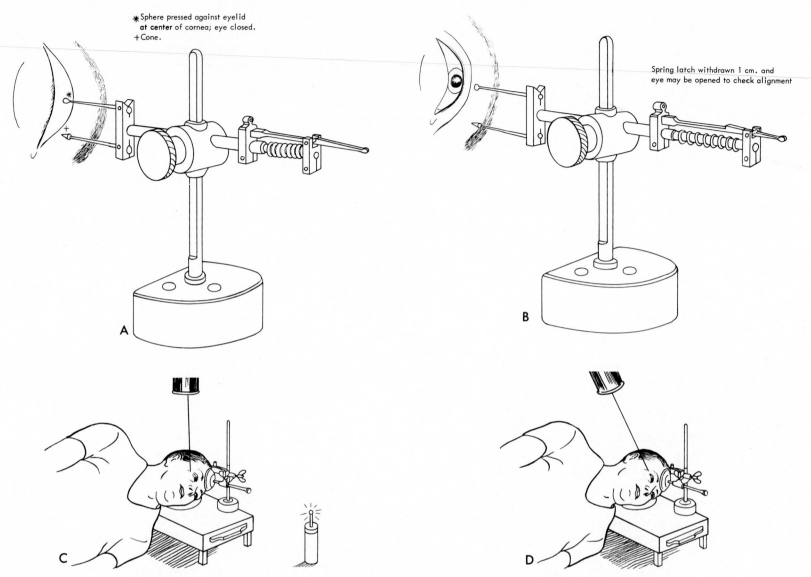

Figure 7–21.   Sweet method for localization of foreign bodies in the eye. The patient's head is placed upon a slide tunnel so constructed that one-half of an 8 by 10 inch cassette is protected while the other half is being exposed. *A.* The indicator ball of the localizer apparatus is adjusted to the center of the eye with the eyelid closed. The cone-shaped metal tip lies directly below the ball. *B.* Upon release of the trigger, both the cone and ball rebound a carefully calibrated distance of 10 millimeters. *C.* The first exposure is made with the central ray of the x-ray beam perpendicular to the plane of the film and parallel to the patient's eyes, passing through both corneas and superimposing the shadows of the indicator ball and cone and their supporting stems. During exposure, the patient is asked to fix his gaze on a small light source or mark on the wall, eyes open, looking straight forward. *D.* For the second exposure the x-ray tube is shifted 4 to 5 inches toward the patient's feet and tilted so that the central ray passes through the ball of the localizer, making an angle of some 10 to 15 degrees with the vertical; the cassette tray is moved to its second position. The films obtained are shown in *E* and *F.*

The method of transferring data from the films to the localizer chart: (1) From straight lateral film #1 the foreign body is indicated in its exact relationship to the superimposed metal ball and cone (F1); (2) a line is drawn horizontally with respect to F1; (3) a line is drawn perpendicularly from F1 to derive point A; (4) a horizontal line is drawn through A across the horizontal plane depiction; (5) from film #2 the perpendicular distance below (or above) the metal cone is measured and plotted (point C); (6) from film #2 the perpendicular distance below (or above) the metal sphere is measured and plotted (point S); (7) line CS is drawn (note here that CS intersects horizontal line #2); (8) a line is drawn perpendicular to intersection of line CS and line #2.

Point F1 indicates position of foreign body behind the center of the cornea and below the horizontal plane. Point F2 indicates the position of the foreign body medial or lateral to the center of the cornea, and thus all three dimensions are noted.

Figure 7–21 continued an the opposite page.

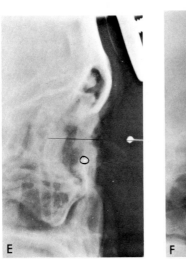

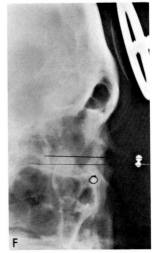

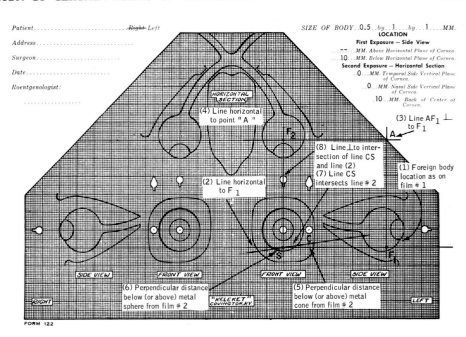

Figure 7-21 Continued. (See opposite page for legend).

4. Demonstration of Foreign Bodies Within the Orbit or Eye

(Figs. 7-21, 7-22). Special techniques are employed. Tangential views of the anterior segment of the eyeball on dental films are very valuable adjuncts in this regard, particularly if obtained with the eye looking upward, downward, to each side, and straight ahead—each on a separate dental-type film. These dental film views are utilized in addition to Sweet localization films, or views of the orbit with a special disk on the anesthetized eye.

5. Orbitography (Fig. 7-23).

Positive contrast orbitography (Hanafee, Hepler, and Coin). The contrast material is prepared as follows: methylglucamine diatrizoate (Renografin 60), 3.3 cc.; distilled water, 5.7 cc.; and 1 per cent Lidocaine, 1 cc. This makes a 20 per cent solution of methylglucamine diatrizoate in a total volume of 10 cc. Injections 3 to 5 mm. in volume are made under local anesthesia through the lower lid at the inferior lateral aspect of the orbit just above the inferior orbital rim, while the patient's gaze is directed upward and nasally. The injection may be made under fluoroscopic control with image amplification to avoid error during injection. Injection of excessive volume of the contrast material can also be avoided. Any localized areas of nonfilling can be confirmed by directing the needle tip to these areas under fluoroscopic control.

When the needle is withdrawn, a compression bandage is applied, and serial roentgenograms are obtained in lateral and Water's projections at intervals of a few minutes. The contrast medium ordinarily disappears slowly after about 15 minutes.

A normal orbitogram with positive contrast media is shown in Figure 7-23. The normal muscle cone has a cloverleaf appearance and notches can be seen along its border. The main impression is the superior rectus muscle. A rounded shadow representing the cross section of the optic nerve is projected into the inferomedial quadrant of the muscle cone.

In the lateral view, the contrast-filled muscle cone appears as a triangular structure whose sides are equidistant from the roof and floor of the orbit. The optic nerve may be seen only rarely in the lateral view but can be identified in the frontal Water's projection.

Negative contrast orbitography (Fig. 7-24). A straight retrobulbar needle is inserted percutaneously into the temporal portion of the upper eyelid toward the center of the muscle cone. Between 15 and 20 ml. of a gaseous contrast agent (either air or oxygen) is injected after ascertaining that no blood vessels have been punctured.

The eyeball, Tenon's capsule, and extraocular muscles divide the orbit into three spaces: (1) an episcleral space, (2) a space inside the muscular cone, and (3) the space peripheral to these. The injected air sometimes enters Tenon's capsule. Tomography is performed after withdrawal of the needle and injection of the air in two planes at right angles.

In the anterior frontal tomogram (Fig. 7-24) the optic nerve is shown in cross section very faintly and a layer of air around the eyeball is well demonstrated.

6. Lacrimal Apparatus and Dacryocystography.

The lacrimal apparatus consists of a lacrimal gland, lacrimal ducts leading to a lacrimal sac, and a nasolacrimal duct that drains into the nose.

The fossa for the lacrimal gland is situated in the roof of the orbit laterally and near its anterior aspect.

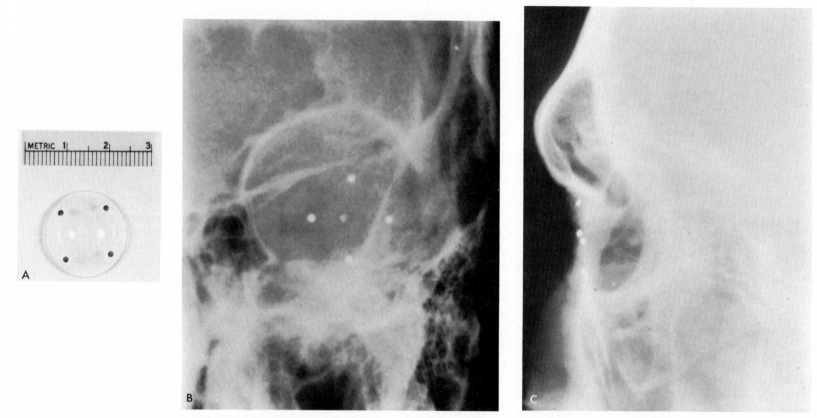

Figure 7–22. Foreign body localization in the eye with the aid of the Thorpe plastic lens. The conjunctiva is anesthetized by the physician, and the lens placed into proper position over the cornea of the eye. Straight posteroanterior and lateral views of the eye are then obtained. *A.* Photograph of the lens. *B.* Posteroanterior radiograph of the eye with the lens in place over the cornea. *C.* Lateral view. The position of the foreign body is noted and measured with respect to the lead markers on the lens. This is a modification of the Pfeiffer-Comberg method. (The plastic lens was obtained from the House of Vision, Inc., Chicago, Illinois—Catalogue No. XP 3611.)

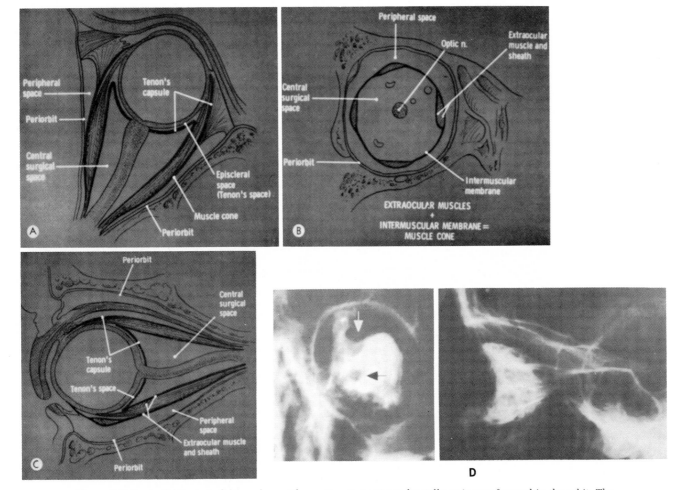

Figure 7–23. *A.* Orbit viewed from above. The optic nerve courses laterally as it goes forward in the orbit. The central surgical space is therefore somewhat conical in shape with its base directed anterior and lateral. Tenon's capsule is shown reflecting off of the muscle cone and enveloping the anterior and posterior margins of the globe. The periosteum covering the bony margin of the orbit forms a thick layer known as the periorbit and is continuous with the dura. *B.* Coronal section of the orbit in the retrobulbar region. The individual muscle bundles are enclosed in a sheath and, in turn, the individual sheaths are united by the intermuscular membrane to form the muscle cone. The cone-shaped enclosed space is called the central surgical space. *C.* Lateral view of the orbit. The central surgical space contains fat, blood vessels, and nerves and surrounds the optic nerve within the orbit. The intermuscular membranes and extraocular muscles surround this central surgical space. The tendons of the extraocular muscles perforate Tenon's capsule anteriorly, thus allowing continuity between the central surgical space and the episcleral space (Tenon's space). Tenon's capsule reflects along the posterior margin of the globe and ends with a very loose attachment at the point of entrance of the optic nerve into the posterior margin of the globe. (From Hanafee, W. N., Hepler, R. S., and Coin, C. G.: Amer. J. Roentgenol., *112*:343, 1971.) *D.* Normal, technically perfect orbitogram. Indentation of superior rectus muscle is indicated by white arrow; optic nerve by black arrow. (From Lombardi, G.: Orbitography. *In* Newton, T. H., and Potts, D. G. (eds.): Radiology of the Skull and Brain. The Skull, Vol. 1, Book 2. St. Louis, The C. V. Mosby Co., 1971.)

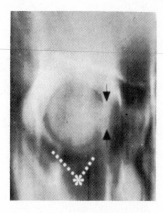

Figure 7-24. Normal orbital pneumotomogram. Frontal view shows layer of air around the eyeball interrupted medially by insertion of the medial rectus muscle (arrows). (From Lombardi, G.: Orbitography. *In* Newton, T. H., and Potts, D. G. (eds.): Radiology of the Skull and Brain. The Skull, Vol. 1, Book 2. St. Louis, The C. V. Mosby Co., 1971; courtesy T. I. Bertelsen, M. D., Bergen, Norway.)

There is a lacrimal lake near the medial angle of the eye, from which small lacrimal passages commence at pores in the upper and lower eyelid and communicate in turn with the lacrimal ducts—small tubes about 10 mm. long paralleling the border of the lacrimal lake. The two ducts pierce the periorbital tissue and unite on a common stem that opens into the lacrimal sac. The latter structure measures about 12 mm. in length and 6 × 3 mm. in diameter, merging below into the nasolacrimal duct. It lies in the anterior medial wall of the orbit known as the *fossa of the lacrimal sac* (Fig. 7–25).

The nasolacrimal duct lies within the bony nasolacrimal canal and communicates with the sac and the nasal cavity. A flap of mucous membrane guards the slitlike opening into the nasal cavity (inferior nasal meatus). The nasolacrimal duct varies in length, averaging about 17 mm., and has a diameter of about 4 mm. There is a slight constriction at its junction with the lacrimal sac. The opening into the inferior meatus of the nose is about

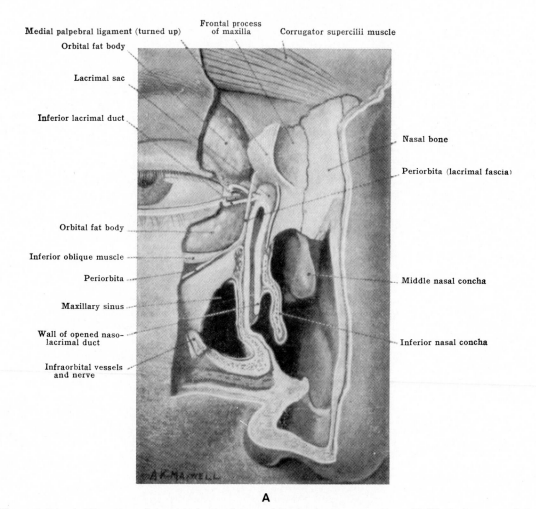

A

Figure 7-25. *A.* Dissection of the right lacrimal sac and its duct system, ×2. (From Wolff, E.: Anatomy of the Eye and Orbit. H. K. Lewis & Co., Ltd.)

Figure 7–25 continued on the opposite page.

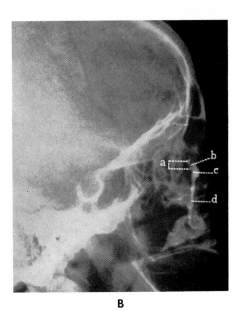

B

35 mm. from the posterior margin of the nostril. The duct contains folds of mucosa in certain locations that have been interpreted as valves although they are inconstant.

7. **Angiography of the Ophthalmic Arterial and Venous Complex** (Figs. 7–26, 7–27). *Arterial complex in angiographic diagnosis.* Opacification of the main portions of the ophthalmic artery usually occurs during normal carotid angiography almost simultaneously with filling of the upper loop of the carotid siphon. The more distal branches may be seen 2 or 3 seconds afterward. At 2 to 5 seconds, the choroid plexus of the eye, supplied mainly by the short posterior ciliary arteries, may be observed as a thin crescent near the anterior third of the orbit. Usually either methylglucamine or sodium diatrizoate (50 per cent) is used as a contrast agent. Direct percutaneous puncture of the internal carotid using 10 to 12 ml. instead of the usual 6 to 8 ml. is most desirable for this additional visualization of the ophthalmic arterial ramifications. Rapid serial exposures are usually necessary, and several exposures in the 2 to 5 second interval are also desirable. The three zones of division of the arterial complex are shown in Figure 7–18.

Orbital venography (Fig. 7–27) usually requires separate injection with approximately 10 ml. of meglumine iothalamate 60

(Text continued on page 319)

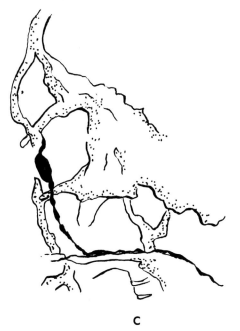

C

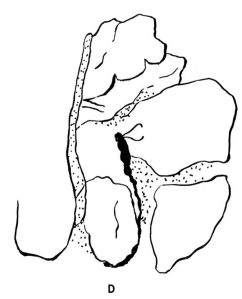

D

Figure 7–25 *Continued.* *B.* Lateral view of nasolacrimal system. (*a*) Lacrimal puncta, (*b*) canaliculi, (*c*) lacrimal sac, (*d*) lacrimal duct. Contrast medium: 1 to 2 cc. warmed Beck's bismuth and oil paste or Sinugrafin. (From Pendergrass, E. P. et al.: The Head and Neck in Roentgen Diagnosis, 2nd ed., 1956. Courtesy of Charles C Thomas, publisher, Springfield, Illinois.) Lateral (*C*) and posteroanterior (*D*) composite drawings from the series of normal roentgenograms. (From Sargent, E. N., and Ebersole, C.: Amer. J. Roentgenol., *102*:831–839, 1968.)

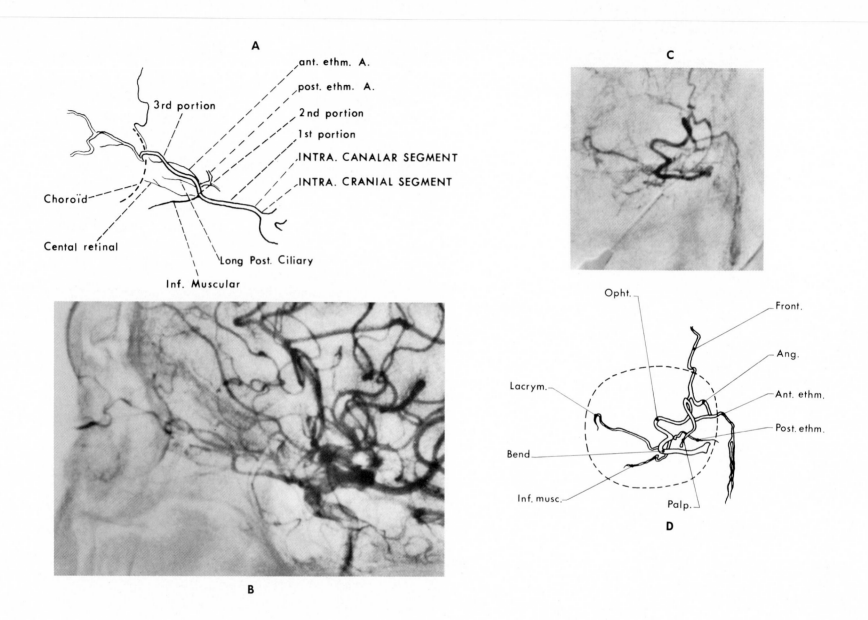

A

ant. ethm. A.

post. ethm. A.

2nd portion

1st portion

INTRA. CANALAR SEGMENT

INTRA. CRANIAL SEGMENT

3rd portion

Choroïd

Cental retinal

Long Post. Ciliary

Inf. Muscular

B

C

D

Opht.

Front.

Ang.

Ant. ethm.

Post. ethm.

Lacrym.

Bend

Inf. musc.

Palp.

Figure 7–26. *A* and *B.* Lateral view of the normal ophthalmic artery. Internal carotid angiography. *C* and *D.* Ophthalmic artery arteriography by catheterization of the exposed angular artery; infra-optic variety; the semi-circle is concave medially. There is good visibility of the ethmoidal arteries. Note the opacification of the mucosa of the medial nasal wall by the anterior ethmoidal artery; and the opacification of the lacrimal artery, the inferior muscular artery, and the medial palpebral artery. No supraorbital artery is demonstrated.

Figure 7–26 continued on the opposite page.

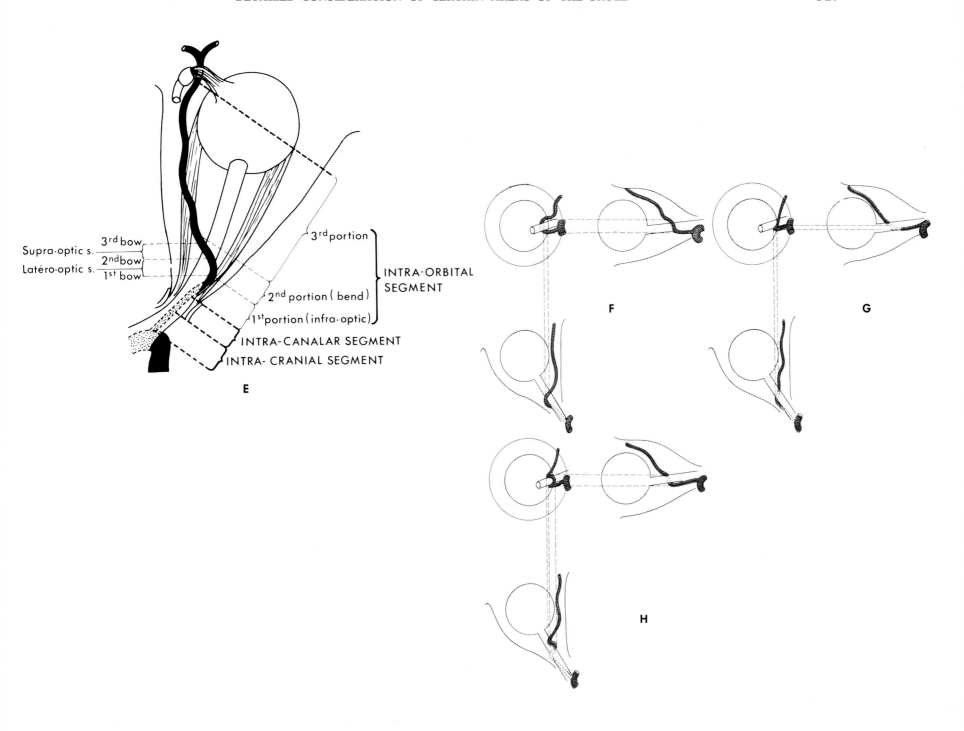

Figure 7–26 *Continued.* *E.* The different segments of the ophthalmic artery. *F, G,* and *H.* Normal variations in configuration of the ophthalmic artery. Frontal, lateral, and axial projections. *F.* Supra-optic variety. *G.* Infra-optic variety, type I. After the infraoptic crossing, the artery remains medial to the optic nerve. *H.* Infra-optic variety, type II. After infra-optic crossing, the artery passes around the medial aspect of the optic nerve, as in *B,* but also makes a hook above the nerve. Notice that only the frontal projection allows recognition of variation in the relation of the artery to the nerve. The semicircle formed around the nerve is concave medially in the infra-optic varieties. (*B* to *H* from Vignard, J., Clay, C., and Aubin, M. L.: Radiol. Clin. N. Amer., *10*(1):39–61, 1972.)

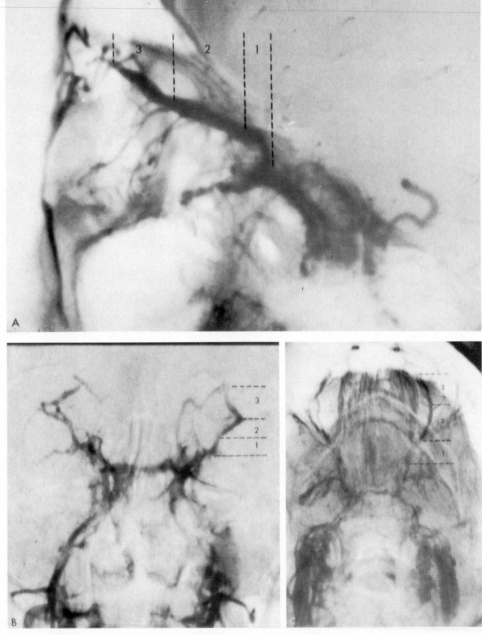

Figure 7–27. Pituitary tumor but normal orbital veins. *A.* Lateral projection; *B.* anteroposterior projection; *C.* exaggerated Water's projection. Normal orbital venogram performed by catheter technique via a frontal vein. Three distinct segments of the superior ophthalmic vein are evident: (1) The posterior segment connecting the superior ophthalmic vein with the cavernous sinus. The superior ophthalmic vein enters the orbit through the superior orbital fissure and enters the muscle cone lateral to the optic nerve. (2) The superior ophthalmic vein lies along the superolateral border of the optic nerve within the muscle cone (central surgical space). (3) The superior ophthalmic vein leaves the muscle cone approximately at the level of the posterior margin of the globe by exiting medial to the levator palpebral superioris to course along the roof of the orbit. It leaves the orbit by passing over the pulley for the superior oblique muscle. (From Hanafee, W. N.: Radiol. Clin. N. Amer., *10*(1):63–81, 1972.)

per cent, with three film series taken at one film per second in anteroposterior, angled anteroposterior, and lateral projections. During the filming in the lateral projection an increase of the intraorbital pressure on the normal side may be obtained by compression of that eye. This allows visualization of an abnormal side without a superimposition. For visualization of the cavernous sinus, an additional film series following a second injection is procured using a basal projection. A total of 30 ml. of contrast agent is usually used. The usual characteristics observed are shown in Figure 7–19A B.

A tracing of the orbital venogram in Water's projection is shown in Figure 7–27.

THE TEMPORAL BONE

The temporal bone is usually divided into three portions: (a) the squamous portion, (b) the tympanic portion, and (c) the petrous portion (Fig. 7–28). These are practical subdivisions in the adult bone, but do not represent separate portions developmentally. Eventually the three parts unite firmly to form a single bone that shows little trace of this complex origin.

The *squamous portion* is largely a bony plate that helps form the calvarium laterally. It also contributes to the mastoid process posterior to the external acoustic meatus.

The *tympanic portion* contributes to the wall of the tympanic cavity and develops in conjunction with the external acoustic meatus; ultimately it constitutes most of the bony wall of this external acoustic passage.

Of the three portions of the temporal bone, the most important is the *petrous portion*, containing the vestibulocochlear organ. Participating in both the lateral wall and the floor of the skull, the petrous element develops originally as an otic capsule. Intracranially, this capsule contains the internal acoustic opening that transmits the facial and vestibulocochlear nerves; on its tympanic surface, it presents the oval and round windows (fenestra vestibuli and fenestra cochleae). The development of the styloid process is closely related to that of the petrous part.

The *mastoid portion* is formed from both the squamous and petrous portions, and this junction is indicated by the petrosquamous suture, which is somewhat variable in appearance and must not be misconstrued as a fracture.

The mastoid process itself is perforated by numerous foramina—the largest being the mastoid foramen, which transmits the mastoid branch of the occipital artery and a vein to the transverse sinus. The sigmoid groove for the transverse sinus is found on the inner aspect of the mastoid process.

The interior of the mastoid process contains numerous air cells opening into a common chamber—the mastoid or tympanic antrum (Fig. 7–29 A). The latter communicates with the upper part of the tympanic cavity or epitympanic recess. There are three groups of cells in the mastoid portion: the anteroposterior, the middle, and the apical. These have been further subdivided according to position into: (1) eustachian, (2) zygomatic, (3) cells along the floor of the middle fossa, (4) sublabyrinthine, (5) squamous, (6) lateral sinus, (7) marginal, (8) retrofacial, and (9) mastoid tip (Fig. 7–29).

The degree of pneumatization is very variable.

The *petrous portion* is a pyramid with two surfaces contained within the cranial cavity and one directed downward at the base of the skull.

On its *posteromedial surface* is situated the internal auditory meatus. At the bottom of this meatus (or canal) is a plate of bone pierced by numerous foramina known as the lamina cribrosa. This canal transmits the facial (seventh), auditory (eighth), and glossopalatine nerves and the internal auditory artery.

The *anterosuperior surface* of the pyramid contains: (1) an impression for the semilunar ganglion of the trigeminal nerve near the apex, (2) the hiatus of the facial canal, (3) the arcuate eminence, under which the superior semicircular canal of the vestibular mechanism lies, and (4) the tegmen tympani laterally, which is a thin bony roof over the tympanic cavity.

The basilar surface of the pyramid is very irregular and presents important structures such as the carotid canal, jugular fossa, stylomastoid process, and foramen. (The medial and posterior walls of the tympanic cavity of the temporal bone are sometimes described as a fourth surface) (Fig. 7–30 B).

The various grooves and sutures of the pyramid that are of radiographic significance are: (1) the *petrosquamous suture,* which varies somewhat in appearance and may be marked by a series of irregular depressions. It is ordinarily directed obliquely and anteroinferiorly; (2) an impression produced by the *insertion of the digastric muscle* just posterior to the mastoid process; (3) a *mastoid foramen,* also somewhat variable in appearance, which transmits the mastoid branches of the occipital artery and vein to the transverse sinus; (4) a layer of *muscular indentation and grooves* representing the occipitofrontal, posterior auricular, sternocleidomastoid, and splenius capitis muscle impressions and indentations; (5) a *temporal line* that represents the continuation onto the squamosa of the superior margin of the zygomatic process; (6) *grooves for the middle temporal artery as seen externally;* (7) a *mandibular fossa* for articulation with the mandibular process of the mandible; (8) a *petrotympanic fissure* immediately beneath the mandibular fossa; (9) a *vaginal process* immediately cephalad to the styloid process.

From its internal aspect, which may also be seen radiologically, other indentations and grooves on the petrous bone must be understood and identified: (1) the *arcuate eminence,* which arches over the vestibular apparatus; (2) the *groove of the superior petrosal sinus;* (3) the *groove for the sigmoid venous sinus;* (4) the *internal acoustic opening;* and (5) *meningeal grooves housing the meningeal arteries and veins.*

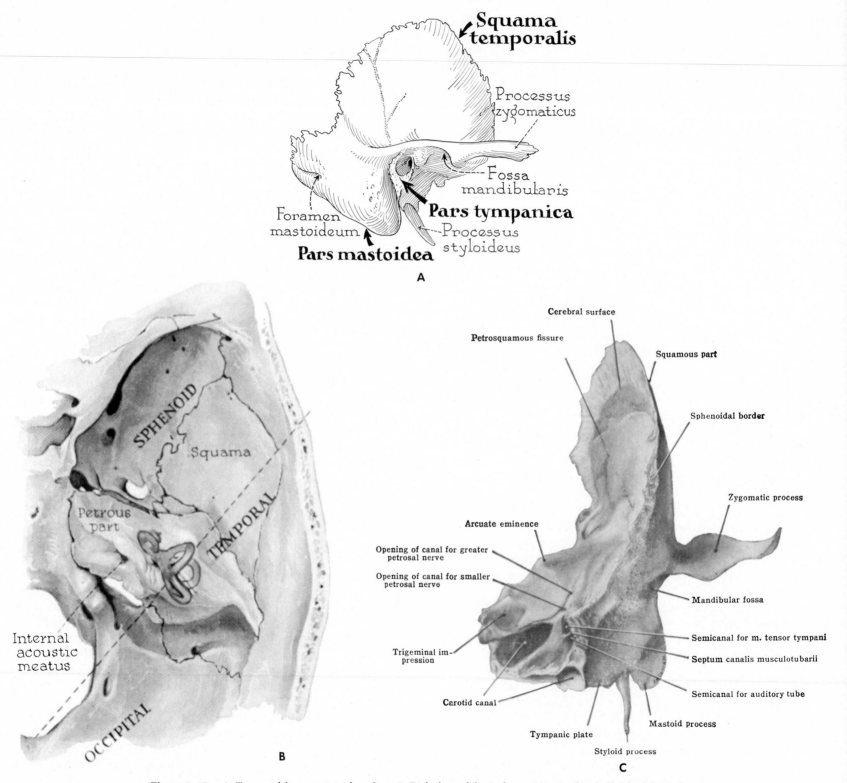

Figure 7–28. *A.* Temporal bone, external surface. *B.* Right bony labyrinth; position in the skull. The labyrinth, drawn from a reconstruction, is shown as if the surrounding part of the temporal bone were transparent. (From Anson, B. J.: An Atlas of Human Anatomy. Philadelphia, W. B. Saunders Co., 1963.) *C.* The left temporal bone, antero-medial view. (From Anson, B. J. (ed.) Morris' Human Anatomy, 12th ed. Copyright © 1966 by McGraw-Hill, Inc., Used by permission of the McGraw-Hill Book Company.)

Figure 7–28 continued on the opposite page.

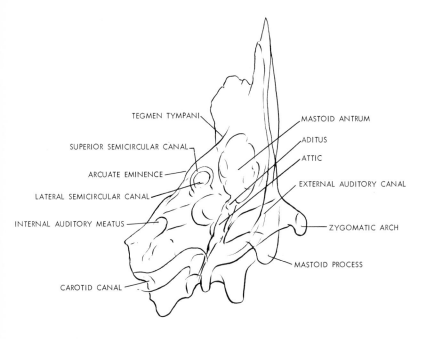

TEGMEN TYMPANI

SUPERIOR SEMICIRCULAR CANAL

ARCUATE EMINENCE

LATERAL SEMICIRCULAR CANAL

INTERNAL AUDITORY MEATUS

CAROTID CANAL

MASTOID ANTRUM

ADITUS

ATTIC

EXTERNAL AUDITORY CANAL

ZYGOMATIC ARCH

MASTOID PROCESS

CHAMBERLAIN - TOWNE VIEW

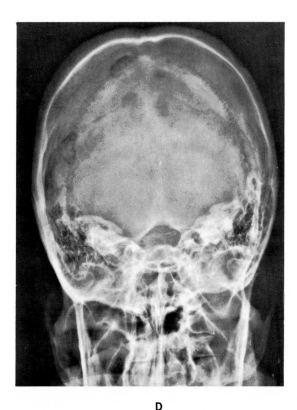

D

Figure 7-28 *Continued.* *D.* Tracing from radiograph of temporal bone, showing component parts (Towne's view).

In the anteromedial view some of these same structures can be further identified, as well as the *carotid canal* and an *impression for the trigeminal nerve* that also lodges the trigeminal ganglion. At times small openings for the greater and lesser petrosal nerves may also be identified (Fig. 7-30).

The apex of the pyramid (of the petrous bone) presents the medial opening of the carotid canal through which the internal carotid artery passes into the skull.

The external auditory meatus is formed partly by the tympanic and partly by the squamous portions. It is an elliptical bony canal which is continuous with a cartilaginous tube to the nasopharynx.

Anatomy of the Adult Ear (Fig. 7-31). The ear consists of three main parts: (1) an external ear containing an auricle, an external acoustic meatus for the conducting tube, and a tympanic membrane at its deep end; (2) a middle ear; and (3) an internal ear.

Middle Ear. The middle ear contains: (1) the tympanic cavity, (2) a tympanic antrum or mastoid antrum that is continuous with the air spaces in the mastoid portion of the temporal bone, and (3) an auditory tube located mostly within the temporal bone that communicates with the nasal part of the pharynx. It also contains the three ear bones that transmit vibrational effects from the tympanic membrane to the inner ear. These structures are shut off from the external ear by the tympanic membrane and from the chambers that form the internal ear by the structures occupying the cochlear and vestibular windows.

The *tympanic cavity* (Fig. 7-29 *A*) may be divided into two regions: a lower region at the level of the tympanic membrane (the tympanic cavity proper), and an upper region known as the *epitympanic recess*. The latter is about half the size of the former. The posterior end of the epitympanic recess communicates with the tympanic antrum via the *aditus ad antrum.* Bounding the tympanic cavity are many vital structures such as the internal jugular vein, the carotid artery, and other structures within the middle and inner ear. Overlying the epitympanic recess is the rooflike *tegmen tympani,* and medially to it are the *semicircular canals and prominence of the facial canal.* Laterally is the *scutum,* which forms a point of attachment for the tympanic membrane; inferiorly is the *fossa for the incus.* The boundary line between the tympanic cavity proper and the epitympanic recess is the prominence of the facial canal medially and the fossa of the incus inferiorly.

Internal Ear. The internal ear, located in the petrous portion of the temporal bone, is composed of three main parts: a membranous portion or *endolymphatic labyrinth;* a *bony labyrinth (perilymphatic);* and the surrounding otic capsule—the core of the petrous part of the temporal bone. It is the bony labyrinth that is so readily detected with polycycloidal tomography.

The Bony Labyrinth. This structure is about 2 cm. long and

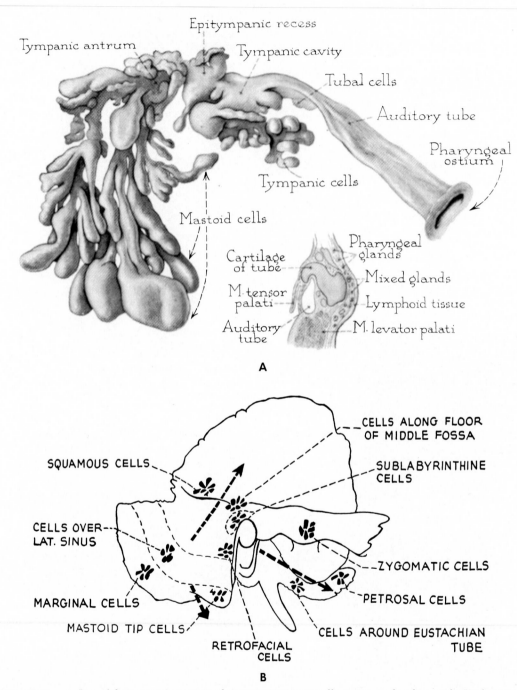

Figure 7-29. *A.* Cast of the tympanic cavity and communicating air cells, recess, and auditory tube (Siebenmann). (From Anson, B. J.: An Atlas of Human Anatomy. Philadelphia, W. B. Saunders Co., 1963.) *B.* Cellular groups within the temporal bone. (Modified from Tremble. Arch. Otolaryngol., *19*, 1934.)

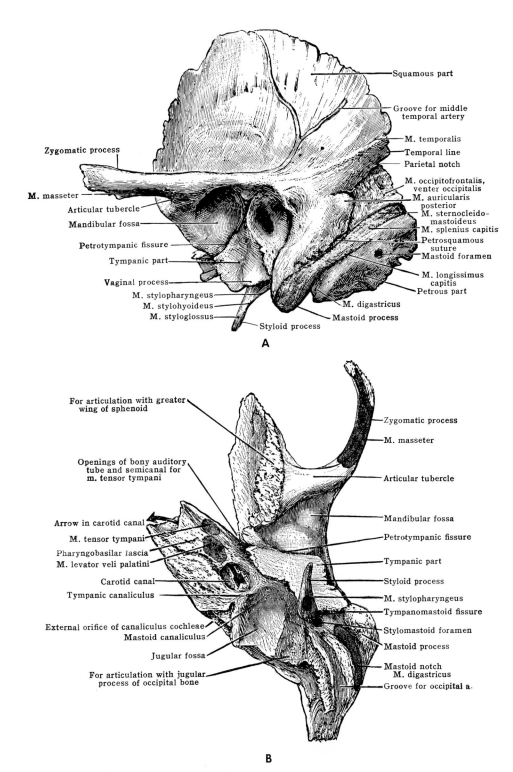

Squamous part

Groove for middle temporal artery

M. temporalis

Temporal line

Parietal notch

M. occipitofrontalis, venter occipitalis

M. auricularis posterior

M. sternocleido-mastoideus

M. splenius capitis

Petrosquamous suture

Mastoid foramen

M. longissimus capitis

Petrous part

M. digastricus

Mastoid process

Zygomatic process

M. masseter

Articular tubercle

Mandibular fossa

Petrotympanic fissure

Tympanic part

Vaginal process

M. stylopharyngeus

M. stylohyoideus

M. styloglossus

Styloid process

A

For articulation with greater wing of sphenoid

Openings of bony auditory tube and semicanal for m. tensor tympani

Arrow in carotid canal

M. tensor tympani

Pharyngobasilar fascia

M. levator veli palatini

Carotid canal

Tympanic canaliculus

External orifice of canaliculus cochleae

Mastoid canaliculus

Jugular fossa

For articulation with jugular process of occipital bone

Zygomatic process

M. masseter

Articular tubercle

Mandibular fossa

Petrotympanic fissure

Tympanic part

Styloid process

M. stylopharyngeus

Tympanomastoid fissure

Stylomastoid foramen

Mastoid process

Mastoid notch M. digastricus

Groove for occipital a.

B

Figure 7–30. Temporal bone, lateral view (*A*), inferior view (*B*). (From Anson, B. J. (ed.): Morris' Human Anatomy, 12th ed. Copyright © 1966 by McGraw-Hill, Inc. Used by permission of McGraw-Hill Book Company.)

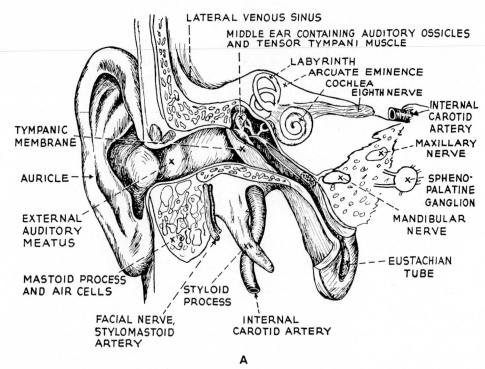

Figure 7–31.   A. Anatomy of the temporal bone.

Figure 7–31 continued on the opposite page.

is divided into three parts: a *vestibule,* containing two sacs, the utricle and the saccule; the *semicircular canals;* and the *cochlea,* which is specialized for hearing. The labyrinth is surrounded by a very hard layer of bone, 2 to 3 mm. thick, known as the *bony labyrinthine capsule.* This is fused with the compact bony substance immediately adjoining.

The bony vestibule is an ovoid chamber, about 4 mm. in diameter, that communicates with the cochlea anteroinferiorly and with the ends of the semicircular canals posterosuperiorly. Also communicating with the semicircular canals is the *oval window* (*fenestra vestibuli*), whereas the *round window* (*fenestra cochleae*) communicates with the cochlea. The oval window is closed by the base of the stapes and the annular ligament.

The Development of the Temporal Bone. Developmentally, there are three parts which differ slightly from the adult subdivisions: the petromastoid portion contains the internal ear; the tympanic portion partially encloses the external auditory canal—with the middle ear lying between the petromastoid and tympanic portions; the squamozygomatic division forms part of the side wall of the skull and the roof of the external auditory canal. In the infant, the petrosquamous suture has considerable clinical significance because it opens directly into the tympanic cavity and affords a pathway for the extension of infections from the middle ear to the meninges and brain. This suture closes slowly until 5 years of age, when it is obliterated in about one-half of the cases.

The mastoid process is not present at birth, at which time the tympanic portion is a thin bony ring incomplete superiorly, and the squamosa is very thin and smooth. At birth, the cavities of the auditory tube, tympanic cavity, and mastoid antrum are filled with mucoid material that is discharged through the auditory tube (eustachian tube) with respiration. Thereafter, pneumatization of the mastoid and petrous pyramids results by evaginations of epithelium from the primary cavities, which all communicate directly or indirectly with the mastoid antrum, middle ear, or eustachian tube. Thus, any infection of the one almost invariably involves the entire temporal bone if it is pneumatized.

The greater part of the process of formation of the air cells occurs in childhood, prior to adolescence, but this is very variable, and may be different on the two sides in the same individual. Thus, a middle ear infection may retard pneumatization on one side considerably; also, it may allow the development of diploic

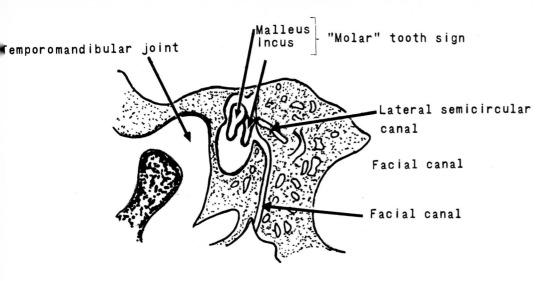

Temporomandibular joint

Malleus
Incus
} "Molar" tooth sign

Lateral semicircular canal

Facial canal

Facial canal

"Molar" tooth sign

Lateral tomogram petrous pyramid

"molar tooth" sign for

identification of ossicles

(malleus and incus)

B

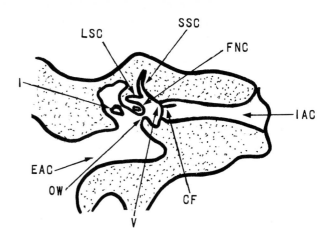

EAC External auditory canal
IAC Internal auditory canal
OW Oval window
LSC Lateral semicircular canal
SSC Superior semicircular canal
V   Vestibule

I   Incus
FNC Facial nerve canal
CF Crista falciformis

C

Figure 7–31 *Continued.* *B.* Diagram of lateral basic tomogram of the middle ear at the level of the middle ear ossicles: the "molar tooth" sign. (From Potter, G. D., Amer. J. Roentgenol., *104*:194, 1968.) *C.* Diagram of antero-posterior tomogram of the middle ear at the level of the crista falciformis. (From Valvassori, G. E.: Amer. J. Roentgenol., *94*:568, 1965.)

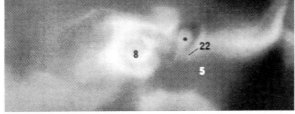

A

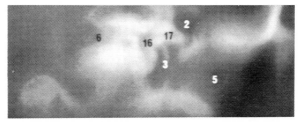

B

Figure 7–32. Anteroposterior tomograms of a normal left ear made in the "cochlear plane" and the "vestibular plane." *A.* Cochlear plane. The turns of the cochlea, the scutum (spur), the head and the handle of the malleus (*asterisk*), and the relation of the malleus to the epitympanic recess are clearly seen. *B.* Vestibular plane (2 mm posterior to *A*). The vestibule, the internal auditory canal, two of the three semicircular canals, and the mastoid antrum are all clearly visible. (From Schaeffer, R. E.: Med. Radiography and Photography, *48(1)*:2–22, 1972. Published by Radiography Markets Division, Eastman Kodak Company.)

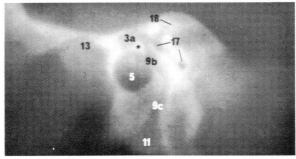

A

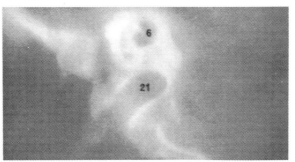

B

Figure 7–33. Lateral tomograms of a normal left ear made in two levels, or planes. *A.* More superficial of the two levels. The facial nerve canal is visible all the way down to its point of exit at the stylomastoid foramen, and the ossicular mass (*asterisk*) can be seen in the epitympanic recess. The two limbs of the lateral semicircular canal are also visible. *B.* Deeper of the two levels (8 mm deeper than *A*). A deep jugular fossa is visible, but the carotid canal is not shown to good advantage. The internal auditory canal is clearly visible. The thin, bony band that stretches across the diameter of the internal auditory canal is an edge-on view of the crista transversa (crista falciformis). (From Schaeffer, R. E.: Med. Radiography and Photography, *48(1)*:2–22, 1972. Published by Radiography Markets Division, Eastman Kodak Company.)

cells only, rather than cells of a mixed type such as occur normally when development is uninterrupted.

CORRELATED ROENTGEN ANATOMY OF THE TEMPORAL BONE

Introduction. Correlated radiographic visualization of the temporal bone is best accomplished by such techniques as sectional anatomy, radiography of 1 mm. sections, and close correlation of these techniques with polycycloidal tomography. These procedures have been carried out in detail by Schaefer and also by Potter, to whom the author is indebted for much of the following material.

In Figure 7–34 *A* six pairs of radiographs and tomograms made in the *anteroposterior projection* are reproduced, the sections progressing from anterior toward the posterior approximately 1 to 1.5 mm. apart. The medial aspect of the temporal bone is on the left, the lateral is on the right.

In *A*, through the anterior part of the external auditory canal, one can see the scutum or spur that forms a point of attachment for the following clearly visible structures: (a) the tympanic membrane, (b) the epitympanic recess or attic, (c) the tegmen tympani, (d) a portion of the facial nerve canal in its petrous segment, (e) the cochlea, and (f) the carotid canal. The mandibular fossa is also shown. The relationships of the epitympanic recess to the tympanic cavity and the external auditory canal are also well demonstrated.

In section *B*, approximately 1 mm. posterior to *A*, somewhat similar structures can be identified, but with minor variations as follows: the spur can be more clearly identified, the facial canal is seen as two small openings and not in continuum, and the mandibular fossa and carotid canal are not at all clearly demonstrated.

The third level, *C*, shows the turn of the cochlea more clearly, the lateral wall of which forms the promontory of the middle ear. The scutum and two portions of the facial nerve canal are once again brought into focus. The most anterior part of the internal auditory canal is just beginning to appear, and the anterior portion of the crista falciformis is just barely visible as it begins to divide the auditory canal into a superior and an inferior channel. The mastoid antrum is found mainly posterior to the tympanic cavity and also slightly above and lateral to it.

In *D*, which coincides with the plane of the internal auditory canal, we now may identify clearly the turns of the cochlea, parts of the superior and lateral semicircular canals, and the oval window (fenestra vestibuli); immediately lateral to the niche for the oval window is the facial nerve canal, which is, however, almost imperceptible. It can be seen better in the radiograph because of the penetration of the x-rays in the latter. This level also shows the epitympanic recess, situated between the middle ear and the mastoid antrum.

The fifth level, *E*, is at a vestibular plane. The superior and lateral semicircular canals, the jugular fossa, the internal auditory canal, and the niche of the oval window are all readily visible. The round window (fenestra cochlea) faces inferolaterally and is often poorly defined; it coincides with the plane of the posterior wall of the external auditory canal.

The final level in this study, *F*, shows the segments of the lateral and the posterior semicircular canals as well as the superior. The jugular fossa may also be seen. Various portions of the mastoid segment of the facial nerve can be visualized as it courses toward its termination at the stylomastoid foramen.

Lateral Projection (Schaefer) (Fig. 7–34 *B*). The lateral projection shows nicely the relationships of the mastoid antrum, the epitympanic recess, the external auditory canal, and the facial nerve canal. The lateral sinus plate is also clearly demonstrated.

The medial relationship of the jugular fossa to these structures is also shown. Proceeding internally, the structures of the internal ear and the carotid canal come into view.

There is no clear-cut boundary between the mastoid antrum, aditus of the antrum, and epitympanic recess as might be expected from previous illustrations. The "molar tooth" configuration of the malleus and incus is clearly demonstrated.

Stenver's Projection (Fig. 7–35). This projection is seldom necessary with good polycycloidal studies in the anteroposterior and lateral views. However, it reveals a number of structures in familiar configuration.

Anteroposterior tomograms of a normal left ear made in the cochlear and vestibular planes have been illustrated for comparison with the specimen study (Fig. 7–32). Lateral tomograms are also very helpful (Fig. 7–33). The following structures are readily identified in these two views: the *scutum* or *spur*, the *handle of the malleus*, the *cochlea*, the *tympanic cavity*, the *mastoid antrum*, the *semicircular canals*, and the *internal auditory canal*. In the lateral view the *facial canal* and its stylomastoid foramen, the *mandibular fossa*, the *epitympanic recess*, and the *jugular fossa* are also clearly seen.

Such clear depictions of minute details of internal anatomy are extremely helpful in the diagnosis of anomalous conditions or abnormalities of the middle ear apparatus, infectious or destructive processes, and neoplasia which may extend from the base of the brain, the internal and middle ear.

ROUTINE STUDY OF THE PETROUS RIDGES AND MASTOID PROCESSES

This is usually a complete study of the temporal bone involving a study of the mastoid process from at least two vantage points, as well as at least two different perspectives of the petrous ridge.

(Text continues on page 330)

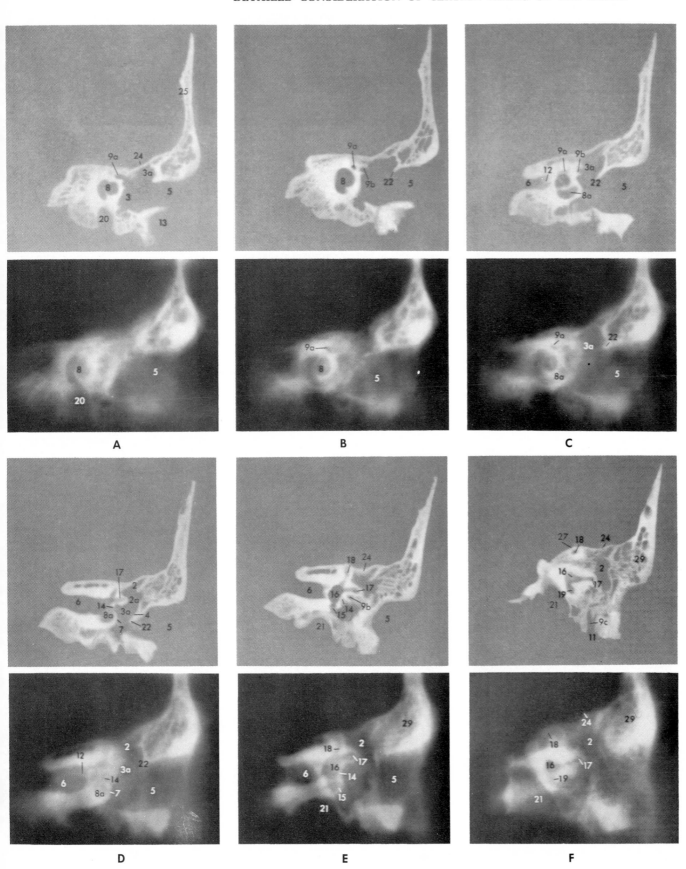

Figure 7–34. A. Anteroposterior (frontal) projection. Six pairs of radiographs (top) and tomograms (bottom) of a dried left temporal bone. Each pair represents a different level, or plane. The progression of levels from left to right is anterior to posterior, and there is about 1 mm to 1.5 mm between levels. The medial aspect of the bone is on the left; the lateral aspect, on the right. Structures seen particularly well in the anteroposterior projection include the internal auditory canal in its long axis and the epitympanic recess (attic).

Legend: (1) Mastoid process, (2) mastoid antrum, (2a) aditus of antrum, (3) middle ear (tympanic cavity), (3a) epitympanic recess (attic), (4) lateral wall of attic, (5) external auditory canal, (6) internal auditory canal, (7) promontory of middle ear, (8) cochlea, (8a) basal turn of cochlea, (9a) facial nerve canal, petrous segment, (9b) facial nerve canal, tympanic segment, (9c) facial nerve canal, mastoid (descending) segment, (10) styloid process, (11) stylomastoid foramen, (12) crista transversa (crista falciformis), (13) mandibular fossa, (14) oval window (fenestra vestibuli), (15) round window (fenestra cochleae), (16) vestibule, (17) lateral semicircular canal, (18) superior semicircular canal, (19) posterior semicircular canal, (20) carotid canal, (21) jugular fossa, (22) scutum (spur), (23) sinus plate, (24) tegmen, (25) squamous portion of temporal bone, (26) crus commune (common limb), (27) arcuate eminence, (28) petrous apex, (29) mastoid air cells. (From Schaeffer, R. E.: Med. Radiography and Photography, 48(1):2–22, 1972. Published by Radiography Markets Division, Eastman Kodak Company.)

Figure 7-34 *Continued.* *B.* Lateral projection. Six pairs of radiographs (*top*) and tomograms (*bottom*) of a dried left temporal bone. Each pair represents a different level, or plane. From left to right, the levels progress from the lateral surface of the bone mediad. The posterior aspect of the bone is on the right. The lateral projection reveals the relation between the epitympanic recess and the mastoid antrum and shows the mastoid (descending) segment of the facial nerve canal. In the specimen used for this projection, the malleus and the incus happened to be present in their normal configuration. The tomogram made in the second level (*B, bottom*) clearly shows these ossicles (*asterisks*); the handle of the malleus is anterior, and the long process of the incus is posterior.

Legend: (*1*) Mastoid process, (*2*) mastoid antrum, (*2a*) aditus of antrum, (*3*) middle ear (tympanic cavity), (*3a*) epitympanic recess (attic), (*4*) lateral wall of attic, (*5*) external auditory canal, (*6*) internal auditory canal, (*7*) promontory of middle ear, (*8*) cochlea, (*8a*) basal turn of cochlea, (*9a*) facial nerve canal, petrous segment, (*9b*) facial nerve canal, tympanic segment, (*9c*) facial nerve canal, mastoid (descending) segment, (*10*) styloid process, (*11*) stylomastoid foramen, (*12*) crista transversa (crista falciformis), (*13*) mandibular fossa, (*14*) oval window (fenestra vestibuli), (*15*) round window (fenestra cochleae), (*16*) vestibule, (*17*) lateral semicircular canal, (*18*) superior semicircular canal, (*19*) posterior semicircular canal, (*20*) carotid canal, (*21*) jugular fossa, (*22*) scutum (spur), (*23*) sinus plate, (*24*) tegmen, (*25*) squamous portion of temporal bone, (*26*) crus commune (common limb), (*27*) arcuate eminence, (*28*) petrous apex, (*29*) mastoid air cells. (From Schaeffer, R. E.: Med. Radiography and Photography, *48*(1):2–22, 1972. Published by Radiography Markets Division, Eastman Kodak Company.)

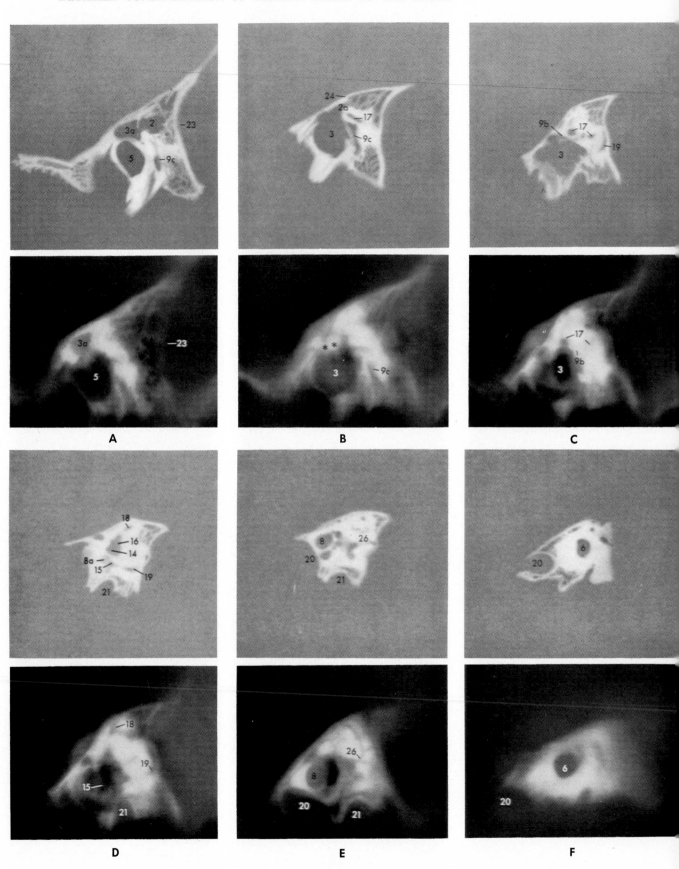

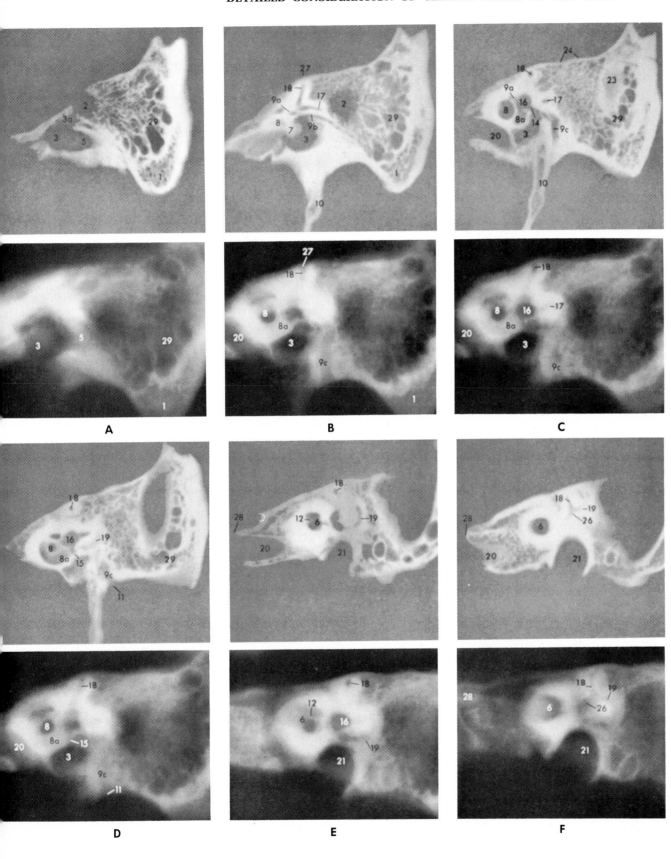

Figure 7-35. Stenver's (oblique posteroanterior) projection. Six pairs of radiographs (*top*) and tomograms (*bottom*) of a dried left temporal bone. Each pair represents a different level, or plane. The progression of levels from left to right is anterior to posterior. The anteromedian aspect of the bone is on the left; the posterolateral aspect is on the right. The jugular fossa, the labyrinth, the course of the facial nerve canal, and the relation of the jugular fossa to the middle ear (tympanic cavity) are shown particularly well in the Stenver's projection.

Legend: (1) Mastoid process, (2) mastoid antrum (2a) aditus of antrum, (3) middle ear (tympanic cavity), (3a) epitympanic recess (attic), (4) lateral wall of attic, (5) external auditory canal, (6) internal auditory canal, (7) promontory of middle ear, (8) cochlea, (8a) basal turn of cochlea, (9a) facial nerve canal, petrous segment, (9b) facial nerve canal, tympanic segment, (9c) facial nerve canal, mastoid (descending) segment, (10) styloid process, (11) stylomastoid foramen, (12) crista transversa (crista falciformis), (13) mandibular fossa, (14) oval window (fenestra vestibuli), (15) round window (fenestra cochleae), (16) vestibule, (17) lateral semicircular canal, (18) superior semicircular canal, (19) posterior semicircular canal, (20) carotid canal, (21) jugular fossa (22) scutum (spur), (23) sinus plate, (24) tegmen, (25) squamous portion of temporal bone, (26) crus commune (common limb), (27) arcuate eminence, (28) petrous apex, (29) mastoid air cells. (From Schaeffer, R. E.: Med. Radiography and Photography, 48(1):2–22, 1972. Published by Radiography Markets Division, Eastman Kodak Company.)

1. **Lateral Projection of the Mastoid Process (Law's Position)** (Fig. 7–36). The various cellular groups are quite clearly delineated, along with a superposition of the internal and external acoustic meatuses, the lateral sinus plate, and the emissary vein posterior to the mastoid process.

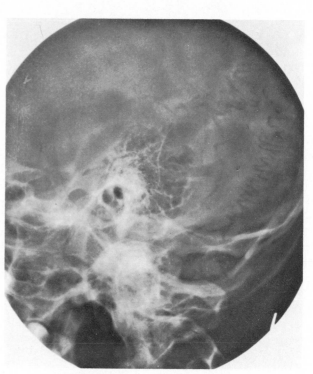

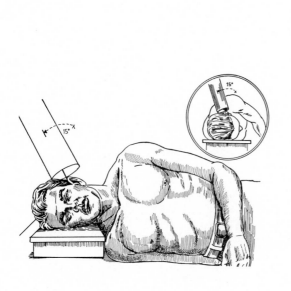

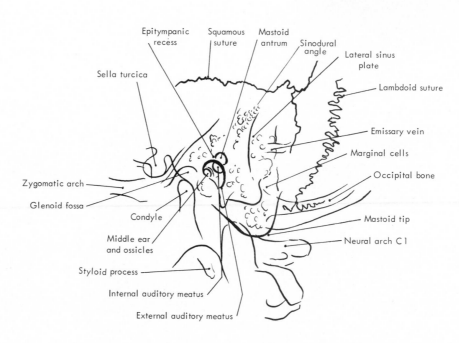

Figure 7–36. Lateral projection of mastoid process (Law's position).

2. **Tangential View of the Mastoid Tips** (Fig. 7–37).   This is virtually an anteroposterior view of the mastoid processes, but shows a particularly clear and unobstructed view of the mastoid air cells in the projecting portion of the mastoid. Other structures of the petrous ridge can also be identified if the exposure is sufficiently penetrating, but ordinarily separate views are obtained for this purpose.

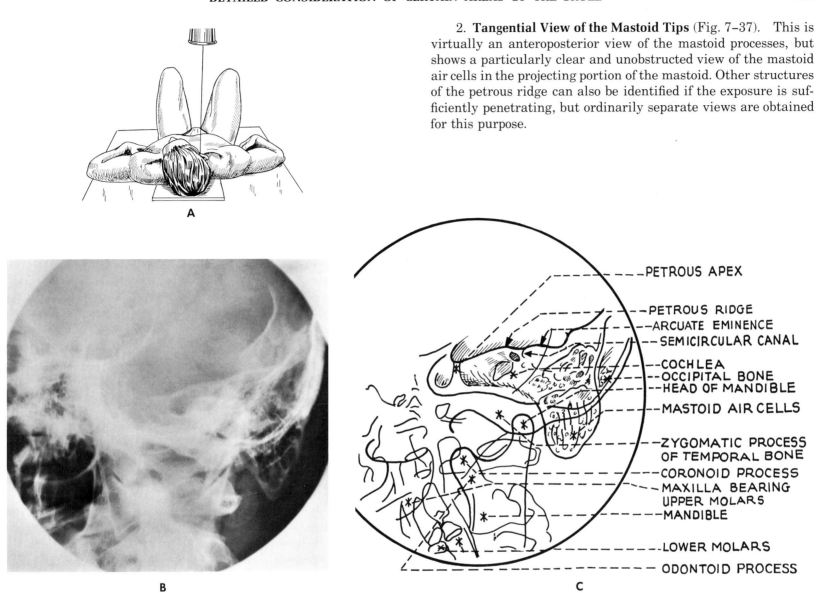

PETROUS APEX

PETROUS RIDGE
ARCUATE EMINENCE
SEMICIRCULAR CANAL

COCHLEA
OCCIPITAL BONE
HEAD OF MANDIBLE

MASTOID AIR CELLS

ZYGOMATIC PROCESS OF TEMPORAL BONE

CORONOID PROCESS
MAXILLA BEARING UPPER MOLARS
MANDIBLE

LOWER MOLARS

ODONTOID PROCESS

Figure 7–37.   Tangential view of mastoid tips. A. Position of patient. B. Radiograph. C. Labeled tracing of B.

Points of Practical Interest with Reference to Figure 7–37

1. The auricles of the ears should be folded forward to avoid the projection of the pinna over the mastoid structures.
2. The smallest possible cone should be employed at a fairly close target-to-film distance (25 to 30 inches). The head is rotated 45 degrees away from the side being radiographed, and the tube is angled 15 degrees caudally, centering over the midpoint of the canthomeatal line.
3. In this view the mastoid process is projected away from the rest of the calvarium, and the mastoid cells in the tip of the process are shown to best advantage. A somewhat lighter exposure technique must be employed to gain this view. This same projection, however, may also be used to visualize the petrous portion of the temporal bone if a somewhat heavier exposure technique is employed.
4. Comparison films between the two mastoids are always obtained.

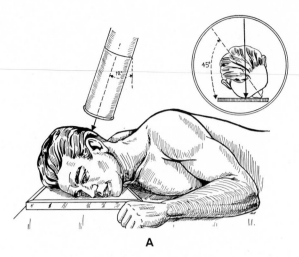

3. **Posteroanterior View of the Petrous Ridge with the Ridge Placed Parallel to the Film (Stenver's Position)** (Fig. 7–38). This is a view of the petrous ridge obtained by placing the skull so that the petrous ridge is parallel with the film. An unobstructed view is thereby obtained of the petrous apex, and the entire bone stands out as a pyramidal structure. Usually the bony labyrinth (semicircular canals, vestibule, and cochlea) can be identified together with the internal auditory meatus and canal. The cellular structure is also clearly seen.

4. **Superoinferior Projection of the Petrous Ridges** (Fig. 6–44). This is obtained by means of Towne's position already described. This is the anteroposterior projection with a 30 to 35 degree tilt of the tube caudally. As previously indicated, an excellent perspective of both petrous ridges is obtained, along with the view of the occipital bone, foramen magnum, and dorsum sellae.

A

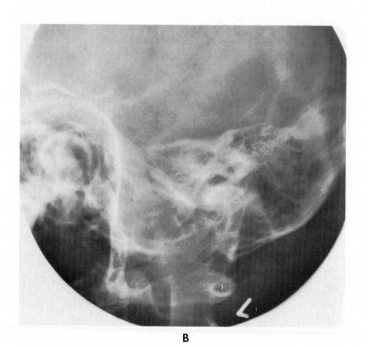

B

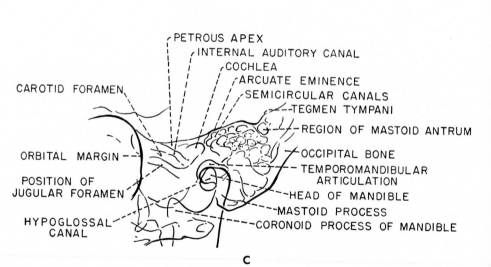

C

Figure 7–38.   Stenver's view of petrous ridge. *A.* Position of patient. *B.* Radiograph. *C.* Tracing of *B.*

5. **Mayer's Position of the Mastoids** (Fig. 7–39). This view is especially useful in separation of the anatomic structures of the middle ear as a prerequisite for fenestration operations. It is difficult to duplicate this view from patient to patient and hence the anatomic depiction is somewhat variable.

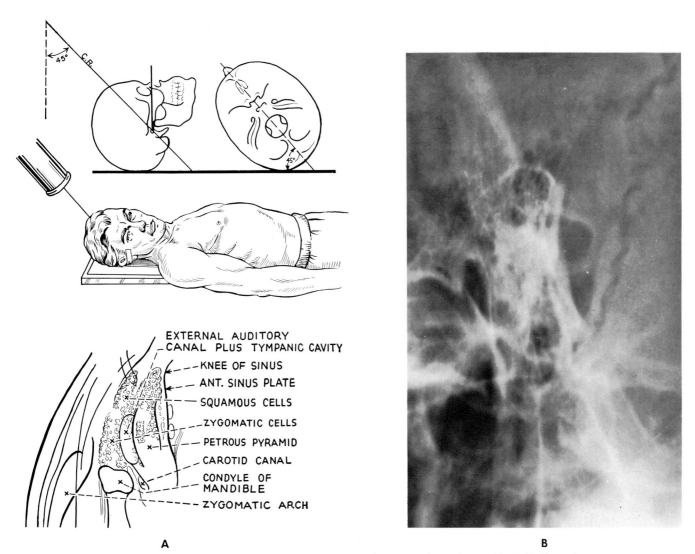

EXTERNAL AUDITORY
CANAL PLUS TYMPANIC CAVITY
KNEE OF SINUS
ANT. SINUS PLATE
SQUAMOUS CELLS
ZYGOMATIC CELLS
PETROUS PYRAMID
CAROTID CANAL
CONDYLE OF MANDIBLE
ZYGOMATIC ARCH

A

B

Figure 7–39. A. Mayer's position for examination of petrous ridge and mastoids. B. Radiograph.

6. **Chaussee III Projection of the Temporal Bone**
(Sansregret) (Fig. 7–40). This view provides a tangential view of
the edge of the epitympanic recess.

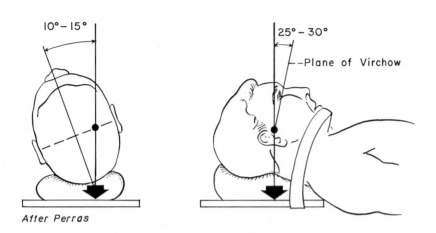

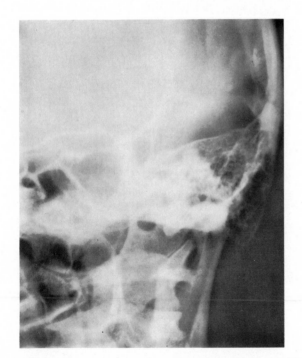

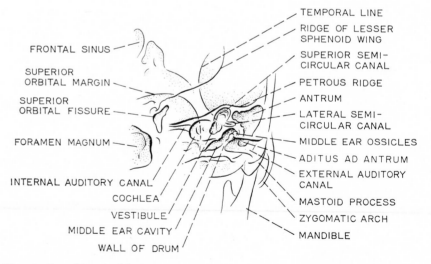

Figure 7–40. Chaussee III projection of temporal bone.

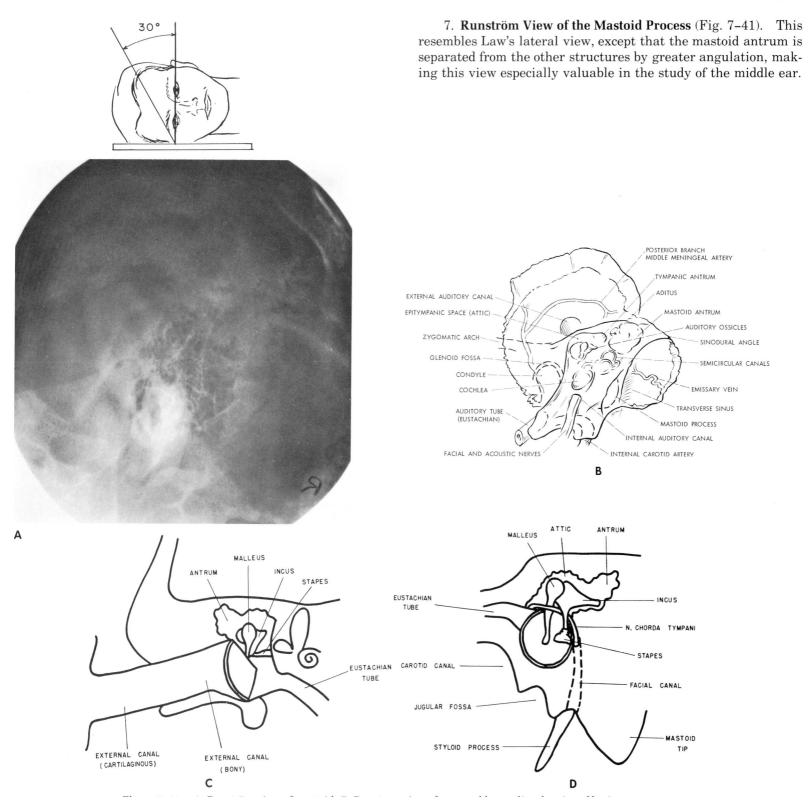

7. Runström View of the Mastoid Process (Fig. 7–41). This resembles Law's lateral view, except that the mastoid antrum is separated from the other structures by greater angulation, making this view especially valuable in the study of the middle ear.

Figure 7–41. *A.* Runström view of mastoid. *B.* Runström view of temporal bone—line drawing of basic anatomy. *C* and *D.* Diagrams showing the relation of the attic and antral area to the middle ear. The coronal section (*C*) is similar to a Stenver's view and the sagittal section (*D*) is similar to a Runström view. (*C* and *D* from Becker, J. A., and Woloshin, H. J.: Amer. J. Roentgenol., *87*:1019, 1962. *D* is adapted from Shambaugh, G. E.: Surgery of the Ear. Philadelphia, W. B. Saunders Co., 1959.)

8. Submentovertical View (to Demonstrate Tympanic Cavity) (Etter and Cross) (Fig. 7–42). The greater angle is usually necessary to display the middle ear separately from the ramus of the mandible.

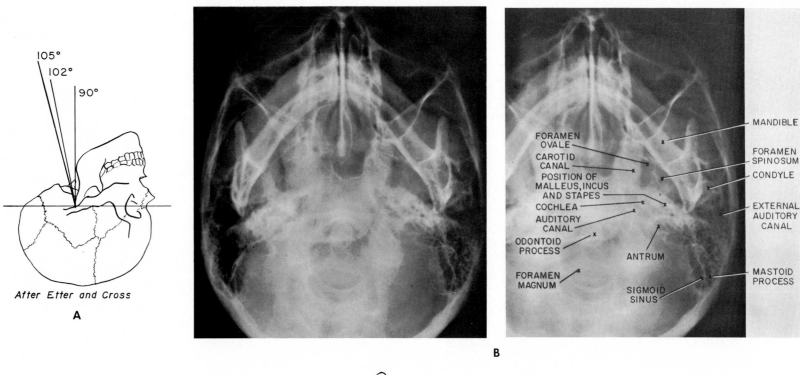

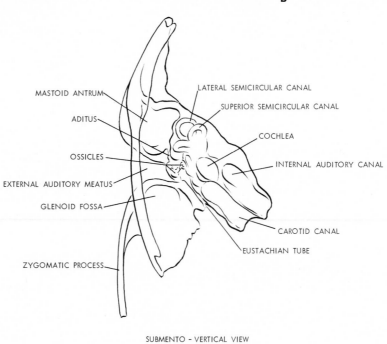

Figure 7–42. *A* and *B*. Submentovertical view to demonstrate tympanic cavity and ossicles. *C*. Line drawing of basic anatomy in submentovertical view of temporal bone.

9. **Laminagraphy of the Ear** (Schaefer; Valvassori). The examination of the small structures of the internal and middle ear has already been previously described (see Figure 7–32). Laminagraphy—polytomography in particular—has made available to the radiologist immense possibilities in the visualization of minute anatomic details. The Massiot polytome (or its equivalent in other apparatus) allows a separating capacity of thicknesses of 1 mm. and a coefficient of distinctness about five times as great as that which can be obtained with linear tomography (Valvassori).

Three projections, occasionally a fourth, are used for polytomography of the ear: lateral, frontal, Stenver's, and occasionally, axial.

Lateral projection. The patient lies prone on the table with the side of the head to be examined turned away from the table top. The structures of the ear extend 2 to 5 cm. from the outer surface as follows: (1) the external auditory canal, $1\frac{1}{2}$ to $2\frac{1}{2}$ cm.; (2) middle ear and its ossicles, $2\frac{1}{2}$ to 3 cm.; (3) vestibule, with most of the semicircular canals and the cochlea, 3 to 4 cm.; and (4) internal auditory canal, 4 to 5 cm.

Frontal projection. For this projection the patient lies either prone or supine. The line between the tragus and the external canthus must be perpendicular to the table top. All the ear structures are included in a 2 cm. thickness extending posteriorly from the anterior wall of the external auditory canal. As previously indicated, the following structures may be visualized, moving from anterior to posterior: cochlea, epitympanic recess, malleus, incus, middle ear cavity, external auditory canal, internal auditory canal, vestibule, oval window, and semicircular canals.

Stenver's projection. The patient lies prone with the head rotated to a 45 degree oblique angle, thus bringing the petrous pyramid parallel to the table top. The head is usually flexed 12 degrees. Here, too, the structures of the ear are included in a 2 cm. thickness extending posteriorly from the external auditory porus. From anterior to posterior the structures best seen are: (1) external and middle ear cavities, (2) round window, (3) vestibule and semicircular canals, (4) cochlea, and (5) internal auditory porus. The relationship of the middle ear to the carotid canal can also be studied accurately in this view.

The normal internal auditory canal (Valvassori and Pierce). These authors define porus as merely the opening of the canal and meatus as either the canal or the opening of the canal.

The internal auditory canal forms a 90 degree angle with the sagittal plane of the skull and an angle of about 45 degrees with the long axis of the petrous pyramids. In cross section, the internal auditory canal is usually ellipsoid, the vertical diameter being slightly larger than the horizontal. The *crista falciformis* divides the lateral part of the internal auditory canal into two unequal portions, with the larger portion in the inferior position.

The frontal and axial views are best for demonstration of the canal in its full length, and the lateral view is best for visualization of the canal in cross section. In Stenver's view, the internal auditory canal is foreshortened. Polytomography is best employed for visualization of the canal and its minute details.

These views demonstrate the longer anterior wall and the shorter posterior wall with its medial concave lip (Fig. 7–42 C). In a study by Valvassori and Pierce, comparison between the posterior walls of the right and left canals of the same patient showed a variation of up to 1 mm. in 86 per cent of the patients and a variation of 1 to 2 mm. in 13 per cent. The variation between the two sides was 2 to 3 mm. in only 1 per cent of the patients.

The anterior wall of the internal auditory canal was also measured. Its greatest length was 19 mm., the shortest was 6 mm., and the average was 12 mm. Comparison between the internal auditory canals of the same patient showed a variation of up to 1 mm. in 85 per cent of the patients, 1 to 2 mm. in 8 per cent, and 2 to 3 mm. in 7 per cent.

In a study of 100 petrous bones for crista falciformis detail, it was noted that in 85 per cent of the patients the crista appeared as a linear density ranging from 1 to 7 mm. Its thickness appeared to decrease progressively from its lateral origin to its medial end. In 15 per cent of the patients only the origin of the crista was detectable as a definite knob of increased density. *The origin of the crista falciformis was located at, or above, the midpoint of the vertical diameter in all of the patients studied.*

Thus, although the length of the crista falciformis is variable, its position in relation to the height of the canal is consistent. *If the crista falciformis can be identified below the midpoint of the canal, an abnormal situation may be identified.* (The above measurements have been corrected for magnification and represent the true anatomic size.)

10. **Positive Contrast Demonstration of Normal Internal Acoustic Meatus, Meckel's Cave, and Jugular Foramen (Posterior Fossa Cisternomyelography)** (Reese and Bull; Baker; Gass; Scanlan). *Method.* Nine ml. of iophendylate (Pantopaque) is introduced into the lumbar subarachnoid space as in myelography. The head is maintained in full extension by a small hard pillow. After all of the oil is pooled in the cervical region and appropriate roentgenograms are made, the table is slowly tilted down with the head in extension, while the oil advances onto the clivus to the base of the dorsum sellae. When the oil is over the tip of the clivus and into the middle fossa, it is irretrievable, so that the head must be carefully controlled at this time. By very carefully turning the head while it is in extension, the oil may be moved from the clivus into the cerebellopontine angle cistern. After anteroposterior and lateral roentgenograms of the clivus have been made, the table is returned to the horizontal position and the oil on the clivus returns to the cervical region (Fig. 7–43).

The head and shoulders are then rotated to one side or the other at least 30 degrees while the head is in hyperextension. The table is tilted downward and the contrast medium is observed closely on the fluoroscope as it flows from the cervical region into

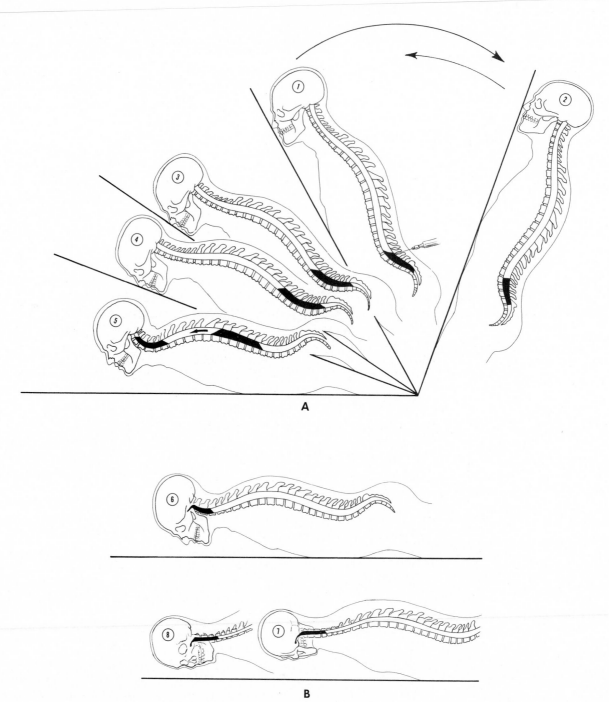

Figure 7–43.   Position of patient during myelography. *A.* Lumbar and cervical. *B.* For visualization of region of clivus and internal acoustic meatus (see text for description).

the cerebellopontine angle cistern. Roentgenograms are then made in the anteroposterior and cross table lateral projections.

Anatomy. The subarachnoid space extends into the internal acoustic meatus to a depth of 7 mm. and forms a rather distinct diverticulum (Fig. 7–44). It arises from the lateral portion of the cerebellopontine angle cistern and extends ventrally and laterally into the petrous bone. It is grooved posteriorly by the seventh and eighth cranial nerves.

The diverticulum-like structure which lies medially and rostrally to the internal acoustic meatus is the *Meckel's cave.* At times there is also a smaller diverticulum just caudal to the internal acoustic meatus and in line with it; this is the extension of the arachnoid space into the jugular foramen (Fig. 7–45).

The *roentgenographic appearance* and appropriate diagrams are shown in Figure 7–45.

11. **Special Views of Jugular Canal** (See Figures 6–29, 6–54, 6–55, and 6–56, and Chapter 6).

12. **Special Views of the Hypoglossal Canal.** *Basic Anatomy* (Kirdani). The hypoglossal canal traverses the occipital condyle, transmitting the twelfth cranial nerve, a meningeal branch of the ascending pharyngeal artery, and a plexus of emissary veins. The canals lie on or very near a line joining the external auditory canal. In oblique views of the skull which place the long axis of the canal perpendicular to the roentgenographic film, the canal is seen as a ring, end-on. Such views are: Stenver's, Law's, and special views for the optic foramina. Body section radiography—polytomography in particular—is essential for visualization of the canal in all three of its dimensions. The level of the tomographic cuts will vary but usually they are quite close to the posterior margin of the mastoid process.

(*Text continues on page 343*)

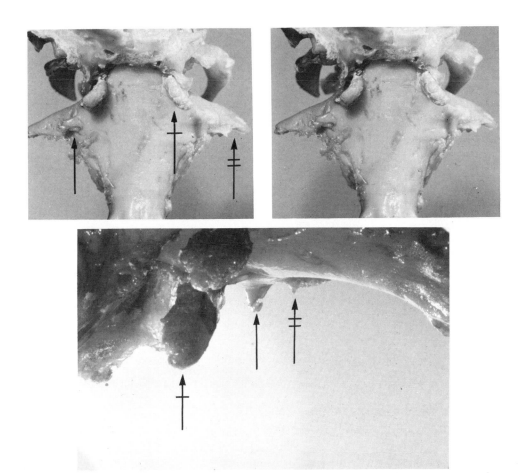

Figure 7–44. Resin-injection casts of the subarachnoid cisterns. *Upper.* Pontine and cerebellopontine angle cisterns seen from below: →, internal auditory canal; ⇢, large Meckel's caves protruding anteriorly; ↔, cerebellopontine angle cisterns. These pictures are a stereoscopic pair. *Lower.* Oblique crosstable lateral view: ↠, bulbous Meckel's cave anteriorly; →, internal auditory canal; ⇢, tiny amount of resin in the jugular foramen. (From Reese, D. F., and Bull, J. W. D.: Amer. J. Roentgenol., *100*:650–655, 1967.)

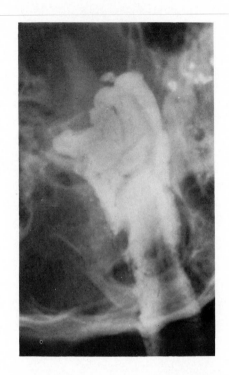

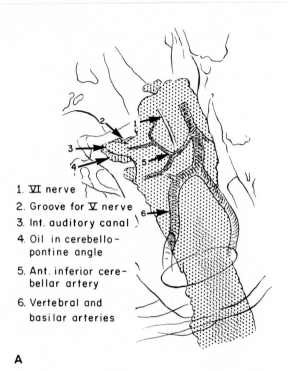

1. VI nerve
2. Groove for V nerve
3. Int. auditory canal
4. Oil in cerebello-
   pontine angle
5. Ant. inferior cere-
   bellar artery
6. Vertebral and
   basilar arteries

A

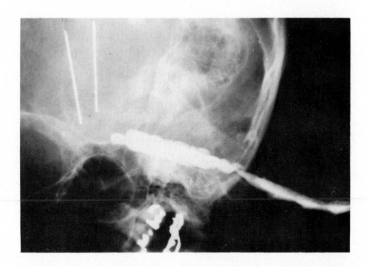

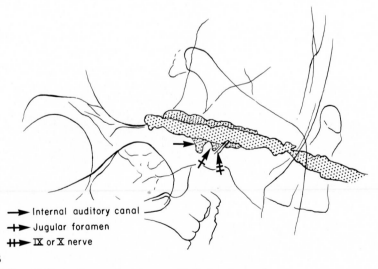

→ Internal auditory canal
+→ Jugular foramen
++→ IX or X nerve

B

Figure 7–45.   *A*. Posteroanterior view of the pontine and left cerebellopontine angle cisterns, with the head turned to the right 45 degrees. The oil in the internal auditory canal is somewhat obscured by oil in the overlying cerebello-pontine angle cistern. *B*. Crosstable lateral view, with head in same position as in *A*. The internal auditory canal and jugular foramen are separated from the oil in the cerebellopontine angle cistern. (From Reese, D. F., and Bull, J. W. D.: Amer. J. Roentgenol., *100*:650–655, 1967.)

Figure 7–45 continued on the opposite page.

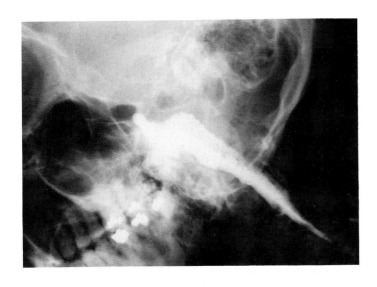

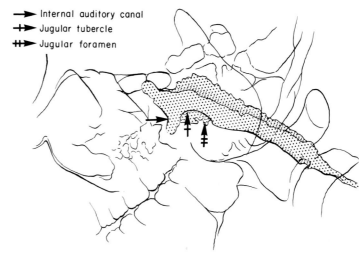

C

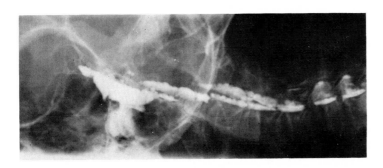

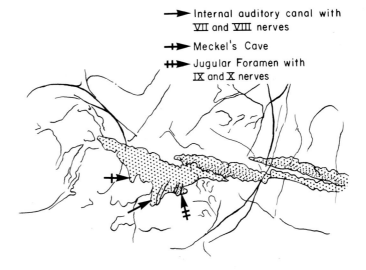

D

Figure 7–45 *Continued.* C. Jugular tubercle is faintly seen, with the internal auditory canal directly in front of and below it. D. Oil is present in Meckel's cave, internal auditory canal, and jugular foramen. In no case to date have we seen such extensive filling of Meckel's cave as found in the resin-injection cast. (From Reese, D. F., and Bull, J. W. D.: Amer. J. Roentgenol., *100*:650–655, 1967.)

Figure 7–45 continued on the following page.

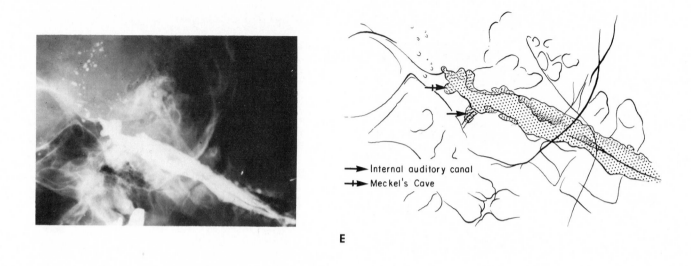

E

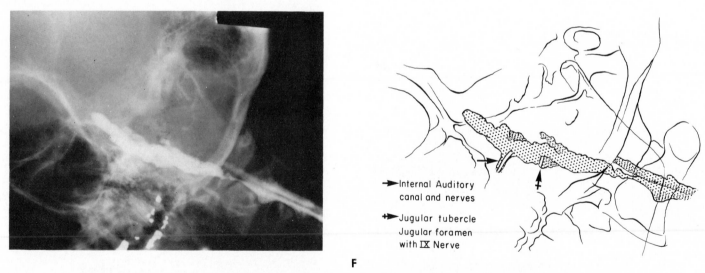

F

Figure 7–45 *Continued.*   E. Meckel's cave and the internal auditory canal are seen. In *D* and *E* the cranial nerves VII and VIII can be seen traversing the posterior portion of the canal. *F.* Jugular foramen and internal auditory canal are filled. The linear shadow in the oil column and the upper cervical part of spinal column is a portion of the dentate ligaments. (From Reese, D. F., and Bull, J. W. D.: Amer. J. Roentgenol., *100*:650–655, 1967.)

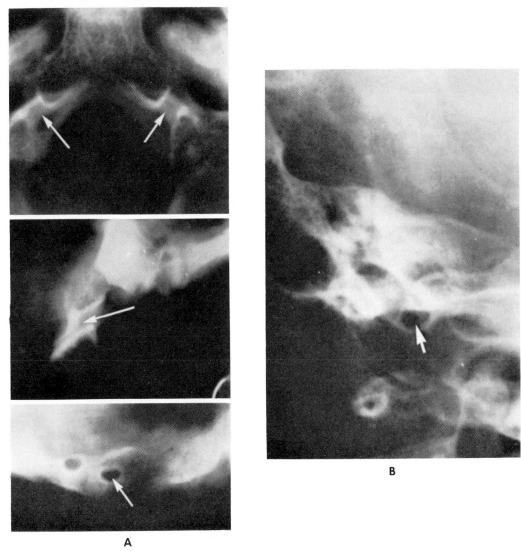

Figure 7–46. *A.* The three projections in a dried skull specimen. *Upper,* Axial laminagram at the level of the hypoglossal canals. *Middle,* Laminagram in the zygomaticomastoid projection showing the hypoglossal canal in its long axis. *Lower,* Laminagram in the zygomatico-occipital projection showing the hypoglossal canal in cross section. Notice another foramen posterior to the hypoglossal canal—the condyloid canal. *B.* Conventional Stenver's view. The hypoglossal canal is seen on end. (From Kirdani, M. A.: Amer. J. Roentgenol., 99:700–704, 1967.)

The canal diameter varies between 4 and 11 mm. with an average of 6 mm. A variation of up to 3 mm. may be found between the two sides of the same skull. The average length of the canal is 11 mm., and a difference between the two canals of the same subject does not usually exceed 5 mm. Occasionally, the hypoglossal canal is septate. Usually, the canal is smooth in contour (Fig. 7–46).

The condyloid foramen may also be demonstrated in the adjoining portion of the occipital bone (Gathier and Bruyn).

THE SELLA TURCICA

Deformity of the sella turcica is often the only clue that abnormality exists within the cranium; hence a familiarity with its anatomy and radiologic appearance is essential.

The sella turcica is the superior saddle-shaped formation on the intracranial aspect of the body of the sphenoid bone. It is bounded anteriorly and posteriorly by the anterior and posterior clinoid processes respectively. The following parts of the sella may be identified (Fig. 7–47): (1) the dorsum sellae, (2) the diaphragma sellae, (3) the tuberculum sellae, (4) the hypophyseal fossa (pituitary fossa), (5) the sulcus chiasmatis or optic groove, (6) the anterior clinoid processes, and (7) the posterior clinoid processes.

The Dorsum Sellae.   This is a square-shaped plate of bone which is situated on the posterior aspect of the sella turcica and which terminates in the two posterior clinoid processes which project laterally and upward. This segment of bone is usually about 1 mm. in thickness when viewed on the lateral radiograph of the skull, with only a slight concavity on its anterosuperior aspect and another slight posterior concavity as it merges into the clivus. Abnormal erosion of the dorsum sellae is of great pathologic significance.

The Diaphragma Sellae.   This is a ring-shaped fold of dura mater covering the pituitary fossa, containing an aperture for the infundibulum. Actually, it is a roof over the hypophyseal fossa which contains the pituitary body.

The Tuberculum Sellae.   The tuberculum sellae is a prominence on the anterosuperior wall of the sella turcica. It lies immediately beneath a prominent variable ridge known as the limbus sphenoidalis. There is usually a groove for the optic chiasma just anterior to the tuberculum sellae, and the optic foramina are situated on either side of it, immediately beneath and medial to the anterior clinoid processes.

The Hypophyseal Fossa.   This is the basal concavity of the sella turcica which houses the pituitary gland. In a straight lateral projection, it appears to form a dense single curved line which lies above the sphenoid sinus. In infants, it tends to be shallow and somewhat prolonged in its anteroposterior dimension owing to the incomplete formation and ossification of the structures in the immediate vicinity of the tuberculum sellae. When the floor of the hypophyseal fossa takes on a double-contoured appearance, this manifestation may have considerable pathologic significance.

The Anterior Clinoid Processes.   The posterior border of the lesser wing of the sphenoid is prolonged medially as the anterior clinoid process on either side. Between the anterior clinoid process and the tuberculum sellae is a notch which marks the termination of the carotid groove for passage of the internal carotid artery. The ophthalmic artery is given off at this point.

The ophthalmic artery accompanies the optic nerve through the optic canal into the orbit.

The *carotid groove* begins at the medial side of the irregular foramen lacerum and ends medial to the anterior clinoid processes as described above. Occasionally there is a bony projection of this groove at its termination with each anterior clinoid process, called the middle clinoid process, which produces the caroticoclinoid foramen. Occasionally the middle clinoid process joins the posterior clinoid process instead, or it may branch and join both the anterior and posterior clinoid processes.

The transverse distance between the anterior clinoid processes is considerably greater than the corresponding distance between the posterior clinoid processes, and occasionally the posterior clinoid processes project forward so that they are situated between them. On the lateral radiograph of the skull, this im-

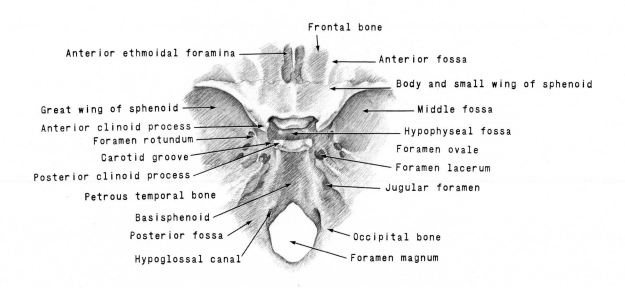

Relations of the Sella Turcica

Figure 7–47.   En face view of sella turcica.

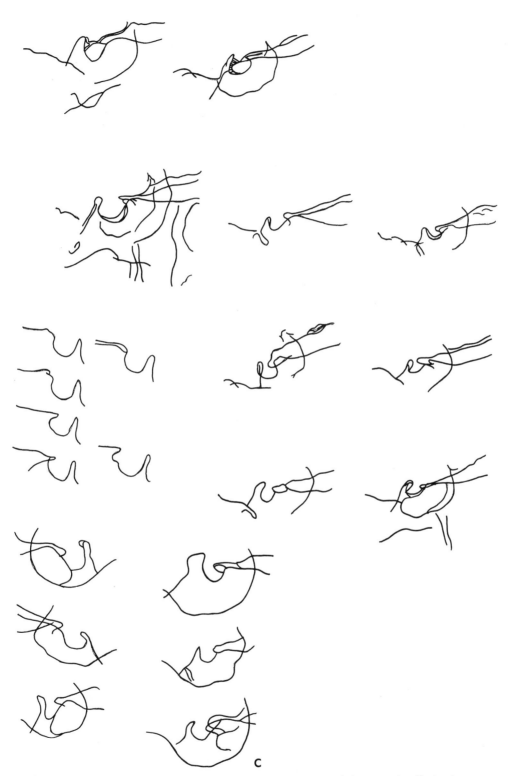

Figure 7–51 *Continued.* C. Variations in sagittal contour of the normal sella turcica.

6. The tuberculum sellae may be unduly prominent.
7. The sulcus chiasmatis (optic groove) may vary in depth and length, and the limbus sphenoidalis just anterior to it may be thick and knoblike.
8. The sella turcica varies considerably in shape, these variations usually being without clinical significance.

An unusually small sella turcica occurs in pituitary dwarfism, but ordinarily it has no pathologic significance.

There is no actual constant relationship between the size of the sella and the size of the hypophysis, although DiChiro and coworkers believe there is such a relationship insofar as it is indicated above.

ROUTINE RADIOGRAPHIC METHODS OF STUDY OF THE SELLA TURCICA

1. **Lateral Stereoscopic Projection of the Sella Turcica** (Fig. 6–45). The technique employed is similar to that used for the lateral view of the skull as a whole, except that a small cone is applied and the central ray is directed over a point approximately midway between the anterior tubercle of the pinna and the outer canthus of the eye. Stereoscopic films are obtained.

2. **Towne's Projection of the Skull** (Fig. 6–44). This view has already been described and should project the dorsum sellae and posterior clinoid processes into the foramen magnum. One can usually also identify the anterior clinoid processes.

3. **Posteroanterior View of the Skull** (Fig. 6–43). In this projection the tuberculum sellae and the anterior clinoid processes are frequently identified, although detail is usually poor in view of the overlying skull structures.

4. **Body Section Radiographs.** This method has not proved as useful here as in other parts of the anatomy, but may on occasion furnish corroborative information which has already been indicated by the other methods of investigation.

5. **Axial View of the Skull** (Fig. 6–46). In this view the floor of the sella turcica and adjoining anatomic structures may be seen to good advantage.

REFERENCES

Acheson, R. M.: Measuring the pituitary fossa from radiographs. Brit. J. Radiol., *29*:76–80, 1956.

Anson, B. J.: An Atlas of Human Anatomy. Philadelphia, W. B. Saunders Co., 1963.

Anson, B. J. (ed.): Morris' Human Anatomy. 12th edition. New York, McGraw-Hill, 1966.

Baker, H. L., Jr.: Myelographic examination of posterior fossa with positive contrast medium. Radiology, *81*:791–801, 1963.

Becker, J. A., and Woloshin, H. J.: Mastoiditis and cholesteatoma. Amer. J. Roentgenol., *87*:1019–1031, 1962.

Camp, J. D.: Normal and pathologic anatomy of the sella turcica as revealed at necropsy. Radiology, *1*:65, 1923.

Camp, J. D.: Normal and pathological anatomy of the sella turcica as revealed by roentgenograms. Amer. J. Roentgenol., *12*:143–155, 1924.

Cunningham, D. J.: Manual of Practical Anatomy. 12th edition. Edited by A. Robinson. London, Oxford University Press, 1959.

DiChiro, G., and Nelson, K. B.: The volume of the sella turcica. Amer. J. Roentgenol., *87*:989–1008, 1962.

Etter, L. E., and Cross, L. C.: Normal and pathologic roentgen anatomy of the middle ear and mastoid process. Amer. J. Roentgenol., *90*:1143–1155, 1963.

Etter, L. E., and Cross, L. C.: Projection angle, variations required to demonstrate the middle ear, antrum and mastoid process. Radiology, *80*:255–257, 1963.

Evans, R. A., Schwartz, J. F., and Chutorian, A. M.: Radiologic diagnosis in pediatric ophthalmology. Radiol. Clin. N. Amer., *1*:459–495, 1963.

Fisher, R. L., and DiChiro, G.: The small sella turcica. Amer. J. Roentgenol., *91*:996–1008, 1964.

Gass, H.: Pantopaque anterior basal cisternography of posterior fossa. Amer. J. Roentgenol., *90*:1197–1204, 1963.

Gathier, J. C., and Bruyn, G. W.: The so-called condyloid foramen. Amer. J. Roentgenol., *107*:515–519, 1969.

Goalwin, H. A.: 1000 optic canals: clinical anatomic, and roentgenologic study. J.A.M.A., *89*:1745–1948, 1927.

Hanafee, W. N., Hepler, R. S., and Coin, C. G.: Positive contrast orbitography. Amer. J. Roentgenol., *112*:342–348, 1971.

Hansman, C. F.: Growth of interorbital distance and skull thickness. Radiology, *86*:87–96, 1966.

Jacobs, J. B., and Grivas, N. E.: Interval cavernous sinography in the evaluation of intrasellar masses. Amer. J. Roentgenol., *107*:589–594, 1969.

Keyes, J. E. L.: Observations on 4000 optic foramina in human skulls of known origin. Arch. Ophthalmol., *13*:538–568, 1935.

Kier, E. L.: Embryology of the normal optic canal and its anomalies. Inves. Radiol., *1*:346–362, 1966.

Kier, E. L.: The infantile sella turcica: new roentgenologic and anatomic concepts based on a developmental study of the sphenoid bone. Amer. J. Roentgenol., *102*:747–767, 1968.

Kirdani, M. A.: The normal hypoglossal canal. Amer. J. Roentgenol., *99*:700–704, 1967.

Kornblum, K., and Kennedy, G. R.: Sphenoidal fissure: anatomic, roentgenologic and clinical studies. Amer. J. Roentgenol., *47*:845–858, 1942.

Lapayowker, M. S., and Cliff, M. M.: Bone changes in acoustic neuromas. Amer. J. Roentgenol., *107*:652–658, 1969.

Last, R. J.: Wolff's Anatomy of the Eye and Orbit. Fifth edition. Philadelphia, W. B. Saunders Co., 1951.

Lee, K. F., and Lin, S-R.: An improved technique in orbital venography with the use of innovar and compression devices. Amer. J. Roentgenol., *112*:339–341, 1971.

Lombardi, G.: Orbitography. *In* Newton, T. H., and Potts, D. G.: Radiology of the Skull and Brain. St. Louis, C. V. Mosby Co., 1971.

Lombardi, G.: Radiology in Neuro-ophthalmology. Baltimore, Williams and Wilkins Co., 1967.

Lombardi, G., and Passerini, A.: Venography of the orbit: technique and anatomy. Brit. J. Radiol., *41*:282–286, 1968.

Meschan, I., and Meschan, R.: Radiographic Positioning and Related Anatomy. Philadelphia, W. B. Saunders Co., 1968.

Meschan, I., and Meschan, R.: Analysis of Roentgen Signs. Philadelphia, W. B. Saunders Co., 1973.

Newton, T. H., and Potts, D. G.: Radiology of the Skull and Brain. The Skull, Vol. 1, Book 1. St. Louis, C. V. Mosby Co., 1971.

Pendergrass, E. P., Hodes, P. J., Tondreau, R., and Marden P.: The tympanic cavity and auditory ossicles—roentgen findings in health and disease. Amer. J. Roentgenol., *76*:327–342, 1956.

Pendergrass, E. P., Schaeffer, J. P., and Hodes, P. J.: The Head and Neck in Roentgen Diagnosis. Second edition. Springfield, Ill., Charles C Thomas, 1956.

Potter, G. D.: The pterygopalatine fossa and canal. Amer. J. Roentgenol., *107*:520–525, 1969.

Potter, quoted by Kieffer, S. A.: Orbit. *In* Newton, T. H., and Potts, D. G.: Radiology of the Skull and Brain. St. Louis, C. V. Mosby Co., 1971.

Potter, G. D., and Trokel, S. L.: Optic canal. *In* Newton, T. H., and Potts, D. G.: Radiology of the Skull and Brain. St. Louis, C. V. Mosby Co., 1971.

Proetz, A. W.: The Displacement Method of Sinus Diagnosis and Treatment. St. Louis, Annals Pub. Co., 1931.

Reese, D. F., and Bull, J. W. D.: Positive contrast demonstration of normal internal acoustic meatus, Meckel's cave and jugular foramen. Amer. J. Roentgenol., *100*:650–655, 1967.

Russell, D. B., and Miller, J. D. R.: Orbital venography. Radiology, *103*:267–273, 1972.

Sansregret, A.: Technique for study of the middle ear. Amer. J. Roentgenol., *90*:1156–1166, 1963.

Sargent, E. N., and Ebersole, C.: Dacrocystography. Amer. J. Roentgenol., *102*:831–839, 1968.

Scanlan, R. L.: Positive contrast medium (Iophendylate) in diagnosis of acoustic neuroma. Arch. Otolaryngol., *80*:698–706, 1964.

Schaefer, R. E.: Roentgen anatomy of the temporal bone: tomographic studies. Med. Radiography and Photography, *48*:2–22, 1972.

Schaeffer, J. P.: The Nose, Paranasal Sinuses, Nasolacrimal Passageway and Olfactory Organ in Man. New York, McGraw-Hill, Blakiston Div., 1920.

Silverman, F.: Roentgen standards for size of the pituitary fossa from infancy through adolescence. Amer. J. Roentgenol., *78*:451–460, 1957.

Valvassori, G. E.: Laminagraphy of the ear. Normal roentgenographic anatomy. Amer. J. Roentgenol., *89*:1155–1167, 1963.

Valvassori, G. E., and Pierce, R. H.: The normal internal auditory canal. Amer. J. Roentgenol., *92*:1232–1241, 1964.

Whalen, J. P., and Berne, A. S.: The roentgen anatomy of the lateral walls of the orbit (orbital line) and the maxillary antrum (antral line) in the submentovertical view. Amer. J. Roentgenol., *91*:1009–1011, 1964.

Wheeler, E. C., and Baker, H. L., Jr.: The ophthalmic arterial complex in angiographic diagnosis. Radiology, *83*:26–35, 1964.

8

The Brain

GROSS ANATOMY OF THE BRAIN AND MENINGES AS RELATED TO RADIOLOGY

The Meninges

The brain is completely enveloped by three fibrous coverings called meninges: (1) a *pia mater,* which is closely applied to the surface of the brain with no structures intervening; (2) an *arachnoid membrane,* separated from the pia mater by the *subarachnoid space* (the pia mater and arachnoid together constitute the *leptomeninges*); and (3) a *dura mater,* the outermost layer, which is very tough and is separated from the arachnoid by a potential *subdural space.* The dura mater has two layers: an outer *endosteal layer,* which adheres tightly to bones for which it serves as periosteum, and an inner *meningeal layer,* which is a smooth mesothelial layer on its inner aspect.

The pia mater covers the entire brain, dipping down between the gyri of the cerebrum and the folia of the cerebellum; it also forms the tela choroidea of the ventricles.

Normally the space between the dura mater and the arachnoid is "potential" and virtually nonexistent, but abnormally the two may be stripped apart, as by hematoma or during a pneumoencephalographic procedure. The subdural space is probably continuous with the tissue spaces of the nerve roots passing through it at spinal cord levels. A small amount of fluid is contained in this space. The outward projection of the subdural space is most marked around the optic and vestibulocochlear nerves.

The two layers of cranial dura mater contain large *blood sinuses* (dural venous sinuses) and *venous lacunae* in certain places.

In the subarachnoid space, there are numerous small and fragile bridges of tissue densely packed over the cerebral convexities (Fig. 8–3).

The thin layer of cells lying in the central canal of the spinal cord as well as the ventricles of the brain is called the *ependymal layer.*

Those aspects of the meninges which are most important to the radiologist are:
1. The reflections or reduplications of the meningeal layer of the dura that form two vertical rigid membranes and two horizontal membranes.
2. The dural venous sinuses.
3. The venous lakes or lacunae into which arachnoidal granulations project.
4. The cerebral spinal fluid cisterns.
5. The meningeal vessels.

Reflections or Reduplications of the Meningeal Layers of the Dura (Fig. 8–1). The two vertical sickle-shaped folds of the dura mater are the falx cerebri and falx cerebelli respectively, and the two horizontal rooflike folds are the tentorium cerebelli and the diaphragma sellae. The *falx cerebri,* separating the two cerebral hemispheres, is attached to the skull at the crista galli and internal occipital protuberance, where it joins the tentorium cerebelli. Its inferior border is free. The *falx cerebelli* divides the cerebellar hemispheres and is attached to the internal occipital crest from the protuberance to the foramen magnum.

The *tentorium cerebelli* separates the cerebellum and cerebrum and is attached posteriorly and laterally along the transverse sinus as well as to the ridge of the petrous bone and posterior clinoid process. It has a free margin called the *incisura tentorii* through which the cerebral peduncles pass. The falx cerebri is attached to its cephalic surface in the midline.

The *diaphragma sellae* forms a roof for the sella turcica and is attached to the clinoid processes; it has a small opening through which the infundibulum passes.

Dural Venous Sinuses. The dural venous sinuses are venous channels lying between the two layers of dura mater in certain regions of the skull (Fig. 8–2).

The *superior sagittal venous sinus* lies in the convexity of the falx cerebri and receives superior cerebral veins, venous lacunae, diploic and dural veins, and parietal emissary veins. It extends from the foramen caecum to the internal occipital protuberance, where it usually deviates toward the right transverse sinus.

The *inferior sagittal venous sinus* lies in the free inferior edge

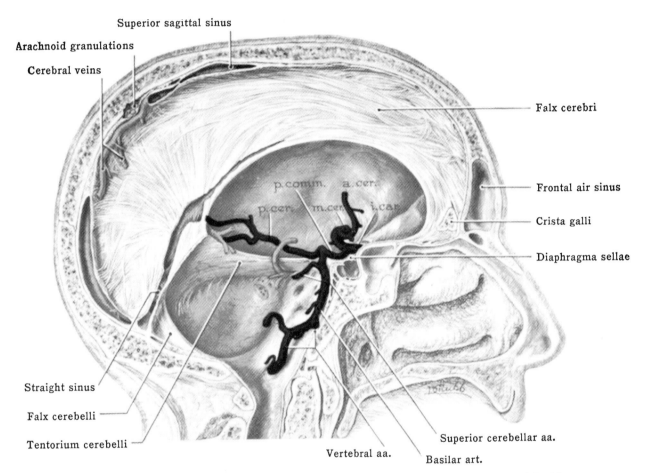

Figure 8–1. Folds of the dura mater. There are two vertical sickle-shaped folds: the falx cerebri and the falx cerebelli, and there are two rooflike folds: the tentorium cerebelli and the diaphragma sellae. (Reproduced by permission from J. C. B. Grant: An Atlas of Anatomy, 5th ed. Copyright © 1962, The Williams & Wilkins Company.)

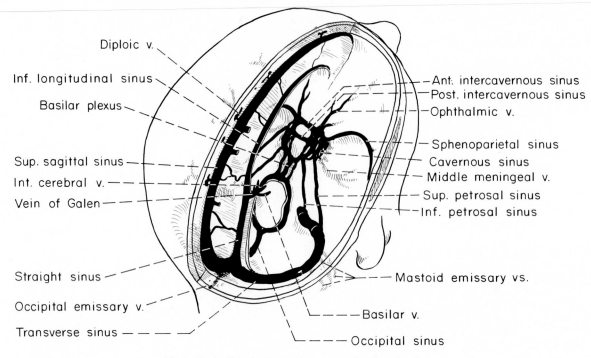

Diploic v.

Inf. longitudinal sinus

Basilar plexus

Sup. sagittal sinus

Int. cerebral v.

Vein of Galen

Straight sinus

Occipital emissary v.

Transverse sinus

Ant. intercavernous sinus
Post. intercavernous sinus
Ophthalmic v.

Sphenoparietal sinus
Cavernous sinus
Middle meningeal v.
Sup. petrosal sinus
Inf. petrosal sinus

Mastoid emissary vs.

Basilar v.

Occipital sinus

Figure 8–2.   Dural venous sinuses as related to the dura.

of the falx cerebri and ends in the straight sinus, receiving veins from the falx cerebri and the medial side of the hemispheres.

The *straight sinus* lies at the attachment of the falx cerebri to the tentorium cerebelli and terminates in the left transverse sinus usually. It receives the great cerebral vein of Galen from the internal aspect of the brain posteriorly, the left transverse sinus (usually), and the superior cerebellar veins.

The *transverse sinuses* (also called *lateral sinuses*) are situated on each side of the midline beginning at the internal occipital protuberance in the margin of the tentorium cerebelli and passing laterally and somewhat caudad to the petrous bone. They then bend caudally and medially to form the sigmoid sinus, which in turn enters the jugular foramina.

The *occipital sinus* is situated in the attached margin of the falx cerebelli, beginning at the foramen magnum and ending at the sinus confluens.

The *sinus confluens* (confluence of sinuses) is situated at the internal occipital protuberance where the superior sagittal, straight, occipital, and transverse sinuses all meet.

The *cavernous sinuses* are situated on each side of the sphenoid bone superiorly and receive the superior ophthalmic and cerebral veins. They communicate with the transverse sinus through the superior petrosal sinus, and with the internal jugular vein

through the inferior petrosal sinus. There are communicating plexuses surrounding the internal carotid and adjoining the sella turcica, as well as the pterygoid venous plexus in the nasopharyngeal region. The cavernous sinus also communicates with the angular vein through the superior ophthalmic vein.

The *intercavernous sinuses* are situated anteriorly and posteriorly around the sella turcica, connecting the cavernous sinuses.

The *superior petrosal sinuses* are situated along the superior border of the petrous bone in the attachment of the tentorium cerebelli; they join the cavernous and transverse sinuses. These sinuses receive the cerebellar, inferior cerebral, and tympanic veins.

The *inferior petrosal sinuses* are situated along the suture between the basilar portion of the occipital and the petrous portion of the temporal bones. They join the cavernous sinuses and internal jugular veins on each side. Additionally, they receive the internal auditory vein, the inferior cerebellar veins, and veins from the medulla.

There is, additionally, a *basilar plexus* situated on the basilar portion of the occipital bone which connects the inferior petrosal sinuses to each other and communicates with the anterior vertebral plexus.

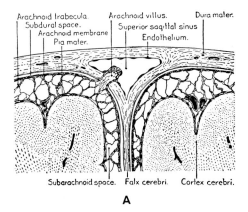

Arachnoid trabecula. Arachnoid villus. Dura mater.
Subdural space. Superior sagittal sinus
Arachnoid membrane. Endothelium.
Pia mater.

Subarachnoid space. Falx cerebri. Cortex cerebri.

A

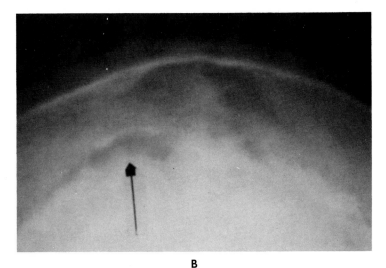

B

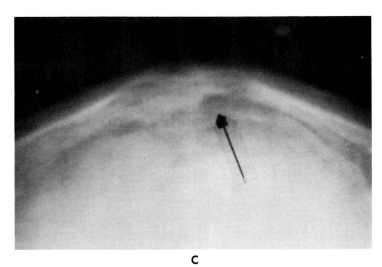

C

Figure 8–3. *A*, Schematic diagram of coronal section of meninges and cortex. (From Weed, Amer. J. Anat., courtesy of Wistar Institute.) *B* and *C*. Close-up view of arachnoid granulations impressing upon the calvarium.

Venous Lacunae (Associated with Arachnoidal Granulations). The venous lacunae are small spaces or clefts that communicate with the meningeal veins and with the blood sinuses. They also communicate with the emissary veins and the diploic veins. The majority of these lie at the sides of the superior sagittal sinus, but others are found in the tentorium associated with the transverse sinuses and the straight sinus.

The *arachnoidal villi or granulations* (pacchionian bodies) are small capillary glomerular tufts of variable size protruding into the venous sinuses or lacunae (Fig. 8–3). These represent an invasion of the dura by the arachnoid membrane; they are covered by a greatly thinned wall of the venous sinus which may consist merely of endothelium. Fluid injected into the subarachnoid space experimentally passes from the villi into the venous sinuses. They are not usually seen in infancy and very rarely until the third year; after the age of 7 they become more common, increasing in number thereafter. As they grow, they absorb the adjoining bone from pressure, producing the pits or depressions on the inner wall of the calvarium that are described in Chapter 6.

Another view of the falx, tentoria, and incisura of the tentorium allowing the brain stem to pass through is shown in Figure 8–4. A detailed view of the tentorial "notch" from its superior aspect is shown in Figure 8–5. The midbrain, surrounded by the subarachnoid space, lies in the tentorial notch as shown. Mass lesions of the brain may cause herniation from one intracranial compartment to another through the tentorial notch. Blockage of the cerebrospinal fluid at the level of the cerebral aqueduct causing increased intracranial pressure results in considerable dilatation above the tentorium cerebelli.

Subarachnoid Cisterns (Fig. 8–6 *A,B*). In certain areas surrounding the brain, especially at its base, the arachnoid and pia are separated by spaces called subarachnoid cisterns. Those usually identified are:

1. A *basal cistern,* divided by the optic chiasm into two parts: (a) the *cisterna chiasmatis,* and (b) the *cisterna interpeduncularis.*

2. The *cisterna pontis* surrounding the pons and continuing anteriorly with the basal cistern and posteriorly with the subarachnoid space around the medulla oblongata.

3. The *cistern of the great cerebral vein of Galen* (connecting with the *cisterna ambiens*), situated between the splenium of the corpus callosum and the superior surfaces of the cerebellum and mesencephalon. It is connected ventrally around the cerebral peduncles with the basal cistern and caudally with the *superior cerebellar cistern* (Fig. 8–7).

4. The *cisterna cerebello-medullaris or cisterna magna,* which is the space between the inferior surface of the cerebellum and the dorsal surface of the medulla oblongata. It continues caudally into the spinal subarachnoid space, and is directly continuous with the fluid in the fourth ventricle by way of the foramen of Magendie in the midline and the foramina of Luschka laterally.

5. Other cisterns of lesser depth are the *cistern of the corpus*

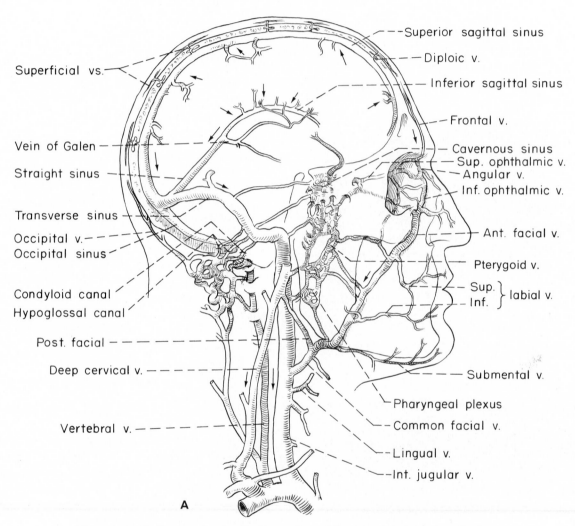

Figure 8–4. A. Diagram showing the flow pattern of the venous drainage from the head.

Figure 8–4 continued on the opposite page.

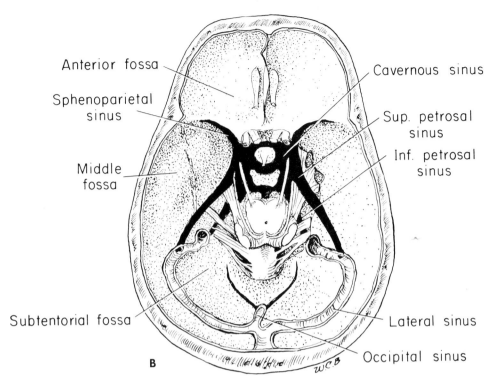

Anterior fossa

Sphenoparietal sinus

Middle fossa

Subtentorial fossa

Cavernous sinus

Sup. petrosal sinus

Inf. petrosal sinus

Lateral sinus

Occipital sinus

B

Figure 8–4 *Continued.* B. Major dural sinuses at the base of the brain seen from above. (Modified from Bailey, P.: Intracranial Tumors, 1933. Courtesy of Charles C Thomas, Publisher, Springfield, Illinois.)

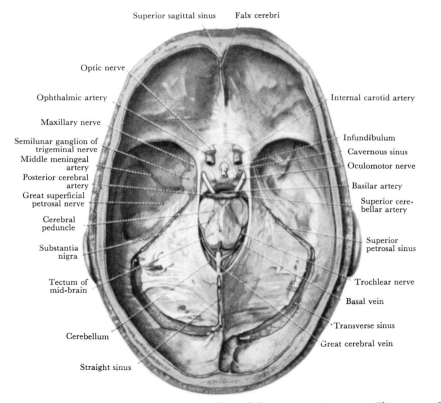

Superior sagittal sinus   Falx cerebri

Optic nerve

Ophthalmic artery

Maxillary nerve

Semilunar ganglion of trigeminal nerve
Middle meningeal artery
Posterior cerebral artery
Great superficial petrosal nerve

Cerebral peduncle

Substantia nigra

Tectum of mid-brain

Cerebellum

Straight sinus

Internal carotid artery

Infundibulum

Cavernous sinus

Oculomotor nerve

Basilar artery

Superior cerebellar artery

Superior petrosal sinus

Trochlear nerve

Basal vein

Transverse sinus

Great cerebral vein

Figure 8–5. Diagram of the skull illustrating the tentorial notch from its superior aspect. The tectum of the midbrain and the floor of the left middle fossa has been exposed by removal of the dura and cerebrum. (From Cunningham's Manual of Practical Anatomy, 12th ed. Vol. 3. London, Oxford University Press, 1958.)

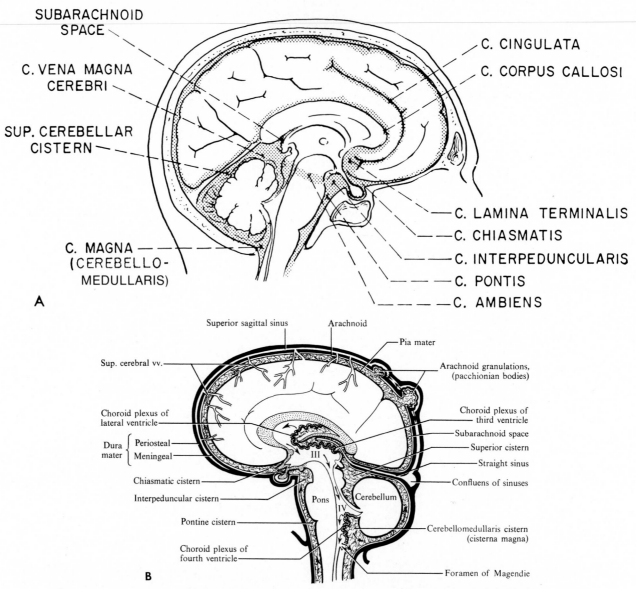

SUBARACHNOID SPACE

C. VENA MAGNA CEREBRI

SUP. CEREBELLAR CISTERN

C. MAGNA (CEREBELLO-MEDULLARIS)

A

C. CINGULATA

C. CORPUS CALLOSI

C. LAMINA TERMINALIS

C. CHIASMATIS

C. INTERPEDUNCULARIS

C. PONTIS

C. AMBIENS

Superior sagittal sinus   Arachnoid

Sup. cerebral vv.

Pia mater

Arachnoid granulations, (pacchionian bodies)

Choroid plexus of lateral ventricle

Choroid plexus of third ventricle

Dura mater { Periosteal / Meningeal

III

Subarachnoid space

Superior cistern

Straight sinus

Chiasmatic cistern

Confluens of sinuses

Interpeduncular cistern

Pons   Cerebellum

Pontine cistern

IV

Cerebellomedullaris cistern (cisterna magna)

Choroid plexus of fourth ventricle

Foramen of Magendie

B

Figure 8–6. *A.* Diagram illustrating subarachnoid cisterns. Not shown: Cisterna fossae lateralis cerebri, and C. laminae terminalis. *B.* Relations of meninges to brain, cord, and cerebrospinal fluids (based on Rasmussen, Principal Nervous Pathways). (From Pansky, B., and House, E. L.: Review of Gross Anatomy, 2nd ed. New York, Macmillan Co. 1969.)

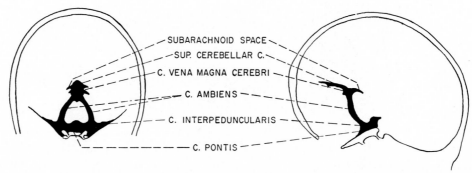

SUBARACHNOID SPACE

SUP. CEREBELLAR C.

C. VENA MAGNA CEREBRI

C. AMBIENS

C. INTERPEDUNCULARIS

C. PONTIS

Figure 8–7. Cisterna ambiens in Towne's and lateral projections. (Modified from Robertson, E. G.: Pneumoencephalography. 1967. Charles C Thomas, Publisher, Springfield, Illinois.)

callosum; the *cistern* of the fossa of the lateral aspect of the cerebrum, *adjoining the sylvian fissure;* and the *cistern of the lamina terminalis,* a shallow structure surrounding the lamina terminalis.

The subarachnoid space as described earlier communicates with the fourth ventricle by means of the foramina of Luschka and Magendie and with the perineural space around the olfactory and optic nerves.

Blood Supply of the Dura. From the radiologic standpoint, it is most convenient to divide the dural blood supply into five regions (Salamon et al., quoted in Wilson) (Table 8–1):

1. The convex dura above the tentorium.
2. The convex dura below the tentorium.
3. Basal dura.
4. Falx cerebri.
5. Tentorium cerebelli.

Meningeal Arteries. Most of the meningeal arteries are very thin and relatively straight (Fig. 8–8). The chief arteries of the dura are shown in Table 8–2 and also in Fig. 6–11 *C).*

There are three main blood vessels supplying the head: (1) the *external carotid* supplies, for the most part, the dura over the convexities of the skull, and also the floor of the anterior, middle, and posterior fossae lateral to the midline; (2) the *internal carotid* supplies those areas, including the midline of the base, from the frontal crest anteriorly to the midclivus posteriorly; (3) the *vertebral artery* supplies the area from the midline of the base from midclivus to occipital crest (Fig. 8–8 *E).*

The falx cerebri and tentorium cerebelli receive branches from all of these three main sources.

The *middle meningeal artery* is the most important branch of the maxillary artery (Fig. 8–8). It enters the cranial cavity by passing through the foramen spinosum in the sphenoid bone and, together with an accompanying vein, lies in grooves in the calvarium as shown. Both it and its accompanying vein are susceptible to injury, resulting in hemorrhage or hematoma. In addition to its anterior and posterior branches, it has the following branches as well: orbital (through the superior orbital fissure, anastomosing with the recurrent meningeal branch of the lacrimal artery); temporal; superior tympanic, extending to the tympanic cavity; ganglionic, supplying the roots and ganglion of the trigeminal nerve; and petrosal, giving twigs to the facial nerve and the tympanic cavity.

These various meningeal arterial vessels enter the collateral circulation of the brain in the presence of intracranial arterial occlusive disease. In this connection the most frequently encountered anastomoses are (Fig. 8–9):

1. Those between the ophthalmic artery and external carotid branches in and around the orbit.
2. Those of the muscular branches of the vertebral artery with those of the external carotid and deep cervical arteries.

TABLE 8–1 BLOOD SUPPLY OF DURA*

1. **Convexity above Tentorium**
   Middle meningeal mainly
   Aslo anterior meningeal of anterior ethmoidal (from ophthalmic)

2. **Convexity below Tentorium**
   Meningeal branches from occipital
   Meningeal branches of vertebral (in midline)

3. **Base of Skull**
   Over Orbits: middle meningeal
   Cribriform Plate: anterior meningeal
   Planium Sphenoidale: anterior meningeal
   Middle Fossa Lateral to Sella Turcica: middle meningeal
   Sella and Upper Clivus: internal carotid
   Lower Clivus and Anterior Half of Foramen Magnum: ascending pharyngeal
   vertebral

4. **Falx Cerebri**
   Deep Falx Cerebri: anterior cerebral
   Outer Falx Cerebri: anterior ethmoidal
   middle meningeal
   posterior meningeal from vertebral

5. **Tentorium Cerebelli**
   Deep Inner: Tentorial artery, branch of internal carotid
   Superior Medial Third: posterior meningeal branch of vertebral
   Posterior Central Third: meningeal twigs from occipital
   Anterior Lateral Third: posterior branch of middle meningeal

*Data from Wilson, M.: The Anatomic Foundation of Neuroradiology of the Brain, 2nd ed. Boston, Little, Brown & Co., 1972.

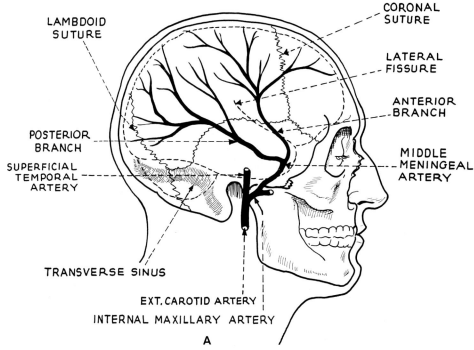

Figure 8–8. A. Projection of middle meningeal artery in relation to the skull.

Figure 8–8 continued on the following page.

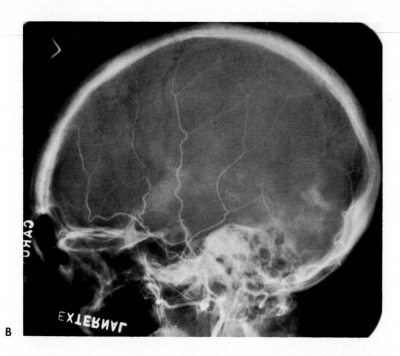

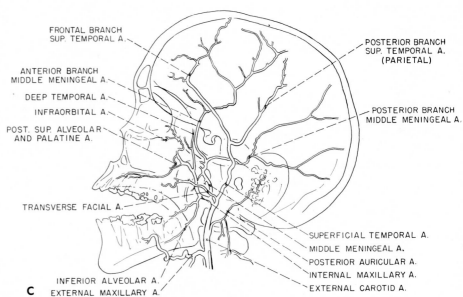

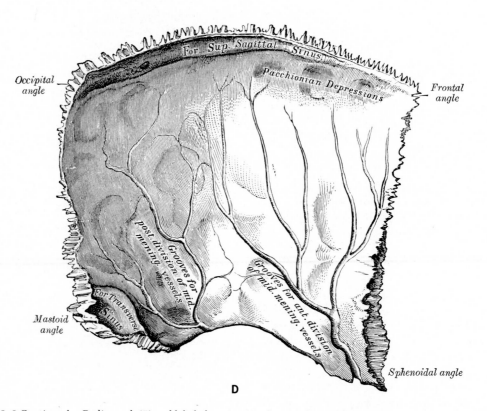

Figure 8–8 Continued.   Radiograph (B) and labeled tracing (C) of external carotid arteriogram. D. Left parietal bone, inner surface.

Figure 8–8 continued on opposite page.

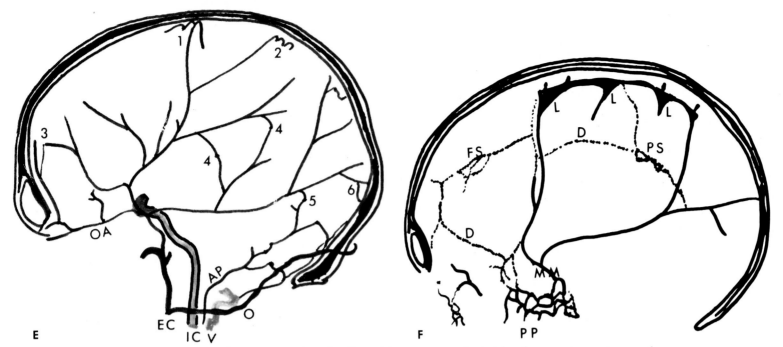

Figure 8-8 *Continued.* Diagrammatic and radiographic appearance of arterial and venous impressions on the bones of the calvarium. (*E*) Diagram of meningeal artery circulation. The middle meningeal artery arises from the external carotid (EC), passes through the foramen spinosum of the sphenoid bone and enters the cranium. It runs forward in a groove on the great wing of the sphenoid bone and divides into two branches, the anterior and posterior. The anterior branch crosses the great wing of the sphenoid and then divides into branches that spread out between the dura mater and internal surface of the cranium. Some of its branches pass upward as far as the vertex of the skull, and others backward to the occipital region. The posterior branch curves backward on the squamous portion of the temporal bone and reaches the parietal, where its branches supply the posterior part of the dura mater and cranium. The various anastomoses of the branches of the middle meningeal are numbered. 1 indicates anastomoses with branches of the pericallosal artery; 2 represents anastomoses with branches of the middle cerebral artery that reach the calvarium; 3 is the site of anastomoses with the meningeal branches of the ophthalmic artery (OA), which arises from the internal carotid artery (IC) at the carotid siphon; 4 represents anastomoses between the posterior and anterior branches of the middle meningeal; 5 indicates anastomoses between the meningeal branches of the ascending pharyngeal artery and the posterior branch of the middle meningeal; 6 is the site of anastomoses between the posterior branch of the middle meningeal and the occipital artery and its meningeal branches (O). The vertebral artery (V) sends out meningeal branches that anastomose with those of the ascending pharyngeal and posterior branch of the middle meningeal. *F.* Diagram showing the main middle meningeal veins. Generally, the middle meningeal veins accompany the middle meningeal arteries and thus there is an anterior and a posterior branch complex, as in Fig. 8–8E. The dotted lines indicate some of the main diploic veins that can be identified on many skull films (D). The "frontal star" (FS) is a cluster of frontal diploic veins that ultimately anastomose with the middle meningeal. The "parietal star" (PS) is a similar collection in the parietal bone that ultimately draws into the middle meningeal, posterior or anterior. The lacunae (L) are venous lakes that communicate with the middle meningeal veins. Arachnoid granulations generally protrude into the lacunae. PP, pharyngeal plexus. (*E* and *F* from Meschan, I.: Seminars in Roentgenology, 9:125, 1974. Used by permission.)

3. Those of meningeal and scalp arteries with distal branches of the cerebral arteries (Wilson).

The ophthalmic-orbital anastomosis alone may take over as much as 20 per cent of the total cerebral blood flow under unusual circumstances (Fazekas et al.).

Meningeal Veins (Fig. 8–8 *F*). The meningeal veins accompany the arteries, usually one vein to each artery. The middle meningeal artery may, however, have two such accompanying veins. These veins communicate with the venous sinuses and with the diploic veins, and drain blood also from the venous lacunae. The lacunae receive meningeal diploic and emissary veins and communicate ultimately with the superior sagittal sinus.

TABLE 8-2 ARTERIES OF THE MENINGES*

Name	Source	Area	Entry
Meningeal br.	Occipital	Post. fossa	Jugular foramen
Post. meningeal	Ascend. pharyngeal	Post. fossa	Jugular foramen
Meningeal br.	Ascend. pharyngeal	Post. fossa	Hypoglossal foramen
Meningeal br.	Vertebral	Post. fossa	Foramen magnum
Meningeal br.	Ascend. Pharyngeal	Middle fossa	Foramen lacerum
Middle meningeal	Maxillary	Middle fossa	Foramen spinosum
Access. meningeal	Maxillary	Middle fossa	Foramen ovale
Recurrent br.	Lacrimal	Ant. fossa	Sup. orbital fissure
Meningeal br.	Ant. ethmoid	Ant. fossa	Ant. ethmoid canal
Meningeal br.	Post. ethmoid	Ant. fossa	Post. ethmoid canal

*From Pansky, B., and House, E. L.: Review of Gross Anatomy. New York, Macmillan Co., 1964, p. 72.

359

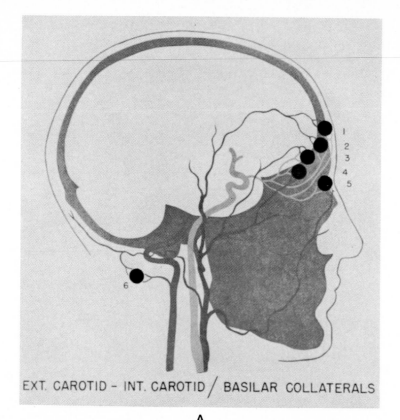

EXT. CAROTID – INT. CAROTID / BASILAR COLLATERALS

A

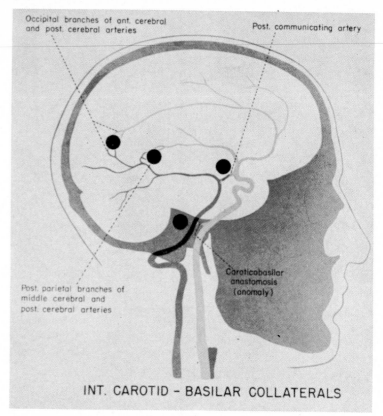

Occipital branches of ant. cerebral and post. cerebral arteries

Post. communicating artery

Post. parietal branches of middle cerebral and post. cerebral arteries

Caroticobasilar anastomosis (anomaly)

INT. CAROTID – BASILAR COLLATERALS

B

Multiple anastomoses on external surface of cerebrum

ANT. CEREBRAL – MIDDLE CEREBRAL COLLATERALS

C

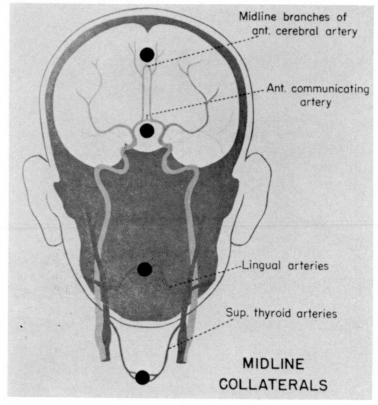

Midline branches of ant. cerebral artery

Ant. communicating artery

Lingual arteries

Sup. thyroid arteries

MIDLINE COLLATERALS

D

Figure 8–9. *A.* Sites of communications around the orbit between branches of the external carotid artery and those of the ophthalmic artery. *B.* Communications that cross the circle of Willis between the internal carotid and the vertebrobasilar system. *C.* Collateral communications over the surface of the cerebral hemispheres between the peripheral branches of the anterior and middle cerebral arteries and also between the distal branches of the posterior cerebral artery and branches of the anterior and middle cerebral group. *D.* The usual collateral channels most often demonstrated by angiography, which cross the midline in head and neck. (From Tatelman, M.: *Radiology, 75:*349–362, 1960.)

Figure 8–9 continued on the opposite page.

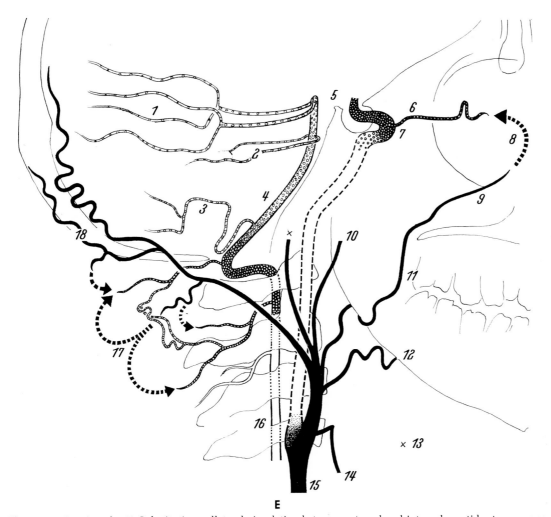

E

Figure 8–9 *Continued.* E. Substituting collateral circulation between external and internal carotid artery on one side and vertebral artery at the level of the atlas on the other side. (1) Posterior cerebral arteries, (2) superior cerebellar arteries, (3) posterior inferior cerebellar artery, (4) basilar artery, (5) dorsum sellae, (6) ophthalmic artery, (7) siphon, (8) anastomoses of the ophthalmic artery, (9) angular artery, (10) maxillary artery, (11) facial artery, (12) lingual artery, (13) superficial temporal artery, (14) superior thyroid artery, (15) common carotid artery. (16) vertebral artery, (17) anastomoses between muscular branches of the vertebral artery and external carotid artery. (From Krayenbühl, H. A., and Yaşargil, M. G.; Zerebrale Angiographie, 2nd ed. Stuttgart, G. Thieme Verlag, 1965.)

Figure 8–9 continued on the following page.

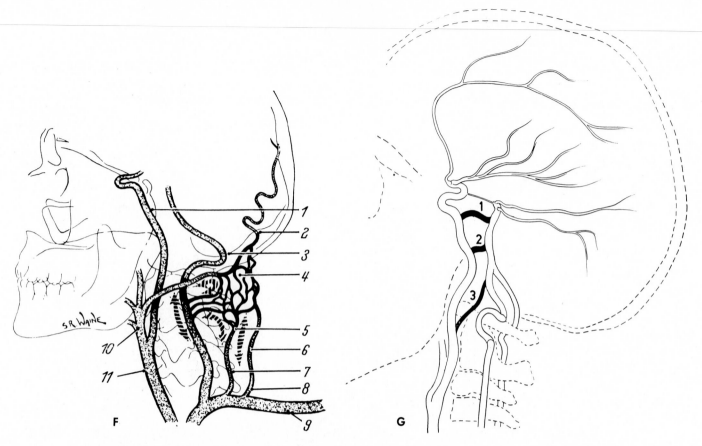

Figure 8-9 *Continued.* *F.* The "cervical arterial collateral network" which joins the carotid, subclavian, and vertebral arteries. (Diagram from Bosniak, Amer. J. Roentgen., 91:1232, 1964.)

(1) Internal carotid artery, (2) occipital artery, (3) vertebral artery, (4) descending cervical artery, (5) ascending cervical artery, (6) deep cervical artery, (7) thyreocervical artery, (8) costocervical artery, (9) subclavian artery, (10) external carotid artery, (11) common carotid artery.

G. Persistent primitive channels between the internal carotid artery and the basilar artery. (1) Primitive trigeminal artery, (2) primitive acoustic artery, (3) primitive hypoglossal artery. (From Krayenbühl, H. A., and Yaşargil, M. G.: Zerebrale Angiographie, 2nd ed. Stuttgart, G. Thieme Verlag, 1965.)

Anatomic Relationships Between Branches of the Middle Meningeal Artery, the Meningeal Veins, the Dura, and the Inner Table of the Skull (Schechter et al.). These variable relationships are illustrated in Figure 8-10. The artery and the adjoining venous channels are often within the diploë; at other times they are together in the grooves on the inner table of the skull, and in certain areas the artery and vein may not accompany one another. This last relationship is extremely important if trauma causes a meningeal vessel to be torn. The superimposition of trauma and the various possibilities are further illustrated in Figure 8-10 *B.*

Jones (1912a) has postulated that the grooves on the inner table of the skull that are commonly related to meningeal arteries and veins actually accommodate the accompanying meningeal veins rather than the arteries themselves.

MENINGEAL STRUCTURES: SPECIAL ANATOMIC FEATURES

Cavernous Sinus. By inserting a percutaneous type of catheter into the internal jugular vein and passing it cephalad into the inferior petrosal sinus, it is possible to study the pattern of the cavernous sinus. The four types of drainage of the inferior petrosal sinus that are encountered by this method are illustrated in Figure 8-11 (Shiu et al.).

The internal carotid artery is situated between the layers of the dura, forming the cavernous sinus (called the "cavernous portion of the internal carotid artery"). This portion of the internal carotid artery supplies branches to the dura at the base of the skull, the cavernous sinus itself, the sella turcica and its contents,

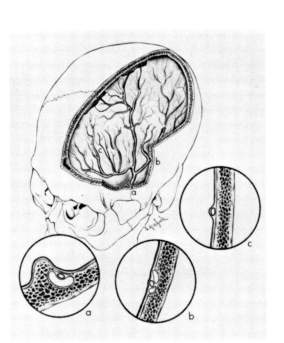

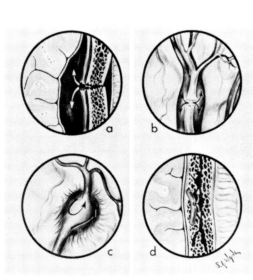

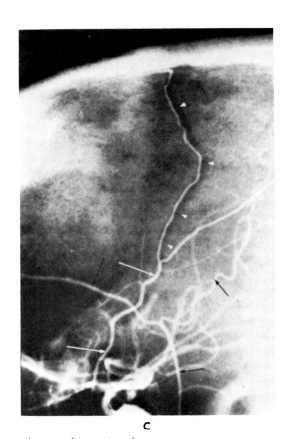

A   C

Figure 8–10.   *A.* The anatomical relationships between branches of the middle meningeal artery, the meningeal veins, the dura, and the inner table of the skull are illustrated here. Note that the middle meningeal artery and its accompanying venous channel are often within the diploe (*a*) in the temporal area. More distally (*b*) the usual situation is that the middle meningeal arteries and veins groove the inner table of the skull. In certain areas more distally (*c*) the middle meningeal artery is not accompanied by venous channels. Note that some of the middle meningeal veins accompanying the middle meningeal artery are shown draining into lacunar channels in the region of the superior sagittal sinus.

Another pathway of drainage is through the sphenoparietal sinus and into the cavernous sinus, or along the floor of the middle fossa toward the foramen ovale, or into the superior petrosal sinus. Some venous channels still more posteriorly situated drain into the transverse sinus. *B.* In drawing *a* as in drawing *c* in the preceding figure (*A*) the middle meningeal artery is not accompanied by a venous channel. A tear in the middle meningeal artery allows the extravasation of blood and contrast material into the epidural space or through the fracture line into the subgaleal space. In drawing *b*, where the middle meningeal artery is accompanied by a venous channel, as in *b* of the preceding figure, blood and contrast material pass out of the torn meningeal artery into the venous channel. This fistula is a type of "protective mechanism." In *c* blood clot has sealed off a tear in the middle meningeal artery, forming a "pseudoaneurysm." This is another type of "protective mechanism." In *d* a tear in the middle meningeal artery as it traverses the diploic space in the temporal area (as in drawing *a*, Part A) allows passage of blood and contrast material into venous diploic channels. *C.* Left common carotid angiogram, lateral view. The small white arrows point to the main stem of the middle meningeal artery. The white arrowheads point to the vascular groove in the skull which is much larger than the lumen of the middle meningeal artery, much larger, in fact, than the lumen and walls of the artery. This is because the groove accommodates venous channels as well as the arterial channel. Note that there are also branches of the middle meningeal artery which do not run in the area of the large venous channels grooving the skull. The small black arrows point to branches of the superficial temporal artery which here are mainly unrelated to the groove in the skull. (From Schechter, M. M., Zingesser, L. H., and Rayport, M.: Radiology, 86:686–695, 1966.)

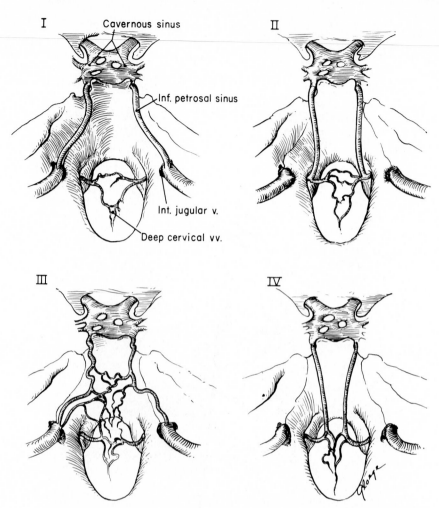

Figure 8–11. The four types of drainage of the inferior petrosal sinus as depicted in our study. Excellent filling of the cavernous sinus and orbital veins can be obtained from Type I and Type II, since the catheter tip can be placed either adjacent to or actually in the orifice of the inferior petrosal sinus. In patients with Type III, the channel is more of a plexus of veins. Even under these circumstances, contrast material injected near the orifice of the inferior petrosal sinus will usually reflux to outline the cavernous sinus. The orbital veins rarely fill in this type of patient. Type IV anatomic configurations of the inferior petrosal sinus draining into the deep cervical plexus are impossible to investigate via the jugular route. (From Shiu, P. C., Hanafee, W. N., Wilson, G. H., and Rand, R. W.: Amer. J. Roentgenol., *104*:57–62, 1968.)

and the tentorium cerebelli. The vessels communicate with identical branches on the opposite side and with meningeal branches of the external carotid, ophthalmic, and vertebral arteries. Thus, there is a network of vessels forming an anastomosis in this region similar to that found in lower animals and occasionally in young patients with long-standing partial obstruction of major vessels in this area, probably in conjunction with slowly occurring arterial obstructive disease or maldevelopment of major tributaries.

An anatomic classification of the cavernous branches of the

carotid artery is presented in Table 8–3 (Wallace et al.). The normal anatomy of this region is shown in Figure 8–12. These individual branches will be discussed more fully in the later description of the internal carotid artery. It will be noted, however, that the meningohypophyseal artery and its tentorial and dorsal meningeal branch are of great significance, especially if a highly vascular meningeal abnormality involves the tentorium cerebelli or the region of the hypophysis.

Vascular Contents of the Subarachnoid Cisterns (Rosen et al.) (Table 8–4). The terminology employed in Table 8–4 varies somewhat from that previously used. The *cisterna pontocerebellaris* is situated in the pontocerebellar recesses laterally. The *cisterna cruralis* is also just lateral to the midline and, as noted from its contents, surrounds the origins of the posterior cerebral arteries, the superior cerebellar arteries, and the branches of the anterior choroidal and medial posterior choroidal arteries as they pass between the uncus of the hippocampus and the cerebral peduncles.

The *cisterna cerebelli superior* lies along the superior surface of the cerebellum.

The *cisterna veli interpositi* lies above the third ventricle and is formed by enfolding the arachnoidal membranes as the blood vessels course rostrally to supply the choroidal plexus in the roof

TABLE 8–3 ANATOMIC CLASSIFICATION OF CAVERNOUS BRANCHES OF CAROTID ARTERY*

Parkinson[a]	Schnürer and Stattin[b]	McConnell[c]
A. Meningohypophyseal Artery	A. Dorsal Main Stem	A. Inferior Hypophyseal Trunk
1. Tentorial branch	1. Basal tentorial branch	
a. Branch to III and IV		
b. Branch to roof of cavernous sinus		
c. Branch to falx and tentorium		
2. Dorsal meningeal branch	2. Clival branches	—posterior branch
a. Clival branch		
b. Branch to VI		
3. Inferior hypophyseal branch		
a. Branch to dura at floor of sella		—inferior hypophyseal branch to posterior hypophysis
b. Branch to dura of post clinoids		
c. Branch to cavernous sinus		
B. Inferior Cavernous Sinus Artery	B. Lateral Main Stem	—anterior branch from inferior hypophyseal trunk
1. Branch to gasserian ganglion	1. Marginal tentorial branch	
2. Anastomosis with middle meningeal and accessory meningeal arteries	2. Branch to gasserian ganglion IV, V, VI	
C. Capsular Arteries	3. Anastomosis with branch of middle meningeal and branch of ophthalmic arteries	C. Capsular
		1. Anterior capsular
		2. Inferior capsular from inferomedial aspect of internal carotid artery halfway along course

*From Wallace S., Goldberg, H. I., Leeds, N. E., and Mishkin, M. M.: The cavernous branches of the internal carotid artery. Amer. J. Roentgenol., *101*:34–46, 1967.

[a]Parkinson, D.: Collateral circulation of cavernous carotid artery: anatomy. Canad. J. Surg., 7, 251–268, 1964.

[b]Schnürer, L. B., and Stattin, S.: Vascular supply of intracranial dura from internal carotid artery with special reference to its angiographic significance. Acta Radiol. (Diag.), 1, 441–450, 1963.

[c]McConnell, E. M.: Arterial blood supply of human hypophysis cerebri. Anat. Rec., *115*, 175–203, 1953.

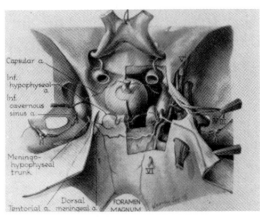

Figure 8–12. The cavernous branches of the internal carotid artery. (From Parkinson, D.: Canad. J. Surg., 7:251–268, 1964.)

of the third ventricle. The internal cerebral veins form within this potential space as paired midline structures.

The cisterna fossae sylvii is formed at the Sylvian fissure.

The term *carotid cistern* has been proposed to designate that portion of the subarachnoid space "enveloping the suprasellar portion of the internal carotid artery" (Lewtas and Jefferson; Rosen et al.).

Importance of the Pericallosal Cistern and Posterior Fossa Sinuses in Diagnosis. Cisternal visualization can be virtually achieved at times during angiography by identifying the vessels appropriate to the anatomic position of the cisterns. Thus, for example, the pericallosal cistern can be readily identified and the corpus callosum postulated by visualizing these branches of the anterior cerebral artery (Fig. 8–13 *A, B, C*). A diagram of the pericallosal pial vessels is shown in Figure 8–13 *D* and *E*. From these representations it can readily be seen that mass effects

TABLE 8–4   VASCULAR CONTENTS OF SUBARACHNOID CISTERNS*

I. Cisterns of Posterior Cranial Fossa
  A. *Cisterna Medullaris*
    1. Anterior spinal arteries
    2. Posterior spinal arteries—rarely seen
    3. Vertebral arteries
    4. Posterior inferior cerebellar arteries
    5. Anterior inferior cerebellar arteries
  B. *Cisterna Magna (Cerebellomedullaris)*
    1. Vertebral arteries
    2. Posterior inferior cerebellar arteries
    3. Inferior cerebellar veins
  C. *Cisterna Pontis*
    1. Basilar artery
    2. Anterior inferior cerebellar artery and its infrequently seen internal auditory branch
    3. Superior cerebellar artery
    4. Posterior cerebral artery in cases of short basilar arteries
    5. Basilar plexus or venous plexus anterior to pons
  D. *Cisternae Pontocerebellaris*
    1. Internal auditory artery—rarely seen
    2. Anterior inferior cerebellar artery
    3. Superficial petrosal veins (veins of cerebellopontine angle)
II. Suprasellar Cisterns
  A. *Cisterna Interpeduncularis*
    1. Basilar artery, superior aspect
    2. Posterior communicating artery
    3. Posterior cerebral arteries, proximal portion
    4. Superior cerebellar artery, proximal portion
    5. Internal carotid artery at level of posterior communicating artery
    6. Basal vein of Rosenthal, proximal portion
  B. *Cisterna Cruralis*
    1. Posterior cerebral artery
    2. Superior cerebellar arteries
    3. Anterior choroidal artery
    4. Medial posterior choroidal artery
    5. Basal vein of Rosenthal, proximal portion

  C. *Cisterna Chiasmatis*
    1. Internal carotid artery, suprasellar portion
    2. Middle cerebral artery, proximal or horizontal portion
    3. Anterior cerebral artery, proximal or horizontal portion
    4. Anterior choroidal artery, proximal portion
  D. *Cisterna Laminae Terminalis*
    1. Pericallosal artery
    2. Anterior communicating artery, variable
    3. Frontopolar artery, proximal portion, variable
III. Cisterns of Tentorial Notch
  A. *Cisterna Corporis Callosi*
    1. Anterior portion
      a. Pericallosal artery, anterior portion
    2. Posterior or splenium portion
      a. Posterior pericallosal artery
      b. Great vein of Galen
      c. Internal cerebral vein, caudalmost aspect
      d. Posterior pericallosal vein
  B. *Cisterna Quadrigeminalis or Cisterna Venae Magnae Galeni*
    1. Great vein of Galen
    2. Medial posterior choroidal artery, distal portion
  C. *Cisterna Ambiens, including Alae Cisterna Ambientium*
    1. Posterior cerebral artery
    2. Superior cerebellar artery
    3. Basal vein of Rosenthal
    4. Medial posterior choroidal artery
    5. Lateral posterior choroidal artery
    6. Anterior choroidal artery
  D. *Cisterna Cerebelli Superior*
    1. Superior cerebellar artery
    2. Superior cerebellar veins
  E. *Cisterna Veli Interpositi*
    1. Internal cerebral vein
IV. Cisterna Fossae Sylvii
  A. *Internal Carotid Artery, Suprasellar Portion*
  B. *Middle Cerebral Artery Complex*

*From Rosen, L., Weidner, W., and Hanafee, W.: Angiographic visualization of the subarachnoid cisterns. Radiology, *85*:1–13, 1965.

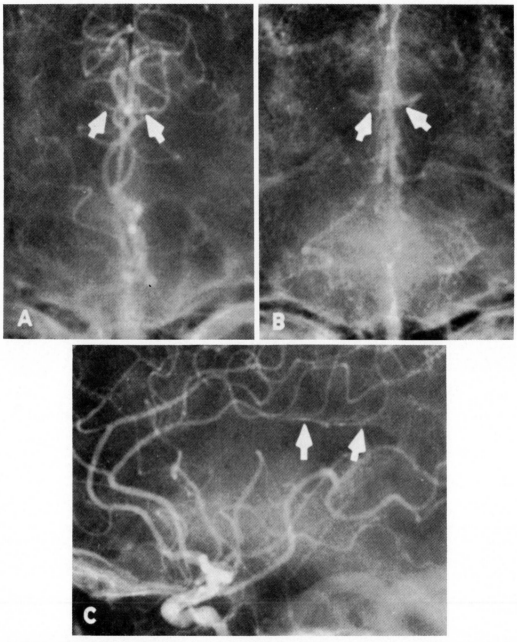

Figure 8–13.   Normal carotid angiograms. *A.* Anteroposterior projection in the arterial phase showing two short transverse vessels (arrows) extending laterally from the midline pericallosal arteries. These vessels are about a centimeter in length and appear to end abruptly. *B.* Venous phase reveals persistent opacification of vessels (arrows) in the same area. They appear to be a little thicker and less sharply outlined. *C.* Lateral projection shows the thin terminal prolongation of the pericallosal artery extending posteriorly over the superior aspect of the posterior part of the corpus callosum (arrows). Note several denser dots within its course (between the arrows) which indicate transverse channels.

Figure 8–13 continued on the opposite page.

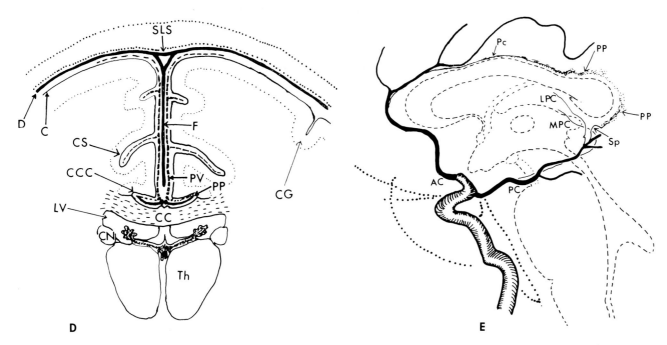

Figure 8-13 *Continued.* Diagrammatic representation of pericallosal pial vessels. *D.* Anteroposterior view. The pericallosal or plexus pial vessels (PP) are located above the corpus callosum (CC) and outline the sulcus or cistern of the corpus callosum (CCC). Pial vessels (PV) are also shown on the medial aspect of the hemispheres, extending into sulci, specifically the sulcus cinguli (CS). The falx (F) extends downward from the superior longitudinal sinus (SLS). Also labeled are the body of the lateral ventricle (LV), the caudate nucleus (CN), the thalamus (Th), the dura (D), the surface of the cortex (C), and the cortical gray matter (CG).

    E. Lateral projection. The pial plexus (PP) around the splenium is supplied by the posterior extension of the pericallosal artery (Pc) and by the splenial branch (Sp) of the posterior cerebral artery (PC). Also labeled are the first portion of the anterior cerebral artery (AC), the medial posterior choroidal artery (MPC), and the lateral posterior choroidal artery (LPC). (*A* to *E* from Huang, V. P., and Wolf, B. S.: Radiology, *82*:14–23, 1964.)

or mass lesions, particularly with displacements from one side to the other, can at times be diagnosed with a knowledge of this basic anatomy (Huang and Wolf).

As noted in Chapter 6, the large venous sinuses produce impressions on the inner table of the calvarium, and their positions can be recognized thereby. Thus, the positions of the lateral sinuses and sinus confluens can be identified. In certain disease entities characterized by a large posterior fossa (Dandy-Walker cyst, communicating hydrocephalus), these structures will be displaced upward. In other entities distinguished by a small posterior fossa, these structures will be lower in position than expected (as with Arnold-Chiari malformation, Chapter 6).

Anatomic Variation of the Height of the Falx Cerebri (Galligioni et al.). By means of measurements made in the venous phase of carotid angiography in the lateral view, the height of the falx cerebri has been determined at different points. In this same investigation the venous angle (to be described later) was

also studied. As noted in the accompanying table (Table 8–5) and Figure 8–14, numerous variations were found: the height of the falx ranges between 28 and 48 mm. anteriorly; between 41 and 62 mm. in the center; and between 40 and 62 mm. at the posterior points designated.

Subdivisions of the Brain

The brain is divided into five principal parts (Figs. 8–15, 8–16): (1) the cerebrum, composed of two cerebral hemispheres, lying above a plane drawn between the internal occipital protuberance, the petrous ridges and the floor of the anterior cranial fossa; (2) the cerebellum, composed of two hemispheres and a small central portion called the vermis, lying in the posterior fossa; (3) the midbrain, which lies between the cerebral hemi-

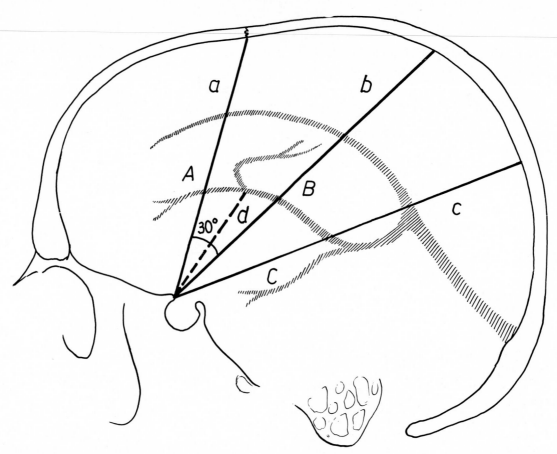

Figure 8–14. Schematic drawing showing the technique of measurements. (A) Distance between the tuberculum sellae (ts.) and the internal surface of the skull at the bregma. (a) Distance from the internal surface of the skull to the inferior longitudinal sinus (ils.) along line A.

(B) Distance between the tuberculum sellae and the internal surface of the skull forming an angle of 30 degrees posterior to line A. (b) Distance from the internal surface of the skull to the ils. along line B.

(C) Distance between the ts. and the internal surface of the skull along a line crossing the proximal end of the vein of Galen. (c) Distance between the internal surface of the skull and the ils. along line C. (d) Distance from the ts. to the venous angle where the thalamostriate and septal veins join the internal cerebral vein. (From Galligioni, F., Bernardi, R., and Mingrino, S.: Amer. J. Roentgenol., 106:273–278, 1969.)

TABLE 8–5   ANATOMIC VARIATION OF THE HEIGHT OF
THE FALX CEREBRI
(as determined from cerebral angiograms)*

	Minimal (cm.)	Maximal (cm.)	Mean (cm.)
Distance from tuberculum sellae to bregma (A)	8.6	11.5	9.9
Distance from ts. to skull (B)	10.5	13.8	8.19
Distance from ts. to skull (C)	11.3	14.3	11.2
Height of falx cerebri in (a)	2.8	4.8	3.58
Height of falx cerebri in (b)	4.1	6.2	5.19
Height of falx cerebri in (c)	4.0	6.2	5.27
Distance from ts. to venous angle (d)	3.2	5.5	3.54

*From Galligioni, F., Bernardi, R., and Mingrino, S.: Anatomic variation in the height of the falx cerebri. Amer. J. Roentgenol., 106:273–278, 1969.

spheres above and the hindbrain below; (4) the pons, lying beneath the fourth ventricle between the cerebral peduncles above and the medulla oblongata below; and (5) the medulla oblongata, which lies immediately above the spinal cord above the level of the foramen magnum.

The Surface of the Brain

CEREBRUM: LATERAL ASPECT

Principal Fissures or Sulci.   The principal gyri and sulci of the cerebrum are shown in Figure 8–15 A. The most important sulci for identification here are: (1) the *lateral (Sylvian) cerebral fissure*, (2) the *central sulcus* (of Rolando), and (3) the smaller *parieto-occipital fissure.*

The *lateral* or *Sylvian fissure* is the oblique cleft passing upward and posteriorly on the lateral aspect of the cerebrum, separating the frontal and temporal lobes on the one hand and the temporal and parietal lobes more posteriorly (Fig. 8–15 *A*). The folds of gray matter making up the margins of the lateral fissure are called the *opercula.*

The *central sulcus* is a prominent fissure that separates the frontal and parietal lobes and extends almost to the lateral fissure.

The *parieto-occipital fissure,* more posteriorly situated and smaller in size, separates the parietal and occipital lobes on the one hand, and the temporal and occipital lobes inferiorly, as shown.

If the folds of the opercula are removed, the *insula* is found beneath it, surrounded by a *circular sulcus* (Fig. 8–15 *C*). The folds of the circular sulcus converge at the base of the brain in a region known as the *limen insulae.* Arteries within these folds are highly significant in cerebral angiography.

The Lobes of the Cerebrum. Thus, we may identify five lobes of the cerebrum: (1) a *frontal lobe* extending from the frontal pole to the central sulcus, (2) a *parietal lobe* extending from the central sulcus to the parieto-occipital fissure, (3) an *occipital lobe* that extends from the occipital pole to the parieto-occipital fissure and inferiorly to a preoccipital notch, (4) a *temporal lobe* extending from the temporal pole to a line extending from the parieto-occipital fissure to the preoccipital notch, and (5) the *insula,* lying at the bottom of the lateral fissure covered by the opercula and encircled by the circular sulcus.

The area of cortex immediately in front of the central sulcus is the motor area, which controls contralateral muscular activity. The body parts are represented in an inverted position in this region, stimulation of the upper part of the motor area causing movements in the lower limb.

The area of cortex behind the central sulcus (posterior central gyrus) is an important primary receptive area to which afferent pathways project by means of relays in the thalamus.

The right and left cerebral hemispheres are separated by the *great longitudinal fissure,* which is occupied by the falx cerebri. In the depth of this fissure centrally is the corpus callosum, which acts as a bridge connecting the two cerebral hemispheres. The falx is rigidly fixed and is virtually indisplaceable except by considerable force or by developmental abnormality in one cerebral lobe.

In the frontal lobes are situated four major gyri, the superior, middle, inferior, and anterior central, each separated by a corresponding sulcus.

The temporal lobes possess three major gyri, the superior, middle, and inferior.

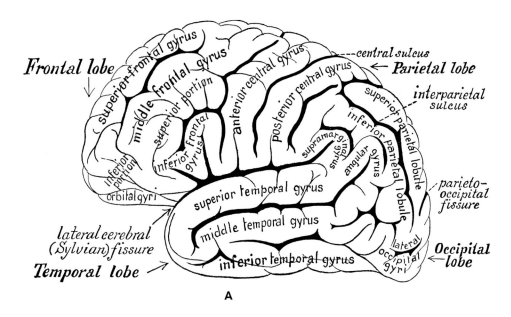

A

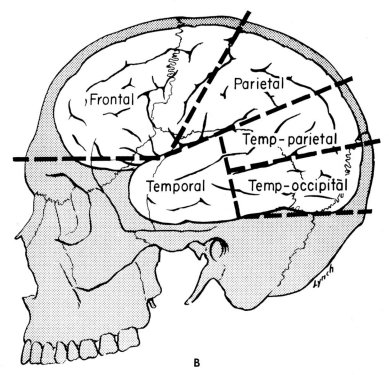

B

Figure 8–15. A. The subdivisions, major sulci and gyri of the lateral aspect of the brain. (From Sobotta, J., and McMurrich, J.: Atlas and Textbook of Human Anatomy.) B. Diagram showing the position of the various subdivisions of the brain as considered clinically and radiologically (supratentorial).

Figure 8–15 continued on the following page.

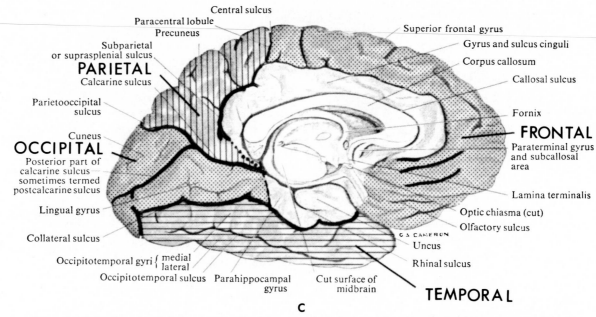

Figure 8-15 *Continued.*   C. Lobes, gyri, and sulci as seen from the sagittal and somewhat inferior aspect of the brain.

Figure 8-15 continued on opposite page.

MEDIAL VIEW OF THE BRAIN (Figs. 8-16, 8-17)

Principal Fissures, Sulci, and Landmarks.   The *corpus callosum* stretches between the two cerebral hemispheres like a bridge over the depth of the great longitudinal fissure; it consists of three parts—the *genu* anteriorly ("knee"), the *body,* and the *splenium.*

The *fornix* arches beneath the corpus callosum (Fig. 8-18), with the *septum pellucidum* stretched between them. The body of the fornix lies above the ependymal roof of the third ventricle (part of the ventricular system soon to be described) and is attached to the undersurface of the corpus callosum. More anteriorly, it is attached to the lower borders of the laminae of the septum pellucidum. The rostrum of the corpus callosum inferiorly blends with the *anterior commissure,* which, like the fornix and the corpus callosum, bridges the two cerebral hemispheres (Fig. 8-16 *A*).

The *hippocampal commissure* is a thin sheet of fibers connecting the medial edges of the crura of the fornix, and it, too, is closely applied to the under aspect of the posterior part of the body of the corpus callosum (Fig. 8-18 *A* and *B*).

The *cingulate sulcus* is usually parallel to the sulcus and body of the corpus callosum to a point dorsal to the central sulcus, where it branches into a Y, forming a marginal ramus and subparietal sulcus. These, for the most part, lie in the parietal lobe (Figs. 8-16 *A* and 8-17).

The *parieto-occipital fissure* begins near the middle of the *calcarine fissure* and runs upward to its superior margin. The *cal-*

carine fissure starts below the splenium of the corpus callosum and curves upward and dorsally toward the occipital pole as shown (Fig. 8-17).

The cerebral lobes identifiable on this medial view of the brain are (Fig. 8-15 *C*):
1. The frontal lobe.
2. The parietal lobe bounded rostrally by the marginal ramus and posteriorly by the parieto-occipital fissure.
3. The occipital lobe, bounded rostrally by the parieto-occipital fissure and a line drawn caudally to the preoccipital notch.
4. The temporal lobe, bounded dorsally by the rostral boundary of the occipital lobe.

The posterior half of the calcarine fissure divides the occipital lobe into the *cuneate* and *lingual* gyri (Fig. 8-15 *C*).

Sagittal Section.   In the medial view of a sagittal section of the brain stem other important structures can be seen (Fig. 8-19): (1) the *choroid plexus of the third ventricle* in its roof, (2) the *pineal body* just posterior to the third ventricle, (3) the *habenular commissure,* (4) the *massa intermedia,* which produces a masslike defect within the third ventricle, (5) the *hypothalamus,* which extends posteriorly from the anterior commissure and inferior to the third ventricle, (6) the *thalamus* on each side of the third ventricle, and (7) the *third ventricle* itself. Note also in the diagram: the lamina terminalis, the optic chiasm, and the cerebral peduncle (Figs. 8-16 *A* and 8-19).

In the midline, the *cerebral aqueduct* can be seen, communicating between the third and fourth ventricles; it lies poste-

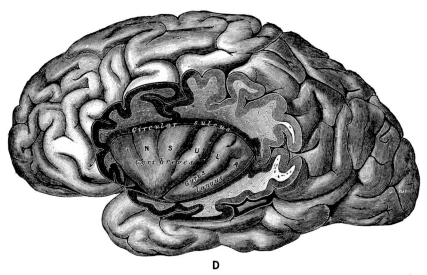

D

Figure 8–15 *Continued.* D. The insula of the left side of the brain, exposed by removing the opercula. (From Gray's Anatomy of the Human Body, 29th ed. Goss, C. M. (ed.) Philadelphia, Lea & Febiger, 1973.)

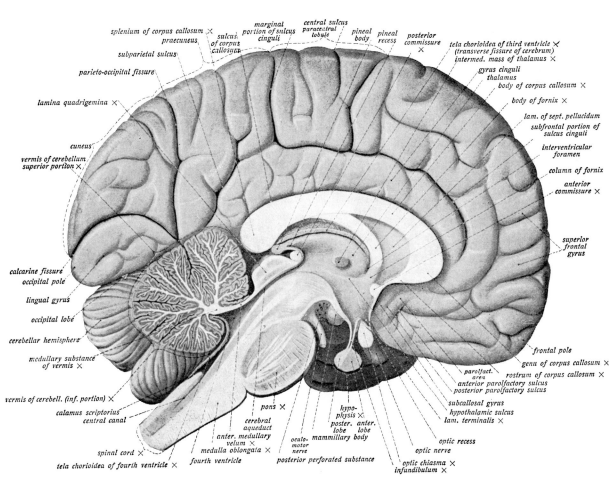

Figure 8–16. Medial sagittal section of the brain. The subdivisions, major sulci, and gyri. (From Sobotta, J., and McMurrich, J.: Atlas and Textbook of Human Anatomy.)

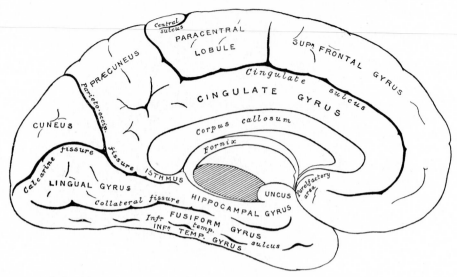

Figure 8–17. Medial surface of left cerebral hemisphere of brain. (From Gray's Anatomy of the Human Body, 29th ed. Goss, C. M. (ed.) Philadelphia, Lea & Febiger, 1973.)

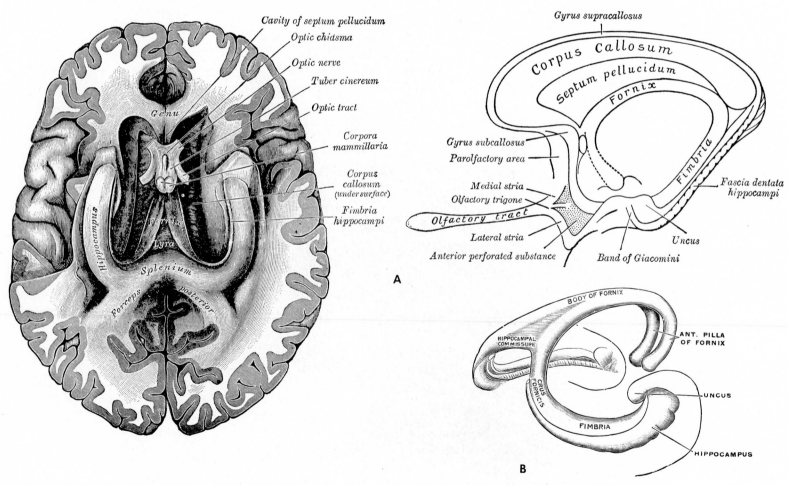

Figure 8–18. A. Relationship of the fornix and hippocampus to the ventricles. B. Diagram of the fornix (Spitzka). (From Gray's Anatomy of the Human Body, 29th ed. Goss, C. M. (ed.) Philadelphia. Lea & Febiger, 1973.)

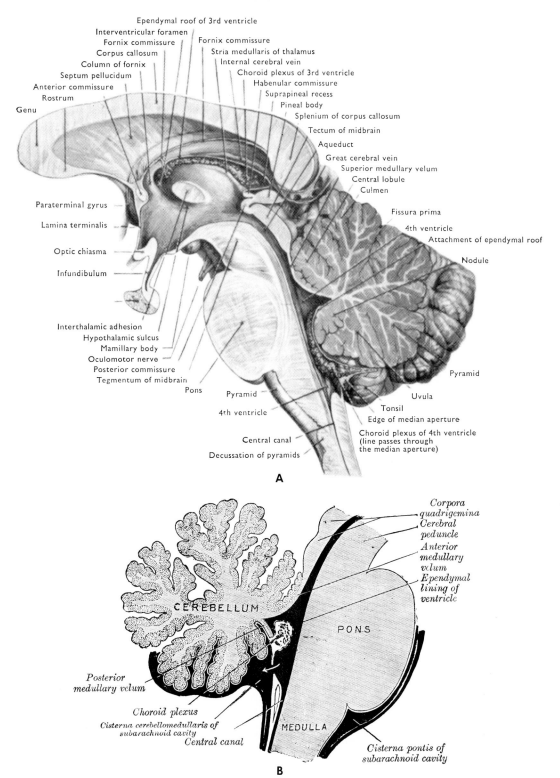

Ependymal roof of 3rd ventricle
Interventricular foramen
Fornix commissure
Corpus callosum
Column of fornix
Septum pellucidum
Anterior commissure
Rostrum
Genu

Fornix commissure
Stria medullaris of thalamus
Internal cerebral vein
Choroid plexus of 3rd ventricle
Habenular commissure
Suprapineal recess
Pineal body
Splenium of corpus callosum
Tectum of midbrain
Aqueduct
Great cerebral vein
Superior medullary velum
Central lobule
Culmen

Paraterminal gyrus
Lamina terminalis
Optic chiasma
Infundibulum

Fissura prima
4th ventricle
Attachment of ependymal roof
Nodule

Interthalamic adhesion
Hypothalamic sulcus
Mamillary body
Oculomotor nerve
Posterior commissure
Tegmentum of midbrain
Pons

Pyramid

Pyramid
4th ventricle

Uvula
Tonsil
Edge of median aperture

Central canal

Choroid plexus of 4th ventricle
(line passes through
the median aperture)

Decussation of pyramids

A

Corpora
quadrigemina
Cerebral
peduncle
Anterior
medullary
velum
Ependymal
lining of
ventricle

CEREBELLUM

PONS

Posterior
medullary velum

Choroid plexus
Cisterna cerebellomedullaris of
subarachnoid cavity
Central canal

MEDULLA

Cisterna pontis of
subarachnoid cavity

B

Figure 8–19. *A.* The parts of the brain cut through in a median section. The side walls of the third and fourth ventricles are also shown. For the medial views of other portions of the brain see Figure 8–15 C. (From Cunningham's Textbook of Anatomy, 10th ed. London, Oxford University Press, 1964.) *B.* Scheme of roof of fourth ventricle. The arrow is in the foramen of Magendie. (From Gray's Anatomy of the Human Body, 24th ed. Lewis, W. H. (ed.) Philadelphia, Lea & Febiger, 1942.)

rior to the cerebral peduncles and anterior to the corpora quadrigemina (Fig. 8–19 *B*).

Proceeding more caudally, the *cerebellum,* the *fourth ventricle,* and the *pons* are readily identified in the brain stem.

In a study of the midline roof of the fourth ventricle, the *anterior medullary velum* is visible as a thin transparent membrane stretching between the superior cerebellar peduncles; it forms the upper part of the fourth ventricle. The *posterior medullary velum* is a rather thin sheet of ependymal epithelium and pia mater that forms the roof of the lower part of the fourth ventricle. This area is rich in choroidal blood vessels.

THE INFERIOR SURFACE OF THE BRAIN (Fig. 8–20)

This view of the brain shows the frontal lobes separated by the longitudinal fissure and anterior extremity of the corpus callosum. The olfactory tracts are embedded in the inferior aspect of the frontal lobes.

Posterior to the rostrum of the corpus callosum and centrally placed are the following structures, proceeding from front to back: (1) the optic chiasm, (2) the hypophysis, (3) the cerebral peduncles (enclosing the tuber cinereum, corpora mammillaria, and posterior perforated substance), (4) the pons, and (5) the medulla.

The temporal lobes and inferior surface of the cerebellum can be seen, and the various cranial nerves as they emerge from the brain substance are shown to good advantage.

The *olfactory tract,* which extends posteriorly from the olfactory bulb, divides into medial and lateral sectors called the *olfactory striae,* and these surround the anterior perforated substance.

At the medial edge of the temporal lobe anteriorly, there is a small portion of gray tissue that protrudes and overlaps the tentorial notch—this is called the *uncus* (Fig. 8–21). The structures at the base of the brain lying between the frontal lobes form the floor of the *diencephalon,* and generally, these structures lie between the medial tips of the two unci. The floor of the diencephalon consists of the following structures: the *optic nerves and chiasm,* the *anterior perforated substance,* and the *limen insulae,* which is continuous more laterally with the cortex of the insula.

Immediately posterior to the two mamillary bodies is the *posterior perforated substance.* Lateral to this are the large cerebral peduncles which are the extensions outside the cerebrum of the right and left internal capsules.

The *cerebral peduncles,* as they continue caudally and medially, become the bulging structures on the base of the *pons.* Caudally the pons merges first into the medulla oblongata and then into the cervical spinal cord at the level of the foramen magnum.

From the pons, there is a large band of white matter called the *middle cerebellar peduncle (brachium pontis)* that extends on each side to enter the cerebellar hemispheres.

The Base of the Brain in the Region of the Diencephalon (Fig. 8–22). Examination of the upper brain stem, if the temporal and occipital lobes of the cerebrum and half of the cerebellum were removed, would reveal the *pulvinar,* which is the most posterior part of the thalamus (Fig. 8–22 *B*). The pulvinar is situated below the splenium of the corpus callosum and protrudes into the subarachnoid space; it lies lateral to the cerebral aqueduct. The *medial geniculate bodies* lie just anterior to the pulvinar. The *lateral geniculate bodies* represent the termination of the optic tracts (Fig. 8–22 *A*).

The *superior and inferior quadrigeminal bodies* (Fig. 8–22 *B*) are situated in the roof of the midbrain just medial to a large fiber tract known as the *lateral lemniscus,* which comes to the surface of the midbrain. This tract ends in the medial geniculate body.

The *massa intermedia* (interthalamic adhesion) bridges the third ventricle and connects the thalami of the two sides in about

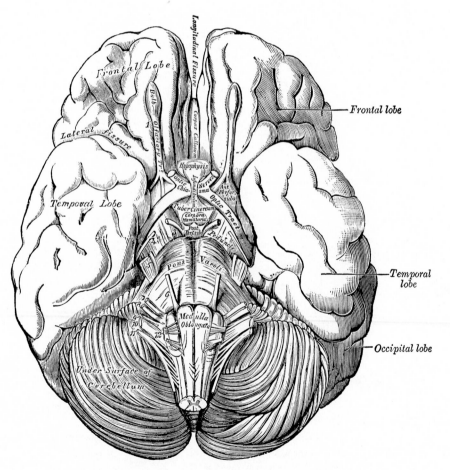

Figure 8–20. View of the base of the brain. (From Gray's Anatomy of the Human Body, 29th ed. Goss, C. M. (ed.) Philadelphia, Lea & Febiger, 1973.)

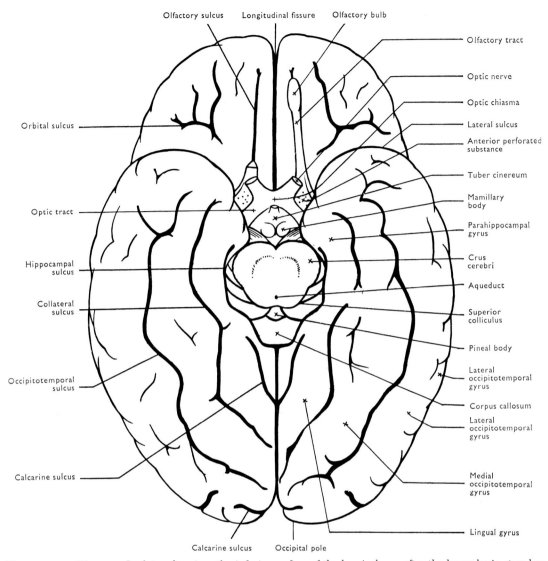

Olfactory sulcus Longitudinal fissure Olfactory bulb

Olfactory tract

Optic nerve

Optic chiasma

Lateral sulcus

Anterior perforated substance

Tuber cinereum

Mamillary body

Parahippocampal gyrus

Crus cerebri

Aqueduct

Superior colliculus

Pineal body

Lateral occipitotemporal gyrus

Corpus callosum

Lateral occipitotemporal gyrus

Medial occipitotemporal gyrus

Lingual gyrus

Orbital sulcus

Optic tract

Hippocampal sulcus

Collateral sulcus

Occipitotemporal sulcus

Calcarine sulcus

Calcarine sulcus Occipital pole

Figure 8–21. Diagram of sulci and gyri on the inferior surface of the hemispheres after the lower brain stem has been removed. (From Cunningham's Textbook of Anatomy, 10th ed. London, Oxford University Press, 1964.)

30 per cent of human brains ("connexis interthalamicus" in Fig. 8–22 *B* and *C*).

Cerebellum

The cerebellum lies in the posterior fossa of the cranial cavity and occupies the deep fossa of the occipital bone. It is attached to the brain stem by *three pairs of peduncles,* and consists of large *lateral hemispheres* on each side and a narrow medial portion, the *vermis.* The numerous grooves for sulci in the surface of the cerebellum vary considerably in depth. The surface folds of the cerebellum are known as the *folia;* they resemble gyri of the cerebral

hemispheres in that they consist of an outer layer of gray substance covering radiating extensions of white substance.

The three pairs of peduncles attaching the cerebellum to the brain stem are:

1. The *inferior cerebellar peduncle,* which connects the cerebellum with the medulla oblongata.
2. The *middle cerebellar peduncle,* which connects the pons and the cerebellum.
3. The *superior cerebellar peduncle,* which connects the cerebellum with the midbrain and the diencephalon.

The inferior cerebellar peduncle is also called the *restiform body;* the middle cerebellar peduncle, the *brachium pontis;* and

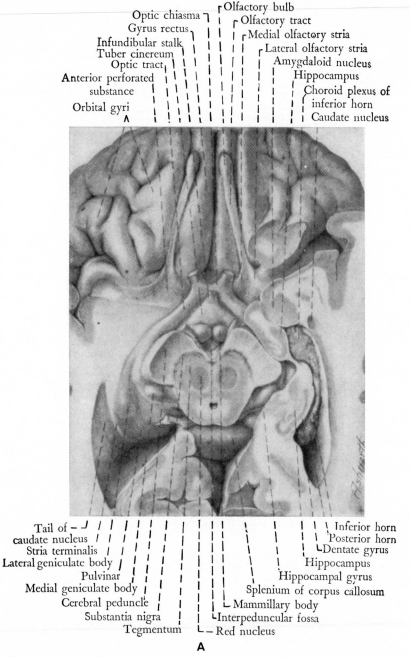

Optic chiasma ┐
Gyrus rectus ╮
Infundibular stalk ╲
Tuber cinereum ╲
Optic tract ╲
Anterior perforated
substance
Orbital gyri

┌Olfactory bulb
│ ┌Olfactory tract
│ │ ┌Medial olfactory stria
│ │ │ ┌Lateral olfactory stria
│ │ │ │ Amygdaloid nucleus
│ │ │ │ Hippocampus
│ │ │ │ ┌Choroid plexus of
│ │ │ │ │inferior horn
│ │ │ │ │Caudate nucleus

A

Tail of –┘
caudate nucleus
Stria terminalis
Lateral geniculate body
Pulvinar
Medial geniculate body
Cerebral peduncle
Substantia nigra
Tegmentum

Inferior horn
Posterior horn
└Dentate gyrus
Hippocampus
Hippocampal gyrus
Splenium of corpus callosum
└ Mammillary body
└Interpeduncular fossa
└ Red nucleus

A

Figure 8–22. A. Dissection of brain exposing optic tract, geniculate bodies, and pulvinar from below on the left side, and inferior horn of lateral ventricle and adjacent structures on the right side. (From Anson, B. J. (ed.): Morris' Human Anatomy, 12th ed. Copyright © 1966 by McGraw-Hill, Inc. Used by permission of the McGraw-Hill Book Company.)

Figure 8–22 continued on the opposite page.

the superior cerebellar peduncle, the *brachium conjunctivum* (Fig. 8–23).

The superior part of the vermis protrudes cephalad into the tentorial notch posteriorly. The caudal parts of the lateral lobes of

the cerebellum are called the *cerebellar tonsils* and lie on each side of the midline just dorsal to the medulla and above the posterior part of the foramen magnum. Thus, with upward displacement, the vermis may protrude through the posterior aspect of the tentorial notch; since caudal displacement of the brain stem must take place through the foramen magnum, increased intracranial pressure may cause the cerebellar tonsils and medulla to be jammed into the rigid bony ring of the foramen magnum. Any upward shift of the contents of the posterior fossa will also jam the pons against the clivus, and compression of the midbrain with obstruction of the cerebral aqueduct may result. The blood vessels delineating such changes will be described subsequently.

Ventricular System

PRELIMINARY STUDY OF THE INTERNAL STRUCTURE OF THE BRAIN

Corpus Callosum. The corpus callosum is the *major transverse pathway connecting the two cerebral hemispheres*. The callosal fibers that cross in the *genu and body* of the corpus callosum lead principally to the frontal, parietal, and anterior temporal lobes on each side and form the roof of the frontal horns, body, and anterior part, respectively, of the temporal horns of the lateral ventricles. Those fibers that cross posterior to the *splenium* generally form the roof and lateral walls of the trigone and occipital horn of each lateral ventricle.

Internal Capsule. The internal capsule is the *great axial projection system* connecting the cerebral cortex with lower centers, and thus, it is intimately related to the *thalamus, caudate nucleus*, and *lentiform nucleus*. A horizontal section of the brain at the level of the interventricular foramen demonstrates the relationships of these and related structures. Similarly, a coronal section of the brain at this same level is very helpful (Fig. 8–24 A, B).

Laterally, the thalamus is bounded by the *posterior limb of the internal capsule* (see *18* in Fig. 8–24 A, and *9* in Fig. 8–24 B). Below the thalamus are the *hypothalamus, anteriorly*, and the *subthalamus, posteriorly*.

The *epithalamus* is a small region in the posterior roof of the diencephalon that contains the *habenular nuclei* connected across the midline by the *habenular commissure*. This latter structure may be seen crossing the posterior wall of the third ventricle just below the suprapineal recess a few millimeters anterior to the pineal body. The habenular commissure will occasionally calcify and is then faintly visible in a lateral skull film as a C-shaped calcific deposit just anterior to the pineal body (see Chapter 6).

The internal capsule has two arms in the form of a V—an anterior limb and a posterior limb. The apex of the V, pointing medially, is named the *genu* (see Fig. 8–24 A).

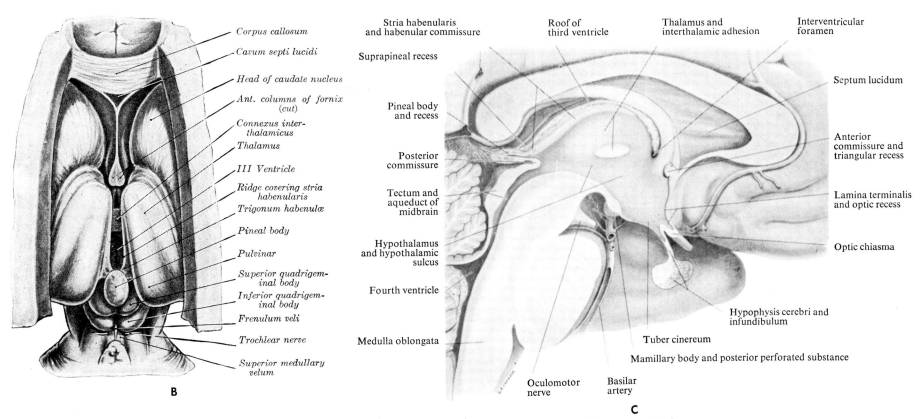

Figure 8–22 *Continued.* B. The thalami, exposed from above. The trunk and splenium of the corpus callosum, most of the septum lucidum, the body of the fornix, the tela chorioidea with its contained plexuses and the epithelial roof of the third ventricle have all been removed. (From Gray's Anatomy of the Human Body, 29th ed. Goss, C. M. (ed.) Philadelphia, Lea & Febiger, 1973.) C. Median sagittal section of the brain, demonstrating massa intermedia (interthalamic adhesion). This varies in size in certain congenital lesions, especially those involving the brain. (Reprinted by permission of Faber and Faber, Ltd. from Anatomy of the Human Body by Lockhart, Hamilton, and Fyfe: Faber and Faber, London; J. B. Lippincott Company, Philadelphia.)

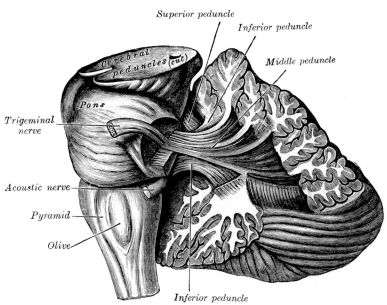

Figure 8–23. Dissection showing the projection fibers of the cerebellum (after E. B. Jamieson). (From Gray's Anatomy of the Human Body, 29th ed. Goss, C. M. (ed.) Philadelphia, Lea & Febiger, 1973.)

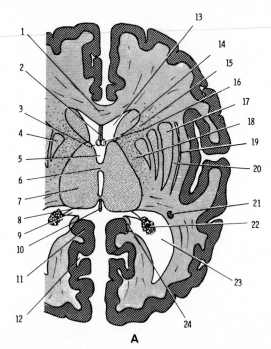

Figure 8-24. A. Horizontal section of the brain at the level of the interventricular foramen. (1) Rostrum of corpus callosum, (2) Septum pellucidum, (3) Interventricular foramen, (4) Globus pallidus, (5) Third ventricle, (6) Massa intermedia, (7) Thalamus, (8) Pulvinar of thalamus, (9) Choroid fissure, (10) Pineal body, (11) Hippocampal gyrus, (12) Calcarine fissure, (13) Anterior horn of lateral ventricle, (14) Head of caudate nucleus, (15) Anterior limb of internal capsule, (16) Anterior pillar of fornix, (17) Putamen, (18) Posterior limb of internal capsule, (19) Claustrum, (20) External capsule, (21) Tail of caudate nucleus, (22) Glomus of choroid plexus, (23) Trigone of lateral ventricle, (24) Posterior pillar of fornix. (From Wilson, M.: The Anatomic Foundation of Neuroradiology of the Brain, 2nd ed. Boston, Little, Brown & Co., 1972.)

Corpus Striatum. The caudate nucleus, lentiform nucleus, and intervening internal capsule are called the *corpus striatum.* The caudate nucleus forms part of the wall of the lateral ventricle throughout its length. The lentiform and caudate nuclei are part of the extrapyramidal motor system.

The *amygdaloid nucleus* (13 on Fig. 8–24 *B*) lies near the medial tip of the temporal lobe and bulges into the tip of the temporal horn. This nucleus is continuous with both the uncus and the tail of the caudate nucleus. The two amygdaloid nuclei are connected by the anterior commissure which crosses the midline in the lamina terminalis immediately in front of the interventricular foramen.

The *external capsule* lies lateral to the lentiform nucleus (20 on Fig. 8–24 *B*).

The *hippocampus* is enfolded into the floor of the temporal horns. The relationship of the hippocampus to the fornix has been previously mentioned (see earlier section on Medial View of the Brain). The fornix connects the hippocampus with the hypothalamus.

The thalamus and hypothalamus merge caudally into the so-called *ventral thalamus,* which is bounded by the right and left internal capsules. More distally, these become the *cerebral peduncles* which form the base of the midbrain.

The *posterior* limb of the internal capsule lies between the thalamus (7 on Fig. 8–24 *A*) and the lentiform nucleus. It contains the fibers controlling movements of the tongue, arms, and legs, respectively. Fibers of the auditory and optic radiation passing to the temporal and occipital cortex are also contained therein.

The *anterior* limb of the internal capsule (15 on Fig. 8–24 *A*) connects the frontal cortex with the thalamus and pons. It also separates the lentiform nucleus from the head of the caudate nucleus (14 on Fig. 8–24 *A*). Strands of gray matter connect the lentiform and caudate nuclei throughout their entire length.

The *lentiform nucleus* is situated in the apex of the V of the internal capsule. Its lateral segment is the *putamen* (17 on Fig. 8–24 *A*), and its medial segment is the *globus pallidus* (4 on Fig. 8–24 *A*).

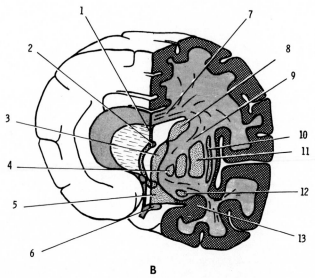

Figure 8-24 *Continued.* B. Coronal section of the brain at the level of the interventricular foramen. (1) Septum pellucidum, (2) Anterior pillar of fornix, (3) Most anterior margin of thalamus, (4) Globus pallidus, (5) Hypothalamus, (6) Anterior portion of optic tract, (7) Corpus callosum, (8) Head of caudate nucleus, (9) Internal capsule, (10) Claustrum, (11) Putamen, (12) Anterior commissure, (13) Amygdaloid nucleus. (From Wilson, M.: The Anatomic Foundation of Neuroradiology of the Brain, 2nd ed. Boston, Little, Brown & Co., 1972.)

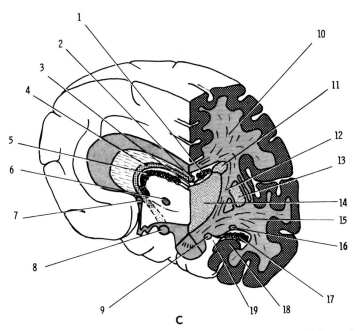

Figure 8-24 *Continued. C.* Coronal section of the brain just behind the middle of the third ventricle. (1) Choroid plexus, (2) Body of fornix, (3) Choroid fissure, (4) Fornix, (5) Choroid plexus of third ventricle, (6) Massa intermedia, (7) Anterior commissure, (8) Mamillary body, (9) Posterior portion of optic tract, (10) White matter, (11) Body of caudate nucleus, (12) Posterior portion of internal capsule, (13) Lentiform nucleus, (14) Thalamus, (15) Sublenticular portion of internal capsule, (16) Tail of caudate nucleus, (17) Choroid plexus in temporal horn, (18) Hippocampus, (19) Choroid fissure. (From Wilson, M.: The Anatomic Foundation of Neuroradiology of the Brain, 2nd ed. Boston, Little, Brown & Co., 1972.)

cerebral aqueduct (of Sylvius), and anteroinferiorly with the central canal of the medulla oblongata.

Lateral Ventricles. Each lateral ventricle is arbitrarily divided into the following parts: (1) *frontal horn* (anteriorly), (2) *body,* (3) *trigone* (isthmus or atrium), (4) *occipital or posterior horns,* and (5) *temporal or inferior horns* (Fig. 8–25).

Anterior Horn. As noted in Figure 8–26 the structures bounding the anterior horn are:

1. WALL AND ROOF: corpus callosum.
2. FLOOR AND LATERAL WALL: head of caudate nucleus.
3. MEDIAL WALL: septum pellucidum.

Body. The structures bounding the body of the lateral ventricle are:

1. ROOF: corpus callosum.
2. MEDIAL AND LATERAL ASPECTS: thalamus medially and body of the caudate nucleus laterally.
3. MEDIAL WALL: septum pellucidum above and fornix below.

The body of the caudate nucleus and corpus callosum meet laterally and superiorly at a rather acute angle, which is usually sharp or slightly rounded. One of the earliest changes in dilata-

BASIC ANATOMY OF THE VENTRICULAR SYSTEM

Ventricles. The ventricles of the brain are a series of communicating cavities lined by ependymal epithelium and containing cerebrospinal fluid (Fig. 8–25). They communicate with the subarachnoid spaces around the brain and around the spinal cord, and with a central canal of the spinal cord.

The *lateral ventricles,* one in each cerebral hemisphere, communicate with one another and with the third ventricle at the interventricular foramina.

The *third ventricle* is a midline slitlike cavity communicating with the lateral ventricles superiorly and laterally, and with the fourth ventricle inferiorly.

The *fourth ventricle* is likewise a midline cavity, diamond-shaped in frontal projection and triangular in lateral cross section. It communicates with the third ventricle superiorly via the

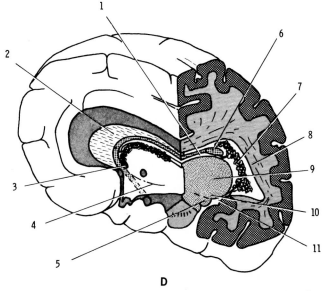

Figure 8-24 *Continued. D.* Coronal section of the brain at the level of the trigone of the lateral ventricle. (1) Choroid fissure, (2) Septum pellucidum, (3) Interventricular foramen, (4) Subthalamic groove, (5) Lateral geniculate body, (6) Posterior pillar of fornix, (7) Glomus of choroid plexus, (8) Optic radiation, (9) Thalamus, (10) Pulvinar of thalamus, (11) Choroid fissure. (From Wilson, M.: The Anatomic Foundation of Neuroradiology of the Brain, 2nd ed. Boston, Little, Brown & Co., 1972.)

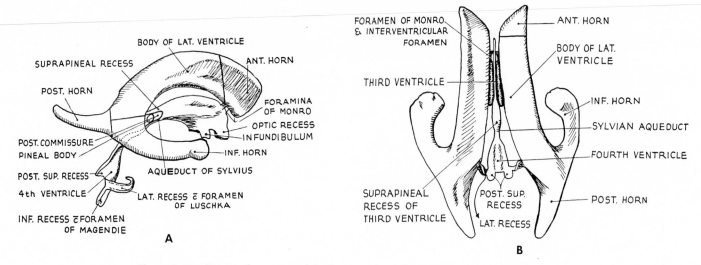

Figure 8–25.   Ventricular system of the brain. *A*. Lateral projection. *B*. Superior projection.

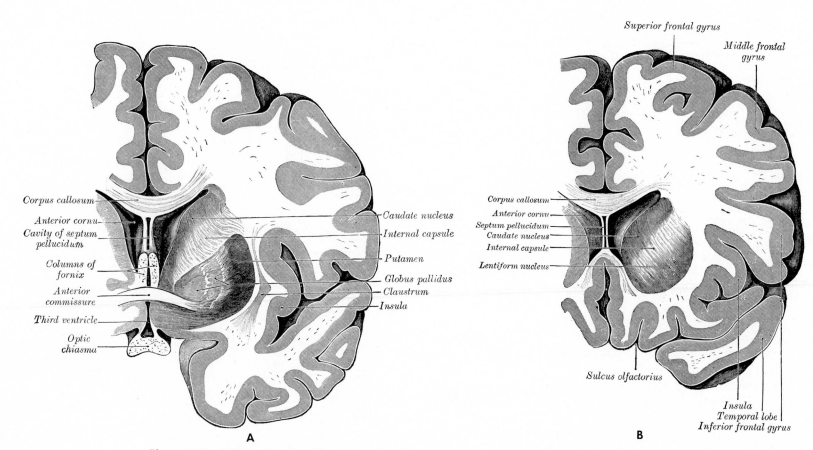

Figure 8–26.   *A*. Coronal section of brain through anterior commissure. *B*. Coronal section through anterior cornua of lateral ventricles. (From Gray's Anatomy of the Human Body, 24th ed. Lewis, W. H. (ed.) Philadelphia, Lea & Febiger, 1942.)

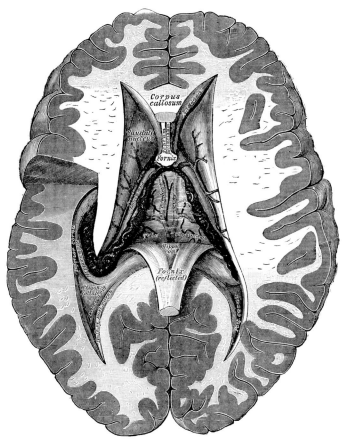

Figure 8–27. Tela chorioidea of the third ventricle, and the choroid plexus of the left lateral ventricle, exposed from above. (From Gray's Anatomy of the Human Body, 29th ed. Goss, C. M. (ed.) Philadelphia, Lea & Febiger, 1973.)

tion of the lateral ventricle is an increased roundness of this acute angle (Fig. 8–26).

4. MEDIAL FLOOR: the choroid plexus lies on the thalamus lateral to the fornix (Fig. 8–27).

Trigone. The *trigone* is the area in which the occipital horn, the body, and the temporal horn merge into a common cavity (Fig. 8–28). Its boundaries are:

1. FLOOR: the *collateral eminence* on the undersurface of the temporal and occipital lobes. Above the collateral eminence, there is a deeper indentation known as the *calcar avis* that is caused by the deep calcarine fissure (Fig. 8–28). (A third indentation on the roof of the trigone just anterior to the calcar avis is called the *bulb* because of the splenium of the corpus callosum [forceps major].)

2. WALL: corpus callosum.

3. ANTERIOR ASPECT: glomus of the choroid plexus.

Lateral to the glomus is the posterior continuation of the caudate nucleus.

Temporal Horn. The temporal or lateral horns extend into each temporal lobe. Anteriorly they become somewhat wider and flatter, with a crescentic or semilunate slit in cross section. The shape of the slit is caused by the indentation of the *hippocampus* bulging inward from the floor (Fig. 8–29). Lateral to the tail of the caudate nucleus, the roof of the temporal horn is formed by the radiating fibers of the internal capsule.

Occipital Horn. The *occipital horns* vary somewhat even from side to side. They extend into the occipital lobes bilaterally. Optic radiation forms the lateral walls of these horns; the other walls are composed of the occipital lobe and the corpus callosum.

Various measurements of the lateral ventricles are indicated in Figure 8–30. Unfortunately, considerable variation in ventricular size may occur at different times even in the same individual. For example, the ventricles may be somewhat larger and more asymmetrical 24 hours after pneumoencephalography (Schatzki et al.).

On occasion there is an air space between the two layers of the septum pellucidum called the "cavum septi pellucidi." The thickness of the septum pellucidum otherwise is usually 2 mm. or less.

Third Ventricle. The *interventricular foramina* are the communicating openings between the lateral ventricles and the third ventricle. They are located near the anterior superior margin of the third ventricle, anterior to the thalamus but posterior to the anterior pillars of the fornix. The third ventricle is bounded as follows (Fig. 8–31):

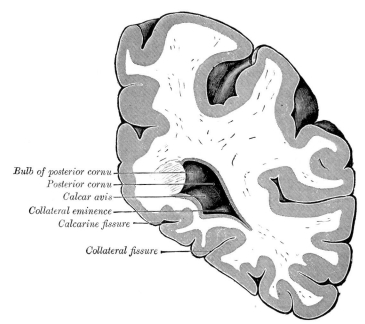

Figure 8–28. Coronal section through posterior cornua of lateral ventricle. (From Gray's Anatomy of the Human Body, 24th ed. Lewis, W. H. (ed.) Philadelphia, Lea & Febiger, 1942.)

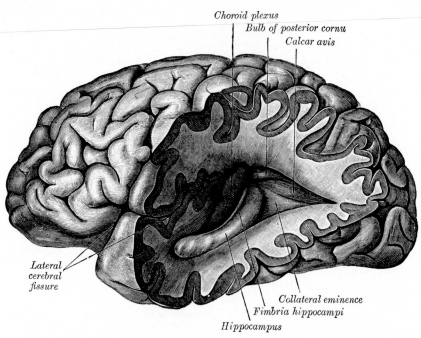

Choroid plexus
Bulb of posterior cornu
Calcar avis
Lateral cerebral fissure
Collateral eminence
Fimbria hippocampi
Hippocampus

Figure 8–29. Posterior and inferior cornua of left lateral ventricle exposed from the side. (From Gray's Anatomy of the Human Body, 29th ed. Goss, C. M. (ed.) Philadelphia, Lea & Febiger, 1973.)

Boundaries of Third Ventricle

1. LATERAL WALLS: the thalamus superiorly and posteriorly.

2. ANTERIOR AND INFERIOR ASPECT: hypothalamus.

The thalamus and hypothalamus are separated by the hypothalamic sulcus or subthalamic groove, which extends along the wall of the third ventricle.

Massa intermedia. The two walls of the third ventricle tend to fuse centrally in an area called the *massa intermedia* (Fig. 8–16). Although called the middle commissure, no fiber tracts actually cross in this area. The massa intermedia appears to link the two thalami across the third ventricle. It appears as a round or oval shadow in the lateral view on ventriculograms. The massa intermedia cannot be assessed reliably from anteroposterior roentgenograms.

Absence of a shadow corresponding to the massa intermedia has been demonstrated in 16.9 per cent of cases studied (Samra and Cooper). A poorly defined border was found in 7.1 per cent, but it was sharply delineated in 75.9 per cent.

The size of the massa intermedia varied in this study. In 20.5 per cent of cases its longest axis was less than 5 mm. In 60.1 per cent, the long axis ranged between 5 and 10 mm., and in 19.3 per cent it was greater than 10 mm.

In 53.2 per cent of cases the massa intermedia was situated in the center of the third ventricle. In 33.8 per cent it was in the upper anterior quadrant; in 8 per cent, in the upper posterior quadrant; in 4.2 per cent, in the inferior anterior quadrant; and in 0.8 per cent, in the inferior posterior quadrant. The most commonly encountered configuration was oval (in 49 per cent of cases), with the long axis in the anteroposterior plane. Thirty per cent were circular.

The *anterior commissure* (Fig. 8–16) is situated just below the anterior pillars of the fornix in the anterior wall of the third ventricle.

3. FLOOR: hypothalamus anteriorly and subthalamus posteriorly. The optic recess is at the most rostral tip of the third ventricle.

Behind the *optic chiasm*, the *hypophyseal stalk* extends down from the floor of the third ventricle through the diaphragma sellae to the sella turcica. The *infundibular or hypothalamic recess* of the third ventricle projects into the infundibulum behind the optic chiasm.

The *tuber cinereum* containing the mamillary bodies lies posterior to the infundibulum.

4. ROOF, BEHIND INTERVENTRICULAR FORAMEN: The roof of the third ventricle is composed largely of a *choroid plexus.* A small diverticulum, called the *suprapineal recess,* evaginates posteriorly at the roof of the third ventricle.

5. POSTERIOR WALL: Indentation by the *pineal gland* occurs beneath the suprapineal recess. The *habenular commissure* is a C-shaped structure identifiable anterior to the pineal gland. The *pineal recess* projects slightly posteriorly. Beneath the pineal recess is the *posterior commissure,* which lies immediately above the origin of the *cerebral aqueduct.*

Width of Third Ventricle

The average width of the third ventricle varies with age (Engeset and Lonnum). It is somewhat wider in older patients, ranging from 6 mm. in children 6 to 15 years of age, to approximately 11 mm. in persons 56 to 65 years of age. The width of the third ventricle is considered a reliable index of general ventricular size.

According to Wilson, "It would seem reasonable to use 7 mm. as the average width of the third ventricle during the second decade of life, and add 1 mm. for each subsequent decade to age 70."

The region of the third ventricle anteriorly between the optic and infundibular recesses has been called the *chiasmal point* by Bull. This may be located up to 17 mm. above the sella turcica.

The angle formed by the floor of the third ventricle and the cerebral aqueduct is more acute in a child than in an adult (Wilson). After 4 or 5 years of age, however, an adult configuration is usually present.

In a perfectly symmetrical anteroposterior film in which the temporal horns as well as the third ventricle can be identified, the

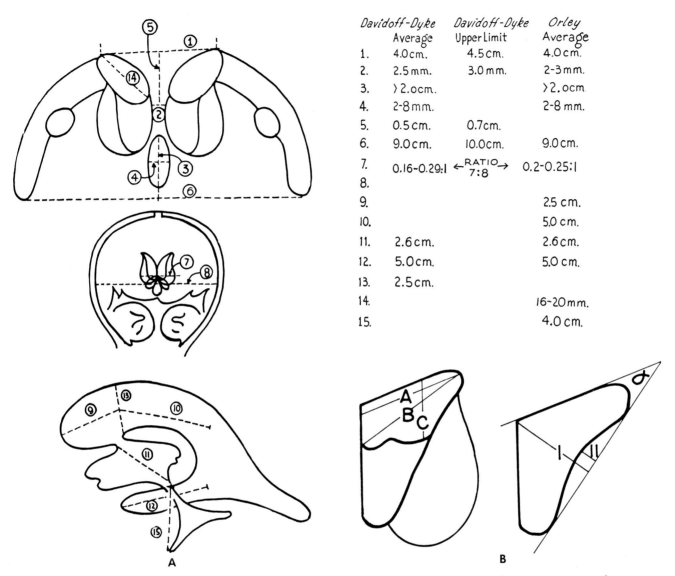

	Davidoff-Dyke Average	Davidoff-Dyke Upper Limit	Orley Average
1.	4.0 cm.	4.5 cm.	4.0 cm.
2.	2.5 mm.	3.0 mm.	2-3 mm.
3.	>2.0 cm.		>2.0 cm.
4.	2-8 mm.		2-8 mm.
5.	0.5 cm.	0.7 cm.	
6.	9.0 cm.	10.0 cm.	9.0 cm.
7.	0.16-0.29:1	←RATIO 7:8→	0.2-0.25:1
8.			
9.			2.5 cm.
10.			5.0 cm.
11.	2.6 cm.		2.6 cm.
12.	5.0 cm.		5.0 cm.
13.	2.5 cm.		
14.			16-20 mm.
15.			4.0 cm.

Figure 8–30. *A.* Average measurements of ventricles as applied to pneumoencephalography. *B.* Measurement of bodies and anterior horns of ventricles. *A* measures distance between septum pellucidum and superolateral angle above caudate nucleus. (Ruler placed parallel to and just below roof of ventricle.) *A* should measure less than 2 cm. Jirout's system of measurements is as follows: When the ventricles are dilated the dimension (I) and the angle alpha increase and the dimension (II) decreases. The dimension (I) is usually smaller than 1.5 to 1.6 cm. Angle alpha is 20 degrees to 35 degrees normally. (From Robertson, E. G.: Pneumoencephalography, 1967. Courtesy of Charles C Thomas, Publisher, Springfield, Illinois.)

Figure 8–30 continued on the following page.

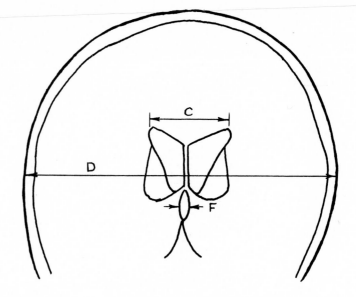

D/C "ventricle index"

Schiersmann's Method of Measurement in Adults
  C = Maximum width of both cellae mediae
  D = Maximum width of skull (outer table to outer table)
  F = Maximum width of third ventricle

D/C< 3 undoubtedly pathological

D/C : 3 to 3.5 moderately dilated

D/C : 3.5-4 normal
                (Engeset and Skraastad believe this should be 4)

D/C>4 undoubtedly normal

F < 5 mm=normal width of third ventricle

CM ≦ 41 mm pathological
    45 mm (2 S.D.)

C   D

Figure 8-30 *Continued.*   C. Method of Engeset and Skraastad (from Bruijn) with further amplification from Burhenne and Davies. (See Bruijn, G. W.: Pneumoencephalography in diagnosis of cerebral atrophy: quantitative study. Thesis, State University of Utrecht, 1959; and Burhenne, H. J., and Davies, H.: Amer. J. Roentgenol., *90:* 1176–1184, 1963.) *D.* Further methods of measurements utilized in encephalography employing the "ventricle index."

Figure 8–30 continued on the opposite page.

distance from the midline of the third ventricle to the lateral border of the temporal horn on the two sides should not vary more than 3 mm. (Lindgren, 1957). Before making this comparison, the examiner must be certain that the two horns contain the same amount of air and that the film is perfectly symmetrical.

The relationship of the floor of the third ventricle to the clivus is indicated by a lining technique devised by Ruggiero and Castellano (Fig. 8–33). As noted, the first line is drawn along the plane of the clivus and is continued upward above the dorsum sellae. The second line is drawn perpendicular to this line, tangent to the most anterior inferior part of the third ventricle. In the normal person, the latter line passes through the rostral end of the cerebral aqueduct or above it. When the floor of the third ventricle or the cerebral aqueduct is displaced upward through the tentorium, this relationship is disturbed.

Cerebral Aqueduct (Fig. 8–32). The cerebral aqueduct is a narrow channel measuring 1.5 to 2.0 cm. in length (or slightly more) and 1 to 2 mm. in diameter, connecting the third and fourth ventricles with a gentle dorsal curvature in the sagittal plane. The roof of the midbrain lies dorsally with respect to the aqueduct

Evan's Method for Children

Line AB = maximum width of anterior horns

Line CD = maximum width skull (inner table to inner table)

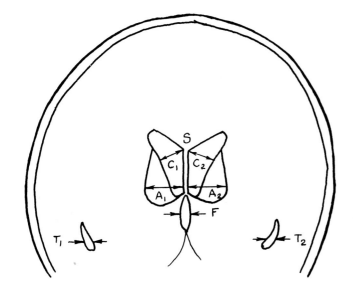

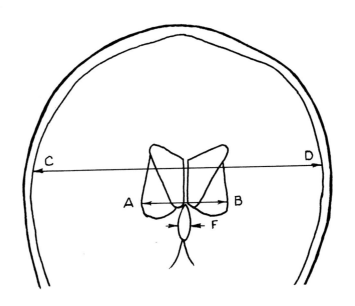

C_1 or $C_2 \lessgtr$ 15 mm pathological   < 12 mm normal*

A_1 or $A_2 \gtrless$ 25 mm pathological   12–14 borderline*

F   = or >   8 mm   > 15 abnormal*

T_1 or $T_2 \lessgtr$ 5 mm

C_1 and C_2 should be within 3 mm of one another

A_1 and A_2 should be within 3 mm of one another

"Supplemental measurements increase the the value of all methods and their correlation"

$$\frac{AB}{CD} - \text{Encephalographic ventricle ratio}$$

$\frac{AB}{CD}$ = 0.2 to 0.24 normal

= 0.25 to 0.29 doubtfully pathological

> 0.3 pathological beyond question (1942 value)

F not > 8 mm normal (Melchior)

E   F

Figure 8–30 *Continued.* E. Further measurements of pneumograms of the brain. (Data based on Jacobsen, H. H., and Melchior, J. C.: Amer. J. Roentgenol., *101*:188–194, 1967; and Engeset, A., and Skraastad, E.: Neurology, *14*:381, 1964.) F. Evan's method for measurement in pneumography of the brain in children.

Figure 8–30 continued on the following page.

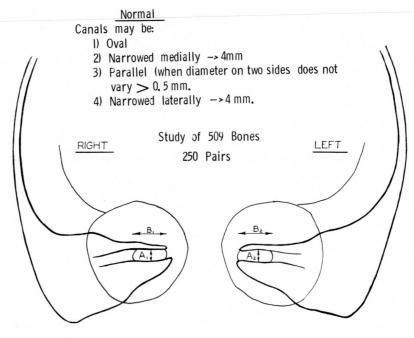

<u>Normal</u>

Canals may be:

1) Oval
2) Narrowed medially $\rightarrow$ 4mm
3) Parallel (when diameter on two sides does not vary $>$ 0.5 mm.
4) Narrowed laterally $\rightarrow$ 4 mm.

Study of 509 Bones
250 Pairs

<u>RIGHT</u>   <u>LEFT</u>

6.1 mm: difference on 2 sides up to 2.5 mm

<u>A</u>   Average : 6.2 mm
     Greatest : 11 mm
     Smallest: 2.5 mm
     Average of both sides: 5.23 mm

<u>B</u>   Average: 7.9 mm   7.8 mm   Greatest variation on 2 sides: 5 mm
     Greatest: 16 mm
     Smallest: 3 mm   usually
                                   4 to 10 mm

Camp, J. D. and Cilley, E. I. L.: The significance of asymmetry of the **pori** acoustici as an aid in the diagnosis of eighth nerve tumors. Amer. J. Roentgenol., <u>41</u>: 713-718, 1939.

Flaring of IAC never normal
Erosion of suprameatal or inframeatal region is abnormal
Different configurations on 2 sides suspicious of abnormality (16% were normal)
(10% quoted by Valvassori)

Diff. of A on 2 sides up to 1.0 mm normal; $>$ 1 mm abnormal

<u>Differential Diagnosis</u>
Acoustic neuroma
Primary cholesteatoma
Meningioma
Glomus jugulare tumor
Metastatic tumor
Invasive nasopharyngeal carcinoma
Eosinophilic granuloma
Carcinoma of middle ear

Diff. of B on 2 sides up to 1.5 mm normal; $>$ 1.5 mm abnormal

Lapayowker and Cliff. Amer. J. Roentgenol., pp 652-658

<u>107</u>, 1969

G

Figure 8–30 *Continued.*   G. Measurements of the internal auditory canal and meatus as related to brain lesions.

and contains the *quadrigeminal plate*. The quadrigeminal plate merges with the *superior cerebellar peduncles* and the *anterior medullary vellum* at its lower end, the latter forming the roof of the upper part of the fourth ventricle. Measurements for the aqueduct (and posterior commissure) are shown in Fig. 8–33 *A* (see legend).

The relationship of the cerebral aqueduct to the third ventricle has been demonstrated by the lining technique just described (Fig. 8–33). Lindgren and DiChiro suggested that the demarcation between the cerebral aqueduct and the fourth ventricle is the point of transition at a level corresponding to the lower border of the quadrigeminal plate.

Another useful line (Fig. 8–33) for demonstration of the relationship of the cerebral aqueduct to the skull is drawn from the superior edge of the dorsum sellae through the lower aqueduct to the inner table of the skull and then divided into three equal segments; the aqueduct should cross this line at about the junction of its anterior and middle thirds (Sahlstedt).

Twining's Line. Twining's line (Fig. 8–33) is obtained by drawing a line from the tuberculum sellae to the internal occipital protuberance. The midpoint of this line should fall near the center of the fourth ventricle or close to its ventral border.

Several authorities have given the length of the aqueduct as 1.5 to 1.8 cm. (Lindgren and DiChiro). The junction of the cerebral aqueduct and third ventricle is called the *iter*.

Ventricular Angle (Fig. 8–33 *A*). A ventricular angle has been suggested by Sutton as follows: if a line is drawn from the iter to the infundibular recess on the one hand (inf), and then from the iter to the midpoint of the floor of the fourth ventricle on the other, a ventricular angle approximating 90 degrees ± 5 degrees is formed.

Fourth Ventricle (Fig. 8–34). The fourth ventricle, as previously noted, is diamond-shaped in frontal view and triangular in lateral view, with boundaries as follows.

Boundaries of Fourth Ventricle

FLOOR: tegmentum of the lower *pons and medulla.*

ROOF: the *anterior medullary vellum* forms the anterior superior portion of the roof and lies between the *superior cerebellar peduncles* and the fourth ventricle. The *posterior medullary vellum* forms the caudal portion of the roof. This latter structure is invaginated by the choroid plexus of the fourth ventricle and the *nodule of the inferior vermis of the cerebellum*. The fourth ventricle communicates with the spinal canal through a midline aperture caudally called the *foramen of Magendie*. Between the anterior and posterior medullary vellum an angle is formed centrally known as the *fastigium*. Somewhat lateral and caudal to the fastigium are the superoposterior recesses of the fourth ventricle on each side.

The size of the fourth ventricle varies considerably, as shown in Figure 8–35. Height varies between 9 and 19 mm. (Oberson et

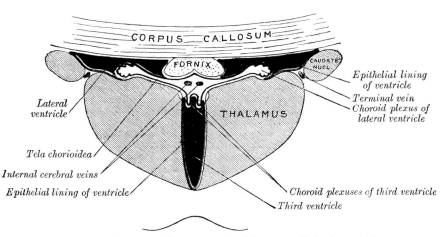

Figure 8–31. Coronal section (diagrammatic) of lateral and third ventricles. (From Gray's Anatomy of the Human Body, 29th ed. Goss, C. M. (ed.) Philadelphia, Lea & Febiger, 1973.)

al.). The position of the fourth ventricle may be accurately delineated by means of Twining's line (Fig. 8–33), as previously described.

Cisterns (Figs. 8–6, 8–36). The cisterns have been previously described in the section on the subarachnoid space. Fur-

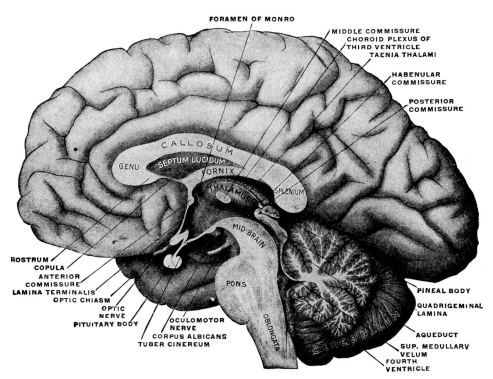

Figure 8–32. Mesial aspect of a brain sectioned in the median sagittal plane. (From Gray's Anatomy of the Human Body, 24th ed. Lewis, W. H. (ed.) Philadelphia, Lea & Febiger, 1942.)

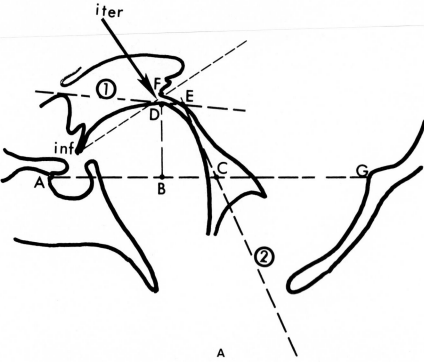

A

Figure 8–33. A. Diagram of the measurements of the cerebral aqueduct and the posterior commissure. The vertical reference line BF and the horizontal line AB are shown along with line 1 and line AG, which are the two tangents on the floor of the aqueduct at its rostral and caudal ends respectively. The distances DE and BC are explained as follows: Line AG is drawn between the tuberculum sellae (A) and the internal occipital protuberance (G). Line 1 is drawn tangent to the cerebral aqueduct as shown, crossing the inferior margin of the cerebral aqueduct superiorly at point D. A tangent to the upper half of the floor of the fourth ventricle is then drawn (line 2) and intersects line 1 at point E. F represents the upper margin of the cerebral aqueduct. Line DB is perpendicular to line AG.

The cerebral aqueduct as demonstrated in this drawing should ordinarily measure no more than 1.5 to 2 cm. in length and 1 to 2 mm. in diameter.

Another useful relationship is indicated on this drawing as follows: If a line is drawn between the infundibular stalk as shown and the junction between the cerebral aqueduct and third ventricle, it should form an angle of approximately $90° \pm 5°$ with a tangent to the floor of the fourth ventricle. (Modified from Hilal, et al.: Acta Radiol. (Diag.), 9:167–182, 1969.)

Figure 8–33 continued on the opposite page.

ther discussion is appropriate in this discussion of the ventricles of the brain because the two structures communicate with each other. Liliequist has classified the cisterns as: (1) ventral, (2) dorsal, (3) communicating, and (4) general subarachnoid space over convexities of the cerebrum and cerebellum.

Ventral Cisterns.   The ventral cisterns are subclassified as follows: (1) medial unpaired cisterns, consisting of medullary, pontine, interpeduncular, and chiasmatic cisterns, and (2) paramedial paired cisterns, consisting of the cerebellopontine angle cistern, crural cistern, and cisterns of the Sylvian fissures.

The ventral cisterns are sometimes called the *basal cisterns* and consist primarily of the pontine, interpeduncular, chiasmatic, and cerebellopontine angle cisterns. The last-named of these are of considerable importance because they may help in demonstrating mass lesions contiguous with the internal acoustic meatus or petrous ridge.

Dorsal Cisterns.   The dorsal cisterns are subclassified as: (1) medial unpaired cisterns, consisting of the superior cerebellar cistern, quadrigeminal cistern or cistern of the great cerebral vein of Galen, and the pericallosal cistern, and (2) paramedial dorsal cisterns, known as the ambient or retrothalamic cisterns.

The quadrigeminal cistern merges into the pericallosal cistern, which in turn runs longitudinally above the corpus callosum. If a *cavum veli interpositi* is present above the roof of the third ventricle, communicating with the third ventricle, it opens into the quadrigeminal cistern. Another ventricular chamber sometimes identified is the *cavum vergae* (a posterior extension of the cavum septi pellucidi), and this, too, may open into the quadrigeminal cistern.

The *ambient cistern,* which encircles the midbrain, communicates between the quadrigeminal cistern or cistern of the great cerebral vein of Galen and the pontine cistern. In most instances there is no clear line of demarcation between one or another of these several contiguous cisterns.

Communicating Cisterns.   The communicating cisterns likewise consist of two unpaired cisterns called (1) the great cistern caudally (cisterna magna), and (2) the cistern of the lamina terminalis rostrally. There is also a single paramedial pair of cisterns around the midbrain called the ambient cisterns.

The great cistern (cisterna magna) lies beneath the cerebellar tonsils, just above and behind the foramen magnum. It is continuous with the cerebral subarachnoid space caudally.

Identification of the ambient cistern is particularly helpful since it contains: the posterior cerebral arteries, the superior cerebellar arteries, the anterior and posterior choroidal arteries, the basal vein of Rosenthal, and the trochlear nerves.

The cistern of the lamina terminalis is continuous around the genu of the corpus callosum with the pericallosal cistern, and the anterior cerebral arteries are contained within it.

The combined images of the quadrigeminal, ambient, crural, and interpeduncular cisterns may clearly outline the midbrain. A visualization of the pericallosal cisterns may be the only indicator of the midline of the brain or superior longitudinal fissure, particularly when other cisterns or ventricles are poorly filled.

CIRCULATION OF CEREBROSPINAL FLUID

The cerebrospinal fluid is formed largely by secretion by the choroid plexus, but other substances enter it, apparently by effusion from the plasma across the ependyma and pia arachnoid. The cerebrospinal fluid is produced mainly inside the ven-

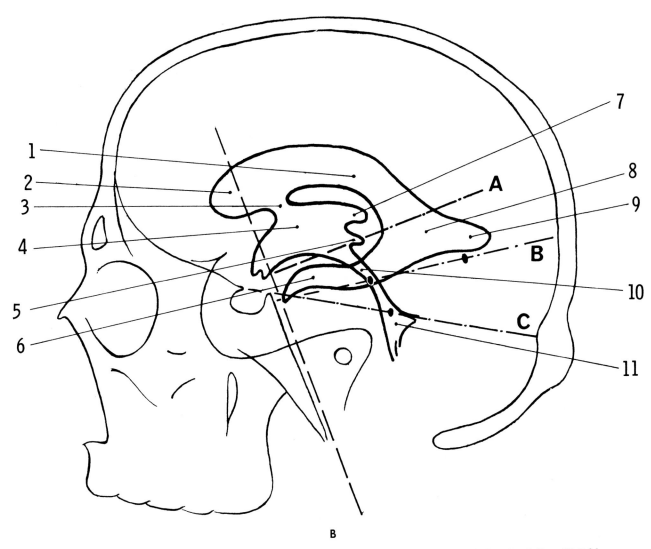

Figure 8–33 *Continued.* B. The ventricular system as seen in the lateral projection. (A) Ruggiero's line, (B) Sahl-stedt's line, and (C) Twining's line. (See text for explanation of these three lines.) The parts of the ventricular system are: (1) Body of the lateral ventricle, (2) Frontal horn, (3) Interventricular foramen, (4) Third ventricle, (5) Pineal recess, (6) Temporal horn, (7) Suprapineal recess, (8) Trigone, (9) Occipital horn, (10) Cerebral aqueduct, (11) Fourth ventricle. (From Wilson, M.: The Anatomic Foundation of Neuroradiology of the Brain, 2nd ed. Boston, Little, Brown & Co., 1972.)

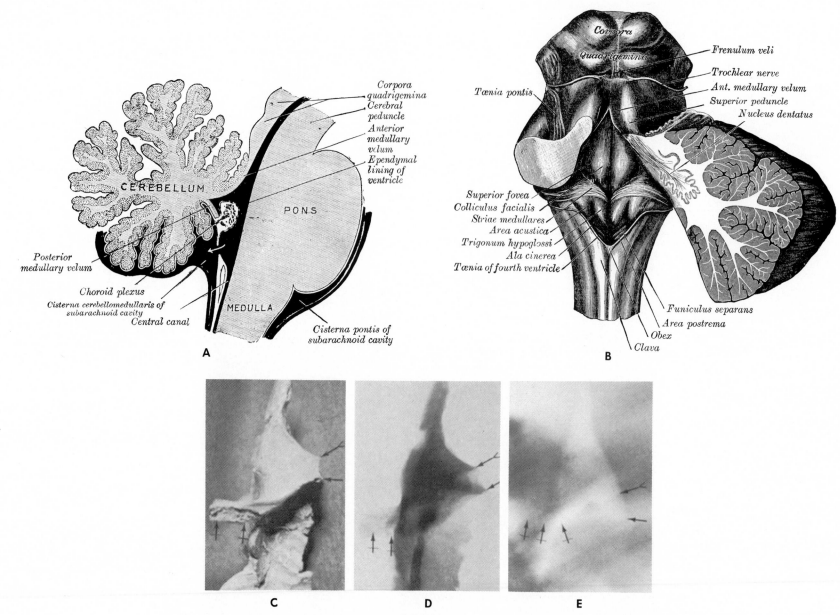

Figure 8–34. *A.* Scheme of roof of fourth ventricle. The arrow is in the foramen of Magendie. *B.* Rhomboid fossa. (From Gray's Anatomy of the Human Body, 29th ed. Goss, C. M. (ed.) Philadelphia, Lea & Febiger, 1973.) *C.* Cast of fourth ventricle. *D.* Its roentgen appearances. *E.* Midline tomogram (zonography) during encephalography in vivo. Fastigium (⟩→), posterior superior recess (⟶), lateral recess (⊦→). (From Corrales, M., and Greitz, T.: Acta Radiol. (Diag.), *12:*113–133, 1972.)

tricular system in the lateral ventricles. There is a flow from the lateral ventricles into the third ventricle, down the cerebral aqueduct into the fourth ventricle, and thereafter out through the foramina of Luschka into the subarachnoid space surrounding the brain. A flow also occurs from the fourth ventricle through the foramen of Magendie down the spinal canal.

Absorption of the cerebrospinal fluid occurs largely over the cerebral hemispheres through the pacchionian villi and arachnoid granulations. There is also a small amount of absorption through the perineural lymphatics.

It is probable that the fluid in the subdural space is produced locally by its own mesothelial cells, but the exact relationship of this fluid to the cerebrospinal fluid is not known (Fig. 8–37).

Approximately 14 per cent of the total blood volume transported through the heart per minute flows to the brain (750 ml., Decker). The volume per minute may be calculated as 50 to 60 ml. per minute for 100 grams of brain substance (Kety and Schmidt). By comparison, the kidneys take in eight times this volume, and the myocardium one and a half times as much per minute per 100 grams of substance. Blood volume flowing through the liver is almost identical to that of the brain. It is estimated that approximately 13 ml. of blood arrive at the brain per heart beat, assuming an average cardiac rate of 70 beats per minute. The volume per minute for both carotid arteries is about 420 to 450 ml. It has been assumed that about 4 ml. per cardiac beat pass into the brain via the vertebral arteries. Careful circulation studies in both normal and pathological states have been carried out by rapid filming in serial angiography (Taveras et al.), as well as by computerized isotopic studies, the latter portending to be of great value.

Increased intracranial pressure may in extreme cases impede intracranial circulation.

If the heart rate is markedly diminished to 40 per minute or even less, the duration of the passage of contrast medium through the brain is generally increased, even with increased arterial blood pressure.

Vasospasm is considered one of the main causes of impeded arterial filling.

Radiography of the Brain by Ventricular and Cisternal Pneumography

The pneumoencephalographic examination is begun with the patient in a sitting position, and the air (or other suitable gaseous medium) is introduced by lumbar puncture. The first fraction of 5 to 8 ml. is injected without withdrawal of cerebrospinal fluid, and the air is trapped in the posterior fossa by carefully flexing the patient's head 90 degrees, as shown in Figure 8–38 A, B C. Ideally, at this juncture, fluoroscopy with the aid of image amplification

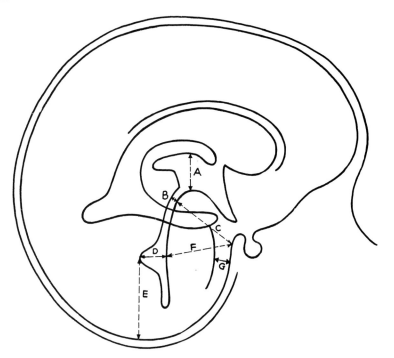

	MINIMUM	MAXIMUM	AVERAGE	ROBERTSON
A	1.10 cm.	1.60 cm.	1.42 cm.	1.3–1.9 cm.
B	0.10 cm.	0.20 cm.	0.15 cm.	0.1–0.2 cm.
C	3.0 cm.	3.9 cm.	3.44 cm.	3.0–3.7 cm.
D	1.0 cm.	1.9 cm.	1.46 cm.	1.1–2.1 cm.
E	3.0 cm.	4.0 cm.	3.26 cm.	————
F	3.3 cm.	4.0 cm.	3.61 cm.	3.1–4.3 cm.
G	0.5 cm.	1.2 cm.	0.82 cm.	0.5 cm.

Figure 8–35. Measurements of ventricles as applied to pneumoencephalography. Further measurements with an indication of range. (From Dyke and Davidoff, Amer. J. Roentgenol., 44:1940; Robertson, E. G.: Pneumoencephalography, 1967, Charles C Thomas, Publisher, Springfield, Illinois; and Oberon, R., et al.: Acta Radiol. (Diag.), 9:193, 1969.)

and closed circuit television will indicate whether the air is in the best position. Films are obtained in posteroanterior and lateral perspectives (Fig. 8–38 D, E). As the degree of flexion of the head is carefully diminished (Fig. 8–38 B, C), air may be seen to rise above the tentorium cerebelli into the third and lateral ventricles. Intermittent injections of small amounts of air, following withdrawal of similar amounts of cerebrospinal fluid, will permit radiographic visualization of the important anatomic detail otherwise obscured by superimposed gas shadows. Intermittent utilization of polytomography also enhances anatomic detail (Fig. 8–39).

If much cerebrospinal fluid must be drained, approximately 80 to 120 ml. of air may be utilized in the course of the study.

In some instances, for reasons usually difficult to explain, the air enters the subdural rather than the subarachnoid space. Since this area has little diagnostic value because of its great variability, the needle should be repositioned or the examination terminated and scheduled for another day (Fig. 8–38 *F*).

The initial films are best for demonstration of the great cistern, fourth ventricle, cerebral aqueduct, and possibly the upper part of the third ventricle. Tomography should be routine at this juncture, since this is the best time for visualization of the posterior fossa. The cerebellum and structures in and around the quadrigeminal plate may also be visualized.

Once visualization of the supratentorial ventricular system has been obtained, it is desirable to inject sufficient air to delin-

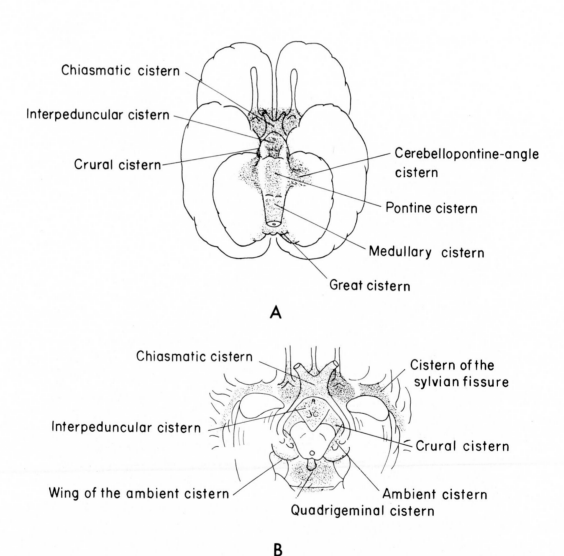

A

B

Figure 8–36. *A.* The subarachnoid cisterns at the base of the brain stem. For purposes of clarity, the cisterns are shown separated. They are, of course, in continuity with each other. *B.* The subarachnoid cisterns about the diencephalon and midbrain, as seen from the ventral aspect. The lower brain stem and the temporal horns have been removed. (*A* and *B* from Wilson, M.: The Anatomic Foundation of Neuroradiology of the Brain, 2nd ed. Boston, Little, Brown & Co., 1972.)

Figure 8–36 continued on opposite page.

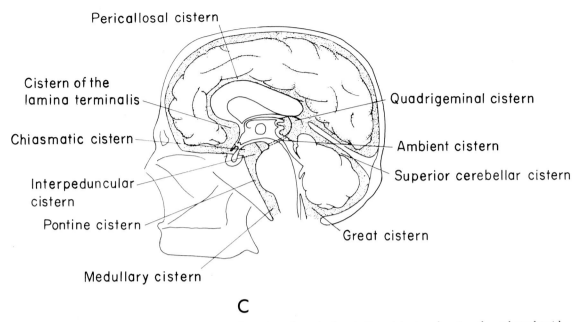

C

Figure 8-36 *Continued.* C. Midline sagittal section through the skull and brain, showing the subarachnoid cisterns. (From Wilson, M.: The Anatomic Foundation of Neuroradiology of the Brain, 2nd ed. Boston, Little, Brown & Co., 1972.)

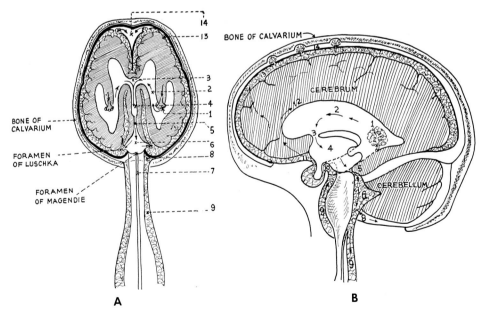

Figure 8-37. Diagrams illustrating the circulation of the cerebrospinal fluid. A. Frontal projection. B. Lateral projection. (See text for explanation.)

eate clearly the borders of the thalamus in the floor of the ventricles, and the basal cisterns and subarachnoid space surrounding the brain. Since different portions of the ventricular system and subarachnoid space are visible in the different projections and positions of the patient, each examiner will develop his own sequence of head positions and views to be obtained for op-

timum demonstration of anatomic detail. Special chairs have been designed for "tumbling" of the patient.

The views and positions usually employed by this author are as follows:

1. Patient sitting, head half-axial at 90 degrees, 65 degrees, or 45 degrees; posteroanterior and lateral views (Fig. 8–38).

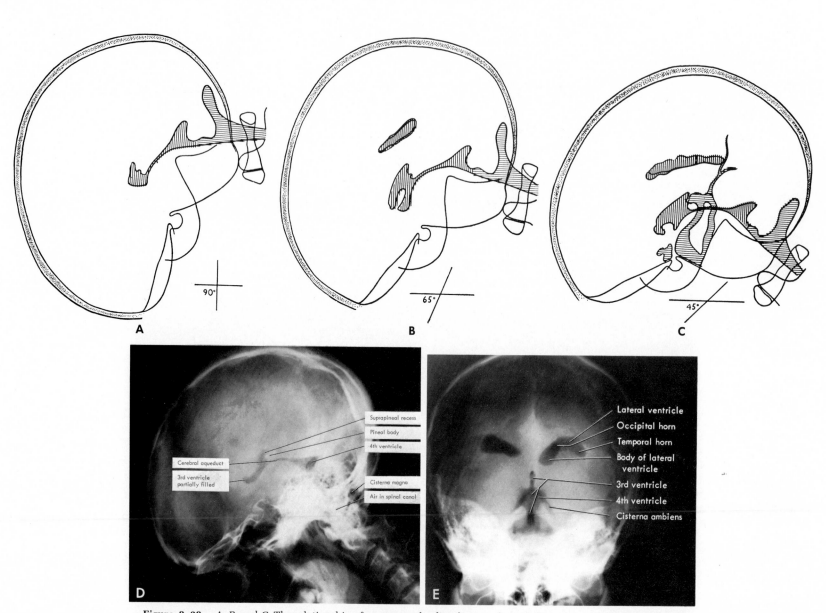

Figure 8–38.   *A, B,* and *C.* The relationship of posture to the distribution of gas in the cadaver. In *A,* the flexion is 90 degrees; in *B,* 65 degrees; in *C,* 45 degrees. (From Robertson, E. G.: Pneumoencephalography, 1967. Courtesy of Charles C Thomas, Publisher, Springfield, Illinois.) *D* and *E.* Radiographs (intensified) obtained by the Robertson-Lindgren technique in posteroanterior and lateral projections (not identical).

Figure 8–38 continued on the opposite page.

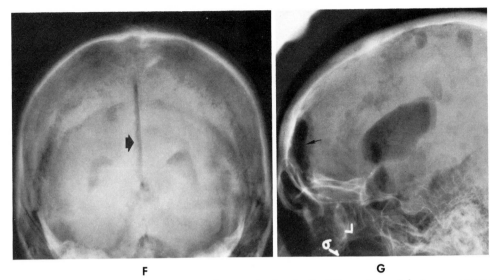

F   G

Figure 8–38 *Continued.* F. Subdural air along the superior longitudinal fissure (arrow) during pneumoencephalography. G. Lateral view of the skull with the patient's head in the supine position and an accumulation of subdural air (arrow) beneath the frontal bone and frontal sinuses.

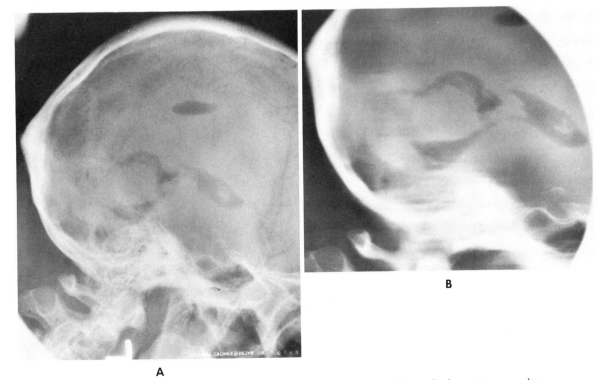

A   B

Figure 8–39. *A* and *B.* Improvement of posterior fossa pneumoencephalography by autotomography.

2. Patient sitting, head erect; lateral and anteroposterior views (Fig. 8–40).

3. Patient sitting, head erect; Towne's view, 15 to 35 degrees as in Figure 8–41, but with the patient erect.

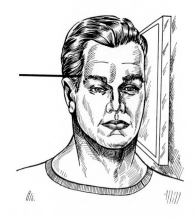

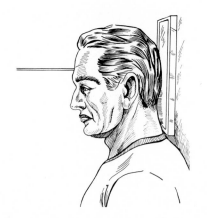

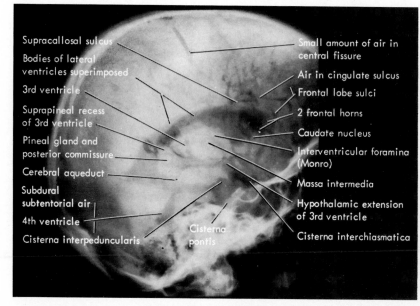

Supracallosal sulcus

Bodies of lateral ventricles superimposed

3rd ventricle

Suprapineal recess of 3rd ventricle

Pineal gland and posterior commissure

Cerebral aqueduct

Subdural subtentorial air

4th ventricle

Cisterna interpeduncularis

Cisterna pontis

Small amount of air in central fissure

Air in cingulate sulcus

Frontal lobe sulci

2 frontal horns

Caudate nucleus

Interventricular foramina (Monro)

Massa intermedia

Hypothalamic extension of 3rd ventricle

Cisterna interchiasmatica

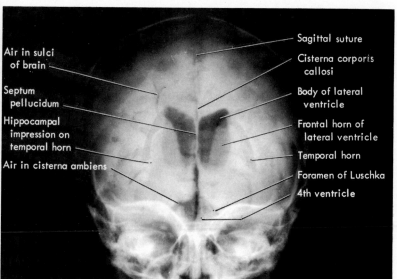

Air in sulci of brain

Septum pellucidum

Hippocampal impression on temporal horn

Air in cisterna ambiens

Sagittal suture

Cisterna corporis callosi

Body of lateral ventricle

Frontal horn of lateral ventricle

Temporal horn

Foramen of Luschka

4th ventricle

Figure 8–40. Positioning for and radiographs (intensified) obtained during pneumoencephalography with patient erect and beam horizontal, lateral and AP projections.

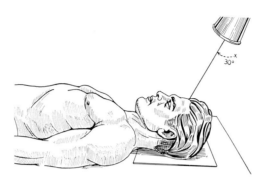

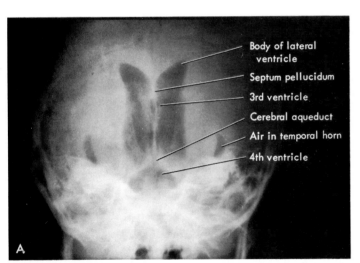

Body of lateral
ventricle

Septum pellucidum

3rd ventricle

Cerebral aqueduct

Air in temporal horn

4th ventricle

A

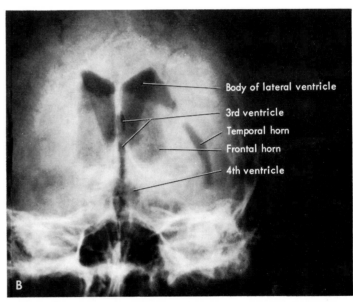

Body of lateral ventricle

3rd ventricle

Temporal horn

Frontal horn

4th ventricle

B

Figure 8–41. Positioning for and radiographs (intensified) obtained during pneumoencephalography with patient supine in Towne's projection. *A.* 30 degree angulation of central ray caudad. *B.* 15 degree angulation of central ray caudad.

4. Patient prone, brow down; posteroanterior and lateral views (Fig. 8–42). (Half-axial views may also be obtained.)

5. Patient supine, brow up; anteroposterior and lateral views

(Fig. 8–43). Half-axial views may be obtained if desired, in Towne's projection (Fig. 8–41).

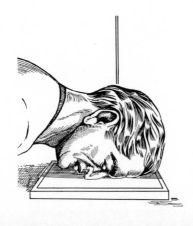

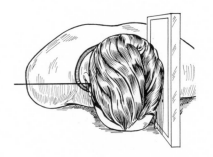

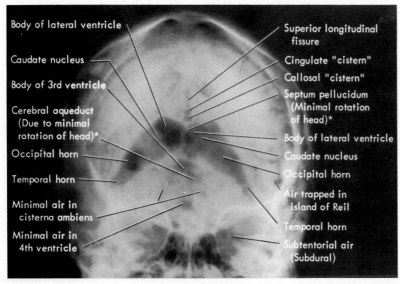

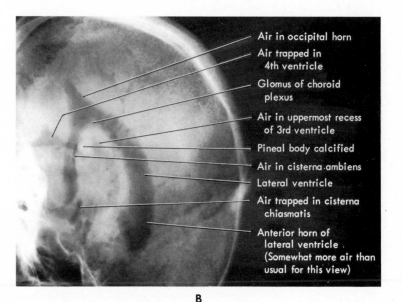

A   **B**

Figure 8–42. Positioning for and radiographs (intensified) obtained during pneumoencephalography with patient prone, brow down. *A.* Vertical beam. *B.* Horizontal beam. *Note that minimal rotation of head as indicated by relationship of mastoid processes with condyloid processes (mandible) may distort the septum pellucidum and third ventricle, as well as make the lateral ventricles appear slightly asymmetrical.

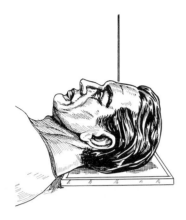

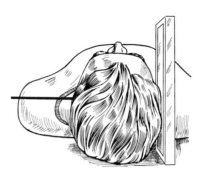

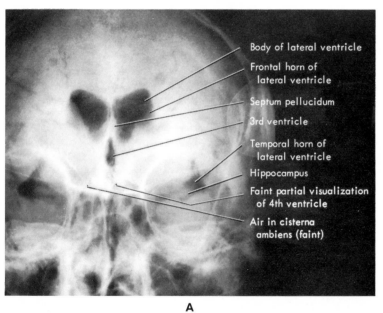

Body of lateral ventricle

Frontal horn of
lateral ventricle

Septum pellucidum

3rd ventricle

Temporal horn of
lateral ventricle

Hippocampus

Faint partial visualization
of 4th ventricle

Air in cisterna
ambiens (faint)

A

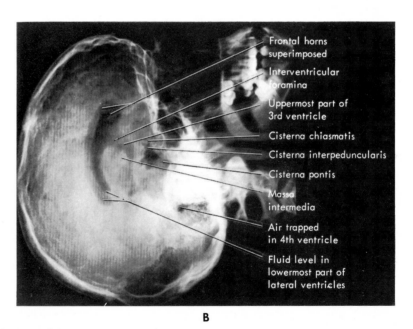

Frontal horns
superimposed

Interventricular
foramina

Uppermost part of
3rd ventricle

Cisterna chiasmatis

Cisterna interpeduncularis

Cisterna pontis

Massa
intermedia

Air trapped
in 4th ventricle

Fluid level in
lowermost part of
lateral ventricles

B

Figure 8–43. Positioning for and radiographs (intensified) obtained during pneumoencephalography with patient recumbent, supine. *A.* Vertical beam, AP. *B.* Horizontal beam, lateral. (Both laterals may be taken.)

6. Patient prone, head turned first to one side and then the other; in each of these two positions, posteroanterior and lateral views are obtained, utilizing a horizontal beam (Fig. 8–44). Views employing a vertical beam, reverse Towne's projection, may also be obtained at this time (Fig. 8–45).

7. A basovertical view with the patient prone, positioned as shown in Figure 8–46, may also be obtained at this time.

8. Body section radiographs and tomograms are utilized whenever a clear view of a given anatomic part is desired. Autotomography is a technique whereby the patient's head is slowly rotated on its vertical axis during a lateral exposure, especially when a view of the midline structures such as the cerebral aqueduct and fourth ventricle is desired. For structures other than those in the midline, special tomographic devices are necessary.

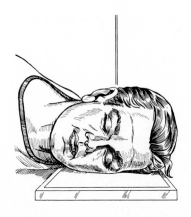

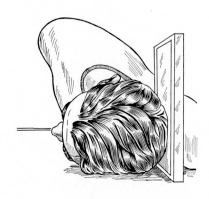

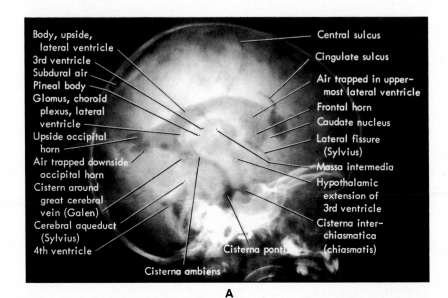

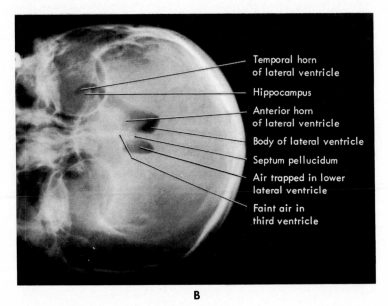

Figure 8–44. Positioning for and radiographs (intensified) obtained during pneumoencephalography with patient lying down, right side of head uppermost. *A.* Vertical beam. *B.* Horizontal beam. A similar set of two films is obtained with the left side of the head uppermost.

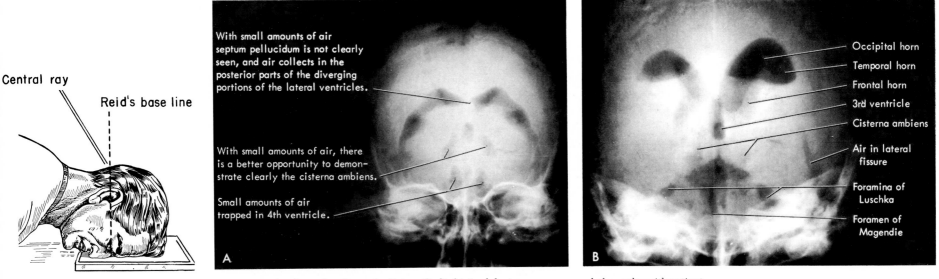

Figure 8–45. Positioning for and radiographs (intensified) obtained during pneumoencephalography with patient prone, reverse Towne's projection. *A.* Central ray angled 12 degrees to Reid's baseline. *B.* Central ray angled 25 degrees to Reid's baseline. (Foramina of Luschka label probable, not certain.)

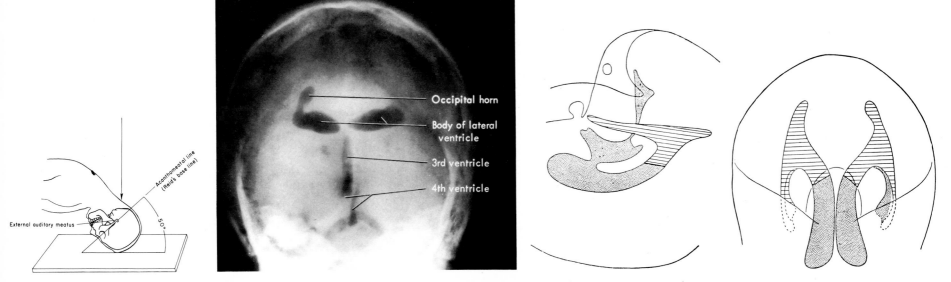

Figure 8–46. Positioning for radiograph (intensified) and tracings of basovertical view; patient prone, beam vertical. A horizontal beam lateral view (diagram, near right) is also obtained with the patient in this position. (Tracings from Robertson, E. G.: Pneumoencephalography, 1967. Courtesy of Charles C Thomas, Publisher, Springfield, Illinois.)

Stereoscopic pairs of films are obtained intermittently in lateral and frontal perspectives. In each instance, frontal and lateral views are obtained at right angles to one another, with the patient in a single position. A three-dimensional perspective is reconstructed in the examiner's eye from the two films.

The student is encouraged to study simplified glass models (Fig. 8–47) of the ventricular system that are partially filled with fluid and air to understand the dynamics of the air and fluid interface under the influence of gravity in these various positions.

The films must be perfectly positioned so that absolute symmetry of structures on the two sides of the head can be obtained.

Ventriculography

If increased intracranial pressure is present, herniation of brain substance through the foramen magnum (resulting in death) may occur at the time lumbar puncture is performed and

cerebrospinal fluid is removed. To prevent this, when air studies of the ventricles are necessary, cerebral puncture is accomplished through the parietal lobes, and cerebrospinal fluid is removed and replaced by air. The same series of films as previously described is obtained. The subarachnoid space outside the ventricular system is ordinarily not well demonstrated by this technique.

On occasion, for better visualization of the cerebral aqueduct or fourth ventricle, 1 to 2 ml. of Pantopaque may be injected into the lateral ventricle (Fig. 8–48). When the patient's head is moved to allow for maximal gravitational flow of the "heavier than spinal fluid oil," the oil, being much heavier than the cerebrospinal fluid, will move downward by gravity toward the cerebral aqueduct and fourth ventricle, and films may be taken to demonstrate the adjoining anatomy. Controversy exists regarding the advisability of injecting such radiopaque substances into the ventricular system, and this method of positive contrast ventriculography is utilized, particularly when other techniques have failed to reveal sufficient detail for an accurate diagnosis.

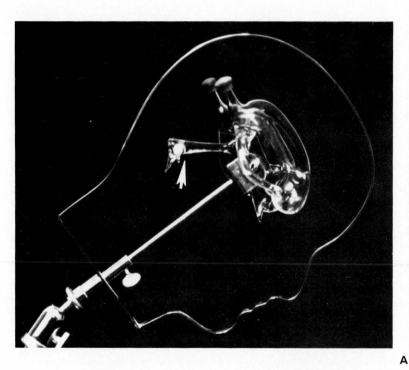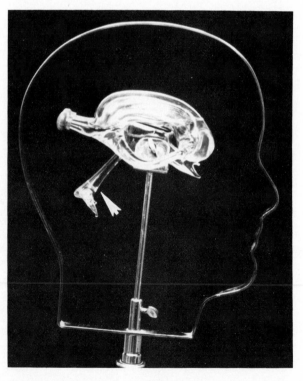

A

Figure 8–47.   *A*. Photographs of glass model of ventricular system, showing how the fluid and air interface may be studied.

Figure 8–47 continued on the opposite page.

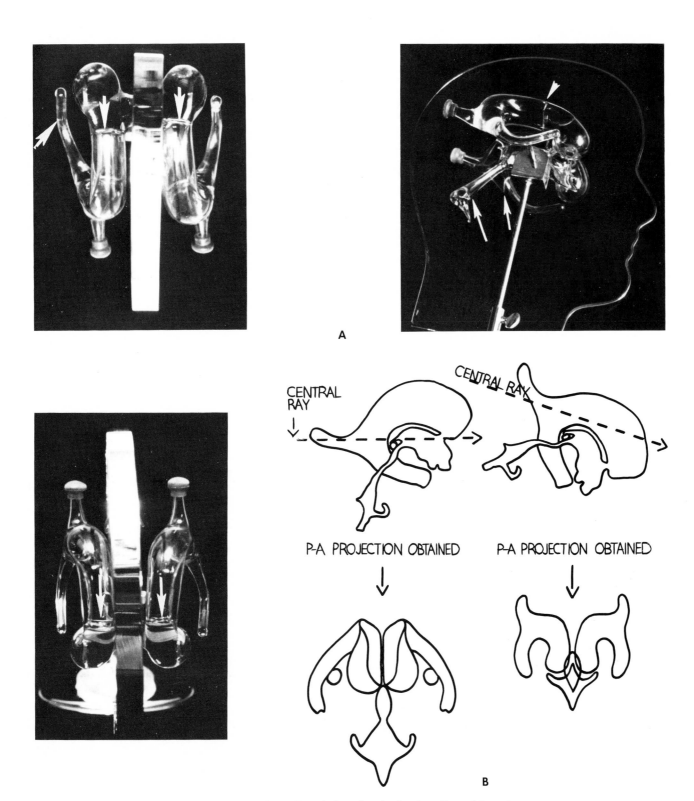

A

B

Figure 8–47 *Continued.* B. Translation of projection to radiographic anatomy.

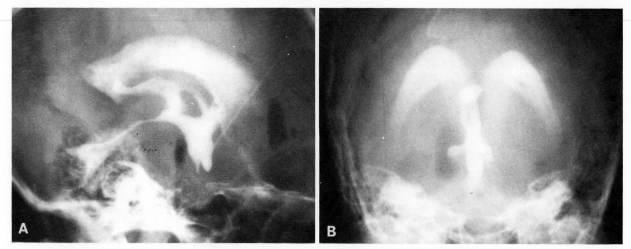

Figure 8–48. *A* and *B*. Positive contrast ventriculograms using water soluble opaque material. This technique results in excellent and detailed visualization of the ventricular system. (Patient was thought to have a small mass, probably a pinealoma, indenting the posterior wall of the third ventricle and encroaching slightly on the upper aqueduct.) (From Wilson, M.: The Anatomic Foundation of Neuroradiology of the Brain, 2nd ed. Boston, Little, Brown & Co., 1972.)

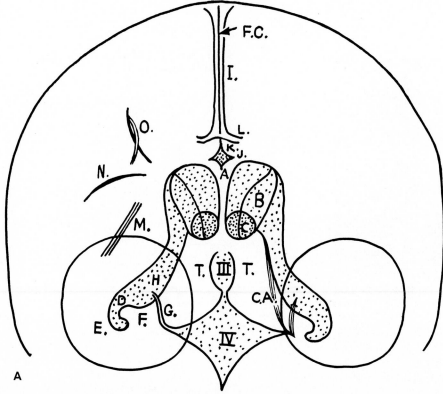

Figure 8–49. Diagram illustrating the various anatomic parts seen in pneumoencephalography. *A*. Anteroposterior projection. (A) Corpus callosum, (B) caudate nucleus, (C) choroid plexus, (D) temporal horns, (E) eminentia collateralis, (F) fornix, (G) lateral recess of fourth ventricle, (H) foramen of Luschka, (I) longitudinal fissure, (J) callosal sulcus, (K) cisterna corpus callosi, (L) cingulate sulcus, (M) air in depths of Sylvian fissure, (N) middle frontal sulcus, (O) interparietal sulcus, (T–T) thalamus, (CA) cisterna ambiens, (FC) falx cerebri.

Figure 8–49 continued on the opposite page.

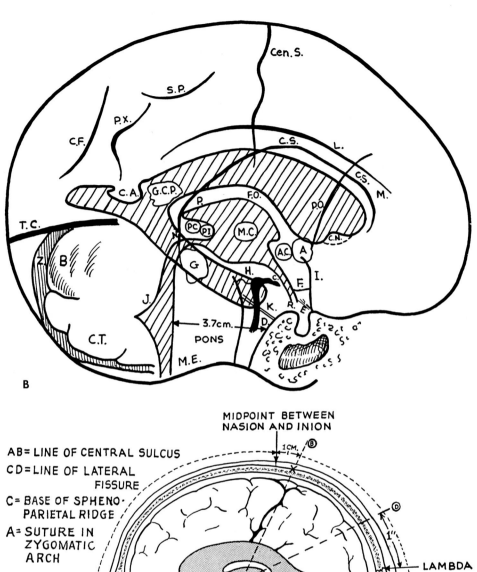

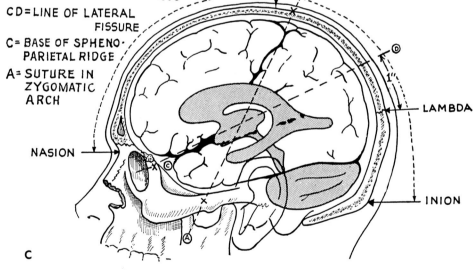

Figure 8–49 *Continued.* B. Lateral projection. (A) Lamina terminalis, (B) cerebellar folia, (C) posterior cerebral artery, (D) basilar artery, (E) optic chiasm, (F) anterior communicating artery, (G) colliculi, (H) cerebral peduncles (mammillary bodies), (I) tuber cinereum, (J) superior medullary velum, (K) oculomotor nerve, (L) cingulate sulcus, (M) cingulate gyrus, (N) cisterna ambiens, (P) pulvinar, (CN) caudate nucleus, (FO) fornix, (AC) anterior commissure, (MC) middle commissure, (PC) posterior commissure, (CA) calcar avis, (PI) pineal, (R) infundibulum, (CS) callosal sulcus-cisterna corpus callosi, (PX) parieto–occipital sulcus, (CF) calcarine fissure, (SP) subparietal sulcus, (PO) parolfactory sulcus, (Cen. S) central sulcus (Rolando), (CT) cerebellar tonsil, (TC) tentorium cerebelli, (Z) air outlining cerebellum, (GCP) glomus of the choroid plexus. C. Medial sagittal section of the brain. Relationship of the central sulcus and lateral fissure to the ventricles and skull.

Special Demonstrations of Pneumoencephalographic Anatomy

Gross demonstrations of pneumoencephalographic anatomy are shown in the following illustrations (Figs. 8–50 to 8–59), but in these several demonstrations, finer detail of brain anatomy can be achieved by polytomography, as indicated in other portions of this chapter.

ANATOMY BASIC TO CEREBRAL ANGIOGRAPHY

The Blood Supply of the Meninges. The arterial supply and venous drainage of the meninges have already been described (Figs. 6–11 and 8–8; Tables 8–1 and 8–2). Anastomoses from side to side as well as intra- and extracranial routes have been covered, and the reader is referred to these previous sections

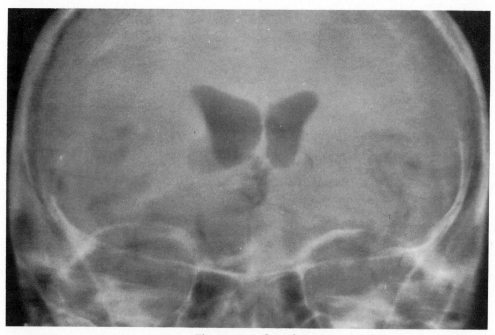

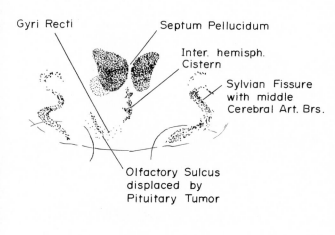

Figures 8–50 through 8–56. Labeled pneumoencephalographic details in a normal person.

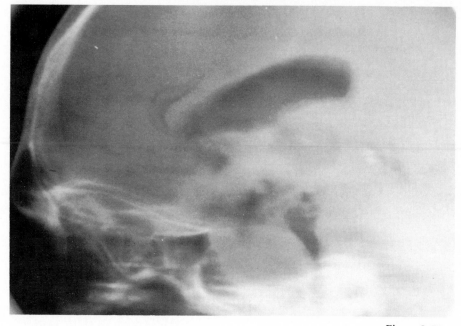

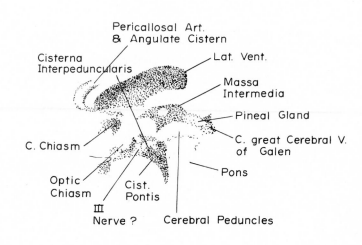

Figure 8–51.

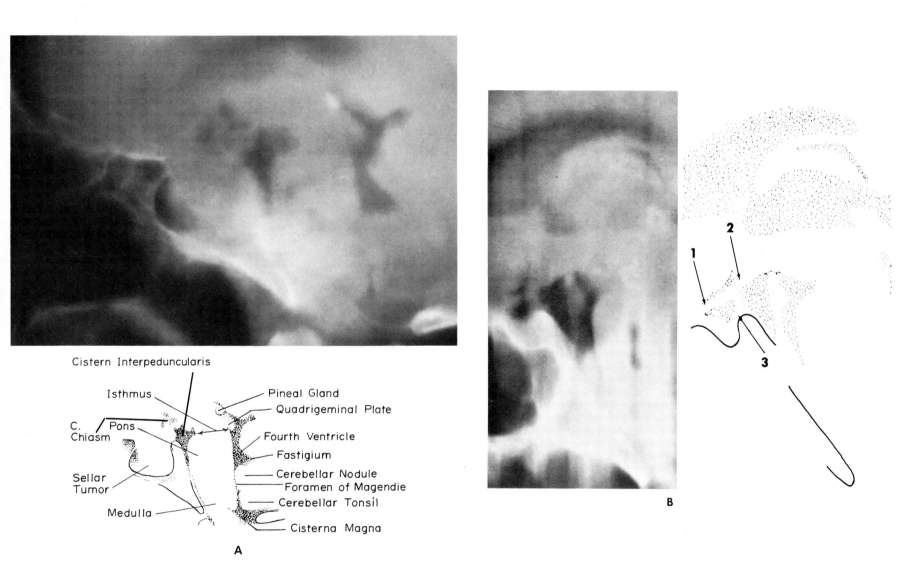

Figure 8–52. A and B. The normal (B) and abnormal (A) appearance of the optic nerves, cistern interchiasmatis, and cistern interpeduncularis. Patient in A had a tumor of the pituitary region. In B: (1) optic nerves (surrounded by c. chiasmatis), (2) optic chiasm, and (3) pituitary stalk. C. interpeduncularis is posterior and above sella. (B from DiChiro, G.: An Atlas of Detailed Normal Pneumoencephalographic Anatomy, 2nd ed. 1971. Courtesy of Charles C Thomas, Publisher, Springfield, Illinois.)

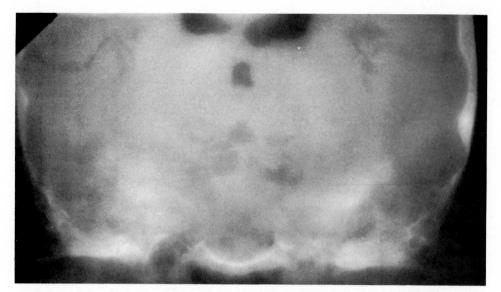

Figure 8–53.

Middle Cerebral A. | Sylvian Point | Island of Reil
Interpeduncular Cistern — Sylvian Fissure
Sup. Cerebellar A — III Ventricle
III Nerve
C. Pontis — Basilar A.
Enlarged Sella with mass

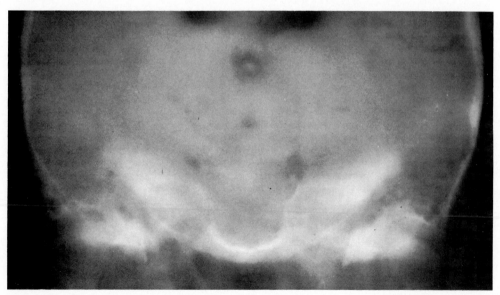

Figure 8–54.

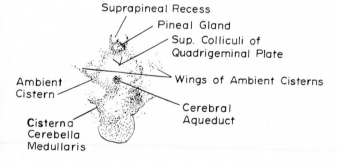

Suprapineal Recess
Pineal Gland
Sup. Colliculi of Quadrigeminal Plate
Ambient Cistern — Wings of Ambient Cisterns
Cerebral Aqueduct
Cisterna Cerebella Medullaris

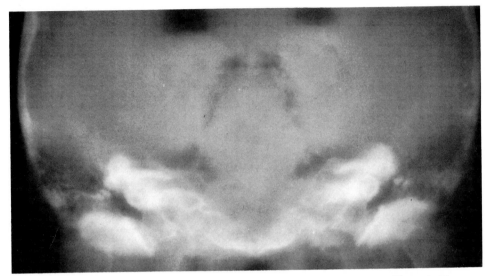

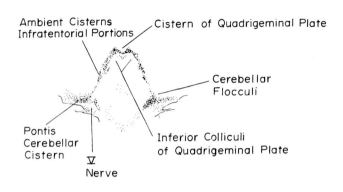

Ambient Cisterns
Infratentorial Portions

Cistern of Quadrigeminal Plate

Cerebellar
Flocculi

Pontis
Cerebellar
Cistern

V
Nerve

Inferior Colliculi
of Quadrigeminal Plate

Figure 8–55.

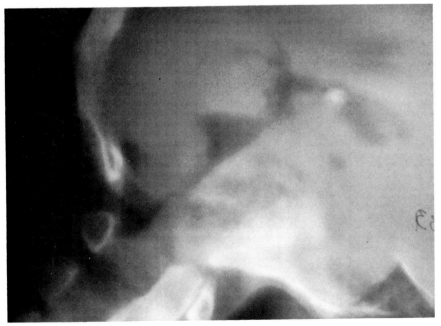

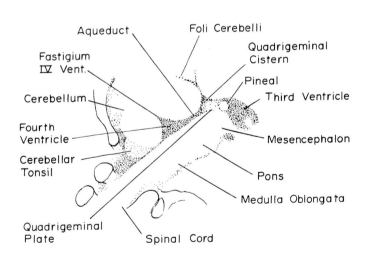

Aqueduct

Foli Cerebelli

Quadrigeminal
Cistern

Fastigium
IV Vent.

Pineal

Cerebellum

Third Ventricle

Fourth
Ventricle

Mesencephalon

Cerebellar
Tonsil

Pons

Medulla Oblongata

Quadrigeminal
Plate

Spinal Cord

Figure 8–56.

for details. The dural supply of the anterior cranial fossa is derived from the middle meningeal artery, recurrent branches of the lacrimal artery entering through the superior orbital fissure, and meningeal branches of the internal carotid and anterior and posterior ethmoidal arteries. That of the middle cranial fossa is supplied by the meningeal branches of the internal carotid artery, as well as branches from the ascending pharyngeal (through the foramen lacerum) and from the maxillary artery (through the foramen ovale). The dura of the posterior cranial fossa is supplied by the vertebral, occipital, and ascending pharyngeal arteries, together with the middle meningeal via the jugular and hypoglossal foramina as well as the foramen magnum.

The veins of the dura anastomose with the diploic veins. Many meningeal veins open directly into venous ampullae on either side of the superior sagittal sinus. Communication is established with the underlying cerebral, emissary, and diploic veins.

The Common Carotid Arteries

The branches of the aortic arch are the *brachiocephalic, left common carotid*, and *left subclavian*. These supply the head, neck,

superior limbs, and part of the thoracic wall. Between the brachiocephalic and left common carotid the *lowest thyroid artery* (thyroidea ima) may arise. Variations of the branches of the aortic arch are indicated in Figure 8–60. The *brachiocephalic trunk* (innominate artery) in turn is usually 3.5 to 5 cm. in length and gives rise to the *right common carotid* and *right subclavian arteries*.

The proximal portion of the left common carotid actually lies within the superior mediastinum, unlike the right carotid. The left carotid, however, may arise from the brachiocephalic trunk (in about 27 per cent of patients).

Near the superior border of the thyroid cartilage, usually on a level with the fourth cervical vertebra, the common carotid arteries divide into *internal* and *external* branches. The point of bifurcation varies. The course of the carotid arteries can be plotted in the neck by extending a line from the sternoclavicular joint to a point just posterior to the neck of the mandible.

The common carotid arteries are contained in sheaths that also contain the internal jugular vein and the vagus nerves.

The *carotid sinus* is that short segment of the carotid artery just below and just above its bifurcation.

External Carotid Artery. The external carotid artery distributes branches to the anterior part of the neck, the pharynx, tongue and oral cavity, face, temporal and infratemporal fossae, nasal cavity, the greater part of the scalp, and the greater part of

(Text continued on page 417.)

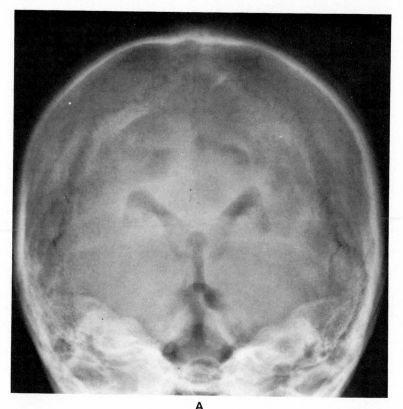

A

Figure 8–57.   *A* and *B*. Labeled and unlabeled posteroanterior pneumoencephalograms in Towne's projection.

Figure 8–57 continued on the opposite page.

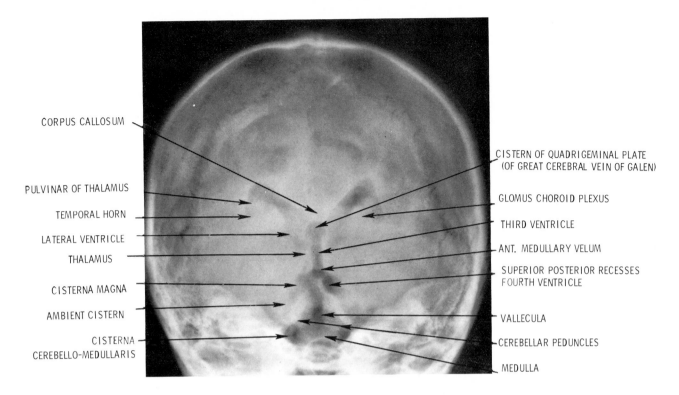

CORPUS CALLOSUM

PULVINAR OF THALAMUS

TEMPORAL HORN

LATERAL VENTRICLE

THALAMUS

CISTERNA MAGNA

AMBIENT CISTERN

CISTERNA
CEREBELLO-MEDULLARIS

CISTERN OF QUADRIGEMINAL PLATE
(OF GREAT CEREBRAL VEIN OF GALEN)

GLOMUS CHOROID PLEXUS

THIRD VENTRICLE

ANT. MEDULLARY VELUM

SUPERIOR POSTERIOR RECESSES
FOURTH VENTRICLE

VALLECULA

CEREBELLAR PEDUNCLES

MEDULLA

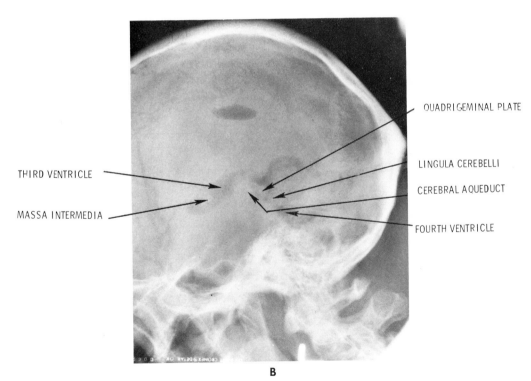

THIRD VENTRICLE

MASSA INTERMEDIA

QUADRIGEMINAL PLATE

LINGULA CEREBELLI

CEREBRAL AQUEDUCT

FOURTH VENTRICLE

B

Figure 8–57. *Continued.*

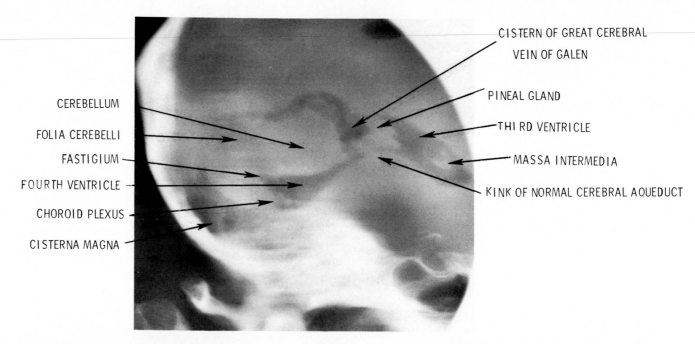

CISTERN OF GREAT CEREBRAL
VEIN OF GALEN

PINEAL GLAND

THIRD VENTRICLE

MASSA INTERMEDIA

KINK OF NORMAL CEREBRAL AQUEDUCT

CEREBELLUM

FOLIA CEREBELLI

FASTIGIUM

FOURTH VENTRICLE

CHOROID PLEXUS

CISTERNA MAGNA

Figure 8–58. Pneumoencephalogram of posterior fossa obtained after autotomography, showing improved detail.

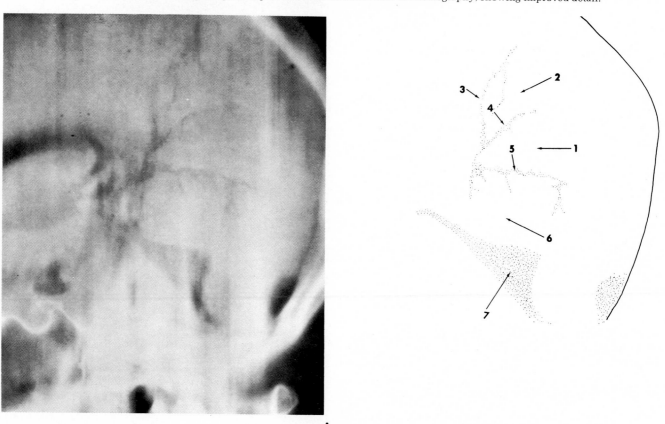

A

Figure 8–59. A. (1) Lobulus lingualis, (2) cuneus, (3) sulcus parieto-occipitalis (parieto-occipital sulcus), (4) fissura calcarina—pars anterior (calcarine fissure—anterior part), (5) cisterna cerebelli superior (superior cerebellar cistern), (6) cerebellum. (7) ventriculus quartus (fourth ventricle). (From DiChiro, G.: An Atlas of Detailed Normal Pneumoencephalographic Anatomy. 2d ed. Springfield, Illinois, Charles C Thomas, Publisher, 1971.)

Figure 8–59 continued on the opposite page.

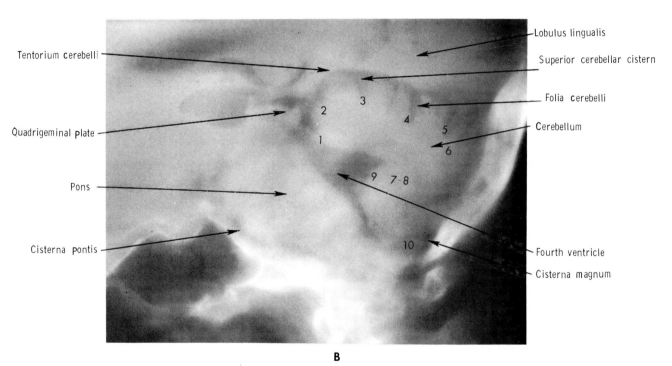

Tentorium cerebelli

Quadrigeminal plate

Pons

Cisterna pontis

Lobulus lingualis

Superior cerebellar cistern

Folia cerebelli

Cerebellum

Fourth ventricle

Cisterna magnum

B

Figure 8–59 *Continued.* *B.* Tomographic view of the posterior fossa with particular emphasis on the detail associated with the cerebellum. Apart from those areas labeled directly there are the following: (1) lingula cerebelli, (2) lobulus cerebelli, (3) culmen, (4) declive, (5) folium vermis, (6) tuber vermis, (7, 8) pyramis and uvula, (9) nodulus, (10) cerebellar tonsil.

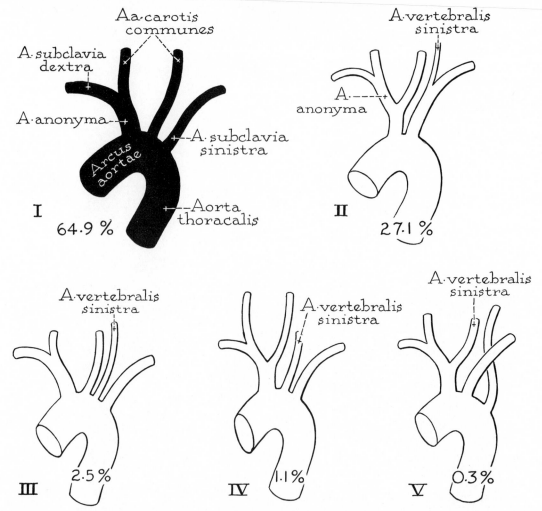

Figure 8–60. Types of branching of the aortic arch encountered in 1000 adult cadavers. (I) The arrangement regarded as "normal" for man is actually encountered more frequently than all other types combined. In specimens of this variety, three branches leave the arch in the following succession, from the specimen's right to left: innominate (with right common carotid and right subclavian as derivatives); left common carotid; left subclavian. (II) An arrangement distinguished by reduction in the number of stems to two, both common carotid arteries arising from the innominate. (III) Here the distinguishing feature is increase, not reduction, in the number of derived branches. The left vertebral artery (usually arising from the subclavian) is the additional vessel. (IV) Differing from the preceding variety, the feature is replacement, the left vertebral artery (not the left common carotid, as in Type I) being the second stem in right-to-left succession. Both common carotid arteries arise from a common stem, as they do in examples of Type II. (V) In this departure from the anatomic norm, the left vertebral artery arises from the innominate, and the order of the left common carotid and left subclavian arteries is reversed. (VI to VIII [facing page]). Three patterns similar in respect to the position of origin of the right subclavian artery; the latter vessel arises as the last branch of the aortic arch, reaching the right upper extremity by passing dorsal to the esophagus. In respect to the origin of the other branches, the types differ. (IX) A bi-innominate sequence, in which paired vessels (in turn having matching main branches) are the only derivatives of the aortic arch. (X and XI) In both these varieties the left vertebral artery arises from an aortic trunk from which the left subclavian is also derived. However, in Type X a regular innominate artery is present (as in Type I), whereas in Type XI the "innominate" (with regular branches) arises from an aortic trunk shared with the common carotid. (XII) Here, as in Type III, an extra vessel arises from the arch between the innominate and the left subclavian, but the added derivative is the *a. thyreoidea ima* instead of the *a. vertebralis*. (XIII) Unification is the distinguishing feature of this departure from the typical scheme of

Figure 8–60 continued on the opposite page.

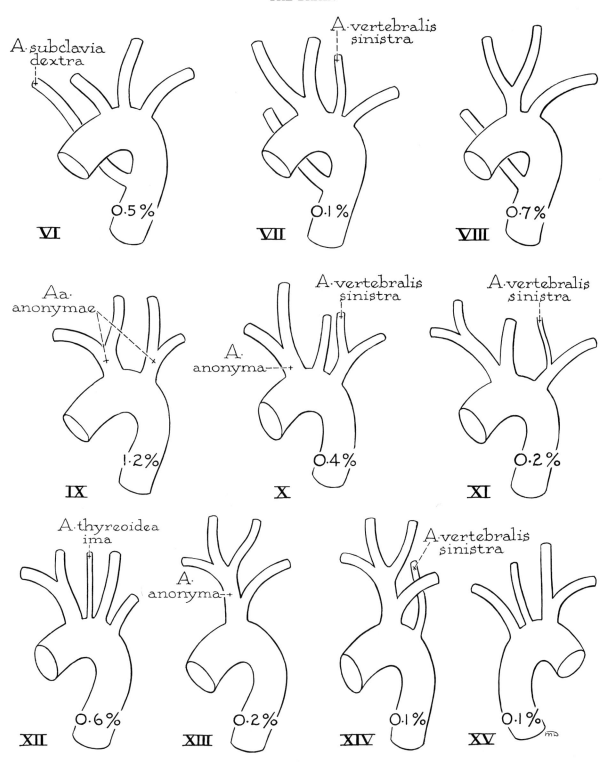

branching; the usual branches (see Type I) take origin from the aortic arch through a single trunk as an intermediary vessel. (XIV) An infrequent variety with all branches derived from a common stem (as in Type XIII) with the exception of the left vertebral, which arises from the arch to the right of the common stem. (XV) In this rare variety, in which the arch passes in a reversed direction from heart to thoracic aorta, the branches maintain a normal succession in relation to the body itself; however, their position on the aortic arch itself is as a mirror image of the "standard" scheme of derivation. (From Anson, B. J.: An Atlas of Human Anatomy, 2nd ed. Philadelphia, W. B. Saunders Co., 1963.)

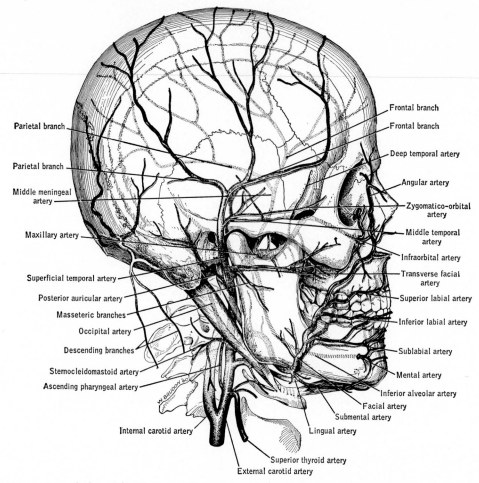

Figure 8–61. General plan of distribution of the branches of the external carotid artery in the head. (From Anson, B. J. (ed.): Morris' Human Anatomy, 12th ed. Copyright © 1966 by McGraw-Hill, Inc. Used by permission of the McGraw-Hill Book Company.)

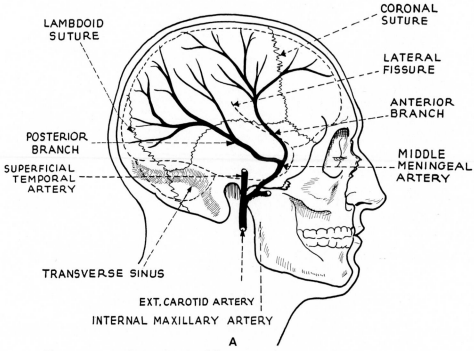

416

Figure 8–62. A. Projection of middle meningeal artery in relation to the skull.

Figure 8–62 continued on the opposite page.

the cranial meninges. From the neuroradiologic standpoint, its most important branches are the *facial*, the *occipital*, the *maxillary*, and the *superficial temporal* arteries. These are indicated diagrammatically in Figure 8–61.

The *facial* and *occipital* arteries arise at approximately the same level, one coursing anteriorly and the other posteriorly.

The two terminal branches of the external carotid are the *superficial temporal* and the *maxillary* arteries; the latter is important neuroradiologically since it gives rise to the *middle meningeal* artery (Fig. 8–62 *A*). The middle meningeal enters the cranial cavity through the *foramen spinosum*, providing a major blood supply through parietal and frontal branches of the meninges. The extent to which branches of the middle meningeal produce grooves in the inner table of the skull varies considerably (see Chapter 6 for a detailed description). Other branches of the internal maxillary artery are indicated in Figure 8–62.

Branches of the occipital and maxillary arteries form important anastomotic communications through numerous channels from outside the cranium to blood vessels within it; these, in the case of the occipital artery, pass through the jugular, hypoglossal, and mastoid foramina. In addition, these branches form anastomoses with muscular branches of the vertebral artery (Fig. 8–63). In the case of the maxillary artery there is considerable anastomosis in and around the orbit with branches of the internal carotid artery. The inferior orbital artery forms anastomoses with the angular and ophthalmic arteries. Other maxillary branches pierce the base of the skull and anastomose with meningeal arteries.

The middle temporal branch of the superficial temporal artery at times produces a groove in the squamous portion of the temporal bone, which by virtue of its straightness may be mistaken for a fracture of this bone (Fig. 8–64). Small twigs of the superficial temporal artery pierce the skull and anastomose with meningeal and cerebral arteries, thus providing further communication between the outside and the inside of the cranium.

Internal Carotid Artery. The proximal portion of the inter-

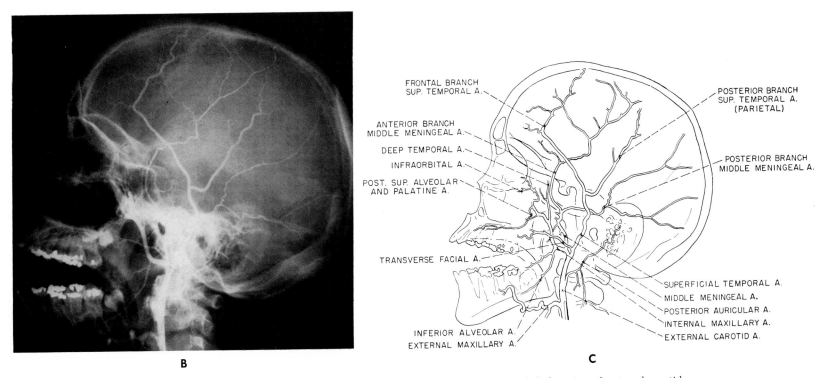

B

C

Figure 8–62 *Continued.* *B.* Radiograph of external carotid arteriogram. *C.* Labeled tracing of external carotid arteriogram.

Figure 8–62 continued on the following page.

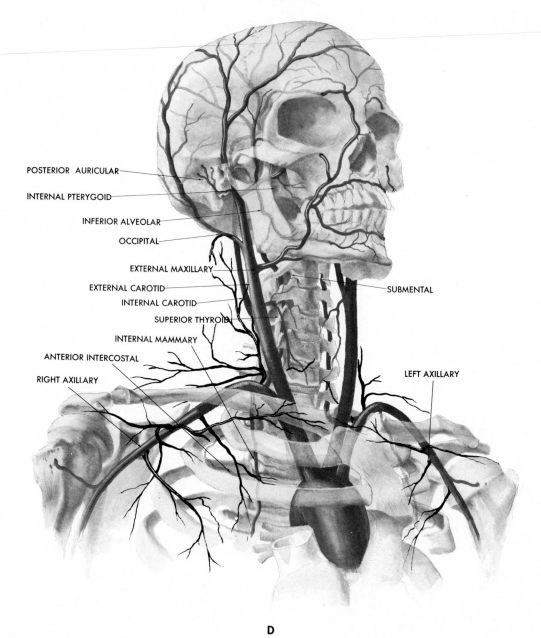

POSTERIOR AURICULAR

INTERNAL PTERYGOID

INFERIOR ALVEOLAR

OCCIPITAL

EXTERNAL MAXILLARY

EXTERNAL CAROTID

INTERNAL CAROTID

SUPERIOR THYROID

INTERNAL MAMMARY

ANTERIOR INTERCOSTAL

RIGHT AXILLARY

SUBMENTAL

LEFT AXILLARY

D

Figure 8–62 *Continued. D.* Deep circulation of the head and neck. (From Bierman, H. C.: Selective Arterial Catheterization, 1969. Courtesy of Charles C Thomas, Publisher, Springfield, Illinois.)

nal carotid artery, as noted previously, is dilated as the *carotid sinus.* At first the internal carotid is usually dorsolateral to the external carotid, and then it ascends within the carotid sheath in the neck that lies on the prevertebral fascia. The internal carotid artery supplies the anterior part of the brain, the orbital contents, the anterior part of the nasal cavity, and the forehead. It is com-

monly divided into four parts: *cervical, petrous, cavernous,* and *intracranial* (Fig. 8–65).

The *cervical segment* of the internal carotid artery has no branches. The internal jugular vein accompanies the artery throughout its cervical course. At first the vein is lateral to the artery so that at the base of the skull it lies dorsolateral to it.

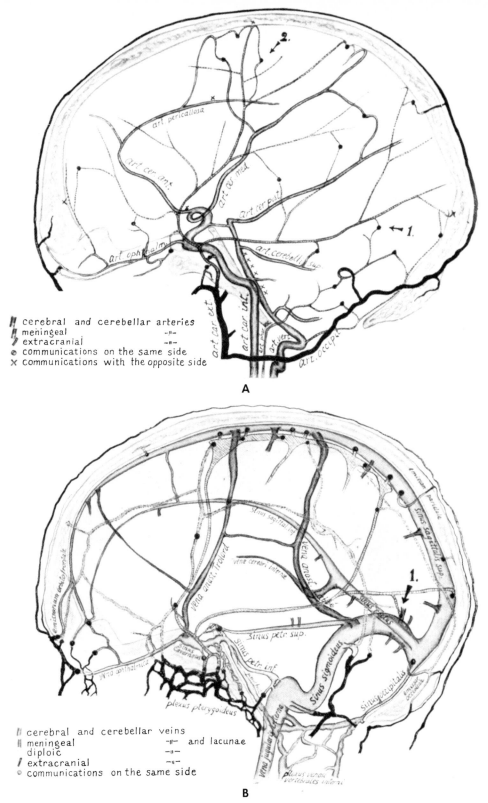

Figure 8–63. *A.* Diagram of the arteries supplying the cranium, with special reference to their communications, indicated by arrows. The arterial system of the auditory apparatus has been omitted from the diagram. *B.* Diagram of the veins and dural sinuses of the cranium and their communications. The venous system of the auditory apparatus has been omitted from the diagram. (From Lindblom, K.: Acta Radiol. (Stockholm), Suppl. 30, 1936.)

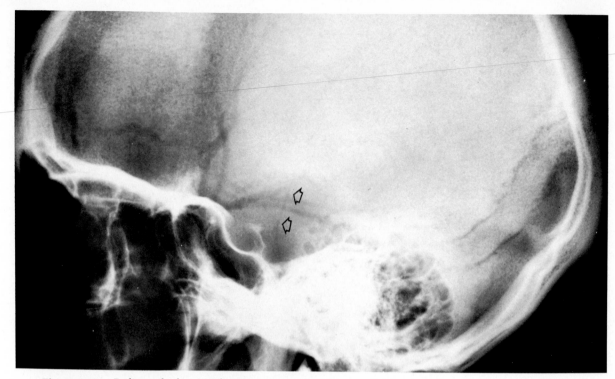

Figure 8-64. Radiograph showing the groove (arrows) of the superficial temporal artery in the squamous portion of the temporal bone. This is a normal finding which, however, may be mistaken for a fracture.

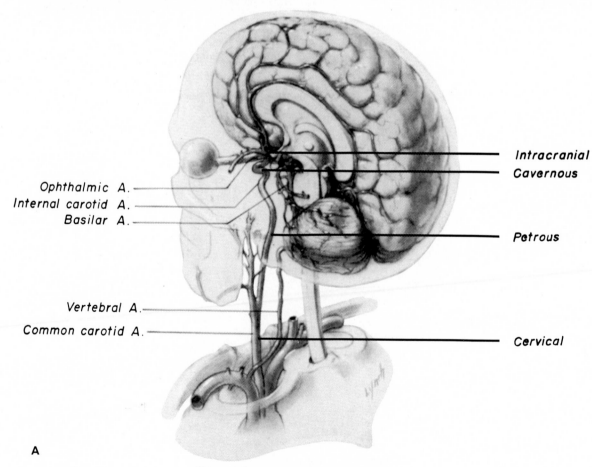

Ophthalmic A.

Internal carotid A.

Basilar A.

Vertebral A.

Common carotid A.

Intracranial

Cavernous

Petrous

Cervical

A

Figure 8-65. *See opposite page for legend.*

The *petrous portion* of the internal carotid artery begins where the vessel enters the external opening of the carotid canal in the base of the skull. There is a downward prolongation of dura mater along the canal that separates the artery from the bone. First the artery is anterior to the tympanum and cochlea (but in close proximity to it), then it turns forward and medially to the auditory tube and enters the middle cranial fossa just deep to the semilunar ganglion and separated from the latter structure by a very thin bony or fibrous plate. It is surrounded by a considerable plexus of nerves, derived from the cervical sympathetic ganglion. The artery crosses the foramen lacerum and swings superiorly to enter the cavernous sinus (Fig. 8–66).

When *intracranial*, the internal carotid artery immediately grooves the medial side of the anterior clinoid process and forms the roof of the cavernous sinus. It passes just below the optic nerve, then between the second and third cranial nerves to the

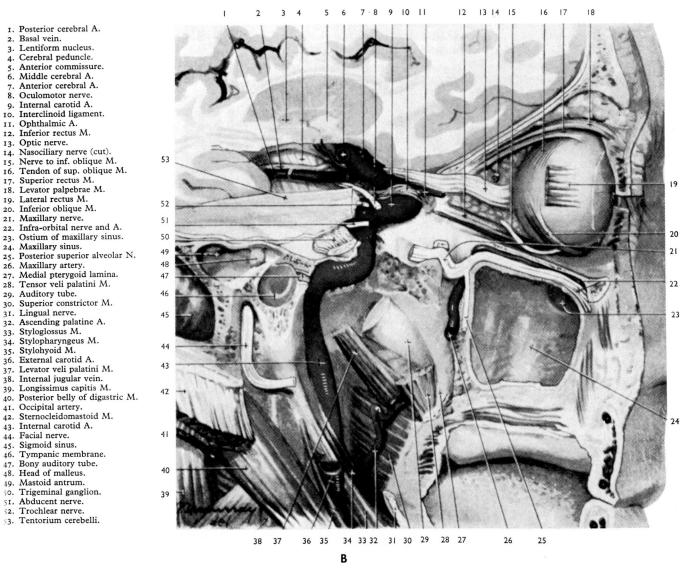

1. Posterior cerebral A.
2. Basal vein.
3. Lentiform nucleus.
4. Cerebral peduncle.
5. Anterior commissure.
6. Middle cerebral A.
7. Anterior cerebral A.
8. Oculomotor nerve.
9. Internal carotid A.
10. Interclinoid ligament.
11. Ophthalmic A.
12. Inferior rectus M.
13. Optic nerve.
14. Nasociliary nerve (cut).
15. Nerve to inf. oblique M.
16. Tendon of sup. oblique M.
17. Superior rectus M.
18. Levator palpebrae M.
19. Lateral rectus M.
20. Inferior oblique M.
21. Maxillary nerve.
22. Infra-orbital nerve and A.
23. Ostium of maxillary sinus.
24. Maxillary sinus.
25. Posterior superior alveolar N.
26. Maxillary artery.
27. Medial pterygoid lamina.
28. Tensor veli palatini M.
29. Auditory tube.
30. Superior constrictor M.
31. Lingual nerve.
32. Ascending palatine A.
33. Styloglossus M.
34. Stylopharyngeus M.
35. Stylohyoid M.
36. External carotid A.
37. Levator veli palatini M.
38. Internal jugular vein.
39. Longissimus capitis M.
40. Posterior belly of digastric M.
41. Occipital artery.
42. Sternocleidomastoid M.
43. Internal carotid A.
44. Facial nerve.
45. Sigmoid sinus.
46. Tympanic membrane.
47. Bony auditory tube.
48. Head of malleus.
49. Mastoid antrum.
50. Trigeminal ganglion.
51. Abducent nerve.
52. Trochlear nerve.
53. Tentorium cerebelli.

Figure 8–65. *A.* Gross indication of the internal carotid artery, its origin, and its various segments in relation to a sagittal section of the brain. (From Toole, J. F., and Patel, A. N.: Cerebrovascular Disorders. Copyright © 1967 by McGraw-Hill, Inc. Used by permission of McGraw-Hill Book Company.) *B.* Dissection showing course and relations of upper part of internal carotid artery, lateral view. The petrous and intracranial portions of the carotid artery are especially well shown. (From Cunningham's Textbook of Anatomy, 10th ed. London, Oxford University Press, 1964.)

anterior perforate substance at the medial end of the lateral cerebral fissure, where it divides into its two terminal branches.

As it passes through the cavernous sinus it gives off a minute but important branch called the *meningohypophyseal* artery (Fig. 8–66), which supplies small twigs to the hypophysis and to the meninges, including the tentorium cerebelli. In neoplasms involving the latter structure this arterial supply grows considerably in size and becomes an important pathologic indicator. (See Table 8–3 for an anatomic classification of cavernous branches of the carotid artery.)

At the point where the internal carotid artery pierces the dura mater, it gives off the *ophthalmic* artery, which passes forward into the orbit via the optic foramen (Fig. 8–67). In the orbit the larger branches of the ophthalmic artery are the *lacrimal, ethmoidal, supraorbital, frontal,* and *dorsal nasal* arteries.

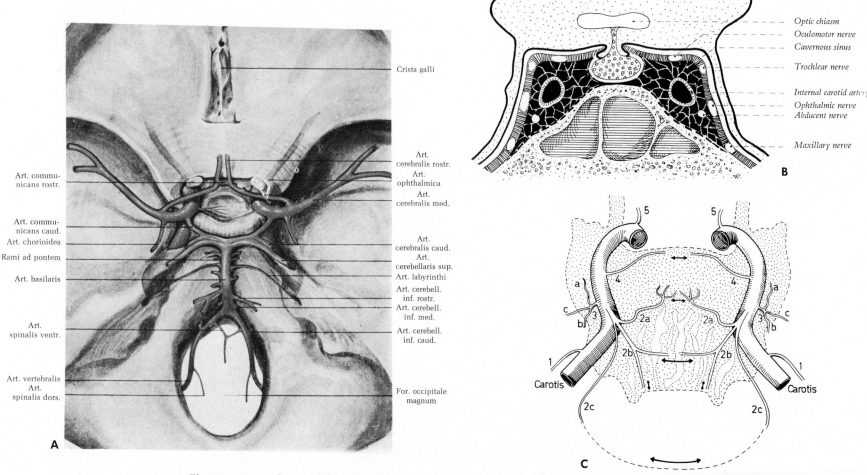

Figure 8–66. *A.* Course of the internal carotid artery at the base of the skull including the circle of Willis (after Clara, 1959). *B.* Diagram of the cavernous sinus (after Ferner, 1959). *C.* Cavernous portion of the carotid artery (2–4) (after Parkinson, 1964).

Anastomoses with opposite side (see arrows)
(1) Carotico-tympanic arteries
(2) Meningohypophyseal trunk
(a) Inferior hypophyseal artery (posterior pituitary lobe, dura of posterior clinoid)
(b) Dorsal meningeal artery (dorsum sellae, clivus, sixth nerve)
(c) Tentorial artery
(3) Inferior cavernous sinus artery
(a) Branches for third, fourth and sixth nerves
(b) Branches for gasserian ganglion
(c) Direct anastomosis with middle meningeal arteries
(4) Capsular arteries (floor of the sella)
(5) Ophthalmic artery

(*A, B,* and *C* from Krayenbühl, H. A., and Yaşargil, M. G.: Zerebrale Angiographie, 2nd ed. Stuttgart, G. Thieme Verlag, 1965.)

Figure 8–66 continued on the opposite page.

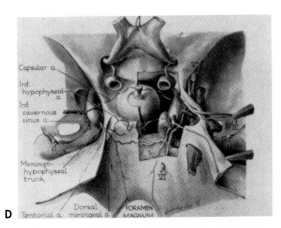

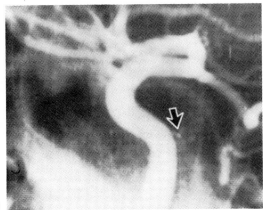

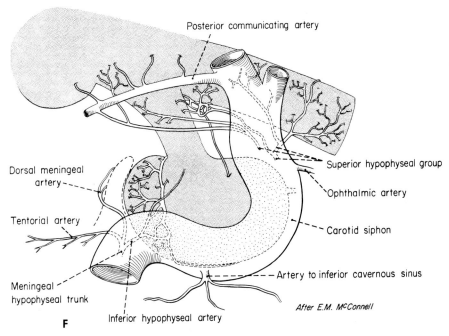

Figure 8-66 *Continued.* *D.* Normal anatomy. (Dissection of the cavernous portion of the internal carotid artery done by Parkinson.) *E.* Meningohypophyseal artery (arrow) in an otherwise normal carotid arteriogram. (*D* and *E* from Parkinson, D.: Canad. J. Surg., 7:251–268, 1964.) *F.* Diagrammatic representation of arterial blood supply to hypophysis, optic apparatus, and parasellar structures. Upper carotid siphon and posterior communicating artery have been elevated to reveal the pituitary stalk. (From Baker, H.: Radiology, 104:67–78, 1972.)

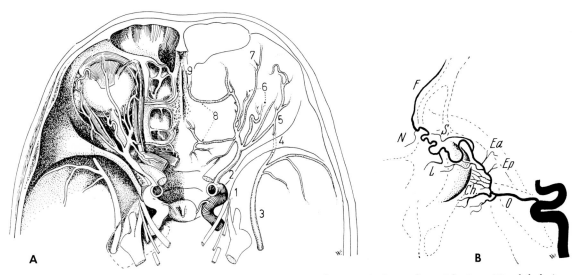

Figure 8-67. *A.* Diagram of orbital arteries (after Rauber-Kopsch, 1948). (1) Internal carotid artery, (2) ophthalmic artery, (3) middle meningeal artery, (4) meningeal branch, (5) lacrimal artery, (6) choroidal and iridal arteries, (7) medial frontal artery, (8) anterior and posterior ethmo arteries, (9) anterior meningeal artery. *B.* Diagram of the orbital arteries as seen in carotid angiography: (O) ophthalmic artery, (Ch) choroidal arteries, (Ea, Ep) anterior and posterior ethmoidal arteries, (S) supraorbital artery, (L) lacrimal artery, (N) dorsal nasal artery, (F) medial frontal artery. (From Krayenbühl, H. A., and Yaşargil, M. G.: Zerebrale Angiographie 2nd ed. Stuttgart, G. Thieme Verlag, 1965.)

The anterior ethmoidal artery (Fig. 8–67 *A*) is of some importance since it gives rise to the anterior meningeal artery, which is of diagnostic significance in pathologic processes affecting the meninges in this location.

The anterior ethmoidal artery also has a small branch to the falx cerebri through the cribriform plate.

The internal carotid artery thereafter swings upward and posteriorly (Fig. 8–68) through the chiasmatic cistern, giving off a *posterior communicating* artery, which joins the *posterior cerebral* artery, and an *anterior choroidal* artery just a few millimeters above the origin of the posterior communicating. The internal carotid terminates in the *anterior* and *middle cerebral* arteries.

Posterior Communicating Artery. The *posterior communicating* artery has a wide range of normal variations. At times the proximal portion of this artery has a funnel-shaped appearance called an *infundibulum* (Fig. 8–74) that simulates an aneurysm. Probably any widening greater than 2 to 3 mm. is of pathologic importance. An infundibulum per se occurs in about 10 per cent of cases (Wilson).

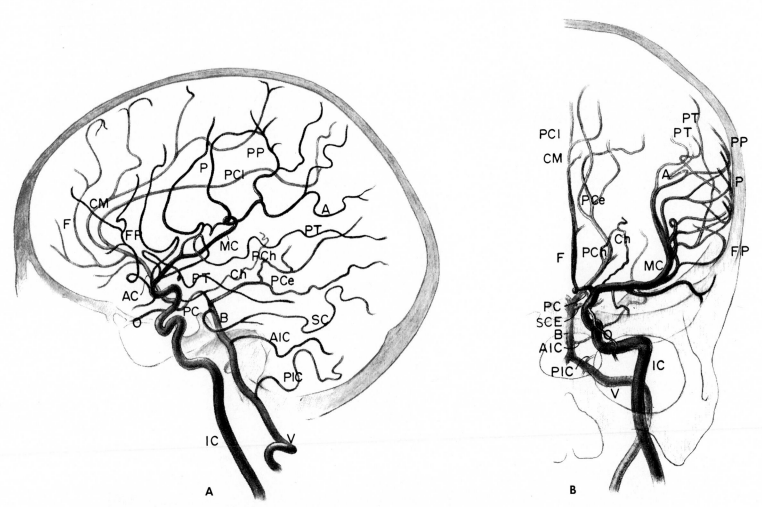

Figure 8–68. Internal carotid and basilar arteriograms. *A.* Diagram of lateral view. *B.* Diagram of AP view. (A) Angular, (AC) anterior cerebral, (AIC) anterior inferior cerebellar, (B) basilar, (Ch) choroidal, (CM) callosomarginal, (F) frontopolar, (FP) frontoparietal, (IC) internal carotid, (MC) middle cerebral, (O) ophthalmic, (P) parietal, (PC) posterior communicating, (PCe) posterior cerebral, (PCh) posterior choroidal, (PCl) pericollosal, (PIC) posterior inferior cerebellar, (PP) posterior parietal, (PT) posterior temporal, (SC) superior cerebellar, (SCE) superior cerebellar, (V) vertebral.

Figure 8–68 continued on the opposite page.

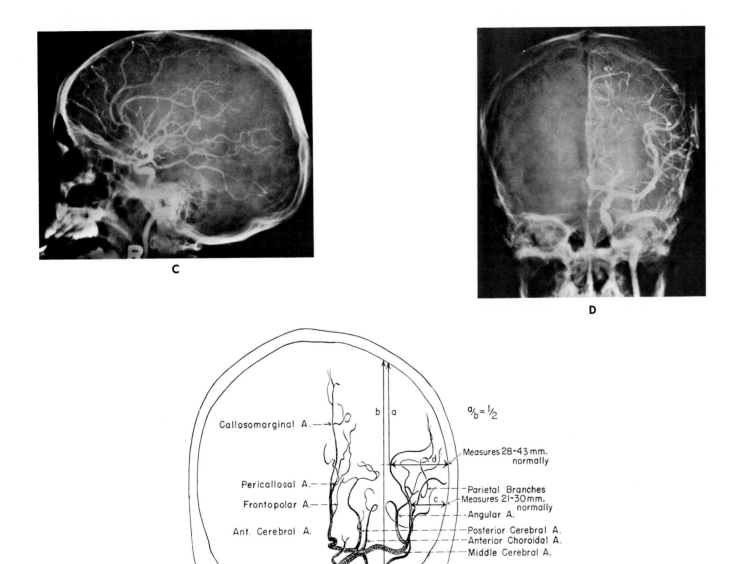

Callosomarginal A.

$\frac{a}{b} = \frac{1}{2}$

b | a

Measures 28-43 mm.
normally

Pericallosal A.

Parietal Branches
Measures 21-30 mm.
normally

Frontopolar A.

Angular A.

Ant. Cerebral A.

Posterior Cerebral A.
Anterior Choroidal A.
Middle Cerebral A.

Internal Carotid A.

Lynch

C

D

E

Figure 8–68 *Continued*. *C*. Lateral radiograph, arterial phase. *D*. Anteroposterior radiograph, arterial phase. *E*. Geometric relationships on anteroposterior view.

Anterior Choroidal Artery. The *anterior choroidal* artery is also a highly variable branch, in both its origin and its course (Fig. 8–69). It may arise from the bifurcation itself or from the middle cerebral or posterior communicating artery (Carpenter et al.). It passes posteriorly and laterally around the brain stem to reach the optic tract above the uncus (Fig. 8–69). In its proximal portion it follows closely a course parallel to the posterior cerebral artery, thus becoming an important indicator of abnormalities in this immediate vicinity. It supplies blood to the hippocampus, amygdaloid nucleus, optic tract, internal capsule, basal ganglia, and upper brain stem and also anastomoses with branches of the *posterior communicating, middle cerebral,* and *lateral posterior choroid* arteries, the last of which arises from the posterior cerebral artery.

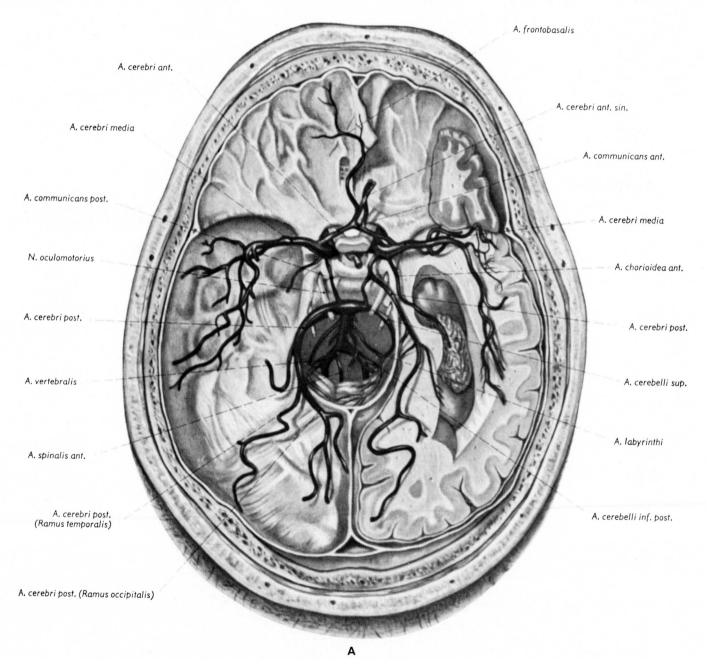

A

Figure 8–69. A. Preparation of the inside of the base of the skull. Exposure of the dural vessels and nerves (*left*); the sinus durae matris has been opened on the right. (Pernkopf, E.: Atlas of Topographical and Applied Human Anatomy. Vol. 1. Philadelphia, W. B. Saunders Co., 1963.)

Figure 8–69 continued on the opposite page.

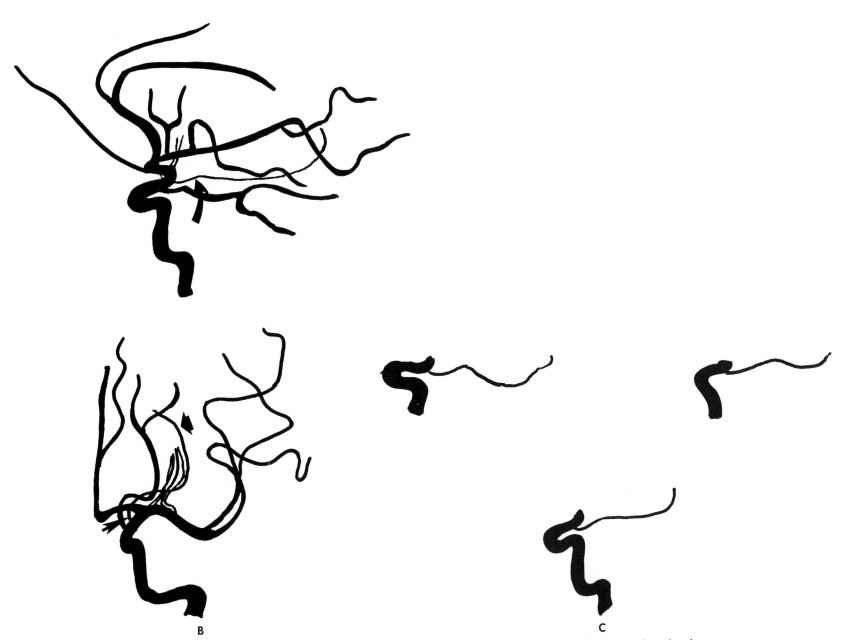

B C

Figure 8–69 *Continued.* B. Line drawings of the main ramifications of the internal carotid artery in frontal and lateral perspective with particular reference to the anterior choroidal artery (arrow). The origin of the anterior choroidal artery can vary as described in the text. C. Variations in the appearance of the anterior choroidal artery in the lateral projection. The details of termination of the anterior choroidal artery will be shown more specifically in relation to the branches of the posterior choroidal artery in a later section (Fig. 8–97).

The terminal bifurcation of the internal carotid artery is usually near the roof of the chiasmatic cistern but immediately lateral to and below the optic chiasm (Fig. 8–70). In frontal perspective the bifurcation has a T-shaped configuration (with variations—see Fig. 8–71) and the Ts usually are symmetrical on both sides. Asymmetry or elevation of the medial limb of the T—the proximal part of the anterior cerebral artery—may be of pathologic importance.

The S-shaped cavernous portion of the internal carotid artery—the *"carotid siphon"*—although highly variable, requires close study since minor variations can be of pathologic significance (Figs. 8–72, 8–73).

Gabrielsen and Greitz have made an extensive study of the normal size of the internal carotid arteries and the middle cerebral and anterior cerebral branches. These tabular values are beyond the scope of this text but the reader may refer to these tables for reference if desired. Changes in relation to sex are also indicated in the tables. It was the conclusion of these authors that "the size of the internal carotid and middle cerebral arteries is somewhat dependent on sex and skull width. In this study of strictly selected, normal carotid angiography, no definite correlation of statistical significance between the size of the cerebral arteries and the variables—site of injection, side of injection, age of patient, blood pressure, and electroencephalographic findings—was evident."

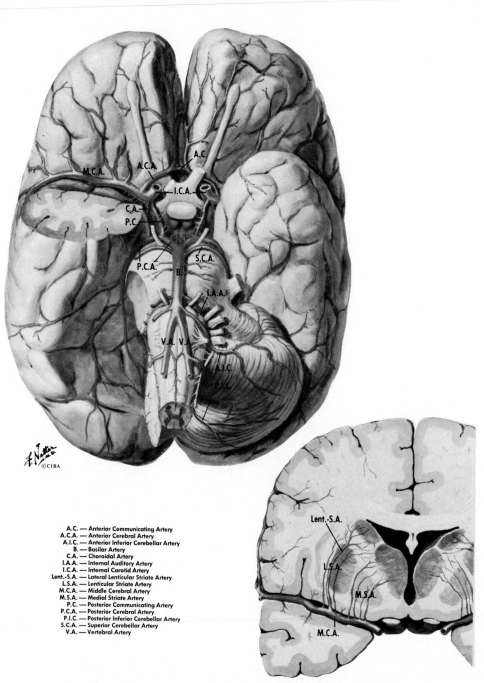

A.C. — Anterior Communicating Artery
A.C.A. — Anterior Cerebral Artery
A.I.C. — Anterior Inferior Cerebellar Artery
B. — Basilar Artery
C.A. — Choroidal Artery
I.A.A. — Internal Auditory Artery
I.C.A. — Internal Carotid Artery
Lent.-S.A. — Lateral Lenticular Striate Artery
L.S.A. — Lenticular Striate Artery
M.C.A. — Middle Cerebral Artery
M.S.A. — Medial Striate Artery
P.C. — Posterior Communicating Artery
P.C.A. — Posterior Cerebral Artery
P.I.C. — Posterior Inferior Cerebellar Artery
S.C.A. — Superior Cerebellar Artery
V.A. — Vertebral Artery

Figure 8–70. Blood supply of the brain. (© Copyright 1953, 1972 Ciba Pharmaceutical Company, Division of Ciba-Geigy Corporation. Reproduced, with permission, from The Ciba Collection of Medical Illustrations by Frank H. Netter, M.D. All rights reserved.)

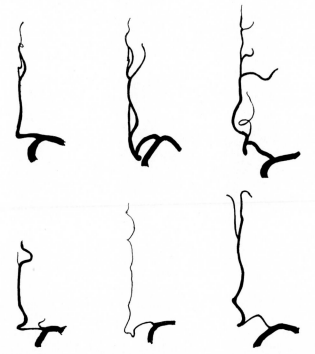

Figure 8–71. Common variations of the anterior cerebral artery. (From Greitz, T., and Lindgren, E.: Cerebral vascular anatomy. In Abrams, H. A. (ed.): Angiography, 2nd ed. Boston, Little, Brown & Co., 1971.)

Anterior Cerebral Artery. The variations in the course of the *anterior cerebral* artery are numerous. Those demonstrated by Wilson are shown in Figure 8–72 *B* and *C*. Those recorded by Krayenbühl and Yaşargil are reproduced in Figure 8–73, along with a table of the statistical occurrence of these variations. It is particularly important to know that looping of the anterior cerebral artery in the immediate vicinity of the anterior communicating artery may give the false impression of a saccular aneurysm. Under these circumstances the half-oblique projection is especially valuable.

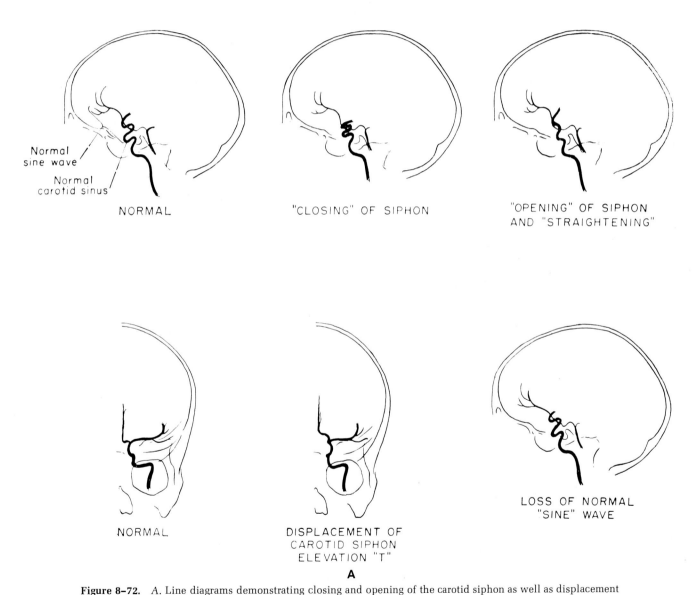

NORMAL

"CLOSING" OF SIPHON

"OPENING" OF SIPHON AND "STRAIGHTENING"

NORMAL

DISPLACEMENT OF CAROTID SIPHON ELEVATION "T"

LOSS OF NORMAL "SINE" WAVE

A

Figure 8–72. *A.* Line diagrams demonstrating closing and opening of the carotid siphon as well as displacement with elevation of the first part of the anterior cerebral artery. The loss of the normal "sine" wave in the anterior artery in lateral perspective is also demonstrated. (From Meschan, I.: Roentgen signs of abnormality in cerebral angiograms. *In* Toole, J. F. (ed.): Special Techniques for Neurologic Diagnosis. Philadelphia, F. A. Davis Co., 1969.)

Figure 8–72 continued on the following page.

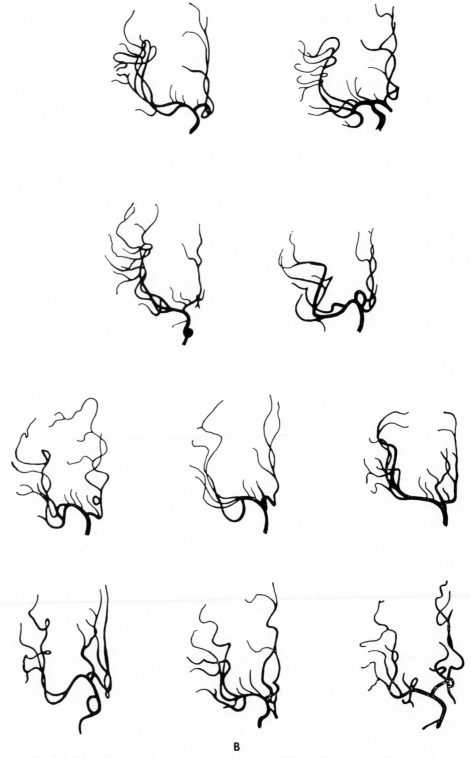

B

Figure 8–72 *Continued.* B. Some variations in the appearance of the cerebral arteries as seen at carotid angiography, frontal projection. In this figure and in Part C, no effort was made to select unusual cases.

Figure 8–72 continued on the opposite page.

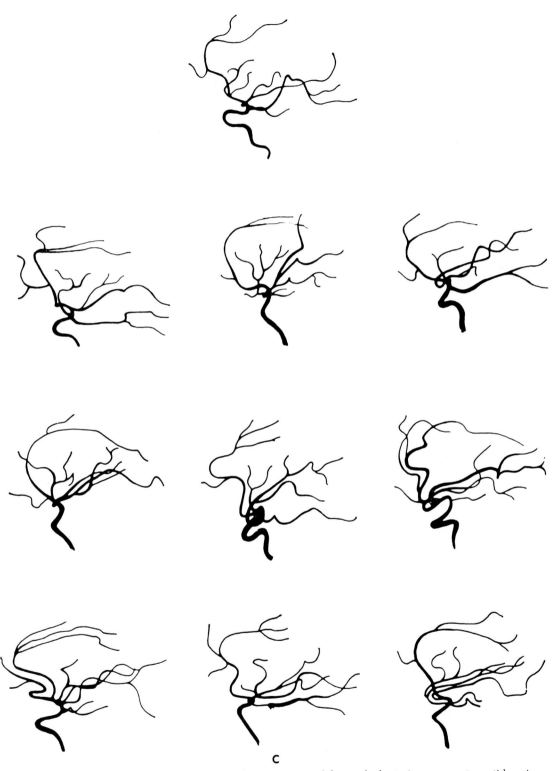

C

Figure 8–72 *Continued.* C. Some variations in the appearance of the cerebral arteries as seen at carotid angiography, lateral projection. (*B* and *C* from Wilson, M.: The Anatomic Foundation of Neuroradiology of the Brain, 2nd ed. Boston, Little, Brown & Co., 1972.)

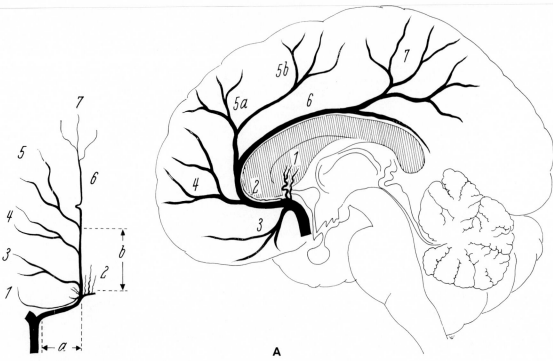

Figure 8–73. A. Regions of vascular supply.

Anterior cerebral artery

(a) Pre-communical segment
(b) Post-communical segment

(1) Anterior striate arteries (Recurrent anterior cerebral artery)
Short diencephalic artery ⎱ lateral segment (8–12 arterioles)
⎰ medial segment (4–8 arterioles)
Long telencephalic artery (Heubner's artery) (1–2 branches)

Paraventricular hypothalamic nuclei
Supra-optic nerve, base of corpus callosum
Head of the caudate nucleus, anterior portion of internal capsule, ventro-oral caudatum and putamen

(2) Medial anterior cerebral artery (issued from anterior communicating artery)

Knee of corpus callosum, septum pellucidum, anterior portion of the fornical column

(3) Frontobasal artery (inferior frontal artery, fronto-orbital artery, orbital artery, inferior medio-frontal artery)

Mediobasal portion, frontal lobe, orbital gyri

(4) Frontopolar artery (anterior frontal artery, anterior internal frontal artery)

Frontal pole, frontal gyrus

(5) Callosomarginal artery (medio-frontal artery)
Pre-frontal artery (medial internal frontal artery)
Cingular artery (posterior internal frontal artery)

Cingular gyrus, medial and dorsal aspect of the superior and medio-frontal gyrus, upper aspects of the central gyrus

(6) Pericallosal artery (artery of corpus callosum)

Anterior ⁴/₅ of the corpus callosum, pre-cuneus

(7) Posterior frontal artery (internal parietal artery, posterior parietal artery)
Pre-central artery
Pre-cuneus artery
Parieto-occipital artery

Pre-cuneus, medial aspect of parietal lobulus

(From Krayenbühl, H. A., and Yaşargil, M. G.: Zerebrale Angiographie, 2nd ed. Stuttgart, G. Thieme Verlag, 1965.)

Figure 8–73 continued on the opposite page.

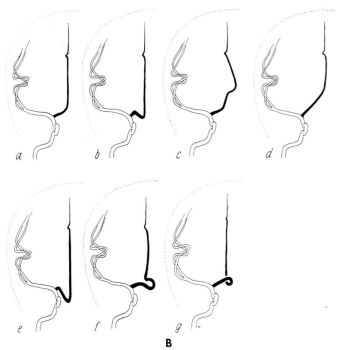

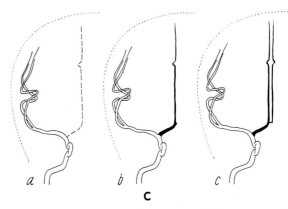

C

Figure 8-73 *Continued.   C.* Angiographic variations of the anterior cerebral artery.

	(a) absent (percentage)	(b) ipsilateral (percentage)	(c) ipsilateral and contralateral (percentage)
Moniz (1940)	—	55	41·85
Ruggiero (1952)	?	80	12·4
Morris and Peck (1955)	?	?	38·0
Curry and Culbreth (1951)	?	?	46·0
			(lateral picture)
Manghi and colleagues (1957)	?	?	25·0
Dilenge (1962)	?	?	41·0
Saltzman (1959a)	?	?	34·7
Tönnis and Schiefer (1959)	0·7	67·9	31·3
Own material	1·3	63·2	34·8

(From Krayenbühl, H. A., and Yaşargil, M. G.: Zerebrale Angiographie, 2nd ed. Stuttgart, G. Thieme Verlag, 1965.)

B

Figure 8-73 *Continued.   B.* Variations of the pre-communical segment of the anterior cerebral artery.

	Own material			Dilenge
	0-20 yrs (percentage)	21-50 yrs (percentage)	51-74 yrs (percentage)	(percentage)
(a) Horizontal course	35·2	20·1	3·0	17
(b) Convex downwards	15·4	30·0	50·0	49
(c) Convex upwards	23·7	19·1	7·0	3
(d) Inclined upwards	24·0	2·8	0·0	10
(e) Inclined downwards	5·0	20·1	25·0	10
(f) Looped	—	5·0	9·0	—
(g) Circles	—	3·0	6·0	—

(From Krayenbühl, H. A., and Yaşargil, M. G.: Zerebrale Angiographie, 2nd ed. Stuttgart, G. Thieme Verlag, 1965.)

The first part of the anterior cerebral artery, proximal to the anterior communicating branch, is ordinarily somewhat horizontally disposed in frontal perspective between the optic chiasm and the olfactory trigone. It then bends in a right angle between the two cerebral hemispheres. The *anterior communicating* artery connects the two anterior cerebral arteries immediately anterior to the lamina terminalis. Aplasia of one of the anterior cerebral arteries may be observed (in approximately 1 per cent of cases) (Fig. 8-73 *C*).

Heubner's Artery.   The branches arising from this portion of the anterior cerebral artery are: (1) *perforating arteries*, which vascularize the front part of the diencephalon, and (2) a *long central artery* which turns laterally back toward the carotid bifurcation approximately parallel to the first part of the anterior cerebral but in an opposite direction—it is called the recurrent artery of Heubner (Fig. 8-75 *A* and *B*). The course and caliber of this artery are highly variable. It supplies the anterior perforated sub-

stance medial to the lateral lenticulostriate of the middle cerebral artery. On angiography, in anteroposterior projection, the horizontal segment of Heubner's artery may be obscured by the horizontal portion of the anterior cerebral artery. Moreover, it is very difficult to distinguish from the other lenticulostriate arteries derived from the middle cerebral artery. Usually it cannot be identified in the lateral perspective.

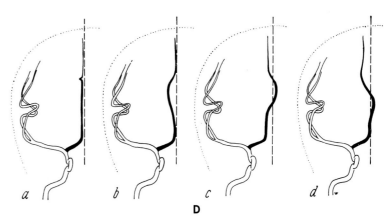

D

Figure 8-73 *Continued.   D.* Variations of the course of the post-communical segment of the anterior cerebral artery: (a) 11 per cent, (b) 7 per cent, (c) 14 per cent, (d) 66 per cent. (From Krayenbühl, H. A., and Yaşargil, M. G.: Zerebrale Angiographie, 2nd ed. Stuttgart, G. Thieme Verlag, 1965.)

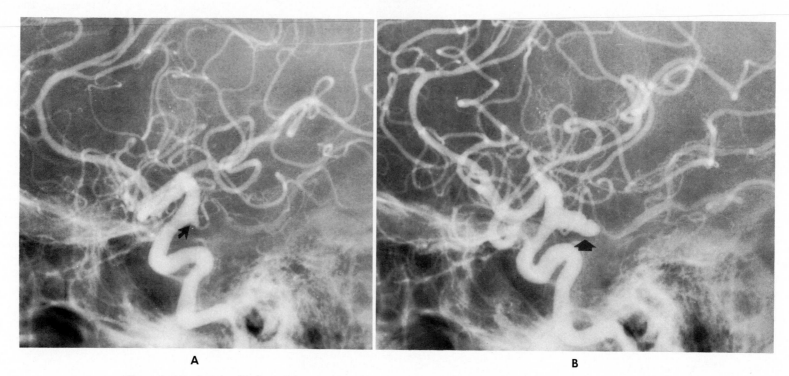

Figure 8–74. *A.* Infundibulum of the posterior communicating artery (arrow). This is a normal variant and must not be confused with an aneurysm (arrow), shown in *B.*

The anterior cerebral thereafter gives rise to the *anterior communicating* artery (Fig. 8–73 *A*), which communicates with the anterior cerebral artery of the opposite side deep in the great longitudinal fissure. The anterior cerebral then follows a course in close relationship to the genu of the corpus callosum.

The various branches of the anterior cerebral artery with their regions of vascular supply are diagrammatically illustrated in Figures 8–76 and 8–73 *A*. The following branches can usually be identified: distal to the anterior communicating artery there is an *orbitofrontal* branch (also called *frontobasilar* or *inferior orbital*), which may have its origin from the next branch in the series, the *frontopolar*. The frontobasilar artery usually is parallel to the olfactory bulb and supplies the medial and basilar portions of the frontal lobe. The frontopolar artery supplies the anterior portion of the frontal cortex. This artery is an important identification point when detecting lesions in the most anterior portion of the frontal lobe. The *callosomarginal* artery originates at the top of the genu (knee) of the corpus callosum and may run in the cingulate sulcus, giving off branches therein. It usually supplies the medial aspect of the frontal lobe above the corpus callosum.

The *pericallosal* artery runs over the corpus callosum and is in fact a continuation of the anterior cerebral artery. It extends to the upper end of the splenium of the corpus callosum, where it may anastomose with dorsal callosal branches of the posterior cerebral artery.

The free rim of the falx cerebri extends from the knee of the corpus callosum to its splenium, directly above the pericallosal artery; it is above it approximately 1 cm. frontally and 1 to 3 cm. posteriorly. The two pericallosal arteries are usually parallel in about 80 per cent of cases; they anastomose with each other as well as with the callosomarginal arteries below the falx and above the midline.

The small branches of the anterior cerebral artery that extend to the corpus callosum in the cingulate gyrus posteriorly beneath the falx cerebri form the so-called "moustache" appearance in about 17 per cent of cases (Fig. 8–76 *D*) (Huang and Wolf, 1964).

In view of the close proximity of the terminal branches of the pericallosal and callosomarginal arteries to the falx cerebri (Fig. 8–76 *E*), herniations of brain beneath the falx will produce a

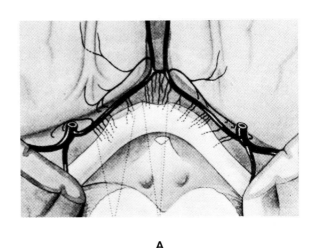

A

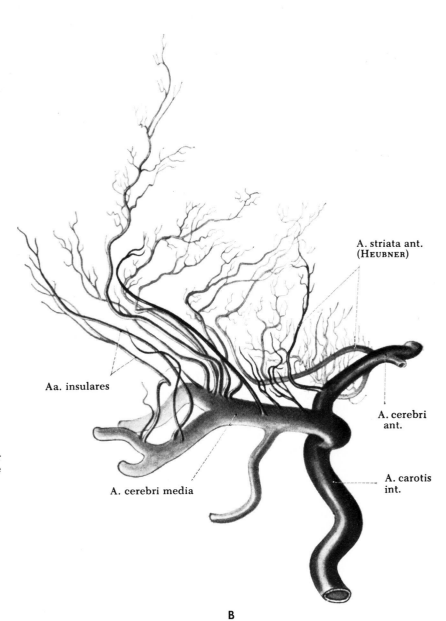

A. striata ant.
(HEUBNER)

Aa. insulares

A. cerebri
ant.

A. cerebri media

A. carotis
int.

B

Figure 8–75. *A* and *B*, Perforating branches and recurrent artery of Heubner (anterior cerebral branch). (From Krayenbühl, H. A., and Yaşargil, M. G.: Zerebrale Angiographie, 2nd ed. Stuttgart, G. Thieme Verlag, 1965.)

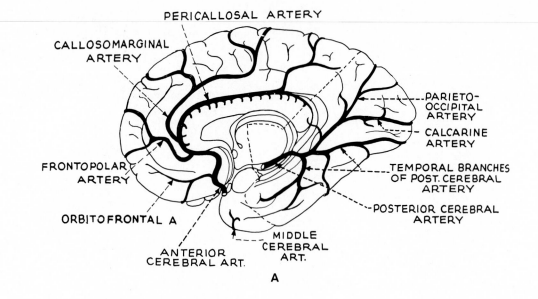

A

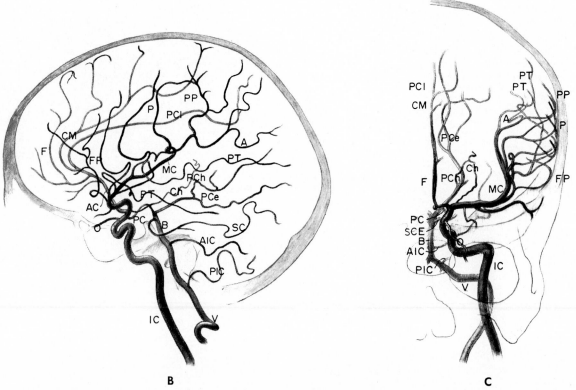

B   **C**

Figure 8–76. *A.* The distribution and major branches of the intracranial portions of the anterior cerebral artery. *B* and *C.* Internal carotid and basilar arteriograms. The branches of the anterior cerebral are shown in a lighter gray tone than those of the middle cerebral but show relationships on the angiograms obtained. *B.* Diagram of lateral view. *C.* Diagram of AP view. (A) Angular, (AC) anterior cerebral, (AIC) anterior inferior cerebellar, (B) basilar, (Ch) choroidal, (CM) callosomarginal, (F) frontopolar, (FP) frontoparietal, (IC) internal carotid, (MC) middle cerebral, (O) ophthalmic, (P) parietal, (PC) posterior communicating, (PCe) posterior cerebral, (PCh) posterior choroidal, (PCl) pericollosal, (PIC) posterior inferior cerebellar, (PP) posterior parietal, (PT) posterior temporal, (SC) superior cerebellar, (SCE) superior cerebellar, (V) vertebral.

Figure 8–76 continued on the opposite page.

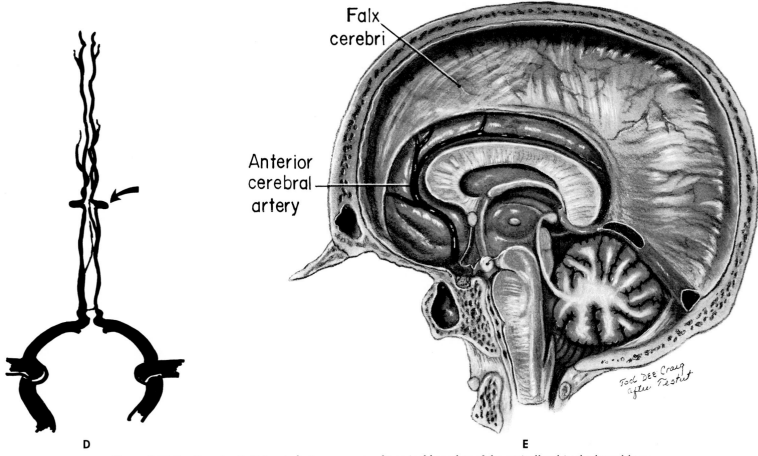

Figure 8–76 *Continued.* D. "Moustache" appearance of terminal branches of the pericallosal in the lateral longitudinal sulcus of the corpus callosum. E. Diagram of longitudinal section of skull and brain. The falx is much
thinner on its anterior aspect and becomes thicker as it goes posteriorly to join the tentorium. The anterior cerebral
artery gives off branches which, as they extend peripherally, go beyond the edge of the falx. Therefore, when these
arteries are displaced, they must return to the midline as they reach the falx edge. (From Taveras, J. M., and Wood,
E. H.: Diagnostic Neuroradiology. Baltimore, The Williams & Wilkins Co., 1964.)

steplike appearance with a bulging of the anterior cerebral to
one or the other side accordingly.

Middle Cerebral Arteries. The middle cerebral artery is the
largest branch of the internal carotid. For purposes of description,
it may be arbitrarily divided into four segments: *sphenoidal,
insular, opercular,* and *terminal* (Fig. 8–68).

Sphenoidal Segment. The sphenoidal segment is usually
horizontal with respect to the sphenoidal wing laterally, varying
in length between 7 and 22 mm. (mean, 14 mm.), and having a diameter of 0.3 to 0.5 cm. (Herman et al.; Jain). In children its
course is more obliquely upward than it is in adults.

The sphenoidal segment may at times give rise to a fronto-orbital artery, or it may consist of two branches for almost its entire
length. Its main branches are *perforating* arteries, (sometimes
called *lenticulostriate* or *thalamostriate* arteries, or *arteries of the*

basal ganglia). These consist of 10 to 20 arterioles of somewhat
variable origin (Fig. 8–77).

Insular Segment. At approximately the level of the lateral
margin of the superior orbital fissure on arteriograms, and at the
beginning of the lateral (Sylvian) fissure at the limen insulae or
boundary line of the island of Reil, the sphenoidal portion of the
middle cerebral divides into two or three main branches. In frontal perspective these appear to alter their course at right angles
to the sphenoidal portion, usually about 3 cm. from the inner
table of the temporal vault of the skull (Chase and Taveras) (Fig.
78 *A*).

From these primary branches there are additionally two or
three cortical branches, both large and small, which lie against
the island of Reil. This group of vessels is designated as the *"Sylvian vessel group."* In straight lateral projection, the inferior

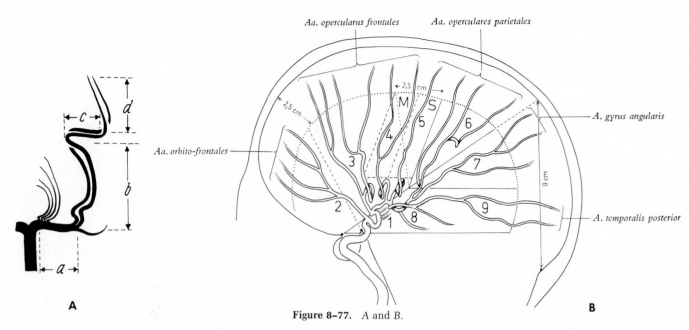

Figure 8–77. A and B.

Middle cerebral artery (after Ring-Waddington, 1967)   Regions of vascular supply

(a) Sphenoidal segment
(b) Insular segment
(c) Opercular segment
(d) Terminal segment

(1) Striate arteries
(perforating arteries, thalamostriate arteries, thala-
molenticular arteries, lenticulostriate arteries)
(10–20 arteries)

Upper, middle aspect of caudate nucleus, middle portion of internal capsule, external capsule, claustrum,
putamen, lateral pallidum, ventrolateral thalamus

(2) Orbitofrontal artery
(lateral frontobasilar artery, lateral inferior frontal
artery)

Middle frontal gyrus, lateral fronto-basilar regions, triangular portion of the inferior frontal gyrus

(3) Precentral artery
(prerolandic artery)

Operculum of the inferior frontal gyrus. Precentral
gyrus, except parasagittal region.

(4) Central artery
(rolandic artery)

Central gyrus, superior parietal lobulus

(5) Anterior parietal artery

Posterior end of the middle frontal gyrus. Central gyrus

(6) Posterior parietal artery

Inferior parietal lobulus

(7) Angular gyrus artery
(artère du pli courbe)

Angular gyrus
Marginal gyrus

(8) Anterior and middle temporal artery

Superior and middle temporal gyrus (anterior and
middle)

(9) Posterior temporal artery

Superior, middle and inferior temporal gyrus (posterior)

(From Krayenbühl, H. A., and Yaşargil, M. G.: Zerebrale Angiographie, 2nd ed. Stuttgart, G. Thieme Verlag, 1965.)

margin of this group of vessels may be aligned in relation to a "clinoparietal" line, which, according to Chase and Taveras, may be traced between the anterior clinoid process and a point 2 cm. above lambda. According to them the Sylvian vessel group lies on this line in the majority of cases; at the most 1 cm. above in adults and 1½ cm. above in children (Fig. 8–78 *D*). I have modified this line by extending it as shown in Figure 8–78 *E*, since the sphenoparietal groove, as projected in a perfect lateral projection, most closely approximates the tip of the temporal lobe and serves as a readily identifiable landmark for these purposes.

On the lateral view, the insular segment is formed by rows of loops of small arteries aligned in a relatively straight line, as shown in Figure 8–79 *B*. The upper loops correspond to the direction of the superior insular sulcus; the lower margins of the loops correspond to the Sylvian fissure and together form the *Sylvian triangle* (Fig. 8–79). Three to five loops may be identified in lateral perspective, and no more than one of these loops should deviate from the straight line pattern normally.

Opercular Segment. These arteries (Fig. 8–80) curve around the operculum like a candelabra and are sometimes called candelabra arteries (see Fig. 8–68 *B*) (Ring and Waddington). The uppermost branch in this group is the posterior parietal artery, and beneath it lies the angular gyrus artery (Fig. 8–80). The uppermost point of the Sylvian triangle formed by the insula as shown previously has been called the "angiographic Sylvian point." The middle cerebral branches leave the Sylvian fissure at this point to surface upon the brain (Fig. 8–70). Measurements provided by Taveras and Wood for the frontal projection of the internal carotid arteriogram in respect to this Sylvian group are shown in Figure 8–79 *D*. These measurements are particularly helpful in the determination of mass lesions of the temporal lobe.

The Sylvian point may also be localized in the lateral projection because at this point one, two, or more vessels may be seen end-on as they emerge straight out toward the surface, parallel to the x-ray beam. Vlahovitch et al. (quoted in Krayenbühl and Yaşargil) have shown that if another line perpendicular to this upper line is drawn from the external acoustic meatus to the

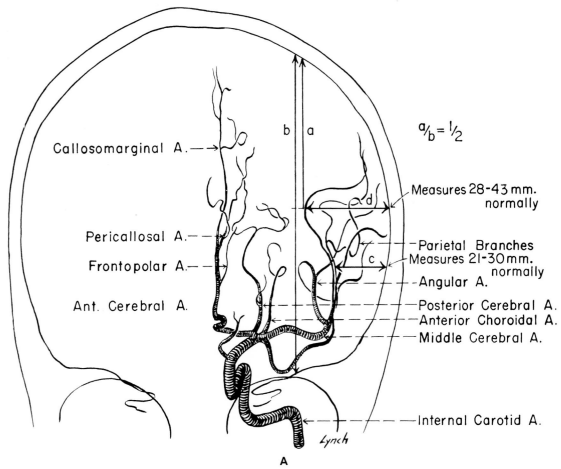

Figure 8–78. A. Various measurements which may be applied to the branches of the middle cerebral artery in frontal perspective. These measurements are based upon those given by Taveras and Wood.

Figure 8–78 continued on the following page.

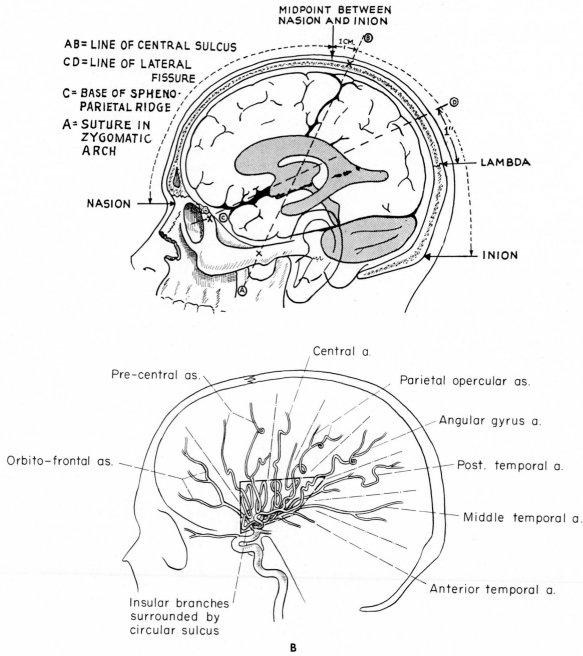

MIDPOINT BETWEEN
NASION AND INION

AB = LINE OF CENTRAL SULCUS

CD = LINE OF LATERAL
FISSURE

C = BASE OF SPHENO-
PARIETAL RIDGE

A = SUTURE IN
ZYGOMATIC
ARCH

NASION

LAMBDA

INION

Central a.

Pre-central as.

Parietal opercular as.

Angular gyrus a.

Orbito-frontal as.

Post. temporal a.

Middle temporal a.

Anterior temporal a.

Insular branches
surrounded by
circular sulcus

B

Figure 8–78 Continued.   B. Medial sagittal section of brain, showing the relationship of the central sulcus and lateral fissures to the ventricles and skull. The Sylvian group of vessels are identified with the Sylvian "lateral" fissure.

Figure 8–78 continued on the opposite page.

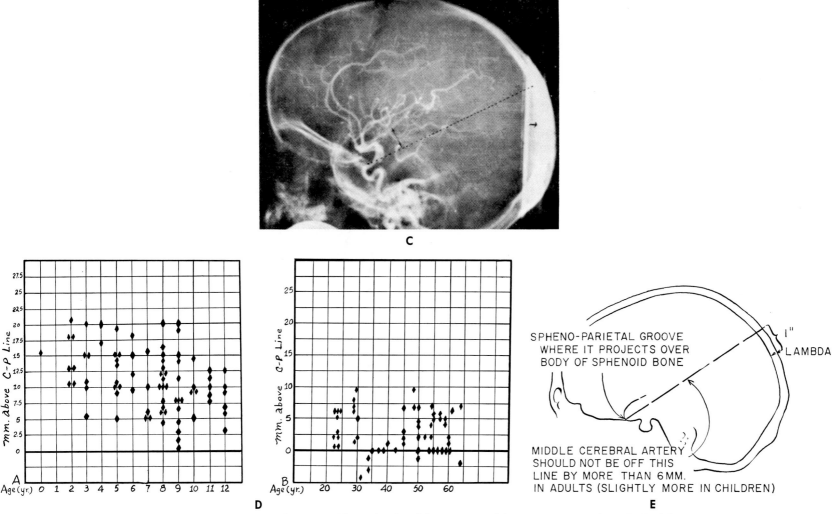

Figure 8–78 *Continued.* C. Clinoparietal line. The dotted line was traced from a point 2 cm. above the lambda (indicated by arrow) to the anterior clinoid process. In the original radiograph of this 2-year-old child, the distance from this line to the lowest major branch of the middle cerebral artery, measured 2 cm. behind the carotid siphon, was 1.4 cm. D. Relation of middle cerebral artery to clinoparietal line. The graphs indicate the relationship of the lower main branch of the middle cerebral artery to the clinoparietal line in children and in adults. The middle cerebral branches seem to become lower with advancing age, as indicated (*left*), but remain stationary after growth is completed (*right*). (C and D from Taveras, J. M., and Wood, E. H.: Diagnostic Neuroradiology. Baltimore, The Williams & Wilkins Co., 1964.) E. Author's technique for illustrating the correct anatomic position of the axis of the middle cerebral artery group of vessels from bony landmarks of the skull provided the lateral projection is a perfect one. The line as noted is drawn from the sphenoparietal groove where it projects over the body of the sphenoid bone to a point 1 inch above lambda. This line is somewhat different from that proposed by Taveras and Wood, but generally we have found that the middle cerebral artery should not vary from this line by more than 6 mm. in adults (slightly more in children).

inner table of the roof of the skull, it should not vary more than 2.5 mm. from the midpoint of this perpendicular line (Fig. 8–80).

Terminal Segment (Fig. 8–80). The anterior temporal and middle temporal arteries pursue a caudal course in relation to the Sylvian fissure; sometimes they are obscured by the Sylvian group. The posterior temporal pursues a course behind the Syl-

vian fissure in the temporo-occipital area. Some overlapping of the posterior cerebral artery branches occurs in this region—the precentral and central branches rise rather vertically upward, and the anterior and posterior parietal branches tend to adjoin the interparietal sulcus.

The *angular gyrus branch* represents a continuation of the

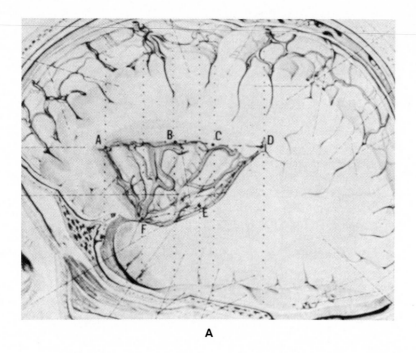

A

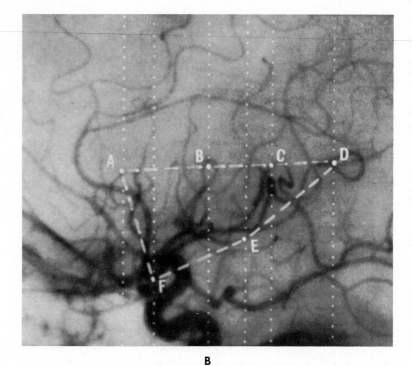

B

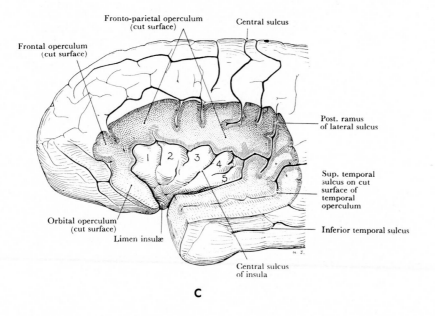

C

Figure 8–79. Position of the insular portion of the middle cerebral artery in the Sylvian triangle. *A.* Lateral diagram. *B.* Radiograph, magnified. The alignment of these points is of considerable diagnostic significance in mass lesions. (From Krayenbühl, H. A., and Yaşargil, M. G.: Zerebrale Angiographie, 2nd ed., Stuttgart, G. Thieme Verlag, 1965.) *C.* Sulci and gyri of the insula. The opercula have been removed to show the surface of the insula surrounded by the circular sulcus. (1, 2, 3) Short gyri on frontal part of insula; (4, 5) long gyrus partly divided. (From Cunningham's Manual of Practical Anatomy, 12th ed. Vol. 3. London, Oxford University Press, 1958.)

middle cerebral artery along the Sylvian fissure as far as the angular gyrus. It ordinarily divides into at least two fusiform branches. In frontal projection it is more laterally disposed than the posterior parietal artery.

There are usually anastomoses between the terminal portions of the posterior parietal, angular, and posterior temporal arteries. Some superimposition of the angular artery's terminal branches and the posterior parietal branch occurs with the terminal branches of the pericallosal and callosomarginal branches of the anterior cerebral.

In frontal perspective the *angular* and *posterior parietal branches* follow closely the arch of the inner table of the vault nearly to the midline.

Also in frontal perspective there may be confusion between

the terminal branches of the middle meningeal or external occipital artery and those of the middle cerebral. The terminal branches of the external carotid artery may appear "tangled" in contrast to the straight appearance of the middle cerebral branches.

The *orbitofrontal artery*, a branch which may or may not arise at the bifurcation or trifurcation near the proximal margin of the Sylvian fissure, passes forward to supply part of the lateral and orbital surface of the frontal lobe anterior to the Sylvian fissure.

Further Comments on the Sylvian Triangle (Gonzalez et al.). The Sylvian triangle is formed as follows: the tops of the insular loops are connected by a straight line tangential to the highest point on each of the loops. A second line is drawn from the last loop along the slope of the nonascending Sylvian branches to the base of the first insular branch. This outlines the base of the triangle. The first insular branch completes the triangle; if it cannot be clearly identified, this line may be formed by connecting the origin of the first ascending insular branch to the most anterosuperior vascular loop.

As previously indicated (Fig. 8–80 *B*), the line developed by Vlahovitch and co-workers allows us to draw a line perpendicular to the top of the Sylvian triangle, extending from the auditory meatus to the inner table of the skull (T). The upper line of the Sylvian triangle exactly bisects the "Vlahovitch line," with a standard deviation of ± 2.5 mm. (two standard deviations: less than 5 mm.).

Alternate Schematic Division of the Middle Cerebral Artery (Ring and Waddington) (Fig. 8–80 *B*). These investigators have chosen to divide the middle cerebral artery into its four main branches: *ascending frontal, posterior parietal*, and *angular and posterior temporal*. The ascending frontal branch is a more variable ramification with divisions which have been named: *orbitofrontal, prerolandic, rolandic*, and *anterior parietal*. Other investigators have described three of these divisions, not four. Ring and Waddington maintain that there are three major and constant subdivisions of the ascending branch which they have called *orbitofrontal*, "*candelabra*," and *artery to the central sulcus*.

The *orbitofrontal* originates either as one trunk or possibly as many as three separate vessels supplying the orbital surface of the brain, the inferior frontal gyrus, and the middle frontal gyrus.

The *candelabra* group is enfolded in the insula and passes directly upward over the lateral aspect of the frontal lobe. The most frequent basic structure is that of two vessels that bifurcate and rebifurcate as they pass upward.

The *artery of the central sulcus* is the one that is remarkably constant. There may be one or two arteries in the central

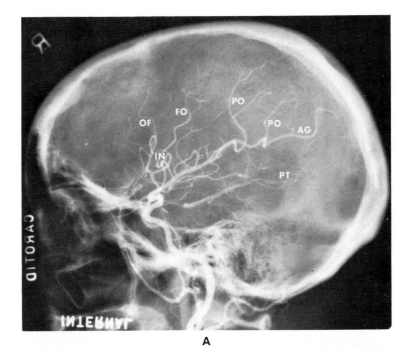

A

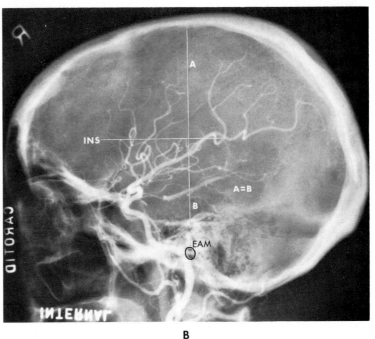

B

Figure 8–80. *A.* Visualization of the middle cerebral artery and its major branches without interference from the anterior cerebral artery. (OF) Orbitofrontal artery, (FO) frontal opercular arteries (precentral artery), (PO) parietal opercular arteries (central artery), (PO) (without the C) is another parietal opercular artery, (AG) the angular gyrus artery, (PT) posterior temporal artery.

B. Diagram for evaluation of the position of the middle cerebral artery in the lateral view (modified from Vlahovitch et al., 1964). (INS) alignment of insular branches. Line AB is drawn perpendicular to this line from the external auditory meatus (EAM). Line A is equal in length to line B, suggesting correct position of the insular branches, and line A divides the frontal branches from the parietal branches.

sulcus—they are the posterior branches of the ascending frontal. The central sulcus artery (or arteries) has only a slight posterior inclination in contrast to the posterior parietal. This vessel usually arises at the level of the radiographic Sylvian point, passing upward and only slightly posterior to its (or their) terminal division.

The Ring and Waddington method of dividing the middle cerebral into its component branches is shown in Figure 8–80 *B*: "First a line is drawn 2½ cm. inside and parallel to the inner table of the skull. A line is drawn from this curve at the point corresponding to the internal occipital protuberance, to the tuberculum sellae. A second line is drawn from the curve down the axis of the Sylvian fissure to the region of the tuberculum sellae. This line, representing the course of the Sylvian vessels, is bisected, and from the midpoint one line is drawn upward parallel to the coronal suture to the inner line, and another posterior [line is drawn] parallel to the line from the tuberculum to the point corresponding to the internal occipital protuberance. This divides the lateral aspect of the film into four sections. The largest and most anterior is the area of the ascending frontal; the posterior superior [is] the area of the posterior parietal. The triangle inferior to this is the area of the angular, and the trapezoidal area at the base is the area of the temporal vessel."

As a variant of the line representing the axis of the Sylvian vessels, a clinoparietal line may be drawn by measuring 9 cm. upward from the internal occipital protuberance and drawing a line from this point to the tuberculum sellae (Chase and Taveras).

"The area assigned to the ascending frontal complex may be further broken down into three components. By measuring anteriorly from the anterior limits of the posterior parietal area 2½ cm. along the outer curved line, drawing a line downward to the midpoint of the Sylvian line, a pie-shaped area is outlined that is the area of central sulcus artery. The subdivision between the candelabra group and orbital frontal vessels is made by measuring the curved line anterior to the central sulcus area to the floor of the anterior fossa and from the midpoint of this curve drawing a line downward to the dorsal sellae. The orbital frontal vessels lie anterior to this line while the largest group, the candelabra, lie between the orbital frontal and the central sulcus areas."

The central sulcus itself may be identified as follows: "... by drawing a line 2½ cm. anteriorly along the axis of the operculum as located by the position of the loops of enfolded vessels. The anterior portion of this line is connected with the curved line at the most anterior portion of the area assigned to the central sulcus artery. The anterior half of this rectangle may be assumed to rep-

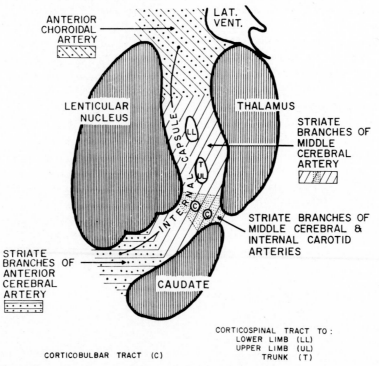

Figure 8–81. Diagram illustrating the vascular supply of the internal capsule of the brain. The territory supplied by the lenticulostriate branches of the middle cerebral artery is indicated. The more lateral lenticulostriates supply the most posterior part of this territory, while the more medial branches supply the most anterior part. The genu of the internal capsule receives some direct branches from the internal carotid artery in addition to the middle cerebral supply. (From Sadek, H., et al.: Radiology, 99:78, 1971. Drawn according to the description and illustrations in Human Neuroanatomy by Truex and Carpenter. 6th ed., Baltimore, Williams & Wilkins Co., 1969.)

resent the motor strip while the posterior portion represents the sensory area."

The Vascular Supply of the Internal Capsule of the Brain. The vascular supply of the internal capsule of the brain is diagrammatically illustrated in Figure 8–81. The internal capsule therefore receives its blood supply not only from the striate branches of the middle cerebral and internal carotid arteries but also from the anterior cerebral and the anterior choroidal arteries as indicated. (Also see Fig. 8–75 A and B.)

Arteries of the Posterior Fossa

Vertebral Artery (Fig. 8–82 A and B).   The vertebral artery is the first branch of the subclavian trunk. It courses upward and backward to the foramen in the transverse process of the sixth cervical vertebra. It is surrounded by the vertebral and internal jugular veins. On the left side, the thoracic duct passes anterior to it.

The artery then courses through the foramina in the transverse processes of the upper six cervical vertebrae, passing obliquely through the transverse process of C2 laterally to the atlas. It then emerges from the foramen in the transverse process of the atlas near the superior articular process on each side of the atlas, enters the suboccipital triangle, and lies in a groove on the upper surface of the arch of the atlas.

Its course then takes it anteriorly past the oblique ligament of the atlas, where it enters the vertebral canal. Finally, it pierces the spinal dura mater and runs upward into the cranial cavity through the foramen magnum. After piercing the arachnoid, it inclines to the front of the medulla oblongata and reaches the lower border of the pons, where it unites with its fellow of the opposite side to form the basilar artery.

We have considered the vertebral artery as belonging more properly to the spine (Chapter 9), but apart from its meningeal, posterior, and anterior spinal branches, the largest branch of the vertebral artery is actually the posterior inferior cerebellar artery which arises a short distance below the pons and passes around the medulla oblongata. This branch will be described in greater detail subsequently, as will the basilar artery and its branches formed by the junction of the two vertebrals.

The *basilar artery* (Fig. 8–84), after giving origin to pontine, internal auditory, anterior inferior cerebellar, and superior cerebellar branches, terminates by dividing into two posterior cerebral arteries, which are connected with the internal carotid arteries by posterior communicating arteries, completing the circle of Willis. It supplies the tentorial surface of the hemisphere, the medial and lateral surfaces of the occipital lobe, and the inferior temporal gyrus. All these vessels will be described in more detail later.

The Circle of Willis (Fig. 8–84).   The two anterior cerebral arteries communicate with one another through the anterior communicating artery; the internal carotid arteries from each side communicate with the vertebral arteries; and the two vertebral arteries unite to form the basilar artery. This circle of vessels at the base of the brain lies in the interpeduncular and chiasmatic subarachnoid cisterns.

Numerous variations on this basic theme will be described subsequently, as they are of great importance in the angiography of the brain.

In rare cases the *vertebral* artery may be entirely missing or replaced by a vessel that emerges from the extradural intracranial part of the internal carotid, connecting the internal carotid and basilar arteries. This is the primitive *trigeminal* artery (Fig. 8–83).

In lateral perspective the *basilar* artery is usually parallel to the clivus, but its upper portion may be elongated or bent posteriorly, with the bifurcation situated as much as 1 cm. from the dorsum sellae. Although the basilar artery is usually located approximately in the midline, it may deviate considerably laterally, particularly in older individuals whose vessels are elongated and redundant. Thus lateral displacement of the basilar artery is of no significance from the standpoint of detection of an expanding lesion at the base of the brain.

At approximately the level of the dorsum sellae or somewhat higher, the basilar artery divides into its two main branches, the *posterior cerebral* arteries, which pass around the cerebral peduncles. These are situated within the medial portion of the ambient cisterns and supply the medial surface of the occipital lobe and inferior portion of the temporal lobe. The *posterior communicating* artery, a branch of the internal carotid at the carotid siphon, produces a communication between the internal carotid and the posterior cerebral arteries. During internal carotid angiography, the entire posterior cerebral artery may be filled because of the internal carotid injection.

From the posterior communicating artery or the proximal portion of the posterior cerebral artery, the *anterior* and *posterior thalamoperforate* arteries emerge, coursing cephalad and somewhat anteriorly; they supply the hypothalamus and posterior parts of the thalamus and adjacent basal ganglia (Westberg).

Branches of the Vertebral Artery.   In the extracranial portion of the vertebral artery there are meningeal branches that anastomose with spinal arteries, and another meningeal branch that enters through the foramen magnum and supplies the dura of the posterior cranial fossa. Occasionally, deep cervical or intercostal arteries also arise from the vertebral artery. Figure 8–82 B demonstrates the intracranial segment of the vertebral artery and its branches as follows:

The *posterior inferior cerebellar* artery is the largest of the intracranial branches of the vertebral artery just prior to its junction point. The various component parts of this vessel are important for the delineation of anatomic structures and will be described separately.

The *anterior spinal* arteries are delicate branches arising just

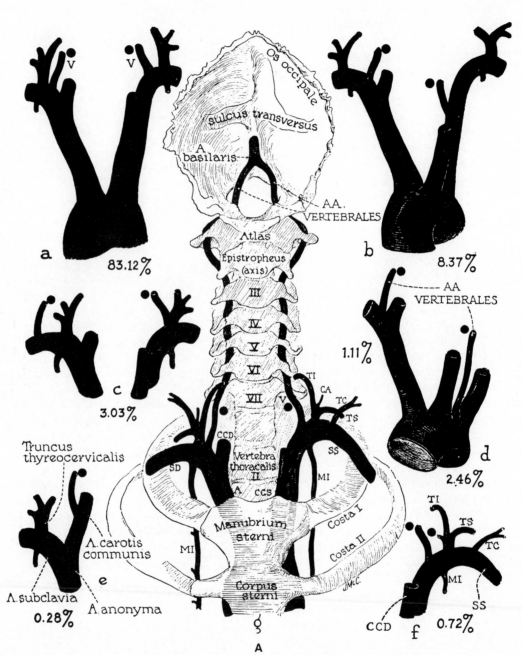

Figure 8–82.   A. Variations in the origin of the vertebral artery. (From Anson, B. J.: Atlas of Human Anatomy, 2nd ed. Philadelphia, W. B. Saunders Co., 1963.)

Figure 8–82 continued on the opposite page.

prior to the union of the two vertebrals to form the basilar. These two twigs unite at the level of the lower border of the olive, and the single vessel thus formed runs caudally along the anterior median fissure throughout the length of the spinal cord.

The *posterior spinal* artery arises from the posterior inferior cerebellar in about three-fourths of patients or from the vertebral artery itself in 20 per cent (Anson, 1966). Near its origin the posterior spinal artery divides into an ascending branch and a descending branch that passes caudally along the dorsal side of the medulla. It descends along the line of the dorsal roots throughout the length of the cord (see Chapter 9).

Posterior Inferior Cerebellar Artery (PICA) (Fig. 8–85). The posterior inferior cerebellar artery (PICA) may arise at various levels of the vertebral artery and occasionally from the basilar artery itself. It is one of the most variable branches of the vertebrobasilar system. The following variations, for example, have been documented:

1. It may arise at the level of the foramen magnum or below.
2. It may arise from either the basilar artery or the anterior inferior cerebellar artery.
3. The size of the vessel may vary considerably.
4. Although in most cases the caudal and cephalic loops indicate the anatomic structures described in the following paragraphs, there is some redundancy of these loops and this designation of anatomy is not absolute. The caudal loop may descend below the foramen magnum in normal cases without necessarily representing tonsillar herniation.

The posterior inferior cerebellar artery follows the sulcus between the rhomboid fossa and the cerebellum toward the inferior cerebellar peduncle where it curves on the undersurface of the cerebellum (Fig. 8–85). It then circumscribes the medial part of the cerebellar tonsil (LM), forming a second loop. Here, it receives *anastomosing branches* of the *inferior anterior cerebellar artery* and bends caudad, sending out small branches to the medial tonsillar surface and to the choroid plexus of the fourth ventricle. As the PICA approaches the lower and lateral edge of the cerebellar tonsil, it terminates in two branches, one *medial* and the other *lateral*.

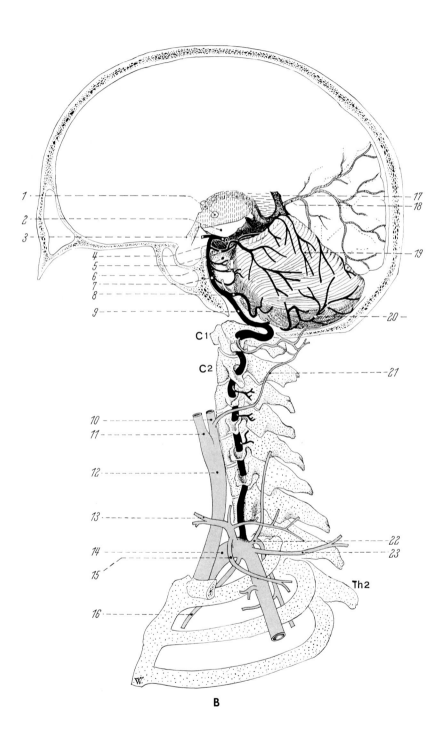

B

Figure 8–82 *Continued.* B. Extracranial and intracranial course of the vertebral artery and its branches. Vascular supply of the posterior portion of the circle of Willis. (From Krayenbühl, H. A., and Yaşargil, M. G.: Zerebrale Angiographie, 2nd ed. Stuttgart, G. Thieme Verlag, 1965.)

(1) Massa intermedia
(2) Cerebral peduncle
(3) Posterior communicating artery
(4) Posterior cerebral artery
(5) Superior cerebellar artery
(6) Pons
(7) Basilar artery
(8) Anterior inferior cerebellar artery
(9) Left vertebral artery
(10) External carotid artery
(11) Internal carotid artery
(12) Common carotid artery
(13) Thyreocervical arteries
(14) Subclavian artery
(15) Suprascapular artery
(16) Internal mammillary artery
(17) Splenium
(18) Right posterior cerebral artery
(19) Superior cerebellar artery
(20) Posterior inferior cerebellar artery
(21) Occipital artery
(22) Costocervical artery
(23) Transverse artery of the neck

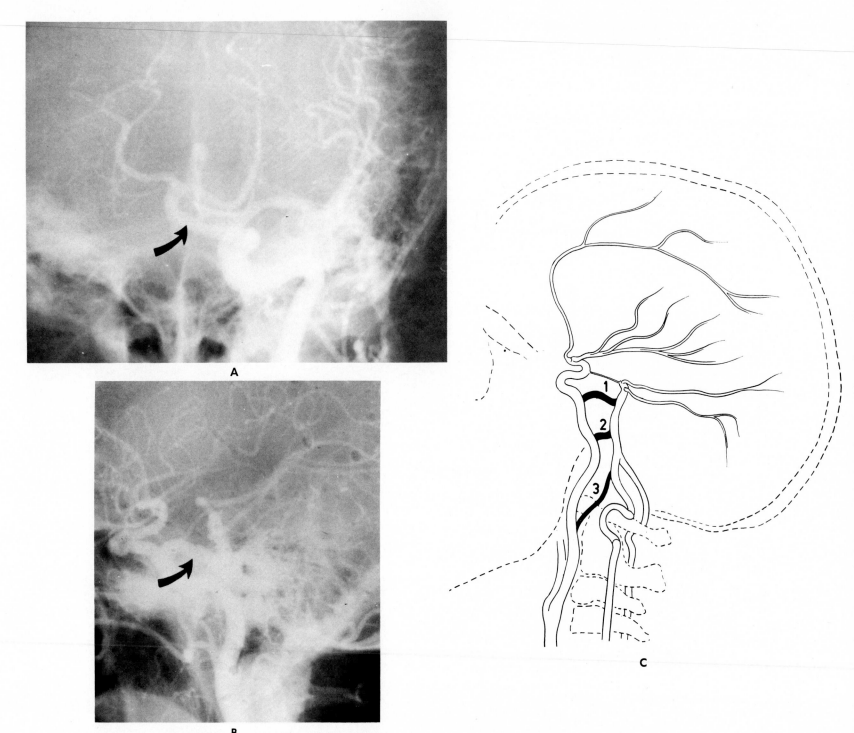

Figure 8–83. *A.* Anteroposterior arteriogram showing the trigeminal artery producing an anomalous communication between the internal carotid artery and the basilar artery. *B.* Lateral view of same patient, demonstrating the trigeminal artery producing a large communication between the internal carotid and basilar arteries. (From Meschan, I.: Roentgen signs of abnormality in cerebral angiograms. *In* Toole, J. F. (ed.): Special Techniques for Neurologic Diagnosis. Philadelphia, F. A. Davis Co., 1969.) *C.* Persistent primitive channels between the internal carotid artery and the basilar artery. (1) Primitive trigeminal artery, (2) Primitive acoustic artery, (3) Primitive hypoglossal artery. (From Krayenbühl, H. A., and Yaşargil, M. G.: Zerebrale Angiographie, 2nd ed. Stuttgart, G. Thieme Verlag, 1965.)

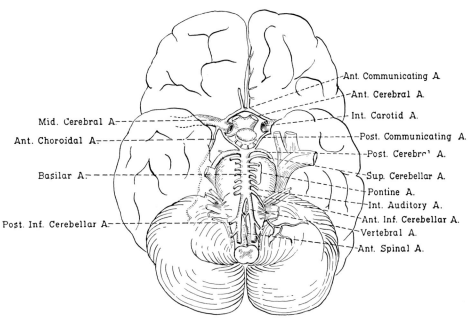

Figure 8–84. Anatomy of the vertebral artery and branches in relation to the base of the brain.

The *medial branch* (V) is situated in the paramedian sulcus and supplies branches to the caudal portion of the vermis, the biventer lobule of the cerebellum, the gracilis, and the superior and inferior semilunar lobules of the cerebellum. The medial branches of the two sides anastomose above the caudal part of the vermis.

The *lateral branch* of the PICA (Th) proceeds to the lateral portions of the tonsils, and anastomoses may occur between this branch and the terminal branches of the anterior inferior cerebellar artery (AICA), and between the lateral branch and the superior cerebellar artery above the cerebellar hemispheres. The detailed anatomy of the PICA has been described by Greitz and Sjögren.

The various segments of the PICA have been described as *anterior medullary* (AM), *lateral medullary* (LM), *supratonsillar* (MSt), *superior retrotonsillary* (SRt), and *vermian* (V). The *anterior medullary segment* is closely related to the medulla oblongata and corresponds to the "cisternal segment of Greitz." This segment courses through the cerebellomedullary fissure around the lateral aspect of the medulla and thus is differentiated here as the *lateral medullary segment*. The loop so formed is often called the "caudal loop" (LM), and this may extend below the inferior pole of the cerebellar tonsil. It is not, however, an absolute indicator of the position of the inferior margin of the cerebellar tonsil. The vessel then turns abruptly cephalad on the posterior surface of the medulla—this portion being called the *posterior medullary segment* (PM). It continues to the level of the incisura of the tonsil, where it reaches the anterior aspect of the superior

pole of the tonsil behind the posterior medullary velum. The further course may vary. The *supratonsillar segment,* also called the *cranial loop* (MSt), which runs over the superior pole of the tonsil, may pass medially or laterally around it (MSt), or it may take a transverse tortuous course (transverse supratonsillar segment). This portion of the vessel is closely associated with the roof of the lower part of the fourth ventricle. The artery then continues posteriorly until it reaches the posterior margin of the tonsil. The segment that courses down the retrotonsillar fissure is called the *superior retrotonsillar segment* (SRt). It forms a convex loop inferiorly as it continues around the anterior and inferior margins of the copula pyramidis. It then courses backward and upward in or near the inferior paravermian sulcus, forming the *vermian segment* (V).

The largest branch of the PICA is the *tonsillohemispheric branch* (Th). It originates typically from the posterior medullary segment, usually coursing posteriorly over or around the superior pole lateral to the supratonsillar segment. It reaches the retrotonsillar fissure (Th) and then runs downward in the retrotonsillar fissure along the lower margin of the biventral lobule near the tonsillobiventral notch and continues on to the inferior surface of the cerebellar hemisphere as the *hemispheric segment* (H). A number of variations in the course of the tonsillohemispheric branch do occur. There are many additional minute branches from these major divisions, as shown in Figure 8–85 *B,* supplying the medulla oblongata and the choroid plexus of the fourth ventricle.

A correlation of the appearance of the posterior inferior

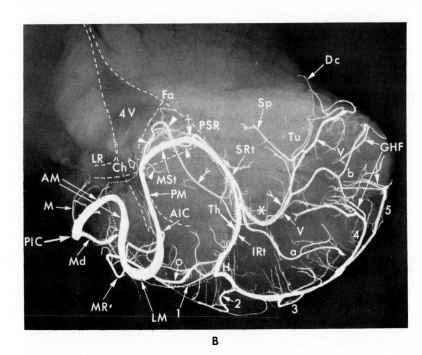

B

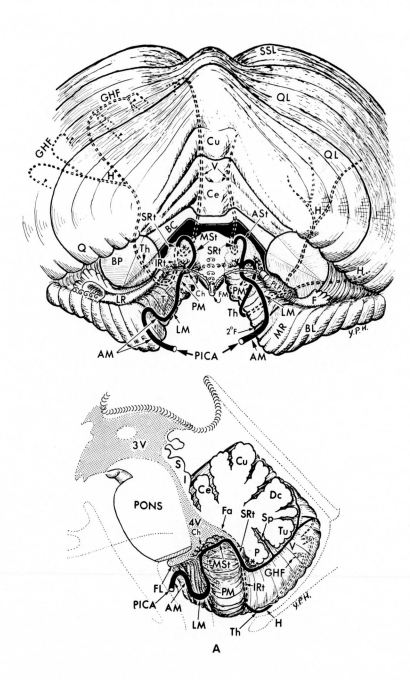

A

Figure 8–85. *A* and *B*. Diagrams showing the anatomic relationships of the posterior inferior cerebellar artery (PICA).

Covered portions of the arteries are shown in dashed fashion. The portions covered by the posterior medullary velum are, however, shown with solid lines. Labeled structures are the anterior medullary segment (AM), apical supratonsillar segment (ASt), brachium conjunctivum (BC), biventral lobule (BL), brachium pontis (BP), central lobule (Ce), choroidal branches (Ch), culmen (Cu), declive (Dc), flocculus (F), fastigium (Fa), foramen of Luschka (FL), foramen of Magendie (FM), great horizontal fissure (GHF), hemispheric segment (H), inferior colliculus (I), inferior retrotonsillar segment (IRt), lateral medullary segment (LM), lateral recess (LR), medullary ridge (MR) of the biventral lobule, medial supratonsillar segment (MSt), pyramid (P), posterior inferior cerebellar artery (PICA), posterolateral fissure (PLF), posterior medullary segment (PM), quadrangular lip (Q), quadrangular lobule (QL), superior colliculus (S), suprapyramidal branch (Sp), superior retrotonsillar segment (SRt), superior semilunar lobule (SSL), cerebellar tonsil (T), tonsillohemispheric branch (Th), tuber (Tu), and vermian segment (V). The location of the copula pyramidis is indicated by an asterisk (*). The secondary fissure (2°F), third and fourth ventricles ($_3$V, $_4$V) are also labeled. (From Huang, Y. P., and Wolf, B. S.: Amer. J. Roentgenol., *107*:543–564, 1969.)

Figure 8–85 continued on the opposite page.

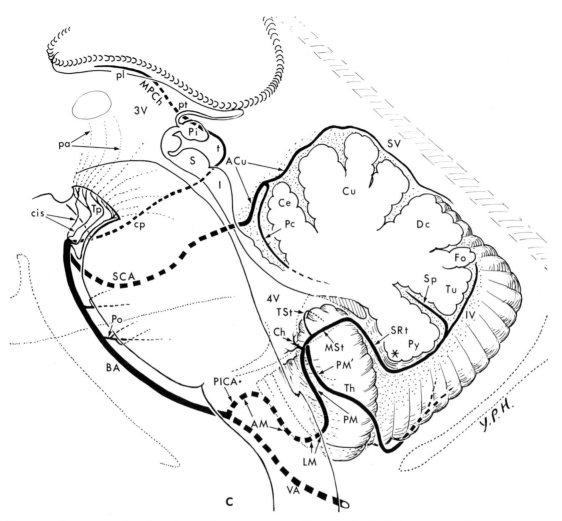

Figure 8–85 *Continued.* C. Diagrammatic representation of "mid-sagittal section" showing the normal course of diagnostically important posterior fossa arteries. The anterior portion of the inferior vermis has been removed to expose the medial aspect of the tonsil. Covered portions of arteries and parenchymal twigs are shown in interrupted fashion.

Labeled structures include the anterior culminate segment (ACu), the anterior medullary segment (AM), basilar artery (BA), central lobule (Ce), choroidal artery (Ch), cisternal segment (cis), circumpeduncular segment (cp), culmen (Cu), declive (Dc), inferior colliculus (I), vermian segment (IV) of the posterior inferior cerebellar artery, the folium (Fo), lateral medullary segment (LM), medial posterior choroidal artery (MPCh), parenchymal segment (pa), precentral cerebellar artery (Pc), pineal gland (Pi), posterior inferior cerebellar artery (PICA), plexal segment (pl), posterior medullary segments (PM, PM′) of the posterior inferior cerebellar artery and its tonsillohemispheric branch, pontine arteries (Po), pretectal segment (pt), pyramid (Py), superior colliculus (S), superior cerebellar artery (SCA), suprapyramidal branch (SP), superior retrotonsillar segment (SRt), medial supratonsillar segment (MSt), and vermian segment (SV) of the superior cerebellar artery, tectal segment (t), tonsillohemispheric branch (Th), transverse supratonsillar branch (TSt), thalamo-perforating arteries (Tp), tuber (Tu), vertebral artery (VA). The copula pyramidis (*), third and fourth ventricles ($_3$V, $_4$V) are also labeled.

The basilar artery may be located anywhere within the pontine cistern, that is, not intimately applied to the brain stem. Small pontine branches (Po), however, form a network directly on the surface of the pons. The thalamo-perforating arteries (Tp) arise in the deep portion of the interpeduncular cistern from the posterior cerebral arteries and assist in outlining the configuration of this cistern.

They may be divided into cisternal (cis) and parenchymal portions (pa). The prepontine and lateral pontine segments of the superior cerebellar artery (SCA) usually show an arcuate course convex inferiorly. The origin of the precentral cerebellar artery (Pc) is variable, but often demonstrates a recurrent course in order to enter the precentral cerebellar fissure. The fissural and parenchymal portions of this vessel are located behind and parallel to the brachium conjunctivum and the upper portion of the roof of the fourth ventricle. The vermian branch (SV) of the superior cerebellar artery (SCA) outlines the apex and tentorial aspect of the superior vermis.

The anterior medullary segment (AM) and the lateral medullary segment (LM) of the posterior inferior cerebellar artery (PICA) vary in their course depending on the site of origin of this vessel. However, the posterior medullary segment (PM) of the artery rather consistently runs adjacent to and behind the floor of the lower portion of the fourth ventricle. The "choroidal point" or junction between the posterior medullary (PM) and the supratonsillar segments (St) is frequently at the site of origin of a major choroidal artery (Ch) of the fourth ventricle. The exact location of the supratonsillar segment in relationship to the superior pole of the tonsil is variable. The superior retrotonsillar segment (SRt) outlines the upper half of the posterior margin of the cerebellar tonsil. The asterisk (*) indicates the copula pyramidis around which the vermian segment (IV) of the posterior inferior cerebellar artery runs. The origin and course of the tonsillohemispheric branch is quite variable. In this diagram, it is shown running a short distance behind the posterior medullary segment (PM′) of the posterior inferior cerebellar artery but still in the cerebello-medullary fissure on the medullary aspect of the tonsil. (From Huang, Y. P., and Wolf, B. S.: Amer. J. Roentgenol., *110*:1–30, 1970.)

cerebellar artery and its branches with the pneumoencephalographic features of the posterior fossa is shown in Figure 8–86. Figures 8–87 and 8–88 show some of the variations in the course of the PICA and its branches and a method of measurement of this artery. In the latter, the upper end of the posterior medullary segment or the beginning of the supratonsillar segment, usually corresponding to the origin of the choroidal artery at or near the in- cisura of the tonsil, may be designated as the choroidal point (C) (Ch on Figure 8–85). This point is located on the average 0.4 mm. behind the "anterior one-third point" of a line connecting the anterior margin of the foramen magnum (F) and the torcular Herophili (T) (Huang and Wolf).

In Figure 8–89, a diagrammatic horizontal section of the cerebellum and brain stem is shown, which illustrates the anatomic

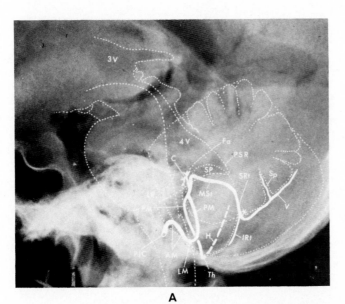

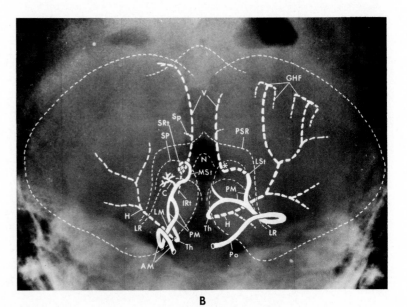

A　　　　　　　　　　　　　　　　　　　　　　　B

Figure 8–86. Correlation of the appearance of the posterior inferior cerebellar artery and its branches with pneumoencephalographic features.

Labeled structures include the anterior medullary segment (AM), choroidal branches (C), fastigium (Fa), great horizontal fissure of the cerebellum (GHF), hemispheric segment (H), inferior retrotonsillar segment (IRt), lateral medullary segment (LM), lateral recess (LR) of the fourth ventricle, lateral supratonsillar segment (LSt), medial supratonsillar segment (MSt), nodulus (N), posterior inferior cerebellar artery (PIC), posterior medullary segment (PM), pontine segment (Po), posterior superior recess (PSR) of the fourth ventricle, superior pole (SP) of the tonsil, suprapyramidal branch (Sp), superior retrotonsillar segment (SRt), tonsillohemispheric branch (Th) and vermian segment (V). Also labeled are the third and fourth ventricles ($_3$V, $_4$V) and the copula pyramidis (*).

A. Lateral view. The posterior medullary segments (PM) of the posterior inferior cerebellar artery (PIC) and of the tonsillohemispheric branch (Th) are located on the posterior surface of the medulla oblongata. The superior retrotonsillar segment (SRt) marks the posterior border of the cerebellar tonsil and anterior border of the copula pyramidis (*). The distance between this segment and posterior medullary segment (PM) indicates the antero- posterior diameter of the body of the cerebellar tonsil and the approximate height of the fourth ventricle. The vermian segment (V) usually runs in the depth of the posterior cerebellar notch.

B. Towne view. On the right side (reader's left), the course of the posterior inferior cerebellar artery is the same as in A. On the left side, an important variation of the posterior inferior cerebellar artery is shown. It originates from the basilar artery and runs laterally on the lower portion of the belly of the pons and brachium pontis (pontine segment–Po). It turns downward, medially, and backward in the upper part of the cerebellomedullary fissure, adjacent to the lateral recess (LR) of the fourth ventricle. The further course of the artery demonstrates an extreme position on the lateral aspect of the superior pole of the tonsil. The artery runs onto the lateral aspect of the superior pole of the cerebellar tonsil (LSt), then a short distance in the retrotonsillar fissure, and emerges beneath the copula pyramidis (*) as the vermian segment (V). The tonsillohemispheric branch (Th) originates in the region of the tonsillar incisura and runs medially and inferiorly on the posterior medullary aspect of the cerebellar tonsil (PM) before coursing onto the inferior surface of the hemisphere (H). The tonsillohemispheric branch turns around the tonsil more posteriorly and medially than on the right. (From Huang, Y. P., and Wolf, B. S.: Amer. J. Roentgenol., 107:543–564, 1969.)

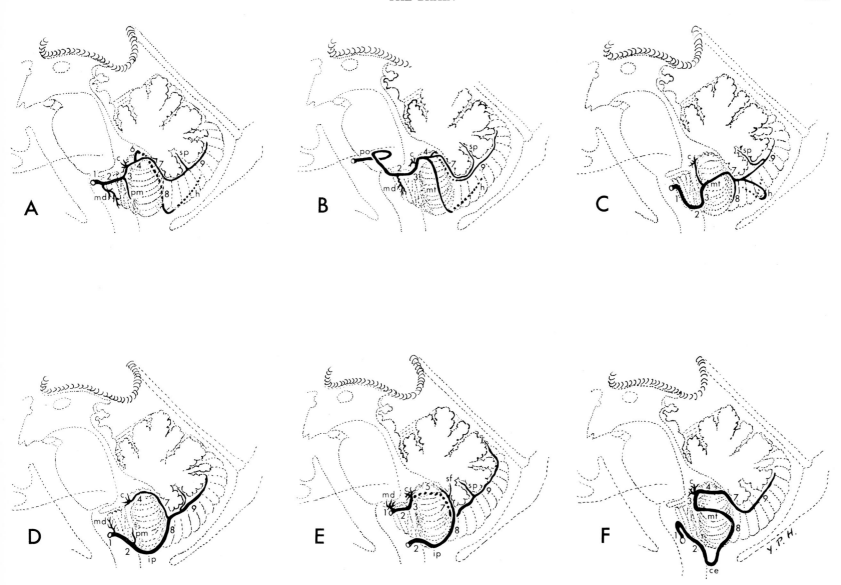

Figure 8–87. Variations in the course of the posterior inferior cerebellar artery and its branches.

Labeled structures include: the anterior medullary segment (1), lateral medullary segment (2), posterior medullary segment (3), medial supratonsillar segment (4), lateral supratonsillar segment (5), transverse supratonsillar segment (6), superior retrotonsillar segment (7), inferior retrotonsillar segment (8) and vermian segment (9). Also labeled are the choroidal branch (c), cervical segment (ce), hemispheric segment (h), inferior polar segment (ip), medullary branch (md), medial tonsillar segment (mt), posterior medullary branch (pm), pontine segment (po), arterial twig in the secondary fissure (sf) behind the uvula, and the suprapyramidal branch (sp).

A. The anterior medullary segment (1) is short and runs horizontally. The lateral medullary segment (2) is therefore located high in the cerebellomedullary fissure. A branch to the medulla (md) is prominent. The medial tonsillar segment (3) is short but the blood supply to the medial surface of the tonsil and posterior aspect of the medulla is reinforced by a small posterior medullary branch (pm). The origin of a tonsillohemispheric branch (6, 7, 8, h) is variable. In this case, it begins at the midportion of the medial supratonsillar segment (4).

B. The posterior inferior cerebellar artery may originate from the basilar artery and runs laterally in relation to the lower portion of the pons and the brachium pontis (po) before turning back and dipping into the upper part of the cerebello-medullary fissure. The tonsillohemispheric branch (mt, h) originates from the supratonsillar segment (4) but runs first in relation to the medial surface of the tonsil (mt) before reaching the inferior surface of the hemisphere (h). Note the origin of the suprapyramidal branch (sp) from the medial supratonsillar segment (4).

C. The supratonsillar segment is replaced by a medial tonsillar segment (mt) which runs on the medial aspect of the cerebellar tonsil considerably below the level of the superior pole. The superior retrotonsillar segment (7) is therefore short. A hemispheric branch (h) originates from the vermian segment (9).

D. The posterior inferior cerebellar artery remains superficial as it runs around the inferior pole (ip) of the tonsil to the region of the tonsillobiventral notch. The main vessel does not enter the medullary portion of the cisterna magna but does send a small branch (pm) into it. The medial supratonsillar branch (4) arises at the tonsillobiventral notch and runs upward (7) and then forward giving off tiny choroidal branches (c).

E. The posterior inferior cerebellar artery is divided into upper and lower trunks with variable branching.

F. The artery is extremely tortuous and dips into the cervical canal (ce). The vermian segment (9) may run not in but at some distance behind the inferior paravermian sulcus in the posterior cerebellar notch.

(From Huang, Y. P., and Wolf, B. S.: Amer. J. Roentgenol., *107*:543–564, 1969.)

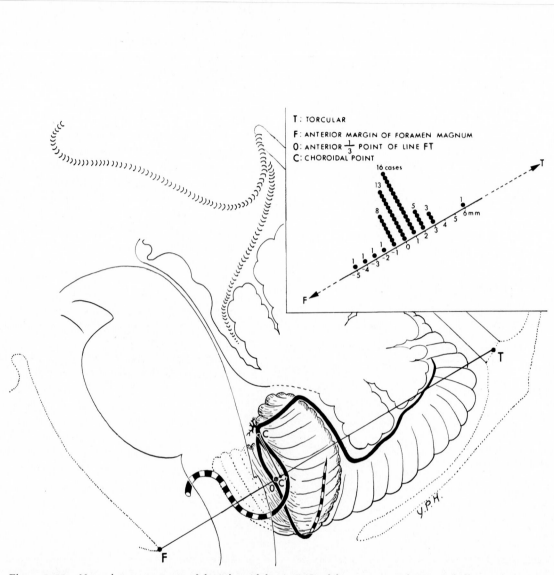

Figure 8–88. Normal measurements of the "choroidal point" (C) of the posterior inferior cerebellar artery in relation to other anatomic landmarks. The choroidal point is chosen as the point at which the posterior medullary segment joins the supratonsillar segment. Geometrically, the slope of the curve begins to decrease at this point or there may be an acute angulation. FT is a line drawn from the anterior margin of the foramen magnum to the torcular.

C′ = the foot of a perpendicular dropped from C to FT. The insert shows the relation of C′ to the anterior one-third point (0) of FT in 50 presumably normal adult cases. In 90 per cent of cases, C′ was located from 1 mm. anterior to 3 mm. posterior to the anterior one-third point. (From Huang, Y. P., and Wolf, B. S.: Amer. J. Roentgenol., 107:543–564, 1969.)

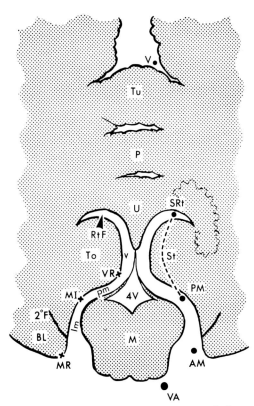

Figure 8-89. Diagrammatic horizontal section of the cerebellum and brain stem showing normal anatomic relationships of various segments of the posterior inferior cerebellar artery. Labelled structures are: anterior medullary segment (AM) of the posterior inferior cerebellar artery, biventral lobule (BL), medulla oblongata (M), medullary impression (MI), medullary ridge (MR) of the biventral lobule, pyramid (P), posterior medullary segment (PM), retrotonsillar fissure (RtF), superior retrotonsillar segment (SRt), supratonsillar segment (St), cerebellar tonsil (Co), tuber (Tu), uvula (U), vermian segment (V), vertebral artery (VA), and vallecular ridge (VR). The fourth ventricle (4V) and part of the hemispheric portion of the secondary fissure (2°F) are also labelled. Cross-sections of the vertebral artery and various segments of the posterior inferior cerebellar artery are shown by black circles. The lateral medullary segment (not shown), which connects the anterior medullary and posterior medullary segments, is located considerably below the level of this section. The supratonsillar segment (St), which runs over the superior pole of the cerebellar tonsil and forms the posterior medullary segment and the superior retrotonsillar segment, is in reality located above the level of the section. The vallecular ridge (VR) is the junction between the vermian and the posterior medullary parts of the medial surface of the tonsil. The depth of the medullary impression (MI) lies opposite the restiform body and separates the posterior medullary from the lateral medullary aspect of the tonsil. The tonsillar incisura lies at the upper end of this impression. (From Huang, Y. P., and Wolf, B. S.: Amer. J. Roentgenol., 107:543–564, 1969.)

relationships of the various segments of the posterior inferior cerebellar artery to these structures.

In another diagram (Fig. 8–90), Greitz and Sjögren have shown schematically the appearances of the three main types of variations in the origin of the posterior inferior cerebellar artery

in the lateral projection and the origin of the three main branches—hemispheric, vermian, and tonsillar.

Basilar Artery (Fig. 8–91). The basilar artery is situated on the ventral surface of the pons and extends to the interpeduncular cistern behind the dorsum sellae. It ends by bifurcating into two terminal branches, the right and left *posterior cerebral arteries.*

The following major branches are derived from the basilar artery: (1) *pontine branches,* (2) the *anterior inferior cerebellar artery,* (3) at times, an *internal auditory artery,* although this may originate from the anterior inferior cerebellar artery, and (4) the *superior cerebellar artery,* located immediately proximal to the termination into the posterior cerebral artery.

The *pontine branches* are arranged in two groups—*median* and *transverse*—that extend laterally.

Anterior Inferior Cerebellar Artery (Fig. 8–92). The *anterior inferior cerebellar artery* arises from the inferior third of the basilar artery. It passes toward the lower margin of the middle cerebellar peduncle into the cerebellopontine angle cistern. It supplies structures in close proximity to the internal auditory meatus but near the meatus it divides into four or five terminal branches that supply the cerebellum and the middle and inferior cerebellar peduncles.

Internal Auditory Artery. An *internal auditory artery* may originate from the basilar artery itself (in 17 per cent of patients) or from the anterior inferior cerebellar artery (in 83 per cent). *This artery passes into the auditory meatus and is an important indicator for structures in this immediate vicinity.*

Superior Cerebellar Artery (Fig. 8–93). The *superior cerebellar artery* arises just proximal to the bifurcation of the basilar and is the most rostral infratentorial vessel originating from the basilar artery. It has been divided into three main parts:

1. An *interpeduncular-crural portion* that encircles the brain stem where it lies inferior to the originating rootlets of the

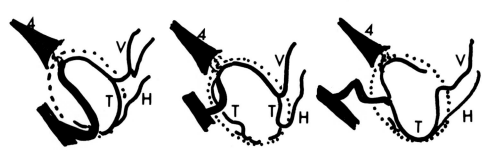

Figure 8-90. Schematic drawings showing the appearance of the three main types of variations in origin and branches of PICA in the lateral projection. Dotted line, tonsil of cerebellum; 4, 4th ventricle; H, hemispheric branch; V, vermian branch; T, tonsillar branch. (Modified from Greitz, T., and Sjögren, S. E.: Acta Radiol. (Diag.), 1:284–297, 1963.)

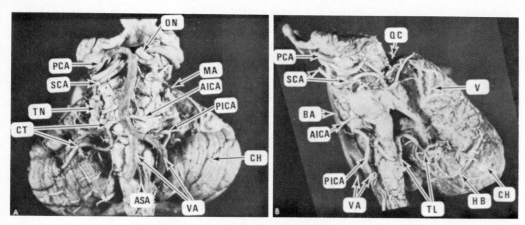

Figure 8–91. Anatomic specimen of the brain stem and cerebellum injected with microbarium. *A.* Frontal projection. (PCA) Posterior cerebral artery, (SCA) superior cerebellar artery, (MA) marginal artery (superior cerebellar branch), (TN) trigeminal nerve, (AICA) anterior inferior cerebellar artery, (PICA) posterior inferior cerebellar artery, (CT) AICA-PICA common trunk, (CH) left cerebellar hemisphere, (VA) vertebral arteries, (ASA) anterior spinal artery, (ON) oculomotor nerve. *B.* Lateral projection. The left cerebellar hemisphere, left tonsil, and left cerebellar peduncles have been removed to expose the vermis (V). (QC) Quadrigeminal plate cistern, (BA) basilar artery, (TL) tonsillar loop (PICA), (HB) hemispheric branch (PICA). Note the bifid superior cerebellar artery (SCA). (From George, A. E.: Radiol. Clin. N. Amer., 12:371–399, August, 1974.)

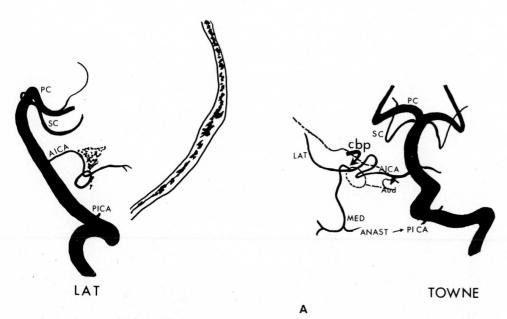

Figure 8–92. *A.* Anterior inferior cerebellar artery (AICA). The lateral and Towne's views are shown diagrammatically. (PC) posterior cerebral artery, (SC) superior cerebellar artery, (Aud) auditory branch, (cbp) cerebellopontine angle. This artery varies and anastomoses with the other two cerebellar arteries, as shown in *B.*

Figure 8–92 continued on the opposite page.

oculomotor nerve, which in turn separates it from the proximal segment of the posterior cerebral artery. It continues anterolaterally around the cerebellar peduncle in the crural cistern.

2. The *second or ambient portion* may be in close proximity with the edge of the tentorium cerebelli in the ambient cistern. The basal vein of Rosenthal and the posterior cerebral artery also lie parallel to the course of this second part of the superior cerebellar artery, *but they are supratentorial structures.*

3. The *third or quadrigeminal portion* lies within the quadrigeminal cistern. The right and left superior cerebellar arteries approach each other closely, giving off anastomotic branches as well as fine branches to the tectum in the region of the inferior colliculus.

The superior cerebellar artery splits into three branches (Fig. 8–93 *A* and *B*): (1) a *marginal branch,* which originates within the ambient cistern and courses first to the anterior surface of the cerebellum and then posterolaterally to the horizontal fissure. This branch demarcates the superior and inferior lobes of the cerebellum. (2) The *hemispheric branches* (Cm) arise distal to the marginal branch within the ambient cistern and course sharply upward to the medial portion of the superior surface of the cerebellar hemisphere. (3) The *superior vermis branch* is the terminal branch of the superior cerebellar artery and originates from the third or quadrigeminal segment. The right and left superior vermis branches anastomose with each other in the quadrigeminal cistern, close to the midline, and also with inferior vermis branches of the posterior inferior cerebellar artery. *These branches are important midline indicators.*

Thus, the main trunk of the superior cerebellar artery outlines the lateral profile of the midbrain at the level of the tentorial notch and indicates the position of the interpeduncular, crural, ambient, and quadrigeminal cisterns.

Generally, *there are three cerebellar arteries on each side.* These tend to anastomose freely and with considerable variation, and when one is relatively small it is usually compensated by increased size in another.

Considerable variation may occur in the appearance of the basilar artery (Fig. 8–94). It may be sinuous; it may be somewhat elongated and extend upward into the interpeduncular cistern in the lateral projection; it may be very close to the clivus or several millimeters behind it. Its length also varies considerably (Greitz and Löfstedt). The bifurcation of the basilar artery varies in respect to the dorsum sellae, tending to be higher and more posterior in older people than in children owing to elongation of the basilar artery from atherosclerosis.

Unfortunately, the internal auditory artery is very difficult to visualize. In about two-thirds of the cases, this artery is a branch of the anterior inferior cerebellar artery (Stopford).

The superior vermian branch of the superior cerebellar artery may be identified in Towne's projections near the midline.

Posterior Cerebral Artery. About 1 cm. from its origin, the

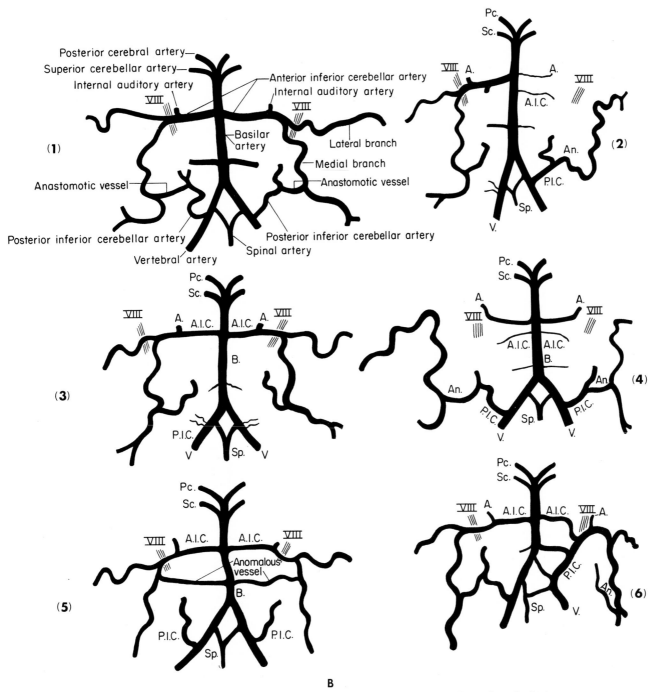

Figure 8–92 *Continued.* B. Variations of the branches of the basilar artery. (1) The "classical" and a fairly common arrangement, (2) the anterior varying inversely with the posterior inferior artery (common), (3) both posterior vessels small, their areas of supply being chiefly fed by the anterior vessels (uncommon), (4) both anterior vessels small, their areas of supply being chiefly from the posterior vessels (uncommon), (5) anomalous importance of vessel from the junction of vertebral arteries, (6) rare—posterior vessel being continuation of vertebral artery.

Pc, posterior cerebral artery; Sc, superior cerebellar artery; AIC, anterior inferior cerebellar artery; PIC, posterior inferior cerebellar artery; B, basilar artery; V, vertebral artery; Sp, spinal artery; A, internal auditory artery; VIII, acoustic nerve; An, anastomotic vessel; Anom, anomalous vessel. (Modified from Atkinson, W. J.: J. Neurol. Neurosurg. Psychiat., *12*:137–151, 1949.)

posterior cerebral artery is connected to the *internal carotid artery* by the *posterior communicating*. It may, as a result, derive its blood supply from either the internal carotid or vertebral systems.

The height or level of bifurcation of the basilar artery into the posterior cerebral arteries may vary considerably, as shown in Figure 8–94. The various segments and branches are illustrated in Figure 8–95. The posterior cerebral artery encircles the brain stem within the ambient cistern near the free edge of the tentorial notch, while giving off numerous *thalamoperforating branches*. It is immediately rostral to the superior cerebellar arte-

ry. At approximately its middle third, it produces *medial and lateral posterior choroid branches* and the *quadrigeminal artery*. The medial posterior choroid artery usually originates near the posterior communicating, whereas the lateral posterior choroid arteries are somewhat more distal. The arteries loop upward around the thalamus to enter the choroid plexus. The quadrigeminal artery is a very small branch arising from the proximal posterior cerebral artery and encircling the brain stem; it supplies the quadrigeminal plate. Small branches of the proximal posterior cerebral artery are also sent to the hippocampus and splenium of the corpus callosum.

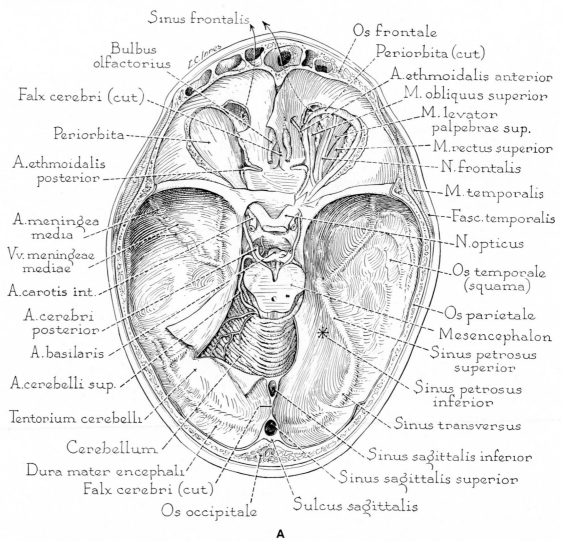

A

Figure 8–93. A. Floor of the cranial cavity demonstrating the en face appearance of the superior cerebellar artery originating from the basilar artery. It parallels the posterior cerebral artery but lies beneath the tentorium cerebelli as is shown in lateral diagram in Figure 8–92. (From Anson, B. J.: An Atlas of Human Anatomy. Philadelphia, W. B. Saunders Co., 1963.)

Figure 8–93 continued on the opposite page.

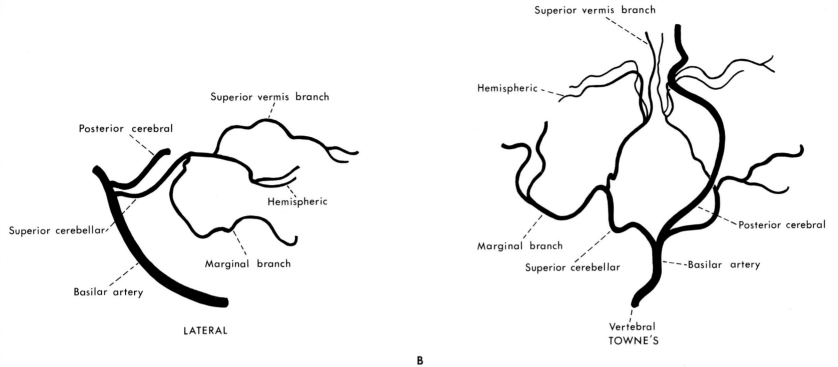

Figure 8–93 *Continued.* *B.* Line diagram demonstrating the superior cerebellar artery and its major branches. (Modified from Mani, R. L., Newton, T. H., and Glickman, M. G.: Radiology, 91:1102–1108, 1968.)

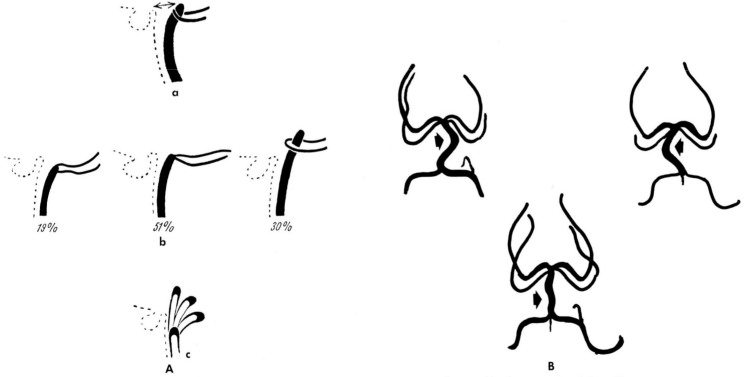

Figure 8–94. *A.* (a) Variations of distance between dorsum sellae and apex of basilar artery: 0.1–0.5 cm 39 per cent; 0.5–0.9 cm 48 per cent; 1 cm and more 18 per cent. (b) Course of apex of basilar artery. (c) Differences in height between dorsum sellae and basilar artery: equally high 51 per cent; below the dorsum sellae 19 per cent; above the dorsum sellae 30 per cent. (From Krayenbühl, H. A., and Yaşargil, M. G.: Zerebrale Angiographie, 2nd ed. Stuttgart, G. Thieme Verlag, 1965.) *B.* Line diagram illustrating some of the variations of curvature of the basilar artery as projected in Towne's view.

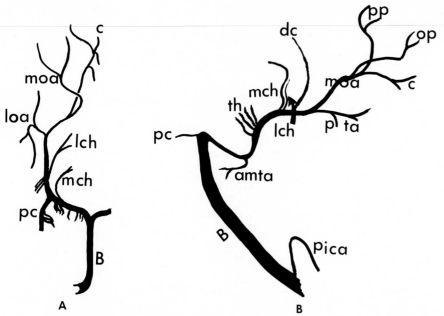

Figure 8-95. Line diagrams of the posterior cerebral arteries in Towne's AP (A) and lateral (B) projections.

(amta) anterior and middle temporal arteries, (B) basilar arteries, (c) calcarine artery, (dc) dorsal callosal artery, (lch) lateral posterior choroidal artery, (loa) lateral occipital artery, (mch) median posterior choroidal artery, (moa) medial occipital artery, (op) occipitoparietal artery, (pc) posterior communicating artery, (pica) posterior inferior cerebellar artery, (pp) posterior parietal artery, (pta) posterior temporal artery, (ta) temporal artery, (th) thalamic artery.

As the posterior cerebral artery continues it gives rise to branches to the inferior and medial cortex of the temporal and occipital lobes. These are called the *cortical branches*. They consist of *anterior and posterior temporal arteries* (sometimes named the middle temporal arteries), and they supply the undersurface of the temporal and occipital lobes.

When the posterior cerebral artery reaches the quadrigeminal cistern it turns medially, and the vessels from each side tend to approach each other or even meet as they pass above the edge of the tentorial notch. Terminally, they enter the parieto-occipital and calcarine fissures, supplying branches with these names.

In frontal perspective the two posterior cerebral arteries have a *flamelike* appearance (Fig. 8-96). Variations of this appearance are of considerable pathologic significance. Some moderate asymmetry between the two sides is common, however.

Usually, the choroid plexus of the lateral ventricles can be identified when the choroid branches are opacified.

Figure 8-97 illustrates diagrammatically the blood supply of the choroid plexus of the lateral ventricle on each side. The anterior choroid artery is usually a branch of the internal carotid artery that progresses posteriorly between the uncus and the brain stem. It usually enters the choroid plexus in the vicinity of the

temporal horn. There are many tributaries in the choroid plexus that anastomose freely with similar vessels arising from the posterior choroid artery. The anterior choroid artery should not exceed 0.1 to 0.5 mm. in diameter (in 85.3 per cent of cases, Wollschlaeger et al.).

Posterior Choroidal Artery. As noted before, the posterior choroidal arteries arise from the posterior cerebral artery (Fig. 8-97) and are generally smaller and not as readily identified. They supply mainly the choroid plexus of the third ventricle and lateral ventricles. There are two main divisions of the posterior choroidal arteries and sometimes they are separate: (1) the *posterior internal* or *medial*, which arises from the proximal portion of the posterior cerebral artery and passes forward around the brain stem and along the roof of the third ventricle to supply the choroid plexus of the third ventricle; and (2) the *posterior external or lateral branch* (sometimes there are two such branches) that supplies the choroid plexus of the body of the lateral ventricle and part of the plexus of the inferior horn (Fig. 8-98).

Measurements. The posterior lateral choroidal arteries, at least two in number, can be differentiated from the posterior medial because they describe a smooth concave curve, whereas the

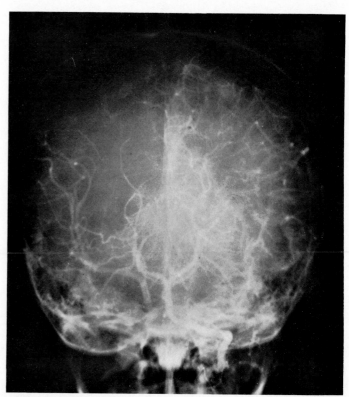

Figure 8-96. Total cerebral angiogram in Towne's projection in the arterial phase. Note the "flamelike" appearance of the posterior cerebral branches as they encircle the brain stem.

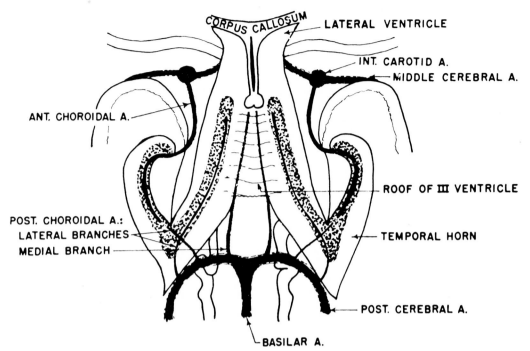

Figure 8–97. Diagram of the blood supply of the choroid plexus of the lateral ventricle. The ventricles are exposed from above. (From Lemay, M. J., and Jackson, D. M.: Amer. J. Roentgenol., 92:776–785, 1964.)

medial arteries form a double curve; also, the posterior medial are usually slightly more anterior than the lateral. Measurements of choroidal vessels made by Löfgren are illustrated in Figure 8–99 *A*. Here we see that the origin of the posterior choroidal vessels in the lateral projection is 25 to 45 mm. posterior to the basilar artery. The medial choroidal artery, after coursing around the brain stem, turns superiorly upon reaching the lateral aspect of the pineal body (Galloway and Greitz) and usually has the shape of a figure 3. It then runs superomedially to reach the roof of the third ventricle. The lateral choroidal arteries run an arcuate course on the pulvinar, enter the choroidal fissure, and anastomose with the anterior choroidal artery (Fig. 8–99 *B*). Two segments are usually recognized (Pachtman et al.).

Measurements have been reported for a group of 68 normal patients (54 normal adults and 14 normal children) in an effort to assist in diagnosis of such entities as hydrocephalus, brain stem tumors, and tumors of the pineal region (Fig. 8–99 *C*).

General Relationships. If a line is drawn between the tuberculum sellae and lambda on the one hand, and the tuberculum sella and the internal occipital protuberance on the other, in the lateral projection of the skull (Fig. 8–99 *C*), practically all of the major ramifications of the posterior cerebral and superior cerebellar arteries are encompassed.

The tentorium cerebelli, however, lies in tentlike fashion between the posterior cerebral artery above and the superior cerebellar below.

According to studies by Von Mitterwallner (quoted by Krayenbühl and Yaşargil), in 19 per cent of cases the posterior cerebral artery arises predominantly from the internal carotid artery either via the posterior communicating (in 17.2 per cent) or via the anterior choroidal (in 1.9 per cent). The posterior cerebral arises predominantly from the basilar artery in 72 per cent of cases and equally from the anterior cerebral as well as the carotid and basilar arteries in 8 per cent. It arises exclusively from the internal carotid artery in 0.3 per cent of cases, and exclusively from the basilar artery in 0.3 per cent also.

By internal carotid angiography it may be visualized in 30.6 to 42.1 per cent of cases. Unfortunately, the origin of the posterior cerebral artery is not constant in angiograms on the same patient or even in angiograms done in quick succession. It arises more frequently from the right side of the internal carotid than from the left (Krayenbühl and Yaşargil).

Bilateral absence of the posterior cerebral artery has been observed in 1.1 per cent of cases; unilateral absence, in 4.6 per cent.

Variations of the Circle of Willis. All components of the circle of Willis are present and normal in diameter in only 18 per cent of specimens (Riggs). The distribution of the various ana-

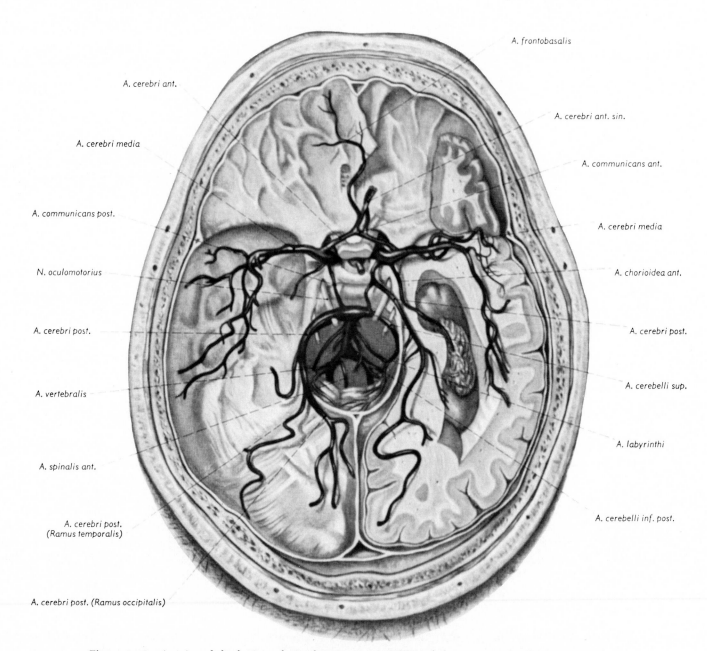

A. frontobasalis

A. cerebri ant.

A. cerebri ant. sin.

A. cerebri media

A. communicans ant.

A. communicans post.

A. cerebri media

N. oculomotorius

A. chorioidea ant.

A. cerebri post.

A. cerebri post.

A. vertebralis

A. cerebelli sup.

A. labyrinthi

A. spinalis ant.

A. cerebri post.
(Ramus temporalis)

A. cerebelli inf. post.

A. cerebri post. (Ramus occipitalis)

Figure 8–98. Arteries of the brain and circulus arteriosus *Willisi* and their topographical relationship to the base of the skull and tentorium. The left hemisphere has been removed, and only portions of the occipital and temporal lobes remain on the right. Through the tentorial notch may be seen the a. basalis and aa. vertebrales with their branches. The right a. cerebri post. arises from the a. carotis int. (frequent variation). (Drawn by K. Endtresser from an illustration in Ferner and Kautzky: Angewandte Anatomie des Gehirns und seiner Hüllen. *In* Handbuch der Neurochirurgie, Springer, Berlin/Göttingen/Heidelberg, 1959.)

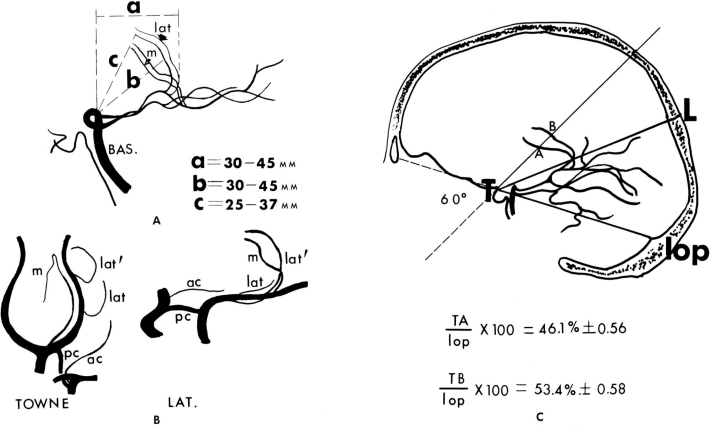

Figure 8–99. *A.* Method of measurement of the medial and lateral branches of the posterior choroidal arteries. Three distances are measured from the bifurcation between the basilar artery and the posterior cerebral artery to the lateral posterior choroid artery forming the largest curve.

(a) the distance to the tangent to the posterior part of the posterior choroid artery as measured along a line parallel to the longitudinal direction of the posterior cerebral artery, (b) the greatest distance to the posterior choroid artery (lateral branch), (c) the distance to the anterior upper part of the posterior choroid artery (lateral branch), (lat) lateral branch, (m) medial branch, (BAS) basilar artery. (After Lofgren, F. O.: Acta Radiol., 50:108–124, 1958.)

B. Diagrams of anterior (ac), lateral (lat), and medial (m) choroidal arteries. The posterior communicating artery (pc) is also shown for orientation. (Modified from Galloway, J. R., and Greitz, T.: Acta Radiol., 53:353–366, 1960.)

C. Line diagram illustrating the relationship of the posterior cerebral and superior cerebellar arteries to a line drawn between the tuberculum sellae and the lambda as well as between the tuberculum sellae and the internal occipital protuberance.

(T) tuberculum sellae, (L) lambda, (Iop) internal occipital protuberance, (A) line TB, drawn 60° from line T–IOP, crosses at A, the medial branch of the posterior choroidal artery in this projection; (B) crossing of the lateral branch of the posterior choroidal artery. (Modified from Pachtman, H., Hilal, F. K., and Wood, E. H.: Radiology, 112:343–352, 1974.)

tomic variants, based on a study of 1647 specimens removed at autopsy, is shown in Figure 8–100. Actually, however, complete absence of a component of the circle is very rare, although one component may be extremely hypoplastic.

Territories of the Brain and Brain Stem Supplied by the Basilar Artery and Its Branches (Fig. 8–101 *A*). The posterior cerebral artery supplies branches not only to the temporal and parietal cortex but also to such deeper areas as the mamillary bodies (Fig. 8–101 *B*), the medial and posterior parts of the thalamus, the tegmentum and central gray matter of the midbrain, the cere-

bral peduncles, the corpora quadrigemina, the geniculate bodies, the posterior limb and portions of the internal capsule, and the choroid plexuses of the third and lateral ventricles.

The numerous variations in origin of the vertebral arteries and variations of the vertebral-basilar system have already been alluded to. For example, the left and right vertebral arteries are of equal caliber in only 25 per cent of patients, the left being larger in 45 per cent and the right in 30 per cent. Indeed, it is not uncommon for the left vertebral artery to be two or three times the size of the right vertebral (Schechter and Zingesser).

The posterior inferior cerebellar artery is absent in 20 per cent of cases; its territory then is supplied by the anterior inferior cerebellar and short circumferential branches of the vertebral artery.

In a small percentage of people a carotid-basilar channel

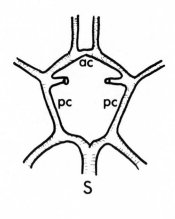

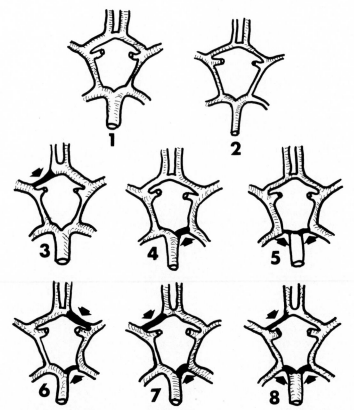

Figure 8–100. Variations of the circle of Willis (after Riggs). (S) standard relationships, (ac) anterior communicating artery, (pc) posterior communicating artery. The blackened segments represent agenesis or absence. Hypoplastic segments are shown narrower in caliber than the others.

such as the trigeminal, acoustic, or hypoglossal artery persists into adult life. (See earlier in Chapter.)

Anastomoses Within the Vertebral-Basilar System. The various routes of *common anastomosis within the vertebral-basilar system* and between this system and the carotid arterial system are indicated in Figure 8–102 *A* and *B*. These anastomoses include the following:

1. Anastomoses between the occipital branch of the external carotid artery and the muscular branches of the vertebral.
2. Leptomeningeal anastomoses between branches of the anterior and middle cerebral with branches of the posterior cerebral artery.
3. Leptomeningeal anastomoses over the cerebellum between the superior and inferior cerebellar arteries.
4. Choroidal anastomoses.
5. Anterior spinal artery connections with the vertebral arteries in several places.

Flow direction and pressure relationships in the vertebral-basilar system may be complex, and reversal of flow with a "stealing of blood" from the basilar system of the brain to an arm gives rise to the so-called "subclavian steal syndrome."

Structures Permitting Assay of the Brain Stem. To summarize, the following structures permit some estimate of anatomic detail in relation to the brain stem: (1) the basilar artery, (2) the anterior inferior cerebellar artery, (3) the posterior cerebral artery, (4) the superior cerebellar artery, (5) the ambient cistern on pneumograms, and (6) (as will be seen later) the basal vein of Rosenthal.

It is well to recall that the posterior cerebral artery becomes a supratentorial structure, whereas the superior cerebellar artery remains subtentorial for its entire length.

Veins of the Brain

The main venous channels of the brain are (Fig. 8–103): (1) a system of *superficial dural sinuses*, (2) deep-lying *encephalic veins*, consisting of relatively straight venous structures as well as a large plexus of veins named the *basilar plexus*, which begins in the anterior perforated substance at the base of the brain and continues downward on the clivus into the spinal canal, communicating with vertebral and soft tissue, thoracic, abdominal, and pelvic veins; (3) *orbital veins*, which empty into the facial and pterygoid veins; and (4) a *rete of veins of the internal carotid artery*. Most of the veins of the brain drain by way of the jugular vein and have been previously illustrated.

There is an unusual confluence of veins in the following strategic areas of this venous system:

1. The *sinus confluens* near the occipital internal protuberance, where the superior longitudinal sinus, straight sinus, and transverse sinus all come together.

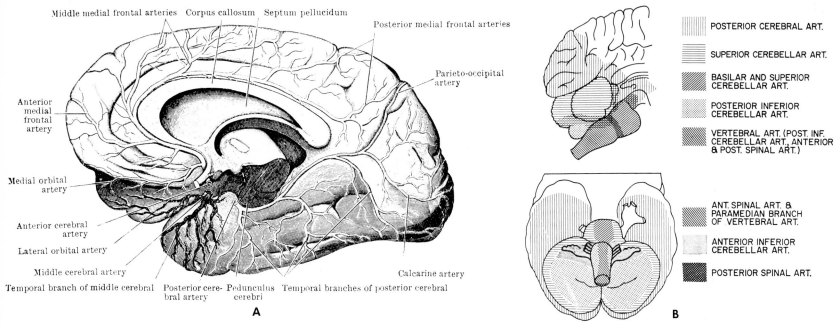

Figure 8–101. *A.* Distribution of the cerebral arteries on the medial and inferior surfaces of the cerebral hemisphere. (From Cunningham's Textbook of Anatomy, 6th ed. London, Oxford University Press, 1931.) *B.* Territories of the brain and brain stem supplied by the basilar artery and its branches. Adapted from Krayenbühl and Yaşargil. (From Schechter, M. M., and Zingesser, L. H.: Radiology, 85:23–32, 1965.)

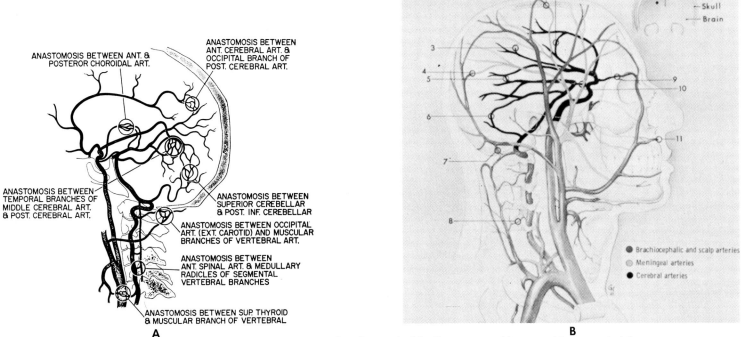

Figure 8–102. *A.* The common anastomoses within the vertebral-basilar system and between this system and the carotid arterial system. (From Wilson, M.: The Anatomic Foundation of Neuroradiology of the Brain. 2nd ed. Boston, Little, Brown & Company, 1972.) *B.* Collateral circulation to the brain. Dark gray vessels, brachiocephalic and scalp arteries; light gray, meningeal arteries; and black, cerebral arteries. The following arterial anastomoses are shown: (1) Scalp artery and meningeal artery, (2) anterior cerebral artery and middle cerebral artery, (3) meningeal artery and middle cerebral artery, (4) scalp artery and meningeal artery, (5) posterior cerebral artery and middle cerebral artery, (6) posterior inferior cerebellar artery and superior cerebellar artery, (7) vertebral artery and scalp artery, (8) vertebral artery and deep cervical artery, (9) ophthalmic artery and orbital artery, (10) Circle of Willis, (11) branches of right and left external carotid arteries. (After Schaeffer, J. P. (ed.): Morris' Human Anatomy, 11th ed., Chapter 6, by B. M. Patten. Copyright 1953 by The Blakiston Company, New York. Used with permission of McGraw-Hill Book Company.

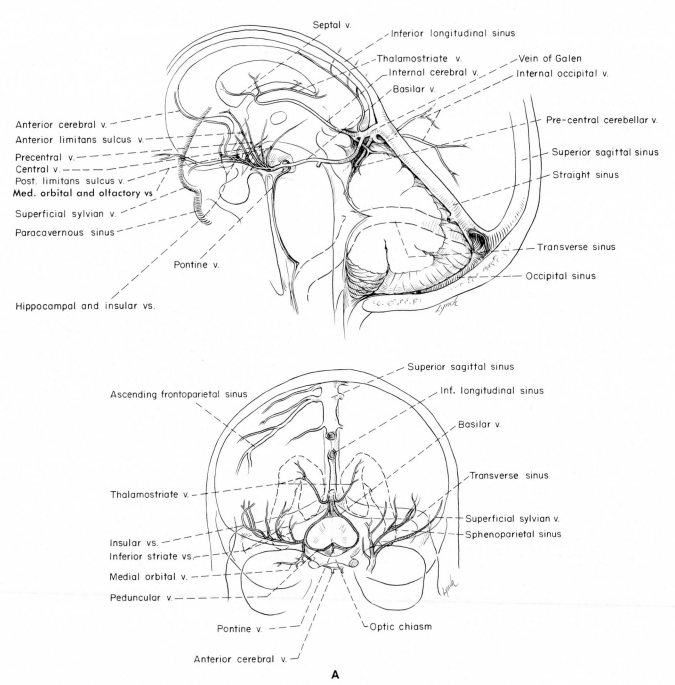

Septal v.

Inferior longitudinal sinus

Thalamostriate v.

Vein of Galen

Internal cerebral v.

Internal occipital v.

Basilar v.

Anterior cerebral v.

Pre-central cerebellar v.

Anterior limitans sulcus v.

Precentral v.

Superior sagittal sinus

Central v.

Straight sinus

Post. limitans sulcus v.

Med. orbital and olfactory vs

Superficial sylvian v.

Paracavernous sinus

Transverse sinus

Pontine v.

Occipital sinus

Hippocampal and insular vs.

Superior sagittal sinus

Ascending frontoparietal sinus

Inf. longitudinal sinus

Basilar v.

Transverse sinus

Thalamostriate v.

Superficial sylvian v.

Insular vs.

Sphenoparietal sinus

Inferior striate vs.

Medial orbital v.

Peduncular v.

Pontine v.

Optic chiasm

Anterior cerebral v.

A

Figure 8–103. A. Diagrammatic illustrations of the venous drainage of the brain.

Figure 8–103 continued on the opposite page.

2. The *confluent area*, where the inferior longitudinal sinus, the great cerebral vein of Galen, superior cerebellar veins, internal occipital veins, and basal vein of Rosenthal all drain into the *straight sinus*.

3. The *veins draining into the great cerebral vein of Galen*, such as the internal cerebral veins, basilar veins of Rosenthal, dorsal callosal veins, and superior cerebellar veins.

4. The *venous angle* at the level of the foramen of Monro, where the striothalamate vein, choroidal veins, and septal veins merge.

5. The area *at the level of the cerebral peduncles*, where the insular veins, deep middle cerebral veins, lenticulostriate veins, hippocampal veins, olfactory veins, anterior cerebral veins, and peduncular veins merge.

6. The area *at the cavernous sinuses*, which lie on either side of the body of the sphenoid bone and receive blood from the superior ophthalmic veins, the sphenoparietal sinuses, a basilar plexus, and at times, the superficial middle cerebral veins from the Sylvian fissures on each side (Fig. 8–103).

DURAL VENOUS SINUSES

The *superior* and *inferior sagittal sinuses* (Fig. 8–103) are midline structures contained within the dura along the superior and inferior margins of the falx cerebri. At the point of junction of the falx and tentorium cerebelli, these two relatively parallel sinuses join the free edge of the tentorium and drain into the straight sinus.

The *straight sinus* is formed by the merging of the inferior sagittal sinus and the great cerebral vein of Galen, which is a major venous drainage channel for the deep structures of the brain.

A small venous sinus—the *occipital sinus*—begins on the inner table of the occipital bone near the posterior margin of the foramen magnum; this runs upward in the line of attachment of the falx cerebri to the occipital bone. It merges with the superior sagittal sinus and straight sinus at a *sinus confluens*. Likewise, there is a confluence of lateral or transverse sinuses at this juncture (the *torcular Herophili*).

The *lateral sinuses* are situated at the line of attachment of the tentorium to the occipital and temporal bones. Upon reaching the petrous ridge, each lateral sinus turns downward to become the sigmoid sinus. The lateral sinus also receives the superior petrosal sinus (Fig. 8–103).

The *sigmoid sinus* runs downward and passes through the jugular foramen to leave the cranial cavity as the internal jugular vein on each side.

All of these sinuses receive blood from numerous cerebral veins adjoining them.

The *cavernous sinuses* lie on each side of the body of the sphenoid bone and sella turcica and communicate with each other

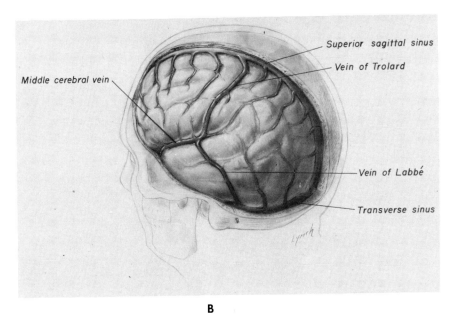

B

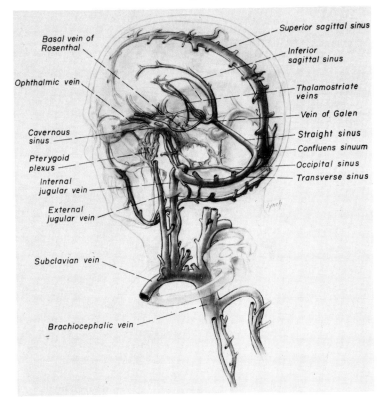

C

Figure 8–103 *Continued.* B. Drawing illustrating the superficial veins of the brain, emphasizing the relationship of the middle cerebral vein to the lateral fissure. Note also the rather regular appearance of the superior cerebral veins as they drain into the superior sagittal sinus. A mass lesion that is superficial in this area will often cause distortion of these superior cerebral veins. C. Labeled drawing illustrating the deep venous drainage of the brain through some of the superior large venous sinuses. (From Toole, J. F., and Patel, A. N.: Cerebrovascular Disorders. Copyright © 1967 by McGraw-Hill, Inc. Used by permission of McGraw-Hill Book Company.)

Figure 8–103 continued on the following page.

by a venous plexus. The cavernous sinuses receive blood from the superior ophthalmic veins, the sphenoparietal sinuses, the basilar plexus, and, at times, superficial middle cerebral veins from the Sylvian fissures on each side.

The *superior* and *inferior petrosal sinuses* extend from each cavernous sinus to the sigmoid sinus on each side. Emissary veins connect the cavernous sinuses with the pterygoid plexuses.

The *inferior petrosal sinuses* lie at the inferior edge of the pe-

trous ridge just lateral to the clivus and join the sigmoid sinuses just before the latter sinuses enter the internal jugular vein. *The cavernous and petrosal sinuses also communicate with spinal veins via the basilar plexus.*

Meningeal veins accompanying meningeal arteries may also drain into the dural sinuses. Likewise, diploic veins in the venous diploë of the bones of the calvarium may drain into adjoining dural sinuses, meningeal veins, or veins of the face and scalp.

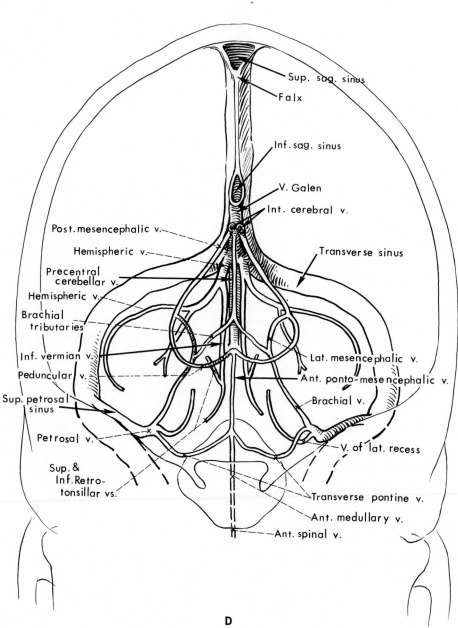

D

Figure 8–103 *Continued.* Diagrams of the basilar vein and its tributaries in Towne's projection (D) and lateral projection (E). (Modified from Wolf, B. S., and Huang, Y. P.: Amer. J. Roentgenol., 90:472–489, 1963.)

Figure 8–103 continued on the opposite page.

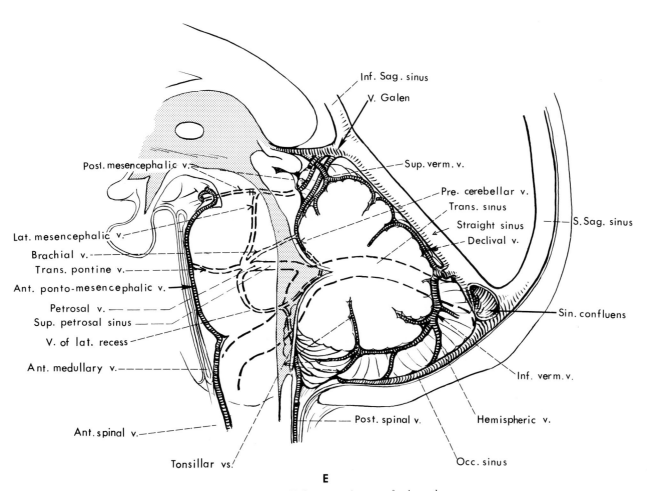

Inf. Sag. sinus

V. Galen

Post. mesencephalic v.

Sup. verm. v.

Pre. cerebellar v.

Trans. sinus

Straight sinus

Declival v.

S. Sag. sinus

Lat. mesencephalic v.

Brachial v.

Trans. pontine v.

Ant. ponto-mesencephalic v.

Petrosal v.

Sup. petrosal sinus

V. of lat. recess

Ant. medullary v.

Sin. confluens

Inf. verm. v.

Ant. spinal v.

Post. spinal v.

Hemispheric v.

Tonsillar vs.

Occ. sinus

E

Figure 8–103. *E. See opposite page for legend.*

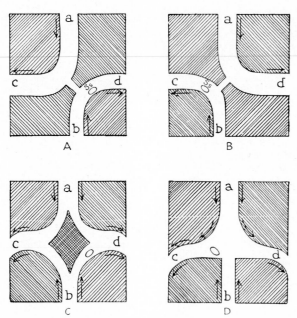

Figure 8–104. Schematic illustration of the sinus confluens, showing variations in its appearance. (From Pendergrass, E. P., Schaeffer, J. P., and Hodes, J. P.: The Head and Neck in Roentgen Diagnosis, 1956. Courtesy of Charles C Thomas, Publisher, Springfield, Illinois.)

Emissary veins connect the dural sinuses with extracranial veins.

Rather constant emissary veins are found in the mastoid and the condyloid regions adjoining the occipital condyles (mastoid and condyloid emissary vein, respectively).

Veins passing through the optic foramen (superior ophthalmic veins) and the foramen ovale or an inconstant foramen of Vesalius also afford a communication between intracranial and extracranial structures.

Variations from the preceding classic anatomic arrangement are common (Browning). Some of the more common variations of the relationship of the sinus confluens and the lateral sinus are shown in Figure 8–104.

ENCEPHALIC VEINS

Encephalic veins may be classified as follows:
1. Superficial cerebral veins.
2. Deep cerebral veins.
3. Cerebellar veins (to be discussed separately).
    (a) Superior group.
    (b) Anterior group.
    (c) Posterior group.

Superficial Cerebral Veins. The superficial cerebral veins lie on the convexity of the cerebral hemispheres in a direction that is almost perpendicular to the superior sagittal sinus; they

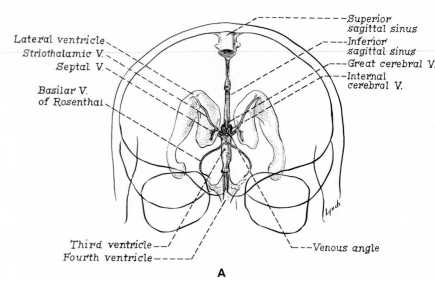

Figure 8–105. A. Diagram of venogram, AP view.

Figure 8–105 continued on the opposite page.

tend to parallel one another fairly closely. An occasional vein may be larger than the others, particularly if they are anastomotic. These are the anastomotic veins of Trolard and Labbé (Fig. 8–105).

The *middle cerebral vein (Sylvian vein)* and the *vein of Labbé* are usually readily distinguished on the surface of the brain (Fig. 8–106). The middle cerebral vein drains the Sylvian fissure and flows into either the sphenoparietal sinus or the cavernous sinus. Occasionally, however, it drains directly into the superior petrosal sinus or even into the transverse sinus. The vein of Labbé usually drains into the transverse sinus in its anterior, middle, or even posterior portion.

In addition, *frontobasal medial veins* draining the anterior two-thirds of the frontal lobe may flow into the sphenoparietal sinus or into the superior ophthalmic vein, or occasionally into the superior petrosal sinus.

Temporal lobe superficial veins drain into the vein of Labbé, into the transverse sinus, or into the superior petrosal veins. Veins on the basal aspect of the temporal lobe drain directly into the basilar vein of Rosenthal via the hippocampal vein.

The veins of the cerebellum will be discussed later.

Deep Cerebral Veins (Fig. 8–107). The two internal cerebral veins are formed at the interventricular foramina on each side by the confluence of the striothalamic, septal, and choroidal veins. These two internal cerebral veins flow along the roof of the third ventricle, separated from one another by a space of 2 to 3 millimeters. The *septal vein* (vein of the septum pellucidum) and the *striothalamic vein* (thalamostriate vein, posterior terminal vein), together with the internal cerebral vein, form the *venous angle* on each side (Krayenbühl and Richter). The normal angle (24.9°)

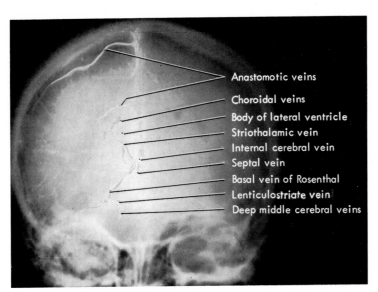

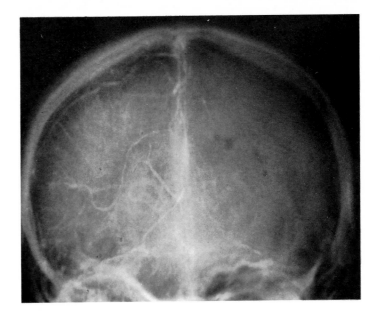

Anastomotic veins
Choroidal veins
Body of lateral ventricle
Striothalamic vein
Internal cerebral vein
Septal vein
Basal vein of Rosenthal
Lenticulostriate vein
Deep middle cerebral veins

B

Figure 8–105 *Continued.* *B.* Representative radiographs (intensified).

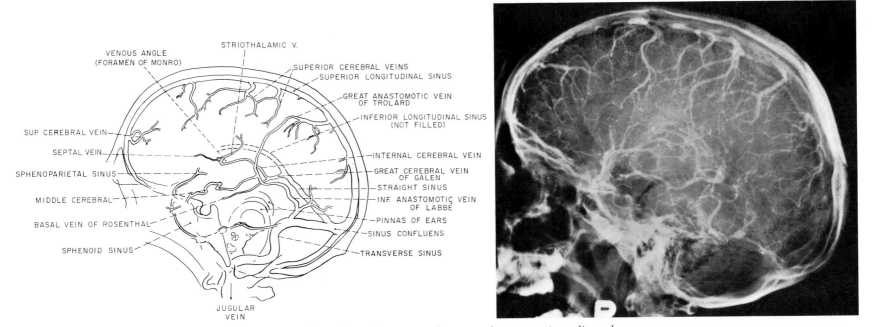

VENOUS ANGLE
(FORAMEN OF MONRO)
STRIOTHALAMIC V.
SUPERIOR CEREBRAL VEINS
SUPERIOR LONGITUDINAL SINUS
GREAT ANASTOMOTIC VEIN
OF TROLARD
INFERIOR LONGITUDINAL SINUS
(NOT FILLED)
SUP CEREBRAL VEIN
SEPTAL VEIN
INTERNAL CEREBRAL VEIN
SPHENOPARIETAL SINUS
GREAT CEREBRAL VEIN
OF GALEN
STRAIGHT SINUS
MIDDLE CEREBRAL
INF. ANASTOMOTIC VEIN
OF LABBÉ
BASAL VEIN OF ROSENTHAL
PINNAS OF EARS
SINUS CONFLUENS
SPHENOID SINUS
TRANSVERSE SINUS
JUGULAR
VEIN

Figure 8–106. Internal carotid venogram diagram and representative radiograph.

TABLE 8–6 NORMAL ANGLES BETWEEN THE INTERNAL
CEREBRAL VEIN AND STRIOTHALAMIC VEIN*

	Half-Axial	Anteroposterior
Mean	24.9 degrees	18.2 degrees
Range	17.3–32.0 degrees	13.5–2.0 degrees
Standard deviation	4.06 degrees	2.45 degrees

Note: The angle varies significantly with projection.
*From Richardson, H. D., and Bednarz, W. W.: The depiction of ventricular size by the striothalamic vein in the anteroposterior phlebogram. Radiology, *81*:604–609, 1963.

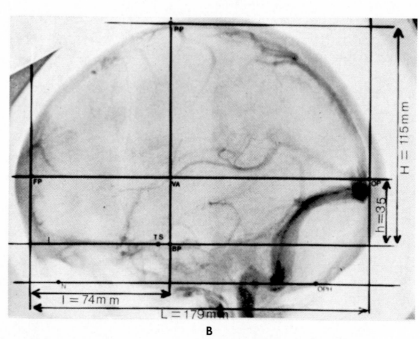

A

B

Figure 8–107. *A.* Diagram showing the method of measurement of the angle between the striothalamic and internal cerebral vein. A vertical line is drawn through the internal cerebral vein perpendicular to the base of the skull. Another line is drawn along the relatively straight laterally inclined segment of the striothalamic vein to intersect the vertical line. The intervening angle is measured.

Normal angles are shown in the table (the angle varies significantly with the projection). (From Richardson, H. D., and Bednarz, W. W.: Radiology, *81*:604–609, 1963.)

B. The Probst method for accurate determination of the venous angle. (VA) venous angle, (TS) tuberculum sellae, (BP) foot point (by dropping a line perpendicular from VA to the basic line drawn between the nasion and the posterior margin of the foramen magnum on the occipital bone).

A line through the tuberculum sellae is drawn parallel to the base line. Another horizontal line drawn parallel to this base line is drawn through the venous angle (VA). A fourth parallel line — the parietal line — is drawn tangentially to the *inner* table of the parietal bone. Thereafter the following lines are drawn perpendicular to the base line: (1) a frontal line which is tangential to the inner table of the frontal bone; (2) a venous angle line drawn perpendicular to the base line through the venous angle; and (3) an occipital line which is drawn tangential to the inner table of the occipital bone.

The following distances are then measured in millimeters and half-millimeters: FP to VA (frontal distance); FP to OP = total length (L); BP to VA = the basal distance (h); and BP to PP = the total height (h).

473

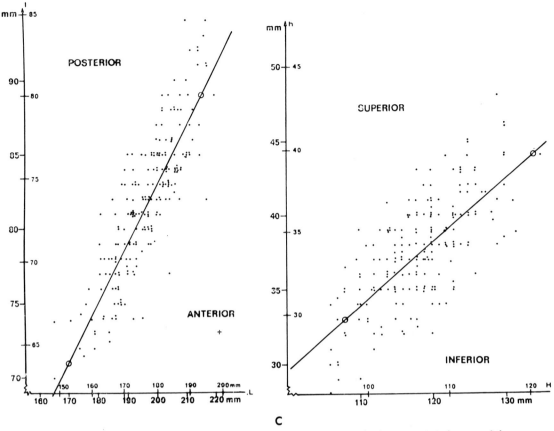

Figure 8–107 *Continued.* *C.* The regression lines are shown here. *Left,* The fronto-occipital range of the venous angles in relation to the inner length of the skull. *Right,* The basovertical range of venous angles in relation to the height of the skull. It is claimed that the maximum ranges of variation in both vertical and horizontal directions are plus or minus 7.35 mm. (99 per cent), and 5.95 mm. (95 per cent), respectively. The maximum distances from the point 0 along the major axis are 8.2 mm. and 6.7 mm., respectively; and along the minor axis 6.6 mm. and 5.25 mm., respectively. (*B* and *C* modified from Probst, F. P.: Acta Radiol. (Diag.), 10:271–288, 1970.)

between the internal cerebral vein and the striothalamic vein in half-axial and anteroposterior projections is shown in Figure 8–107 *B* with its adjoining table.

The position of the "venous angle" in the median sagittal plane has been given very extensive study by Probst. The venous angle apparently appears in about 80 per cent of all carotid angiography studies and usually marks the apex of the posterior superior limits of the interventricular foramen. It is, of course, extremely important to know whether a "false venous angle" is present, since misleading diagnoses may result otherwise. These false venous angles are caused by the confluence of veins other than the striothalamic vein entering the anterior third of the internal cerebral vein. Overlying veins, especially in the superficial aspects of the brain, may likewise make visualization of the venous angle difficult. Probst has summarized and illustrated the various methods for localization of the venous angle. Unfortunately, many of these methods depend upon craniometric points which are not readily visualized on the usual films that are obtained. The site of the tuberculum sellae probably varies least

and is more readily determined than other sites. This, therefore, is probably the most useful foot point for the base line of any coordinate system. The methods of Lin et al. (1955) and Mokrohisky et al. (1956), which have been previously mentioned, resemble the chart given by Vastine and Kinney for orientation of the pineal body. The base line in these techniques, as illustrated, was drawn through the tuberculum sellae to the nasion. A perpendicular line, the Y-axis, was drawn from this base line through the convexity point along the venous angle to the inner table of the vault. The position of the venous angle in the anteroposterior view was measured along a line passing through A, which was the longest fronto-occipital distance between the inner tables.

Unfortunately, these techniques have had a restricted application. The reader is referred to Probst's original article for an exhaustive review of the subject and to Figure 8–107 *B* and *C*, which are included for reference. A method based upon 250 consecutive carotid angiographic studies from adults judged to be normal was proposed by Probst. In each of these he required that the venous angle and the internal cerebral vein be distinctly visible, and angiographs not fulfilling these conditions were discarded. Thus, of the 250 cases, 216 angiographic films were available for study. They found an incidence of 5 per cent of false venous angles when comparing the angles on the two sides.

The *septal veins* receive blood from the septum pellucidum, the anterior end of the corpus callosum, and the head of the caudate nucleus. The *striothalamic vein* flows along the terminal stria from back to front, lying above and almost parallel to the internal cerebral vein. It drains the thalamus, the internal capsule, and the stria.

The choroidal vein follows the edge of the choroid plexus in the lateral ventricle and drains the blood from it. It has a corkscrew appearance.

The Septal Vein as an Indicator of Space-Occupying Lesions in the Anterior Cranial Fossa (Zimmer and Annes).   The septal veins are of particular value in corroborating the nature and presence of space-occupying lesions on the anterior cranial fossa. As noted before, these are paired subependymal veins that receive blood from the anterior frontal lobe. The septal tributaries pass medially along the flared rostral portion of the frontal horns and then posteriorly in the paired leaflets of the septum pellucidum, around the anterior columns of the fornix, and finally into the internal cerebral veins. In the anteroposterior projection an angular configuration demarcates the plane of the rostral portion of the septum pellucidum (Fig. 8–108 *A*). Zimmer and Annes have proposed that this angular apex be called the *septal point*. This

point permits an evaluation of the anterior midline similar to the anterior cerebral artery. *Thus, anteriorly the septal point and posteriorly the internal cerebral vein become excellent indicators of the midline.* Variations in the appearance of the septal vein in accordance with tube angulation are shown in Figure 8–108 *B*.

The septal vein usually begins to opacify on carotid angiograms 5 seconds after injection but is best seen 8 to 10 seconds after injection and after the superficial cortical veins and basal vein have emptied. A slight caudad angulation of the x-ray tube of about 20 to 25 degrees may help separate the septal vein from other superimposed structures in the frontal projection. Usually, the distance between the septal points demonstrates the normal width of the septum pellucidum (2 to 3 mm.). The *subependymal branches of the septal vein* are good indicators of the position of the margins of the frontal horns.

Septal veins usually lie 38 mm. or less above a theoretical baseline (Fig. 8–108 *C*). The anomalies most frequently associated with greater measurements are absent or false venous angles and a posterior junction of the septal and internal cerebral veins.

Great Cerebral Vein of Galen (Fig. 8–109 *A, B,* and *C*).   The internal cerebral veins flow in the roof of the third ventricle between the two layers of the vellum interpositum and beneath the fornix, uniting beneath the pineal gland to form the great cerebral vein of Galen. This large-calibered short vein is situated between the undersurface of the corpus callosum (splenium) and the section of the quadrigeminal plate extending to the anterior free edge of the tentorium cerebelli It enters the inferior longi-

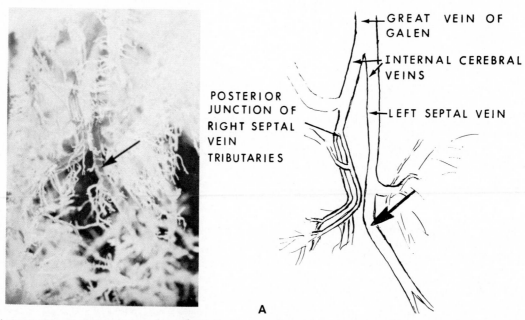

Figure 8–108.   A. Anterior view of a case of injection-corrosion of the venous system. The septal point demarcates the apex of the angle formed by the change in course of the septal vein (arrow). (From Zimmer, A. E., and Annes, G. P.: Radiology, 87:813–823, 1966.)

Figure 8–108 continued on the opposite page.

tudinal sinus during its transition into the straight sinus and receives branches from the superior cerebellar veins, the dorsal callosal vein, precentral cerebellar vein, and internal occipital vein.

Tributaries of the Great Cerebral Vein. The *basilar vein of Rosenthal* drains the blood from the base of the brain. It receives tributaries from the olfactory bulb, insula, hippocampus, cerebral peduncles, and also lenticulostriate branches. Anastomoses are formed with the opposite side of the brain in the interpeduncular fossa. This vein curves around the cerebral peduncle and drains into the great cerebral vein of Galen or directly into the straight sinus.

The *posterior dorsal pericallosal vein* (Fig. 8–107 *A*) is a small vein that runs from the superior surface of the corpus callosum downward around the splenium and into the great cerebral vein.

Other small tributaries also flow into the great cerebral vein from the hippocampal gyrus and from the posterior temporal and occipital cortices. The *superior and precentral cerebellar veins* also drain into the great cerebral vein. (See posterior fossa veins.)

Moving forward in the brain once again, a number of small venous channels on the insula that form the *deep middle cerebral vein* in the Sylvian fissure can be seen. This vein passes medially to the roof of the *chiasmatic cistern*. The deep middle cerebral vein runs medially and posteriorly to reach the optic tract and then laterally over the cerebral peduncles to become the basal vein of Rosenthal (Fig. 8–109 *C*). The basal vein follows the optic tract around the cerebral peduncles and brain stem, traversing the ambient cisterns, and enters the quadrigeminal cistern, where it

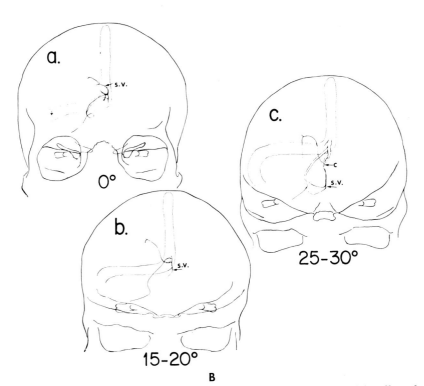

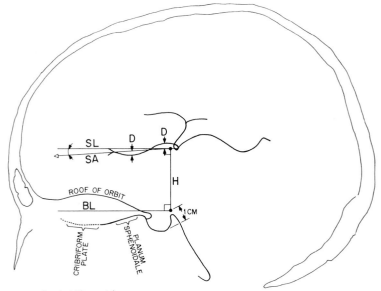

BL = Septal Base Line
H = Height of Axis of Septal Vein
SA = Axis of Septal Vein
SL = Septal Line
D = Deviations of Septal Vein from Septal Axis
∤ = Angle of Septal Axis to Septal Line

Figure 8–108 *Continued.* *B.* Diagrams of the effect of x-ray projection and tube angulation on visualization of the septal vein; 20 to 25 degrees caudal angulation usually suffices to demonstrate it. (SV) septal vein, (C) curve lateral to anterior column of fornix. *C.* *To analyze these septal veins: (1) A line *SA* is drawn through axis of the septal vein. (2) A septal baseline *BL* is constructed passing from the dorsum sellae at a point 1 cm above the floor of the pituitary fossa through or above the tuberculum sellae so that the line lies midway between the roof of orbit and cribriform plate. (3) A second line *H* is erected perpendicularly to intersect the septal axis and measured. (4) The septal line *SL* is then erected at right angles to line *H* as shown. (5) The angle *SL-SA* between the septal line and septal axis is measured. (6) The deviation *D* or excursions of the septal vein above and below the septal axis are measured. The measurements in our cases are based on a straight lateral projection, with the lateral cassette changer next to the patient's shoulders and a target-to-film distance of 52 inches. Seven of 117 angiograms were satisfactory for *H* measurements but unsuited for other measurements because of poor detail or other technical reasons. (From Zimmer, A. E., and Annes, G. P.: Radiology, *87*:813–823, 1966.)

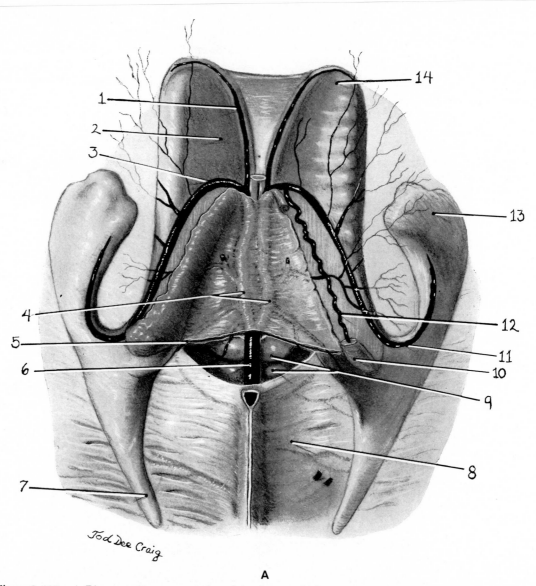

A

Figure 8–109.   A. Diagrammatic representation of the deep cerebral veins.

The two thalamostriate veins are seen to join the septal vein to form the internal cerebral vein on each side. The internal cerebral veins are contained within the velum interpositum and join posteriorly to form the vein of Galen. The chorioid plexus was removed on the right side to show the chorioid vein. The thalamostriate vein is drawn to the temporal horn. This is seen sometimes but is by no means a constant feature. Variation in the configuration of the veins is, of course, the rule.

(1) Septal vein, (2) anterior horn at the junction with the body of the lateral ventricle, (3) thalamostriate vein, (4) internal cerebral veins, (5) the two leaves of the velum interpositum, (6) vein of Galen, (7) occipital horn, (8) tentorium, (9) quadrigeminal tubercles, (10) chorioid plexus, (11) initial segment of the thalamostriate vein or terminal vein, (12) chorioidal vein, (13) temporal horn, (14) frontal horn of the lateral ventricle. See also Part B.

Medial to the thalamostriate vein is the thalamus and anterolaterally is the caudate nucleus.

Figure 8–109 continued on the opposite page.

joins the great cerebral vein of Galen (or sometimes, the internal cerebral prior to its junction with the great cerebral). The basal vein, as noted earlier, may also receive drainage veins from the cerebellum and brain stem. The subependymal veins of each lateral ventricle drain into either the internal cerebral vein or the basal vein of Rosenthal.

The septal veins delineate the frontal horns of the lateral ventricles medially (Fig. 8–109 A) by draining the head of the caudate nucleus forceps minor of the corpus callosum. *Transverse caudate veins* from the caudate nucleus drain into the striothalamic veins.

Veins from the temporal horns communicate with the basal vein of Rosenthal both anteriorly and posteriorly. Veins from the occipital horn drain into either the medial or the lateral atrial vein or the basal vein of Rosenthal.

The *true venous angle,* as noted earlier, identifies the position of the interventricular foramen. Several methods (for instance, that of Probst) have been devised for determining whether this angle is displaced from its normal position (Fig. 8–110) as seen in the lateral projection during angiography. It is not only the exact position that is important but also the configuration. At times a *"false venous angle"* appears, when the striothalamic vein runs a shorter course than usual and joins the internal cerebral vein proximal to the interventricular foramen. The methods of Lin et al. and Laini et. al. are also shown.

Some variations of the relationship of the striothalamic vein,

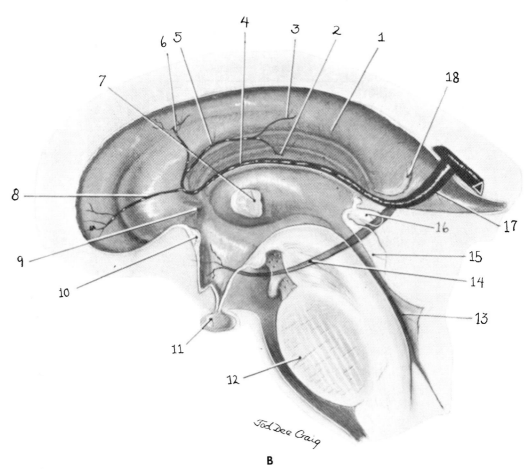

B

Figure 8–109 *Continued.* B. Diagrammatic representation of the deep cerebral veins and their relation with the adjacent brain structures in lateral projection.

(1) Lateral ventricle, (2) terminal branch of thalamostriate vein, (3) posterior caudate veins, (4) internal cerebral vein, (5) thalamostriate vein, (6) anterior caudate vein, (7) massa intermedia, (8) septal vein, (9) foramen of Monro, (10) anterior commissure, (11) hypophysis, (12) pons, (13) fourth ventricle, (14) basilar vein passing schematically behind the midbrain, (15) quadrigeminal plate, (16) pineal, (17) vein of Galen, (18) splenium of corpus callosum. (A and B from Taveras, J. M., and Wood, E. H.: Diagnostic Neuroradiology. Baltimore, The Williams & Wilkins Co., 1964.)

Figure 8–109 continued on the following page.

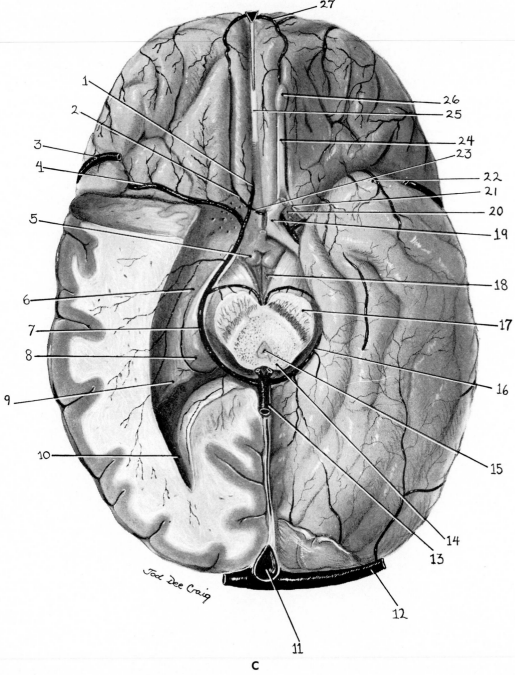

C

Figure 8–109 *Continued.* C. Diagram depicting the basal vein, its origins and relations with the midbrain. The tip of the temporal lobe on the right side has been removed and a horizontal cross section of the temporal and occipital lobes has been done to open the temporal horn, occipital horn, and atrium of the ventricle. (1) Anterior cerebral vein, (2) olfactory vein, (3) superficial middle cerebral vein, (4) deep middle cerebral vein, (5) mammillary body, (6) temporal horn of the lateral ventricle, (7) basilar vein, (8) hippocampus major, (9) collateral eminence, (10) posterior horn of the lateral ventricle, (11) superior sagittal sinus joining (12) transverse sinus, (13) vein of Galen, (14) quadrigeminal plate, (15) aqueduct of Sylvius, (16) basilar vein, (17) cerebral peduncle, (18) posterior perforated substance, (19) optic chiasm, (20) anterior perforated substance, (21) lateral olfactory striae, (22) anterior tip of the temporal lobe, (23) anterior communicating vein, (24) olfactory tract, (25) longitudinal (interhemispheric) fissure, (26) olfactory bulb, (27) superficial cerebral vein. (From Taveras, J. M., and Wood, E. H.: Diagnostic Neuroradiology. Baltimore, The Williams & Wilkins Co., 1964.)

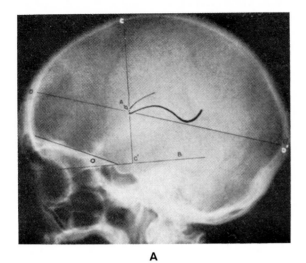

A

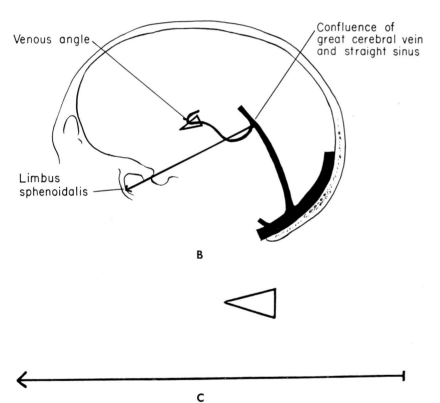

Venous angle

Confluence of
great cerebral vein
and straight sinus

Limbus
sphenoidalis

B

C

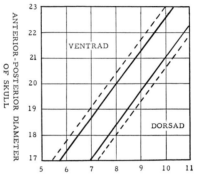

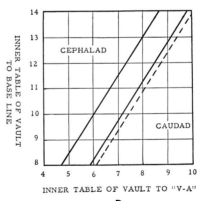

D

Figure 8–110. *A.* Method of orientation of the "venous angle." Base line, *B,* passes through the nasion and tuberculum sellae. Orientation in the cephalocaudad direction: measure *C–A* against *C–C'.* Orientation in the ventrodorsad direction: measure the longest anteroposterior diameter *D–D',* against *D–A.* (From Lin, P., Mokrohisky, J., Stauffer, H., and Scott, M.: J. Neurosurg., *12:*256–277, 1955.) *B.* Template method for demonstrating normal position of the venous angle. In a normal full-sized adult, the venous angle should fall within the triangle if the relations as shown are carried forward, to a straight line drawn as shown from the limbus sphenoidalis to the point of confluence of the great cerebral vein (of Galen) and the straight sinus. *C.* Normal full-sized topogram (adult). Arrow from confluence of great cerebral vein and straight sinus to limbus sphenoidalis. The venous angle is inside the normal topogram. (From Laine, E., et al.: Acta Radiol., *46:*203–213, 1956.) *D.* The diagnostic importance of normal variants in deep cerebral phlebography is shown by an orientation chart for localizing the foramen of Monro or the "venous angle" of the brain. The normal range of variation of the "venous angle" in the ventrodorsad direction is represented by the broken lines; in the cephalocaudad direction the normal range of variation is shown by the anterior solid line and the posterior broken line. (From Mokrohisky, J. F., et al.: Radiology, *67:*34–47, 1956.)

septal vein, and internal cerebral vein in frontal and lateral projections are shown in Figure 8–111 *A* and *B*. *In general, the relationship of the striothalamic vein to the internal cerebral vein as it appears in the frontal view gives a reasonably accurate picture of the oblique sectional pattern of the body of the lateral ventricle.* When the lateral ventricle is dilated, the concave medial relationship of the striothalamic vein is disturbed; it extends outward convexly with an increased circumference that can be readily detected in a venogram (Fig. 8–112).

Medullary Veins of the Cerebral Hemisphere (Huang and Wolf) (Fig. 8–113). The medullary veins are those lying within the white matter of the cerebral hemispheres. They consist essentially of two groups:

1. *Short venous channels* that begin in the white matter about 1 or 2 cm. below the gray cortex and run directly through the cortex to join the pial veins on the surface of the cortex.

2. Relatively *long venous channels* originating in approximately the same region of the white matter, 1 or 2 cm. below the gray cortex, but converging toward the lateral ventricle. They first drain into subependymal veins and thereafter into the internal cerebral or the basal vein of Rosenthal (Fig. 8–113 *A, B, C*).

The deep medullary veins tend to concentrate above the head and body of the caudate nucleus and are sometimes called "longitudinal caudate veins." The deep medullary veins elsewhere run downward and medially toward the superior and lateral corner of the frontal horn and body of the lateral ventricle, ultimately draining into the striothalamic vein and the subependymal veins. Under normal conditions, medullary veins rarely can be clearly identified on carotid angiograms (Huang and Wolf). Faint visualization, however, may be obtained (Fig. 8–113 *D* to *I*).

Choroid Plexus and the Choroid Vein of the Lateral Ventricle (Takahashi and Okudera) (Fig. 8–114). The choroid plexus of the lateral ventricle consists of small vessels containing arterioles, capillaries, and venules. It extends posteriorly along the floor of the lateral ventricle to the atrium, where it enlarges and forms the *glomus*. Thereafter it courses anteriorly and inferiorly along the roof of the temporal horn.

The anterior and posterior choroid arteries (lateral and medial branches of the latter) have been previously described.

The choroid plexus of the lateral ventricle is drained by the *superior choroid vein* and *choroid branches of the veins of the posterior and inferior horns*. The superior choroid vein is located in the floor of the trigone and body of the lateral ventricle, embedded in the choroid plexus (Fig. 8–111). It usually drains into the thalamostriate vein, although occasionally it drains into the internal cerebral near the foramen of Monro. There may be other small veins draining directly into the posterior horn or into the medial atrial vein. Angiographically, these veins occasionally may be seen following the capillary phase; they are contiguous with the internal cerebral vein at the foramen of Monro.

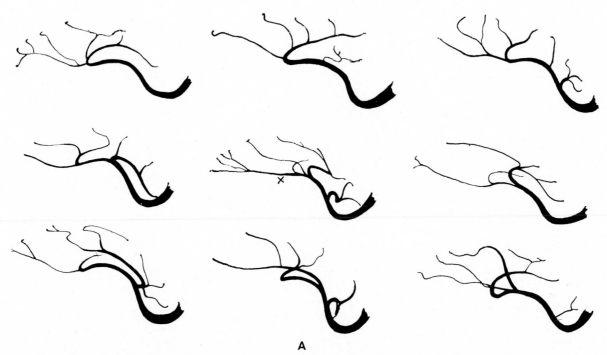

A

Figure 8–111. A. The most common variations of the tributaries to the internal cerebral vein. Cross in center drawing indicates foramen of Monro.

Figure 8–111 continued on the opposite page.

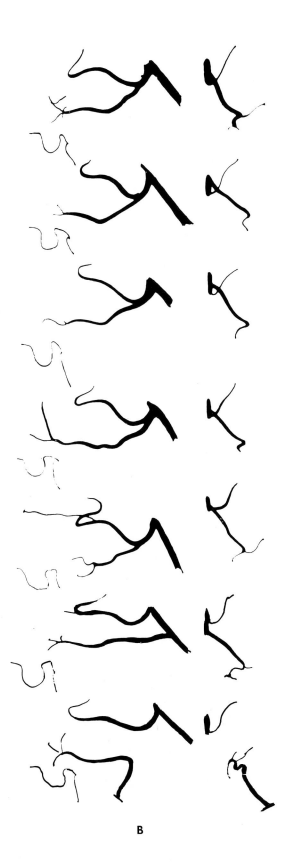

B

Subependymal Veins of the Lateral Ventricles (Wolf and Huang) (Figs. 8–113 and 8–115).   The ability to determine the position of the ventricular walls during angiography, especially the walls of the lateral ventricles, depends to a great extent on the recognition of the subependymal veins. The striothalamic vein is situated in the striothalamic sulcus in the anterior portion of the body of the lateral ventricle, joining the internal cerebral vein as previously indicated. The vein of the septum pellucidum joins the striothalamic at the venous angle along the posterior superior margin of the foramen of Monro. The superior choroidal vein also joins the venous angle at this site. There are tributaries of the striothalamic vein such as the posterior terminal vein and a vein from the surface of the head of the caudate nucleus, called by some the "anterior terminal vein." Wolf has called the vein along the stria terminalis the "posterior terminal vein," and the anterior tributary the "anterior caudate vein." There are numerous other tributaries. The veins in the roof and medial wall of the lateral ventricle form an entirely separate group unrelated to the stria terminalis (Fig. 8–116).

The subependymal veins of the lateral ventricles are classified into two main groups, a *medial* group and a *lateral* group (Fig. 8–115 *A* to *D*). These groups in turn can be subdivided into those related to the frontal horn, body, and atrium, and the inferior horn of the lateral ventricle. The vessels in each of these areas are sufficiently characteristic for probable identification. The reader is referred to the original careful descriptions by Wolf and Huang, 1964 (Fig. 8–115).

Special Comment: Deep Middle Cerebral Venous Drainage in Relation to the Insula.   A simplified representation of the appearance of the veins draining into the Sylvian vallecula is shown in Figures 8–116 and 8–117 (Wolf and Huang). Generally, four insula veins are shown. These converge in a common trunk, which in turn empties into the basal vein of Rosenthal. The inferior striate veins join this major trunk at the anterior perforated space lateral to the optic chiasm and optic tract. The cisterns of the Sylvian fossa, Sylvian vallecula, peduncular fossa, and pons are shown by dotted lines. The superficial Sylvian vein extends into the sphenoparietal and paracavernous sinuses.

In the anteroposterior projection, the classic drainage of the insular veins, inferior striate veins, orbital vein, and anterior cerebral vein into the basal vein of Rosenthal is shown. The peduncular vein is also shown, joining the basal vein at the most medial point. On the left side a common vertical trunk is shown with the

Figure 8–111 *Continued*.   B. Variations of the basilar vein. Lateral and half-axial projections. Bottom drawings show anomalous drainage to straight or superior petrosal sinuses. (A and B from Greitz, T., and Lindgren, E.: Cerebral vascular anatomy. *In* Abrams, H. A.: Angiography, 2nd ed. Boston, Little, Brown & Company, 1971.)

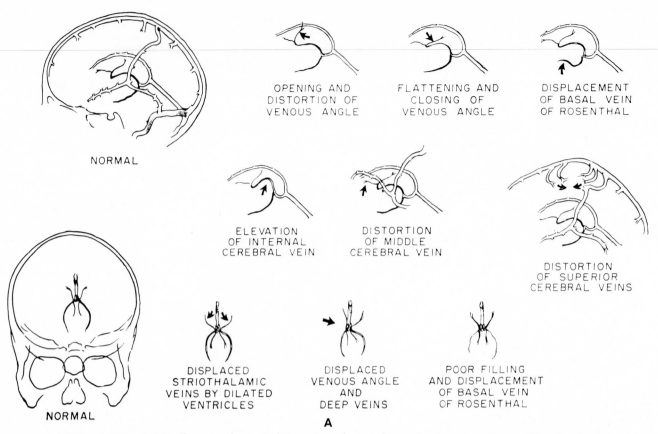

NORMAL

OPENING AND
DISTORTION OF
VENOUS ANGLE

FLATTENING AND
CLOSING OF
VENOUS ANGLE

DISPLACEMENT
OF BASAL VEIN
OF ROSENTHAL

ELEVATION
OF INTERNAL
CEREBRAL VEIN

DISTORTION
OF MIDDLE
CEREBRAL VEIN

DISTORTION
OF SUPERIOR
CEREBRAL VEINS

NORMAL

DISPLACED
STRIOTHALAMIC
VEINS BY DILATED
VENTRICLES

DISPLACED
VENOUS ANGLE
AND
DEEP VEINS

POOR FILLING
AND DISPLACEMENT
OF BASAL VEIN
OF ROSENTHAL

A

Figure 8–112. *A.* Line diagrams demonstrating various deep and superficial venous abnormalities in lateral and frontal perspectives.

Figure 8–112 continued on the opposite page.

uncal vein that drains into the sphenoparietal and paracavernous sinuses. The superficial Sylvian vein is directly continuous with the sphenoparietal sinus.

For a more detailed description see Wolf and Huang, 1963.

VEINS OF THE CEREBELLUM AND BRAIN STEM
(Fig. 8–117 *A, B*)

The veins of the posterior fossa have been conveniently divided into a *superior group,* which drains into the internal cerebral veins or the straight sinus; an *anterior group,* which drains into the superior or inferior petrosal sinuses; and a *posterior group,* which drains into the lateral or straight sinuses.

Superior Group of Veins. The superior group consists of a precentral cerebellar vein, superior vermian veins, and posterior and lateral mesencephalic veins. These may unite to form a single large vessel before entering the great cerebral vein, in which case it is called the *superior cerebellar vein.*

The precentral cerebellar vein flows in the subarachnoid space from the anterior medullary velum and the superior cerebellar

peduncles upward between the superior vermis of the cerebellum and the tectum of the midbrain, across the quadrigeminal cistern into the great cerebral vein. It describes an S-shaped curve in the sagittal plane but is almost straight otherwise.

The *superior vermian vein* originates in the superior cerebellar vermis, passes upward and forward in the quadrigeminal cistern, and joins the great cerebral vein anterior to the precentral cerebellar vein.

The *lateral mesencephalic vein* may also be named the lateral anastomotic mesencephalic vein since it forms an anastomosis between the superior anterior groups.

The *posterior mesencephalic vein* is a major channel that arises on the lateral aspect of the cerebral peduncle and passes around the midbrain to join the great cerebral vein or a tributary such as the basal vein. It is usually closely associated with the basal vein of Rosenthal. This vein receives an *anterior pontomesencephalic vein,* originating anterior to the pons, and a *lateral mesencephalic vein,* which originates on the lateral mesencephalic sulcus and may join either the posterior mesencephalic vein or the basal vein.

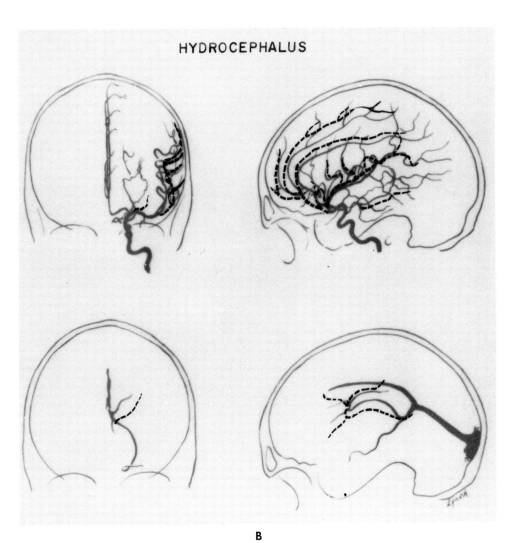

HYDROCEPHALUS

B

Figure 8–112 *Continued.* *B.* Superimposed composite line diagrams showing the arterial and venous changes that may occur in association with hydrocephalus. The anterior cerebral artery demonstrates the sweep sign (dotted lines), and in frontal view, the middle cerebral artery is displaced outward. In frontal view of the venogram phase, the striothalamic vein is displaced outward and is converted from its normal convex appearance medially to a concave tendency medially. (*A* and *B* from Meschan, I.: Roentgen signs of abnormality in cerebral angiograms. *In* Toole, J. F. (ed.): Special Techniques for Neurological Diagnosis. Philadelphia, F. A. Davis Co., 1969.)

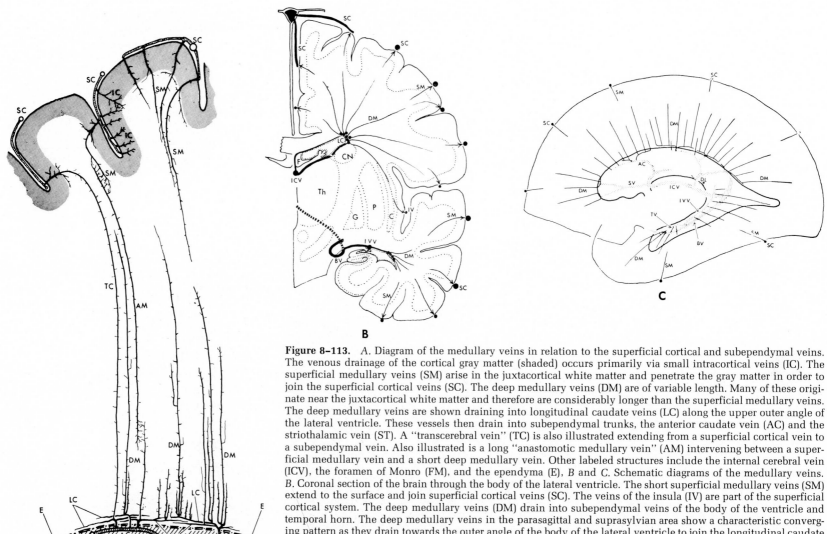

Figure 8–113. *A.* Diagram of the medullary veins in relation to the superficial cortical and subependymal veins. The venous drainage of the cortical gray matter (shaded) occurs primarily via small intracortical veins (IC). The superficial medullary veins (SM) arise in the juxtacortical white matter and penetrate the gray matter in order to join the superficial cortical veins (SC). The deep medullary veins (DM) are of variable length. Many of these originate near the juxtacortical white matter and therefore are considerably longer than the superficial medullary veins. The deep medullary veins are shown draining into longitudinal caudate veins (LC) along the upper outer angle of the lateral ventricle. These vessels then drain into subependymal trunks, the anterior caudate vein (AC) and the striothalamic vein (ST). A "transcerebral vein" (TC) is also illustrated extending from a superficial cortical vein to a subependymal vein. Also illustrated is a long "anastomotic medullary vein" (AM) intervening between a superficial medullary vein and a short deep medullary vein. Other labeled structures include the internal cerebral vein (ICV), the foramen of Monro (FM), and the ependyma (E), *B* and *C.* Schematic diagrams of the medullary veins. *B.* Coronal section of the brain through the body of the lateral ventricle. The short superficial medullary veins (SM) extend to the surface and join superficial cortical veins (SC). The veins of the insula (IV) are part of the superficial cortical system. The deep medullary veins (DM) drain into subependymal veins of the body of the ventricle and temporal horn. The deep medullary veins in the parasagittal and suprasylvian area show a characteristic converging pattern as they drain towards the outer angle of the body of the lateral ventricle to join the longitudinal caudate veins (LC). The deep medullary veins of the temporal lobe are smaller and converge to subependymal veins in the roof of the temporal horn and, via these vessels, into the inferior ventricular vein (IVV). This latter vein joins the basal vein (BV). Other labeled structures include the fornix (F), the internal cerebral vein (ICV), the thalamus (Th), the caudate nucleus (CN), the globus pallidus (G), the putamen (P), and the claustrum (C).

C. Lateral view. The deep medullary veins (DM) run toward the superior lateral corner of the lateral ventricle and drain into the septal vein (SV), the anterior caudate vein (AC), the direct lateral vein (DL), the tip veins of the temporal horn (TV) and the inferior ventricular vein (IVV). The line of junction between the deep medullary veins and the subependymal venous trunks serves as a landmark to indicate the border of the lateral ventricle. Other structures shown are the internal cerebral vein (ICV), the basal vein of Rosenthal (BV), superficial medullary (SM) and superficial cortical (SC) veins. (From Huang, Y. P., and Wolf, B. S.: Amer. J. Roentgenol., 92:739, 1964.)

Figure 8–113 continued on the opposite page.

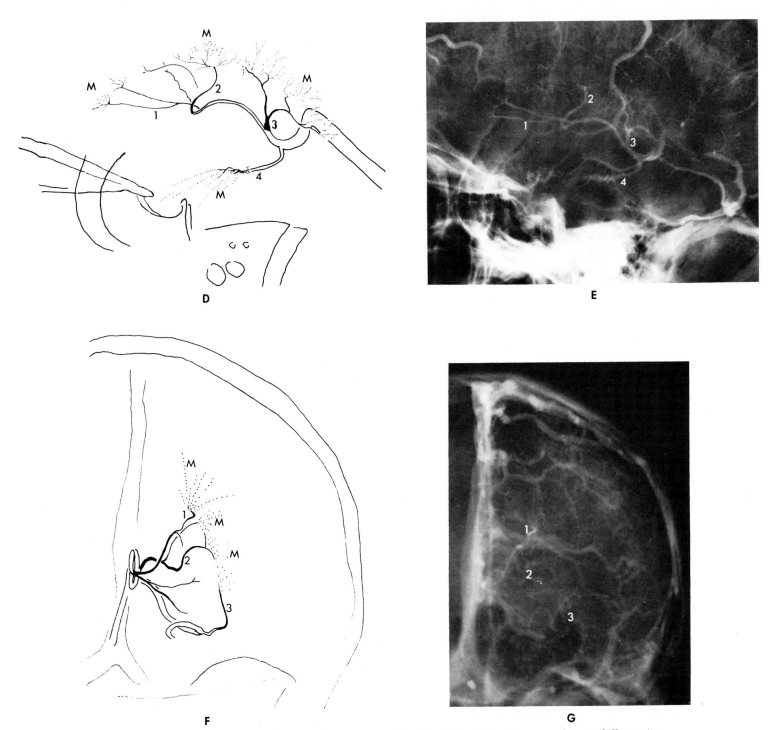

D

E

F

G

Figure 8–113 *Continued.* *D* and *E.* Normal appearance. *D.* Tracing of lateral view. Numerous deep medullary veins (M) enter the vein of the septum pellucidum (1), the striothalamic stem (2), and an atrial subependymal vein (3). In addition, small anterior temporal deep medullary veins (M) enter the basal vein (4) via small temporal tip subependymal veins. *E.* Corresponding roentgenogram. *F* and *G.* Normal appearance. *F.* Tracing of anteroposterior view. A large number of veins—superficial, cortical, subependymal, galenic and intracerebral—overlap one another in this projection. The smallest of these vessels can be identified as deep medullary veins (M) by their convergence and drainage into subependymal venous channels. Deep medullary veins join longitudinal caudate (1) and striothalamic veins, the direct lateral (2) and the inferior ventricular (3) subependymal veins. *G.* Corresponding roentgenogram. (*D−G* from Huang, Y. P., and Wolf, B. S.: Amer. J. Roentgenol., *92:*739, 1964.)

Figure 8–113 continued on the following page.

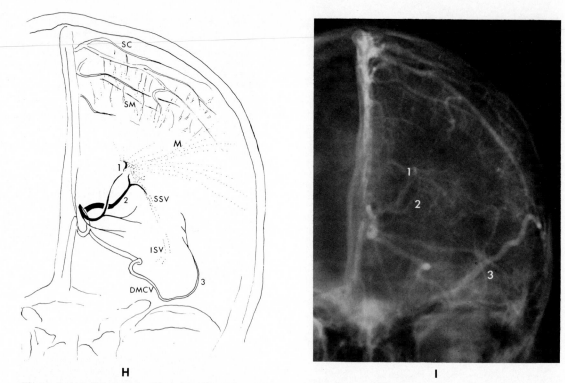

H   **I**

Figure 8–113 *Continued. H* and *I.* Normal appearance. *H.* Tracing of anteroposterior view. A spray of deep medullary veins (M) traverses almost the entire thickness of the cerebral hemisphere to enter longitudinal caudate (1), striothalamic and direct lateral (2) subependymal veins. Superior striate veins (SSV) run upward to join longitudinal caudate veins. Portions of inferior striate veins (ISV) are also indicated. A large insular vein (3) continues directly into the deep middle cerebral vein (DMCV). Many short fine superficial medullary veins (SM) enter superficial cortical veins (SC) at a right angle. The boundary between superficial medullary and superficial cortical veins is rarely clear roentgenographically. *I.* Corresponding roentgenogram. (From Huang, Y. P., and Wolf, B. S.: Amer. J. Roentgenol., *92:*739, 1964.)

The posterior mesencephalic vein also receives the precentral cerebellar vein which, as previously indicated, originates on the central lobulus of the vermis.

Each *brachial vein* draining the superior and middle cerebellar peduncles runs medially and superiorly to join the precentral cerebellar vein, or laterally and inferiorly to drain into the petrosal vein.

The *marginal vein* is somewhat similar in that it connects the superior vermian vein with either the lateral mesencephalic vein or the petrosal vein.

Roentgen Significance of the Pontomesencephalic Veins (Gabrielsen and Amundsen). Anatomically there is usually a plexus of longitudinal veins on the side of the pons a few millimeters from the midline and parallel to the basilar artery. This venous plexus anterior to the pons is continuous with a plexus in the interpeduncular fossa and is anterior to the medulla oblongata and spinal cord. The *pontomesencephalic veins* in most cases drain primarily into (a) the *superior petrosal sinuses* through the petrosal veins, and (b) the *peduncular veins* that pass

laterally around the upper margin of the cerebral peduncles and empty into the basal veins of Rosenthal or the posterior mesencephalic veins. Some venous drainage into the inferior petrosal sinuses also occurs, and some bridging veins drain into the basilar venous plexus along the clivus. Sometimes the pontomesencephalic veins empty into the *uncal vein,* which usually drains into the cavernous sinus or the lateral anastomotic mesencephalic vein. Subtraction is usually necessary for the best evaluation of the pontomesencephalic veins in the half-axial anteroposterior projection. These veins, however, are well demonstrated in lateral projection without subtraction.

The site of the anterior border of the brain stem relative to the clivus can be estimated by locating the posterior margins of the pontomesencephalic veins in lateral projections. These, in turn, may be compared with their appearance on pneumoencephalograms for greatest accuracy. In the lateral projection, the pontomesencephalic veins have the appearance of a single longitudinal vein outlining the anterior border of the brain stem, despite the anatomic findings of a plexus of veins in this location.

The pontomesencephalic veins can usually be studied best during the venous phase of vertebral angiograms. *These veins mark the location of the anterior border of the pons and the roof of the interpeduncular fossa.* Actually, the distance between the pontomesencephalic veins and the colliculocentral point of the precentral cerebellar vein should enable the radiologist to make a fairly accurate estimate of the anteroposterior diameter of the pons.

Anterior Group of Veins. These include the petrosal (anterior) cerebellar vein, the anterior pontomesencephalic vein, the transverse pontine veins, and several superior and inferior hemispheric veins.

As previously noted, the brachial vein and the lateral anastomotic mesencephalic vein may drain into either the anterior or the superior group of veins.

The *petrosal veins* are rather large, and are usually identified as they pass anteriorly and laterally to join the superior petrosal sinus, usually in its medial third. The *petrosal vein is an indicator of structures in the immediate vicinity of the internal acoustic meatus.*

The *petrosal (or great anterior inferior cerebellar) vein* is formed in the cerebellopontine angle and receives tributaries from the anterior part of the cerebellar hemisphere as well as from the anterolateral aspect of the pons and medulla. The petrosal vein anastomoses with veins on the lower surface of the cerebellar hemisphere.

The *anterior pontomesencephalic vein* or plexus of veins originates near the optic chiasm and interpeduncular fossa and passes posteriorly between the cerebral peduncles. It loops anteriorly on the superior edge of the pons and follows the ventral surface of

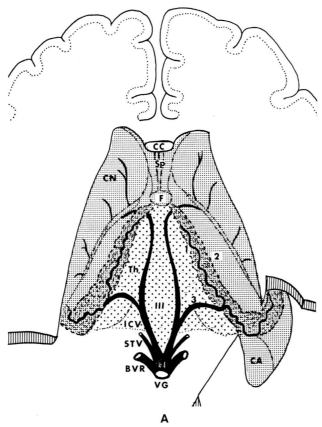

A

Figure 8–114. A. Diagram of the choroid plexus of the lateral ventricle exposed from above. The choroid plexus is attached to the tela choroidea projecting between the crus fornicis (removed) and the thalamus. The choroid vein is tortuous and courses through the choroid plexus in the floor of the lateral ventricle. A large connecting vein arises from the choroid plexus and enters the choroid fissure. This vein usually enters the distal portion of the internal cerebral vein.

(1) Superior choroid vein; (2) choroid plexus; (3) connecting vein; (III) third ventricle; (Th) thalamus; (ICV) internal cerebral vein; (STV) superior thalamic vein; (BVR) basal vein of Rosenthal; (VG) vein of Galen; (F) fornix; (SP) septum pellucidum; (CC) corpus callosum; (CN) caudate nucleus; (CA) calcar avis. (From Takahashi, M., and Okudera, T.: Radiology, *103*:113–120, 1972.)

Figure 8–114 continued on the following page.

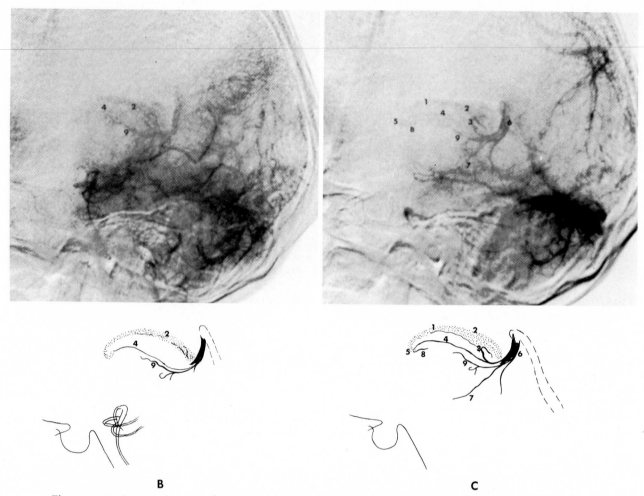

B   **C**

Figure 8–114 *Continued.* Normal supratentorial venous system by vertebral artery injection. *B.* Capillary phase in lateral projection. *C.* Venous phase in lateral projection. (From Takahashi, M., and Okudera, T.: Radiology, *103*:113–120, 1972.)

Figure 8–114 continued on the opposite page.

the pons closely. It may drain into the petrosal vein or into the inferior petrosal sinus. It may, on occasion, drain into the lateral anastomotic mesencephalic vein.

Transverse pontine veins sweep across the ventral pontine surface and middle cerebellar peduncles, joining the anterior pontomesencephalic vein to the petrosal vein. The anterior pontomesencephalic veins are continuous with veins on the ventral aspect of the medulla.

The *inferior vermian veins* arise near the cerebellar tonsils and pass superiorly near the midline on either side of the inferior vermis, emptying into the sinus confluens or closely adjacent parts.

The venous anatomy of the posterior fossa has become increasingly important in view of the relation of these structures to mass lesions. Of special interest in this connection are *the precentral cerebellar vein, the superior vermian vein, the posterior mesen-*

cephalic veins, and the anterior pontomesencephalic veins. The precentral cerebral vein and the anterior pontomesencephalic vein are midline structures. The petrosal vein, as indicated previously, is a guide to the structures near or adjoining the internal acoustic meatus. The petrosal vein usually lies on the superior posterior edge of the medial third of the petrous ridge.

Posterior Group of Veins. The *posterior, superior, and inferior veins* draining the cerebellar hemisphere join to form a large vein on the posterior aspect of the cerebellar hemisphere called the *posterior cerebellar vein.* This runs medially, parallel to, and slightly above the transverse sinus toward the sinus confluens. The veins that belong to this posterior system include the *superior and inferior hemispheric veins,* the *inferior veins of the vermis,* and the *medial superior cerebellar veins* from the posterior part of the vermis adjacent to the tentorium.

Summarizing these venous groups we can say that the three

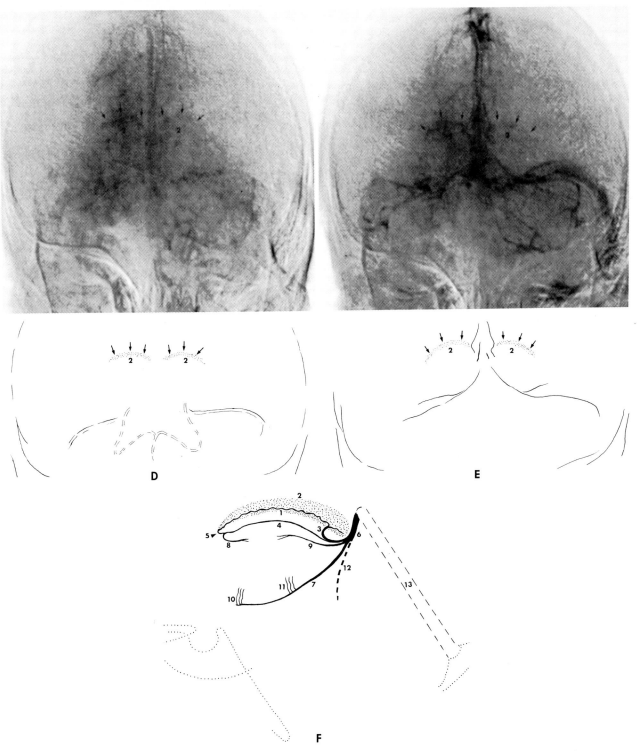

Figure 8–114 *Continued.* *D.* Capillary phase in Towne projection. *E.* Venous phase in Towne projection. The numbers indicate the following veins: (1) superior choroid vein, (2) choroid plexus, (3) connecting vein, (4) internal cerebral vein, (5) venous angle, (6) great vein of Galen, (7) basal vein of Rosenthal or posterior mesencephalic vein, (8) anterior thalamic vein, (9) superior thalamic vein. *F.* Schematic illustration of the supratentorial venous system by vertebral artery injection. The numbers indicate the following veins and their percentage visualization: (1) superior choroid vein (97%), (2) choroid plexus (lateral 84%, Towne 29%), (3) connecting vein (63%), (4) internal cerebral vein (97%), (5) venous angle, (6) great vein of Galen (100%), (7) basal vein of Rosenthal or posterior mesencephalic vein (67%), (8) anterior thalamic vein (78%), (9) superior thalamic vein (95%), (10) inferior thalamic vein (13%), (11) posterior thalamic vein (19%), (12) precentral cerebral vein, (13) straight sinus. (*D–F* from Takahashi, M., and Okudera, T.: *Radiology, 103:*113–120, 1972.)

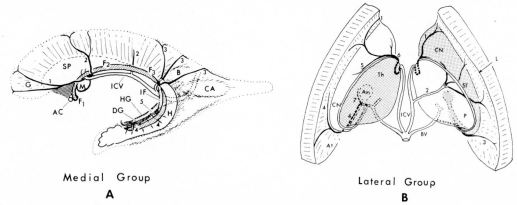

Medial Group

A

Lateral Group

B

Figure 8–115. *A* and *B.* Diagrammatic representation of the two groups of subependymal veins of the lateral ventricles. The intraventricular portions of these veins are drawn in solid fashion and the extraventricular portions, unshaded.

A. Medial group. The vein of the septum pellucidum (1), two posterior septal, callosal, or direct medial veins (2, 2), the medial atrial vein composed of three main tributaries (3, 3, 3), and small veins of the hippocampus (4) are illustrated. The larger and more anterior of the two septal veins runs downward lateral to the column of the fornix to join the internal cerebral vein behind the foramen of Monro. The smaller posterior septal vein runs downward between the two halves of the body of the fornix to join the internal cerebral vein. The most posterior of the tributaries of the medial atrial vein arises in the medial wall and roof of the posterior horn. The tributaries of the medial atrial vein leave the ventricle, *i.e.,* the subependymal region, to enter the subarachnoid space, along the medial attached border of the fornix. A common stem is formed outside the ventricle. The multiple small transverse veins of the hippocampus leave by passing through the medial attached border of the fimbria of the fornix and join a longitudinal collecting vein (5) adjacent to the dentate gyrus. This vein is shown joining the posterior end of the internal cerebral vein or the vein of Galen. Labeled structures include the genu of the corpus callosum (G), the septum pellucidum (SP), the anterior commissure (AC), the interventricular foramen (M), the four portions of the fornix (shaded)—column (F_1), body (F_2), posterior pillar (F_3), and fimbria (F_4), the internal cerebral vein (ICV), the bulb in the atrium and posterior horn (B), the calcar avis (CA), the hippocampus (H), the dentate gyrus (DG), the hippocampal gyrus (HG), and the inferior fasciculus of the forceps major (IF). The inferior fasciculus includes those fibers of the forceps major extending from the lower inferior portion of the splenium to the lingual gyrus. The hatched triangular area below the stem of the vein of the septum pellucidum lies between the lamina rostralis of the genu and the column of the fornix. It is composed of the so-called peduncles of the corpus callosum and septum pellucidum and the septum per se is attached along its upper margin.

B. Lateral group. The medial wall and the roof of all portions of the lateral ventricles have been removed. The structures remaining are shown as viewed from behind and above. The caudate and amygdaloid nuclei are shaded on the right; the thalamus is shaded on the left. On the right side, three veins of the lateral group are shown —an anterior caudate vein (1), the direct lateral vein (2), and the lateral atrial vein (3). On the left side, the anterior caudate vein (1) runs above the head of the caudate nucleus and joins the posterior terminal vein (5) to form the striothalamic stem (6). On this side, a large inferior ventricular vein (4, 4) is shown arising along the upper or lateral border of the tail of the caudate nucleus and extending into the temporal horn. This vein receives small twigs from the tip of the temporal horn (7) as it turns medially to enter the basal vein. Note that all the veins of the lateral group run deep to the stria terminalis. Labeled structures include the caudate nucleus (CN), the stria terminalis (ST), the pulvinar of the thalamus (P), the thalamus (Th), the amygdaloid nucleus (Am), the lateral wall of the atrium (At), the basal vein (BV), the internal cerebral vein (ICV), and the superior lateral corner of the body of the ventricle (L). (From Wolf, B. S., and Huang, Y. P.: Amer. J. Roentgenol., **91:**406–426, 1964.)

Figure 8–115 continued on the opposite page.

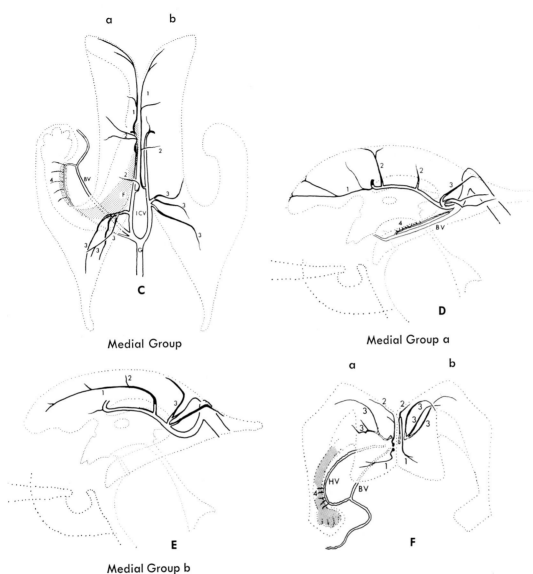

Medial Group

Medial Group a

Medial Group b

Figure 8–115 *Continued.* *C* to *F*. Idealized appearance of the medial group of subependymal veins as they might be seen on an angiogram. The intraventricular portions are drawn in solid fashion and the extraventricular unshaded.

C. Base view. Two different arrangements are illustrated (*a* and *b*). In *a*, the fornix (F) is shaded. On this side, the typical appearances of the vein of the septum pellucidum (1), posterior septal or callosal veins (2,2), medial atrial tributaries from the roof and medial wall of the atrium and posterior horn (3,3,3), and veins of the hippocampus (4) are shown. The veins of the hippocampus join the extraventricular longitudinal hippocampal vein along the dentate gyrus. The usual course of the basal vein (BV) is also indicated. In *b*, a long anomalous vein of the septum pellucidum (1) is illustrated entering the posterior portion of the internal cerebral vein. A small posterior septal vein (2) joins the main septal vessel. On this side, the tributaries (3,3,3) making up the medial atrial vein are shown as draining a larger area, including a portion of the body of the ventricle. The internal cerebral vein (ICV) and the vein of Galen (G) are also labeled.

D. Lateral view of arrangement *a* of the medial group of subependymal veins.

The same vessels shown in the base view are illustrated in this projection. The small transverse hippocampal veins (4) are seen almost on end. The longitudinal hippocampal vein is shown as joining the basal vein (BV) both anteriorly and posteriorly.

E. Lateral view of arrangement *b*. The anomalous vein of the septum pellucidum (1) has a striking appearance in this projection. The anterior tributary of the medial atrial vein (3) arises in the roof of the posterior portion of the body of the ventricle.

F. Anteroposterior view of the two sides. In *a*, the hippocampus is shaded and the longitudinal hippocampal vein (HV) and basal vein (BV) are indicated. The internal cerebral vein and the vein of Galen (not drawn) ordinarily obscure the central portions of the veins of the septum pellucidum (1,1) and posterior septal veins (2,2). The medial atrial venous tributaries (3) shown in *a*, begin more posteriorly than those shown in *b*, and therefore differ somewhat in appearance. (From Wolf, B. S., and Huang, Y. P.: Amer. J. Roentgenol., 91:406–426, 1964.)

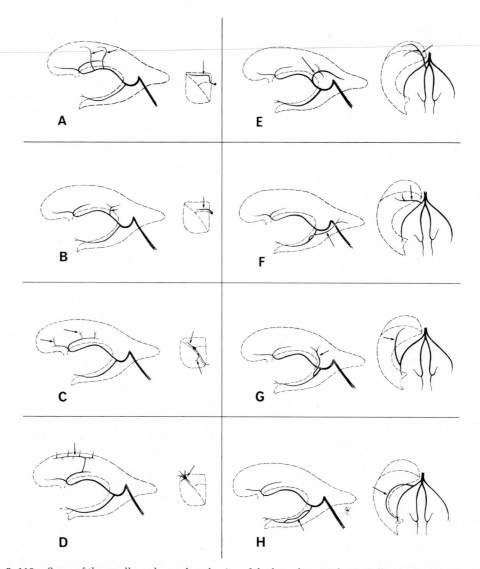

Figure 8–116. Some of the smaller subependymal veins of the lateral ventricle. *A.* Callosal veins. *B.* Direct lateral vein. *C.* Anterior and transverse caudate veins. *D.* Longitudinal caudate vein. *E.* Medial atrial vein. *F.* Lateral atrial vein. *G.* Inferior ventricular vein. *H.* Vein of temporal horn. (From Wilson, M.: The Anatomic Foundation of Neuroradiology of the Brain, 2nd ed. Boston, Little, Brown & Company, 1972.)

major venous drainage systems in the posterior fossa are: (1) the *superior cerebellar vein,* (2) the *posterior cerebellar vein,* and (3) the *great anterior cerebellar vein or petrosal vein.*

The *superior cerebellar vein* flows into the great cerebral vein of Galen or the straight sinus. It drains the superior and anterior surface of the cerebellum via the superior vermian vein and the precentral cerebellar vein, as well as the brain stem via the posterior mesencephalic vein and the anterior pontomesencephalic vein.

The *posterior cerebellar vein* drains two major venous groups: (1) a superior group that drains the superior posterior surface of

the cerebellum, and (2) an inferior group that drains the inferior posterior surface of the cerebellum. Some of the posterior cerebellar veins form a single channel on the posterior aspect of the cerebellar hemisphere, running medially parallel to and slightly cephalad to the lateral sinus toward the sinus confluens. Other posterior cerebellar veins may drain directly into the lateral sinus or the sinus confluens. The major tributaries of the inferior group of posterior cerebellar veins are: (a) the lateral inferior cerebellar vein, and (b) the medial inferior cerebellar vein.

The *great anterior cerebellar vein or petrosal vein* lies in the cerebellopontine angle below the fifth nerve and drains into the superior petrosal sinus just above the internal auditory meatus. There are usually three or four major tributaries of this vein; the most constant is the anastomotic channel between the petrosal vein and the basilar vein of Rosenthal, which runs in the lateral mesencephalic sulcus of the pons within the ambient cistern. This vein is called the *lateral mesencephalic vein.* The second largest tributary is the vein running from the pontomedullary venous plexus. The third tributary drains the anterior inferior cerebellar hemisphere.

The petrosal vein is not well visualized when the posterior inferior cerebellar artery is itself not opacified, since it is this area that is drained largely by the petrosal vein. Branches of the anterior inferior cerebellar artery and superior cerebellar artery also contribute to the regions of the brain drained by the petrosal vein, but to a lesser extent. The half-axial projection is the best view for demonstration of the petrosal vein (Fig. 8–117).

Special Comment. *The Significance of the Petrosal Vein.* The petrosal vein is one of the three major venous drainage systems of the posterior fossa, as indicated above. It runs within the cerebellopontine angle, draining the anterior aspect of the cerebellum and the venous plexus of the pons (Takahashi et al.). It is thought to have an important diagnostic significance in the evaluation of mass lesions in the region of the cerebellopontine angle.

ANGIOGRAPHIC DIAGNOSIS OF POSTERIOR FOSSA MASS LESIONS (Davis and Roberson, George) (Fig. 8–119 *E*)

It is not our purpose in this text to emphasize abnormalities, but it is important to illustrate, when possible, those aspects of normal radiographic anatomy that have an important part in the diagnosis of morphologic abnormality. Thus, avascular mass lesions in the posterior fossa in angiographic diagnosis are arbitrarily divided into two kinds: (1) anterior, and (2) posterior. Accurate identification of the compartment in which a mass arises helps in predicting the type of lesion which may be encountered.

The anterior compartment consists of an intra-axial component—namely, the brain stem, and an extra-axial component consisting of a prestem subarachnoid cistern and a precerebellar subarachnoid cistern. The anterior compartment can be established on the lateral view by drawing an imaginary line between the precentral cerebellar vein and the choroidal portion of the posterior inferior cerebellar artery (Fig. 8–88).

The posterior compartment consists of an intra-axial component, the cerebellum, and an extra-axial component consisting of the posterior and lateral subarachnoid spaces and the prevermis regions, both superiorly and inferiorly, including the fourth ventricle.

The precentral cerebellar vein is a most important landmark in this system. It can be related accurately to the position of the fourth ventricle by utilizing Twining's line. It will be recalled that Twining's line is drawn between the tuberculum sellae and the torcular Herophili. If a second line is drawn tangentially to the knee of the precentral vein and perpendicular to Twining's line, this line should meet Twining's line at its midpoint plus or minus 5 per cent of its length. Posterior displacement of the precentral cerebellar vein, therefore, indicates a mass in the anterior compartment, whereas anterior displacement indicates a mass in the posterior compartment. However, if the mass is very low, one must depend on the choroidal loop of the posterior inferior cerebellar artery and its identification just anterior and inferior to the inferior vermis. Unfortunately, its location is more variable. Again, anterior displacement of this choroidal loop indicates a posterior compartmental mass, whereas posterior displacement indicates an anterior one.

The further division of an anterior compartmental mass into extra- and intra-axial components is made as follows. Although the basilar artery is highly variable, as indicated in previous illustrations, marked posterior displacement from the clivus is a good indicator of a mass in the extra-axial portion of the anterior compartment. However, the pontomesencephalic vein or prepontine veins run at or near the midline of the pons about 6 mm. from the clivus. The pontomesencephalic vein is very closely applied to the brain stem, as shown in Figure 8–117, and is actually a better indicator of the position of the anterior surface of the pons than is the basilar artery. Its position relative to the clivus is also an accurate indicator of the cisterns in this immediate vicinity. Posterior displacement, therefore, of the pontomesencephalic vein has the same significance as posterior displacement of the basilar artery: it indicates an anterior extra-axial mass. Anterior displacement means a mass in either the brain stem or the cerebellum.

In summary, therefore, the precentral cerebellar vein and the pontomesencephalic vein, as well as the choroidal branch of the posterior inferior cerebellar artery, are extremely important indicators.

Having established from the lateral view the posterior fossa compartment in which a mass is present, one then turns to the anteroposterior view to determine, if possible, the side on which the mass is located. The most important indicator for this purpose is the vermis branch of each posterior inferior cerebellar artery (PICA). The vermis branch of the PICA arises in the vallecula just behind the fourth ventricle, and courses around the vermis to anastomose eventually with the vermis branch of the superior cerebellar artery. This vessel is normally at or within about 2 millimeters of the midline and normally courses ipsilaterally, never contralaterally, to the side of its origin. Lateral or cerebellar hemisphere mass lesions displace it contralaterally. If a lesion, however, is situated in the inferior portion of the cerebellar hemisphere, it may not affect the vermian branches of PICA but only the distal PICA in the region of the choroidal loop,

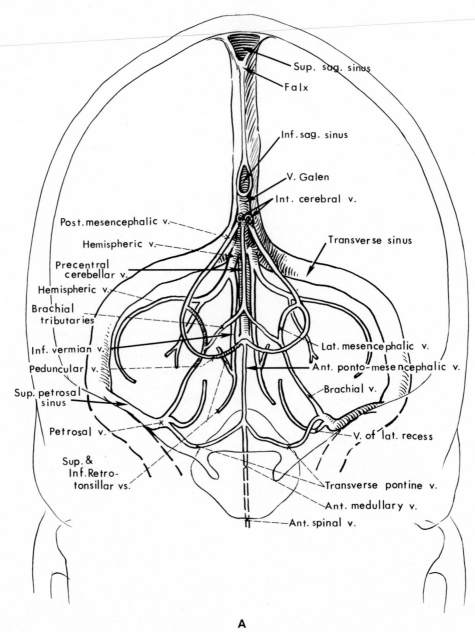

Sup. sag. sinus

Falx

Inf. sag. sinus

V. Galen

Int. cerebral v.

Post. mesencephalic v.

Hemispheric v.

Transverse sinus

Precentral cerebellar v.

Hemispheric v.

Brachial tributaries

Lat. mesencephalic v.

Inf. vermian v.

Ant. ponto-mesencephalic v.

Peduncular v.

Brachial v.

Sup. petrosal sinus

Petrosal v.

V. of lat. recess

Sup. & Inf. Retro-tonsillar vs.

Transverse pontine v.

Ant. medullary v.

Ant. spinal v.

A

Figure 8–117.   Line drawings demonstrating the major venous drainage of the cerebellum and brain stem in lateral (B) and Towne's projections (A). Half-axial projection is best for demonstration of the petrosal vein.

Figure 8–117 continued on the opposite page.

just proximal to the origin of the vermian artery. Therefore, one must carefully evaluate the entire course of the PICA to ascertain this factor. It must be added that if a lesion is bilateral it may not have an effect on the vermian artery, and other indicators such as herniation of important arterial or venous components toward the spinal canal are important. Actually, if the angio-gram indicates hydrocephalus from a posterior fossa mass lesion and the PICA loops and vermis artery branches are well seen in normal positions, a midline mass may be suspected; such a mass may give direct evidence of its presence by spreading the chor-oidal loops of the PICA.

The anterior inferior cerebellar artery (AICA) passes, as

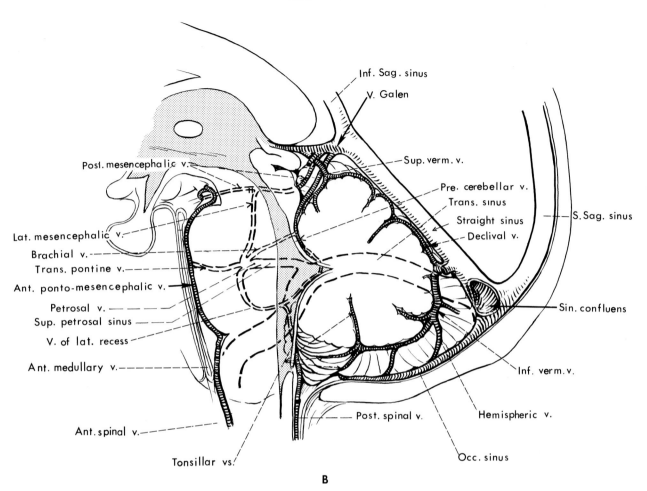

B

Figure 8–117 *Continued.* B.

has been previously shown, through the ipsilateral cerebello-pontine angle cistern, looping near the porus of the internal auditory canal and then coursing around the anterior surface of the cerebellum. Its displacement in the region of the internal acoustic canal is of great importance in indicating a local mass.

Thus far it would appear that the posterior cerebral and superior cerebellar arteries are of little help in evaluating posterior fossa mass lesions except in unusual situations. Upward herniation is certainly an important indicator, and these arteries should be studied with this in mind. If the posterior cerebral and superior cerebral arteries are widely separated and have lost their normal undulations as they course around the brain stem, enlargement of the brain stem is suggested.

The superior vermian veins, unfortunately, are apparently not displaced significantly from their essentially midline position even with large masses in the posterior fossa.

The petrosal vein, located as described in Figure 8–117 between the cerebellum and the superior petrosal sinus, may perhaps be useful in a negative fashion. If it is not seen in the pres-

ence of good filling of the ipsilateral PICA, a mass in the angle cistern is suggested. The reverse should also be true. The clinical usefulness, however, of this latter sign is not fully established.

Wolf and Huang have addressed themselves generally to the diagnostic value of cerebral veins in mass lesions of the brain. From their extensive experience they have drawn the following conclusions:

1. For the diagnosis of expanding or mass lesions, the dural sinuses are least useful since they are fixed in their position by firm attachments.

2. Displacements of superficial cortical veins are of some significance in relation to such processes as subdural hematomas or epidural mass lesions. However, premature visualization of a cortical vein may be the most important evidence of a vascular intracerebral mass lesion. In contrast to the superficial veins the subependymal veins within the walls of a lateral ventricle often show marked displacement and deformity and are therefore of great value in diagnosis.

3. The usefulness of the deep veins is of course particularly evident in cases of displacement and deformity of the internal cerebral vein. The internal cerebral vein adjoins the midline in the roof of the third ventricle and its displacement is an indicator of a mass lesion.

4. Displacement of the striothalamic veins toward the periphery of the skull is also significant because it points toward a dilated lateral ventricular system that may be indicative of either unilateral or bilateral obstructive hydrocephalus.

5. Displacement of the basal vein of Rosenthal inferiorly is a common feature of downward tentorial herniation. Apparently such herniation underneath the falx can sometimes be recognized even in the absence of contralateral displacement of the anterior cerebral artery.

6. Abnormalities of the frontal lobe may be recognized by posterior displacement of the inferior striate and uncal veins.

7. As pointed out by Davis and Roberson, the precentral cerebellar vein is of special significance since it is located in the cleft between the upper portion of the cerebellum and the brain stem.

8. Displacements of the petrosal vein or the great anterior cerebellar vein have been demonstrated with masses in the cerebellopontine angles—specifically, acoustic neuromas.

One can hardly leave this subject of cerebral angiography without emphasizing its importance in the evaluation of patients with cerebrovascular disease generally (Chase and Kricheff). Abnormalities of blood vessels are outside the scope of this text, but arteriosclerotic cerebrovascular disease is indeed one of the leading causes of death in the United States and is probably more frequently the underlying cause of neurologic deficit than all other disease processes combined. It is therefore important to identify not only the position of the vessels but also their size, degree of filling, contour alterations, and abnormalities of the intima. The blood supply of the brain by way of both carotid arteries and the vertebral arteries forms a communicating network of potential collateral channels in the neck, the face, the scalp, the base of the brain, and over the cerebral surface, as we have already emphasized.

Occlusions and stenoses may occur virtually anywhere in this network of vessels but the areas where vessels originate are the most common sites of atheromatous plaque formation, and these are the areas which must be studied most closely. Stenosis of the vertebral artery is particularly important at the site of its origin from the subclavian; the next most frequent site of vertebral artery narrowness occurs at its entrance to the foramen magnum. Osteophytic encroachment upon the vertebral artery may also take on clinical significance.

A study of extracranial collaterals is therefore clinically important, and it is for that reason that such careful attention has been paid to this aspect of radiologic anatomy.

Intracranial vascular disease may, of course, manifest itself by multiple areas of irregularity, narrowness of vessels, and occlusion of major or minor branches. Arteriosclerotic plaques are common in certain areas such as the carotid siphon and in the basilar artery.

A word of caution is advisable: one cannot make a diagnosis on the basis of a single study without seeing collaterals in reference to posterior cerebral arterial occlusion. The posterior cerebral may arise from a variety of origins—either from the carotid artery or from the basilar. Similarly, an anterior cerebral occlusion may be discovered only by bilateral carotid studies or by the presence of leptomeningeal collaterals filling the anterior cerebral territory.

TECHNIQUE OF CEREBRAL ANGIOGRAPHY

Basically, this method of examination involves the direct or indirect introduction of a suitable contrast agent into the major blood vessels of the brain. This may be accomplished by needle puncture of the carotid arteries (rarely, the vertebral artery); by threading a catheter through the brachial or femoral artery to an appropriate position in the arch of the aorta for direct injection of any of the four major vessels supplying blood to the brain, as well as for an "arch injection"; or by retrograde injection of the contrast agent directly into the brachial or axillary artery. On the left side this retrograde injection will demonstrate primarily the vertebral basilar circulation.

If the injection is made directly into the carotid artery, usually 6 to 8 ml. injected rapidly by hand will suffice; if the injection is made into the arch of the aorta or more peripherally, a greater volume of 30 to 40 ml. may be necessary, injected by a mechanical injector syringe.

The position of the needle or catheter in the appropriate carotid artery should always be checked by a small test injection, either by taking a single film after this injection or by cinefluoroscopy. If an intramural injection has been made, the examination should be interrupted and continued on a later occasion.

Direct needle puncture of the carotid sinus should be avoided, since this may elicit a sinus reflex producing blood pressure changes in the patient.

At times compression of the opposite artery may be used to fill the intracranial vessels across the midline.

Serial exposures are routinely made in anteroposterior half-axial (Fig. 8–117) and lateral projections employing a horizontal beam, simultaneously at two per second for 3 seconds, and one per second for 4 to 10 seconds thereafter (Figs. 8–118 and 8–119). Rapid film changing is necessary not only to evaluate circulation time but to reveal the very existence of a tumor or vascular malformation.

The lateral projection should always be made with the patient in the supine position and the x-ray beam horizontal. The anteroposterior and lateral views may be made simultaneously with appropriate timing sequences in the changer programmer. Stereoscopic films may be taken as necessary (Figs. 8–118, 8–119).

Subtraction techniques are especially valuable in cerebral angiography, as are techniques of magnification (Fig. 8–119 *A* and *B*).

In the presence of an arterial aneurysm, supplementary views are taken to show the neck of the aneurysm. Oblique projections are particularly useful for this purpose (Fig. 8–120). In the oblique supraorbital projection, with the central beam parallel to the floor of the anterior fossa and the head turned 30 degrees toward the noninjected side, the region of the *anterior communicating artery* is shown to best advantage. When a straight intraorbital projection is utilized, the *middle cerebral artery* is shown to best advantage. Here the middle cerebral artery is projected within the orbit. *In some cases a submentovertical projection is necessary to analyze the neck of an aneurysm.*

The half-axial angulation is 15 to 20 degrees for carotid angiography and 30 degrees for vertebral angiography. Occasionally, an angulation of 30 degrees for basilar views is also employed.

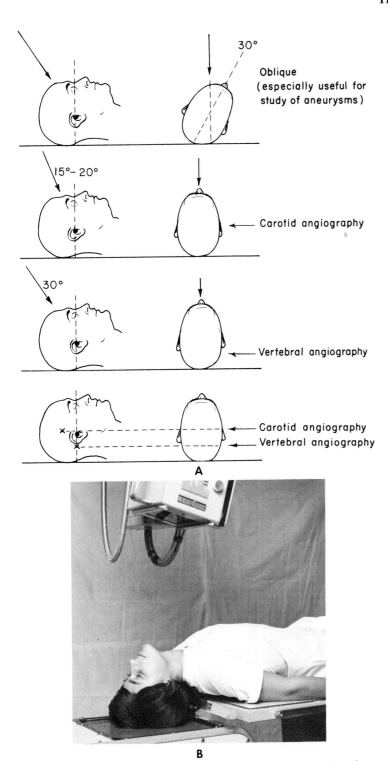

Oblique
(especially useful for study of aneurysms)

Carotid angiography

Vertebral angiography

Carotid angiography
Vertebral angiography

A

B

Figure 8–118. *A.* Positioning for carotid and vertebral angiography. The axial view may also be used on occasion to demonstrate the basilar artery and its branches. *B.* The patient's head is extended beyond the level of the table top and rests directly on the film changer. *The orbitomeatal line is angled approximately 15° from the horizontal and the roentgen tube is angled 15° toward the head,* bringing the roentgen beam perpendicular to the orbitomeatal line. A small foam pad is placed under the patient's shoulders.

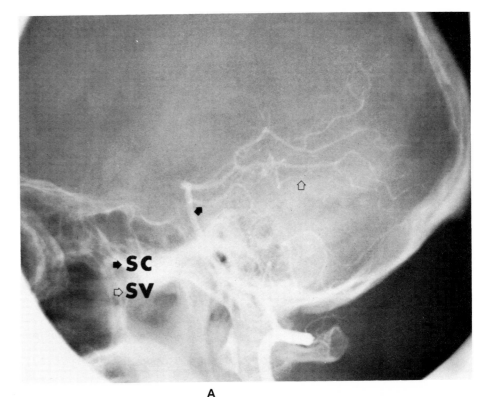

A

Figure 8–119. *A.* Lateral vertebral arteriogram, (SC) superior cerebellar, (SV) superior vermian. The detail is considerably enhanced by "subtraction technique" (see Chapter 1) as shown in *B.*

Figure 8–119 continued on the following page.

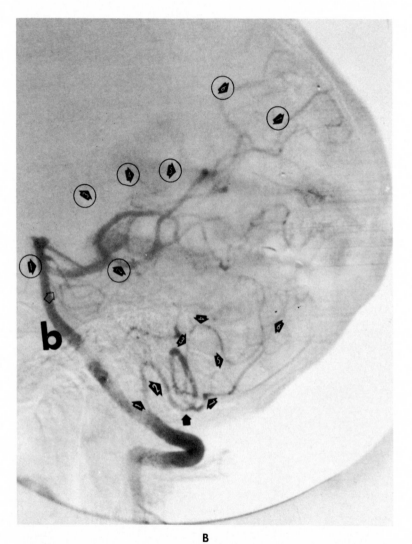

B

Figure 8–119 Continued.   B. Subtraction study of 8–119 A. Open arrow, superior cerebellar; circled arrows: (1) posterior cerebral, (2) temporal occipital, (3) medial branch of posterior choroidal, (4) lateral branch of posterior choroidal, (5) dorsal callosal, (6) occipital branch, (7) calcarine artery; plain arrows: (1) anterior medullary segment of PICA, (2) lateral medullary segment of PICA, (3) posterior medullary segment of PICA, (4) choroidal point, (5) retrotonsillar segment, (6) inferior vermian branch, (7) tonsillohemispheric branch; black arrow, caudal loop: b, basilar artery.

Figure 8–119 continued on the opposite page.

Water soluble iodine containing the contrast media is employed in this technique. The agents usually used are the diatrizoate, the metrizoate, and the iothalamate salts (Renografin or Hypaque, Isopaque, and Conray, respectively). These apparently have less influence on both the local and systemic circulations than do other compounds. Generally, the methylglucamine salts are less toxic but more viscous than the corresponding sodium salts.

These media usually produce increased blood flow, a slight decrease in blood pressure, and tachycardia. Generally, the capacity of the internal carotid artery is estimated to be 6 ml.; that of the external carotid, 4 ml.; and that of the vertebral artery, 4 ml. These quantities may at times be exceeded by 2 ml. The patient is observed by electrocardiographic control after each injection so that the examination may be interrupted at any point if the patient's symptoms warrant it.

If the injection is made below the bifurcation of the common carotid artery, the external carotid artery may also be visualized, although its circulation is a few seconds slower than that of the internal carotid. Carotid angiography is especially helpful in demonstration of certain pathologic entities such as meningiomas that receive their blood supply mainly from the external carotid circulation. If the injection is made into the subclavian artery, the vertebral artery on that side is visualized simultaneously, along with its flow pattern in relation to the basilar artery and its major ramifications.

The ideal frontal perspective in most instances is one in which the supraorbital ridge is directly superimposed over the petrous ridge (Fig. 8–118). *The condyloid processes of the mandible must be absolutely symmetrical with respect to the mastoid processes. In the lateral views, there must be a perfect superimposition of the rami of the mandible and the temporomandibular joints.*

It will be noted that if emphasis on the vertebral circulation is required, the horizontal x-ray beam should be centered 3 cm. below the external auditory meatus for the lateral views. In carotid angiography, the horizontal beam is centered 3 cm. above and 1 cm. anterior to the meatus (Fig. 8–118).

The exposures are begun near the end of the injection period. Injections may be repeated with somewhat different timing after the initial films are seen. In general (Krayenbühl and Yasargil), the arterial phase occurs within the first 1.5 to 3 seconds (median, 2.3 seconds); the capillary phase occurs 0.5 second thereafter; and the venous phase takes place in the final 1.5 to 4.5 seconds (median, 3.5 seconds). These sequences (4 to 8 seconds) may have to be varied depending upon individual requirements (median value, 6.3 seconds).

In most cases neither the intramural injection of the contrast agent nor an associated hematoma produces neurologic complications, especially if symptoms are recognized immediately and the examination is stopped. However, embolization from an atheromatous plaque may occur if a needle puncture or catheter has dislodged a plaque from the wall of the vessel. Atheromatous

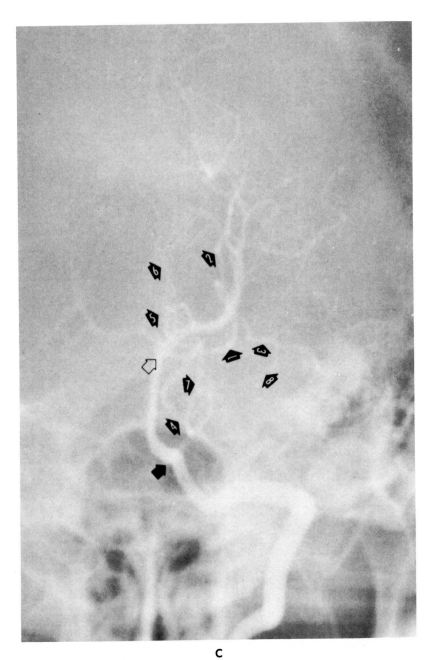

C

Figure 8–119 *Continued.* C. Towne's view of posterior fossa (vertebral arteriogram). Black arrow, posterior inferior cerebellar artery; open arrow, internal peduncular segment of superior cerebellum; 1, crural artery; 2, ambient artery; 3, marginal branch; 4, caudal loop; 5, cephalic point (choroidal point); 6, inferior vermian artery; 7, tonsillohemispheric branch; 8, inferior hemispheric branch.

Figure 8–119 continued on the following page.

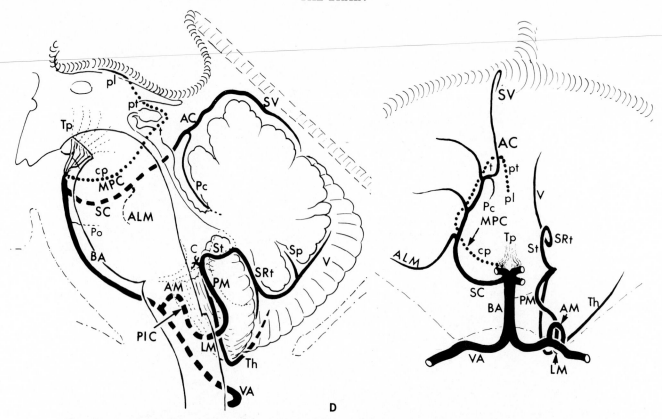

D

Figure 8–119 *Continued.*   Schematic diagram of the major arteries in the posterior fossa. *D.* Lateral projection (left), Towne's projection (right). (AC) Anterior culminate segment. (ALM) anterior lateral marginal branch, (AM) anterior medullary segment, (BA) basilar artery, (C) choroidal arteries, (cp) circumpeduncular segment, (LM) lateral medullary segment, (MPC) medial posterior choroidal artery, (No) nodular branch, (Pc) precentral cerebellar artery, (PIC) posterior inferior cerebellar artery, (pl) plexal segment, (PM) posterior medullary segment, (Po) pontine artery, (pt) pretectal segment, (SC) superior cerebellar artery, (Sp) suprapyramidal branch of the posterior inferior cerebellar artery, (SRt) superior retrotonsillar segment of the posterior inferior cerebellar artery, (St) supratonsillar segment of the posterior inferior cerebellar artery, (SV) vermian segment, (Th) tonsillohemispheric branch, (Tp) thalamoperforate anteries, (V) vermian segment, (VA) vertebral artery, (t) tectal segment. (From Huang, Y. P., and Wolf, B. S.: Neuroradiology, 1:4, 1970.)

Figure 8–119 continued on the opposite page.

plaques are especially common at the bifurcation of vessels, and care must be exercised at these sites.

An arteriovenous fistula may occasionally also develop.

Embolization may result from thrombus formation on the catheter, and this is possibly one of the major sources of complications in catheter angiography. *To help avoid this complication, the catheter should be flushed in heparinized normal saline at frequent intervals and the examination should not continue much longer than 1 hour.* It has been shown that other causes of embolization may be talc from surgical gloves, or cotton fibers from draping towels (Kutt et al.). Another complication of catheter angiography is intravascular breakage of a defective tip on the guidewire; hence, the guidewire must be thoroughly tested before use.

Normal Topography of the Cerebral Vessels in Childhood (Bergstrom et al.).   Various changes appear to occur during the growth of the child up to the age of 5 to 7 years which reflect themselves in angiograms of the brain. These are summarized as follows: The frontal lobe tends to grow; the carotid siphon tends to become somewhat more tortuous and elongated; the Syl-

vian group is displaced downward toward the clinoparietal line; and the pericallosal artery appears to become somewhat tortuous as the frontal lobe grows larger in the lateral projection.

Also, over the age of 10 the basilar artery appears to be displaced somewhat caudad. The posterior cerebral artery becomes somewhat more tortuous and its proximal portion tends to fall below a line drawn between the tuberculum sellae and lambda after the age of 7.

The venous angle is displaced very slightly in a basal direction and there is only a very minimal change in the position of the sinus confluens.

The most rapid phase of development of the ventricular system is mainly completed by the age of 2 years, after which only minor changes occur in its absolute and relative size.

Some changes are also reflected in the size of the basal cisterns. The depth of the suprasellar cistern decreases, the interpeduncular cistern increases, and the depth and lateral extension of the pontocerebellar cisterns decrease at the same rate as the volume in the pons increases. The absolute depth of the pontine cistern and the relative size of the cisterna magna do not

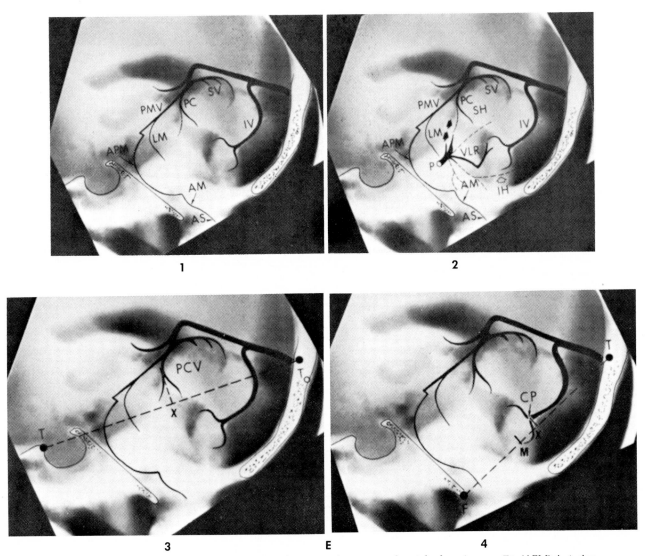

Figure 8–119 *Continued.* E. Schematic. Lateral venous phase, normal vertebral angiogram. *E1.* (APM) Anterior pontomesencephalic vein, (AM) anterior medullary vein, (AS) anterior spinal vein, (PMV) posterior mesencephalic vein, (LM) lateral mesencephalic vein, (PC) precentral cerebellar vein, (SV) superior vermian vein, (IV) inferior vermian vein. *E2.* The petrosal vein (P) and its tributaries have been added to the basic venous diagram. (VLR) Vein of the lateral recess, (IH) inferior hemispheric vein, (SH) superior hemispheric vein. A brachial tributary of the petrosal vein joins the brachial tributary of the precentral cerebellar vein (arrows).

E3. The relationship of the precentral cerebellar vein to Twining's line. (T) Tuberculum, (To) torcula, (X) point of perpendicular intersection. (TX) = XTo ± 5 per cent.

E4. The relationship of the copular point (CP) to the F-T line. Note that the copular point itself should lie 3 or 4 mm. above or below the F-T line. (F) Anterior lip of the foramen magnum, (T) torcula, (X) point of perpendicular intersection, (M) midpoint of the F-T line. (MX) = approximately 4 mm. (*E1–4* from George, A. E.: Radiol. Clin. N. Amer., *12*:371–399, August, 1974.)

Figure 8–119 continued on the opposite page.

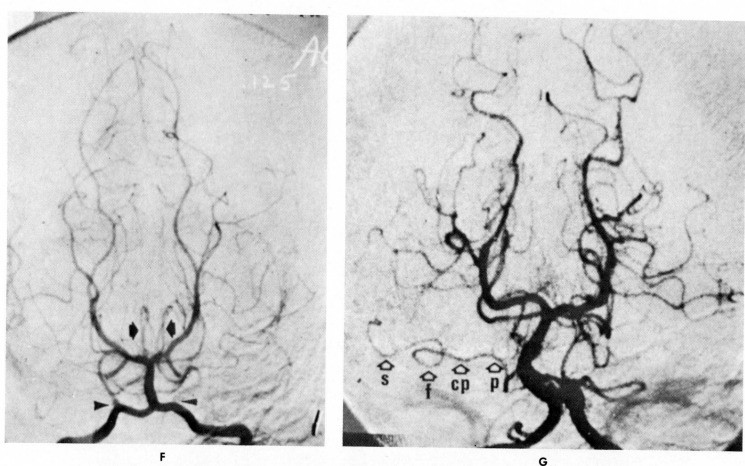

Figure 8–119 *Continued.* F. Normal vertebral angiogram, anteroposterior arterial phase. Both PICA's are opacified (lower arrows). The posterior medullary segments (upper arrows) delineate the lateral walls of the vallecula. G. Normal vertebral angiogram, anteroposterior arterial phase. The posterior cerebral, superior cerebellar and right anterior inferior cerebellar (arrows) arteries are well demonstrated. (p) Pontine segment, (cp) cerebellopontine angle segment, (f) floccular segment, (s) semilunar segment. (From George, A. E.: Radiol. Clin. N. Amer., 12:371–399, August, 1974.)

Figure 8–119 continued on the following page.

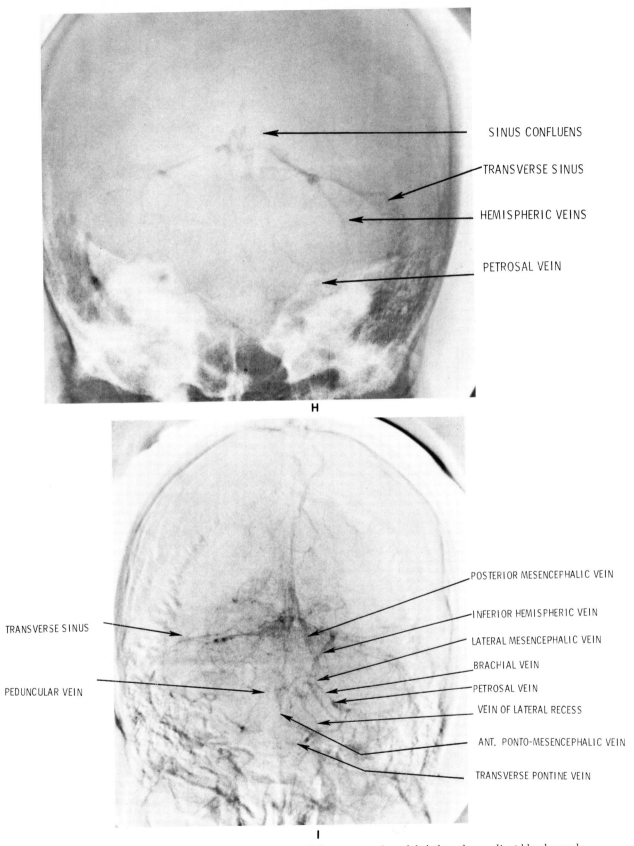

SINUS CONFLUENS

TRANSVERSE SINUS

HEMISPHERIC VEINS

PETROSAL VEIN

H

TRANSVERSE SINUS

PEDUNCULAR VEIN

POSTERIOR MESENCEPHALIC VEIN

INFERIOR HEMISPHERIC VEIN

LATERAL MESENCEPHALIC VEIN

BRACHIAL VEIN

PETROSAL VEIN

VEIN OF LATERAL RECESS

ANT. PONTO-MESENCEPHALIC VEIN

TRANSVERSE PONTINE VEIN

I

Figure 8–119 *Continued.*   *H* through *K*. Venograms of the posterior fossa labeled to show salient blood vessels.

Figure 8–119 continued on the following page.

503

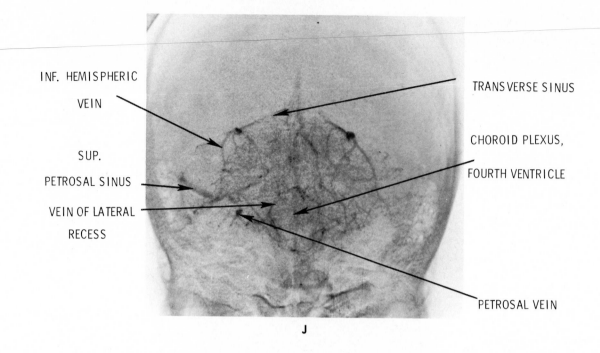

INF. HEMISPHERIC
VEIN

SUP.
PETROSAL SINUS

VEIN OF LATERAL
RECESS

TRANSVERSE SINUS

CHOROID PLEXUS,
FOURTH VENTRICLE

PETROSAL VEIN

J

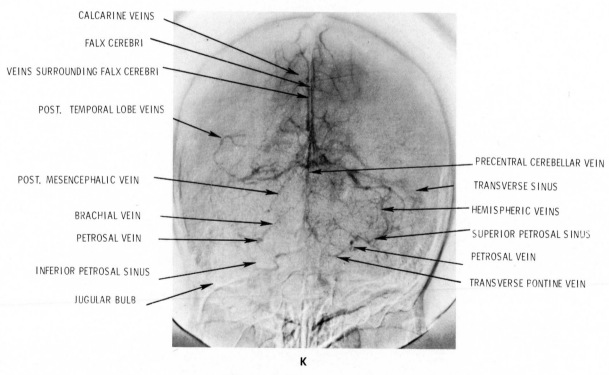

CALCARINE VEINS

FALX CEREBRI

VEINS SURROUNDING FALX CEREBRI

POST. TEMPORAL LOBE VEINS

POST. MESENCEPHALIC VEIN

BRACHIAL VEIN

PETROSAL VEIN

INFERIOR PETROSAL SINUS

JUGULAR BULB

PRECENTRAL CEREBELLAR VEIN

TRANSVERSE SINUS

HEMISPHERIC VEINS

SUPERIOR PETROSAL SINUS

PETROSAL VEIN

TRANSVERSE PONTINE VEIN

K

Figure 8–119 Continued. J and K.

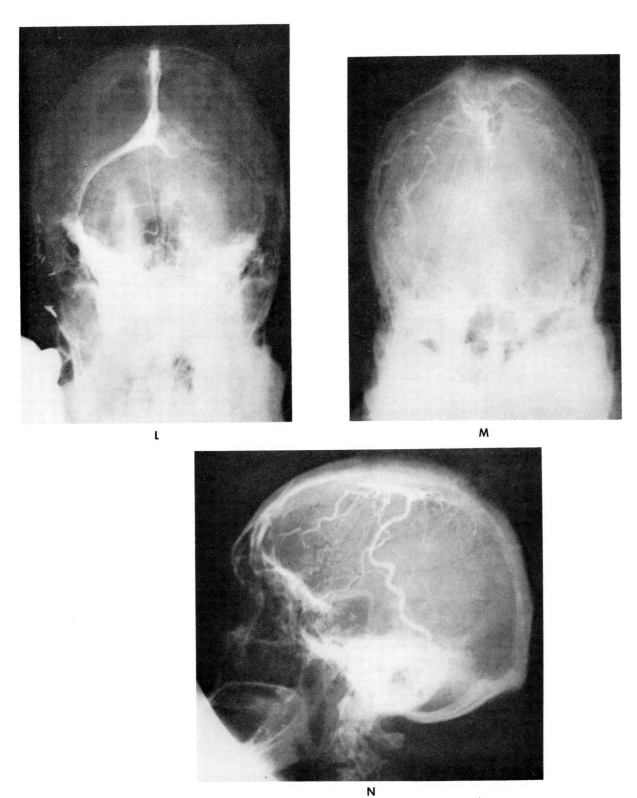

Figure 8–119 *Continued.* *L.* Normal superior sagittal sinus venogram. *M.* Superior sagittal sinus venogram, Towne's view, obstruction by meningioma. *N.* Superior sagittal sinus venogram, obstruction by meningioma, lateral view.

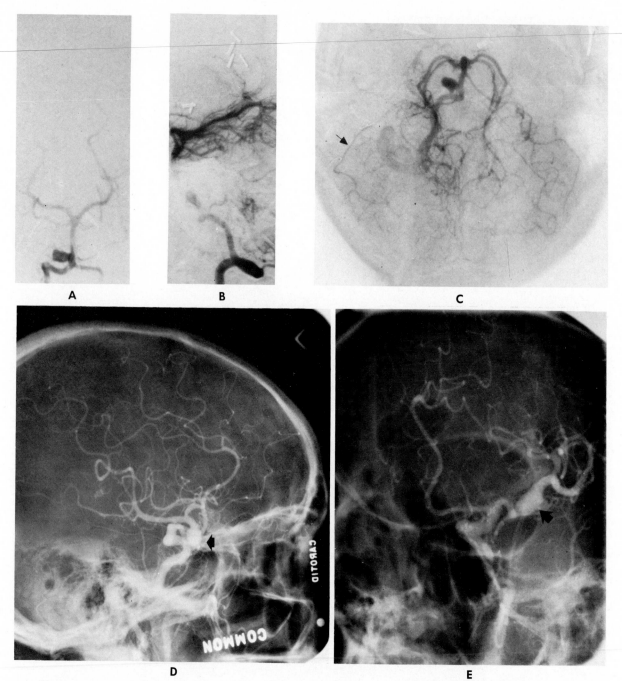

Figure 8–120.   A. Right vertebral angiogram. Towne's projection shows an aneurysm projected to the right, originating from the basilar artery. It is superimposed upon the origin of the right anterior inferior cerebellar artery and may originate at that point. The neck of the aneurysm is not shown clearly.

B. The aneurysm is not seen clearly in the lateral projection. Surgical clips are present from the previous correction of bilateral posterior communicating artery aneurysms.

C. In the basal projection, the presence of the aneurysm is verified and its neck is demonstrated. The neck originates 7 mm. proximal to the origin of the anterior inferior cerebellar artery. Note the normal appearance (arrow) of the marginal branch of the right superior cerebellar artery as it courses parallel and slightly posterior to the petrous ridge. (From Glickman, M. G., Gletne, J. S., and Mainzer, F.: Radiology, 98:611–618, 1971.)

D and E. Representative oblique angiographic studies of an aneurysm, showing the importance of oblique studies for this disease entity. In frontal perspective an aneurysm may be readily overlooked or not seen to best advantage, and it is important from the surgical standpoint to be able to see the exact size, configuration, and neck of origin of the aneurysm.

themselves change. Most of these alterations are complete by the age of 5 to 7 years.

Dural Sinus Venography. In an attempt to study the intracranial venous system more satisfactorily than in the end phase of an arterial injection, the following procedures have been employed: (1) direct injection through a catheter introduced into the anterior third of the superior sagittal sinus, (2) retrograde injection through a catheter introduced into the basilar vein of the arm and passed upward to the superior bulb of the internal jugular vein, and (3) direct measurement of venous pressure in the superior sagittal sinus. These are seldom employed with the best subtraction techniques.

1. The superior sagittal sinus venogram is performed by passing a catheter into the superior sagittal sinus through a small burr hole. Fifteen cc. of 30 per cent diatrizoate (Renografin or Hypaque) or its equivalent is rapidly injected and the x-ray exposure made at the termination of the injection; alternatively, serial films may be obtained. A slightly oblique Towne's view and a lateral view are obtained (Fig. 8–120). In the normal subject, the contrast medium passes backward to the torcular Herophili and thence into the transverse sinuses and internal jugular veins (Fig. 8–120 *A*). The other dural sinuses ordinarily do not fill, although occasionally a scalp or diploic vein or the orbital and facial veins anteriorly may be seen. Jugular compression, even if prolonged, never causes filling of the superior cerebral veins, but rather results in extensive filling of the vertebral and occipital plexuses of veins.

In about half or more of the cases, only one of the transverse sinuses will fill, apparently with no particular predominance of one side or the other.

Venous pressure in the superior sagittal sinus in the normal person varies between 100 and 150 mm. of saline. Abnormal patterns are obtained when the superior sagittal sinus or transverse sinus is invaded or obstructed (Fig. 8–120 *B, C*) by tumor or when either sinus is thrombosed.

Improved techniques combined with subtraction have virtually eliminated the necessity for dural sinus venography, which is very seldom employed as such for morphologic visualization of the dural sinus structures.

2. Retrograde jugular venograms are performed by passing a cardiac catheter from the antecubital vein to the superior jugular bulb, applying compression or pressure on both jugular veins and injecting 25 cc. of 50 per cent Renografin or Hypaque or its equivalent rapidly. A film or serial films are made in the lateral projection at the termination of the injection.

This procedure will cause the superior and inferior petrosal sinuses to fill, and sometimes also the cavernous sinus and transverse sinus of the same side. The pterygoid and vertebral plexuses are apparently usually filled and occasionally the orbital and facial veins also.

REFERENCES

Anderson, P. E.: The lenticulostriate arteries and their diagnostic value. Acta Radiol., *50*:84, 1958.

Anson, B. J.: An Atlas of Human Anatomy. Second edition. Philadelphia, W. B. Saunders Co., 1963.

Anson, B. J. (ed.): Morris' Human Anatomy. 12th edition. New York, McGraw Hill, 1966.

Atkinson, W. J.: The anterior inferior cerebellar artery. J. Neurol. Neurosurg. Psychiat., *12* 137–151, 1949.

Baker, H.: Delineation of sellar and parasellar masses. Radiology, *104*:67–78, 1972.

Bergstrom, K., Lodin, H., and Ottander, H. G.: Normal topography of the cerebral vessels in childhood. Acta Radiol. (Diag.) 8:146–160, 1969.

Bierman, H. C.: Selective Arterial Catheterization. Springfield, Ill., Charles C Thomas, 1969.

Browning, H.: The confluence of dural venous sinuses. Amer. J. Anat., *93*:307, 1953.

Bruijn, G. W.: Pneumoencephalography in diagnosis of cerebral atrophy: quantitative studies. Thesis, State University of Utrecht, 1959.

Bull, J.: The normal variations in the position of the optic recess of the third ventricle. Acta Radiol., *46*:72, 1956.

Burhenne, H. J., and Davies, H.: The ventricular span in cerebral pneumography. Amer. J. Roentgenol., *90*:1176–1184, 1963.

Camp, J. D., and Cilley, E. I. L.: Significance of asymmetry of the pori acoustici as an aid in the diagnosis of eighth nerve tumors. Amer. J. Roentgenol., *41*:713–718, 1939.

Carpenter, M. B., Noback, C. R., and Moss, M. L.: The anterior choroid artery (its origin, course, distribution and variations). Arch. Neurol. Psychiat., *71*:714, 1954.

Chase, N. E., and Kricheff, I. I.: Cerebral angiography in the evaluation of patients with cerebrovascular disease. Radiol. Clin. N. Amer., *4*:131–144, 1966.

Chase, N. E., and Taveras, J. M.: Temporal tumors studied by cineangiography—a review of 150 cases. Acta Radiol., *1*:225–238, 1963.

Corrales, M., and Greitz, T.: Fourth ventricle: 1. A morphologic and radiologic investigation of the normal anatomy. Acta Radiol. (Diag.), *12*:113–133, 1972.

Cunningham, D. G.: Manual of Practical Anatomy. Vol. 3, 12th edition. London, Oxford University Press, 1958.

Daseler, E. H., and Anson, B. J.: Surgical anatomy of the subclavian artery and its branches. Surg. Gyn. Obst., *108*:149–174, 1959.

Davis, D. O., Roberson, G. H.: Angiographic diagnosis of posterior fossa mass lesions. Seminars in Roentgenol., *6*:89–102, 1971.

Decker, K.: Clinical Neuroradiology. New York, McGraw Hill, 1966.

Dyke, C. G., and Davidoff, L. M.: The pneumoencephalographic appearance of hemangioblastoma of the cerebellum. Amer. J. Roentgenol., *44*:1–8, 1940.

Engeset, A., and Lonnum, A.: Third ventricles of 12 mm. width or more. Acta Radiol., *50*:5, 1958.

Engeset, A., and Skraastad, E.: Methods of measurement in encephalography. Neurology, *14*:381, 1964.

Fazekas, J. F., Yuan, R. H., Callow, A. D., Paul, R. E., and Alman, R. W.: Studies of cerebral hemodynamics in aortocranial disease. New Eng. J. Med., *266*:224, 1962.

Gabrielsen, T. O., and Amundsen, P.: The pontomesencephalic vein: a roentgenographic study. Radiology, *92*:889–896, 1969.

Gabrielsen, T. O., and Greitz, T.: Normal size of the internal carotid, middle cerebral and anterior cerebral arteries. Acta Radiol. (Diag.), *10*:1–10, 1970.

Galligioni, F., Bernardi, R., and Mingrino, S.: Anatomic variation in the height of the falx cerebri. Amer. J. Roentgenol., *106*:273–278, 1969.

Galloway, J. R., and Greitz, T.: The medial and lateral choroid arteries. An anatomic and roentgenographic study. Acta Radiol., *53*:353–366, 1960.

Gardner, E., Gray, D. J., and O'Rahilly, R.: Anatomy. A Regional Study of Human Structures. Third edition. Philadelphia, W. B. Saunders Co., 1969.

George, A. E.: A systematic approach to the interpretation of posterior fossa angiography. Rad. Clin. N. Amer., *12*:371–400, 1974.

Gonzalez, C., Kricheff, I. I., Lin, J. P., and Lorber, S.: Evaluation of the Vlahovitch system for the measurement of the Sylvian triangle. Radiology, *94*:535–539, 1970.

Grant, J. C. B.: Atlas of Anatomy. Fifth edition. Baltimore, Williams and Wilkins Co., 1962.

Gray, H.: Gray's Anatomy of the Human Body. 29th edition. Philadelphia, Lea and Febiger, 1973.

Greitz, T., and Lindgren, E.: Cerebral vascular anatomy. *In* Abrams, H. L. (ed.): Angiography. Second edition. Vol. 1. Boston, Little, Brown and Co., 1971.

Greitz, T., and Löfstedt, S.: The relationship between the third ventricle and the basilar artery. Acta Radiol., *42*:85, 1954.

Greitz, T., and Sjögren, S. E.: The posterior inferior cerebellar artery. Acta Radiol. (Diag.), *1*:284–297, 1963.

Herman, L. H., Ostrowski, A. Z., and Geurdjian, E. S.: Perforating branches of the middle cerebral artery. Arch. Neurol., *8*:32–35, 1963.

Hilal, S. K., Solomon, G. E., Gold, A. P., and Carter, S.: Primary cerebral occlusive disease in children. Radiology, *99*:86, 1971.

Hilal, S. K., Tookoran, H., and Wood, E. H.: Displacement of aqueduct of Sylvius by posterior fossa tumors. Acta Radiol. (Diag.), *9*:167–182, 1969.

Huang, Y. P., and Wolf, B. S.: Angiographic features of brain stem tumors and differential diagnosis from fourth ventricle tumors. Amer. J. Roentgenol., *110*:1–30, 1970.

Huang, Y. P., and Wolf, B. S.: Angiographic features of fourth ventricle tumors with special reference to the posterior inferior cerebellar artery. Amer. J. Roentgenol., *107*:543–564, 1969.

Huang, Y. P., and Wolf, B. S.: Angiographic features of the pericallosal cistern. Radiology, *82*:14–23, 1964.

Huang, Y. P., and Wolf, B. S.: Precentral cerebellar vein in angiography. Acta Radiol. (Diag.), *5*:250, 1966.

Huang, Y. P., and Wolf, B. S.: The veins of the lateral recess of the fourth ventricle and its tributaries: roentgen appearance and anatomic relationship. Amer. J. Roentgenol., *101*:1–21, 1967.

Huang, Y. P., and Wolf, B. S.: The veins of the posterior fossa—superior or galenic drainage group. Amer. J. Roentgenol., *95*:808–821, 1965.

Huang, Y. P., and Wolf, B. S.: Veins of the white matter of the cerebral hemispheres (the medullary veins). Amer. J. Roentgenol., *92*:739–755, 1964.

Huang, Y. P., Wolf, B. S., and Okudera, T.: Angiographic anatomy of the inferior vermian vein of the cerebellum. Acta Radiol. (Diag.), *9*:327, 1969.

Huang, Y. P., Wolf, B. S., Antin, S. P., and Okudera, T.: The veins of the posterior fossa—anterior or petrosal drainage group. Amer. J. Roentgenol., *104*:36–56, 1968.

Jacobsen, H. H., and Melchior, J. C.: On pneumoencephalographic measuring methods in children. Amer. J. Roentgenol., *101*:188–194, 1967.

Jain, K. K.: Some observations on the anatomy of the middle cerebral artery. Canad. J. Surg., *7*:134, 1964.

Jones, F. W.: Grooves upon ossa parietalia commonly said to be caused by arteria meningea media. J. Anat. Physiol., *46*:228–238, 1912a.

Jones, F. W.: Vascular lesion in some cases of middle meningeal hemorrhage. Lancet, *2*:7–12, 1912b.

Kety, S. S., and Schmidt, C. F.: Determination of cerebral blood flow in man by use of nitrous oxide in low concentrations. Amer. J. Physiol., *143*:53–66, 1945.

Krayenbühl, H. A., and Richter, H. R.: Die Zerebrale Arteriographie. Stuttgart, Georg Thieme, 1952.

Krayenbühl, H. A., and Yaşargil, M. D.: Cerebral Angiography. Philadelphia, J. B. Lippincott Co., 1968.

Kutt, H., Verebely, K., Bang, N., Streuli, F., and McDowell, F.: Possible mechanisms of complications of angiography. Acta Radiol. (Diag.), 5:276, 1966.

Lapayowker, M. S., and Cliff, M. M.: Bone changes in acoustic neuromas. Amer. J. Roentgenol., 107:652–658, 1969.

LeMay, M. J., and Jackson, D. M.: Changes in the anterior choroidal artery in intracranial lesions. Amer. J. Roentgenol., 92:776–785, 1964.

Lewtas, N. A., and Jefferson, A. A.: The carotid cistern—a source of diagnostic difficulties with suprasellar extension of pituitary adenomata. Symposium Neuroradiologicum VII, New York, N.Y., September 20–25, 1964.

Liliequist, B.: The subarachnoid cisterns. Acta Radiol. (Suppl.), 185, 1959.

Lindblom, K.: A roentgenographic study of the vascular channels of the skull. Acta Radiol. (Stockholm), Suppl. 30, 1936.

Lindgren, E., and DiChiro, G.: The roentgenologic appearance of the aqueduct of Sylvius. Acta Radiol., 39:117–125, 1953.

Lindgren, E.: Radiologic examination of the brain and spinal cord. Acta Radiol. (Suppl.) 151, 1957.

Löfgren, F. O.: Vertebral angiography in the diagnosis of tumors in the pineal region. Acta Radiol., 50:108–124, 1958.

Mani, R. L., Newton, T. H., and Glickman, M. G.: The superior cerebellar artery: an anatomic-roentgenographic correlation. Radiology, 91:1102–1108, 1968.

Meschan, I.: Roentgen signs of abnormality in cerebral angiograms. In Toole, J. F. (ed.): Special Techniques for Neurologic Diagnosis. Philadelphia, F. A. Davis, 1969.

Netter, F. H.: Nervous System. Vol. 1. Ciba Collection of Medical Illustration, 1957.

Oberson, R., Candardjis, G., and Raad, N.: Height of fourth ventricle. Acta Radiol (Diag.), 9:193, 1969.

Pachtman, H., Hilal, F. K., and Wood, E. H.: The posterior choroidal arteries: normal measurement and displacement by hydrocephalus or tumors of the pineal region or brain stem. Radiology, 112:343–352, 1974.

Padget, D. H.: Cranial venous system in man in reference to development, adult configuration and relation to arteries. Amer. J. Anat., 98:307, 1956.

Pansky, B., and House, E. L.: Review of Gross Anatomy. New York, Macmillan Co., 1964.

Pendergrass, E. P., Schaeffer, J. P., and Hodes, J. P.: The Head and Neck in Roentgen Diagnosis. Springfield, Illinois, Charles C Thomas, 1956.

Pernkopf, E.: Atlas of Topographical and Applied Human Anatomy. Vol. 1. Philadelphia, W. B. Saunders Co., 1963.

Probst, F. P.: Position of the "venous angle" in the median sagittal plane: a new topometric method. Acta Radiol. (Diag.), 10:271–288, 1970.

Richardson, H. D., and Bednarz, W. W.: The depiction of ventricular size by the striothalamic vein in the anteroposterior phlebogram. Radiology, 81:604–609, 1963.

Riggs, H. E.: Anomalies of circle of Willis. Trans. Phila. Neurol. Soc., December, 1937.

Ring, A. B., and Waddington, M.: Ascending frontal branch of middle cerebral artery. Acta Radiol. (Diag.), 6:209–220, 1967.

Robertson, E. G.: Pneumoencephalography. Second edition. Springfield, Ill., Charles C Thomas, 1967.

Rosen, L., Weidner, W., and Hanafee, W.: Angiographic visualization of the subarachnoid cisterns. Radiology, 85:1–13, 1965.

Ruggiero, G., and Castellano, F.: Upward displacement of the posterior part of the third ventricle. Acta Radiol., 39:377, 1953.

Sahlstedt, H. Quoted in Lisholm, E.: Das Ventrikulogramm. Acta Radiol. (Suppl.), 24, 1935.

Samra, K. A., and Cooper, I. S.: Radiology of the massa intermedia. Radiology, 91:1124–1128, 1968.

Schatzki, R., Baxter, D. H., and Trolard, C. E.: Second day encephalography with particular reference to the size of the ventricles. New Eng. J. Med., 236:419, 1947.

Schechter, M. M., and Zingesser, L. H.: The anterior spinal artery. Acta Radiol (Diag.), 3:489, 1965.

Schechter, M. M., and Zingesser, L. H.: The radiology of basilar thrombosis. Radiology, 85:23–32, 1965.

Schechter, M. M., Zingesser, L. H., and Rayport, M.: Torn meningeal vessels, an evaluation of a clinical spectrum through the use of angiography. Radiology, 86:686–695, 1966.

Shiu, P. C., Hanafee, W. N., Wilson, G. H., and Rand, R. W.: Cavernous sinus venography. Amer. J. Roentgenol., 104:57–62, 1968.

Stopford, J. S. B.: The arteries of the pons and medulla oblongata. J. Anat., 50:131, 1916a.

Stopford, J. S. B.: Arteries of the pons and medulla oblongata. Part 3. J. Anat., 50:255, 1916b.

Sutton, D.: The radiological assessment of the normal aqueduct and fourth ventricle. Brit. J. Radiol., 23:208, 1950.

Takahashi, M., and Okudera, T.: The choroid plexus and the choroid vein of the lateral ventricle. Radiology, 103:113–120, 1972.

Takahashi, M., Wilson, G., and Hanafee, W.: The significance of the petrosal vein in the diagnosis of cerebellopontine angle tumors. Radiology, 89:834–840, 1967.

Taveras, J. M., and Poser, C. M.: Roentgenologic aspects of cerebral angiography in children. Amer. J. Roentgenol., *82*:371–391, 1959.

Taveras, J. M., and Wood, E. H.: Diagnostic Neuroradiology. Baltimore, Williams and Wilkins Co., 1954.

Toole, J. F., and Patel, A. N.: Cerebrovascular Disorders. New York, McGraw Hill, 1967.

Wallace, S., Goldberg, H. I., Leeds, N. E., and Mishkin, M. M.: The cavernous branches of the internal carotid artery. Amer. J. Roentgenol., *101*:34–46, 1967.

Westberg, G.: Arteries of the basal ganglia. Acta Radiol. (Diag.), *5*:581, 1966.

Wilson, M.: The Anatomic Foundation of Neuroradiology of the Brain. Second edition. Boston, Little, Brown and Co., 1963.

Wolf, B. S., and Huang, Y. P.: The insula and deep middle cerebral venous drainage system, normal anatomy and angiography. Amer. J. Roentgenol., *90*:472–489, 1963.

Wolf, B. S., and Huang, Y. P.: The subependymal veins of the lateral ventricles. Amer. J. Roentgenol., *91*:406–426, 1964.

Wolf, B. S., Huang, Y. P., and Newman, C. M.: The lateral anastomotic mesencephalic vein and other variations in drainage of the basal cerebral vein. Amer. J. Roentgenol., *89*:411–422, 1963.

Wolf, B. S., and Huang, Y. P.: Diagnostic value of cerebral veins in mass lesions of the brain. Radiol. Clin. N. Amer., *4*:117–130, 1966.

Wollschlaeger, G., Wollschlaeger, P. B., Meyer, P. G., and Krautmann, J. J.: Widening or hyperplasia of the anterior choroidal artery. Radiology, *93*:1079–1083, 1969.

Zajgner, J.: Normal relationship between basal vein and posterior cerebral artery. Acta Radiol. (Diag.), *9*:549–552, 1969.

Zatz, L. M., and Iannone, A. M.: Cerebral emboli complicating cerebral angiography. Acta Radiol. (Diag.), *5*:621, 1966.

Zimmer, A. E., and Annes, G. P.: The septal vein: an indicator of space-occupying lesions in the anterior cranial fossa. Radiology, *87*:813–823, 1966.

9

The Vertebral Column and Spinal Cord

THE VERTEBRAL COLUMN

The vertebral column is composed of separate articulating segments called vertebrae. These are 33 in number and are distributed as follows: 7 cervical, 12 thoracic, 5 lumbar, 5 sacral, and 4 coccygeal.

Occasionally there is an extra vertebra in either the thoracic or lumbar spine regions, or there may be one less vertebra than normal, particularly in the lumbar spine. In the latter case, an extra vertebra may be fused with the coccyx, either completely or partially.

At birth the vertebral column has only two curves, with a figure 3 configuration (Fig. 9–1). It is a very asymmetrical 3 because the central angle is at the junction of the last lumbar and the first sacral segment, the so-called sacral-vertebral or lumbosacral angle. The cervical curvature starts to take shape 2 or 3 months after birth, when the child begins to lift its head significantly, and develops further when he begins to sit upright, at 7 to 9 months of age. The lumbar curvature first appears at about 1 year of age, when walking is begun. The thoracic and sacral curves are the true primary curves of the spine. With advancing years the column loses its flexibility and resilience, and variable amounts of calcification occur at the junction of the vertebral bodies with the paraspinous ligaments. The fused sacrum and also the coccyx are

CHANGES IN SPINAL CURVATURE WITH AGE

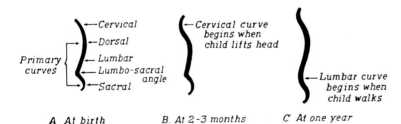

A At birth   B. At 2-3 months   C At one year

Figure 9–1. Changes in spinal curvature with age. (From Meschan, I., and Farrer-Meschan, R. M. F.: Radiology, 70:1958.)

hollowed out anteriorly, and this configuration of the sacrum is particularly important in the female when the pelvis is converted to a birth canal. A flattened sacrum encroaches upon the midpelvic dimension, usually making parturition more difficult.

The coccyx is extremely variable in its configuration, making it virtually impossible to describe its normal contour. Its development follows no definite scheme.

Anatomy of a Normal Vertebra. A vertebra consists of the following parts (Fig. 9–2): (1) the body, (2) the transverse processes on each side, (3) the pedicles, (4) the laminae, (5) the superior articular processes, (6) the inferior articular processes, (7) the spinous process, and (8) the partes interarticulares, situated between the two articular processes.

This basic anatomy is modified (Fig. 9–2) in certain parts of the spine to serve particular functions. In the cervical area, the vertebral bodies tend to be small, and the true transverse process unites with the costal process laterally, enclosing the transverse foramen. The two processes together comprise the lateral mass and are situated in a more anterior position than comparable portions of other vertebrae. In the thoracic spine, the costal process is separate from the transverse process and participates in the formation of the head and neck of the rib with which it articulates. There are costal pits on both the body and the transverse process for this articulation. In the lumbar and sacral spine, the costal and transverse processes are completely fused. The vertebral bodies become stouter and larger toward the bottom of the spinal column. The costal elements tend to occupy the greater part of the lateral mass in the sacrum.

Joints of the Vertebral Column. In the adult spine, there are two major types of joints and a third ancillary system of joints: (1) the amphiarthrodial joint between vertebral bodies, the intermediate area being occupied by the intervertebral disk (Fig. 9–3); (2) two diarthrodial joints which are true synovial joints between the articular processes of adjoining vertebrae; (3) diarthrodial joints in association with the costal facets of the thoracic spine; and (4) synovial joints (diarthroses) between the posterolateral margins of the lower five cervical bodies (joints of Luschka) (Fig. 9–4)

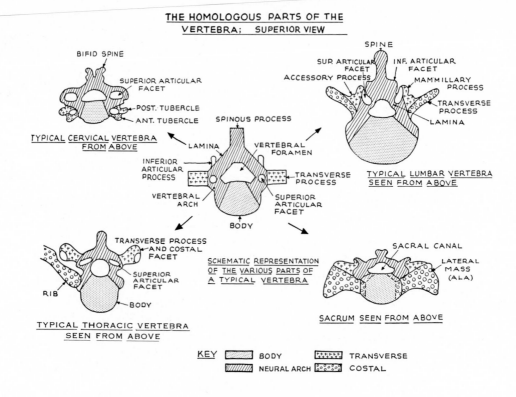

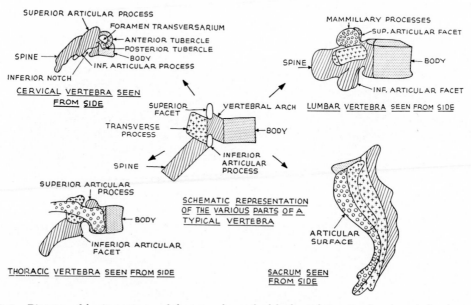

Figure 9–2. Diagram of basic anatomy of the normal vertebral body and its neural arch and development of homologous parts in various portions of the spine. Superior and lateral views.

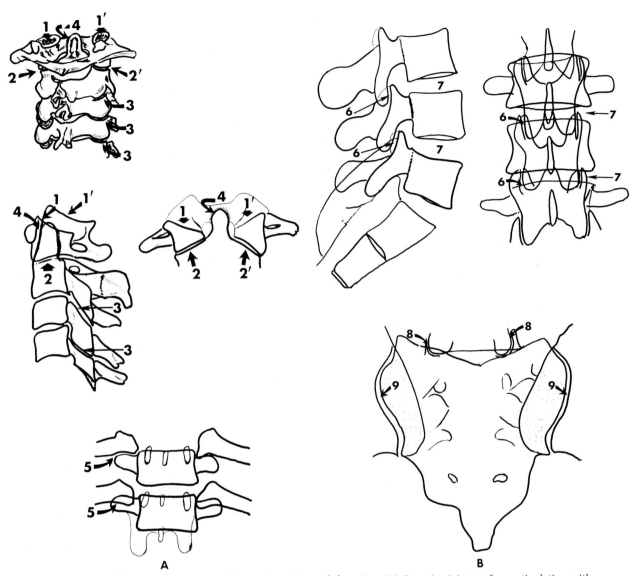

Figure 9–3. *A* and *B.* Diagrams of the various joints of the spine. (1) Superior joint surface articulating with occipital condyles, (2) apophyseal joint between the atlas and the axis (C1 and C2), (3) apophyseal joint of the rest of the cervical spine, (4) joint between the anterior tubercle of C1 and the odontoid process of C2, (5) costovertebral joint, (6) apophyseal joints of the lumbar region, (7) intervertebral joint, (8) the synovial joints between L5 and the superior sacrum, (9) sacroiliac joint.

Figure 9–3 continued on the following page.

(Boreadis et al.). These latter joints are located anteromedially to the mixed nerve root and posteromedially to the vertebral artery, vein, and sympathetics as these pass through the vertebral foramen (Fig. 9–5). On the anteroposterior projection of the cervical spine radiograph, the elements of the Luschka joints are formed by spurlike projections near the upper lateral margins of the lower five cervical vertebral bodies, and the corresponding undersurfaces of the inferior margins of the vertebral bodies above. In oblique projections, the margins of these joints are seen close to the lower anterior portion of the intervertebral foramen (Fig. 9–6).

The significance of disease in Luschka joints is based on the anatomic relationship of these joints to the neighboring structures — especially the mixed nerve roots, vessels, sympathetics, and ligaments. There has been no observation of damage to the spinal cord resulting from disease in Luschka joints.

The true intervertebral joints (between the articular processes) are frequently called "apophyseal joints." These apophy-

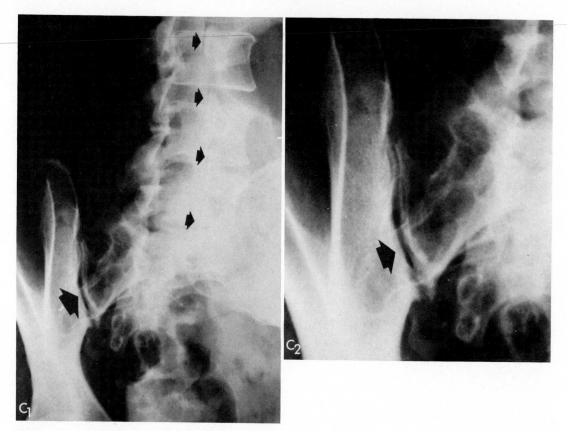

Figure 9–3 *Continued.* *C1.* Left anteroposterior oblique view of lumbosacral spine. Small arrows point to left apophyseal joints viewed in tangent. Large arrow points to right sacroiliac joint similarly viewed. *C2.* Close-up view of right sacroiliac joint.

Figure 9–3 continued on the opposite page.

seal joints have an oblique configuration that varies somewhat in different parts of the spine and between individuals, but on one side in the lumbar region they tend to be parallel, with their plane perpendicular to the corresponding sacroiliac joint. The planes of the apophyseal joints of both sides tend to meet anteriorly at an angle of 60 to 90 degrees, whereas the planes of the two sacroiliac joints tend to approach one another posteriorly at a similar angle. The diarthrodial articulations between the last lumbar and first sacral segment (lumbosacral joints) are apophyseal joints like the rest, but their obliquity differs on occasion from the others (Fig. 9–7). There are no apophyseal joints in the sacrum owing to fusion of segments.

Development of the Vertebral Column as a Whole. The primitive axial support of all vertebrates is the notochord. In humans, the notochord is only a transient structure except in the intervertebral disks where it persists as the nucleus pulposus (Fig. 9–8).

The axial skeleton differentiates from the mesenchyme, most of which occurs in serially arranged pairs of mesodermal seg-

ments, designated sclerotomes. The sclerotomes migrate to lie in paired segmental masses alongside the notochord. Each sclerotome differentiates into a caudal compact portion and a cranial less dense half. At alternate segments there is an intersegmental artery between the less dense and a compact portion. The denser caudal part of each sclerotome mass then unites with the looser cranial half and thus forms the substance of the definitive vertebra. The intervertebral disk differentiates from the denser caudal region.

Cartilaginous Stage. This so-called membranous vertebral column is succeeded at about the fourth week of fetal life by the cartilaginous vertebral column. Two cartilaginous centers appear on either side of the notochord and rapidly extend around it, thereby forming the bodies of the cartilaginous vertebrae (Figs. 9–8, 9–9). Second pairs of cartilaginous foci appear in the lateral parts of the vertebral arch and extend backward on either side of the neural tube to form the cartilaginous vertebral arch. Still different cartilaginous centers appear for each costal arch.

During the cartilaginous stage the notochord is progressively

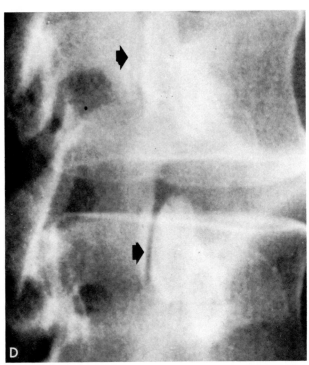

Figure 9-3 *Continued.   D.* Close-up view of lumbar apophysial joint as shown in *C1*.

compressed into the central regions of the dense intervertebral disks. Eventually it disappears completely except as the nucleus pulposus of the intervertebral cartilage. The intersegmental artery persists as a narrow channeled anterior portal into the central portion of the vertebral body (Fig. 9-10). This appearance of the intersegmental artery produces an anterior notching of the vertebral bodies centrally, which may persist into adult life. Such persistence is probably without pathologic significance.

The anterior and posterior longitudinal spinal ligaments develop during the cartilaginous stage. In the ninth week of fetal life, anterior and posterior indentations into the cartilaginous body are produced by periosteal vessels, which form ventral and dorsal blood lakes (Fig. 9-11). These correspond with the arterial and venous supply to the vertebral bodies, as shown in the illustration.

Ossification Stage.   There is considerable disagreement as to the exact changes that occur during the ossification stage. Ossification centers are said to form either dorsally and ventrally, or superiorly and inferiorly, in the vertebral body and are separated by cartilaginous septa, which soon disappear (Fig. 9-9). In either instance, the primary ossification center is shaped like an hourglass, and abnormalities in ossification account for various unusual wedged appearances of the vertebral bodies. Such wedging

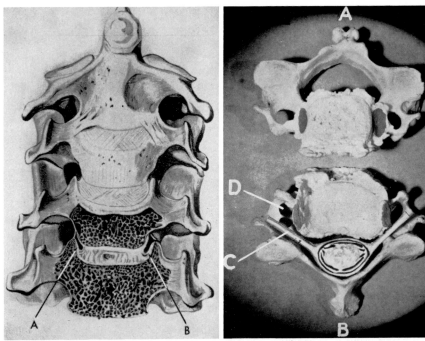

Figure 9-4.   Figure 9-5.

Figure 9-4.   Reproduction from Luschka's "Monograph," showing the joints (*A* and *B*) between the posterolateral aspects of the sectioned lower cervical vertebral bodies.

Figure 9-5.   Photograph of the fifth (*A*) and sixth (*B*) cervical vertebrae showing Luschka joints in relationship to the mixed nerve roots and vertebral foramina. The joints are painted for contrast; the female segment is seen on *A* and the male part on *B*. It is apparent that Luschka joints are situated ventromedial to the nerves (*C*) which emerge through the intervertebral foramina and also medial to the vertebral vessels and sympathetics which pass through the vertebral foramina (*D*). (From Boreadis, A. G., and Gershon-Cohen, J.: Radiology, 66:1956.)

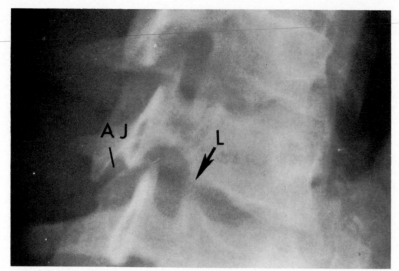

Figure 9–6. Oblique cervical spine radiograph demonstrating joints of Luschka. (AJ) Apophyseal joint, (L) Luschka joint.

can usually be differentiated from traumatic or infectious wedging on the basis of the overdevelopment that is often discernible in contiguous vertebrae.

There are also separate ossification centers on each side that enter into the formation of the neural arch. Thus, for each vertebral segment there are three separate ossification centers.

Aberrations in the further development of the neural arch are usually considered defects in the development of the ossification rather than abnormalities in the centers per se. Figure 9–12 demonstrates the various areas of defective ossification that can occur in the formation of the neural arch.

At approximately the fifth to the sixth month of fetal life, the ossification center of the vertebral body has separated the carti-

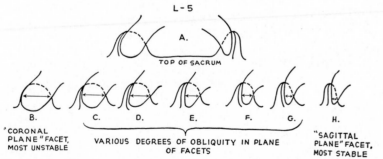

PATIENT WITH ASYMMETRICAL FACETS

Figure 9–7. The plane of the lumbosacral facets in relation to stability. (Modified from Ferguson, A. B.: Roentgen Diagnosis of Extremities and Spine. New York, Paul B. Hoeber, Inc., 1949.)

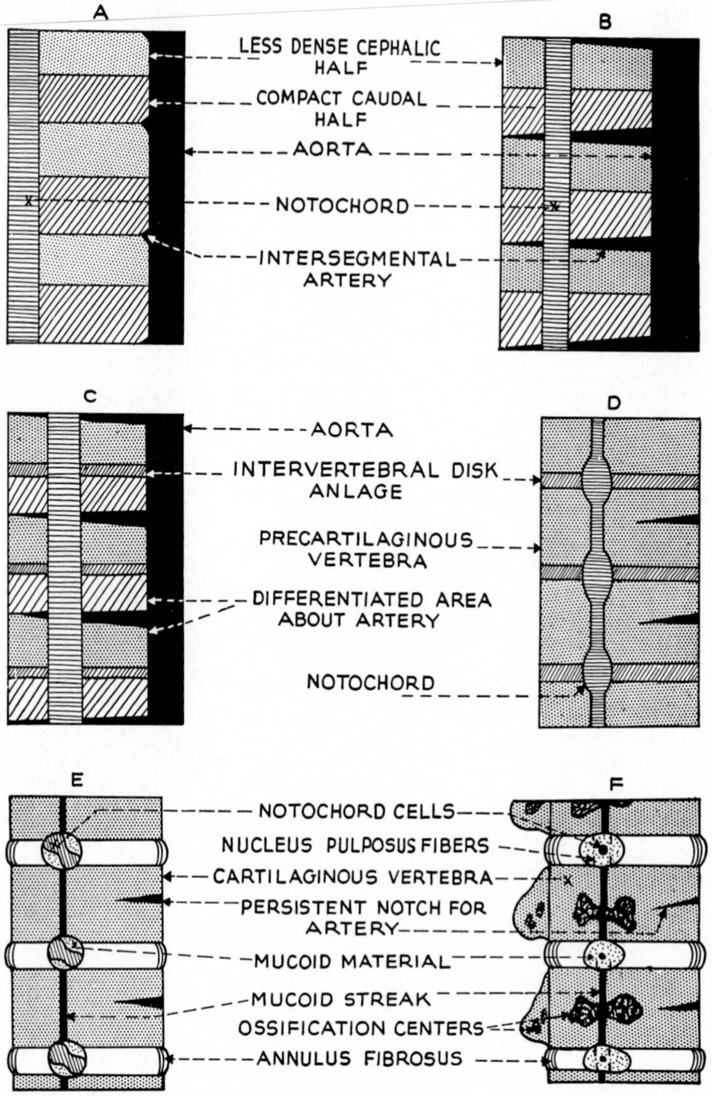

Figure 9–8. Development of the vertebral column as a whole, demonstrating the membranous cartilaginous and early ossification stages. (After Bradford, F. K., and Spurling, C. G.: The Intervertebral Disc.)

laginous body into two thick catilaginous plates showing endochondral ossification toward the intervertebral disk side. Along the anterior and lateral periphery of the vertebral bodies, horseshoe-shaped cartilaginous plates appear, respresenting cartilaginous ring apophyses (Fig. 9–9 C). Later, these form the anlage of the bony ring apophysis that appears in adolescent life, usually by 16 years but occasionally much earlier (Hindman and Poole). These apophyses fit into notches in the superior and inferior portions of the vertebral bodies so that, prior to the ossification of the ring apophysis, the vertebral body has a notched appearance (Fig. 9–10). The rami of the lumbar neural arches unite

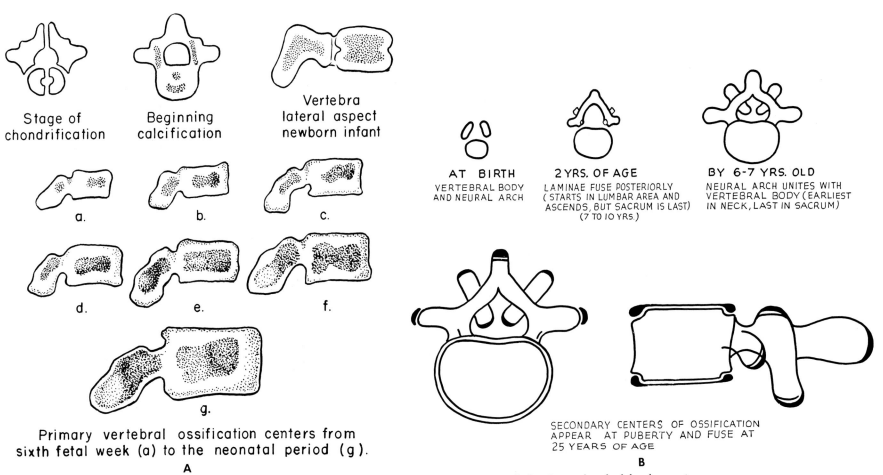

Stage of chondrification

Beginning calcification

Vertebra lateral aspect newborn infant

a.

b.

c.

d.

e.

f.

g.

Primary vertebral ossification centers from sixth fetal week (a) to the neonatal period (g).

A

AT BIRTH
VERTEBRAL BODY AND NEURAL ARCH

2 YRS. OF AGE
LAMINAE FUSE POSTERIORLY (STARTS IN LUMBAR AREA AND ASCENDS, BUT SACRUM IS LAST) (7 TO 10 YRS.)

BY 6-7 YRS. OLD
NEURAL ARCH UNITES WITH VERTEBRAL BODY (EARLIEST IN NECK, LAST IN SACRUM)

SECONDARY CENTERS OF OSSIFICATION APPEAR AT PUBERTY AND FUSE AT 25 YEARS OF AGE

B

Figure 9–9. *A.* Further diagrams of the stage of chondrification, beginning calcification, and gradual development of ossification in the vertebral body of the newborn. *B.* Diagrams illustrating time of union of the laminae and the joining of the neural arches with the body. The secondary centers of ossification are also illustrated.

during the first year of life, and similar changes follow in the neural arches of the thoracic and cervical regions. The tips of the transverse and spinous processes remain cartilaginous in the years before puberty. At about the 16th year, secondary centers appear at the tips of the transverse processes, the tips of the spinous processes, and at the upper and lower surfaces of the vertebral body (Fig. 9–9). These fuse with the rest of the vertebral body by age 25.

Aberrations of Development. Other aberrations of development in relation to the vertebral body and the intervertebral disk are noteworthy. Very often there is a posterior wedging of the fifth lumbar vertebra (Fig. 9–13) which persists even into adult life. Such posterior wedging is a relatively normal contour variation and has no pathologic significance. It is related to the junction of the lumbar curvature with the sacral curvature. Also, the intervertebral disk between L5 and S1 may be narrowed through-

out life. This likewise is related to the junction point between the lumbar and sacral curvature. *Narrowness of the interspace between L5 and S1, therefore, is without pathologic significance unless there are some other radiographic criteria, such as sclerosis of the end plates, irregularities of the end plates, or changes in the adjoining ligamentous structures.*

Congenital absence of the odontoid process is a rare anomaly, and very few cases have been reported in the literature (Gwinn and Smith). The odontoid process is an upward extension of the body of the second cervical vertebra that is formed from three ossification centers: two that appear in the base at approximately the sixth fetal month and fuse at the time of birth, and a third that appears behind the anterior tubercle of the atlas and ossifies downward to join the two ossification centers at the base. This apical ossification center of the odontoid process cannot be visualized roentgenographically until the second year of life, and

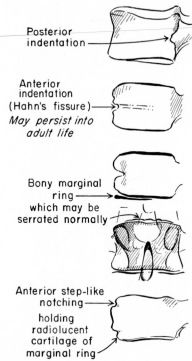

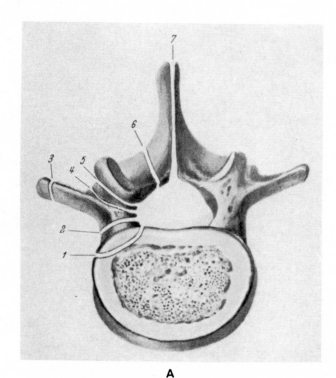

Posterior
indentation

Anterior
indentation
(Hahn's fissure)
*May persist into
adult life*

Bony marginal
ring
which may be
serrated normally

Anterior step-like
notching
holding
radiolucent
cartilage of
marginal ring

Figure 9–10. The normal appearance of posterior and anterior indentations on vertebral bodies in relation to blood supply and venous drainage. The anterior steplike notching changes the contour in relation to the cartilaginous end plates of the vertebral body.

A

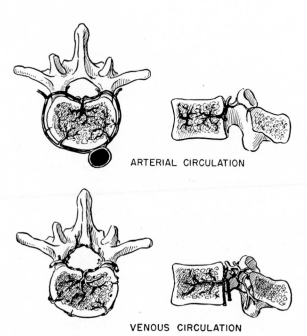

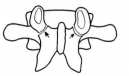

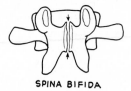

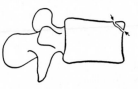

ARTERIAL CIRCULATION

VENOUS CIRCULATION

Figure 9–11. Diagrams illustrating the arterial and venous circulation of a vertebral body and its neural arch.

DEFECTS IN OSSIFICATION OF VERTEBRAE

DEFECTS IN PARS INTERARTICULARIS

EXTRA-APOPHYSES

SPINA BIFIDA

B

Figure 9–12. A. Diagram illustrating the various areas for defective ossification in the neural arch and pedicles: (1) Retrosomatic hiatus, (2) hiatus in the pedicle, (3) persistent epiphysis of the transverse process, (4 and 5) defects in the pars interarticularis, (6) retroisthmic hiatus, (7) bifid posterior spinous process. (From Köhler, A. and Zimmer, E. A.: Borderlands of the Normal and Early Pathologic in Skeletal Roentgenology. 11th ed. New York, Grune & Stratton, 1968. Used by permission.)

B. Further tracings demonstrating defects in the pars interarticularis, spina bifida, and extra-apophyses as they may appear on various roentgenographic views.

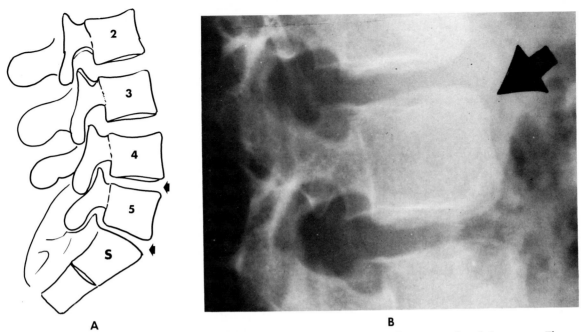

Figure 9–13. Some variations of normal lumbar vertebrae. *A.* The lumbar vertebrae are numbered; S = sacrum. The arrows point to the narrowed interspaces between L4 and L5 and between L5 and S1. The narrowed interspace between L5 and S1 may be normal. Usually a narrowed interspace between L4 and L5 represents a degenerative process. Degeneration of the intervertebral disk between L5 and S1 is usually (but not always) accompanied by marked sclerosis of the adjoining end plates. *B.* Radiograph showing the anterior notching of vertebrae of a young adolescent where the unossified end plates, at this point cartilaginous, are situated. These become the secondary ossification centers in these sites.

fusion of the base and apex usually occurs by the age of 12 years. The odontoid process remains separated from the body of C2 by a cartilaginous disk and does not normally fuse until adulthood. If the odontoid fails to fuse with the body of C2 it is called an "os odontoideum" or "third condyle." Occasionally the apical ossification center of the odontoid process fails to appear and hence, ossification of this area does not proceed normally.

This area of the spine, then, is supported totally by the associated ligamentous structures. Other anomalies in this immediate vicinity may also result. For example, anomalies of fusion of the occipital bone and C1 may result in an extra partially fused vertebral segment between the formed occipital bone and atlas. This has been called by some the "pro-atlas" (Epstein; Wollin).

Various other abnormalities of the foramen magnum may occur as the result of anomalies of fusion of the occipital vertebrae. There may be an anterior condyle or lateral paracondyloid and basilar processes. Accessory bony elements may be fused with the rim of the foramen magnum. If the space for the cord is not compromised by extra bony elements or if the mobility of the upper cervical spine with respect to the skull and upper cord is not excessive because of these bony aberrations, such malformations are of little clinical importance. If there is encroachment or excessive mobility, surgical intervention is necessary.

At times an assimilation of the atlas and axis may occur, with complete or partial circumferential union of the first cervical vertebrae with the foramen magnum. In this instance also an instability of the atlas and axis or abnormal mobility of the dens may result, requiring surgical intervention.

Simultaneous congenital defects in both the anterior and posterior arches of the atlas have been reported (Budin and Sondheimer). Differentiation of these congenital defects from fractures of the ring of the atlas is essential. The anterior arch of the atlas commonly develops from a single midline ossification center which may, however, be bipartite—rarely, tripartite, or even entirely absent. Anterior spina bifida results when double centers fail to fuse as they normally should by the age of 8 or 9 years. Isolated spina bifida of the posterior arch of the atlas is a relatively common anomaly found in about 3 per cent of the largest series of investigations. This defect results from deficient posterior growth of the lateral mass epiphyses of this segment. Closure of the first neural arch normally occurs between the ages of 3 and 7 years.

The *union of laminae* begins in the lumbar region soon after birth (Fig. 9–9 *B*) and, spreading upward, is completed in the cervical region early in the second year, but not in the sacrum until the seventh to tenth years. After fusion of the laminae there is a

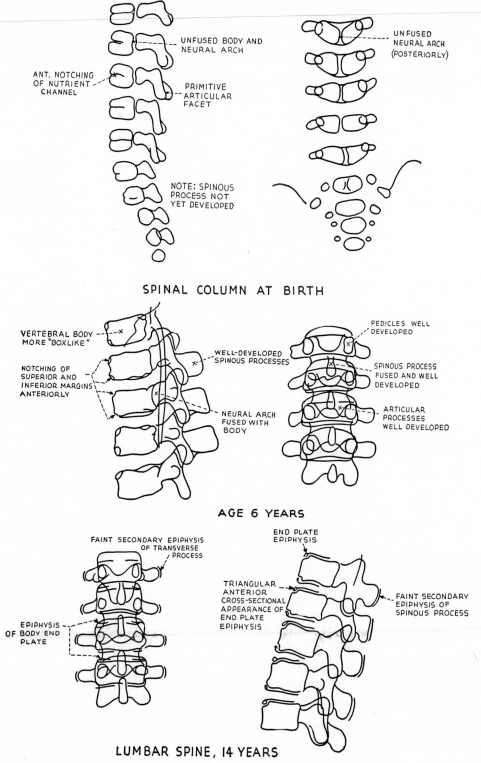

Figure 9-14. Spinal column at various stages of development.

gradual extension of the ossification process into the spinous processes.

The *bony union of the neural arch and the vertebral body* begins in the cervical area at the age of 3, and the process spreads downward in the spine to reach the sacrum in the sixth or seventh year (Fig. 9–14).

The growth pattern of vertebral bodies from T12 to L3 was studied by Brandner et al. in children of both sexes as well as adults; tabular values (see Tables 9–1 to 9–6) were presented for the ratio of the vertical diameter of these vertebral bodies to their sagittal diameters. Likewise, tabular values of the ratio of the intervertebral disk thickness to the vertical diameter of vertebral bodies were also presented (Tables 9–2, 9–3). It was demonstrated in this study that the index of the vertical to the sagittal diameter of T12 to L2 was significantly higher in the second month of life than in newborn, but after 18 months this index decreased and was stable. There was another rise from the fourth to the twelfth year. A sex difference was found in T12 and L1 in children 4 to 12 years old and in children at the age of puberty in that the index of vertical to sagittal diameter was higher in girls than in boys. This

TABLE 9–1 A

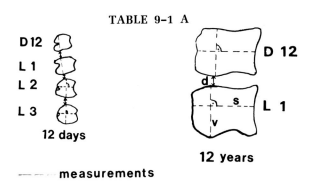

D 12
L 1
L 2
L 3

12 days

D 12
L 1

12 years

- - - - measurements

L 1
L 2
L 3

$\dfrac{v}{s} = I_{vb}$

$\dfrac{d}{v} = I_d$

9 days

Method of measuring vertebral bodies and disk spaces. Only dotted lines were measurable. This is the method used to form the indices.

TABLE 9–1   AGE GROUPS*

Group	I	II	III	IV	V
Age	0–1 month	2–18 months	19–36 months	4–12 years	13 years and more

*From Brandner, M. E.: Normal values of vertebral body and intervertebral disk index during growth. Amer. J. Roentgenol., *110*:618–627, 1970.

TABLE 9–2 $I_{vb}(v/s)$ OF DIFFERENT VERTEBRAL BODIES*

Vertebral Body	Age Group	n	Mean v/s	s	Range x ± 2s	p
D 12	I	13	0.81	0.061	0.69–0.93	<0.005
	II	26	0.91	0.077	0.75–1.06	
	III	22	0.86	0.066	0.73–0.99	≅0.10
	IV f	18	0.86	0.062	0.74–0.98	<0.001
	IV m	35	0.78	0.052	0.67–0.88	
	V f	7	0.93	0.148	0.64–1.23	<0.05
	V m	20	0.84	0.116	0.60–1.07	
L1	I	16	0.87	0.060	0.76–0.99	<0.001
	II f	11	1.02	0.066	0.88–1.15	<0.02
	II m	16	0.96	0.043	0.87–1.05	
	II m + f	27	0.98	0.055	0.87–1.09	<0.001
	III	23	0.89	0.080	0.73–1.05	
	IV f	20	0.87	0.068	0.73–1.00	<0.001 (IV f/m)
	IV m	40	0.80	0.048	0.70–0.90	<0.001 (IV f/Vf)
	V f	19	1.03	0.095	0.88–1.22	<0.001 (IV m/Vm)
	V m	27	0.87	0.063	0.74–0.99	<0.001 (V f/m)
L2	I	10	0.92	0.060	0.80–1.04	<0.01
	II	21	1.01	0.090	0.83–1.19	<0.001
	III	20	0.91	0.060	0.79–1.03	<0.001
	IV	49	0.82	0.076	0.67–0.97	<0.001
	V f	15	1.03	0.096	0.84–1.22	<0.001
	V m	25	0.88	0.086	0.70–1.05	
L3	I	11	0.95	0.068	0.81–1.08	<0.25
	II	17	0.98	0.084	0.81–1.15	<0.005
	III	16	0.88	0.081	0.72–1.04	<0.001
	IV	35	0.79	0.072	0.67–0.91	<0.001
	V f	11	1.00	0.101	0.80–1.20	<0.001
	V m	17	0.87	0.094	0.68–1.03	

*From Brandner, M. E.: Normal values of vertebral body and intervertebral disk index during growth. Amer. J. Roentgenol., *110*:618–627, 1970.
f = girls; m = boys; *n* = number; *v/s* = vertical/sagittal.

TABLE 9–3 $I_d(d/v)$ OF DIFFERENT VERTEBRAL SEGMENTS*

	Age Group	n	Mean d/v	s	Range x ± 2s	p
D 11/12	I	12	0.37	0.060	0.25–0.49	<0.005
	II	26	0.30	0.065	0.16–0.43	
	III	19	0.25	0.089	0.08–0.43	
	IV	49	0.24	0.053	0.13–0.34	≤0.001
	V	21	0.18	0.042	0.10–0.26	
D 12/L1	I	17	0.35	0.063	0.22–0.48	<0.01
	II	27	0.28	0.068	0.14–0.41	
	III	20	0.26	0.057	0.14–0.37	
	IV	53	0.25	0.050	0.15–0.35	≤0.001
	V	37	0.19	0.043	0.10–0.28	
L 1/2	I	15	0.35	0.046	0.26–0.44	<0.001
	II	26	0.26	0.073	0.12–0.41	
	III	19	0.27	0.055	0.15–0.38	>0.25
	IV	44	0.28	0.047	0.18–0.37	≤0.001
	V	37	0.20	0.056	0.09–0.31	
L 2/3	I	9	0.38	0.075	0.23–0.53	~0.01
	II	18	0.28	0.089	0.10–0.46	
	III	15	0.30	0.083	0.13–0.47	
	IV	32	0.30	0.049	0.20–0.40	≤0.001
	V	22	0.21	0.051	0.11–0.31	

*From Brandner, M. E.: Normal values of vertebral body and intervertebral disk index during growth. Amer. J. Roentgenol., *110*:618–627, 1970.
n = number; d/v = disk thickness/vertical; *s* = sagittal.

TABLE 9–4 VERTEBRAL AND INTERVERTEBRAL DISK SPACE MEASUREMENTS IN TEN YOUNG AND TEN OLDER WOMEN PATIENTS*

Vertebrae	Mean Intervertebral Disk Space (mm.)	Mean Height of Anterior Vertebral Border (mm.)	Mean Height of Posterior Vertebral Border (mm.)	Mean Midline Height of Vertebra (mm.)	Mean Width of Superior Border of Vertebra (mm.)	Mean Width of Inferior Border of Vertebra (mm.)	Range in Disk Space (mm.)	Mean Distance between Anterior Borders (mm.)	Mean Distance between Posterior Borders (mm.)	Mean Midline Width of Vertebra (mm.)	Mean Intervertebral Disk Space of Older Group (mm.)
L5–4 + L5	11.0	35.4	32.2	31.0	37.8	39.6	8–14	10.5	7.3	36.8	10.5
L4–3 + L4	10.2	35.1	33.7	28.0	39.0	38.3	7–17	12.4	6.8	36.8	11.7
L3–2 + L3	10.2	34.7	34.3	34.0	37.0	37.6	6–16	10.6	6.4	36.4	12.0
L2–1 + L2	7.9	32.9	33.7	29.0	34.9	36.5	3–10	8.0	4.4	34.2	10.3
L1–D12 + L1	6.9	31.7	32.4	31.0	35.8	33.3	5–12	6.8	4.7	34.3	8.8
D12–11 + D12	6.4	28.7	28.5	31.5	35.5	34.0	4–12	5.4	3.8	34.3	7.3
D11–10 + D11	4.7	26.7	27.1	28.5	35.2	35.2	4–8	4.5	3.7	33.9	6.5
D10–9 + D10	4.4	26.5	26.0	25.0	35.0	35.1	4–7	3.2	3.2	35.9	5.4
D9–8 + D9	4.4	24.8	24.9	25.0	33.8	33.8	4–5	2.9	2.6	36.5	4.7
D8–7 + D8	4.4	23.3	24.0	23.0	31.1	31.7	4–1	2.4	2.0	31.1	4.1
D7–6 + D7	4.0	23.5	23.7	22.0	29.6	31.4	3–8	2.5	2.3	29.4	3.8
Totals in mm. (to nearest integral)											
Younger group	75	323	321	308	386	388	3–17	69	47	379	
Older group[a]	84	321	337	316	386	395	3–14	63	40	374	

Mean age			Mean height	
Younger group	22 years (15–30)		Younger group	63.2 inches
Older group	62 years (47–75)		Older group	63.2 inches

*From Hurxthal, Z. M.: Measurement of anterior vertebral compressions and bioconcave vertebrae. Amer. J. Roentgenol., *103*:642, 1968.

[a]In order to save space, only the totals of the above columns are given (except for the last) for comparison purposes.

The disk space heights recorded here closely parallel those reported elsewhere, namely, 4–5 mm. for upper dorsal area, 6–8 mm. for lower dorsal area and 10–12 mm. for lumbar area.

was explained by the higher vertical diameters in girls older than 12 years or taller than 140 cm. and by higher sagittal diameters in boys. The intervertebral disk index (height of the intervertebral disk related to the height of the vertebral body just below it) decreased significantly after the first month of life and was almost stable until 12 years of age, when it decreased once more. No significant sex differences were found in this index. A comparable study in adults showed that the index for the vertebral bodies proved to be significantly higher in adult women than in men and was comparable to that of adolescents. The sexual difference was explained by the greater sagittal diameter of the vertebral bodies in men.

It has been shown that these indices are of some value in differentiation of different types of mucopolysaccharidoses. Somewhat comparable measurements by Hurxthal are also indicated in Table 9–4. This table presents the vertebral and intervertebral disk space measurements in 10 young women and 10 older women.

TABLE 9–5 $I_{vb}(v/s)$ OF DIFFERENT VERTEBRAL BODIES*

	Sex Group	n	Mean I_{vb}	s	Range $x \pm 2s$	p
D 12	♀	14	1.00	0.073	0.86–1.15	
	♂	—	—	—	—	
L 1	♀	15	1.03	0.057	0.92–1.15	$p < 0.001$
	♂	14	0.90	0.072	0.75–1.04	
L 2	♀	15	1.03	0.085	0.86–1.20	$p \sim 0.2$
	♂	9	0.96	0.091	0.78–1.14	
L 3	♀	12	0.97	0.081	0.81–1.13	
	♂	—	—	—	—	

*From Brandner, M. E.: Normal values of the vertebral body and intervertebral disk index in adults. Amer. J. Roentgenol., *114*:411–414, 1972.
♀Girls aged 18–24 years.
♂Men aged 18–27 years.
n = number; s = standard deviation.

TABLE 9-6 $I_d(d/v)$ OF DIFFERENT VERTEBRAL BODIES*

| | | Mean | | Range | |
	n	I_d	s	$x \pm 2s$	
D 11/12	10	0.14	0.026	0.09-0.19	♀ : $n = 10$
D 12/L 1	14	0.16	0.027	0.11-0.22	♀ : $n = 12$; ♂ : $n = 2$
L 1/2	12	0.19	0.035	0.12-0.26	♀ : $n = 10$; ♂ : $n = 2$
L 2/3	—	—	—	—	

*From Brandner, M. E.: Normal values of the vertebral body and intervertebral disk index in adults. Amer. J. Roentgenol., *114*:411–414, 1972.
♀ Girls aged 18–24 years.
♂ Men aged 18–27 years.
n = number; s = standard deviation.

Normal Interpediculate Distances in Children and Adults. A concept of the width of the spinal canal may be obtained by measurement of the distances between the inner margins of the pedicle as portrayed on the anteroposterior films of the spine. These have been plotted for individuals of different ages (Fig. 9-15). A gradual diminution has been noted in the dorsal spine to approximately T4 through T6, and thereafter a gradual increase in the measurement down to the lower lumbar region. Variations of 2 mm. or more are considered of significance. The most accurate concept of pediculate erosion is obtained by body section tomography (Fig. 9-16). Actually, the pedicles in the cervical

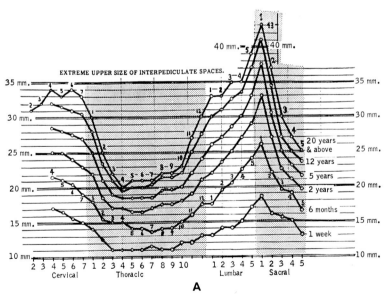

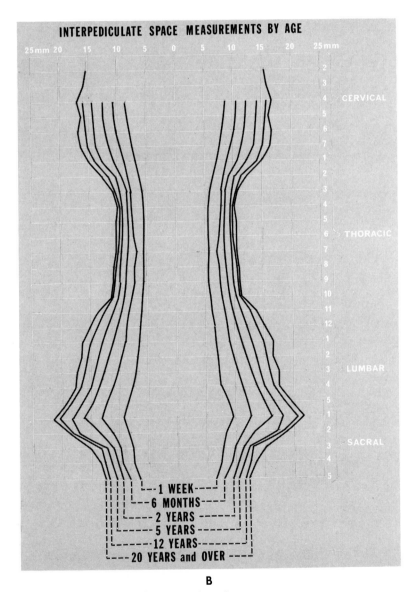

Figure 9–15. A. Composite graph showing extreme upper measurements of interpediculate spaces in various age groups. Variations of 2 mm. or more are considered significant, suggesting a mass lesion of the spinal canal. (From Schwarz, G. S.: Amer. J. Roentgenol., 76:476, 1956.) B. Chart for determination of interpedicular distances of the spine, adapted from chart in A.

region are difficult to identify, especially in a child, and the graph shows these values for children only to the level of C4 vertebra.

Hinck, Clark, and Hopkins (1966) published refined maximum and minimum interpediculate distances in children and adults, exploring particularly the possibility of minimum measurements as well as maximal. They pointed out that the subject of spinal canal stenosis caused by a decrease of interpediculate distances is virtually unexplored and is possibly as important as the increased interpediculate measurement (see Tables 9–7 to 9–10).

Motion Studies of the Spine. Cineradiography lends itself to the study of the spine in motion as it does with other moving parts of the body. Somewhat similar information, although not nearly as extensive, may be derived by attaining flexion, neutral, and extension studies of the various parts of the spine and making appropriate measurements. Thus, for example, flexion and extension studies of the cervical and lumbar spine are shown in Figure 9–17. A lateral view of the lumbar spine with tracings

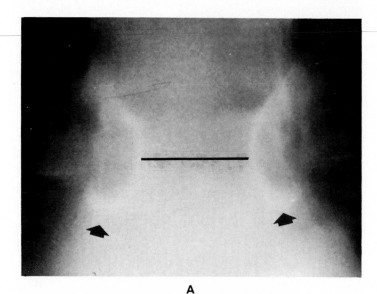

A

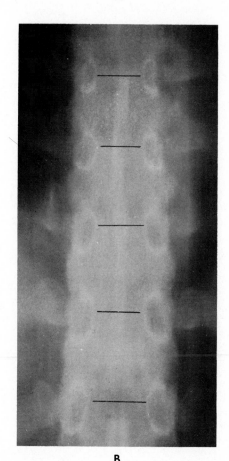

B

Figure 9–16. *A* and *B*. Radiographs showing advantage of tomography for demonstration of pedicles.

TABLE 9–7 MEAN INTERPEDICULATE DISTANCE (IPD) OF EACH VERTEBRA BY AGE (Male [mm.])*

	Age Group (yr.)							
	3, 4, 5	*6, 7, 8*	*9, 10*	*11, 12*	*13, 14*	*15, 16*	*17, 18*	*Adult*
Age (yr.)	4.0	7.0	9.4	11.6	13.5	15.6	17.4	>18
Vertebra								
C3	24.3	26.3	26.9	26.0	26.9	27.9	28.6	28.6
4	25.5	27.4	27.3	27.8	28.0	28.8	29.5	29.5
5	26.1	27.8	27.5	27.0	28.4	29.3	29.9	30.3
6	25.8	28.2	27.3	27.2	28.4	29.2	30.1	30.2
7	24.8	27.1	26.2	26.0	27.3	28.0	28.8	29.3
T1	22.5	22.7	23.8	23.8	24.2	25.2	24.5	25.1
2	19.4	19.7	20.4	20.6	20.6	21.7	21.2	21.4
3	17.9	18.1	19.0	18.8	19.1	19.2	19.4	19.6
4	16.9	17.6	18.2	17.6	18.3	18.0	18.7	18.8
5	16.4	17.3	17.4	17.4	18.3	17.7	18.4	18.2
6	16.5	17.3	18.8	17.4	18.3	17.3	18.2	17.8
7	16.7	17.5	16.5	17.4	18.5	17.6	17.9	17.8
8	17.0	18.1	16.7	17.6	18.9	18.3	18.4	18.0
9	17.0	18.5	17.0	17.8	19.3	18.6	18.7	18.6
10	16.9	18.8	17.3	18.1	19.5	18.1	18.9	19.1
11	18.2	20.1	18.8	19.2	20.9	19.8	20.2	20.4
12	20.4	22.5	21.3	21.8	23.5	23.2	23.4	23.5
L1	20.7	22.5	23.3	23.9	23.8	24.5	25.1	25.9
2	20.7	22.4	23.5	24.2	23.3	24.6	24.8	26.5
3	21.2	23.0	24.1	24.6	23.6	25.1	25.2	26.8
4	21.9	23.6	24.8	23.6	24.7	26.0	26.6	27.6
5	24.7	26.9	28.4	28.9	28.0	30.1	29.9	30.7

*From Hinck, V. C., Clark, W. M., and Hopkins, C. E.: Normal interpediculate distances (minimum and maximum) in children and adults. Amer. J. Roentgenol., *97*:141–153, 1966.

TABLE 9–8 MEAN INTERPEDICULATE DISTANCE (IPD) OF EACH VERTEBRA BY AGE (Female [mm.])*

Age Group (yr.)

Vertebra	3, 4, 5	6, 7, 8	9, 10	11, 12	13, 14	15, 16	17, 18	Adult
Age (yr.)	4.2	7.2	9.6	11.6	13.7	15.5	17.6	>18
C3	22.1	25.5	24.8	26.6	27.5	26.6	26.6	27.4
4	22.2	26.0	25.6	27.4	28.4	27.7	27.5	28.2
5	22.3	26.4	25.9	28.0	28.7	28.1	27.9	28.7
6	23.6	26.7	26.0	27.3	28.6	27.5	28.0	28.6
7	24.0	25.5	26.3	25.8	27.1	26.1	26.1	27.1
T1	19.8	22.1	23.1	23.0	22.6	22.3	22.4	23.1
2	16.6	18.2	19.7	18.8	19.6	18.9	19.1	19.8
3	15.2	17.0	17.9	17.5	18.3	17.6	17.9	18.2
4	14.6	16.3	17.1	16.6	17.8	16.9	17.4	17.4
5	14.6	16.3	16.6	16.0	17.2	16.8	17.1	17.1
6	14.5	16.1	16.3	15.9	17.4	16.5	16.9	16.9
7	14.7	16.3	16.5	16.1	17.8	16.6	17.4	17.0
8	15.0	16.9	16.6	16.4	18.0	16.8	17.8	17.4
9	15.1	17.1	16.9	16.8	18.1	17.3	18.2	17.9
10	15.4	17.3	17.1	17.1	18.2	17.7	18.7	18.4
11	16.5	18.0	18.2	18.4	19.8	19.2	19.9	20.0
12	19.1	20.2	21.1	20.9	22.8	21.7	22.5	22.9
L1	20.1	21.0	22.5	22.2	23.7	23.6	24.1	24.3
2	20.0	21.1	22.6	22.3	23.6	23.6	24.2	24.9
3	20.2	21.7	23.2	22.8	24.6	24.4	24.5	25.4
4	21.1	23.0	24.7	24.2	26.9	25.4	25.8	26.4
5	23.9	26.1	28.2	28.5	30.4	28.6	29.5	29.0

*From Hinck, V. C., Clark, W. M., and Hopkins, C. E.: Normal interpediculate distances (minimum and maximum) in children and adults. Amer. J. Roentgenol., 97:141–153, 1966.

superimposed in flexion, neutral, and extension positions enables the radiologist to plot angles of movement in these various positions so that any change in the smoothness of the curvature may be apparent in localizing altered mobility from any cause. The relative movement of various elements of the spine may also be studied by bending the patient from right to left as shown in the accompanying illustration (Fig. 9–18). This method of analysis is important in measuring the degree of curvature in scoliosis. When the spine is bent, the primary curvature remains relatively constant, whereas the secondary curvature tends to correct itself. By drawing lines as shown before and after the tilt test, the primary curvature can be determined first, the secondary curvature next, and finally the degree of correction required. Both Cobb's method and Ferguson's method are outlined.

Various techniques have been devised for analyzing the curvature at the lumbosacral junction and also the degree of slippage of one vertebral body with another when this occurs (spondylolisthesis). The method utilized by the author in analysis of spon-

dylolisthesis is shown in Figure 9–19. The angle drawn should not exceed 2 or 3 degrees, as shown, or, if the lines are parallel, it should not exceed 3 mm., in our experience. Greater angulation indicates an abnormal state. This method is particularly applicable to the study of vertebral slippage and to changes evident in progression from the erect to the recumbent positions, when similar projections are available with the patient first recumbent and then erect (Fig. 9–20). Hyperextension and hyperflexion of the spine may thereby be studied also. Variations of normal in respect to the lumbosacral junction are shown in Figure 9–21. When L5 is projected slightly in front of the sacrum and yet has not actually slipped and has no defect in the pars interarticularis, this is called a pseudospondylolisthesis. At times, projection phenomena will produce the appearance of reverse spondylolisthesis. Reverse spondylolisthesis may actually exist but it is probable that no pathologic significance can be attributed to this.

The lumbosacral angle has also been measured by what is called Ferguson's angle. In the upright position this angle has been shown to measure 41.1 degrees $\pm$ 7.7 degrees (Hellems and Keats), in contrast with the recumbent angle demonstrated by Ferguson (34°).

The normal mechanism of movement between the lower cer-

TABLE 9–9 STANDARD DEVIATION OF INTERPEDICULATE DISTANCE (IPD) OF EACH VERTEBRA BY AGE (Male and Female Combined [mm.])*

Age Group (yr.)

Vertebra	3, 4, 5	6, 7, 8	9, 10	11, 12	13, 14	15, 16	17, 18	Adult
			Standard Deviation in mm. (Sample Size, N)					
Age (yr.)	.09 (35)	.08 (52)	.05 (30)	.05 (46)	.05 (59)	.05 (63)	.05 (68)	—(121)
C3	1.7 (8)	1.5 (18)	1.7 (8)	2.6 (18)	1.2 (22)	1.8 (17)	1.9 (21)	1.5 (36)
4	1.7 (8)	1.5 (18)	1.3 (8)	2.5 (18)	1.5 (23)	1.6 (18)	2.0 (22)	1.5 (43)
5	1.7 (8)	1.7 (18)	1.6 (8)	2.6 (19)	1.7 (23)	1.6 (18)	2.1 (22)	1.7 (44)
6	1.7 (9)	1.7 (18)	1.7 (8)	2.7 (20)	2.1 (23)	1.8 (20)	2.2 (24)	1.8 (50)
7	1.4 (9)	2.0 (19)	2.1 (8)	2.8 (21)	1.8 (25)	2.4 (21)	2.1 (24)	2.0 (60)
T1	2.5 (12)	1.9 (14)	1.4 (10)	2.2 (22)	1.5 (17)	2.3 (19)	1.6 (27)	1.8 (53)
2	2.2 (12)	1.6 (14)	1.2 (10)	2.0 (23)	1.8 (17)	2.4 (21)	1.4 (27)	1.7 (53)
3	1.6 (12)	1.5 (14)	0.9 (9)	1.6 (23)	1.6 (17)	1.5 (20)	1.3 (27)	1.5 (50)
4	1.5 (12)	1.4 (14)	1.0 (9)	1.7 (23)	1.8 (15)	1.3 (19)	1.3 (26)	1.6 (43)
5	1.4 (13)	1.2 (14)	0.8 (9)	1.6 (22)	1.8 (15)	1.4 (19)	1.3 (25)	1.7 (42)
6	1.6 (13)	1.2 (13)	1.0 (9)	1.5 (22)	1.8 (15)	1.3 (19)	1.6 (25)	1.5 (42)
7	1.6 (12)	1.2 (13)	1.3 (9)	1.4 (22)	1.9 (15)	1.6 (19)	1.5 (26)	1.5 (42)
8	1.6 (13)	1.4 (14)	1.0 (9)	1.5 (22)	1.9 (15)	1.6 (19)	1.5 (25)	1.5 (41)
9	1.5 (13)	1.3 (15)	1.3 (10)	1.6 (23)	1.8 (15)	1.8 (19)	1.6 (26)	1.5 (43)
10	1.3 (14)	1.4 (17)	1.6 (10)	1.7 (23)	2.0 (17)	1.6 (20)	1.5 (26)	1.6 (44)
11	1.5 (15)	1.9 (17)	1.8 (10)	1.8 (23)	2.3 (18)	1.7 (24)	1.7 (30)	1.8 (53)
12	1.5 (17)	2.1 (17)	1.6 (11)	1.8 (24)	2.3 (20)	1.7 (28)	1.7 (31)	2.0 (59)
L1	1.6 (26)	1.9 (33)	1.8 (20)	1.7 (26)	1.6 (35)	2.0 (40)	2.4 (37)	2.2 (59)
2	1.5 (26)	2.0 (32)	1.6 (20)	1.8 (25)	1.6 (35)	1.8 (40)	2.2 (36)	2.3 (57)
3	1.6 (26)	2.1 (33)	1.7 (20)	1.9 (25)	2.0 (35)	1.9 (40)	2.3 (36)	2.7 (53)
4	1.7 (26)	2.1 (33)	2.3 (20)	3.1 (24)	3.3 (34)	2.4 (39)	2.9 (36)	3.0 (52)
5	1.9 (26)	3.1 (33)	2.7 (20)	3.1 (23)	3.6 (34)	2.9 (38)	3.6 (35)	3.7 (50)

*From Hinck, V. C., Clark, W. M., and Hopkins, C. E.: Normal interpediculate distances (minimum and maximum) in children and adults. Amer. J. Roentgenol., 97:141–153, 1966.

TABLE 9–10 TOLERANCE RANGE (90 PER CENT) OF INTERPEDICULATE DISTANCE (IPD) OF EACH VERTEBRA BY AGE (Male and Female Combined [mm.])*

			Age Group (yr.)										Age Group (yr.)					
	3, 4, 5	6, 7, 8	9, 10	11, 12	13, 14	15, 16	17, 18	Adult		3, 4, 5	6, 7, 8	9, 10	11, 12	13, 14	15, 16	17, 18	Adult
Vertebra									*Vertebra*								
C3	18–29	22–30	21–32	20–32	24–31	23–31	23–32	25–31	T7	12–20	13–21	14–20	13–20	14–22	13–21	15–21	14–20
4	19–30	23–31	21–32	21–33	25–32	24–32	24–33	26–32	8	12–21	14–21	14–20	13–21	14–23	14–21	15–21	15–21
5	20–31	23–31	22–32	21–32	25–32	25–32	25–34	26–33	9	12–21	14–21	13–21	14–21	15–23	14–22	15–21	15–21
6	20–31	24–31	22–32	21–33	25–32	24–33	25–34	26–33	10	12–21	15–22	13–21	14–21	15–23	14–22	16–22	16–22
7	19–30	23–31	21–32	20–32	24–31	21–32	23–32	24–32	11	13–22	16–23	14–23	15–22	16–25	16–23	17–23	17–24
									12	16–24	18–25	17–25	18–25	19–27	18–26	20–26	19–27
T1	17–26	19–26	20–27	20–27	19–28	18–29	20–26	20–28									
2	14–22	15–22	17–24	16–24	16–24	14–25	17–23	17–24	L1	17–24	17–27	19–28	19–27	20–27	20–28	20–29	21–29
3	13–21	14–21	15–21	14–22	15–23	15–22	15–21	16–22	2	17–24	17–27	19–28	19–27	20–27	20–28	20–29	21–30
4	12–20	14–21	15–21	14–21	14–22	14–20	15–21	15–21	3	17–24	17–27	19–28	20–27	21–28	21–29	20–29	21–31
5	12–20	13–20	14–20	13–21	14–22	14–21	15–21	14–21	4	18–25	18–28	20–29	20–28	19–33	21–30	19–33	21–33
6	12–20	13–20	14–20	13–20	14–22	13–20	14–20	14–20	5	21–28	22–32	24–33	24–34	22–36	23–35	23–37	23–37

*From Hinck, V. C., Clark, W. M., and Hopkins, C. E.: Normal interpediculate distances (minimum and maximum) in children and adults. Amer. J. Roentgenol., *97*:141–153, 1966.

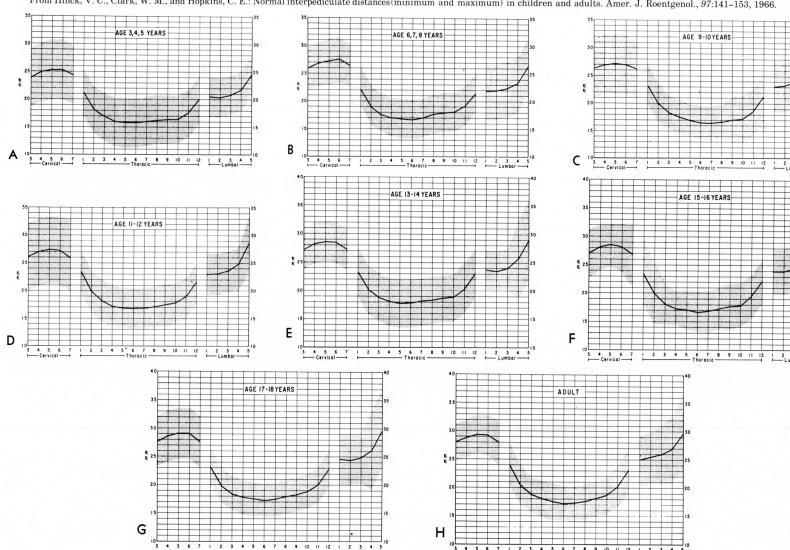

TABLE 9–10A. Tolerance range (90 per cent) of interpediculate distance (IPD). each vertebra, male and female combined. (*A*) Age 3–5 years, (*B*) age 6–8 years, (*C*) age 9–10 years, (*D*) age 11–12 years, (*E*) age 13–14 years, (*F*) age 15–16 years, (*G*) age 17–18 years, (*H*) adult.

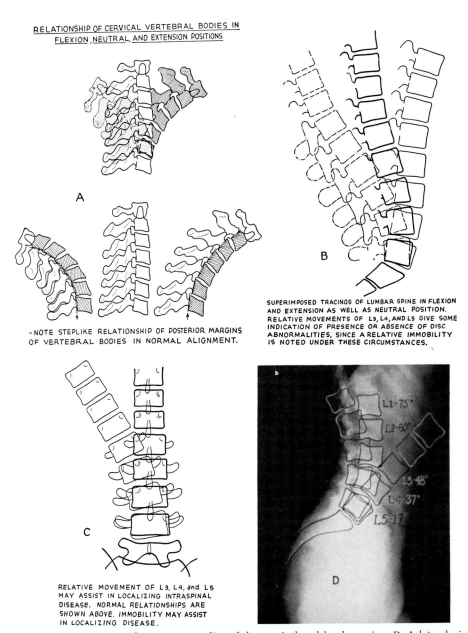

RELATIONSHIP OF CERVICAL VERTEBRAL BODIES IN
FLEXION, NEUTRAL, AND EXTENSION POSITIONS

A

-NOTE STEPLIKE RELATIONSHIP OF POSTERIOR MARGINS
OF VERTEBRAL BODIES IN NORMAL ALIGNMENT.

B

SUPERIMPOSED TRACINGS OF LUMBAR SPINE IN FLEXION
AND EXTENSION AS WELL AS NEUTRAL POSITION.
RELATIVE MOVEMENTS OF L3, L4, AND L5 GIVE SOME
INDICATION OF PRESENCE OR ABSENCE OF DISC
ABNORMALITIES, SINCE A RELATIVE IMMOBILITY
IS NOTED UNDER THESE CIRCUMSTANCES.

C

RELATIVE MOVEMENT OF L3, L4, and L5
MAY ASSIST IN LOCALIZING INTRASPINAL
DISEASE. NORMAL RELATIONSHIPS ARE
SHOWN ABOVE. IMMOBILITY MAY ASSIST
IN LOCALIZING DISEASE.

L1-75°
L2-60°
L3-48°
L4-37°
L5-17°

D

Figure 9–17. A to C. Flexion and extension studies of the cervical and lumbar spine. D. A lateral view of the lumbar spine with tracing superimposed on the lumbar spine in flexion, neutral position, and extension. A method is devised for determining the total change of angulation of each vertebral body. If these angles were plotted, a smooth curve would be obtained. Any change in the smoothness of this curve may be significant in localizing altered mobility from any cause.

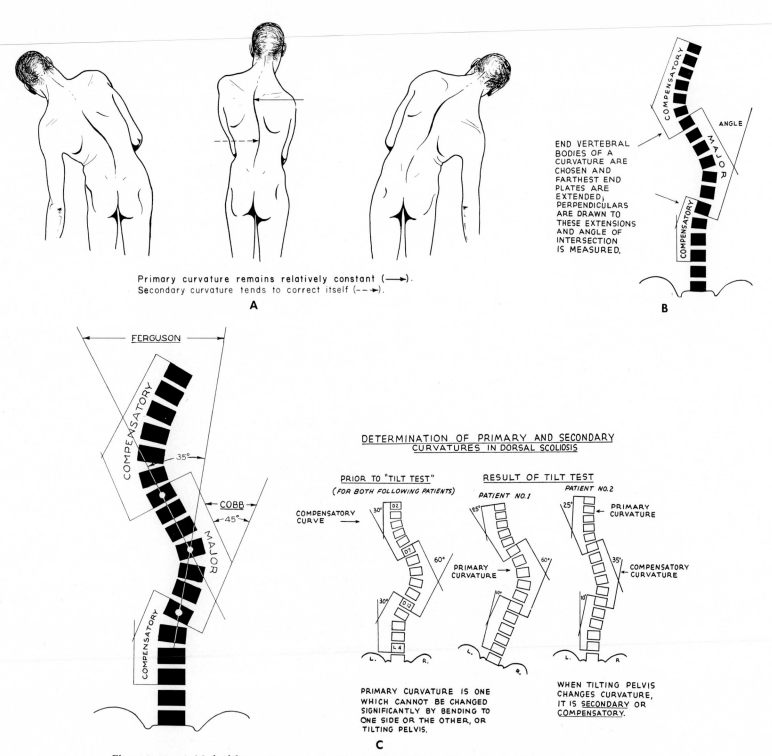

Primary curvature remains relatively constant (———➤).
Secondary curvature tends to correct itself (— —➤).

A

END VERTEBRAL BODIES OF A CURVATURE ARE CHOSEN AND FARTHEST END PLATES ARE EXTENDED; PERPENDICULARS ARE DRAWN TO THESE EXTENSIONS AND ANGLE OF INTERSECTION IS MEASURED.

B

DETERMINATION OF PRIMARY AND SECONDARY CURVATURES IN DORSAL SCOLIOSIS

PRIOR TO "TILT TEST" (FOR BOTH FOLLOWING PATIENTS)

RESULT OF TILT TEST

PATIENT NO.1

PATIENT NO.2

COMPENSATORY CURVE

PRIMARY CURVATURE

PRIMARY CURVATURE

PRIMARY CURVATURE

COMPENSATORY CURVATURE

PRIMARY CURVATURE IS ONE WHICH CANNOT BE CHANGED SIGNIFICANTLY BY BENDING TO ONE SIDE OR THE OTHER, OR TILTING PELVIS.

WHEN TILTING PELVIS CHANGES CURVATURE, IT IS SECONDARY OR COMPENSATORY.

C

Figure 9–18. *A.* Method for positioning patient for study of scoliosis of the spine. *B.* Method of measuring scoliosis. *C.* Methods of measuring dorsal spine scoliosis. *Left,* Modified to show Cobb's method of measurement as well as Ferguson's. *Right,* Tilt test in determination of curvature of spine. (Modified from Ferguson, A. B.: Roentgen Diagnosis of Extremities and Spine. New York, Paul B. Hoeber, Inc., 1949.)

A RADIOGRAPHIC ANALYSIS OF SPONDYLOLISTHESIS

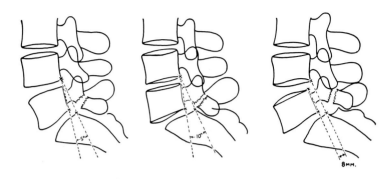

TRACINGS OF RADIOGRAPHS OF SUBJECTS WITH SPONDYLOLISTHESIS. THE LINES EITHER INTERSECT ABOVE THE FIFTH LUMBAR VERTEBRA AND FORM AN ANGLE EXCEEDING 2° (A and B) OR REMAIN PARALLEL, BUT ARE MORE THAN 3 MM. APART (C).

[A]

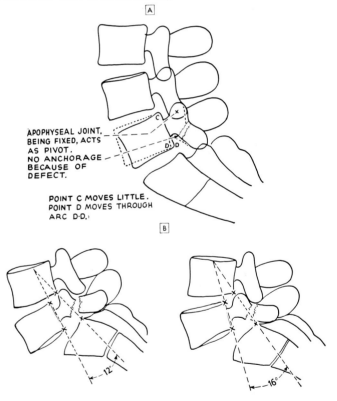

APOPHYSEAL JOINT, BEING FIXED, ACTS AS PIVOT. NO ANCHORAGE BECAUSE OF DEFECT.

POINT C MOVES LITTLE. POINT D MOVES THROUGH ARC D-D₁

[B]

SPONDYLOLISTHESIS AFFECTING THE FIFTH LUMBAR VERTEBRA. TRACINGS OF RADIOGRAPHS TO DEMONSTRATE AN INSTABILITY OF 4° (16° MINUS 12°); (A) WEIGHT-BEARING FLEXION - THE MINIMUM DEGREE OF SLIPPING IS FREQUENTLY FOUND IN FLEXION.

(B) WEIGHT-BEARING EXTENSION - THE MAXIMUM DEGREE OF SLIPPING IS FOUND IN EXTENSION.

[C]

Figure 9–19. *A.* Radiographic analysis of spondylolisthesis showing a method of lining and detection. *B.* Diagram illustrating the usual mechanism of spondylolisthesis. *C.* Tracings demonstrating method of measuring instability at the lumbosacral region in erect flexion and extension with spondylolisthesis.

vical and upper thoracic vertebrae in various extreme postures of the vertebral column was studied by Penning in both nonpathologic and pathologic relationships. He pointed out that in flexion the dorsal borders of the cervical bodies are arranged like a flight of steps (Fig. 9–17 *A*), while in extension this arrangement resembles a washboard. The gliding motion of the articular facets was also investigated by his method (Fig. 9–23).

The Cervical Spine (Fig. 9–24)

The atlas and axis differ with regard to development from the rest of the vertebrae in that the ossification center for the body of C1 separates from the rest of this vertebra and unites with the body of C2 to form the odontoid process. An epiphysis for the top of the odontoid process appears between the second and sixth years and unites with the others usually before 12 years of age. The base of the odontoid process is formed from two ossification centers, which appear at approximately the sixth fetal month and fuse at the time of birth. This fusion creates a wedge-shaped process that extends superiorly behind the anterior ring of the atlas, to unite ultimately with the separate ossification center for the odontoid process near its apex. The latter does not appear roentgenographically until at least 2 years of age. Fusion of the base and the apex usually occurs by 12 years of age. The spine of the atlas is represented by the tubercle on the posterior arch. (Spines are absent below the level of the third sacral segment.) The articular process of the atlas and the superior articular process of the axis are not truly homologous with the articular processes of the other vertebrae, and are virtually absent as such in these segments—the articular function in the atlas and superior articular process of the axis being taken over by a modification of the costal pits. *The articular surfaces of C1 and the upper articular surface of C2 are thus more anteriorly situated than the other articulations in the cervical spine.*

Occasionally occipitalization of the atlas will occur as previously described.

The alignment of C1 with respect to the foramen magnum of the skull is illustrated in Figure 9–25 *A.* When a straight line is drawn along the front of the odontoid process, it meets the anterior margin of the foramen magnum, and a line drawn above the inner margin of the posterior arch of C1 will meet the posterior margin of the foramen magnum. Lines drawn along the anterior margins and posterior margins of the vertebral bodies are practically parallel. A line connecting the anterior margins of the spinous processes forms a gentle continuous curvature, meeting the posterior margin of the foramen magnum. The curvature of the cervical spine virtually disappears when the neck is flexed, but these linear relationships persist, and a deviation is definitely significant.

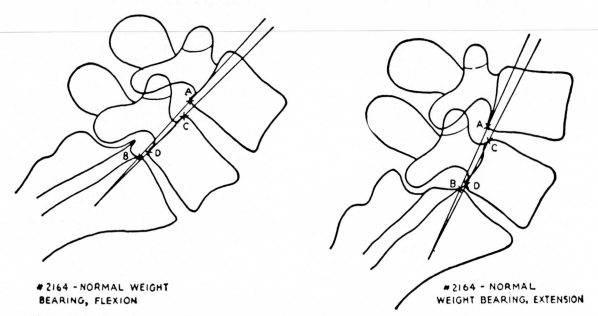

#2164 - NORMAL WEIGHT
BEARING, FLEXION

#2164 - NORMAL
WEIGHT BEARING, EXTENSION

Figure 9–20. Special views utilized for detecting degree of mobility of the lumbosacral spine in flexion and extension.

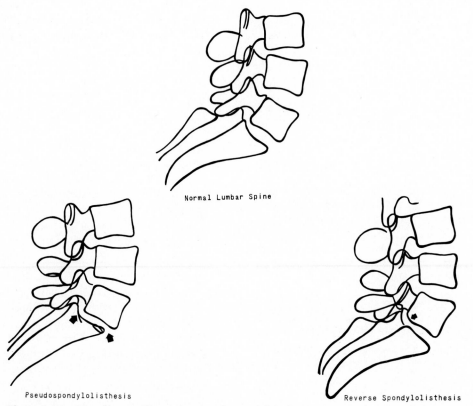

Normal Lumbar Spine

Pseudospondylolisthesis

Reverse Spondylolisthesis

Figure 9–21. Line diagram illustrating pseudospondylolisthesis and reverse spondylolisthesis.

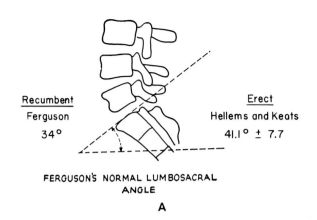

Recumbent
Ferguson
34°

Erect
Hellems and Keats
41.1° ± 7.7

FERGUSON'S NORMAL LUMBOSACRAL ANGLE

A

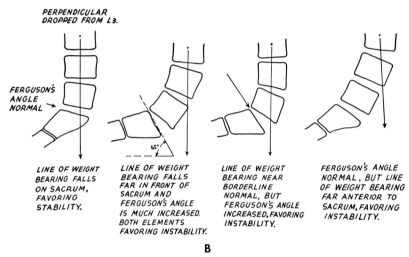

PERPENDICULAR DROPPED FROM L3.

FERGUSON'S ANGLE NORMAL →

65°

LINE OF WEIGHT BEARING FALLS ON SACRUM, FAVORING STABILITY.

LINE OF WEIGHT BEARING FALLS FAR IN FRONT OF SACRUM AND FERGUSON'S ANGLE IS MUCH INCREASED. BOTH ELEMENTS FAVORING INSTABILITY.

LINE OF WEIGHT BEARING NEAR BORDERLINE NORMAL, BUT FERGUSON'S ANGLE INCREASED, FAVORING INSTABILITY.

FERGUSON'S ANGLE NORMAL, BUT LINE OF WEIGHT BEARING FAR ANTERIOR TO SACRUM, FAVORING INSTABILITY.

B

Figure 9–22. Analysis of two factors in lumbosacral instability. (Modified from Ferguson, A. B.: Roentgen Diagnosis of Extremities and Spine. New York, Paul B. Hoeber, Inc., 1949.)

Another mode of alignment of the cervical spine with respect to the skull is referred to as "Chamberlain's line" (Fig. 9–25 A): Normally, a line drawn from the hard palate to the inner table of the occipital bone will fall just above the odontoid process. An abnormality (basilar impression) usually exists if this does not occur. Other relationships of the odontoid process to the foramen magnum and base of the skull are illustrated in Figure 9–25 C. Whereas Chamberlain's line is drawn from the superior margin of the hard palate to the inner table aspect of the posterior margin of the foramen magnum, McGregor's line is drawn from the hard palate to the external aspect of the posterior margin of the foramen magnum. Thus, whereas the tip of the dens to Chamberlain's line equals 1 ± 3.6 mm., the tip of the dens to McGregor's line equals 1.3 ± 2.6 mm. The maximum allowable distance for

the dens to project above these lines normally is approximately 4.5 mm., according to McGregor.

Another line of interest is one drawn from the tuberculum sellae to the internal occipital protuberance, as shown in Figure 9–25 C. Usually, the distance of the tip of the dens to this line is 30 mm. or more. Anything less than 30 mm. may be regarded as abnormal. Other lines that evaluate the relationship of the odontoid process are Fischgold's biventor line and Fischgold's bimastoid line, as shown. A line drawn between the tips of the mastoid processes usually will intersect the tip of the dens, and the biventor line will usually lie more than 1 cm. above this line. For reference purposes the relationship of the foramen magnum to the inner aspect of the clivus is also shown as Boogaard's angle; it should measure between 119 and 136 degrees.

The undeflected contour of the line joining the posterior margins of the vertebral bodies is most important (Fig. 9–25 A).

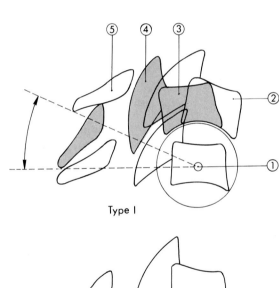

Type I

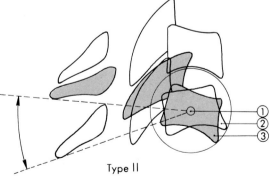

Type II

Figure 9–23. Diagrams of two types of motor function indicating the relative movement in the sagittal plane of a pair of lower cervical vertebrae. In Type I, the superior vertebra is supposed to be fixed, while the inferior vertebra is in the extreme flexion and extension positions. In Type II the reverse is presumed. (1) Motor axis, (2) flexed position of the mobile vertebra, (3) extended position, (4) articular process, (5) spinous process. Total movement range 29 degrees. (Reproduced with permission from J. Bone Joint Surg., 45A:1671–1678, 1963.)

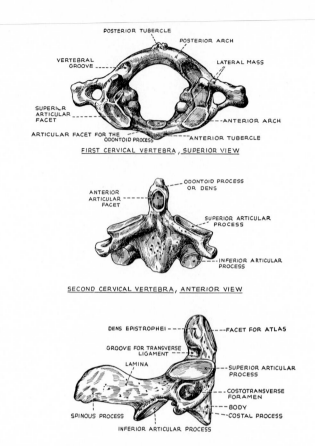

FIRST CERVICAL VERTEBRA, SUPERIOR VIEW

SECOND CERVICAL VERTEBRA, ANTERIOR VIEW

THE EPISTROPHEUS OR AXIS

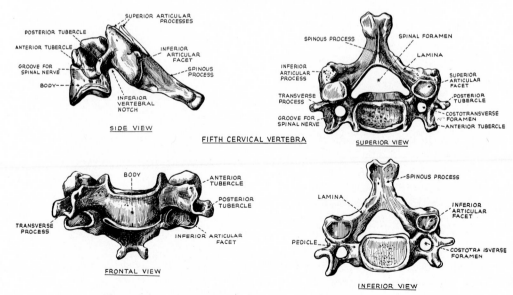

SIDE VIEW

FIFTH CERVICAL VERTEBRA

SUPERIOR VIEW

FRONTAL VIEW

INFERIOR VIEW

Figure 9–24. Distinguishing characteristics of cervical vertebrae.

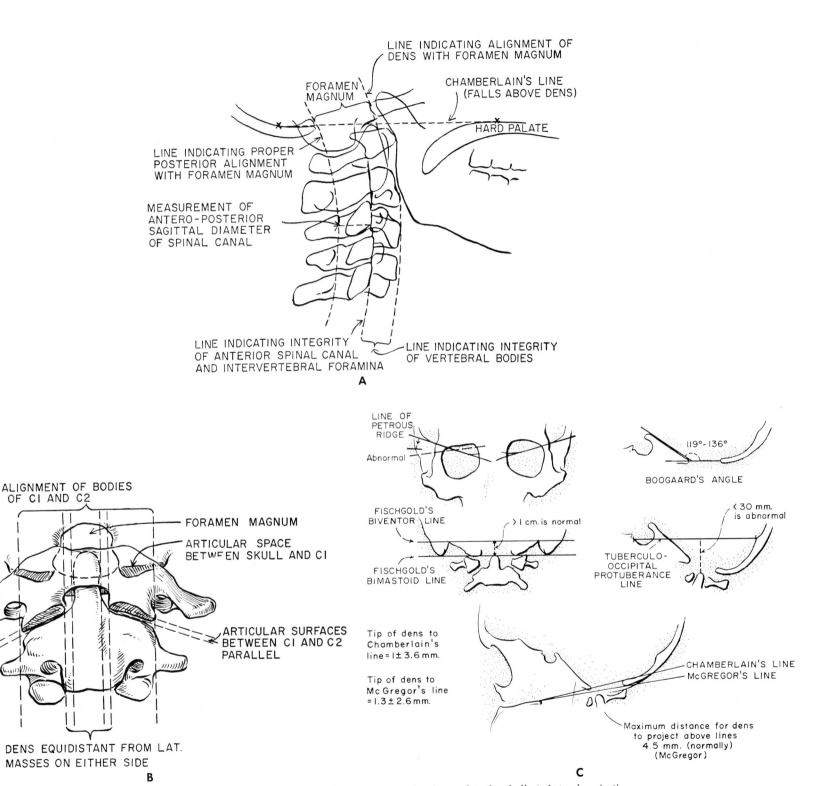

LINE INDICATING ALIGNMENT OF DENS WITH FORAMEN MAGNUM

FORAMEN MAGNUM

CHAMBERLAIN'S LINE (FALLS ABOVE DENS)

HARD PALATE

LINE INDICATING PROPER POSTERIOR ALIGNMENT WITH FORAMEN MAGNUM

MEASUREMENT OF ANTERO-POSTERIOR SAGITTAL DIAMETER OF SPINAL CANAL

LINE INDICATING INTEGRITY OF ANTERIOR SPINAL CANAL AND INTERVERTEBRAL FORAMINA

LINE INDICATING INTEGRITY OF VERTEBRAL BODIES

A

ALIGNMENT OF BODIES OF CI AND C2

FORAMEN MAGNUM

ARTICULAR SPACE BETWEEN SKULL AND CI

ARTICULAR SURFACES BETWEEN CI AND C2 PARALLEL

DENS EQUIDISTANT FROM LAT. MASSES ON EITHER SIDE

B

LINE OF PETROUS RIDGE

Abnormal

FISCHGOLD'S BIVENTOR LINE

> 1 cm. is normal

FISCHGOLD'S BIMASTOID LINE

Tip of dens to Chamberlain's line = 1 ± 3.6 mm.

Tip of dens to McGregor's line = 1.3 ± 2.6 mm.

119°-136°

BOOGAARD'S ANGLE

< 30 mm. is abnormal

TUBERCULO-OCCIPITAL PROTUBERANCE LINE

CHAMBERLAIN'S LINE
McGREGOR'S LINE

Maximum distance for dens to project above lines 4.5 mm. (normally) (McGregor)

C

Figure 9–25. Alignment of cervical segments with respect to each other and to the skull. A. Lateral projection. B. Odontoid projection. C. Various roentgen criteria for platybasia and basilar impression.

Deflections usually indicate small spurs that may encroach upon the spinal canal or intervertebral foramina.

The visualization of the odontoid process in the anteroposterior projection requires special techniques (Fig. 9–29). This is accomplished either by opening the mouth, by moving the mandible while the exposure is made (so that it does not obscure the upper cervical spine), or by body section radiography. Also, a short film-target distance is employed to distort the mandible out of clear view.

The symmetrical appearance of the odontoid with respect to the surrounding articulation is clearly demonstrated by the lines drawn as illustrated (Fig. 9–25).

The vertebral bodies below C2 level are very regular and similar in appearance, with the exception of C5, which very frequently normally appears somewhat narrowed anteriorly. This variation of normal must not be misinterpreted.

With the exception of C1 and C7, all of the vertebrae have somewhat bifid spinous processes. The transverse processes of C7 may be considerably elongated, and its costal element may actu-

ally form a complete rib, in which case it is known as a cervical rib.

In the anteroposterior projection the lateral mass and the articular processes are projected over one another. To visualize the two separately, the lateral projection is obtained, on which the articular processes are projected posteriorly (Fig. 9–26).

The intervertebral foramina are best shown in the oblique projection (Fig. 9–26). These are ovoid in shape, and tend to diminish slightly in size between the levels of C2 and C5, and then to increase slightly. Great variations in size are of definite significance from the standpoint of possible encroachment on nerve structures contained therein.

Measurements of the anteroposterior diameter of the bony cervical canal as well as of the adjoining soft tissue spaces assume considerable clinical significance. The measurements of Wolf et al. and those of Wholey et al. agree fundamentally and are shown in the accompanying illustration (Fig. 9–27). Wolf et al. concluded that a sagittal diameter of 10 mm. or less anywhere in the cervical spinal canal is likely to be associated with cord compres-

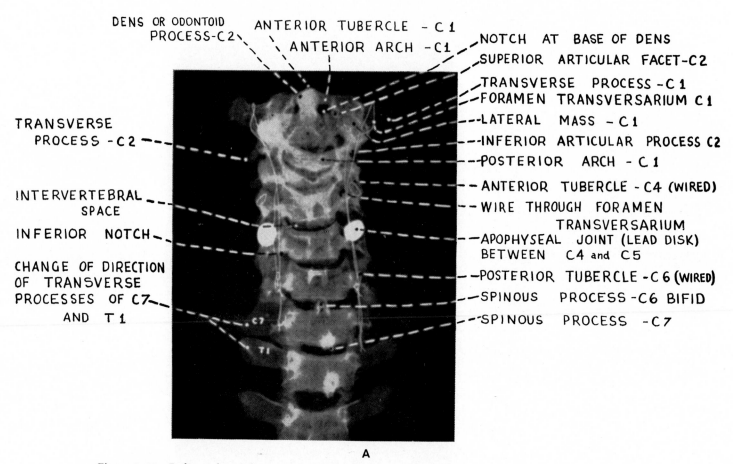

A

Figure 9–26. Radiographs of the cervical spine with certain anatomic features indicated. A. Anteroposterior projection.

Figure 9–26 continued on the opposite page.

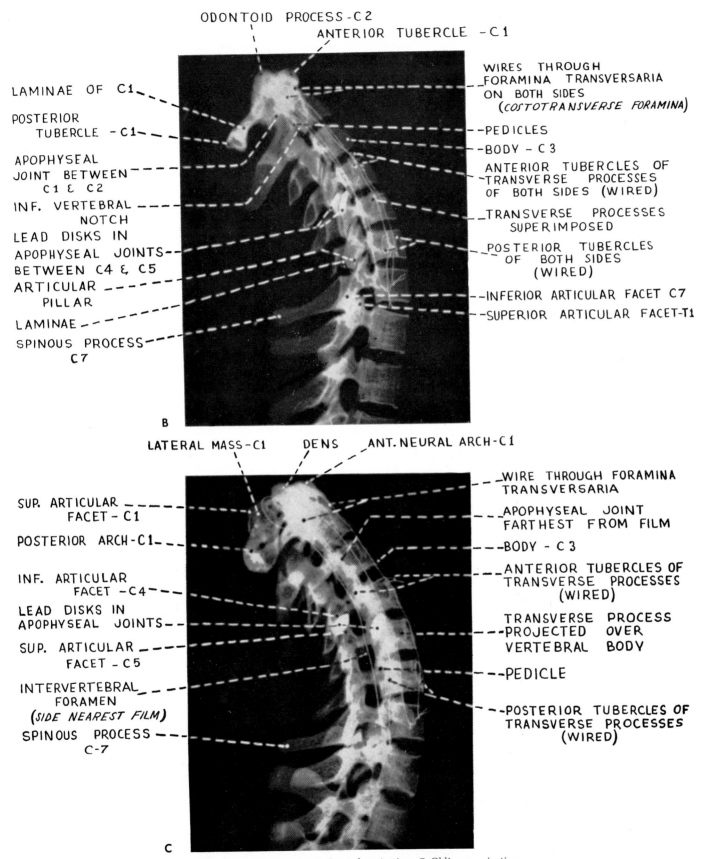

ODONTOID PROCESS - C 2

ANTERIOR TUBERCLE - C 1

WIRES THROUGH
FORAMINA TRANSVERSARIA
ON BOTH SIDES
(COSTOTRANSVERSE FORAMINA)

LAMINAE OF C 1

POSTERIOR
TUBERCLE - C 1

PEDICLES

BODY - C 3

APOPHYSEAL
JOINT BETWEEN
C 1 & C 2

ANTERIOR TUBERCLES OF
TRANSVERSE PROCESSES
OF BOTH SIDES (WIRED)

INF. VERTEBRAL
NOTCH

TRANSVERSE PROCESSES
SUPERIMPOSED

LEAD DISKS IN
APOPHYSEAL JOINTS
BETWEEN C4 & C5

POSTERIOR TUBERCLES
OF BOTH SIDES
(WIRED)

ARTICULAR
PILLAR

INFERIOR ARTICULAR FACET C7

SUPERIOR ARTICULAR FACET-T1

LAMINAE

SPINOUS PROCESS
C 7

B

LATERAL MASS - C 1   DENS   ANT. NEURAL ARCH - C 1

WIRE THROUGH FORAMINA
TRANSVERSARIA

SUP. ARTICULAR
FACET - C 1

APOPHYSEAL JOINT
FARTHEST FROM FILM

POSTERIOR ARCH - C 1

BODY - C 3

INF. ARTICULAR
FACET - C 4

ANTERIOR TUBERCLES OF
TRANSVERSE PROCESSES
(WIRED)

LEAD DISKS IN
APOPHYSEAL JOINTS

TRANSVERSE PROCESS
PROJECTED OVER
VERTEBRAL BODY

SUP. ARTICULAR
FACET - C 5

PEDICLE

INTERVERTEBRAL
FORAMEN
(SIDE NEAREST FILM)

SPINOUS PROCESS
C-7

POSTERIOR TUBERCLES OF
TRANSVERSE PROCESSES
(WIRED)

C

Figure 9-26 Continued.   B. Lateral projection. C. Oblique projection.

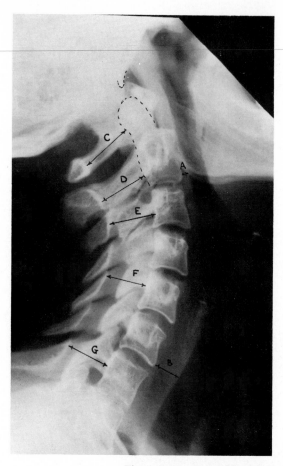

NORMAL SAGITTAL MEASUREMENTS

Region Evaluated	Normal Sagittal Measurements for Children 15 Years and Under (120 cases)		Normal Sagittal Measurements for Adults (480 cases)	
	Average (mm.)	Range (mm.)	Average (mm.)	Range (mm.)
Retropharyngeal space	3.5	2–7	3.4	1–7
Retrotracheal space	7.9	5–14	14.0	9–22
Cervical spinal canal:				
At first cervical vertebra	21.9	18–27	21.4	16–30
At second cervical vertebra	20.9	18–25	19.2	16–28
At third cervical vertebra	17.4	14–21	19.1	14–25
At fifth cervical vertebra	16.5	14–21	18.5	14–25
At seventh cervical vertebra	16.0	15–20	17.5	13–24

Figure 9–27. Normal lateral view of neck indicating regions evaluated. (A) Retropharyngeal space, second cervical vertebra, (B) retrotracheal space, sixth cervical vertebra, (C to G) cervical spinal canal. (C) First cervical vertebra, (D) second cervical vertebra, (E) third cervical vertebra, (F) fifth cervical vertebra, (G) seventh cervical vertebra. (From Wholey, M. H. et al.: Radiology, 71:350, 1958.)

sion. Also, a minimum sagittal diameter greater than 13 mm. suggests that any adjoining spur formation probably is not responsible for cord compression in this area, although nerve compression is certainly not excluded. Averages and ranges of normal sagittal measurements for children 15 years and under as well as for adults are given in the accompanying table (Fig. 9–27).

Difficulty in evaluating the cervical prevertebral soft tissues is well known, and measurements for these that have been devised are illustrated (Fig. 9–27). Whalen and Woodruff (1970) have called attention to the cervical prevertebral fat stripe noted on lateral roentgenograms of the cervical spine that lies anterior to the anterior spinal ligament and in close proximity to the anterior surfaces of the cervical vertebrae down to the level of C6 (Fig. 9–28). Expansion of the prevertebral space by inflammation or fractures of the cervical spine region will alter the appearance of this fat stripe.

Hinck et al. (1962) also measured and defined the sagittal diameter of the cervical spinal canal in children between the ages of 3 and 18 years (Fig. 9–29). They advocated the use of normal

minimal sagittal measurements as described in this investigation, and also the use of normal minimal interpediculate distances lower in the spine, so that the small spinal canal could be adequately detected. In Figure 9–29 C the measurements are given for the sagittal diameters of C1 to C5 in boys and girls from 3 to 18 years of age within a 90 per cent tolerance limit. In Figure 9–29 D, the differences in sagittal diameter of C1 to C5 between adjacent vertebrae are plotted. The differences between C2 and C1 are significantly greater than those between the other vertebrae, while only moderate differences are noted between C4 and C5. The actual measurements of C1 for boys were greater than those for girls of comparable ages, but the differences between C2 and C1 were less for the boys.

These sagittal diameter measurements may be compared with absolute measurements of the transverse diameter of the spinal cord between C3 and T3, which were made by Elsburg and Dyke from 80 normal myelograms (Fig. 9–30). Generally, the interpediculate measurements according to Elsburg and Dyke were slightly higher than the averages obtained by others but did not ordinarily exceed 22.5 mm. at C6 level. The average diameter of the cervical cord was greatest between C5 and C6, with a maximum of approximately 25 mm. and a minimum of some 17 mm. at this level. The cord diminishes greatly in size toward the upper thoracic spinal canal region (Fig. 9–30).

In the interpretation of the myelographic spinal cord measurements, Khilnani and Wolf indicated that abnormality was suggested by a difference of more than 3 mm. between adjacent cervical segments and a cord diameter of 80 per cent more or 50 per cent less than the diameter of the subarachnoid space.

The interval between the posterior margin of the anterior tubercle of the atlas and the anterior margin of the odontoid process has been called the atlantodental interval (ADI). The mean value for the ADI in adults is 0.93 ± 0.36 mm (Hinck and Hopkins). As a rule of thumb these investigators suggested that the ADI ranges between 0.5 and 3 mm. in the adult, with a slightly larger range in younger age groups.

The ADI was measured in children by Locke et al., who noted that no significant age or sex difference was found in four groups of children aged 3 to 5, 6 to 8, 9 to 11, and 12 to 15 years. Changes in position, film-to-tube distance, and variance in reader mea-

surements interacted in such a way that specific conclusions regarding these factors were difficult to make. Generally, however, in the supine roentgenograms with a 40 inch tube-to-film distance, no child had an ADI of more than 4 mm. Using the 72 inch tube-to-film distance in the upright neutral position, one normal child had an ADI of 5 mm., which was the largest ADI found in a normal child in any position. Generally, flexion tended to increase the ADI, as did extension. However, extension at the 72 inch film-to-tube distance tended to decrease the interval. It was recommended that films be exposed with the patient in a neutral position. The magnification factor usually may be ruled out by taking teleroentgenograms at 5 or 6 feet. The actual line measured by Locke et al. is shown in Figure 9–31.

Encroachment upon the intervertebral foramina is visualized in the oblique views and is not measured by this expedient.

Changes with Growth and Development. The distinguishing developmental characteristics of the atlas and axis have been described already. With regard to the other cervical vertebrae, at birth the laminae are united only by cartilage, and there is likewise no osseous union of the neural arch with the body (Fig. 9–26). Union does not occur until the second or third

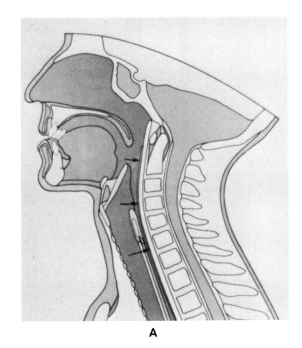

A

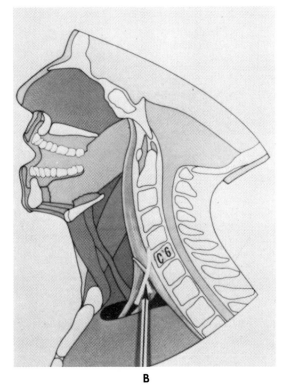

B

Figure 9–28. *A.* Drawing of sagittal section of neck illustrating the prevertebral fat (arrows). *B.* Drawing demonstrating anterior reflection of fat over scalenus muscles. (From Whalen, P., and Woodruff, C. L.: Amer. J. Roentgenol., *109:*445–451, 1970.)

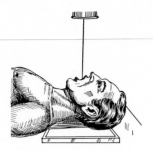

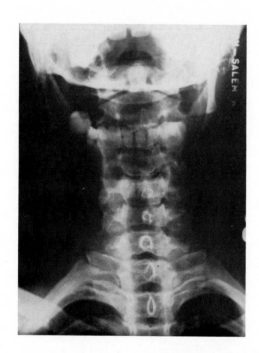

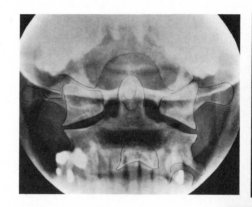

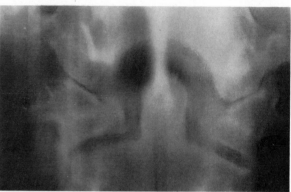

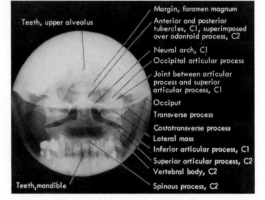

A

Figure 9–29. *A.* Anteroposterior view (*left*) of the cervical spine obtained with a rhythmic motion of the lower jaw during the exposure. The head, of course, is rigidly immobilized to prevent movement of the cervical spine. When a view is obtained in this manner a concept of the upper two cervical segments may be obtained which otherwise is not possible in this projection, since these segments are invariably obscured by the shadow of the mandible (Ottonello method). Anteroposterior view (*right* and *center*) of upper cervical spine with mouth open particularly to show odontoid process. (Radiograph intensified.)

Figure 9–29 continued on the opposite page.

year. A faint cartilaginous line may persist until 6 or 7 years of age, particularly at the base of the odontoid process. Such cartilaginous lines may readily be confused with fractures.

The vertebral body does not take on its more definitive appearance until long after puberty, and particularly in the cervical region the anterior margins of the bodies tend to be slightly narrowed in comparison with the posterior margins. This configura-

tion must not be misinterpreted as compression (Fig. 9–32 *E*). The vertebral bodies that may persistently retain this infantile contour are C5 and, less frequently, C6. The secondary centers of ossification do not appear until puberty, uniting at about 25 years of age.

The change in curvature of the cervical spine with the changing posture of the growing individual has already been described.

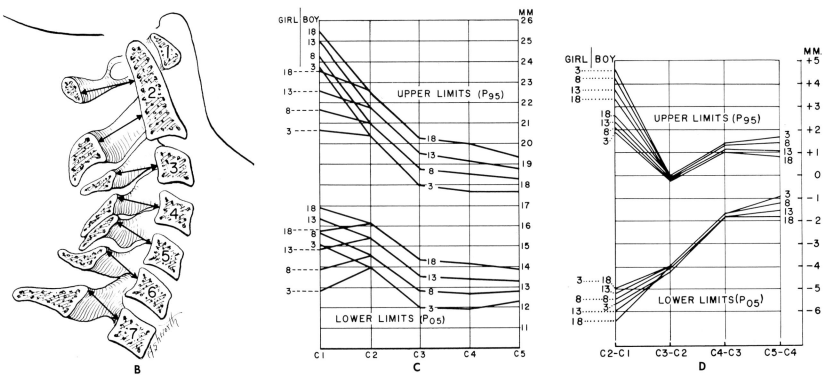

Figure 9–29 *Continued.* *B.* The sagittal diameter was measured from the middle of the posterior surface of the vertebral body to the nearest point on the ventral line of the cortex seen at the junction of spinous processes and laminae (arrows), as described by previous investigators. *C.* Ninety per cent tolerance limits for sagittal diameters of C1 to C5, in boys and girls from 3 to 18 years of age. *D.* Ninety per cent tolerance limits for sagittal diameter differences between adjacent vertebrae, C1 to C5, in boys and girls, from 3 to 18 years of age. (*B, C,* and *D* from Hinck, V. C., Hopkins, C. E., and Savara, B. S.: Radiology, *79*:97–108, 1962.)

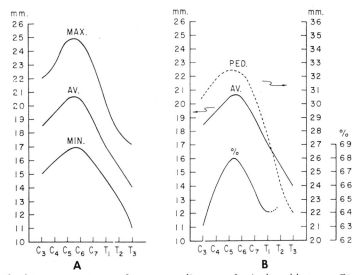

Figure 9–30. *A.* Absolute measurements of transverse diameter of spinal cord between C3 and T3 in 80 normal myelograms. It will be noted that the usual upper limits of interpediculate measurements according to Elsburg and Dyke are for the most part slightly higher than the average, but do not ordinarily exceed 22.5 mm. at C6 level. *B.* Curve PED is of the usual upper limits of interpediculate measurements, according to Elsburg and Dyke. The millimeter scale for this curve is on the right of the graph. The average curve is taken from *A.* The percentage curve gives the average ratios of the width of the cord to the width of the subarachnoid space. (From Khilnani, M. T., and Wolf, B. S.: J. Neurosurg., *20*:660, 1963.) (For method of measurement of sagittal dimension of cervical canal see Figure 9–27.)

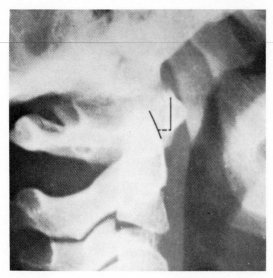

Figure 9–31. A normal cervical spine showing the distance measured (broken line) between the posterior inferior portion of the anterior arch of the atlas and the anterior border of the dens. (From Locke, G. R., Gardner, J. I., and Van Epps, E. F.: Amer. J. Roentgenol., 97:135–140, 1966.)

ROUTINE RADIOGRAPHIC POSITIONS FOR STUDY OF THE CERVICAL SPINE

1. **Anteroposterior Views of the Cervical Spine** (Fig. 9–32). In this view, only the vertebrae below C3 level are visualized unless the view is obtained with the mandible in motion. The lateral mass, consisting of the costal process, the transverse process and the costotransverse foramen, overlaps the articular process, and the anatomic parts are therefore difficult to distinguish. A mind's eye three-dimensional concept is most important to visualize these structures.

2. **Anteroposterior View of the Upper Cervical Spine Through the Open Mouth or with the Mandible in Motion** (Fig. 9–33). In this view, care must be taken to obtain a view of the entire odontoid process. The base of the skull may obscure it in part. The relationship of the dens to its adjoining articulations has already been described (Fig. 9–25 B).

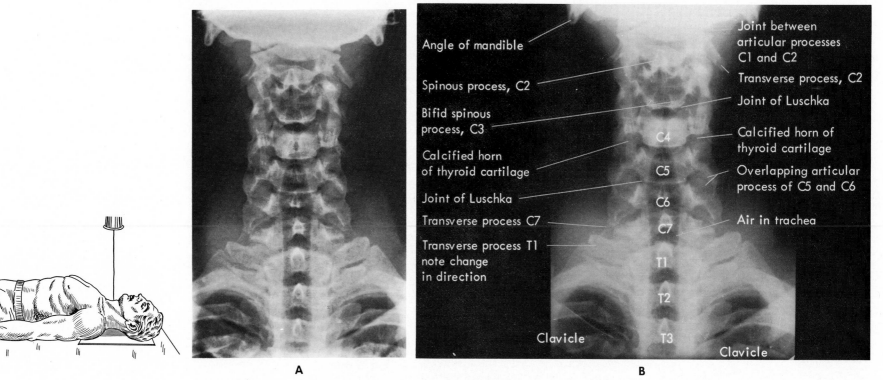

Figure 9–32. A and B. Anteroposterior views of cervical spine.

Figure 9–32 continued on the opposite page.

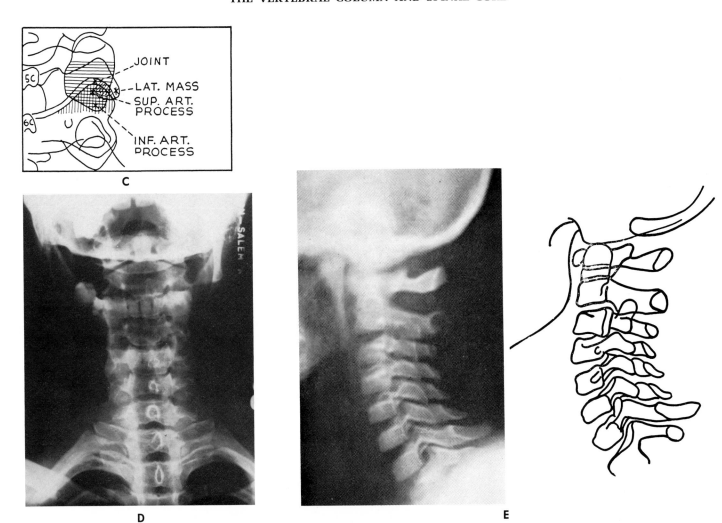

Figure 9–32 *Continued.* *C.* Labeled tracing of *B. D.* Anteroposterior view of the cervical spine obtained with a rhythmic motion of the lower jaw during exposure. This illustration virtually combines the anatomic features of Figures 9–32 *B* and 9–33. For anatomic detail, study these latter two illustrations. *E.* Radiograph and tracing of child's cervical spine to demonstrate irregularity and anterior narrowness of the vertebral bodies.

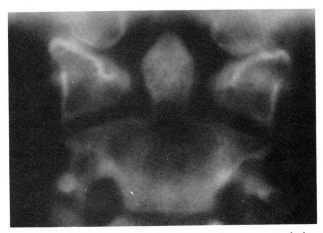

Figure 9–33. Anteroposterior view of upper cervical spine with mouth open, particularly to show odontoid process.

3. **Lateral View of the Cervical Spine** (Fig. 9–34). In order to obtain a good visualization of C7, the patient sits up and drops his shoulders as much as possible. Traction on the arms by means of heavy weights in the hands helps in lowering the shoulders. In order to obtain a true lateral projection, the patient's neck must be perfectly perpendicular to his shoulders, and also to the central ray. This places the cervical spine a considerable distance from the film. *Distortion and magnification are very considerable under*

these circumstances, unless a long film-target distance is employed (6 feet). Every effort is made to preserve the normal curvature of the cervical spine, but frequently this curvature disappears in the event of muscular spasm. The normal alignment previously described is only slightly disturbed under these circumstances.

In this projection, the lateral mass is projected in part over the vertebral body, particularly in its costal element. The articular processes, however, are shown very clearly.

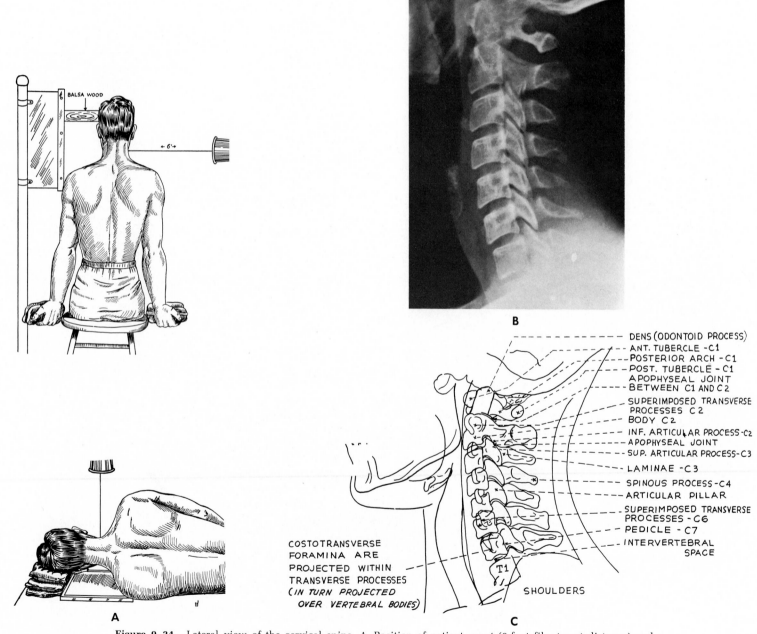

Figure 9–34. Lateral view of the cervical spine. *A.* Position of patient; erect (6-foot film-target distance) and recumbent views. *B.* Radiograph. *C.* Labeled tracing of *B.*

4. **Oblique View of the Cervical Spine** (Fig. 9–35). In order to obtain comparable views of the intervertebral foramina, care must be taken to rotate the entire body 45 degrees, not just the cervical spine. Actually, in this oblique projection, the head, neck, and torso are in perfectly straight alignment. The anatomy so projected is shown in Figure 9–35.

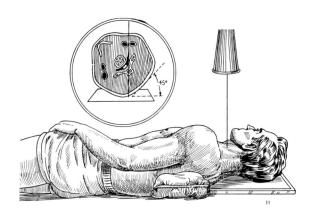

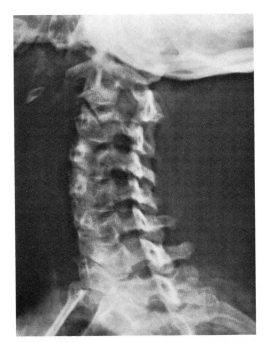
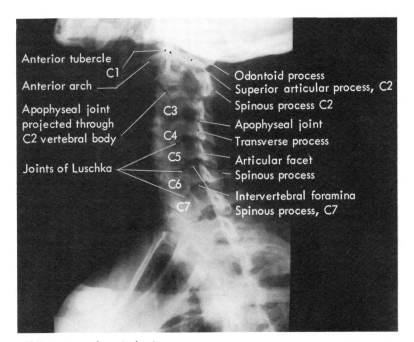

Figure 9–35. Oblique view of cervical spine.

The Thoracic or Dorsal Spine

There are several distinguishing characteristics of the thoracic spine (Fig. 9–36 A). The vertebral bodies of the upper eight segments articulate with two ribs on each side, and the lower four articulate with only the one rib with which they are numerically associated. There are also small costal facets on each transverse process of the upper ten thoracic vertebrae. The two different joints formed are called the costovertebral and costotransverse joints, respectively, with separate synovial cavities and joint capsules in each instance (Fig. 9–36 B and C).

The superior and inferior surfaces of these bodies are ordinarily quite flat. Occasionally notches appear in the center. These notches, when central and not too clearly defined, occur sufficiently frequently (in approximately 40 per cent of adult spines) to be considered without special signficance, although Schmorl believed them to be caused by congenital defects in the end plates of the vertebra (hence called "Schmorl's nodes"). However, when these nodes are eccentric, or associated with an undulating appearance of the superior or inferior surfaces of the vertebral bodies, they may well be of definite pathologic significance (Fig. 9–36 D).

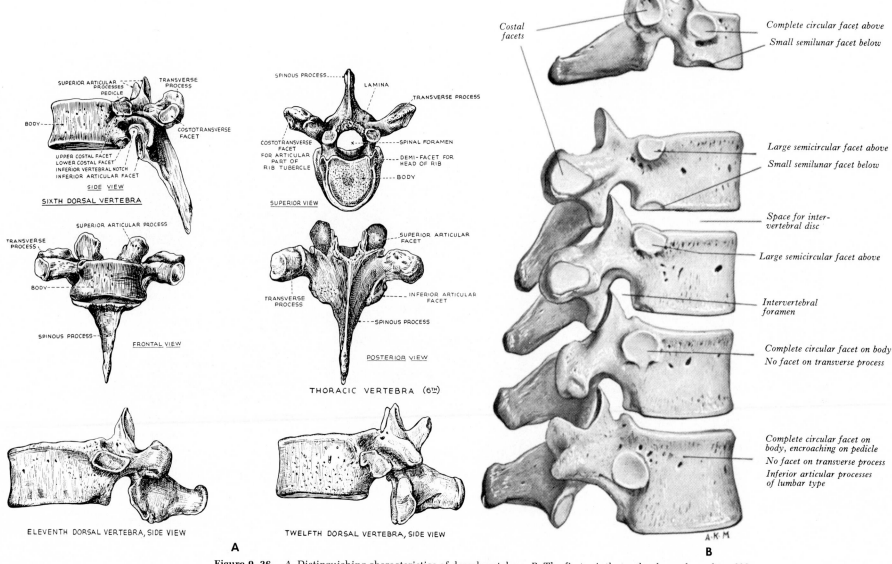

Figure 9–36. A. Distinguishing characteristics of dorsal vertebrae. B. The first, ninth, tenth, eleventh, and twelfth thoracic vertebrae. Right lateral aspect. (B from Warwick, R., and Williams, P. L.: Gray's Anatomy. 35th British edition. London, Longman [for Churchill-Livingstone], 1973.)

Figure 9–36 continued on the opposite page.

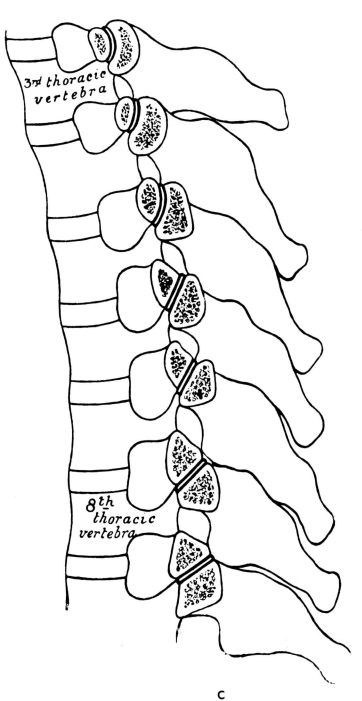

3rd thoracic vertebra

8th thoracic vertebra

C

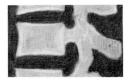

NORMAL

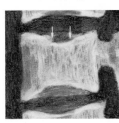

STEP-LIKE INDENTATION
END PLATES
(SICKLE CELL ANEMIA)

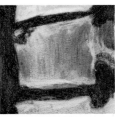

EPIPHYSITIS
SCHEUERMANN'S DISEASE

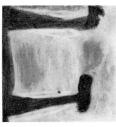

INCREASE HEIGHT
(ACROMEGALY)

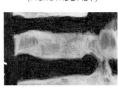

FLATTENED OSTEO-
CHONDRODYSTROPHY

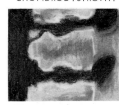

EPIPHYSITIS ADVANCED
WEDGED AND
UNDULATING END-PLATES
(ADVANCED
SCHEUERMANN'S DISEASE)

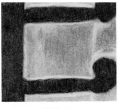

SQUARED
(TURNER'S SYNDROME)

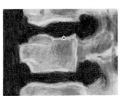

PERSISTANT EPIPHYSIS
INCREASED INTERSPACES
(CRETINISM
HYPOTHYROIDISM)

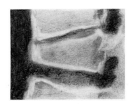

VERTEBRA PLANA
RETICULOENDOTHELIOSIS
EOSINOPHILIC GRANULOMA

D

Figure 9–36 *Continued.* C. A section through the costotransverse joints from the third to the ninth inclusive. Contrast the concave facets on the upper with the flattened facets on the inferior transverse processes. (From Warwick, R., and Williams, P. L.: Gray's Anatomy. 35th British edition. London, Longman [for Churchill-Livingstone], 1973.) D. Varying normal and abnormal appearances of the vertebral end plates. Schmorl's node is not illustrated but resembles the end plate shown for sickle cell anemia—except that in the latter the edges of the nodal indentation are vertical rather than rounded.

The posterior surfaces of these vertebral bodies are slightly concave from side to side, producing a somewhat double contoured appearance on the radiograph.

There is a gradual increase in size from top to bottom in the vertebral supero-inferior dimensions, both anteriorly and posteriorly. The posterior dimension tends to be slightly greater than the anterior. Diminution in size of a vertebra in relation to the adjoining vertebral bodies, therefore, becomes of definite significance.

The twelfth thoracic vertebra differs from the others (Fig. 9–36) in that its transverse processes are each replaced by three tubercles, and its inferior apophyseal joint faces in a more lateral direction than do the joints above it.

The spinous processes are long and slender, being steepest in the middle of the thoracic spine (Figs. 9–36 *C* and 9–39). These structures are to a great extent obscured by the ribs which curve backward and overlie them. The laminae overlap one another (this is called imbrication), further obscuring detail. The intervertebral foramina are circular, and are smaller than in the cervical or lumbar areas.

The paraspinal line (paravertebral soft tissue shadows), which is well delineated in frontal radiographs of the thoracic spine, must be differentiated from manifestations of disease. A left paraspinal shadow delimited by the left pleura reflection is commonly visualized on films of the thoracic spine. It roughly parallels the left margin of the vertebral column and the aorta and lies between these two structures (Fig. 9–37).

Above the level of the aortic arch the two pleural layers lie almost in contact with each other anterior to the vertebral column, and because of the superposition of the tracheal air column the pleural air shadows are difficult to define radiographically. The right mediastinal shadow parallels the dorsal spine in corresponding fashion and lies between the dorsal spine and the right margin of the cardiac silhouette.

When there is a diffuse dilatation of the descending thoracic aorta, the left pleural reflection is pulled laterally, producing an apparent widening of the left paraspinal shadow, but at the same time this still maintains a relative symmetry in contour with the aorta.

Any bony changes may also alter the paraspinal shadow. Hypertrophic spurs on the lateral aspects of the vertebral bodies may reach a size sufficient to deflect the pleura on either or both sides. Inflammatory masses or neoplasms involving the vertebrae may likewise extend into the soft tissues and displace the pleura to the right or left at the affected levels.

In the absence of demonstrable vertebral body disease and in the presence of an apparently normal aorta, other soft tissue abnormalities may be presumed to alter the paraspinal shadow. These may be related to tumors of nerve tissue origin, metastatic carcinoma, and other neoplasms, particularly those involving the mediastinum.

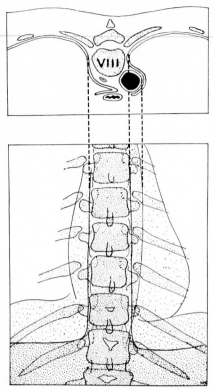

Figure 9–37. *Upper,* Cross section through the posterior mediastinum at the level of the eighth thoracic vertebra. *Lower,* Diagram taken from a roentgenogram depicting the posterior portions of the visceral or parietal pleura as lines along the vertebral column. Dotted lines indicate anatomic substrates of pleural lines and aortic lines in cross section. (From Lachman, E.: Anat. Rec., 83, 1942.)

Changes with Growth and Development. As in the case of the cervical spine, at birth the laminae are not yet united, and the neural arch has not yet joined with the vertebral body. These small ossified segments therefore stand out clearly (see tracing of radiograph in Fig. 9–14). The laminae unite at about 1 year of age, when a more definitive appearance is obtained. The vertebral bodies do have a boxlike appearance in this region despite the lack of the secondary centers of ossification, unlike the cervical spine. The secondary centers of ossification appear at about the age of puberty, the epiphyseal rings on the upper and lower margins of the vertebral body standing out most clearly. Occasionally, these do not appear to be homogeneously ossified, and this appearance must be differentiated from outright fragmentation, which is an indication of abnormality. The secondary centers unite at about 25 years of age (or somewhat sooner), at which time growth in height ceases completely.

ROUTINE RADIOGRAPHIC POSITIONS AND
RADIOGRAPHIC ANATOMY OF THE THORACIC SPINE

1. **Anteroposterior View of the Thoracic Spine** (Fig. 9–38)
In view of the primary curvature of the thoracic spine, some of the
vertebral bodies are seen obliquely in the anteroposterior projection. The posterior and anterior margins of the vertebral body are
projected separately, and will overlap the adjoining vertebral surface, producing a diminution in anatomic detail.

The transverse processes, though prominent, are obscured by
the heads and necks of the ribs to a considerable degree.

The pedicles stand out prominently as ovoid structures, and
their inner margins bear a rather definite relationship to one
another. The distance between their inner margins is called the
interpedicular distance.

The charts for the interpedicular distance between the lower
cervical and the lumbar spine have been previously presented (see
Figure 9–15 *B* and also Tables 9–7 to 9–10). It will be noted that
the interpedicular distances diminish down to the fourth or fifth
thoracic vertebra, and then gradually increase after a relatively
stationary period. In view of the fact that the intervertebral
foramina of the thoracic spine are smaller than those of the cervical or lumbar areas, a space-occupying lesion located in this
area is more apt to erode the pedicle along with the margins of
the intervertebral foramina. This is manifest by a sudden and
inordinate increase in the interpedicular distance on this projection. Erosion of the pedicle will alter the normal ovoid contour of
the pedicle as seen in frontal perspective, so that it will appear
"semi-lunate" and concave medially. As previously shown (Fig.
9–16) such erosion is best demonstrated by tomography.

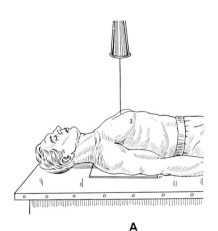

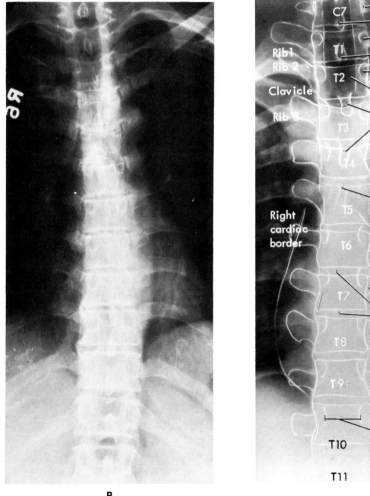

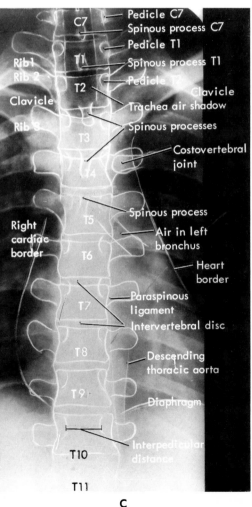

A   B   C

Figure 9–38.   Anteroposterior view of the thoracic spine. *A.* Position of patient. *B.* Radiograph. *C.* Labeled tracing
of *B.*

2. **Lateral View of the Thoracic Spine** (Fig. 9–39) The lateral projection gives an excellent perspective of the vertebral bodies and spinal canal. The various processes and synovial joints are obscured to a great extent by the overlapping laminae, spinous processes, and ribs.

The gas shadows of the lung structures overlie the vertebral bodies of the thoracic spine and frequently make the interpretation of minimal trabecular abnormality virtually impossible. In cases of doubt, body section radiographs are of considerable help.

It is not usually satisfactory to attempt to include the lower dorsal vertebrae with lumbar vertebrae on a single exposure, since separate techniques are required for maximum clarity.

The uppermost two or three vertebrae are usually not seen in the routine lateral radiograph, in view of the interference caused by the shoulder shadows. This portion of the spine is most difficult to radiograph. Ordinarily a routine study does not include this small section unless specifically requested or desired.

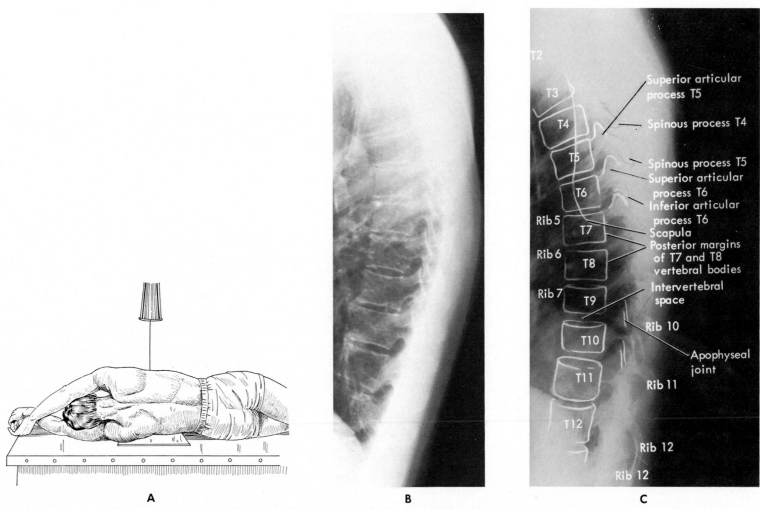

Figure 9–39. Lateral view of the thoracic spine. *A.* Position of patient. *B.* Radiograph. *C.* Labeled radiograph.

3. **Lateral (Slightly Oblique) View of the Upper Two Thoracic Segments** (Fig. 9–40) The accompanying illustration demonstrates the manner in which this projection is used to obtain a clear view of these segments. The exposure factors must likewise be different from those for the remainder of the dorsal spine. Usually factors similar to those utilized in radiography of the lumbar spine are employed. The anatomic detail is somewhat distorted but usually sufficiently clear.

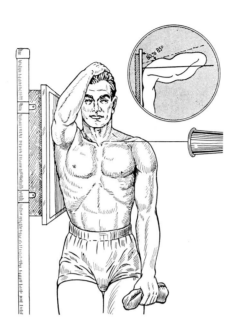

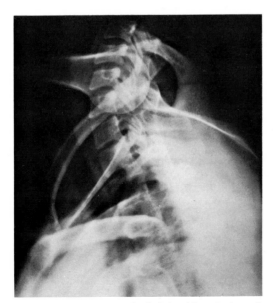
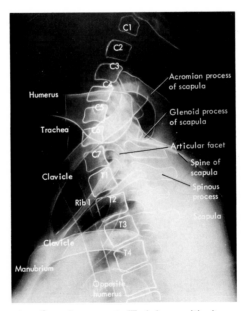

Figure 9–40. Lateral (slightly oblique) view of upper two thoracic segments (Twining position).

SECOND LUMBAR VERTEBRA

SUPERIOR VERTEBRAL NOTCH
SUPERIOR ARTICULAR PROCESS
MAMMILLARY PROCESS
TRANSVERSE PROCESS
SPINOUS PROCESS
INFERIOR VERTEBRAL NOTCH
INFERIOR ARTICULAR FACET

SIDE VIEW

MAMMILLARY PROCESS
SUPERIOR ARTICULAR FACET
ACCESSORY PROCESS
BODY
TRANSVERSE PROCESS
SPINOUS PROCESS
INFERIOR ARTICULAR FACET

POSTERIOR VIEW

SPINOUS PROCESS
LAMINA
MAMMILLARY PROCESS
SUPERIOR ARTICULAR PROCESS
ACCESSORY PROCESS
PEDICLE
TRANSVERSE PROCESS
SPINAL FORAMEN

SUPERIOR VIEW

INTERVERTEBRAL DISK
BODY
PEDICLE
INTERVERTEBRAL FORAMEN

SUPERIOR ARTICULAR PROCESS
MAMMILLARY PROCESS
TRANSVERSE PROCESS
INFERIOR ARTICULAR PROCESS
SPINOUS PROCESSES
INFERIOR VERTEBRAL NOTCH
SUPERIOR VERTEBRAL NOTCH

FIFTH LUMBAR VERTEBRA, SIDE VIEW

LUMBAR VERTEBRAE, SIDE VIEW

A

SUPERIOR ARTICULAR PROCESS
LATERAL MASS (ALA)
SACRAL PORTION OF THE BRIM OF THE PELVIS
ANTERIOR SACRAL FORAMEN
TRANSVERSE RIDGES
APEX OF SACRUM

MALE SACRUM, ANTERIOR VIEW

BASE OF SACRUM
SUPERIOR ARTICULAR PROCESS
FIRST SACRAL VERTEBRA
SACRAL CANAL
APEX OF SACRUM
FIFTH SACRAL VERTEBRA
SACRAL CORNU
COCCYGEAL CORNU
FIRST COCCYGEAL VERTEBRA

SACRUM AND COCCYX IN SAGITTAL SECTION THROUGH MEDIAN LINE

B

The Lumbar Spine (Fig. 9–41 A)

The lumbar curvature is secondary to the erect posture of the human and does not develop until the child learns to walk. Lumbar vertebrae differ from cervical and thoracic vertebrae in that they have no foramen in the transverse process and no facets for ribs. They are considerably larger than the other vertebrae.

The transition from the lower dorsal vertebrae to the lumbar is frequently very gradual, and the last ribs may have the appearance of transverse processes. Occasionally the last lumbar vertebra is fused in whole or in part with the sacrum, or the first sacral segment becomes a separate segment and has the appearance of the last lumbar. Its transverse processes may be partially or wholly fused with those of the sacrum, or an articulation in this location may exist.

Defects in the neural arch of the lower lumbar segments are particularly frequent (they are found in 5 to 10 per cent of the adult population), but these abnormalities are not within the scope of the present text.

In the lateral projection, there may be a progressive increase in the height of the vertebral bodies or the height remains the same, descending the spine, except in the case of the fifth lumbar, which may vary somewhat. The *fifth lumbar interspace is usually narrower than adjoining interspaces, and this is without special significance when unaccompanied by other findings.* Otherwise the interspaces are equal in width, and variations are of special significance.

The posterior margins of the vertebral bodies ordinarily form a smooth curved line. Occasionally, the superior margin of the lower lumbar vertebra will deviate from this line. The author's method of drawing lines described in Figure 9–42 has proved of value in determining whether or not this alignment is normal. When these lines are drawn as described, it has been found in studying a large series of normal cases that they fall into certain definite categories, whereas the anteriorly slipped vertebral body (spondylolisthesis) produces a definite variation in the arrangement of these lines.

Occasionally, it will appear that a margin is posteriorly displaced. This appearance may be caused by the phenomenon of projection or by deformity in the posterior margin of the sacrum, but it is possible that a true posterior spondylolisthesis may exist, although the existence of this entity is doubted by some (Fig. 9–43).

Ferguson (Fig. 9–44 A) has defined the lumbosacral angle as the angle formed between a horizontal line and the plane of the superior margin of the sacrum. This is an index of the angle be-

Figure 9–41. Lumbar spine and sacrum. *A.* Distinguishing characteristics of the lumbar spine. *B.* Sacrum (frontal and lateral projections).

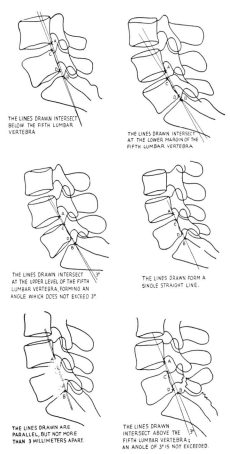

THE LINES DRAWN INTERSECT
BELOW THE FIFTH LUMBAR
VERTEBRA

THE LINES DRAWN INTERSECT
AT THE LOWER MARGIN OF THE
FIFTH LUMBAR VERTEBRA

THE LINES DRAWN INTERSECT
AT THE UPPER LEVEL OF THE FIFTH
LUMBAR VERTEBRA, FORMING AN
ANGLE WHICH DOES NOT EXCEED 3°.

THE LINES DRAWN FORM A
SINGLE STRAIGHT LINE.

THE LINES DRAWN ARE
PARALLEL, BUT NOT MORE
THAN 3 MILLIMETERS APART.

THE LINES DRAWN
INTERSECT ABOVE THE
FIFTH LUMBAR VERTEBRA;
AN ANGLE OF 3° IS NOT EXCEEDED.

Figure 9–42. Lines demonstrating various types of alignment in the lumbosacral lateral projection. A line AB is drawn between the posterior-inferior margin of L4 and the posterior-superior margin of S1. A second line CD is drawn between the posterior-superior and posterior-inferior margins of L5. These two lines form the six definite normal configuration patterns as shown.

The presence of a defect in the pars interarticularis is not always associated with a "slipping" forward, but predisposes to such a condition (called spondylolisthesis) (From Meschan, I.: Radiology, 47, 1945.)

tween the lumbar and sacral spine, and this author believes that when it exceeds 34 degrees, an abnormality in stability exists. In the erect position with weight bearing, Hellems and Keats have shown the lumbosacral angle to measure 41.1 degrees, with a standard deviation of 7.7 degrees.

Weight-bearing films in the lateral projection in flexion and extension may also be utilized to determine the stability at the lumbosacral junction as shown in Figure 9–44 *B*.

Occasionally extra ossicles form along the superior anterior margins of lumbar bodies. These are called extra-apophyses and are important only because they must be differentiated from fractures; otherwise they have no pathologic significance (Fig. 9–12 *B*).

The pars interarticularis (Fig. 9–45) is that slender, bony segment between the superior and inferior articular processes. Not infrequently (in about 5 per cent of the population) its

cartilage or fibrous tissue remains unossified, a predisposition to the condition already described as spondylolisthesis.

The apophyseal joints of the lumbar area are more frequently affected in atrophic arthritic disease than are the higher portions of the spine, and it is indeed fortunate that they can be so clearly demonstrated. The obliquity of these joints will vary, and occasionally several oblique views must be obtained before definite abnormality can be excluded.

As previously indicated, the plane of the apophyseal joints is perpendicular to the plane of the sacroiliac joint on the same side, and it is the sacroiliac joint of the side that is *farthest* from the film (anteroposterior oblique) which is seen clearly, whereas the apophyseal joint of the side *closest* to the film is seen to best advantage.

Changes with Growth and Development in the Lumbosacral Spine. The development of the lumbar vertebrae closely parallels that of the thoracic vertebrae, with minor differences. However, that of the sacral spine is significantly different.

In addition to the centers for the vertebral body and neural arches (Fig. 9–14) in the sacrum there are also centers for the costal processes present at birth. The costal parts fuse with the arches at the fifth year. The arch fuses with the body 2 or 3 years later, and the halves of the arches unite posteriorly between 7 and 10 years of age. The secondary centers of ossification that adjoin the wings of the sacrum on each side appear at 15 to 18 years of age and fuse in the early twenties. *Before their appearance, the sacroiliac joints appear somewhat wider than might be expected, and this appearance must be considered normal.*

The vertebral arches are incomplete below the third and fourth sacral segments and are wholly absent from the lower coccyx.

The coccyx is cartilaginous at birth, and each segment ordi-

SIGNS OF POSTERIOR DISPLACEMENT OF THE LUMBAR VERTEBRAE

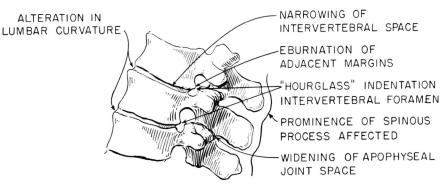

ALTERATION IN
LUMBAR CURVATURE

NARROWING OF
INTERVERTEBRAL SPACE

EBURNATION OF
ADJACENT MARGINS

"HOURGLASS" INDENTATION
INTERVERTEBRAL FORAMEN

PROMINENCE OF SPINOUS
PROCESS AFFECTED

WIDENING OF APOPHYSEAL
JOINT SPACE

OTHER CRITERIA:
ANTERIOR AND POSTERIOR MARGINS MUST BE DISPLACED
WITH REFERENCE TO UNDERLYING VERTEBRA

OTHER SIGNS OF DISC DEGENERATION MAY BE PRESENT

Figure 9–43. Criteria for backward displacement of the lumbar vertebrae.

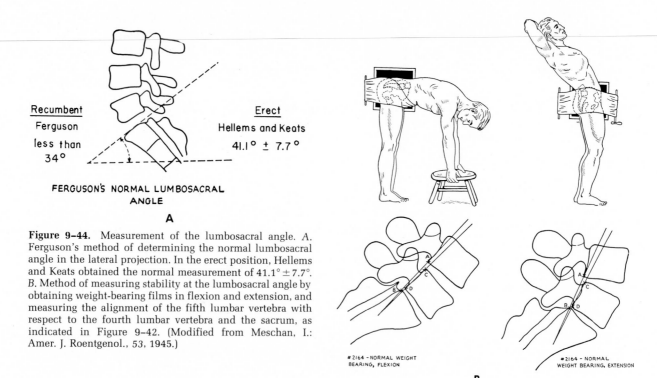

Recumbent
Ferguson
less than
34°

FERGUSON'S NORMAL LUMBOSACRAL
ANGLE

A

Erect
Hellems and Keats
41.1° ± 7.7°

#2164 - NORMAL WEIGHT
BEARING, FLEXION

#2164 - NORMAL
WEIGHT BEARING, EXTENSION

B

Figure 9-44. Measurement of the lumbosacral angle. *A.* Ferguson's method of determining the normal lumbosacral angle in the lateral projection. In the erect position, Hellems and Keats obtained the normal measurement of 41.1° ± 7.7°. *B.* Method of measuring stability at the lumbosacral angle by obtaining weight-bearing films in flexion and extension, and measuring the alignment of the fifth lumbar vertebra with respect to the fourth lumbar vertebra and the sacrum, as indicated in Figure 9-42. (Modified from Meschan, I.: Amer. J. Roentgenol., *53,* 1945.)

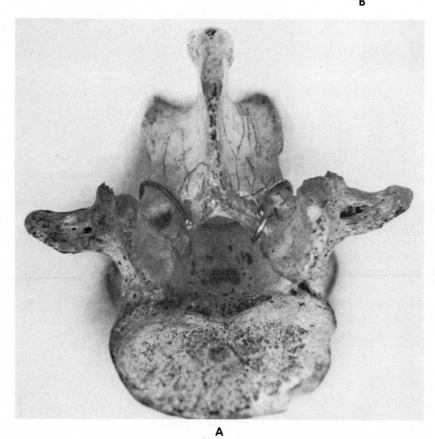

A

Figure 9-45. Vertebral body with wire delineating the pars interarticularis. *A.* Photograph.

Figure 9-45 continued on the opposite page.

narily has only one primary center. The segments appear from top to bottom from birth to puberty. Fusion is variable and usually occurs from bottom to top. The coccyx is one of the most variable bones in the human body, and interpretation of abnor-mality is frequently very difficult. In the female the coccyx is more freely movable and less likely to be fused with the sacrum, and its first segment more often than not fails to fuse with the second.

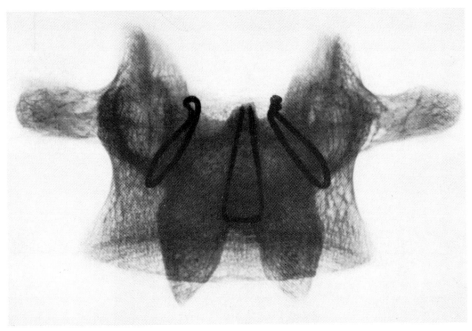

B

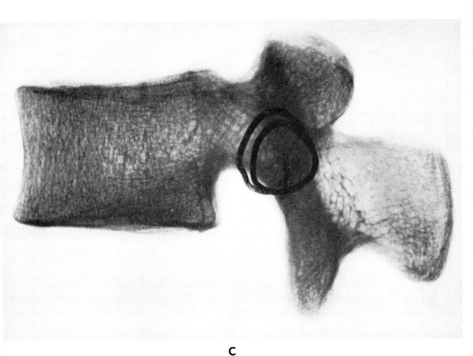

C

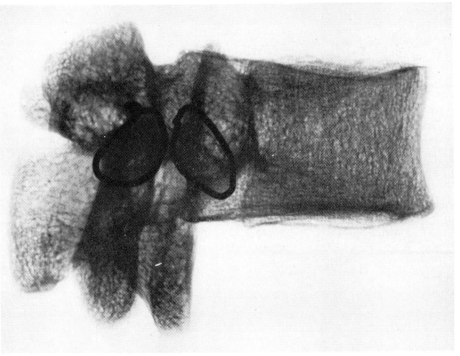

D

Figure 9–45 *Continued.* B. Radiograph in anteroposterior projection. C. Radiograph in lateral projection. D. Radiograph in oblique projection.

Table 9-13. As noted in this table, scalloping is ordinarily a roentgen sign of abnormality, and as such, is beyond the scope of this text. However, minimal to moderate scalloping may be seen in as much as 56 per cent of adult cases (Mitchell et al.), and in these instances, it is always limited to the lumbar spine, best identified in the lateral projection. Physiologic scalloping is never associated with widened interpediculate distances. Scalloping in areas other than the lumbar spine warrants investigation in the probability that abnormality is present.

Vertebral scalloping has also been noted in acromegaly (Stuber and Palacios, 1966), which is also outside the scope of this text.

Vertebral Body and Intervertebral Disk Indices (see Tables 9-1 through 9-6). These indices have been previously described in this chapter. The vertebral body index divides the greatest vertical diameter by the smallest sagittal diameter of each body from the twelfth thoracic through the third lumbar. The intervertebral disk index divides the minimal width of the intervertebral disk from T11 to T12 through L2 and L3 by the vertical diameter of the immediately subjacent vertebral body. These indices are particularly valuable in certain disorders and are especially important in the lower thoracic and upper lumbar regions. Tracings of newborn vertebrae both in a normal group and in a mongoloid group are presented in Figure 9-47 to indicate the practical significance of this index in the mucopolysaccharidoses (Rabinowitz and Moseley). (This congenital abnormality is outside the scope of this text and is included here only to show the application of this index.)

Sagittal Diameter of the Lumbar Spinal Canal in Children and Adults (Hinck, Hopkins, and Clark, 1965). Age group means and 90 per cent tolerance limits for the sagittal diameter of the spinal canal of each lumbar vertebra, male and female combined, are shown in Figure 9-48. As a rule of thumb it is recommended that any lumbar sagittal diameter below 15 mm. or above 25 mm. be regarded with suspicion. Measurements accumulated by these authors are shown in Tables 9-11 and 9-12.

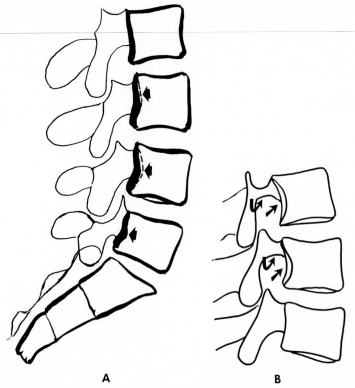

A   **B**

Figure 9-46. *A.* Occasional posterior "physiologic scalloping." The pedicles are normal. For the importance of this sign in pathologic circumstances see Mitchell et al. *B.* Scalloping of the posterior margins of vertebral bodies which may be abnormal in view of the thinness of the adjoining pedicles. When associated pedicular erosion is present, the scalloping of the vertebral bodies posteriorly takes on pathologic significance.

Scalloped Vertebrae. Scalloping is the term used to describe an exaggeration of the normal slight concavity of the dorsal surface of the vertebral body (Fig. 9-46). Such scalloping may result from local expansion of a mass lesion in the spinal canal. There are many other causes, however, and these are shown in

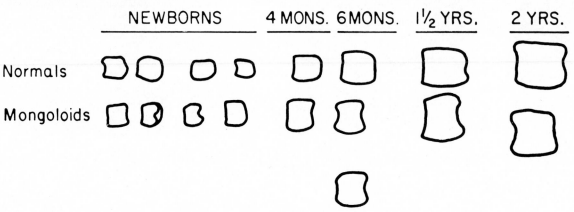

Figure 9-47. Tracings of the outline of the lumbar vertebral bodies of nonmongoloid and mongoloid children at the same age. (From Rabinowitz, J. G., and Moseley, J. F.: Radiology, 83:74-79, 1964.)

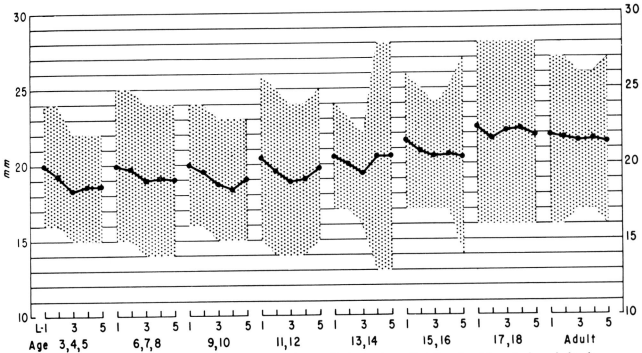

Figure 9–48. Age group means and 90 per cent tolerance limits for the sagittal diameter of the spinal canal of each lumbar vertebra, male and female combined. (From Hinck, V. C., Hopkins, C. E., and Clark, W. M.: Radiology, 85:929–937, 1965.)

TABLE 9–11 AGE-GROUP MEANS AND STANDARD DEVIATIONS, BY SEX (mm.)*

Vertebra	Male N	Mean	S.D.	Female N	Mean	S.D.	Male N	Mean	S.D.	Female N	Mean	S.D.
		Age 3, 4, 5 years						Age 6, 7, 8 years				
L1	15	20.3	1.8	9	19.8	1.2	14	20.3	1.9	10	19.3	2.6
2	15	19.6	1.2	9	18.9	1.4	15	19.9	1.7	9	19.5	1.6
3	15	18.4	1.4	9	18.1	1.4	15	19.1	1.8	10	18.4	1.6
4	15	18.8	1.1	9	18.0	1.5	15	19.0	1.7	10	19.1	1.8
5	14	19.0	1.6	9	17.5	1.4	15	19.0	2.4	10	19.1	2.3
		Age 9, 10 years						Age 11, 12 years				
L1	8	20.1	1.0	4	19.8	1.9	5	22.6	2.0	11	19.6	1.1
2	8	19.6	1.0	5	19.6	1.7	5	21.2	2.7	11	18.9	1.7
3	8	18.8	1.6	5	18.9	1.3	5	19.9	2.9	11	18.4	1.4
4	8	18.6	1.7	5	18.6	1.2	5	18.8	3.0	11	19.1	1.7
5	8	19.1	1.9	5	18.9	1.1	5	19.7	2.7	11	19.8	2.4
		Age 13, 14 years						Age 15, 16 years				
L1	14	20.5	1.5	10	20.8	1.4	10	21.6	2.2	18	21.6	2.2
2	14	19.7	1.4	10	20.1	0.9	11	20.8	2.1	18	20.9	1.8
3	14	18.9	1.7	10	20.0	1.3	11	20.5	1.6	18	20.7	1.6
4	14	20.4	4.1	10	20.2	2.5	11	20.0	1.7	18	21.0	2.1
5	14	20.8	4.2	10	20.1	3.2	10	20.1	2.9	18	20.8	3.4
		Age 17, 18 years						Adult				
L1	11	23.9	1.9	17	21.7	1.7	22	22.2	3.1	25	21.3	2.3
2	11	22.4	2.3	17	21.3	1.9	23	22.3	2.7	26	21.2	2.1
3	12	22.6	2.3	18	22.0	3.1	23	21.7	2.6	26	21.3	2.1
4	12	22.9	2.8	18	21.9	2.6	23	21.8	2.4	26	21.3	1.9
5	12	22.6	3.4	18	21.4	2.2	21	22.6	2.7	25	20.4	2.4

*From Hinck, V. C., Hopkins, C. E., and Clark, W. M.: Sagittal diameter of the lumbar spinal canal in children and adults. Radiology, 85:929–937, 1965.

TABLE 9-12 AGE-GROUP MEANS, STANDARD DEVIATIONS AND 90 PER CENT TOLERANCE LIMITS, EACH LUMBAR VERTEBRA (SAGITTAL), MALE AND FEMALE COMBINED (mm.)*

Vertebra	N	Mean	S.D.	90% Tolerance Min.	90% Tolerance Max.	N	Mean	S.D.	90% Tolerance Min.	90% Tolerance Max.
		Age 3, 4, 5 years					Age 6, 7, 8 years			
L1	24	20.1	1.6	16	24	24	19.9	2.2	15	25
2	24	19.4	1.2	16	24	24	19.7	1.7	15	25
3	24	18.4	1.3	15	22	25	18.8	1.7	14	24
4	24	18.6	1.2	15	22	25	19.1	1.7	14	24
5	23	18.6	1.5	15	22	25	19.0	2.3	14	24
		Age 9, 10 years					Age 11, 12 years			
L1	12	20.0	1.3	16	24	16	20.6	2.0	15	26
2	13	19.6	1.2	16	24	16	19.6	2.3	14	25
3	13	18.8	1.4	15	23	16	18.9	2.0	14	24
4	13	18.6	1.5	15	23	16	19.0	2.1	14	24
5	13	19.0	1.6	15	23	16	19.8	2.4	15	25
		Age 13, 14 years					Age 15, 16 years			
L1	24	20.6	1.4	17	24	28	21.6	2.2	17	26
2	24	19.9	1.2	17	23	29	20.9	1.9	17	25
3	24	19.4	1.6	16	22	29	20.6	1.6	17	24
4	24	20.4	3.5	13	28	29	20.7	2.0	17	25
5	24	20.5	3.7	13	28	28	20.6	3.2	14	27
		Age 17, 18 years					Adult			
L1	28	22.5	2.1	16	28	47	21.8	2.7	16	27
2	28	21.7	2.1	16	28	49	21.7	2.5	16	27
3	30	22.2	2.7	16	28	49	21.5	2.3	17	26
4	30	22.3	2.7	16	28	49	21.6	2.2	17	26
5	30	21.9	2.8	16	28	49	21.4	2.7	16	27

*From Hinck, V. C., Hopkins, C. E., and Clark, W. M.: Sagittal diameter of the lumbar spinal canal in children and adults. Radiology, *85*:929–937, 1965.

TABLE 9-13 CLASSIFICATION OF SCALLOPED VERTEBRAE ACCORDING TO PATHOGENIC MECHANISMS*

Increased Intraspinal Pressure
A. Localized
  (1) Intradural neoplasms
  (2) Intraspinal cysts
  (3) Syringomyelia and hydromyelia
B. Generalized increased intraspinal pressure
  (1) Uncontrolled communicating hydrocephalus
Dural "Ectasia"
A. Marfan's syndrome
B. Ehlers-Danlos syndrome
C. Neurofibromatosis
Small Spinal Canal
A. Achondroplasia
Congenital Skeletal Disorders
A. Morquio's disease ⎫
B. Hurler syndrome ⎬ mucopolysaccharidoses
Normal variants — "Physiologic Scalloping"

*From Mitchell, G. E., Lourie, H., and Berne, A. S.: The various causes of scalloped vertebrae with notes on their pathogenesis. Radiology, *89*:67–74, 1967.

ROUTINE RADIOGRAPHIC POSITIONS AND
RADIOGRAPHIC ANATOMY OF THE LUMBAR SPINE

1. **Anteroposterior View of the Lumbosacral Spine** (Fig. 9–49). Because the lumbar curvature will impose a degree of distortion and magnification on those lumbar vertebrae farthest from the film, the patient's knees should be flexed in order to diminish this effect by straightening the lumbar spine to some extent.

When interpreting the radiographic anatomy, the radiologist can see through the vertebral body and delineate the laminae, spinous processes, and articular processes. The transverse processes are irregular in appearance, and are frequently asymmetrical.

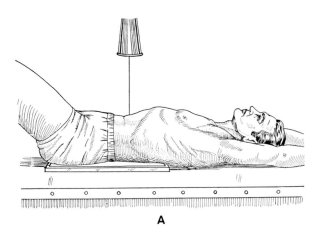

A

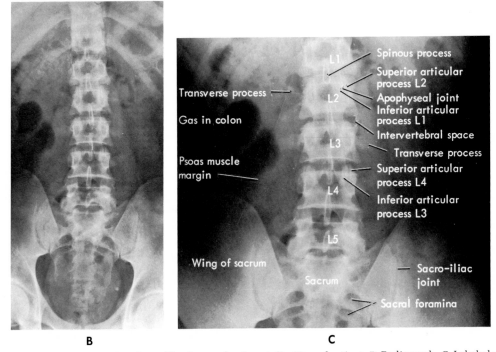

B C

Figure 9–49. Anteroposterior view of lumbosacral spine. *A.* Position of patient. *B.* Radiograph. *C.* Labeled radiograph.

2. **Lateral View of the Lumbosacral Spine** (Fig. 9–50). When a 36 inch film-target distance is employed the usual lumbar sag is quite permissible, in that it forms part of the arc of a circle with a 36 inch radius, and the vertebral surfaces are parallel to the rays from the target. However, if a longer film-to-target distance is employed, it is best to eliminate the lumbar sag (with a balsa wood block), especially in women, so that an undistorted view of the lumbar spine can be obtained.

This area requires special exposure factors to penetrate the structures present, and the less dense structures such as the spinous processes frequently require a bright light source for visualization.

Occasionally the sacrum cannot be included satisfactorily in this study, because exposure factors for some sacra are excessively high (Fig. 9–51).

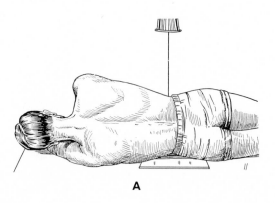

A

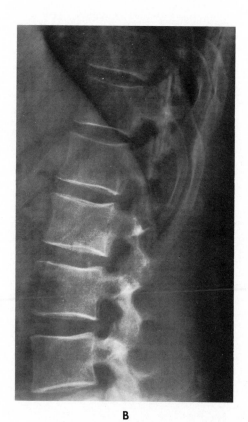

B

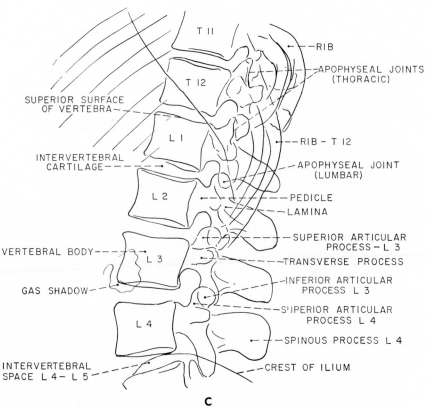

C

Figure 9–50.   Lateral view of the lumbosacral spine. A. Position of patient. B. Radiograph (intensified). C. Labeled tracing of B.

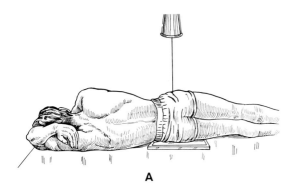

A

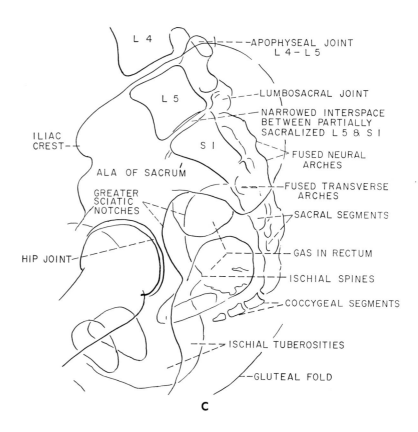

L 4

—APOPHYSEAL JOINT
L 4 - L 5

L 5

—LUMBOSACRAL JOINT

—NARROWED INTERSPACE
BETWEEN PARTIALLY
SACRALIZED L 5 & S I

ILIAC
CREST—

S I

—FUSED NEURAL
ARCHES

ALA OF SACRUM

—FUSED TRANSVERSE
ARCHES

GREATER
SCIATIC
NOTCHES

—SACRAL SEGMENTS

HIP JOINT—

—GAS IN RECTUM

—ISCHIAL SPINES

—COCCYGEAL SEGMENTS

—ISCHIAL TUBEROSITIES

—GLUTEAL FOLD

C

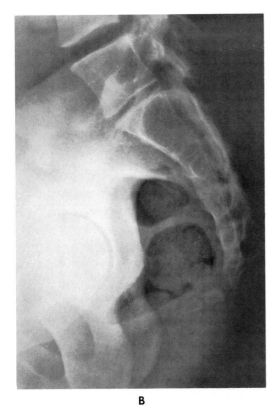

B

Figure 9–51. Special lateral view of sacrum and coccyx. *A.* Position of patient. *B.* Radiograph. *C.* Labeled tracing of *B.*

Points of Practical Interest with Reference to Figure 9–51

1. The patient's hips and knees are flexed to a comfortable position to help immobilize the patient.
2. The coronal plane passing 3 inches posterior to the midaxillary line is adjusted to the longitudinal axis of the table.
3. It is usually desirable to place folded sheets or balsa wood blocks in the depression above the iliac crest to maintain the lower thoracic spine in a perfectly parallel relationship with the table top.
4. Although the film here is demonstrated immediately beneath the patient, a Potter-Bucky diaphragm is always employed.
5. If it is the coccyx which is the major interest, a somewhat lighter exposure technique would have to be employed and lesser detail with regard to the sacrum would then be obtained.

3. **Oblique View of the Lumbosacral Spine** (Fig. 9–52). This view is obtained as shown. It has particular value in demonstrating the partes interarticulares and the apophyseal joints to best advantage. It has already been described as a means of delineating the sacroiliac joints (Chapter 5).

The pars interarticularis coupled with the superior articular process of this vertebra has the appearance of the neck and head of a "Scotty dog" in profile (Fig. 9–53). If the collar on the Scotty dog can be visualized as the area of potential defect of ossification, it is a very helpful sign in detecting potential spondylolysis interarticularis. This is almost universally found in association with spondylolisthesis—slipped vertebral body due to defective ossification of the pars interarticularis.

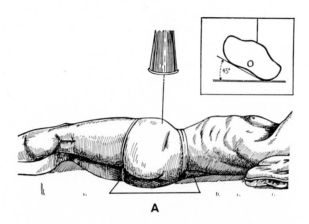

A

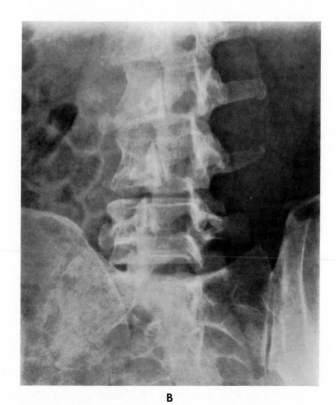

B

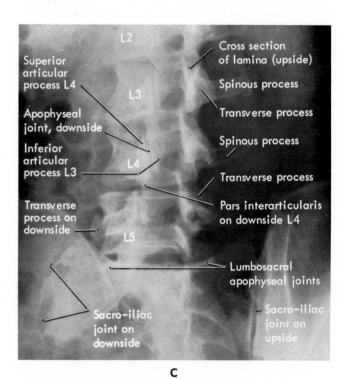

C

Figure 9–52. Oblique view of lumbosacral spine. A. Position of patient. B. Radiograph. C. Labeled radiograph.

Points of Practical Interest with Reference to Figure 9–52

1. The patient's body is placed obliquely with respect to the table top at an angle of 25 to 45 degrees. The coronal plane passing through the spinous processes is centered to the midline of the table.
2. If the lower lumbar apophyseal joints are of greatest interest the central ray passes through the level of the raised iliac crest. If a view of the upper lumbar apophyseal joints is desired, the central ray passes through a point about 1 inch above the raised iliac crest.
3. The apophyseal joints closest to the film will be shown to best advantage, but occasionally it will require several attempts with varying degrees of angulation to obtain a clear view of all of the apophyseal joints. This may be necessary since the plane of the joint varies somewhat as one descends the lumbar spine.
4. The sacroiliac joint which is farthest from the film will be opened up to best advantage. An angle of approximately 25 degrees is usually most satisfactory for depiction of the sacroiliac joint.

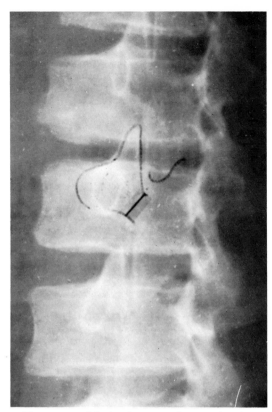

Figure 9–53. Oblique view of the lumbar spine showing the "Scotty dog" appearance of the transverse process, superior articular process, and pars interarticularis. The collar on the "Scotty dog" is the area of defective ossification most frequently encountered in association with spondylolisthesis.

Sacralization or Lumbarization. Sacralization of the fifth lumbar vertebra means that is is incorporated in whole or in part into the sacrum. Lumbarization of the first sacral segment refers to the segmentation and incorporation of the first sacral segment into the lumbar spine. Actually, a full count of the entire spine is usually necessary to determine either of these entities, but usually if the last rib can be detected, it can be assumed that four distinct lumbar vertebrae without the fifth suggests sacralization, whereas six vertebral bodies counted below the last rib suggests lumbarization. At times, unilateral sacralization or lumbarization may also occur, in which case primarily the transverse process of the involved vertebra is affected either on one or both sides (Fig. 9–54).

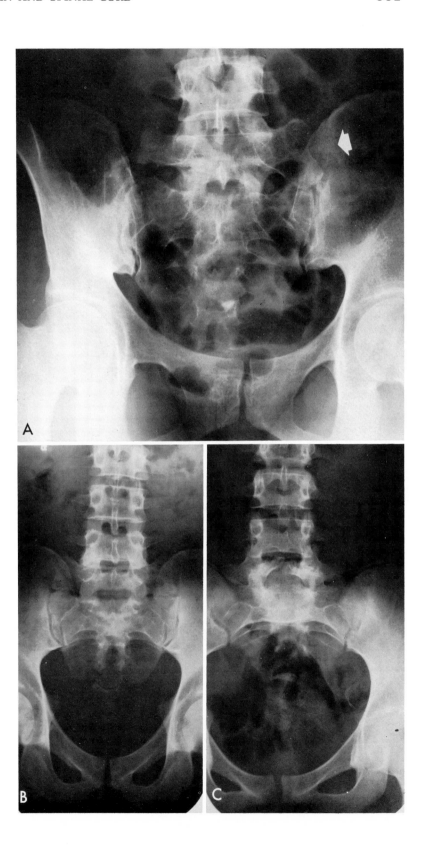

Figure 9–54. Sacralization of the fifth lumbar vertebra and lumbarization of the first sacral segment. *A.* Sacralization of the left lateral transverse process of L5 vertebral body (arrow). *B.* Bilateral sacralization of the transverse process of L5 vertebral body. *C.* Lumbarization of the first sacral segment, also demonstrating a spina bifida of this segment.

The Sacrococcygeal Segment

The special radiographic anatomy of the sacrum and coccyx has already been described (Chapter 5). The coccyx is ordinarily not seen to best advantage on the routine lateral view of the lumbosacral spine, and special lateral views are therefore obtained (Fig. 9–51). The great normal variability of the coccyx makes interpretation of this structure extremely difficult, and indeed, usually impossible. In the anteroposterior projection gas and fecal material in the rectum and sigmoid colon add to the confusion. Special tilted views of the sacrum (Chapter 5) may be obtained as described to partially overcome this difficulty.

The configuration of the anterior margin of the sacrum is of great importance obstetrically, in that a flat sacrum (one that has lost its concavity developmentally) diminishes the available space in the midpelvis (Chapter 17).

The secondary epiphyses projected in the sacroiliac joints (covering the auricular or alar surfaces of the sacrum) do not appear until puberty, and until then the sacroiliac joints may have a somewhat "fuzzy" and widened appearance. This is a normal variation that one must learn to recognize.

The special views of the sacroiliac joint in oblique projection to show distortion of the sacrum have been described in Chapter 5.

STRUCTURE OF THE INTERVERTEBRAL DISK (Fig. 9–55)

There is an intervertebral disk between each vertebral body between the second cervical and first sacral segments. Its devel-

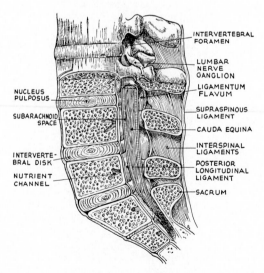

NUCLEUS PULPOSUS

SUBARACHNOID SPACE

INTERVERTE-BRAL DISK

NUTRIENT CHANNEL

INTERVERTEBRAL FORAMEN

LUMBAR NERVE GANGLION

LIGAMENTUM FLAVUM

SUPRASPINOUS LIGAMENT

CAUDA EQUINA

INTERSPINAL LIGAMENTS

POSTERIOR LONGITUDINAL LIGAMENT

SACRUM

Figure 9–55. Structure of intervertebral disk and its relationship to the subarachnoid space and adjoining ligamentous structures.

opment has already been described. This structure is described here in considerable detail, as it may cause compression of the spinal cord when degenerated and posteriorly herniated.

The annulus fibrosus forms the major portion of the disk, and is composed of lamellated fibrocartilage intimately attached to the epiphyseal bony ring of the adjacent vertebral bodies. Its periphery is reinforced by the longitudinal ligaments.

The nucleus pulposus is the residuum of the notochord, and is composed of gelatinous matrix interspersed with fibers from the inner zone of the annulus fibrosus, with which it blends. Its apparent function is to distribute the pressure evenly over the vertebral bodies.

There is a cartilaginous plate cemented to the adjoining surface of the vertebral body, which fuses with the epiphyseal ring of the body. There are vacuolated spaces in this calcified cartilage through which nutrition diffuses for maintenance of the intervertebral disk.

There are numerous places of congenital weakness in the intervertebral disks and cartilaginous end plates which are residua of small vascular channels that have disintegrated and become filled by cartilage as the individual grows and develops. These weaknesses in both the cartilaginous end plates and the disks permit the nucleus pulposus to protrude in one direction or another. When this protrusion occurs into the adjoining vertebral bodies centrally, the phenomenon is referred to as a "Schmorl's node." When, however, the protrusion is posterior or lateral, a compression of a nerve structure may result. Thus, simple Schmorl's nodes of a central type are relatively frequent and asymptomatic. However, protrusion elsewhere may be of definite pathologic significance, producing clinical symptoms and signs.

Other abnormalities in the configuration and dimensions of the intervertebral disk are related to the underlying bone. Thus, for example, when osteoporotic bone is compressed the central portion of the intervertebral disk is in turn depressed; this produces the so-called "fish vertebra," an ellipsoid expansion of the intervertebral disk. In many cases of sickle cell disease or thalassemia, a cuplike defect is produced as shown in Figure 9–56.

THE VERTEBRAL CANAL AND SPINAL SUBARACHNOID SPACE

Radiographic Anatomy. The vertebral canal tends to be triangular in shape, relatively large in the cervical and lumbar areas and small and ovoid in the thoracic area. It is bounded by the following structures: (1) Anteriorly lie the posterior longitudinal ligament, the posterior portions of the vertebral bodies, and the posterior margins of the intervertebral disks. (2) Laterally are situated the pedicles of the vertebral bodies, the intervertebral foramina, and the articulating facets. (3) Posteriorly lie

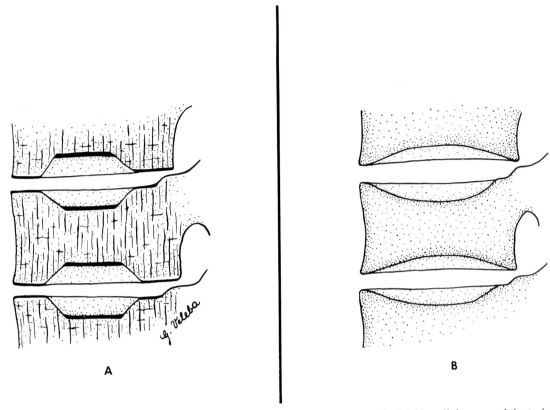

A

B

Figure 9–56. The morphologic differences between the cuplike defect typical of sickle cell disease and the truly concave deformity produced by the compression of osteoporotic bone are illustrated diagrammatically. A. The lesion of sickle cell disease. Note that only the central portion of the end plate is depressed and that the "floor" of the depression is formed by a flat plate of thickened bone. B. The biconcave deformity caused by the collapse of soft bone. Note that the entire surface of the end plate is altered to form a continuous curve across the width of the centrum. The depression is smoothly rounded; no flat surfaces remain. (Reproduced with permission from Reynolds, J.: The Roentgenological Features of Sickle Cell Disease and Related Hemoglobinopathies. 1965, pp. 99–105. Courtesy of Charles C Thomas, Publisher, Springfield, Illinois.)

the laminae, the ligamenta flava, and the spinous processes. The vertebral canal contains the following structures (Fig. 9–57): (*a*) Centrally, the spinal cord and its meninges are longitudinally placed. (*b*) The spinal nerves and vessels traverse the intervertebral foramina. (*c*) Between the inner margins of the vertebral canal and the meninges is the epidural space. This contains considerable fat, venous plexuses, and nerves (supplying the meninges, intervertebral disks, and ligaments). The fat is most abundant in the thoracic region. There is a small recurrent nerve from the spinal nerves adjoining the division of the latter into anterior and posterior rami that supplies the structures within the vertebral canal.

All of these structures are important in that their aberrations may cause encroachment on the vertebral canal; the site of involvement may be easily determined, but the exact nature of anatomic and pathologic processes may remain obscure.

It will be recalled that the spinal cord lies loosely within its meninges and extends from the foramen magnum to the lower border of the first lumbar vertebra. It has two bulbous enlargements innervating the upper and lower extremities respectively, and below the lower enlargement, it narrows to a cone-shaped structure, the conus medullaris, from which a slender filament, the filum terminale, extends downward to the first segment of the coccyx.

As in the case of the brain, the dura is normally closely applied to the arachnoid, with only a potential subdural space between them. The dura ends in a cone-shaped cul-de-sac, usually in the vicinity of the first or second sacral segment, occasionally somewhat higher. The space between the arachnoid and pia mater investing the cord, the subarachnoid space, is bathed in spinal fluid and is in direct communication with the ventricles of the brain and its surrounding spaces.

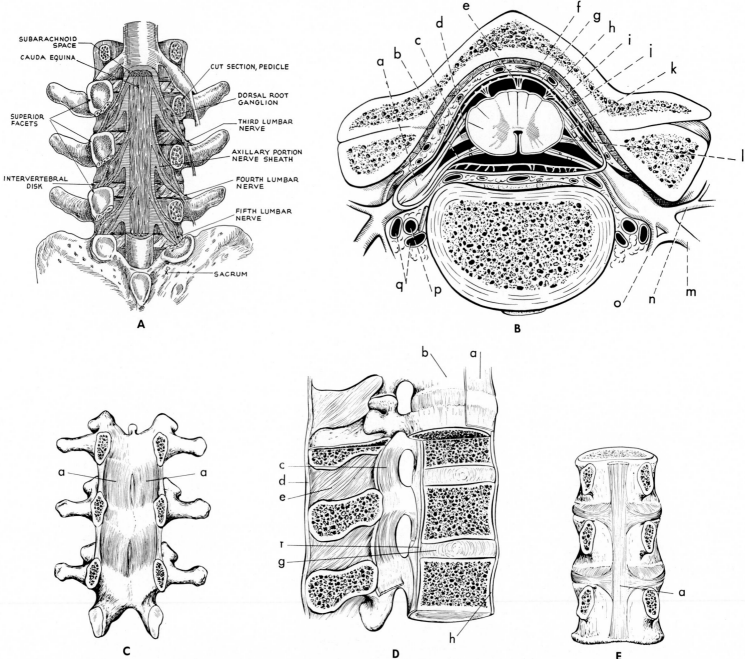

Figure 9–57. *A.* Relationship of spinal nerve roots to axillary pouches of the subarachnoid space. *B.* Diagram demonstrates the cross section of the spinal canal showing its meningeal coverings and the manner of exit of the spinal nerves (after Rauber in Buchana's *Functional Anatomy.*) (a) Dorsal root ganglia, (b) ventral root, (c) lig. denticulum, (d) dorsal root, (e) dorsal arachnoid septum, (f) epidural space, (g) dura mater, (h) subdural space, (i) arachnoid, (j) SAS (subarachnoid space), (k) dorsal root with pial covering, (l) pia mater, (m) ventral primary division, (n) dorsal primary division, (o) ramus communicans, (p) vertebral art., (q) vertebral vein. *C.* (a) Shows ligamentum flavum adherent to the lamina of adjacent vertebrae. *D.* The ligaments of the spine are demonstrated on this diagram. (a) Ant. longitudinal ligament, (b) vertebral body, (c) ligamentum flavum, (d) supraspinous ligament, (e) interspinal ligament, (f) post. long. ligament, (g) intervertebral disk, (h) ant. long. ligament. *E.* (a) Posterior longitudinal ligament, (*B* to *E* from Vakili, H.: *The Spinal Cord.* New York, Intercontinental Medical Book Corporation, 1967.)

The spinal nerves arise at considerably higher levels than their corresponding intervertebral foramina. The cauda equina is formed by the spinal nerves extending below the termination of the spinal cord at L1 level, and these nerves lie free in the subarachnoid space with one exception: just as they leave the vertebral canal they are invested for a short distance by the meningeal covering of the cord, called the nerve sheath. There is a small pouch on the inferior aspect of the nerve sheath near the point of exit called the axillary pouch or subarachnoid pouch (Fig. 9–57 A). In the lumbar region, the nerve sheath curves under the vertebral pedicle to reach its exit, and thus has a relatively long extradural but intravertebral course compared with other regions of the spine. The point of exit is below the inferior margin of the intervertebral disk, a fact that is of considerable importance when an aberration of the disk exists because it allows pressure upon the nerve in this vulnerable location.

Pockets of the subarachnoid and dural membranes appear to extend through the intervertebral foramina, accompanying the anterior and posterior roof of the foramina. The arachnoid membrane thus participates in the formation of a posterior ligament. This ligament, coupled with the ligamentum denticulum, serves to keep the cord in the midline and to prevent its undue rotation. The ligamentum denticulum divides the spinal subarachnoid space into anterior and posterior compartments, but these interconnect considerably. The various nerve roots, both anterior and posterior, cross through the spinal subarachnoid space, receiving a prolongation of the arachnoidal membrane down to a level below the intervertebral foramina.

The posterior part of the spinal subarachnoid space in both the cervical and dorsal regions is subdivided into lateral parts by means of a posterior septum of the arachnoidal membrane. This septum may not be complete and may indeed be very thin and hardly detectable (Fig. 9–57 B).

The various ligaments of the spine are:

1. An anterior longitudinal ligament from C2 to the front of the superior segment of the sacrum.

2. A posterior longitudinal ligament on the posterior aspect of the vertebral bodies within the spinal canal, extending from C2 to the sacrum. The anterior and posterior longitudinal ligaments are attached to each intervertebral disk (Fig. 9–57 C, D and E). In the dorsolumbar areas, the width of the posterior ligament is considerably decreased at the level of each vertebral body, and there is a series of dentate projections along both of its margins. In the cervical region, the width of the ligament is more uniform.

3. Articular ligaments and capsules of the joints at each vertebral arch level.

4. Ligamentum flavum, a paired ligament, is composed of elastic connective tissue and extends between the laminae of adjoining vertebrae on each side. This closes the vertebral canal between the laminae.

5. Interspinous ligaments passing from the tip of the spinous processes of one vertebra to the base of the spinous process of the other below it.

6. Supraspinous ligaments extending from tip to tip of adjacent vertebral processes.

7. Lateral lumbosacral ligaments extending from the transverse processes of L5 to the base of the sacrum.

Cerebrospinal Fluid. The circulation of the cerebrospinal fluid was discussed previously in Chapter 8. It is estimated that there are about 125 to 200 ml. of cerebrospinal fluid investing the brain and spinal cord. In the erect position, cerebrospinal fluid exerts pressure of about 100 to 300 mm. in the lumbar region, whereas in the horizontal position pressure is applied from about 70 to 180 ml. of cerebrospinal fluid. Changes in posture and venous pressure will significantly alter the pressure. Ordinarily, the pressure of cerebrospinal fluid is very slightly above that of venous pressure. Cerebrospinal fluid is seen in the fetus as early as 18 weeks of intrauterine life.

General Features of the Spinal Cord

The spinal cord is approximately 45 cm. long on the average in the adult male, and 43 cm. in the adult female. Until the third month of intrauterine life it occupies the entire length of the vertebral canal. However, since the spinal canal grows faster than the spinal cord, the cord terminates at various levels, ranging from the middle of the body of T12 to the superior border of the body of L3; usually, however, it ends somewhere between the inferior border of the body of L1 and the superior border of the body of L2. At birth the lower end of the cord is at the level of the body of L3.

In certain abnormal states, the lower end of the spinal cord remains tethered to the lowest portion of the spinal canal, giving rise to the so-called "tethered cord syndrome."

The spinal cord remains suspended within the spinal canal by lateral ligaments called ligamenta denticulata. There is also a cushion of adipose tissue between the dura and spinal cord that contains a considerable venous plexus.

The cord contains an ellipsoid expansion or bulge in its contour in the lower half of the cervical spine to accommodate the brachial plexus, and in the region of the lumbosacral to accommodate the lumbosacral plexus. These bulges correspond with the nerve supply of the upper and lower extremities. The greatest dimension of the cord is opposite C5, where it measures 12 to 14 mm. In the lumbar region the cord is enlarged from T10 to T12, with the greatest dimension at T12, where it measures approximately 11 to 13 mm. The cord tapers to its conus medullaris below this level.

The *filum terminalus* is about 6 inches long from the lowest portion of the spinal cord to approximately the level of L2. Generally, it adheres to the posterior aspect of the coccyx. There are two parts to the filum terminalus, internal and external. The internal part is a simple fibrous thread strengthened by dura mater, and the external part is composed largely of pia mater. The latter encloses the terminal part of the central spinal canal in its superior half.

As implied before, the nerves are largest when they form the trunks of the upper and lower limbs and smallest in the coccyx. The thoracic nerves, except for the first, are slender. The cervical nerve roots diminish in size from bottom to top.

METHOD OF STUDY OF THE SPINAL SUBARACHNOID SPACE

Contrast Myelography. The contents of the vertebral canal are studied radiographically by introducing contrast media into either the subarachnoid space or the epidural space (usually the former). The two major methods of study involve the use of either negative or positive contrast media in the subarachnoid space. Dandy (1919) first advocated the use of air, and Sicard and Forestier (1922, 1926) introduced the use of iodized oil (Lipiodol, iodized poppy-seed oil). Various other media have been used, and oxygen has to a large extent replaced air as the negative contrast medium of choice. Aqueous media like Thorotrast have been used, but they are irritating, and the removal of Thorotrast is very tedious. It has an inherent radioactivity and cannot be left in the

vertebral canal; its use in the United States is now forbidden by the Food and Drug Administration. Skiodan is another aqueous contrast medium, but it is irritating and does not produce as satisfactory contrast as do the iodized oils.

The best results have been obtained with the oil-type media. Among these, Pantopaque (ethyl-iodophenylundecylenate, discovered in 1944) has been found most satisfactory. It is absorbed at the rate of about 1 cc. per year if left in the vertebral canal, and it may be slightly less irritating than Lipiodol. Ordinarily it is removed following the examination.

Technique. With the patient in the prone position, 3 to 15 ml. of the iodized oil is introduced at the level of the third or fourth lumbar interspace (Fig. 9–59 A). It is desirable if possible to avoid the interspace in which the pathologic condition is suspected, since the introduction of the needle at this level may introduce a small area of hemorrhage that may complicate the interpretation of the findings. The needle is usually left in place to facilitate removal of the contrast medium after completion of the examination, unless it is desired to examine the thoracic subarachnoid space particularly.

First the patient is almost erect, so that the caudal sac may be studied in posterior, anterior, oblique, and lateral decubitus projections. The patient is then slowly moved into a horizontal position (Fig. 9–59 B), with each interspace studied fully. The horizontal beam study is particularly valuable, because it may outline a posteriorly herniated disk with the patient prone,

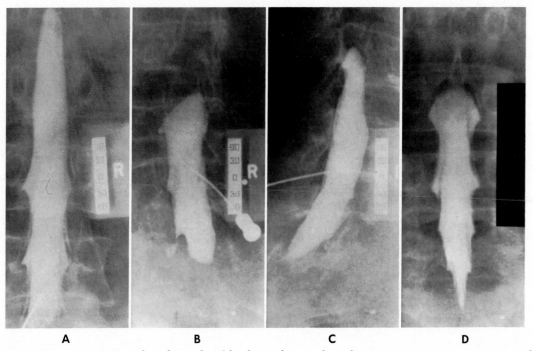

     A   B   C   D

Figure 9–58. *A* to *G.* Example radiographs of lumbar and cervical myelograms. *A* to *D.* Anteroposterior and oblique projections of lumbar myelograms.

Figure 9–58 continued on the opposite page.

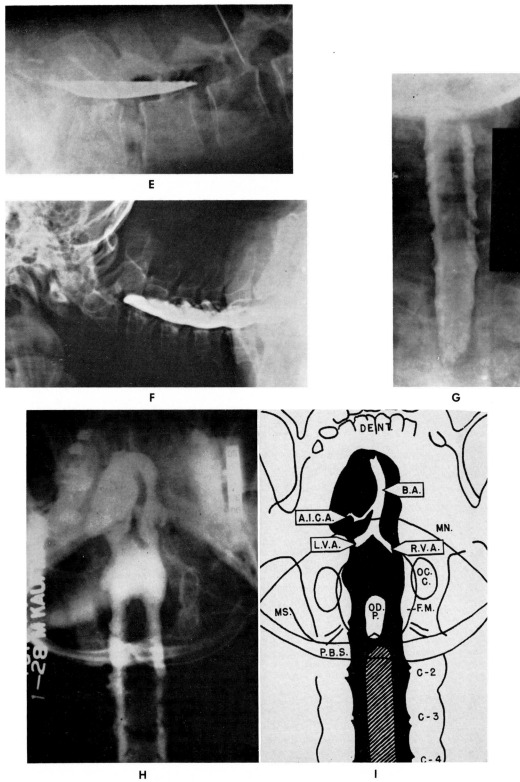

Figure 9–58 *Continued.* E. Lateral horizontal beam study of lumbosacral myelogram. F. Lateral horizontal beam study of cervical myelogram. G. Anteroposterior view of cervical myelogram. H and I. Normal anteroposterior view of the foramen magnum and clivus myelogram. (H and I from Malis, L. I.: Radiology, 70:196–221, 1958.)

Figure 9–58 continued on the following page.

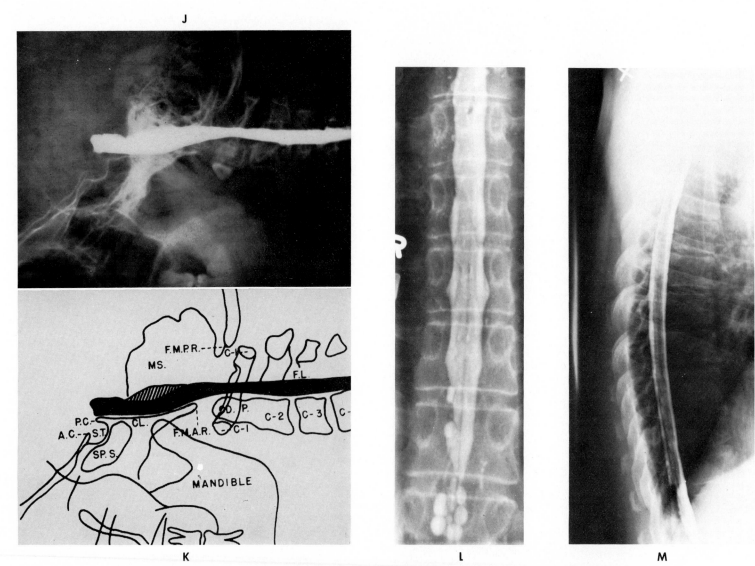

J

K   L   M

Figure *9-58 Continued.*   *J* and *K*. Normal cross-table (horizontal beam) lateral view, in same position as Figure 9–58 ᴶ. (B.A.) Basilar artery, (A.I.C.A.) ant. inferior cerebellar artery, (L.V.A.) left vertebral artery, (R.V.A.) right vertebral artery, OC. C.) occipital condyle, OD. P.) odontoid process, (MS.) mastoids, (F.M.) foramen magnum, (P.B.S.) posterior base of skull, (F.M.P.R.) foramen magnum posterior rim, (F.M.A.R.) foramen magnum anterior rim, (CL) clivus, (A.C.) anterior clinoids, (P.C.) posterior clinoids, (S.T.) sella turcica, (SP.S.) sphenoid sinus, (F.L.) fluid level of Pantopaque. (From Malis, L. I.: Radiology, *70*:196–221, 1958.) *L* and *M.* Thoracic myelograms of a herniated disk. *L.* Anteroposterior view. *M.* Lateral view. (*L, M,* and *N,* courtesy of Dr. Dixon Moody.)

Figure 9–58 continued on the opposite page.

is known, the aberration in anatomy in terms of pathology can be predicted with fair accuracy.

In cisternal myelography, a globule of oil may persist between the two cerebellar tonsils and fail to descend. The column of iodized oil in the cervical spine is thinner (and hence more radiolucent) anteroposteriorly and is relatively broader than the column elsewhere. The axillary nerve sheath peaks point at right angles to the spinal column and are more closely spaced, and the superior and inferior margins tend to be symmetrical. These differences may be explained anatomically by the shorter, more direct course of the cervical nerves. The spinal cord usually can be faintly delineated in both cervical and thoracic myelography (Fig. 9–58).

Although thoracic myelography is ordinarily not very satisfactory in the prone position because the iodized oil column breaks up into small globules in the region of the thoracic curvature, this examination can be carried forward satisfactorily if the patient lies supine or if a definite point of obstruction is encountered. In the latter instance, because the passage of the globules is impeded they tend to coalesce, thus improving the diagnostic value of the procedure and demonstrating a point of complete or almost complete obstruction. The nature of the obstruction is then studied in posteroanterior and lateral perspectives.

CERVICAL MYELOGRAPHY

Cervical Myelograms. In this procedure, the lumbar puncture and the instillation of the oil are performed in the usual manner, with the patient lying either on his side or prone with a pillow under the abdomen to hyperextend the back. A short beveled 18- or 19-gauge needle is employed to reduce the incidence of subdural or epidural injection. In the absence of a complete block, 9 to 12 cc. of Pantopaque is employed. If a complete block has been demonstrated by a Queckenstedt test, only 2 to 3 cc. of contrast media need be employed to demonstrate the level of the block.

Following the appropriate examination of the lumbar and thoracic areas, the examiner's assistant assumes a position at the head of the table and takes complete control of the patient's head. The patient is instructed to keep the head perfectly prone at all times and fully hyperextended unless otherwise moved by the examiner's assistant. With the patient's head fully hyperextended, the table is tilted head downward about 50 degrees from the horizontal, so that most of the oil trickles over the dorsal hump into the cervical region. The hyperextension of the head will keep the oil from going beyond the foramen magnum.

The table is then returned to a horizontal position, with the patient's head still hyperextended. Under fluoroscopic control and at the direction of the examiner, the assistant slowly flexes the patient's head until the oil column rises to C2 level. The table may then be tilted downward slowly about 10 to 15 degrees, which will ordinarily allow the oil to run in along the clivus. *Under no circumstances is rotation of the head permitted.*

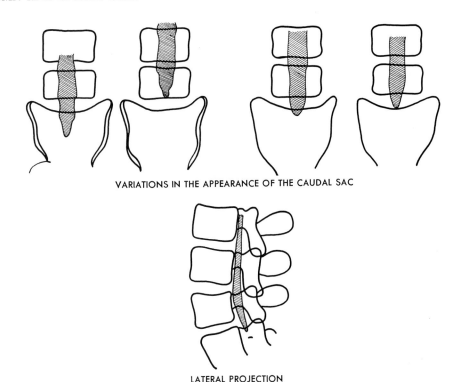

VARIATIONS IN THE APPEARANCE OF THE CAUDAL SAC

LATERAL PROJECTION

Figure 9–60. Variations in appearance of the terminal theca.

Appropriate anteroposterior spot films and lateral horizontal beam studies are taken with the shoulder rest removed.

Measurements of the Spinal Cord on Myelography (Vakili). The average diameter of the cervical cord is 1.4 to 1.7 cm.; when greater than 1.8 cm. it is suspicious of pathologic enlargement. The lower limit of the normal diameter is not well identified. The spinal canal is large in the cervical area from C7 or T1, decreasing in width to T5. Then, from T5 down to and including T9 the width is rather constant; this is the narrowest part of the spinal canal. From T10 to L5 the width again increases. Landmesser and Heubleun (quoted in Vakili) believe that the T4 to T8 level of the spinal canal reaches its maximum width at 4 years of age; the L1 to L5 level at 13 years of age; and the T1 to T3 level at 7 years of age. Generally, the midthoracic area shows the slowest rate of growth.

Lindgren believes that the measurement of the sagittal diameter on the lateral view in the cervical area is reliable—more so than the transverse diameter. If a line is drawn from the middorsal surface of the vertebral body to the nearest point of the spinal process, a measurement that may be called the sagittal diameter of the spinal canal is obtained. This is greatest at C1 level, decreasing gradually but remaining constant at C5 to C7 level.

Chamberlain (quoted in Vakili) thinks that the subarachnoid space should fill one-third and the cord two-thirds of the spinal canal, the cord ranging between 11 and 8 mm. normally. Vakili's findings are slightly different. The upper and lower limits of the cord are 18 and 7 mm. respectively, and the dorsal cord is often the smaller area.

Air Contrast Studies of the Spinal Subarachnoid Space. Air in the spinal subarachnoid space for diagnosis and localization of spinal cord lesions has been utilized since 1925 (Dandy). The method of Girout has probably achieved the widest use, with some modifications (Girout; Lindgren; Murtagh et al.; Wende and Beer). The procedure is performed as follows: the patient is placed in a sitting position with the cervical spine anteflexed so that the cervical spinal cord is at the highest level of the cerebrospinal fluid pathway (Fig. 9–61A). This position is maintained by a head rest under the forehead of the patient. A lumbar puncture is performed in a routine manner, but no fluid is withdrawn. Next, 20 cubic cm. of air are slowly injected and an upright roentgenogram is taken in the lateral projection. Additional air is then injected in 20 cubic cm. increments until the upper cervical spinal cord is completely visualized. An average volume of 40 cc. of air is used for cervical air myelography, but volumes of 80 cc. or more are occasionally required. High kilovoltage technique and tomography are essential for best results. Murtagh et al. tilted the patient in different positions for visualization of different parts of the spinal cord.

The anterior and posterior margins of the cervical cord are well illustrated in this technique. The diameter of the cord can be estimated by it—information that is of considerable value in certain disorders of the cervical cord. The normal cervical and thoracic cord are illustrated (Fig. 9–61 *B, C, D, E*), and an abnormal lumbar myelogram is illustrated in Figure 9–61 *F* and *G*. Wende and Beer emphasized that tomography is the only technique that provides optimum visualization, since interfering shadows are excluded by this method of examination. The great advantage of this method as compared with opaque myelography of the subarachnoid space is the fact that in the latter procedure the spinal cord may be obliterated by the heavy density positive contrast medium. One cannot with opaque contrast obtain an exact diameter of the spinal cord visually. Air, however, is completely absorbed in a relatively short period of time without the potential danger of stirring up adhesions by residual contrast material remaining in the spinal subarachnoid space.

Cervical Diskography. Diskography has been developed on the premise that neck, shoulder, or other pain due to disease of intervertebral disks is not satisfactorily demonstrated by conventional roentgenographic techniques. It is defined as roentgenographic visualization of an intervertebral disk after the injection of an opaque solution into it (Meyer). Diskography was first used in the lumbar region (Cloward, 1952) but has also been used in the cervical spine, with some conflicting results. A needle is inserted into the disk in the cervical region from its anterolateral surface, using a two-needle technique. A No. 20 gauge needle is

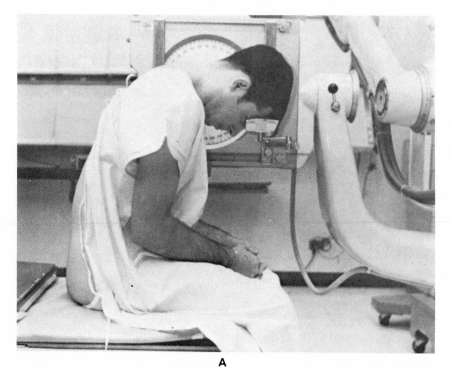

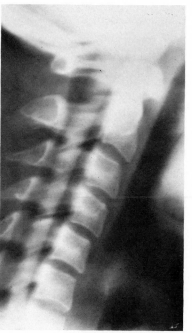

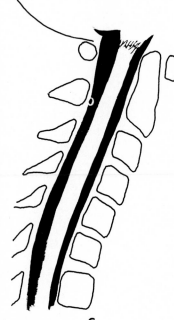

A   B   C

Figure 9–61. *A.* Position of patient for lumbar puncture and cervical air myelography. (From Southworth et al.: Amer. J. Roentgenol., *104*:487, 1969.) *B* and *C.* Normal cervical cord. (From Wende, S., and Beer, K.: Amer. J. Roentgenol., *104*:213–218, 1968.)

Figure 9–61 continued on the opposite page.

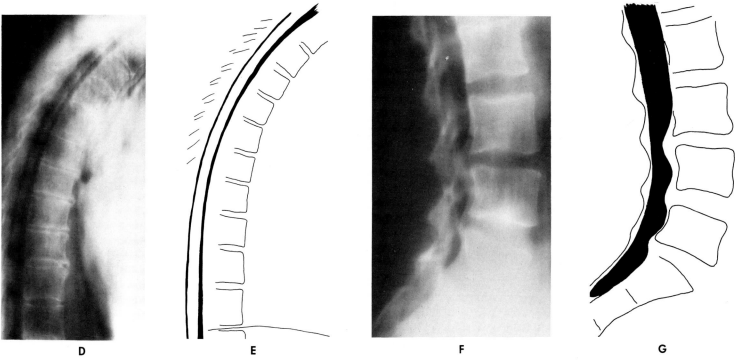

D   E   F   G

Figure 9–61 *Continued.*   *D* and *E.* Normal thoracic cord. *F* and *G.* Protruding disk at L4–L5. (From Wende, S., and Beer, K.: Amer. J. Roentgenol., *104:*213–218, 1968.)

first placed diagonally into the outer anterolateral fibers of the angulus. Through this guide a No. 25 gauge needle is inserted into the nucleus pulposus, which lies in the center of the disk. The position of the needle is determined by roentgenograms in two planes, using anteroposterior and cross-table lateral views. When the tip of the needle is satisfactorily placed in the center of the disk, the contrast medium is injected. Usually Hypaque 50 per cent or Renografin 60 (diatrizoate) are employed. Generally, no less than 0.2 cc. nor more than 1 cc. of the contrast agent is used. After injection, anteroposterior and cross-table lateral roentgenograms are taken with the needle in place. If the roentgenograms are satisfactory, the needles are withdrawn. A somewhat similar technique may be employed in the lumbar region, where the disk may be approached from the midline of the back rather than anterolaterally. Normal diskograms are shown in Figure 9–62.

THE BLOOD SUPPLY OF THE SPINAL CORD

The arterial blood supply of the spinal cord is derived from the following major vessels:

1. Two posterior spinal arteries, each derived from the corresponding vertebral arteries or posterior inferior cerebellar branches of the vertebral arteries.

2. A single anterior spinal artery formed by the union of the branches of each vertebral artery crossing throughout the anterior median fissure of the spinal cord.

3. Segmental arteries derived from ascending cervical, supreme intercostal, posterior intercostal, subcostal, lumbar segmental, ileolumbar, and lateral and medial sacral arteries.

The posterior spinal arteries pass downward through the whole length of the cord, lying either in front of or behind the posterior nerve roots. Each of the segmental arteries divides into three branches: (1) postcentral, (2) prelaminar, and (3) neural (Fig. 9–63 *A, B*). Each postcentral branch divides on the lateral part of the posterior longitudinal ligament into an ascending and a descending branch, by which means a bilateral series of anastomosing arches is formed throughout the length of the canal. From the concavities of the opposite arches, transverse connecting stems are again connected by a median longitudinal channel.

The prelaminar branches also divide and form an anastomosis central to the laminae and ligamentum flavum. This is similar in character to the postcentral anastomosis but much less regular in configuration.

The neural branches enter the dura mater and send small branches into the spinal cord in various ways. In general, the neural branches tend to bifurcate, sending a small artery along each dorsal and ventral route. These are known as the anterior and posterior radicular arteries. At any given segmental level, ei-

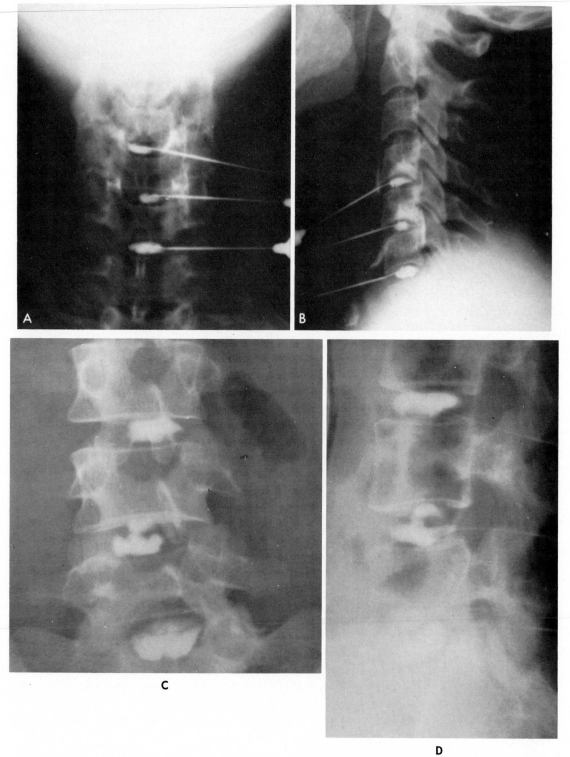

Figure 9–62.　*A* and *B*. Case J.E., age 28. Cervical diskograms illustrating normal nuclei at all three disk levels. The level at C6 and C7 shows a normal disk. C4 and C5 level and C5 and C6 level show dissemination of contrast medium outside of the disks anteriorly, laterally, and posteriorly, interpreted as possible disk disorganization at C4 to C5, and C5 to C6. (From Mayer, R. R.: Amer. J. Roentgenol., *90*:1208–1215, 1963.) *C*. Normal diskogram in anteroposterior projection. *D*. Normal diskogram of the lumbar region in lateral projection.

ther or both of these radicular branches may be represented only by twigs ending on the nerve root. The posterior radiculars regularly give off ganglionic branches to the dorsal root ganglia. Occasionally, a posterior radicular branch may extend to the spinal cord and join the posterior pial plexus. At certain levels, only a second and separate anterior or posterior artery accompanies the nerve root and goes directly to join the anterior medial spinal artery or posterior spinal artery derived from the vertebral arteries, or the posterior inferior cerebellar arteries described earlier. These may be called segmental medullary arteries in order to distinguish them from radicular arteries supplying only nerve roots.

Two anterior segmental medullary arteries occur at cervical levels. Two or three are found in the upper thoracic level, and a great anterior medullary artery enters at the first or second lumbar level, prior to a long course on the spinal root. There may be six to eight posterior medullary arteries on a side, two rather large ones being found at lumbar levels.

There is no predicting the segments in which these large branches will occur. In the entire length of the spinal cord there are usually no more than six or eight segments that possess large medullary arteries. These arise asymmetrically and are more frequent on the left.

Thus, in summary, the main blood supply of the spinal cord is formed by: (1) the *anterior spinal artery,* beginning at the junction of the corresponding branches of the vertebral arteries; (2) the *posterior spinal arteries,* which are continuations of the posterior spinal branches of the vertebral arteries; and (3) extensive *segmental anastomoses between the anterior and posterior spinal arteries* through their pial branches as described earlier. The anterior spinal artery extends the length of the spinal cord in the anterior longitudinal fissure, and the posterior spinal arteries run the length of the cord in the posterolateral sulci. There are additional *radicular arteries* as described.

The major supplying vessel of the dorsal and lumbar cord is the *artery of Adamkiewicz* (also called the arterioradicularis magna [ARM]). In 75 per cent of cases it arises on the left between the ninth and the twelfth thoracic nerve roots. An intercostal artery in this area branches into the artery of the dorsal lumbar enlargement, which in turn divides into two rami, one supplying the posterior spinal artery and the other the artery of Adamkiewicz, with an anterior destination.

The ARM has a characteristic hairpin-like appearance and a slender ascending branch that joins the thoracic portion of the anterior spinal artery (Fig. 9–64). It has a somewhat larger descending branch that anastomoses with the posterior spinal arteries and the lumbosacral radicular arteries to form the vascular terminal conus. During arteriography, subtraction techniques are often necessary to demonstrate these delicate and sinuous arteries.

It should be emphasized that the ARM represents the major segmental arterial supply to the lower dorsal and lumbar seg-

ments of the spinal cord. The relationship of spinal cord complications following aortography and aortic surgery to injury of the ARM is well recognized. The ARM arises as the largest anterior radicular branch from one of the lower intercostal or upper lumbar (T8 to L4) segmental arteries. Unusual origins from as high as T5 or as low as L5 have been reported. In over 60 per cent of cases it is left-sided and passes through the intervertebral foramen with a corresponding anterior nerve root. It turns cranially and ascends along the lateral and anterior surface of the cord to the anterior median sulcus, where it bifurcates into a small ascending and a large descending branch. These branches become the anterior spinal artery at this cord level, usually anastomosing with a very small descending branch in the midthoracic area. As it turns into the anterior spinal region to become the anterior spinal artery of the lower cord and conus, the hairpin configuration is very noticeable.

The posterior radicular arteries are generally smaller than the anterior, and they are actually irregular anastomosing chan-

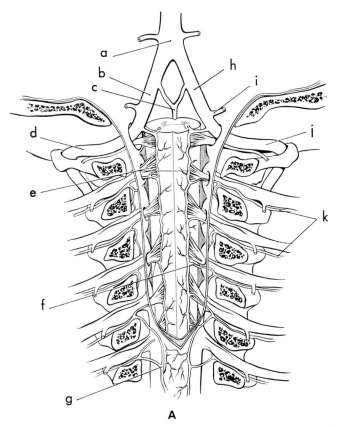

Figure 9–63. A. Arteries of the spinal cord. (a) Basil. art., (b) vert art., (c) ant. spinal art., (d) vert. art., (e) post. spinal art., (f) post. radicular art., (g) prelaminar br., (h) vert. art., (i) PICA, (j) vert. art., (k) spinal ramus. (From Vakili, H. The Spinal Cord. New York, Intercontinental Medical Book Corporation, 1967.)

Figure 9–63 continued on the following page.

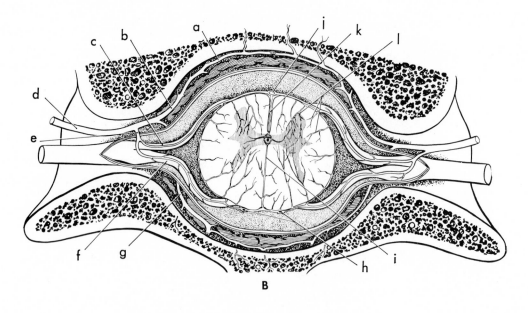

B

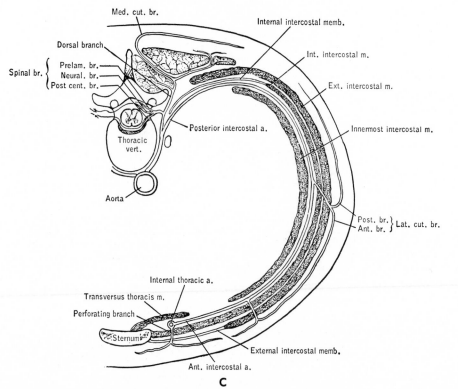

C

Figure 9–63 *Continued.* B. Arteries of spinal cord diagrammatically shown in horizontal section. (a) Post. central br., (b) post. central br., (c) ant. radicular art., (d) spinal ramus, (e) neural br., (f) post. radicular art., (g) prelaminar br., (h) post. spinal art., (i) post. central art., (j) ant. spinal art., (k) ant. central art., (l) internal spinal art. (From Vakili, H.: The Spinal Cord. New York, Intercontinental Medical Book Corporation, 1967.)

Figure 9–63 continued on the opposite page.

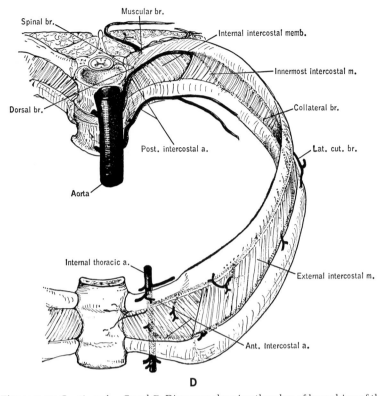

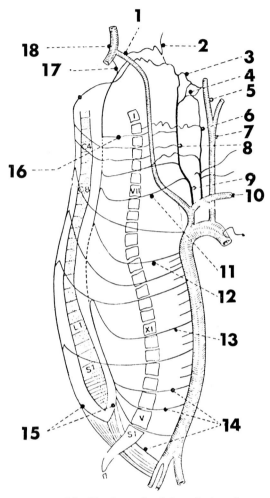

Figure 9–63 *Continued.* *C* and *D.* Diagrams showing the plan of branching of the anterior and posterior intercostal arteries. (*C* and *D* from Anson, B. J. (ed.): Morris's Human Anatomy, 12th ed. Copyright © 1966 by McGraw-Hill, Inc. Used by permission of McGraw-Hill Book Company.)

Figure 9–64. Drawing of the blood supply of the spinal cord.
1. Vertebral artery.
2. Posterior inferior cerebellar artery.
3. External occipital artery.
4. Retro-atlanto-axial anastomotic knot.
5. External carotid artery.
6. Ascending cervical artery.
7. Common carotid artery.
8. Deep cervical artery.
9. Costocervical trunk.
10. Subclavian artery.
11. Cervical enlargement artery.
12. Dorsal segment artery.
13. Lumbar enlargement artery which gives rise to the artery of Adamkiewicz.
14. Lumbosacral radicular arteries.
15. Terminal vascular conus.
16. Radicular artery at C3.
17. Posterior spinal artery.
18. Basilar artery.
(From Djindjian, R.: Amer. J. Roentgenol., *107*:461–478, 1969.)

nels. To a large degree they retain their embryonic plexiform pattern, covering the posterior cord surface like a net.

The *vertebral veins* (Fig. 9–65) are derived from the substance of the spinal cord and terminate in a plexus in the pia mater, in which six longitudinal channels have been described. There are anterior components in front of the vertebral bodies and posterior components that surround the spinous and transverse processes. The internal plexuses include the dural and spinal veins, the longitudinal sinuses, and the basivertebral veins that drain the vertebral bodies. The internal and external plexuses communicate with the intervertebral veins, which in turn terminate in the lumbar veins; these in turn are connected both with the inferior vena cava and the ascending lumbar veins. Segmental veins pass outward along the nerve roots to join the internal vertebral venous plexus and upward to join the intracranial venous sinuses (Fig. 9–65). In the sacral region the sacral plexuses are continuous with the major veins from the lower extremities. The common iliac and internal iliac veins communicate by innumerable channels with vertebral and ascending lumbar veins. The inferior vena cava throughout the lumbar region communicates with lumbar veins at every level and hence, with as-

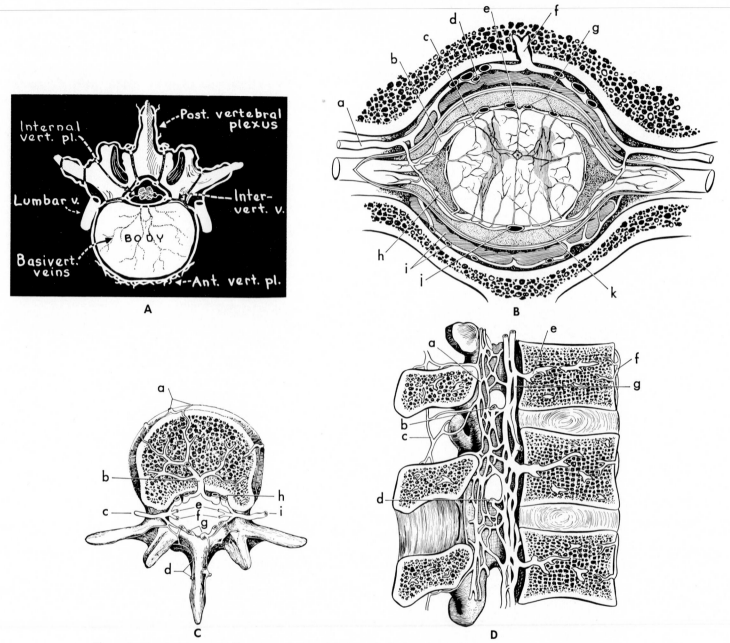

Figure 9–65. *A.* Diagrammatic representation of the vertebral plexuses at the lumbar level (seen from above). The external plexuses include anterior components in front of the vertebral bodies and posterior components, which surround the spinous and transverse processes. The internal plexuses include the dural and spinal veins; the longitudinal sinuses; and the basivertebral veins, which drain the vertebral bodies. The internal and external plexuses communicate with the intervertebral veins, which terminate in the lumbar veins. The lumbar veins are connected both with the inferior vena cava and the ascending lumbar veins. (From Abrams, H. L.: Angiography, 2nd ed. Vol. 1. Boston, Little, Brown & Co., 1971.)

B. (a) Intervertebral vein, (b) ant. radicular vein, (c) int. spinal vein, (d) ant. internal vertebral plexus, (e) ant. central vein, (f) basivertebral vein, (g) ant. external vertebral plexus, (h) post-radicular vein, (i) post. internal vertebral plexus, (j) post. external vertebral plexus, (k) post. central vein.

C. (a) Ant. external vertebral plexus, (b) basivertebral vein, (c) intervertebral vein, (d) post. external vertebral plexus, (e) ant. radicular vein, (f) post. radicular vein, (g) post. internal vertebral plexus, (h) ant. internal vertebral plexus, (i) int. vertebral vein. (From Vakili, H.: The Spinal Cord. New York, Intercontinental Medical Book Corp., 1967.)

D. (a) Ant. internal vertebral plexus, (b) intervertebral vein, (c) post. external vertebral plexus, (d) intervertebral vein, (e) basivertebral vein, (f) ant. external vertebral plexus, (g) ant. internal vertebral plexus.

cending lumbar trunks (Abrams). The plexiform nature of these veins is illustrated in Figure 9–65.

According to Batson, who has performed classical experiments regarding the function of the vertebral veins and their role in the spread of metastases, "the entire system of epidural and vertebral veins has a free and rich anastomosis at each spinal segment with the veins of the thoracico-abdominal cavity. It is a system of veins without valves except in minor connecting channels."

From these experiments, it would appear that there is an easy communication from the venous system of the intra-abdominal contents with that contained in the spinal canal and extending caudad or cephalad on a gravitational basis. A similar pressure effect upon the flow of blood in the spinal veins has long been demonstrated by means of the Valsalva maneuver—an accompaniment of almost every spinal puncture. Coughing may exert a similar effect.

Batson also found that superficial injections in a breast region may likewise give rise to retrograde flow in the vertebral venous system via the intercostal veins to the vertebral veins. This entire concept is, of course, of great importance in respect to the transport of tumor cells from their sites of origin to the spinal cord and remainder of the central nervous system.

The vertebral veins are sometimes called the meningorachidian veins (Batson, 1940). It is also extremely important to recognize that, in the head and neck in man, the veins ordinarily have no valves except at the point where the internal jugular veins empty; there are rich anastomoses throughout.

The vertebral veins and its system communicate with the segmental intercostal veins of the thoracico-abdominal wall (including those of the breast) and with the azygos system of veins; through the azygos veins there are free communications with the posterior bronchial vein and the parietal pleural veins. There are, of course, rich communications with pelvic viscera.

Batson proposed that, in addition to the recognized systems of veins, such as the pulmonary, the caval, and the portal, the vertebral veins be considered a venous system having a very important physiopathologic significance.

TECHNIQUE OF SPINAL CORD ARTERIOGRAPHY
(Djindjian)

Arteriography of the cervical region of the spinal cord may be accomplished by either of the following methods:

1. Direct puncture of the subclavian, axillary, or brachial artery with subsequent opacification of the vertebral artery and its medullary branches.

2. Selective opacification of the costocervical trunk, the vertebral artery, or the ascending cervical artery via a catheter introduced percutaneously into the femoral artery.

Arteriography of the dorsal and lumbar regions may be achieved by aortography or by selective lumbar or intercostal arteriography.

REFERENCES

Abrams, H. L.: Angiography. Second edition. Boston, Little, Brown and Co., 1971.

Anson, B. (ed.): Morris' Human Anatomy. 12th edition. New York, Mcgraw-Hill, 1966.

Batson, O. V.: The function of the vertebral veins and their role in the spread of metastases. Ann. Surg., *112*:138–149, 1940.

Boreadis, A. G., et al.: Luschka joints of the cervical spine. Radiology, *66*:181–187, 1956.

Brandner, M. E.: Normal values of the vertebral body and intervertebral disc in adults. Amer. J. Roentgenol., *114*:411–414, 1972.

Brandner, M. E.: Normal values of the vertebral body and intervertebral disc index during growth. Amer. J. Roentgenol., *110*:618–627, 1970.

Brandner, M. E., Maroteaux, P., Rampini, J. D., and Nussle, D.: Ann. Radiol., *14*:321–328, 1971.

Budin, E., and Sondheimer, F.: Lateral spread of the atlas without fracture. Radiology, *87*:1095–1098, 1966.

Cloward, R. B.: Cervical diskography: contribution to etiology and mechanism of neck, shoulder and arm pain. Ann. Surg., *150*:1052–1064, 1959.

Cloward, R. B.: Cervical diskography: technique, indications and use in diagnosis of ruptured cervical disks. Amer. J. Roentgenol., *79*:563–574, 1968.

Cloward, R. B., and Buzaid, L. L.: Diskography: technique, indications and evaluations of normal and abnormal intervertebral disk. Amer. J. Roentgenol., *68*:552–564, 1952.

Dandy, W. E.: Diagnosis and localization of spinal cord tumors. Ann. Surg., *81*:223–254, 1925.

DiChiro, G., Doppman, J., and Ommaya, A. K.: Selective arteriography of arteriovenous aneurysms of the spinal cord. Radiology, *88*:1065–1077, 1965.

Djindjian, R.: Arteriography of the spinal cord. Amer. J. Roentgenol., *107*:461–478, 1969.

Elsburg and Dyke, quoted in Khilnani, M. T., and Wolf, B. S.: Transverse diameter of cervical spinal cord on Pantopaque myelography. J. Neurosurg., *20*:660, 1963.

Epstein, B. S.: The Spine: A Radiologic Text and Atlas. Third edition. Philadelphia, Lea & Febiger, 1969.

Girout, J.: Pneumographic investigation of cervical spine. Acta Radiol., 50:221–225, 1958.

Gwinn, J. L., and Smith, J. L.: Acquired and congenital absence of the odontoid process. Amer. J. Roentgenol., 88:424, 1962.

Hellems, H. K., and Keats, T. E.: Measurement of the normal lumbosacral angle. Amer. J. Roentgenol., 113:642–645, 1971.

Hinck, V. C., Clark, W. M., and Hopkins, C. E.: Normal interpediculate distances (minimum and maximum) in children and adults. Amer. J. Roentgenol., 97:141–153, 1966.

Hinck, V. C., and Hopkins, C. E.: Measurement of the atlantodental interval in the adult. Amer. J. Roentgenol., 84:945–951, 1960.

Hinck, V. C., Hopkins, C. E., and Clark, W. M.: Sagittal diameter of the lumbar spinal canal in children and adults. Radiology, 85:929–937, 1966.

Hinck, V. C., Hopkins, C. E., and Savara, B. S.: Sagittal diameter of the cervical spinal canal in children. Radiology, 79:97–108, 1962.

Hindman, B. W., and Poole, C. A.: Early appearance of secondary vertebral ossification centers. Radiology, 95:359–361, 1970.

Hurxthal, L. M.: Measurement of vertebrae. Amer. J. Roentgenol., 103:642, 1968.

Jacobaeus, H.: On insufflation of air in the spinal canal for diagnostic purposes in cases of tumors in the spinal canal. Acta Med. Scand., 55:555–564, 1921.

Khilnani, M. T., and Wolf, B. S.: Transverse diameter of cervical spinal cord on Pantopaque myelography. J. Neurosurg., 20:660, 1963.

Lindgren, E.: Radiological examination of brain and spinal cord. Acta Radiol. (Suppl.) 151:25–33, 1957.

Locke, G. R., Gardner, J. I., and Van Epps, E. F.: Atlas-dens interval in children. Amer. J. Roentgenol., 97:135–140, 1966.

Meyer, R. R.: Cervical diskography: A help or hindrance in evaluating neck, shoulder, or arm pain? Amer. J. Roentgenol., 90:1208–1215, 1963.

Mitchell, G. E., Lourie, H., and Berne, A. S.: The various causes of scalloped vertebrae with notes on their pathogenesis. Radiology, 89:67–74, 1967.

Murtagh, F., Chamberlain, W. E., Scott, M., and Wycis, H. T.: Cervical air myelography: Review of 130 cases. Amer. J. Roentgenol., 74:1–21, 1955.

Penning, L.: Nonpathologic and pathologic relationships between the lower cervical vertebrae. Amer. J. Roentgenol., 91:1036–1049, 1964.

Rabinowitz, J. G., and Moseley, J. E.: Lateral lumbar spine in Down's syndrome: a new roentgen feature. Radiology, 83:74–79, 1964.

Reynolds, J.: The "fish vertebra" sign. Amer. J. Roentgenol., 97:693–707, 1966.

Sicard, J. A., and Forestier, J. E.: Roentgenological exploration of spinal and cerebral spaces, genitourinary organs and other organic cavities with iodized oil. Radiology., 7:385, 1926.

Stuber, J. L., and Palacios, E.: Vertebral scalloping in acromegaly. Amer. J. Roentgenol., 112:397–400, 1971.

Stuck, R. M.: Cervical diskography. Amer. J. Roentgenol., 86:975–982, 1961.

Teng, P.: Arterial anomalies of the spinal cord. Myelographic diagnosis and treatment by section of dentate ligament. Arch. Neurol. Psychiat., 80:577–586, 1958.

Teng, P.: Multiple arachnoid diverticula. Arch. Neurol., 2:348–356, 1960.

Teng, P.: Myelographic identification of dentate ligament. Radiology, 74:944–946, 1960.

Tureen, L. L.: Circulation of the spinal cord and effect of vascular occlusion. In Cobb, S., et al. (eds.): The Circulation of the Spinal Cord. Baltimore, Williams and Wilkins Co., 1938.

Vakili, H.: The Spinal Cord. Intercontinental Medical Book Corp., 1967.

Wende, S., and Beer, K.: The diagnostic value of gas myelography. Amer. J. Roentgenol., 104:213–218, 1968.

Whalen, J. P., and Woodruff, C. L.: The cervical prevertebral fat stipe: a new aid in evaluating the cervical prevertebral soft tissue space. Amer. J. Roentgenol., 109:445–451, 1970.

Wholey, M. H., Bruwer, A. J., and Baker, H. L., Jr.: Lateral roentgenogram of neck; with comments on atlanto-odontoid-basion relationship. Radiology, 71:350–356, 1958.

Wolf, B. S., Khilnani, M., and Malis, L.: Sagittal diameter of bony cervical spinal canal and its significance. J. Mt. Sinai Hosp.,23:283–292, 1956.

Wollin, D. G.: The os odontoideum. J. Bone Joint Surg., 45-A:1459–1471, 1963.

10

The Respiratory System

The respiratory tract can be conveniently subdivided for purposes of discussion into: (1) the upper air passages, (2) the larynx, (3) the trachea and bronchi, (4) the lung parenchyma, (5) the vascular supply, venous drainage, and lymphatics of the respiratory tract, (6) the lung hili, and (7) the thoracic cage, pleura and diaphragm.

THE UPPER AIR PASSAGES

The upper air passages are usually amenable to direct and indirect inspection to such a great extent that radiography need not often be employed. Nevertheless, because considerable useful information can be obtained by fluoroscopic and radiographic methods, a consideration of this subject is worthwhile.

Apart from the nasal air passages, which have already been described in Chapter 7, the upper air passages are referred to anatomically as the pharynx. This, in turn, consists of three fundamental areas: (1) the nasopharynx, which extends from the nasal cavity anteriorly and the base of the skull superiorly to the tip of the uvula and margin of the soft palate below; (2) the oropharynx, which extends from the soft palate above to the epiglottis and its pharyngo-epiglottic folds, opposite the hyoid bone; and (3) the laryngeal pharynx, which extends from the hyoid bone above to the upper boundary of the esophagus below, opposite the sixth cervical vertebra (posterior to the larynx). The larynx itself is considered separately.

The pharynx is approximately 12 cm. in length. It communicates with the nasal cavity, the oral cavity, the middle ear via the auditory (eustachian) tube, the esophagus, and the trachea. The vital structures on either side of the pharynx are: the carotid arteries, the jugular veins, the ninth, tenth, eleventh, and twelfth cranial nerves, the cervical sympathetic chain, important lymph nodal chains, and important fascial planes which may extend into the mediastinum.

Nasopharynx (Fig. 10-1). The anterior boundary of the nasopharynx is formed by the choanae, with the vomer of the nasal septum between them. The posterior wall lies above the level of the anterior arch or tubercle of the atlas of the cervical spine and usually contains considerable lymphatic tissue, which is continuous with a ring of lymphatic tissue around the circumference of the pharynx. The posterior wall is separated from the anterior arch of the atlas by the superior pharyngeal constrictor and longus capitis muscles (Fig. 10-1 *B*). The lateral nasopharyngeal walls are concave outward or sigmoidal in contour, a configuration due to the soft tissue prominence surrounding the nasopharyngeal opening of the eustachian tube, the *torus tubarius*. Posterolateral to the torus tubarius is the fossa of Rosenmüller or pharyngeal recess. The normal nasopharyngeal air shadow on basal projection does not project beyond the bony pterygoids owing to muscular structures in its lateral walls as well as its attachment to the skull base. These structures are indicated radiographically in Figure 10-1 *C* and *D*. The shadows of the oropharynx and pyriform sinuses may be superimposed upon the nasopharyngeal air column (Fig. 10-1 *E* and *F*); they may project behind the anterior arch of C1 or extend beyond the bony pterygoids, usually presenting a convex border laterally. The uvula is often identified as a nodular structure surrounded by oropharyngeal air (Fig. 10-1 *E*).

The adenoids of children are composed of the lymphatic tissue on the posterior wall of the nasopharynx, which tends to become atrophic in adults. As a result, the soft tissue width of the nasopharyngeal posterior wall is considerably greater in children than in adults, and tends to swell forward and downward toward the soft palate in the very young. The extent of this swelling is readily visualized on the lateral radiograph of the child's neck (Fig. 10-2) and furnishes an accurate means of evaluating the extent of adenoid hypertrophy.

Below and in front of the fossa of Rosenmüller are found the orifices of the auditive (eustachian) or auditory tubes. The elevated boundaries of the latter structures can usually be identified on the lateral radiograph of the neck.

Oropharynx. The oropharynx is the common passageway of both the digestive tract (mouth to esophagus) and the respiratory tract (nasopharynx to larynx). It is bounded anteriorly by the posterior third of the tongue, which contains lymphoid follicles, and posteriorly by the soft tissue covering of the upper three cervical spine segments.

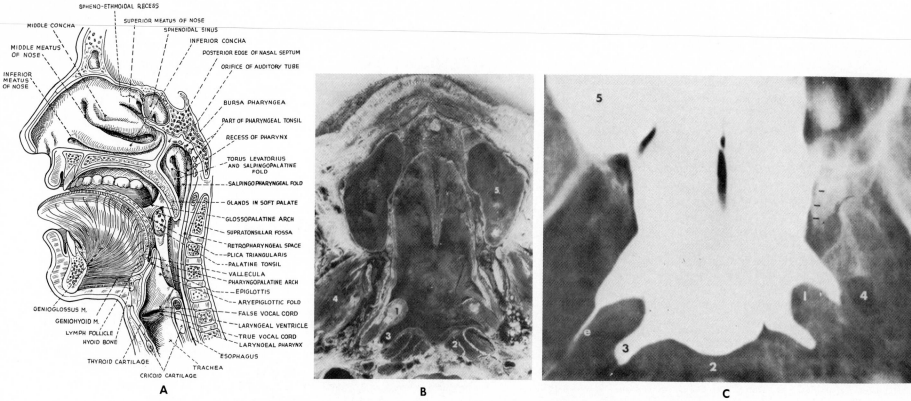

Figure 10–1. *A.* Sagittal section of the head and neck demonstrating the structure of the nasopharynx and larynx. *B,* Horizontal cross section in a postmortem specimen at the level of the nasopharynx. (1) Torus tubarius; (2) prevertebral musculature; (3) fossa of Rosenmüller; (4) internal pterygoid muscle; (5) maxillary atrium.

C. Postmortem positive contrast radiographic examination in the base view, outlining the soft tissue structures of the lateral and posterior nasopharyngeal walls. Barium enters the eustachian tube (*e*). The right maxillary antrum is also opacified. Note the relationship of the barium-filled nasopharynx to the designated bony structures. (1) Torus tubarius; (2) prevertebral soft tissues; (3) fossa of Rosenmüller; (4) foramen ovale; (5) right maxillary antrum; black lines, medial pterygoid plate.

Figure 10–1 continued on the opposite page.

On each lateral wall of the oropharynx is the tonsillar fossa with its anterior and posterior pillars. Embedded between these pillars is the palatine or faucial tonsil.

Laryngeal Pharynx (Fig. 10–3). The laryngeal pharynx connects with the oropharynx above and the esophagus below. It is bounded posteriorly by the soft tissues overlying the fourth, fifth, and sixth cervical vertebrae, and anteriorly by the posterior wall of the larynx. The posterior wall of the larynx contains the arytenoid cartilages and the lamina of the cricoid cartilage. The lateral walls of this area are attached to the thyroid cartilage and to the hyoid bone. The epiglottis is situated anteriorly and superiorly, in the median plane, with the aryepiglottic folds extending posteriorly and inferiorly from the epiglottis to the arytenoids. Beneath the level of these folds on each side are the pyriform sinuses. The valleculae are hollow pockets situated between the epiglottis and the dorsal aspect of the tongue just lateral to the median plane.

THE LARYNX

The cartilaginous framework is illustrated in Figure 10–4. This consists of three large single cartilages: the thyroid, cricoid, and epiglottis; and three paired cartilages: the corniculate, cuneiform, and arytenoids.

The thyroid cartilage is composed of two wings or laminae, and two superior and two inferior horns or cornua. The superior margins of the two wings are convex and meet at the superior thyroid notch at an angle of 90 degrees in the male and 120

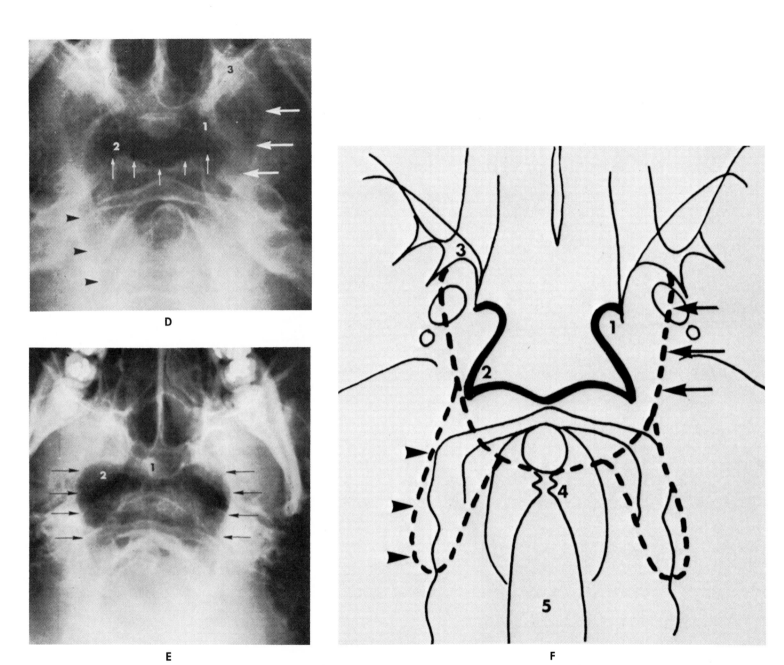

Figure 10–1 *Continued.*   D. Clinical examination of the skull in the base view clearly demonstrating the outline of the nasopharynx. (1) Torus tubarius; (2) fossa of Rosenmuller; (3) pterygoid process; vertical arrows, posterior wall.

The oropharynx is convex outward and laterally situated (horizontal arrows). Arrowheads define piriform sinus.

E. Clinical radiograph in the base view. The oropharyngeal air shadow (horizontal arrows) is seen with its convex lateral margins projecting beyond the lateral pterygoid processes. The uvula (1) is surrounded by oropharyngeal air. The lateral concavity formed by the torus tubarius (2) is outlined by nasopharyngeal air and is seen apart from the more inferiorly related oropharynx.

F. Composite schematic drawing of B to E. (1) Torus tubarius; (2) fossa of Rosenmüller; (3) pterygoid process; (4) vocal cords; (5) trachea; bold line, nasopharynx; arrows, oropharynx; arrowheads, piriform sinus. (B to F from Rizzuti, R. J., and Whalen, J. P.: Radiology, *104*:537–540, 1972.)

degrees in the female, which explains the greater laryngeal prominence in the male.

The cricoid cartilage attaches to and rests upon the first cartilaginous ring of the trachea, below the thyroid cartilage. It has the shape of a signet ring, being expanded posteriorly. This broad posterior aspect, or lamina, has a ridge centrally for attachment to the esophagus, an upper elliptical surface for attachment to the arytenoid cartilages, and inner impressions for attachment of the crico-arytenoid muscles. The inferior horns of the thyroid cartilage articulate with the lateral aspect of the cricoid ring.

The arytenoid cartilages are paired pyramidal cartilages surmounting the laminae of the cricoid posteriorly, while the corniculate cartilages are mounted superiorly on the arytenoids. The cuneiform cartilages are embedded in the aryepiglottic folds.

The epiglottic cartilage is situated behind the root of the tongue above the thyroid cartilage and behind the body of the hyoid bone. It lies in front of and above the superior opening of the larynx and acts to deflect the swallowed bolus of food to either side into the pyriform fossae. The aryepiglottic folds act as a sphincter, preventing the food bolus from entering the larynx and trachea.

The thyroid, cricoid, and the greater part of the arytenoid cartilages are composed of hyaline cartilage that tends to calcify late in life and may be transformed into bone. The rest of the cartilages are composed for the most part of fibrocartilage, and do not calcify. The calcification may be irregular, and these open spaces must not be misinterpreted as erosion of the cartilage. Also, these areas of calcification must not be misinterpreted as foreign bodies in the esophagus or larynx. This distinction is

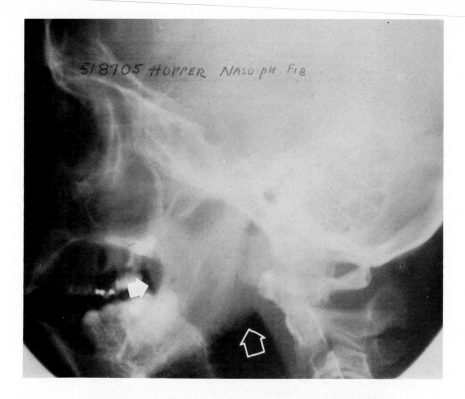

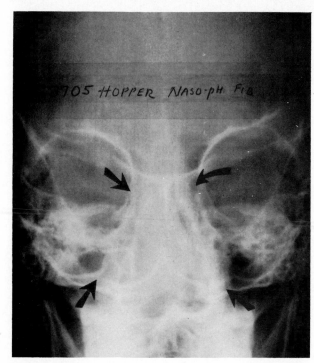

Figure 10–2   Nasopharyngeal tumor (an angiofibroma) in a child, producing a notable swelling of the posterior wall of the oropharynx and nasopharynx. A deformity (bowing) of the pterygopalatine processes is also visible.

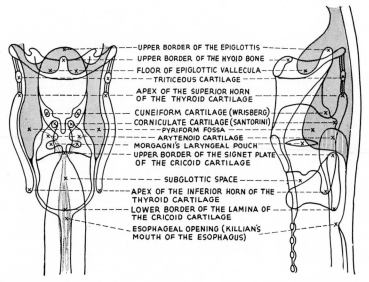

UPPER BORDER OF THE EPIGLOTTIS
UPPER BORDER OF THE HYOID BONE
FLOOR OF EPIGLOTTIC VALLECULA
TRITICEOUS CARTILAGE
APEX OF THE SUPERIOR HORN OF THE THYROID CARTILAGE
CUNEIFORM CARTILAGE (WRISBERG)
CORNICULATE CARTILAGE (SANTORINI)
PYRIFORM FOSSA
ARYTENOID CARTILAGE
MORGAGNI'S LARYNGEAL POUCH
UPPER BORDER OF THE SIGNET PLATE OF THE CRICOID CARTILAGE
SUBGLOTTIC SPACE
APEX OF THE INFERIOR HORN OF THE THYROID CARTILAGE
LOWER BORDER OF THE LAMINA OF THE CRICOID CARTILAGE
ESOPHAGEAL OPENING (KILLIAN'S MOUTH OF THE ESOPHAGUS)

Figure 10–3.   General schematic representation of the roentgen anatomy of the larynx and pharynx.

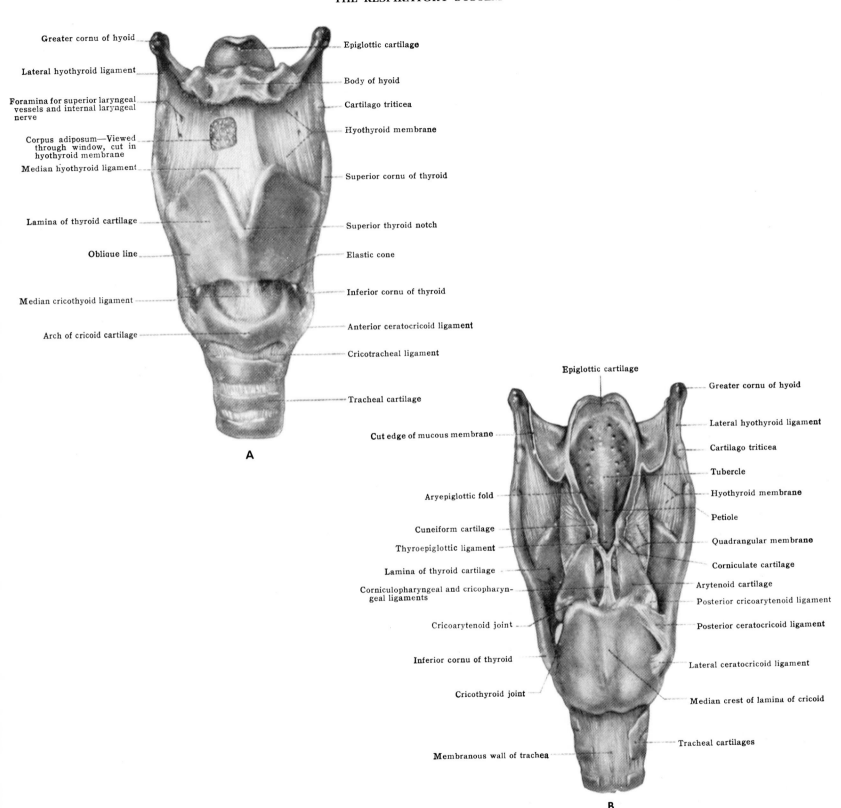

Greater cornu of hyoid

Lateral hyothyroid ligament

Foramina for superior laryngeal vessels and internal laryngeal nerve

Corpus adiposum—Viewed through window, cut in hyothyroid membrane

Median hyothyroid ligament

Lamina of thyroid cartilage

Oblique line

Median cricothyroid ligament

Arch of cricoid cartilage

Epiglottic cartilage

Body of hyoid

Cartilago triticea

Hyothyroid membrane

Superior cornu of thyroid

Superior thyroid notch

Elastic cone

Inferior cornu of thyroid

Anterior ceratocricoid ligament

Cricotracheal ligament

Tracheal cartilage

A

Epiglottic cartilage

Cut edge of mucous membrane

Aryepiglottic fold

Cuneiform cartilage

Thyroepiglottic ligament

Lamina of thyroid cartilage

Corniculopharyngeal and cricopharyngeal ligaments

Cricoarytenoid joint

Inferior cornu of thyroid

Cricothyroid joint

Membranous wall of trachea

Greater cornu of hyoid

Lateral hyothyroid ligament

Cartilago triticea

Tubercle

Hyothyroid membrane

Petiole

Quadrangular membrane

Corniculate cartilage

Arytenoid cartilage

Posterior cricoarytenoid ligament

Posterior ceratocricoid ligament

Lateral ceratocricoid ligament

Median crest of lamina of cricoid

Tracheal cartilages

B

Figure 10-4. Laryngeal skeleton. *A.* Ventral view. *B.* Dorsal view. (From Anson, B. J. (ed.): Morris' Human Anatomy, 12th ed. Copyright © 1966, by McGraw-Hill, Inc. Used by permission of McGraw-Hill Book Company.)

with the base of the triangle formed by the ventricular folds and arytenoid cartilages posteriorly. The anterior margin of this triangle is formed by the aryepiglottic folds, and the posterior by the epiglottis.

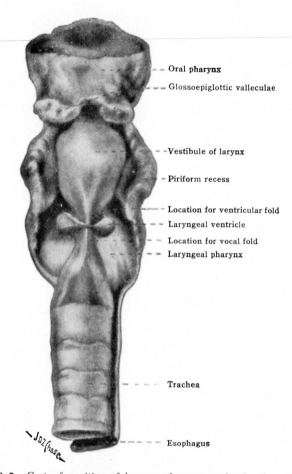

Oral pharynx

Glossoepiglottic valleculae

Vestibule of larynx

Piriform recess

Location for ventricular fold

Laryngeal ventricle

Location for vocal fold

Laryngeal pharynx

Trachea

Esophagus

Figure 10-5. Cast of cavities of larynx, pharynx, and related parts (ventral aspect). (From a cast by J. P. Schaeffer in The Daniel Baugh Institute of Anatomy of The Jefferson Medical College.) (From Anson, B. J. (ed.): Morris' Human Anatomy, 12th ed. Copyright © 1966 by McGraw-Hill, Inc. Used by permission of McGraw-Hill Book Company.)

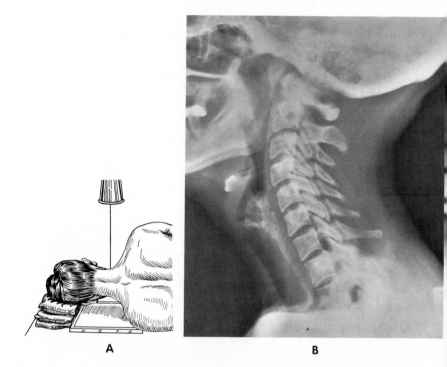

A   B

readily made if barium is administered to the patient and the barium column is then seen to go behind the larynx.

Cavity of the Larynx. The laryngeal aditus or superior laryngeal aperture or inlet is readily identified on the soft tissue films of the larynx (Fig. 10-5) as an opening bounded by the epiglottis in front and the aryepiglottic folds on each side. The pyriform recess or sinus is identified just outside the aditus on either side, between the aryepiglottic fold and the inner wall of the thyroid cartilage.

The vestibule or upper laryngeal compartment of the larynx extends from the laryngeal aditus to the ventricular folds (false vocal cords). The narrow opening between the ventricular folds is the vestibular slit. As seen on the lateral radiograph of the neck (Fig. 10-6), the vestibule of the larynx is triangular in shape,

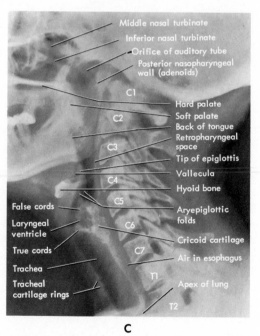

Middle nasal turbinate

Inferior nasal turbinate

Orifice of auditory tube

Posterior nasopharyngeal wall (adenoids)

C1

C2

C3

C4

C5

C6

C7

T1

T2

Hard palate

Soft palate

Back of tongue

Retropharyngeal space

Tip of epiglottis

Vallecula

Hyoid bone

Aryepiglottic folds

Cricoid cartilage

Air in esophagus

Apex of lung

False cords

Laryngeal ventricle

True cords

Trachea

Tracheal cartilage rings

C

Figure 10-6. Lateral soft tissue film of the neck. A. Position of patient. B. Radiograph. C. Labeled film of B.

The middle laryngeal compartment is situated between the ventricular folds above and the vocal folds (true vocal cords) below. The ventricular folds are undermined on each side by a small lateral outpouching forming the laryngeal ventricle.

The "rima glottidis" is an elongated slitlike opening between the true vocal folds. This is the narrowest part of the laryngeal cavity.

The portion of the laryngeal cavity below the level of the vocal folds is the lower laryngeal compartment and is the inferior entrance to the glottis. It changes from a slit to a rounded cavity surrounded by the cricoid cartilage below, and is continuous with the trachea. This portion is a favorable site for the development of edema because of its loose connective tissue.

The sensory nerve supply of the larynx above the true vocal folds is carried by the superior laryngeal nerve and below the vocal folds by the recurrent laryngeal; the motor nerve supply (with the exception of the cricothyroid muscle) is carried by the recurrent laryngeal. The cricothyroid muscle is supplied by the superior laryngeal nerve.

Articulations of the Laryngeal Cartilages. The cricothyroid articulation is lined with synovial membrane and is a typical arthrodial joint. As such it is subject to all of the diseases of the synovial joints and is of particular importance in rheumatoid arthritis or collagen diseases in which cricothyroid articular disease may occur, with esophageal cricothyroid pseudobulbar palsy and adjoining esophageal spasm. The cricoarytenoid articulation is also a typical arthrodial joint.

Position of the Larynx in the Neck. In fetal and infantile life the larynx is situated high in the neck, descending in later life. In a fetus of 6 months, the organ is in a position two vertebrae higher than in the adult. The larynx in general follows the thoracic viscera in their subsidence, which continues until old age.

At birth the space between the hyoid bone and the thyroid cartilage is relatively small and increases but little during early life.

The Normal Swallowing Function. The process of deglutition has been thoroughly studied by cineradiography in recent times. Briefly, the sequence of events is as follows:

1. There is a forward and upward movement of the tongue, which displaces the contents of the mouth backward.

2. The larynx rises and the pharyngeal space is obliterated for a fraction of a second.

3. With a backward thrust, the base of the tongue forces the bolus downward.

4. Once the bolus has passed the epiglottis, filled the pyriform recesses, and entered the esophagus, air begins to enter the nasopharynx, the soft palate relaxes, and the epiglottis and larynx begin to return to their resting position.

5. In frontal projection, the epiglottis produces the appearance of a central ovoid filling defect during the act of swallowing.

6. According to Barclay, the chief function of the epiglottis is to form, along with the vallecula, a trap for saliva running down over the back of the tongue between the acts of deglutition. When food is trapped by the epiglottis, it is forced into the vallecula, thereafter to be swallowed.

7. Below the level of the upper third of the esophagus, peristaltic action carries the food bolus down into the stomach. Peristalsis begins in the posterior pharynx and is shallow in nature, not occlusive.

8. The function of the gastroesophageal segment is complex, and will be described later in relation to the esophagus and stomach.

The laryngeal structures return to their resting position after the bolus has passed into the esophagus.

Comparison of Width of the Retro-epilaryngeal Space with the Retrotracheal Space. Figure 10–7 *A* shows the relationship of the soft tissues of the child and the adult in the specified regions at the levels of the fifth and sixth cervical vertebrae respectively. Roughly, up to the age of 1 year, the widths of these tissues equal one another and are approximately 1½ to 2 times the anteroposterior dimension of the fourth cervical vertebral body (C); however, in the adult this ratio changes so that the retropharyngeal space measured at C5 level is about one-third the width of the retrolaryngeal space measured at C6 level. Immediately below the middle compartment of the larynx, the retrolaryngeal space is considerably wider than the retrotracheal space, and this measurement is related to the junction with the esophagus. More recent measurements as proposed by Oon are shown in Figure 10–7 *B*. Here, the posterior wall of the nasopharynx, roof of the nasopharynx, postpharyngeal space, posttracheal space, as well as diameter measurements for the trachea, are given in terms of range, mean, and standard deviation as shown.

Eller et al., on the other hand, carried out a careful statistical study of the nasopharyngeal soft tissues in males and females and plotted these against age with upper and lower tolerance limits. It was clear from this study that the amount of nasopharyngeal soft tissue in adults decreased with age and varied slightly between the sexes. However, the range of variation was so great that these investigators found this knowledge of little practical significance. It was also suggested that the involution of nasopharyngeal tissue was not complete by age 25 but continued throughout life. They recommended that other features of the nasopharynx should be regarded as more important than the measurements of the nasopharyngeal soft tissues. For example, there were two consistent features: (1) the roof thickness of the nasopharynx was always less than the thickness of the posterior wall (with one exception in which they were equal); and (2) there was a smooth concave contour of the soft tissue outline of the nasopharynx. Changes in these relationships should be regarded as significant.

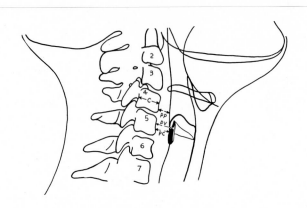

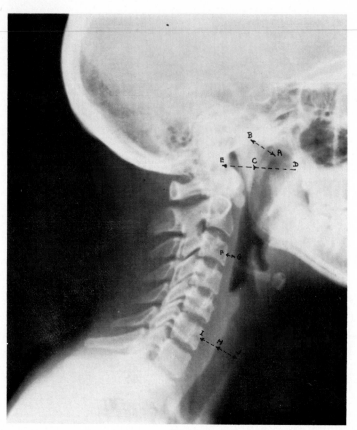

UPPER NORMAL LIMITS OF SOFT TISSUE SPACES OF NECK					
AGE	POSTPHARYNGEAL SOFT TISSUE		POSTLARYNGEAL SOFT TISSUE		
0 - 1	1.5c		2.c		
1 - 2	.5c		1.5c		POSTVENTRICULAR
2 - 3	.5c		1.2c		
3 - 6	.4c		1.2c		
6 - 14	.3c		1.2c		
ADULT	MALE .3c	FEMALE .3c	MALE .7c	FEMALE .6c	POSTCRICOID

PV = POSTVENTRICULAR SOFT TISSUE
PP = POSTPHARYNGEAL SOFT TISSUE   PC = POSTCRICOID SOFT TISSUE
C = ANTERO-POSTERIOR DIMENSION OF C-4 VERTEBRAL BODY AT ITS MIDDLE

A   **B**

MEASUREMENTS SHOWN IN FIGURE 10–7B

		Range (in mm.)	Mean (in mm.)	Standard Deviation (in mm.)
A-B	Posterior wall of nasopharynx	12–24	18.4	2.5
C-D	Roof of nasopharynx	2–10.5	5.9	2.2
F-G	Postpharyngeal space	1.5–4.5	3.1	0.7
H-I	Post-tracheal space	8–17	12.4	1.9
J-H	Anteroposterior diameter of trachea (male)	15–23.5	19.2	1.8
	Anteroposterior diameter of trachea (female)	11.5–18	14.5	1.3

Figure 10–7.   A. Relative width of the posterior oropharynx to the soft tissues of the neck posterior to the larynx. (After Hay.) B. Posterior wall of nasopharynx (*A–B*): (*A*) Posterior edge of the bony plate forming the nasopharynx. (*B*) Anterior lip of foramen magnum (basion). Soft tissue measurement is basion to posterior limit of nasopharyngeal air space.
Roof of nasopharynx (method of Ho).
      Measure along line of posterior border of lateral pterygoid plates from the skull base to the uppermost limit of the nasopharynx (*E–C*).
Postpharyngeal space. Midpoint of anterior border of C3 to posterior pharyngeal wall (*F–G*).
Post-tracheal space. From a point immediately below the inferior horns of the thyroid cartilage to the anterior border of the body of the adjacent cervical vertebra (usually C6) (*I–H*).
Trachea. Anteroposterior diameter in the same transverse plane as the post-tracheal space (*H–J*).
(Print without line overlay courtesy of Thomas Thompson, M.D., modified from Oon, C. L.: Brit. J. Radiol., *37*: 674–677, 1964.)

Radiographic Methods of Study

The air passages are moderately well demonstrated by the fluoroscope and radiograph.

In addition to identifying the anatomic structures already described, the *fluoroscopic adjunct permits visualization of the movement of the vocal cords* in the anteroposterior projection, with phonation.

1. **Soft Tissue Lateral Film of the Neck (with and without Barium)** (Fig. 10–6). Visualization of the larynx is enhanced if the hypopharynx is distended with air by an effort at expiration with the mouth and nostrils closed. It is also helpful to extend the tongue. The technique is very similar to that employed for demonstration of the cervical spine, except that a "soft exposure" technique is employed. Barium may or may not be employed in the pharynx as desired.

The structures best visualized on the lateral film of the neck are: (1) the epiglottis, (2) the aryepiglottic folds, (3) the superior laryngeal compartment, (4) the ventricular and vocal folds, with the laryngeal ventricle between, (5) the thyroid, cricoid, and arytenoid cartilages, (6) the retropharyngeal and laryngeal soft tissue spaces, and (7) the trachea, thyroid, and surrounding soft tissue structures.

At the posterior margin of the laryngeal ventricle is a spherical soft tissue mass produced by the arytenoids.

The pyriform sinuses and vallecula are best studied with the aid of barium in the pharynx.

Xeroradiography has proved to be particularly helpful in the study of the soft tissues of the neck. The vocal cords, cartilage, soft tissues, bone, and tumors, if present, have a slightly different appearance of density in this method of representation (Fig. 10–8).

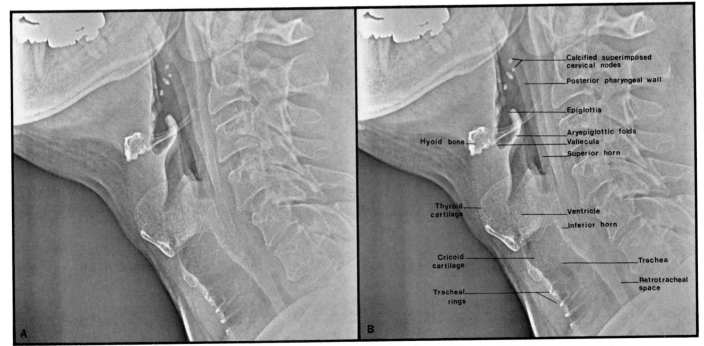

Figure 10–8. Normal larynx and trachea of a 55-year-old man is shown by (A) with structures of same xeroradiogram identified by (B). (From Xeroradiography, published by Xerox Corporation, Pasadena, California 91107. Courtesy of Dr. P. Holinger.)

2. **Soft Palate Movement Studies with Phonation** (Fig. 10–9). Soft palate movements with phonation can be studied in considerable detail to assist in analysis of speech defects. In its simplest form, these studies consist of four views, all in the lateral projection centering over the soft palate: (1) the resting state with normal breathing and no phonation; (2) the patient making the sound "ssss"; (3) the patient speaking the long vowel "eeeeee"; and (4) the patient speaking the long vowel "aaaaaa." These views can, of course, be supplemented by cineradiographic studies and special film examinations of the swallowing function, although this extra radiation exposure is a disadvantage.

3. **Anteroposterior Body Section Radiograph of the Larynx** (Fig. 10–10). If a section through the middle of the larynx in the coronal plane is obtained, the vestibule and the "zeppelin-shaped" laryngeal ventricle are clearly demonstrated, along with the true and false vocal cords. Ordinarily, such radiographs are obtained

with the larynx at rest (Fig. 10–10 *A, B*); and during phonation (Fig. 10–10 *C, D*).

The laryngogram (Fig. 10–10 *F* and *G*) contributes significantly to the management of malignant laryngeal tumors by permitting an accurate classification of the lesion (Fig. 10–10 *E* [Lehman and Fletcher]).

4. **Laryngograms.** Laryngograms may also be obtained using opaque media with and without phonation. In this procedure, a topical anesthetic such as 0.5 per cent Dyclone is sprayed onto and into the pharynx and larynx, and 10 to 20 ml. of Dionosil oily is dropped slowly over the tongue during quiet inspiration. Frontal and lateral spot film radiographs are made while the patient performs nasal inspiration and phonation, strains down against a closed glottis, and breathes in against a closed glottis (Fig. 10–11). Powdered tantalum has also been utilized as a medium for human laryngography (Zamel et al.).

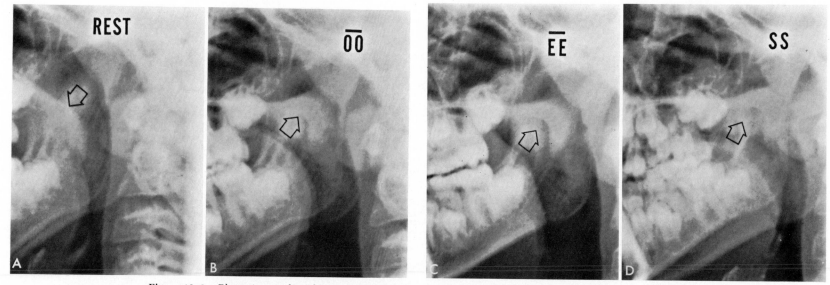

Figure 10–9. Phonation studies showing good mobility of the soft palate. *A.* Resting state. *B.* $\overline{\text{Oo}}$. *C.* $\overline{\text{Ee}}$. *D.* Ss. Note the complete approximation of the soft palate with the posterior nasopharyngeal wall in *D.*

These studies may be supplemented by cineradiographic examination and by an associated study of the swallowing function.

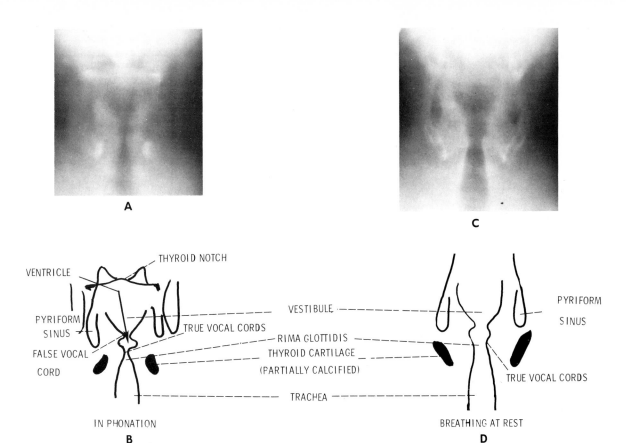

A

C

VENTRICLE — THYROID NOTCH

PYRIFORM
SINUS

FALSE VOCAL
CORD

TRUE VOCAL CORDS

VESTIBULE

RIMA GLOTTIDIS

THYROID CARTILAGE
(PARTIALLY CALCIFIED)

TRACHEA

PYRIFORM
SINUS

TRUE VOCAL CORDS

IN PHONATION

B

BREATHING AT REST

D

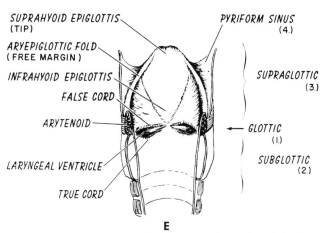

SUPRAHYOID EPIGLOTTIS
(TIP)

ARYEPIGLOTTIC FOLD
(FREE MARGIN)

INFRAHYOID EPIGLOTTIS

FALSE CORD

ARYTENOID

LARYNGEAL VENTRICLE

TRUE CORD

PYRIFORM SINUS
(4.)

SUPRAGLOTTIC
(3.)

GLOTTIC
(1.)

SUBGLOTTIC
(2.)

E

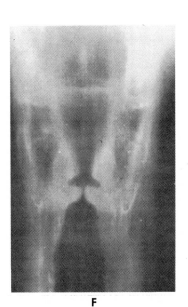

F

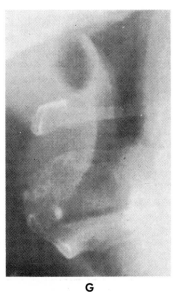

G

Figure 10–10. *A–D.* Anteroposterior body section radiographs of the larynx. *A.* During rest. *B.* Labeled tracing of *A. C.* During phonation. *D.* Labeled tracing of *C.*

E. Classification of laryngeal carcinoma. (1) *Glottic:* Tumors arising on any surface of the true vocal cord; (2) *True Subglottic:* Excluding subglottic extension from tumors of vocal cord origin; (3) *Supraglottic:* Tumors arising above the ventricles—on the epiglottis, false cords, or aryepiglottic folds: (4) *Laryngopharyngeal:* Tumors arising from the walls of the pyriform sinuses, adjacent pharyngeal wall, or posterior surface of the arytenoid and cricoid cartilages. *F* and *G.* Larynx tumor survey. *F. Tomogram:* The laryngopharyngeal walls, formed by the thin aryepiglottic fold above and the thicker false cord below, separate the vestibule

from the pyriform sinuses. The vocal cords, approximating in the midline, delineate the ventricles above from the subglottic space below. The air-filled valleculae and midline glosso-epiglottic fold can be seen above the hyoid bone.

G. Lateral Soft-Tissue View: The hyoid bone divides the epiglottis into supra- and infrahyoid portions. The vertical position of the epiglottis during phonation may cause bulging of its lower portion, which should not be mistaken for a tumor. Air contrast outlines the valleculae, the free margin of the aryepiglottic folds, the laryngeal ventricle, and the subglottic space. Thyroid cartilage calcification and pre-epiglottic soft tissues are readily studied. (*E, F* and *G* from Lehmann, Q. H., and Fletcher, G. H.: Radiology, *83:*486–500, 1964.)

591

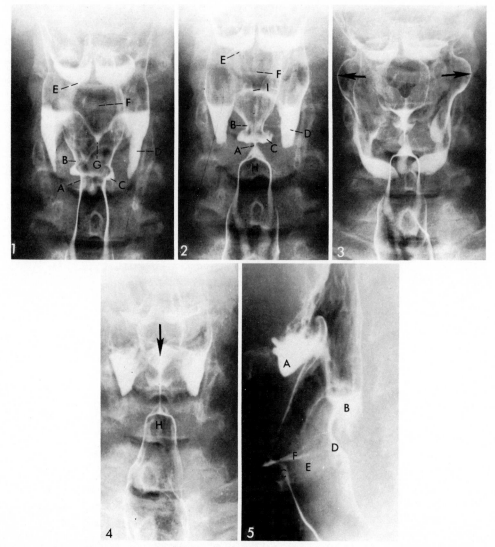

Figure 10–11.   Laryngograms of a normal larynx employing Dionosil oily after local anesthesia of the pharynx and larynx: 1, Inspiration. 2, Phonation. 3, Modified Valsalva maneuver (forceful blowing against the cheek with lips closed as for blowing a horn). 4, True Valsalva maneuver (straining down against the closed glottis). 5, Lateral view in inspiration.

In parts 1, 2, 3, and 4: (*A*) true cords; (*B*) false cords; (*C*) collapsed ventricles; (*D*) pyriform sinuses; (*E*) valleculae; (*F*) laryngeal vestibules; (*G*) arytenoid groove; (*H*) subglottic angle; (*I*) postcricoid line. In 3, arrows point to lateral pharyngeal walls that balloon outward. In 4, arrow points to contrast material pooling above the contracted vestibule and pyriform sinuses.

In part 5, lateral view: (*A*) valleculae; (*B*) pyriform sinuses; (*C*) anterior commissure; (*D*) posterior commissure; (*E*) vocal cords; (*F*) collapsed ventricle; (*G*) hyoid bone; (*H*) epiglottis; (*I*) aryepiglottic folds. (From Fletcher, G. H., and Jing, B-S.: The Head and Neck. Chicago, Year Book Medical Publishers, 1968. Courtesy of Dr. Bao-Shen Jing, Department of Diagnostic Radiology, University of Texas; M. D. Anderson Hospital and Tumor Institute, Houston, Texas.)

THE TRACHEA AND BRONCHI

The Trachea. The trachea consists of a framework of cartilaginous C-shaped rings that are connected posteriorly by a dense layer of connective tissue and muscle. The cartilages present marked irregularities, and they may be partially fused with adjoining cartilage rings. The carinal cartilage is formed by the fusion of tracheal and left bronchial cartilages, and the carina tracheae is a prominent ridge running anteroposteriorly across the bottom of the trachea between the origin of the bronchi. There is very little distinction between the epithelium lining the trachea and that lining the bronchi, and four types of epithelial cells are identified: (1) basal cells, (2) intermediate cells, (3) ciliated cells, and (4) goblet cells. The latter two types predominate.

The trachea begins at the level of the cricoid cartilage (sixth or seventh cervical vertebra). It extends downward through the neck, into the superior mediastinum, and ends at the upper border of the fifth to the eighth thoracic vertebra by bifurcating into the right and left bronchi. Bifurcation is lower in the adult than in the child (Fig. 10–12), in which it usually occurs at the level of the fourth costal cartilage. The trachea moves upward upon swallowing, and downward in deep inspiration.

The trachea adheres to the midline, except toward its termination where it deviates slightly to the right. As it passes downward, it recedes from the surface, following the curvature of the vertebral column from which it is separated by the esophagus.

In the infant, the trachea may normally deviate to the right (Fig. 10–13), and tracheal shift in the infant must be interpreted with great caution. This is related to a relative redundancy of the trachea at this stage, and also to some irregularity in the position of the thymus. Lateral deviation of the trachea at the thoracic inlet occurs normally in infants and children up to 5 years of age. Since the deviation to the right is opposite the aortic arch, it is thought that the aortic arch, too, may be a major cause of this occurrence (Chang et al.). The trachea in the infant is roughly one-third the length of the adult's, growing from approximately 4 cm. in the infant to 12 cm. in the adult.

The isthmus of the thyroid gland is closely connected ventrally with the trachea, usually covering the second, third, and fourth cartilages of the trachea. More caudally, the trachea is close to the peritracheal lymph nodule and, especially in children, to the thymus gland. The innominate artery occasionally crosses the trachea obliquely in the root of the neck.

On the dorsal aspect of the trachea is the esophagus. The great vessels of the neck lie on each side of the trachea, and the inferior laryngeal nerve lies between the esophagus and the trachea.

Within the thorax, the trachea is located in the mediastinum and fixed with strong fibrous connections to the central tendon of the diaphragm. The innominate and left common carotid arteries are in close proximity to the trachea, at first ventral and then lateral to it. The left innominate vein and the thymus are situated

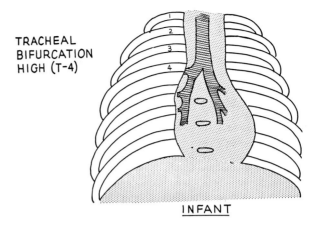

TRACHEAL BIFURCATION HIGH (T-4)

INFANT

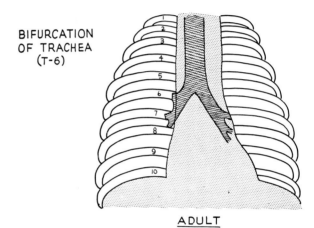

BIFURCATION OF TRACHEA (T-6)

ADULT

Figure 10–12. Comparison of level of bifurcation of trachea in adult and child. (After Pediatric X-ray Diagnosis, 6th ed., by Caffey, J. Copyright © 1972 by Year Book Medical Publishers, Inc., Chicago. Used by permission.)

farther away ventrally. The aortic arch is in contact with the ventral surface of the trachea near the bifurcation. On the right is the vagus nerve, the arch of the azygos vein, the superior vena cava, and the mediastinal pleura. On the left, the arch of the aorta continues, followed by the origin of the left subclavian artery and the inferior laryngeal nerve. Bronchial and peribronchial lymph nodes lie caudal to the angle of the bifurcation. As it descends, the esophagus extends toward the left and dorsal aspect of the trachea.

Calcification of the tracheal rings may occur normally in the adult.

The Bronchi. The angle which the two bronchi form with the trachea varies according to the age of the individual (Kobler and Hovorka, quoted in Miller) as follows:

Age	Right Bronchus	Left Bronchus
Newborn	10–35 degrees	30–65 degrees
Adult male	20 degrees	40 degrees
Adult female	19 degrees	51 degrees

Thus, the angle of divergence of the two bronchi from each other ranges around 60 degrees in the adult male and 70 degrees in the adult female in autopsy investigations.

Measurements made from living patients on teleroentgenograms of the chest (using a 40 inch distance for patients under 1 year of age), showed that the angle decreased uniformly up to 16 years of age and leveled off after that age. There was considerable difference in the measurements obtained from the supine and upright posteroanterior or anteroposterior positions. The 95 per cent confidence band for people under 16 years of age is shown in Figure 10–14.

In a summary of patients over 16 years of age, the mean value of the angle between the two bronchi for males was 56.40 degrees ± 5.664 degrees. The range for 95 per cent of all values was 45.298 degrees to 67.502 degrees. The mean value of this angle for females was 57.73 degrees ± 6.375 degrees; with the 95 per cent confidence limits ranging between 45.24 degrees and 70.23 degrees. Males and females, when calculated together, had a mean value of the angle of 57.16 degrees ± 6.06 degrees. The 90 per cent confidence limits for both males and females ranged between 45.28 degrees and 69.04 degrees (Alavi, Keats, O'Brien).

From each main bronchus, lateral branches are given off. The dorsal branches are usually more slender than the ventral branches.

The right main bronchus is more nearly continuous with the trachea than the left but is shorter and soon divides into two main branches—one above, and the other below the right pulmonary artery (Fig. 10–15): (1) the upper lobe bronchus (eparterial), and (2) the continuation of the main stem (hyparterial).

The right upper lobe bronchus (Fig. 10–16) has three main branches: (1) the *apical*, which in turn divides into an anterior and a posterior component; (2) the *posterior*, which supplies a pyramidal region along the axillary and posterior surface of the upper lobe; and (3) an *anterior*, which supplies the anterior segment of the upper lobe.

The right lower main stem ("intermediate bronchus") thereafter subdivides into the *middle lobe bronchus* and the *lower lobe bronchus*.

The right middle lobe bronchus has two main branches: (1) a *medial* branch that supplies the sternocardiac region of the middle lobe, and (2) a *lateral* branch that supplies the outer portion.

The *right lower lobe bronchus* has five main branches ordinarily: (1) the *superior basal branch*, which supplies the upper posterior and outer part of the apex of the lower lobe (this is sometimes an accessory lobe); (2) the *medial basal branch*, which arises directly from the inner side of the main stem and supplies the inner side of the right lower lobe. This branch arises just below the superior basal branch and above the level of the three other basal branches; (3) the *anterior basal branch*, which subdivides and supplies the anterior basal portion of the lower lobe; (4) the *posterior basal branch*, which supplies the posterior basal part of the right lower lobe; and (5) the *lateral basal branch*,

which supplies the axillary portion of the basal part of the right lower lobe. After the superior and medial basal branches have been identified the other three can be readily identified in every projection, using as a guide to orientation the first letters of the words anterior, lateral, and posterior, which spell the word "ALP."

The absence of the middle lobe modifies the pattern of the bronchi in the left side. The left main bronchus is larger than the right but leaves the trachea at a more acute angle. Opposite the inner end of the third anterior interspace, it divides into an *upper lobe branch* and a *lower lobe branch*, which continues the line of the main stem. Above the curve of the bronchus, a shadow can be seen with a free crescentic upper margin—this is the left pulmonary artery.

The *upper lobe bronchus* divides into upper and lower divisions, which almost immediately subdivide. The *upper division* has two main branches: (1) the *apical-posterior branch*, which supplies the apical and posterior portions of the left upper lobe; and (2) an *anterior branch*, which supplies the anterior portion of

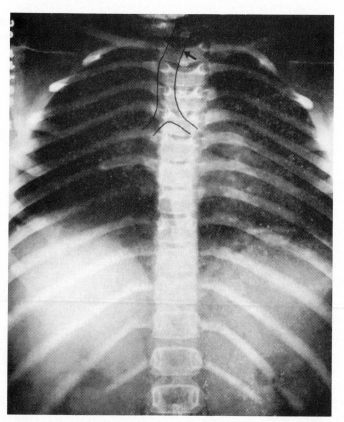

Figure 10–13. Radiograph (posteroanterior) of chest of infant to demonstrate slight normal deviation of trachea to the right, which occasionally occurs. This may result from a slight rotation of the infant's head, which may be very difficult to control, redundancy of the trachea, or slight thymic enlargement.

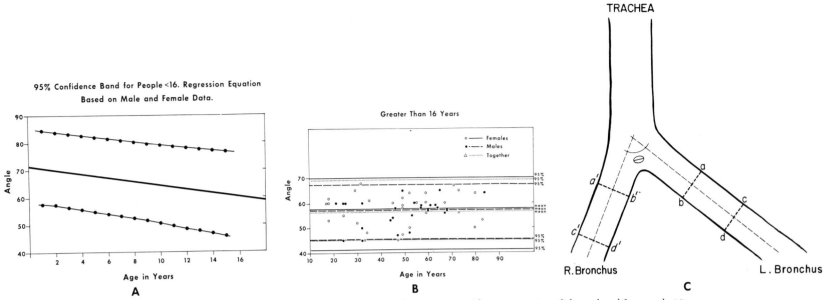

Figure 10–14. *A.* Angle of tracheal bifurcation plotted against age with 95 per cent confidence band for people 16 years old or younger. *B.* Angle of tracheal bifurcation plotted against age demonstrates a plateau plus the 95 per cent confidence band. *C.* Diagram demonstrating the method for obtaining the most consistent angle of bifurcation. (From Alavi, S. M., Keats, T. E., and O'Brien, W. M.: Amer. J. Roentgenol., *108*:546–549, 1970.)

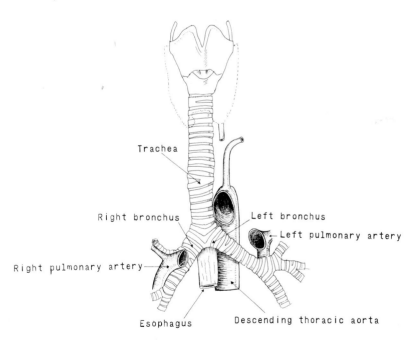

(Note differences between artery-bronchial relationships

on right and left sides)

Figure 10–15. Relationships of tracheobronchial tree to the main ramifications of the pulmonary artery.

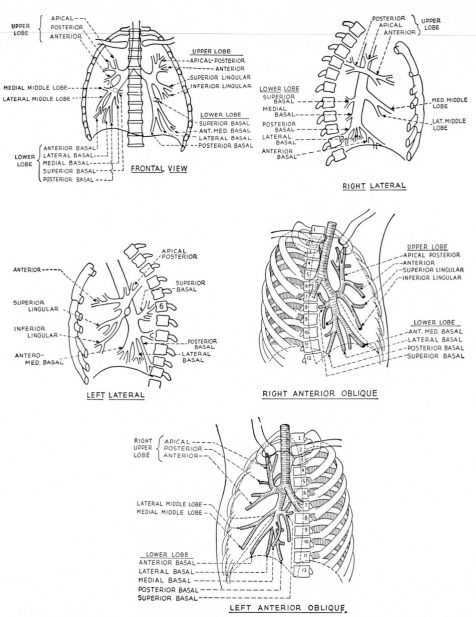

Figure 10–16.   Bronchial distribution of the lung.

terior basal, posterior basal, and lateral basal branches are the same.

Bronchial Segments (Fig. 10–17).   The regions supplied by individual bronchi represent definite and separate bronchopulmonary segments of the lung that are combined according to a rather definite scheme into lobes. These are important to identify and are fully illustrated in Figure 10–17. Orientation of the lobes and fissures of the lung can be seen in Figure 10–18.

BRONCHOGRAPHY

Methods and Materials.   There are various methods and contrast media useful in visualizing the bronchi. Most methods require that the pharynx and larynx be anesthetized locally. Once that is accomplished, the simplest technique is to allow the contrast media to flow down over the back of the tongue with the tongue drawn forward and the patient leaning forward. The patient is then rotated in various positions to distribute the contrast media in the various bronchial branches. It is usually difficult to obtain a satisfactory visualization of the upper lobe in this manner, but ordinarily the lower lobe bronchi are well delineated. It is our preference to visualize the entire bronchial tree if possible—hence the catheter technique illustrated in Figure 10–19 is recommended.

Another method involves puncturing the trachea with a suitable needle and injecting the contrast media directly. Occasionally this allows considerable leakage of air into the surrounding subcutaneous tissues, causing respiratory embarrassment to the patient; this is the main disadvantage of this method.

The most suitable technique we have found for visualization of the entire bronchial tree requires the introduction of a catheter into the trachea after completely anesthetizing the throat, larynx, and upper trachea (Fig. 10–19). Small quantities of contrast media are then introduced into each major lung sector by positioning the patient as shown during the introduction of the media (Churchill's maneuvers) (see Fig. 10–19).

A variant of this technique that usually gives satisfactory results requires the injection of 20 cc. of the media while the patient is in position *B* (Fig. 10–19), instructing the patient to inspire deeply immediately thereafter; then another 20 cc. is injected in position *G,* and the patient is similarly instructed to inspire deeply once again. Thereafter posteroanterior stereoscopic erect films, both oblique projections, and a recumbent anteroposterior film are obtained in rapid sequence.

Lateral Decubitus Bronchography.   Lateral decubitus bronchography with a single bolus is illustrated in Figure 10–20 and is described as follows: The catheter is placed in either the right or the left main stem bronchus with a small amount of topical anesthetic in the usual fashion. A scout film is obtained to assure proper radiographic exposure. The patient is placed in the

the apical area. The *lower division* divides into two branches, similar to those of the right middle lobe but slightly different in direction: (1) a *superior branch* and (2) an *inferior branch,* which supply the corresponding parts of the lingula portion of the left upper lobe.

The *left lower lobe bronchus* is almost identical to its counterpart on the right side except that the medial basal branch arises from the anterior basal branch rather than as a direct off-shoot from the left lower lobe bronchus. Otherwise, the superior, an-

lateral decubitus position (Fig. 10–20) with the side to be examined dependent. He is instructed to exhale, and an additional small amount of local anesthetic is injected; he is then instructed to inhale. There should no longer be any coughing. The syringe containing the contrast medium is connected to the catheter, and once again the patient is instructed to exhale forcefully. The contrast medium is then injected rapidly under fluoroscopic control until the entire bronchial tree is outlined as a solid cast. Seven to 15 ml. should be adequate. A spot film is obtained. The patient is then instructed to breathe normally. This results in further peripheral aspiration of the contrast medium and a double contrast visualization of the bronchi. Additional spot films are obtained as required in the lateral and oblique positions. The overhead films are taken in the following sequence: lateral decubitus, posterior oblique, and anteroposterior. Generally, the films are uniformly excellent, since the opaque medium runs into various major divisions of the bronchi, which are all dependent. The patient's breathing forces the contrast bolus farther into the periphery and results in a double contrast visualization of the entire bronchial tree (Amplatz and Haut).

The ideal contrast agent has not as yet been developed for this purpose. Ideally, the agent should be nonirritating and nonsensitizing; it should be readily absorbed or expectorated so that it does not remain in the lungs for any significant period of time after the examination; if absorbed, it should not be toxic; and if any of it remains even in microscopic quantities in the lung, it should not produce any irritant or granulomatous reactions within the lung. For many years the nonabsorbable iodized oils such as Lipiodol or Iodochlorol were used, even though they clouded the lung fields for years afterward, and occasionally produced granulomas or iodine sensitivity. In more recent times, Dionosil, either aqueous or in oil suspension, has been favored by us, although this, too, is not ideal. The aqueous Dionosil is very irritating and requires a general anesthetic, which in turn makes film-making more difficult, and the procedure more time-consuming, expensive, and hazardous. Dionosil in oil suspension leaves the lungs in about 4 days, but mild pneumonitis, granulomas, and other manifestations of irritation can result.

Delayed irritative effects of contrast medium persisting in the lungs following bronchography have been well documented. Oil retention for more than 90 days in humans was regularly followed by granuloma formation in the lungs (Fischer). Granuloma formation was noted by other researchers in rats and humans and attributed to the presence of carboxy-methylcellulose following the introduction of water soluble contrast media (Werthemann and Vischer). Dionosil oily in rabbits produced foreign body granulomas in the lungs after bronchography, and this was attributed to the arachis oil in this medium (Dionosil oily is a suspension of propyliodone in arachis oil) (Bjork and Lodin). In a long-term study, Holden and Cowdell recorded the results of bronchography after 5 years of continuous use of Dionosil oily; they found: (1) no clinical evidence of long-term ill

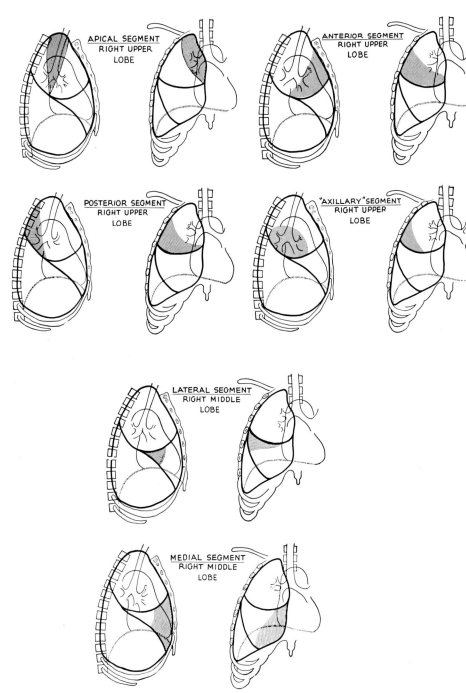

Figure 10–17. Bronchial segments of the lung.

Figure 10–17 continued on the following page.

effects; (2) immediate clinical reactions were most unusual; (3) in the survey of all resected lung tissue, no unusual reactions directly attributable to the examination were noted; (4) in only five cases was there much acute inflammatory change, in the form of either ulcerative bronchitis or small areas of bronchopneumonia.

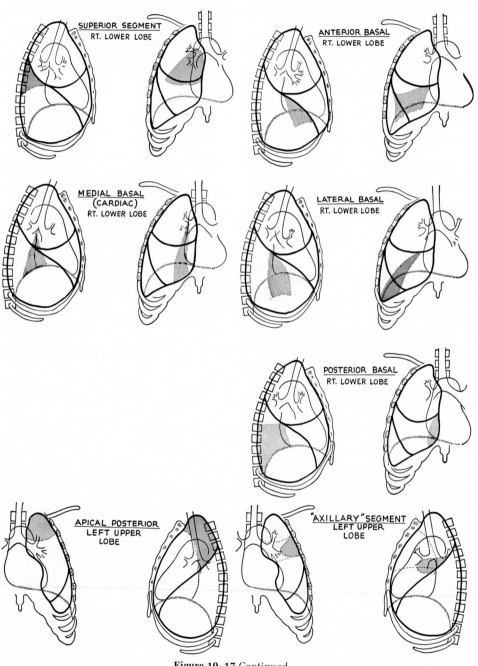

Figure 10-17 Continued.

Figure 10-17 continued on the opposite page.

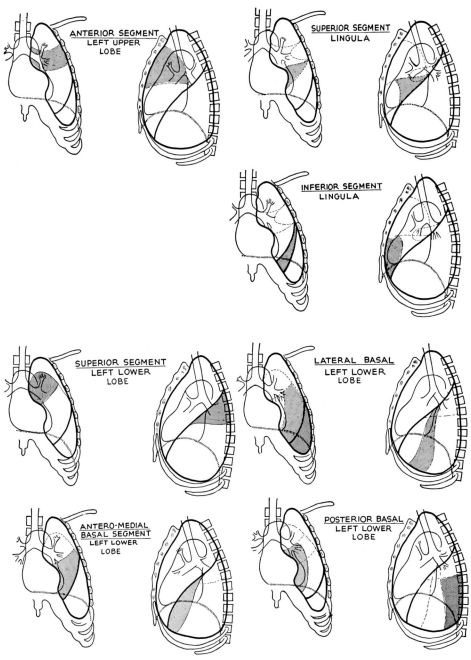

Figure 10-17 *Continued.*

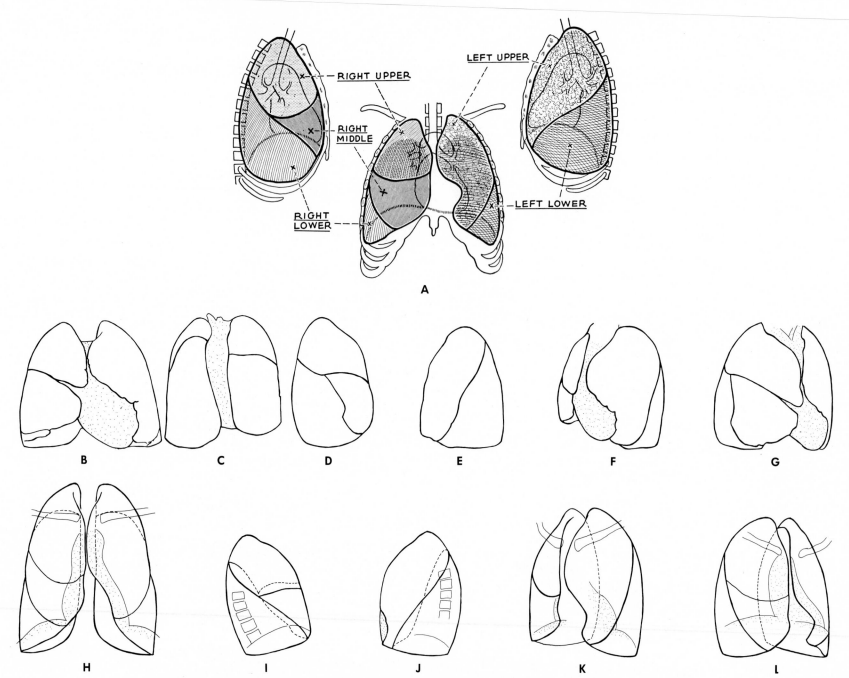

Figure 10–18. A. Lobes and fissures of the lung. B to L. Line diagrams illustrating the pleural demarcation zones anteriorly and posteriorly. (Also see the fissures and lobes of the lungs.) B through G: Frontal, posterior, lateral and oblique views of lungs. H through L: Similar "transparent views" with "out of view" zones projected over one another.

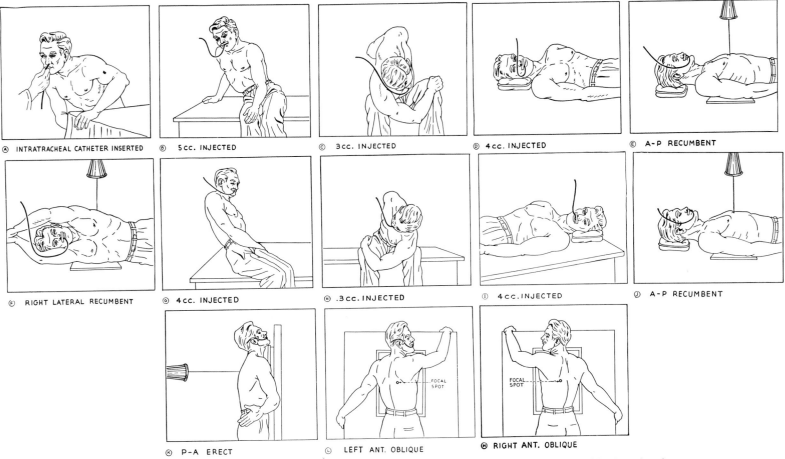

Figure 10-19. Technique of bronchography. In positions *A*, *B*, *C*, *G* and *H* the patient is rocked backward and forward, still maintaining the general position as indicated in the diagram. In positions *D* and *I*, the patient is rolled slightly from side to side, likewise still maintaining the general position as indicated in the diagram. This rocking or rolling motion is efficacious in obtaining a better distribution of the iodized oil medium in the bronchi.

In these five cases no evidence of granulomatous reaction to foreign material was noted more than 1 month after study. It was the belief of these investigators that these acute inflammatory changes could not be attributed to the contrast medium; (5) in no case was fatty material demonstrated in a granuloma.

The rate of elimination of the contrast material varied. In most cases, the lungs were radiologically clear within 2 days, although occasionally some remained for longer periods in cases of bronchial abnormalities. This study, however, consisted of human material already in part diseased so that interpretations were at times difficult.

Some experiments with 50 per cent colloidal barium in saline plus a 2 per cent methylcarboxycellulose mixture would appear to offer some promise but experience with this latter medium is still too limited.

Our own preference at this time is Dionosil in oil suspension, although admittedly this is not ideal in either contrast or benignity of reaction.

The following film studies are obtained after the injection of the contrast media:

1. Anteroposterior recumbent and lateral views of the side first injected, immediately after injection and before the second side is injected (Fig. 10-21 *A*, and *B* or *E*).

2. An anteroposterior view of the chest after both sides are injected.

3. An erect posteroanterior view of the chest after both sides are injected (Fig. 10-21 *D*).

4. Both oblique views after both sides are injected (stereoscopic views may be obtained if desired) (Fig. 10-21 *C* and *F*).

The above study may be combined with fluoroscopy, if a good

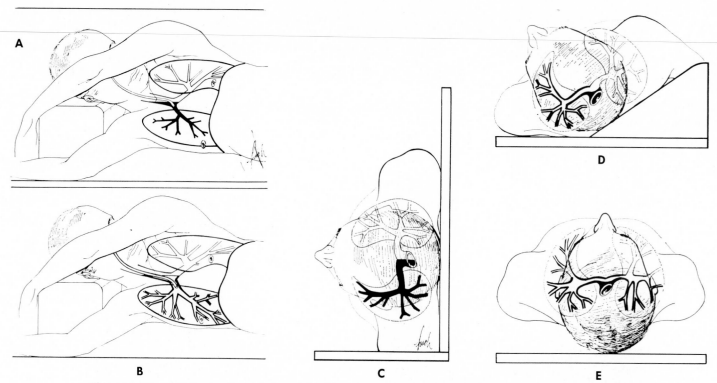

Figure 10–20. *A.* Patient reclining in lateral decubitus position. Contrast medium injected during forceful expiration allows filling of all proximal radicles with a single bolus injection. Orifices of all major bronchi are occluded by contrast medium, but distal radicles are not filled.

B. Following inhalation, the air pushes the contrast medium into peripheral radicles, resulting in double contrast visualization.

Spot-films and first overhead films made in lateral decubitus position (*C*) to be followed by posterior oblique (*D*). Last film made in supine position may result in spillage of contrast medium into contralateral lung, which is not objectionable in this view (*E*). (From Amplatz, K., and Haut, G.: Radiology, *95*:439–440, 1970.)

spot-film apparatus is available that will give detail as good as the conventional studies. One advantage of the fluoroscopic examination is that it permits visualization of the filling as it occurs, so that the examiner knows immediately whether or not further filling is required. Moreover, a concept of the physiologic function of the bronchial tree is also thereby acquired. Balanced against this great advantage, however, is the fact that spot films are seldom as satisfactory in minute detail as are conventional long distance and small focal spot-film studies. The examiner must therefore adapt the technique to his requirements.

Ordinarily, both sides of the lung are injected at the same examination if the patient's respiratory capacity will permit it. In many patients, injection of only one side at a single sitting is possible.

The radiographic anatomy of the bronchi and their distribution have been illustrated in previous diagrams (see Fig. 10–16).

Bronchial Brush Biopsy and Selective Bronchography. A bronchial abrasion technique for cytologic study of peripheral

bronchial lesions was described some years ago (MacLean, 1958a). In more recent times controllable brushes, telescoping catheters, and fibroscopes have provided a means not only for obtaining microbiopsies or cytologic study of peripheral lesions, but also for segmental bronchography of these regions (Fennessy, 1967; Sovak; Bean et al., 1968; Willson and Eskridge). The most recent technique, advocated by Willson and Eskridge, is carried out as follows: The patient is given a topical anesthetic as for bronchography. The outside larger catheter of a telescoping catheter (a 45 cm. No. 16 French radiopaque polyvinyl tube) is positioned with the tip in the trachea just above the carina. Through it is inserted a specially molded telescoping bronchial catheter of radiopaque polyethylene with a precurved tip to fit the desired lobar bronchus. A controllable guidewire is used to guide this catheter into the correct position under fluoroscopic control (Fig. 10–22). Once the inner catheter is in position a special brush is passed through it to the desired location under fluoroscopic control and moved in a clockwise direction so that a scraping of the bronchial mucosa or a specimen of the lesion in question is obtained. This brush is then withdrawn back into the telescoping catheter and removed. Various specimens may be obtained by this method, including: (1) a smear of the tissue on a slide, (2) a microbiopsy specimen, or (3) cultures.

Following the procurement of satisfactory specimens, selective bronchography is carried out by injection through the catheter into the desired areas of lung, and spot films are taken of the areas in question.

Fiberoptic Bronchoscopy (Schoenbaum et al.; Kahn). A flexible bronchofiberscope was introduced by Ikeda in 1968. This instrument was inserted originally through a bronchoscope or an endotracheal tube under general anesthesia, but since that time commercial flexible fiberoptic bronchoscopes have become available.*

---

*Olympus Bronchofiberscope, Type 5 B; Olympus Bronchofiberscope, Type 5 B2, Olympus Corporation of America, 2 Nevada Drive, New Hyde Park, New York, 11040; Fiber-Bronchoscope FBS-6T with associated instruments, American Optical Machida Company, Southbridge, Mass.

These instruments vary somewhat but generally consist of a flexible tube which contains numerous bundles of thread-size glass fibers as image and light guides (Fig. 10–22 *B*). The hard tip at the end of this scope has an outer diameter of 5.2 mm. and its bending section is flexible through an angle of 160 degrees. The angle is controlled by a lever in the handle or control unit. The outer diameter of the bending section is 5.4 mm., and the flexible tube has an outer diameter of 5.7 mm. and a working length of 600 mm. A biopsy forceps or a cytology brush can be inserted through the hollow suction channel from the control unit on the handle. Photographs may be taken with the attachable Olympus camera. Various other attachments are available for teaching and evaluation by groups of two or more physicians.

Patients are given premedication with a suitable sedative, atropine, and topical anesthesia. A No. 36 French nasopharyngeal airway is passed through the nose into the oropharynx and, in most instances, the fiberoptic bronchoscope is then passed through the airway into the trachea under direct visualization.

Biopsies may be made of centrally located lesions, which may be brushed under direct visualization through the scope.

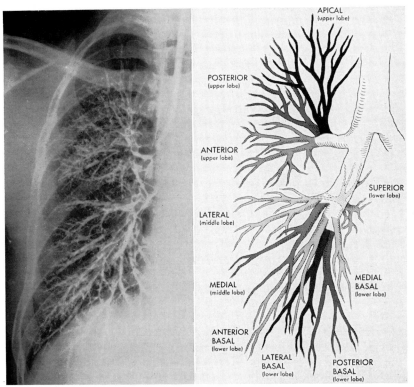
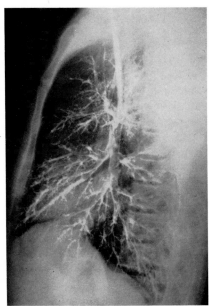
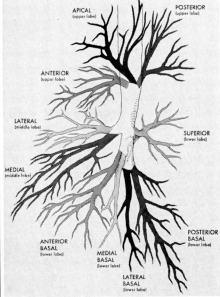

Figure 10–21. The normal human bronchial tree. *A.* Right posteroanterior projection. *B.* Right lateral projection.
(From Lehman, J. S., and Crellin, J. A.: Medical Radiology and Photography, *31,* 1955.)

Figure 10–21 continued on the following page.

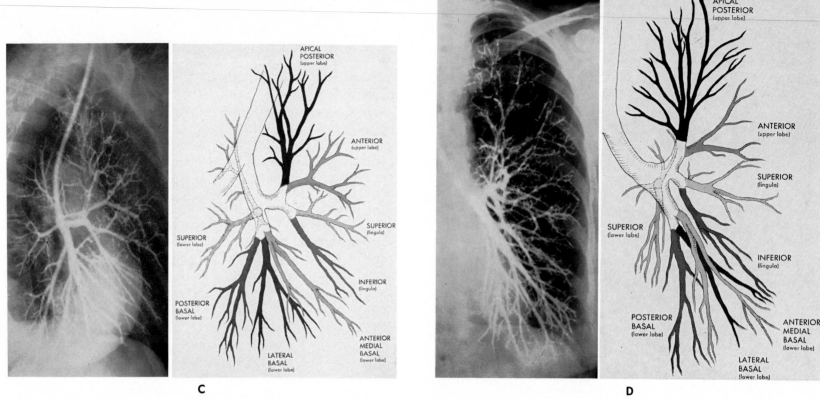

Figure 10–21 *Continued.*   C. Right anterior oblique projection. D. Left posteroanterior projection.

Figure 10–21 continued on the opposite page.

The specimen obtained is smeared on a slide coated with egg albumin and immersed immediately in 70 per cent alcohol, and is then sent for cytologic examination together with washings from the appropriate area. Biopsy specimens may be immersed in formalin and sent for histologic examination.

The fiberoptic bronchoscope may be guided to a lesion under suspicion by image-amplified fluoroscopy; bronchial brush biopsy, smears, and cultures may thereby be obtained. If a bronchogram is indicated, the fiberoptic bronchoscope is exchanged under fluoroscopic control over an appropriate angiographic guidewire for a polyethylene tube, the bronchogram then being obtained through the polyethylene catheter.

Generally, patients with heart failure, chronic obstructive pulmonary disease, asthma, pneumonia or other pulmonary problems may be studied only after careful arterial blood gas samples have been analyzed. Even the premedication should not be given to patients with borderline pulmonary functions, hypoxemia requiring oxygen, or respiratory failure.

The control handle of the instrument cannot be immersed in any liquid sterilization substance since damage may result, but the flexible section of the scope may be sterilized by soaking it in Betadine and then rinsing in isopropyl alcohol 70 per cent followed by sterile water. Cold gas sterilization may also be used, but unfortunately this procedure takes 17 to 24 hours and is not practical when more than one patient must be examined in a day.

Many investigators have used modifications of the above procedure (Smiddy et al.).

Faber et al. reported the use of the flexible fiberoptic bronchoscope in 205 cases of suspected malignancy. A positive diagnosis was obtained by brush biopsy in 76 per cent of 170 patients with proven pulmonary carcinoma. This represented an increase of 28 per cent as compared with their fixed catheter technique of obtaining such specimens.

Tracheobronchial secretion management, selective bronchography, bacteriology, and many other applications have been described for this technique. With approximately 1200 cases reported in the literature to date, there have been no reported complications (Kahn).

Schoenbaum et al. have reported the use of this technique

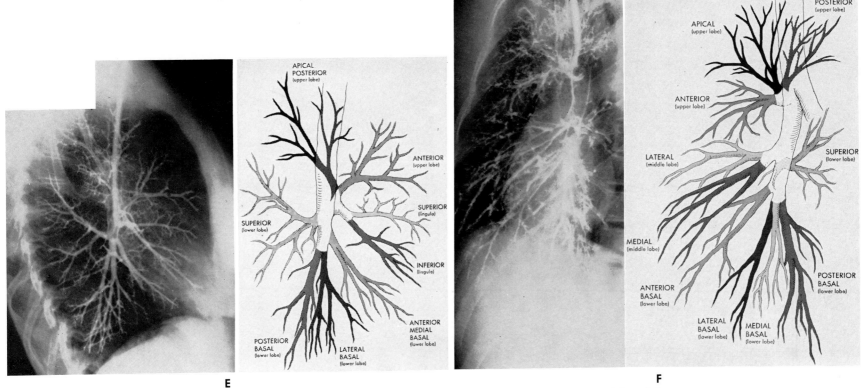

Figure 10–21 *Continued.* *E.* Left lateral projection. *F.* Left anterior oblique projection. (*C* to *F* from Lehman, J. S., and Crellin, J. A.: Medical Radiography and Photography, *31*, 1955.)

in patients with primary bronchial carcinoma and many other diseases such as bronchiectasis, tuberculosis, pneumonia, and other infections.

Selective Wedge Bronchography (Sargent and Sherwin). In this technique a radiopaque thin-walled polyethylene tube with a distal tip slightly tapered to an external diameter of approximately 0.5 mm. is used to enter airways with the smallest diameters. This small catheter is inserted through the lumen of a larger one, thus facilitating entry into a distal selective small airway. The opaque medium is then instilled through the smaller inner catheter, and the material is allowed to enter the airway by gravity and respiratory motion.

When this study was performed on experimental animals a wide variety of opaque materials were evaluated, including: powders such as tantalum, Dionosil, micropaque (barium sulfate in an emulsion mixture), calcium tungstate, and Renografin. Oil base suspensions, such as Dionosil oily and Lipiodol, were also used. Aqueous suspensions, including aqueous Dionosil, Dionosil suspended in buffered and dextrose solutions, tantalum sus-

pended in human serum albumin, calcium tungstate suspended in reconstituted human serum albumin, stereopaque barium, Renografin-60, and Urografin in an adhesive mixture, were evaluated also.

The aqueous preparations, except for the very viscous Urografin adhesive mixtures, were the most satisfactory for ease of instillation. The powdered materials clogged the internal lumen of the small catheters used. Likewise, the oily media with their greater viscosity were not satisfactory. The tantalum and calcium tungstate suspensions in human serum albumin were the only two media extending into the periphery of the lobule that usefully filled alveolar ducts and alveoli. The commercial aqueous Dionosil preparations extended into the terminal bronchioles but rarely beyond. Oily Dionosil and Lipiodol failed to extend beyond the terminal bronchioles and a few kinds of respiratory bronchioles, and did not enter the alveoli at all. When higher pressures were used, however, bronchiolar and alveolar wall disruption occurred, resulting in loss of recognizable histologic anatomy. Thus, the best agent for demonstration of the smallest airways was found to

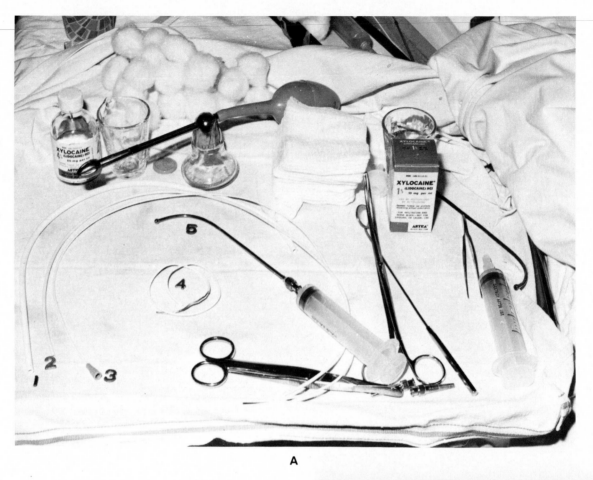

A

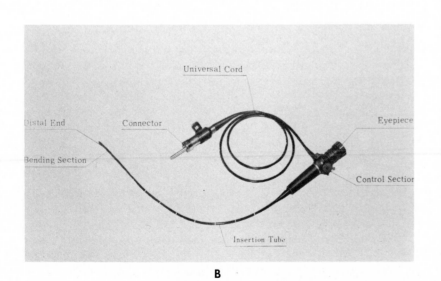

B

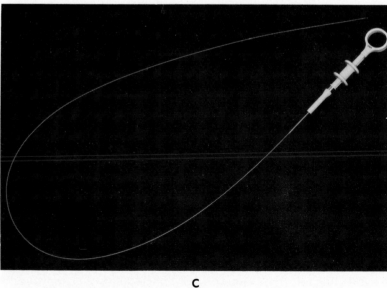

C

Figure 10–22.   *A.* Tray usually employed for bronchial brush biopsy when the bronchofiberscope is not available. This tray consists of three different sizes of plastic tubes and local anesthetic devices. The largest tube is passed through the nares to the larynx. A smaller tube goes through the larger one into the trachea and bronchus, and a spiral wire with a cutting helix on its end passes through the smallest tube to be used for cytologic or biopsy specimens. A very small caliber tube may also be passed for segmental or wedge bronchoscopy at this time. *B.* Olympic bronchofiberscope. *C.* Biopsy wire of bronchofiberscope which can be inserted to protrude through the distal end.

Figure 10–22 continued on the opposite page.

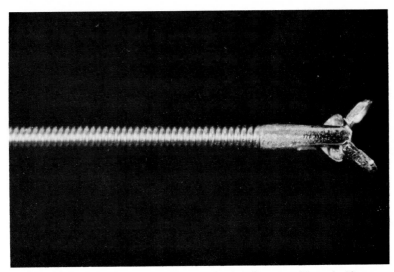

Figure 10–22 *Continued.* D. Close-up of claw mechanism of bronchofiberscope used for biopsy.

be tantalum suspended in human serum albumin. The technique of selective wedge bronchography is designed to limit the filling of selective portions of the lung so that only one or a few secondary lobules are filled, and superimposition of filling in adjacent areas is avoided.

From this study it was concluded that, in the normal lung, oily suspensions immediately fill airways beyond the first order respiratory bronchioles up to the alveolar region without using excessive tissue disruptive pressures. However, with the more viscous oily substances, no filling beyond the terminal bronchioles occurred unless excessive pressures were applied. The longer the media were permitted to remain in the distal airways, the greater the chance of alveolar filling.

The "alveolar image" seen on the usual bronchogram in clinical practice is actually a conglomeration of shadows with superimposition of secondary lobules which probably cannot be accurately correlated morphologically.

Unfortunately, tantalum has been demonstrated in experiments to remain in the lung as long as 12 months after bronchography (Nadel et al.). The long-term retention of tantalum in experimental bronchography is about 20 per cent of the administered tantalum dose (Upham et al.). Unfortunately also, the diatrizoates can produce pulmonary edema, and barium sulfate suspensions can obstruct airways by a mechanical inspissation (Reich).

Dionosil has the advantage of being only slightly soluble in saline and serum. It is hydrolized enzymatically in the body, and the resulting organic iodopyracet is not further metabolized or degraded but is secreted rapidly by the kidneys (Fischer and Balug). Oily Dionosil, which contains peanut oil, can cause changes resembling those produced by Lipiodol, such as late pulmonary granuloma and fibrotic alterations. Aqueous Dionosil

contains carboxymethylcellulose, which is said to be the source of granuloma formation, particularly in emphysematous lungs. Although emulsified Ethiodol has been suggested as a bronchographic medium, toxicity studies are not available at this time (L'Heureux and Baltaxe). Thus, it was concluded in this study that of all the media tried, aqueous Dionosil might fulfill the ideal requirement for human use. However, aqueous tantalum suspended in human serum albumin was superior for roentgenographic opacification of the smallest airways (Sargent and Sherwin).

THE LUNG PARENCHYMA; THE AIR SPACES

The Primary Lobule (Fig. 10–23). The bronchi continue to ramify until a point is reached when the walls no longer contain cartilage. forming the tubular bronchioli. Eventually the tubular character changes, and small projections appear on all sides of the bronchiolus known as alveolar ducts (Fig. 10–23). At the distal end of each alveolar duct, there are three to six spherical cavities called atria. These atria, in turn, communicate with a variable number of larger and more irregularly shaped cavities called air sacs. Projecting from the wall of each air sac and atrium there are a number of smaller spaces called pulmonary alveoli This entire

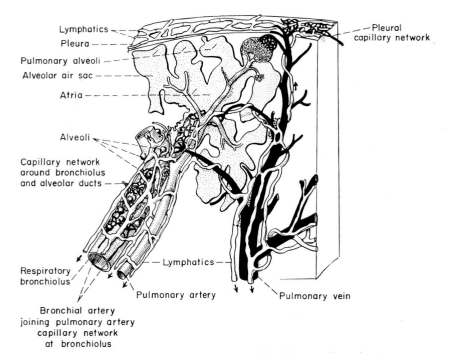

Figure 10–23. Primary lobule of the lung. (Modified from Miller, The Lung. Courtesy of Charles C Thomas, Publishers, Springfield, Illinois.)

group of structures together with the accompanying blood vessels, lymph vessels, and nerves forms a primary lobule. The primary lobules are grouped into bronchial segments, in accordance with the pattern previously described.

The epithelium of the alveoli, like that of the bronchi and bronchioli rests upon a network of reticulum, which is of some importance in connection with interstitial disease processes of the lungs.

The interchange of gases takes place in the alveoli, and the entire structure of the lungs is subservient to this end.

Secondary Lobule. When a bronchial pathway is followed to its end, a point is reached where branching of parallel walls of the pathway occurs about every 0.5 to 1.0 cm. After three or four such branchings an abrupt transition takes place after which the branching patterns occur much more frequently—at 2 to 3 mm. intervals. Reid and Simon have called these the centimeter and

millimeter patterns respectively. The centimeter pattern represents small bronchi and bronchioles; the millimeter pattern represents terminal bronchioles. A cluster of 3 to 5 terminal bronchioles in this millimeter pattern, together with the respiratory tissue that they supply, constitutes one *secondary lobule*. Generally, a secondary lobule is a unit with a diameter of about 1.0 to 1.5 cm., allowing 2 mm. as the distance between terminal bronchiolar branches and 5 mm. as the depth of respiratory tissue beyond the terminal bronchiole.

This concept of the secondary lobule is different from that of a lung unit demarcated by septal connective tissue passing into the lung from the pleura (Miller; VonHayek).

The secondary lobule as defined by Reid and Simon is morphologically recognizable on films, particularly following bronchographic study, or when this sector of the lung contains a water density material. A "mulberry-like" shadow is produced (Fig. 10–24 and 10–26 *B, C*).

The *acinus* represents that portion of the lung parenchyma encompassing all the tissues distal to one terminal bronchiole, i.e., all of the respiratory bronchioles, alveolar ducts, and alveoli (Fig. 10–25). Thus, a secondary lobule contains a cluster of three to five terminal bronchioles supplying three to five acini. Very likely, then, an acinus measures 5 to 7 mm. in diameter, in contrast to a secondary lobule which is approximately 1.0 to 1.5 cm. in diameter.

Each alveolar duct, in contrast, supplies a family of approximately 20 to 25 alveoli. The primary lobule of Miller comprises only the air spaces supplied by one alveolar duct and is probably 1.0 to 1.5 mm. in diameter; it is not to be confused with the much larger secondary lobule recognizable macroscopically.

Various histologic measurements of airway passages and alveoli are given for reference (Davies; Weibel; Pump).

The secondary pulmonary lobule furnishes a practical concept for interpretation of both normal and abnormal chest radiographs (Heitzman et al.).

Canals of Lambert. In the distal portions of the bronchiolar tree there are a number of epithelium-lined tubular communications that apparently provide an accessory route for the passage of air directly from the bronchioles into the alveoli. These are known as the *canals of Lambert* (Lambert).

Alveolar Pores (the Pores of Kohn). These pores in the alveoli are openings or discontinuities of the alveolar wall that measure about 10 to 15 microns in diameter. These apparently permit the transfer of gases, fluids, or particulate matter between lobules. They exist only between segments of a lobe; the total lobe remains an isolated unit with no collateral channel communications with adjacent lobes. However, if segmental or sub-

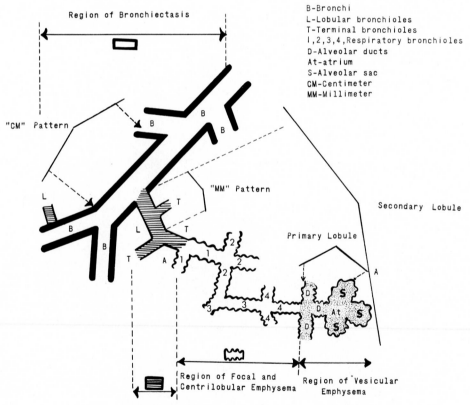

B-Bronchi
L-Lobular bronchioles
T-Terminal bronchioles
1,2,3,4,Respiratory bronchioles
D-Alveolar ducts
At-atrium
S-Alveolar sac
CM-Centimeter
MM-Millimeter

Figure 10–24.   The "secondary lobule" (diagram).

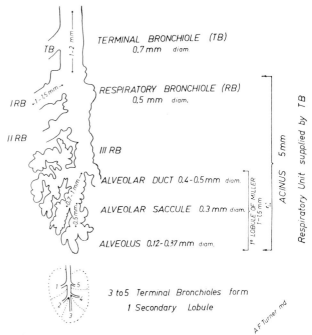

Figure 10–25. Anatomic drawing of terminal bronchiole and components of one acinus. (From Sargent, E. N., and Sherwin, R.: Amer. J. Roentgenol., 113:660–679, 1971.)

segmental bronchial occlusion exists, ventilation of the occluded segment may be brought about through these collateral channels. Hence, this is known as "collateral air drift." McLean has suggested that the positive pressure of expiration produces a collapse of the pores of Kohn and that this causes a check-valve mechanism to operate at each of these collateral pathways. Reich and co-workers have referred to this as "an interalveolar air drift," and represent this as an integral part of the mechanism of coughing. They have discussed these anatomic structures in relation to various pathologic entities (Fig. 10–26 *A, B, C*) (Macklin).

Fissures and Lobes of the Lungs (Fig. 10–18 *A*). The right lung is subdivided into three lobes, an upper, middle, and lower, by two interlobar fissures. The major fissure separates the lower lobe from the middle and upper lobes. With minor differences to be described soon, this fissure corresponds to the major fissure on the left side. The other fissure, or minor fissure, separates the upper from the middle lobe.

The left lung contains only a major fissure, and is subdivided into two lobes, an upper and a lower.

Each lobe of the lung is almost completely covered by visceral pleura, and each interlobar fissure is composed, therefore, of the visceral pleura of the two adjoining lobes that have extended down the fissure.

There is a considerable variation in the normal configuration and exact position of each fissure. From the radiologic point of view, the configuration of the entire surface of the interlobar fissure is of great importance. Each fissure must be visualized not as it is projected onto the surface of the thorax, but rather as a three-dimensional structure (Figs. 10–18, and 10–27).

Shape of the Interlobar Surfaces (Figs. 10–18, 10–27). The major fissure on the right side has the shape of an elongated and concave semi-ellipse. On the left side, it is rather crescentic. The major fissures reach to a variable distance from the hilus, and the minor (middle lobe) fissure is closed on the hilar surface.

Pleural bridges unite the various surfaces. There are also parenchymatous bridges uniting the various lobes with one another, particularly on the hilar and posterior aspects.

The right minor or middle lobe fissure is triangular, with the apex directed anteriorly. The base of the triangle is formed by the junction of the middle lobe fissure and the major fissure.

The upper part of the interlobar surface of the lower lobe faces anteriorly and somewhat laterally, while the lower part of this surface faces anteriorly and inward. This gives this surface a somewhat spiral appearance (resembling a propeller).

The minor (middle lobe) fissure on the right side is horizontal, at the level of the fourth costal cartilage.

The upper limit of the lower lobe posteriorly is at the vertebral end of the third rib or medial end of the spine of the scapula. The lower end is opposite the lateral part of the sixth costal cartilage.

The left upper lobe forms about one-eighth of the diaphragmatic surface of the left lung in its anteromedian portion. On the right side, a rather large part of the middle lobe is in contact with the diaphragm (as much as one-half).

The major fissure is steeper on the left side than on the right, forming an angle of about 60 degrees with the horizontal as against 50 degrees on the right side.

In addition to the spiral curvature of the major fissure, there is an upward convexity of the surface as well.

Radiographic Visualization of the Fissures. The interlobar fissures are areas in which the visceral pleura can be visualized on roentgenograms owing to the double thickness of the investing pleura of adjacent lobes and the contrasting air on either side of the fissure line (Felson; Fleischner et al.; Robbins and Hale, 1945a). Fairly large planes of the fissures must be parallel with the roentgen ray beam in order to permit visualization. Thus the interlobar fissure between the upper and middle lobes on the right is seen often, since much of its surface is thrown into tangential projection in the posteroanterior projection. In the straight lateral projection, the major fissure may likewise be seen at least in part for the same reason. It is conceivable that if one were to try carefully to obtain a good surface tangential view of the various portions of the surface of any of the fissures, it would

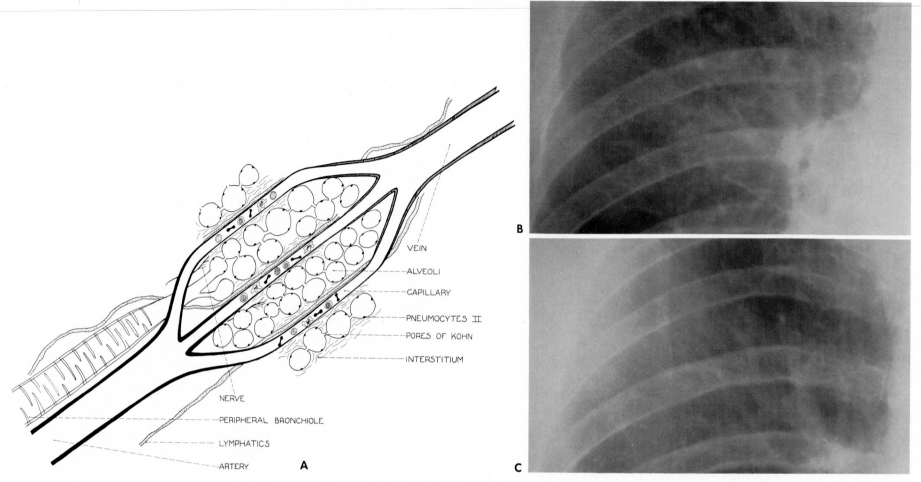

Figure 10-26. *A.* Diagram showing interrelationship of component parts of peripheral lung. *B* and *C.* Magnified view of air space consolidation in acute pulmonary edema before and after diuresis. Some discrete acinar shadows are shown before diuresis.

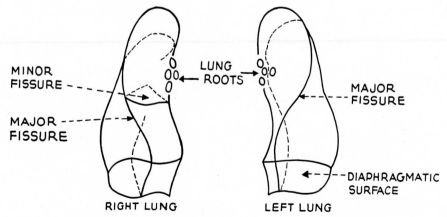

Figure 10-27. Three-dimensional concept of interlobar fissures.

be possible to demonstrate successively the various portions of the fissures.

Visualization of the fissures is helpful in detecting and localizing disease, and in determining its nature. Bean et al. found that approximately 70 per cent of normal chest roentgenograms in the newborn demonstrate fissure lines. This percentage decreases to about 50 per cent at 1 month, and then progressively increases with age, reaching 70 per cent at about 9 years, and about 100 per cent beyond 20 years of age. In the presence of acute inflammatory diseases of the chest the fissures are accentuated, either by fluid in the pleural space or in the lung adjacent to the pleura. After the acute phase, this accentuated appearance disappears and the per cent of visualization returns to the expected normal. This return to normal, however, does not occur in children with tuberculosis or cystic fibrosis.

In the adult, fissure lines are accentuated when a tumor adjoins an interlobar fissure.

The Pleura. The pleura is a thin continuous layer of endothelial cells resting on a thin membrane of connective tissue, which in turn contains blood vessels, lymphatics, and nerves. This lining membrane covers the entire inner aspect of the thoracic cavity as a closed space and also invests the lungs as well. That portion lining the thoracic cavity is called the *parietal* pleura, and that investing the lungs is called the *visceral* pleura. The interlobar fissures are formed by invagination into the lungs of two closely approximated layers of visceral pleura.

Ordinarily the pleura is not visualized unless it contains excessive fluid or foreign tissue as with inflammation or neoplasm. When the pleural shadow can be identified it is usually indicative of an active or previous abnormality.

The costophrenic and cardiophrenic angles are ordinarily rather sharply delineated also. Since the costophrenic angles represent the most dependent portions of the chest when the patient is in the erect position, it is in this location that excessive fluid accumulates first. The cardiophrenic angles vary considerably in appearance, depending on the variable appearance of the pericardial fat pad (to be described later with the heart).

Segments of the Lungs (Fig. 10–17). Although the segments of the lung do not have definite visceral pleural subdivisions as do the various lobes of the lungs, there is a certain amount of separability of these segments within the lung parenchyma. Each segment is supplied by a separate bronchial and arterial subdivision (see Fig. 10–34), and thus is a separate entity surgically.

Accessory Lobes of the Lungs

Inferior Accessory Lobe (Fig. 10–28). The segment of lung supplied by the medial basilar branch of the lower lobe bronchus on the right or the corresponding medial basilar branch of the anterior basilar branch of the left lower lobe bronchus may exist wholly or partially as a separate lobe. Schaffner found it in 45 per cent of 210 postmortem examinations, and radiologically it may be found in about 8 per cent of chest films (Twining). Fleischner has noted the variation in direction of the fissure of this lobe, and hence its variable appearance must be constantly borne in mind. It resembles closely at times an abnormally large pericardial fat pad in the right cardiophrenic angle, or any other abnormality that may be projected in this location.

Posterior Accessory Lobe. The segment supplied by the superior branch of the lower lobe bronchus may not infrequently be an accessory lobe. It is probable, however, that it need not necessarily be a separate lobe even if it is shown sharply demarcated from the surrounding lung in disease, since the segmental distribution of the bronchi is discrete in any event.

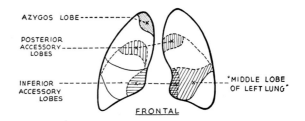

OCCASIONAL ACCESSORY LOBES OF LUNGS

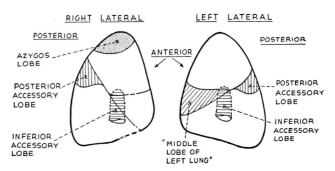

Figure 10–28. Diagrammatic presentation of accessory lobes of the lungs.

Middle Lobe of Left Lung. Although the lingular portion of the left upper lobe is separated from the rest of the upper lobe by a relatively avascular portion and occasionally by an incomplete fissure, it is practically never a completely separate accessory lobe as in the case of the other lobes.

Accessory Azygos Lobe (Figs. 10–28 *B*, and 10–29). Embryologically the azygos vein runs just lateral to the apex of the right upper lobe. As the apex grows upward, the azygos vein ordinarily glides medially so that it lies medial to the right lung apex.

If this gliding movement is interrupted as the apex of the right upper lobe grows upward, the azygos vein produces an indentation into the right upper lobe medially, carrying with it a fold of both visceral and parietal pleura. Thus, unlike the true fissures between lobes that consist of two layers of visceral pleura, this artificial fissure consists of four layers, two visceral and two parietal.

This false fissure appears radiologically as a thin, outwardly convex line, always in the right upper lobe medially. It is usually thicker at its lower end, a characteristic probably related to the fact that the azygos vein is situated in this location, or possibly this is to be associated with a fold of pleura. This thicker area must be carefully differentiated from any abnormality in the lung.

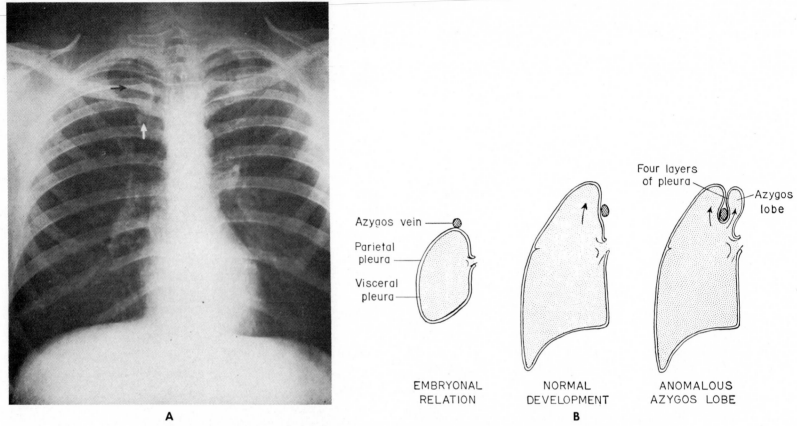

Figure 10–29. *A.* Radiograph of chest showing position and appearance of the azygos lobe. *B.* Anatomic concept of "azygos" lobe. Normally the azygos vein migrates into its normal suprahilar position by moving "around" the apex of the right upper lobe. In some cases it takes a shorter route, and indents both the parietal and the visceral pleura, producing the anomalous "fissure." Unlike a true interlobar fissure, this one consists of four mesothelial layers—two from the parietal and two from the visceral pleura. The true interlobar fissure consists of only two layers of visceral pleura.

VASCULAR SUPPLY, VENOUS DRAINAGE, AND LYMPHATICS OF THE RESPIRATORY TRACT

Blood Vessels of the Lungs. *Pulmonary Artery.* The pulmonary artery (Figs. 10–15, 10–30) follows closely the subdivisions of the bronchial tree. It arches over the right main-stem bronchus and lies dorsal and slightly lateral to the bronchus. The artery diminishes more rapidly in size than the bronchus it accompanies, and by the time it reaches the primary lobule, it is about one-fourth or one-fifth the size of the ductulus alveolaris. It finally ends in a capillary network surrounding the alveolus. The pulmonary vein takes origin from the latter capillary network.

The common pulmonary artery divides into right and left pulmonary arteries (Fig. 10–31). The right pulmonary artery passes under the aortic arch below the tracheal bifurcation and crosses in front of the right bronchus between its upper lobe and lower division branches. It divides into three branches, two going to the upper lobe, and one supplying the middle and lower lobes. Each of the branches of these subdivisions follows the corresponding branches of the bronchial tree rather closely, with the artery lying along the upper side of the bronchus most of the way. The left pulmonary artery is seen just below the aortic knob as it arches posteriorly into the left lung, forming the crescentic shadow of the left hilus above the downward curving left bronchus. It enters the hilus as three branches and then subdivides into nine principal branches, five of which go to the upper lobe and four to the lower lobe following corresponding bronchial branches. (The relationships of the heart, major vessels, and other structures of the mediastinum will be discussed in greater detail in Chapters 11 and 12.)

Capillaries. The network of capillaries is situated in the walls of the alveoli, and each capillary is common to two alveoli.

The mesh of capillaries in the walls of the alveoli situated beneath the pleura is much coarser than that within the lung. The same holds true for the capillaries situated near the fibrous septa and larger blood vessels.

Pulmonary Veins. Unlike the pulmonary artery, which is virtually in the same sheath as the bronchus, the more peripheral pulmonary veins are situated far removed from the corresponding bronchus in the septa that unite several lobules. The pulmonary veins have four sources of origin: (1) the capillary network of the pleura, which is derived from the bronchial artery; (2) the capillary network of the alveoli; (3) the bronchopulmonary veins, which are situated on either side of the junction of two bronchi or

bronchioli; and (4) the capillary network in the alveolar ducts, which gives origin to two venous radicles, one on either side of the duct.

The veins and arteries come closer together at about the fourth bronchial bifurcation, the veins lying anterior to and below the arteries. As they approach the hilum, they again become dissociated, the veins lying below and anterior to the arteries and diverging from them to enter the left atrium.

THE ESTIMATION OF PULMONARY VENOUS AND ARTERIAL PRESSURES FROM ROUTINE CHEST ROENTGENOGRAMS. There have been many attempts to estimate pulmonary vascular pressures from routine chest radiographs (Davies et al.; Jacobson et al.; Milne;

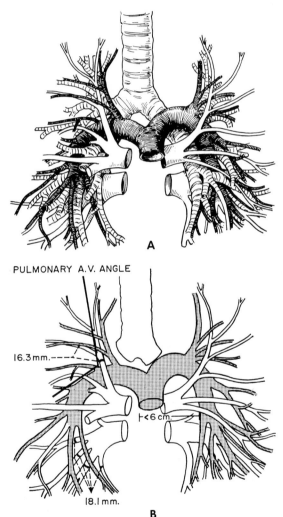

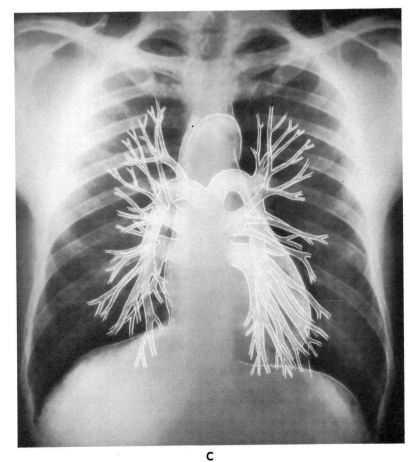

Figure 10–30. *A.* Relationship of major ramifications of pulmonary artery and tracheobronchial tree to one another, also showing the relationship to major pulmonary veins. Note that left pulmonary artery is slightly more cephalad than right. *B.* The pulmonary arteriovenous angle, which becomes more obtuse with passive hyperemia of the lungs. Also shown are several measurements which are occasionally quoted in the literature (after Logue et al.). The measurement 16.3 mm. indicates the sum of the diameters of the apical vein of the right upper lobe at the level of the right upper lobe bronchus, and the posterior segmental vein of the right upper lobe at the point at which it is crossed by the anterior segmental artery. The 18.1 mm. is the sum of the diameters of the superior and inferior basal veins of the right lower lobe measured 1 cm. from their junction. (From Lavendar et al.: Brit. J. Radiol., 35:413, 1962.) *C.* Diagrammatic intensification of pulmonary arteries and veins on a routine posteroanterior radiograph.

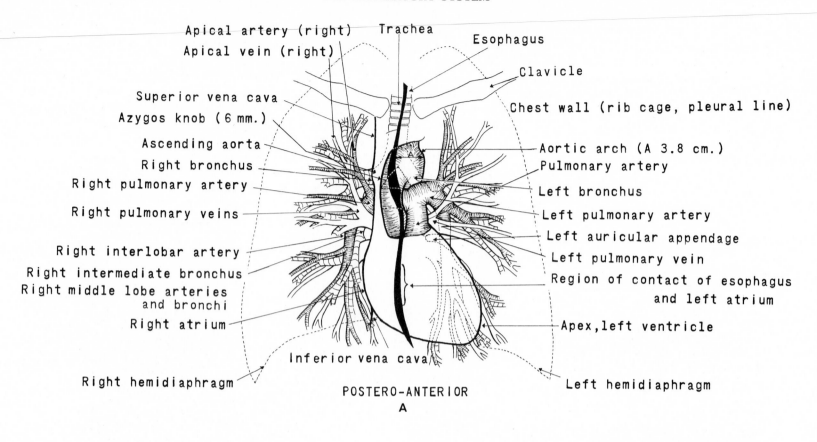

Apical artery (right)   Trachea   Esophagus

Apical vein (right)

Clavicle

Superior vena cava

Chest wall (rib cage, pleural line)

Azygos knob (6 mm.)

Ascending aorta   Aortic arch (A 3.8 cm.)

Right bronchus   Pulmonary artery

Right pulmonary artery   Left bronchus

Right pulmonary veins   Left pulmonary artery

Left auricular appendage

Right interlobar artery   Left pulmonary vein

Right intermediate bronchus   Region of contact of esophagus

Right middle lobe arteries   and left atrium
and bronchi

Right atrium   Apex, left ventricle

Inferior vena cava

POSTERO-ANTERIOR

A

Right hemidiaphragm   Left hemidiaphragm

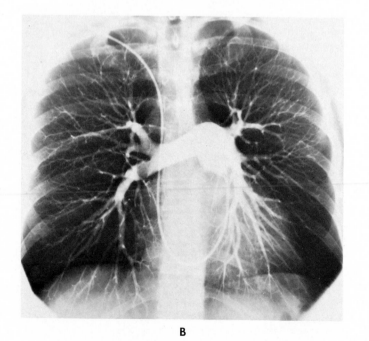

B

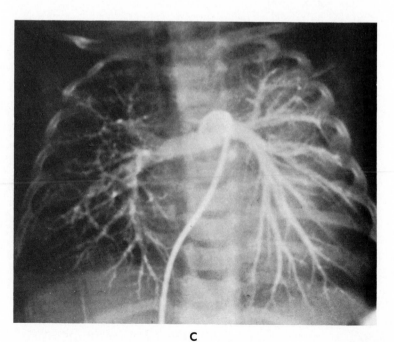

C

Figure 10–31. *A.* Diagram of chest film showing arteries, veins, and relationships to bronchi. *B.* Pulmonary arteriogram, arterial phase. *C.* Pulmonary arteriogram in an infant, arterial phase.

Simon, 1963; Steiner; Turner et al.). Since the pulmonary vascular bed is a low resistance bed, it can be readily surmised that in pulmonary circulation the blood flows forward across the capillary bed for oxygenation, and returns to the left atrium by means of a postcapillary or pulmonary venous pressure component. The precapillary pressure requirements are assessed by changes in the main pulmonary artery and its visualized major branches. The pulmonary venous pressure or postcapillary component is evaluated by studying the regional distribution of pulmonary blood flow.

Considerable change in blood-flow through the lungs occurs as body position changes, since, normally, blood-flow is directed into the lower lung zones largely by gravity. Normally, the size and number of vessels per unit area in the lower lung are greater than they are in the upper zones in the upright position. Normally, the pulmonary vessels show an orderly tapering and branching toward the periphery, so that for perhaps 2 or 3 cm. in the immediate subpleural area the vessels become virtually invisible. Moreover, the distribution of vessels is considerably greater in the lower lung in the erect position by at least a factor of 3. Various methods of studying redistribution of the numbers of vessels in the lower and upper lung have been devised (Turner et al.). Redistribution is then interpreted in terms of postcapillary pressure.

ASSESSMENT OF PRECAPILLARY OR ARTERIAL PRESSURE. Precapillary or arterial pressure is assessed by: (1) studying the *size of the main pulmonary artery* and its major branches, and (2) studying the *degree of tapering* of the vessels as they branch in the midzone of the lungs. Experience and correlation with cardiac catheterization values is remarkably good. Unfortunately, pulmonary parenchymal disease and increased total pulmonary blood-flow are the major sources of inaccurate estimations.

The upper lobe pulmonary veins are most consistently visualized at the main pulmonary artery level. Superimposition of artery and vein occurs in about 40 to 50 per cent of examinations, but otherwise the vein is almost invariably lateral to the artery. The pulmonary vessels are usually vertical in the left upper lobe and either vertical or oblique in the right upper lobe. Considerable significance can be ascribed to the detection of a change in diameter of upper lobe pulmonary veins in serial chest roentgenograms (Burko et al.).

Doppman and Lavender proposed a careful study of the hilum on the right as an indicator of left atrial pressure (Fig. 10-32). In the normal individual an angle of approximately 120 degrees is formed by the intersection of the superior pulmonary vein and the descending pulmonary artery (Figs. 10-30, 10-32 *A*). This concave hilar angle is obliterated early with rising left atrial pressure (Fig. 10-32 *B*).

Bronchial Artery. The bronchial arteries vary in number and origin. They may arise from the aorta (in over 90 per cent of cases), or from any of the first three intercostal subclavian or internal mammary arteries. In about 80 per cent of cases, their level of origin is opposite the fifth and sixth dorsal vertebrae. They supply the bronchi, visceral pleura, walls of pulmonary vessels, and interstitial supporting structures of alveoli. No precapillary anastomoses are present between pulmonary and bronchial arteries in normal lungs. The middle third of the esophagus, the hilar lymph nodes, vagus nerve, and mediastinal fascia are also nourished by bronchial arterial circulation. Anastomoses with other systemic arteries may occur.

The variations in origin of the bronchial arteries have been carefully cataloged by Cauldwell et al. In 74 per cent of their dissections, the right and left bronchial arteries arose independently, while in the remainder, a common trunk divided into right and left bronchial arteries. Rarely, the bronchial artery originated from the subclavian. The bronchial arteries are embedded in the connective tissue surrounding the bronchi and usually form an acute angle with the aorta at their origin, coursing upward and anteriorly initially, and following the course of the bronchi closely. The vessels end in an arterial plexus that anastomoses with the pulmonary capillary plexus (Newton and Preger; Viamonte et al.; Cudkowicz and Armstrong) (Fig. 10-33). The capillaries in the alveolar walls are derived from the pulmonary artery and not from the bronchial artery. (It is interesting to note that this point of transition from the bronchial to the pulmonary circulation is a favorite site for tubercle formation.)

Bronchial Veins. True bronchial veins are found only at the hilus of the lung. These arise from the first or first two dividing points of the bronchial tree, and receive branches from part of the pleura close to the hilus. These bronchial veins empty into the azygos, the hemiazygos, or one of the intercostal veins. Communications exist between the bronchial arteries and pulmonary veins via the capillaries, but Guillor (Miller) could not demonstrate such communication with the pulmonary artery directly. These vascular phenomena are of considerable importance from the standpoint of much of the circulatory pathology of the lungs.

Lymphatics of the Lungs (Figs. 10-34, 10-35). The lung is provided with a great abundance of lymphatics, more than the liver, spleen, or kidney (Miller). They may be divided grossly into a superficial set and a deep set. The superficial lymphatics are situated in the pleura; the deep group are situated along the pulmonary artery, veins, and bronchi, and form a dense network between the secondary lobules in the connective tissue septa. These two sets of lymphatics communicate with one another at the pleura and in the hilus. The pleural lymphatics have unusually large diameters and are arranged in the form of irregular polyhedral rings. Numerous valves, 1 to 2 mm. apart, direct the flow of lymph in both pleural and intrapulmonary lymphatics.

Normal lymph nodes may be found in the substance of the lung far from the hilum (Trapnell, 1964).

Lymphatics of the Bronchi. The larger bronchi have two sets of lymphatics which intercommunicate with one another, but

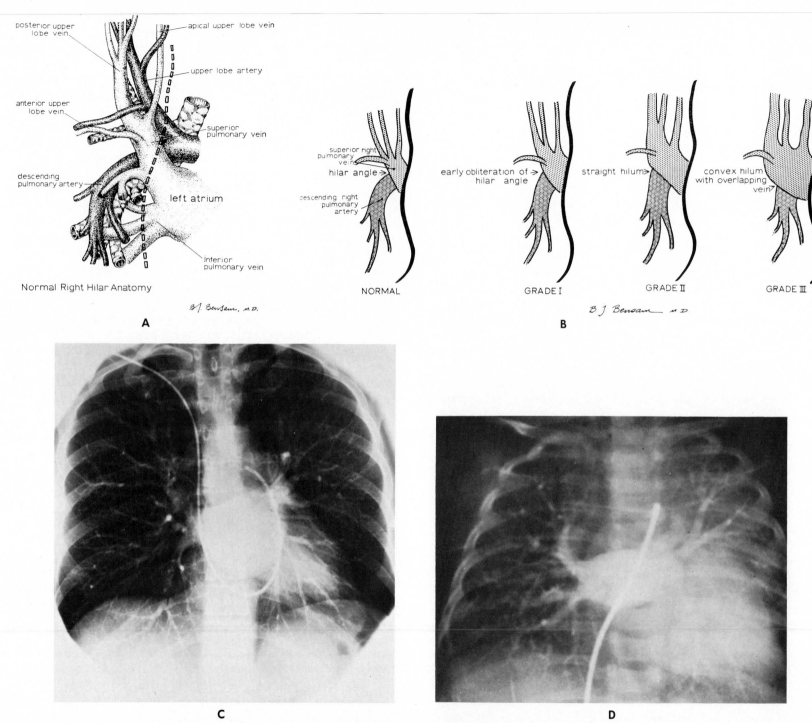

Figure 10–32.   *A.* Diagrammatic representation of vasculature of right lung. Note the concave hilar angle formed by the intersection of the superior pulmonary vein and the descending pulmonary artery. *B.* Progressive changes in hilar contour with rising left atrial pressure. Grade I shows partial obliteration of the hilar angle by the enlarging upper lobe vein. Grade II shows complete effacement of the hilar angle with a straight lateral border to the hilum. The clear space between descending pulmonary artery and right atrium is encroached upon. Grade III shows a convex hilum with the horizontal inferior margin of the upper lobe vein crossing the artery. (From Doppman, J. L., and Lavender, J. P.: Radiology, *80:*931–936, 1963.) *C.* Pulmonary arteriogram, venous phase. Note that the major veins which return blood to the left atrium are situated partially over the spine and are concealed by the cardiac silhouette. *D.* Venogram phase of a pulmonary arteriogram in a normal infant.

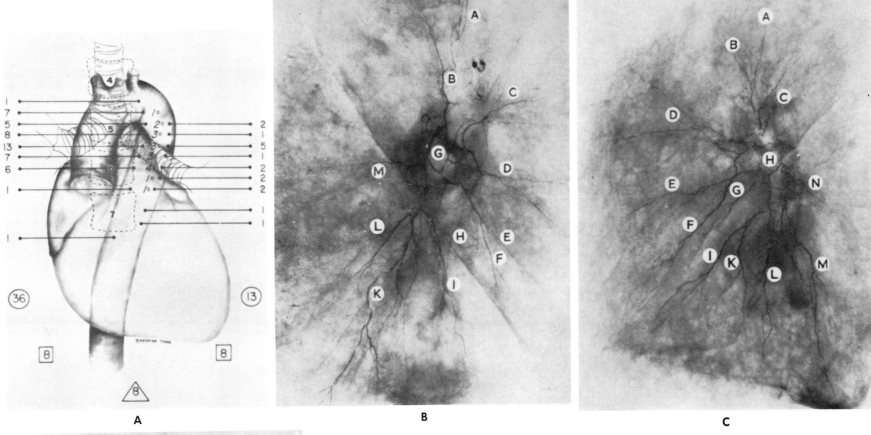

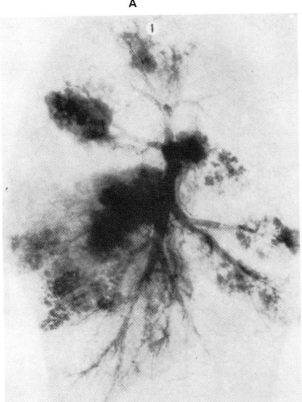

Figure 10–33. *A.* Diagram showing levels of origin of the right and left bronchial arteries and of common trunks (central circles) that were studied. Lateral circles indicate the number of lesions studied on each side. In the squares are the number of bilateral lesions. In the triangle, the number of midline lesions is indicated.

Note: First 71 studies. (From Viamonte, M., Parks, R. E., and Smoak, W. M. III: Radiology, *85:205–230,* 1965.)

B. Standard pattern of left bronchial arteries seen in a lateral view of a left lung (Case 6). (Hilum faces x-ray tube.)

Upper lobe: (A) apical pleural branch, (B) posterior branch, (C) apical branch, (D) anterior branch, (E) superior lingual branch, (F) inferior lingular branch, (G) annulus. *Lower lobe:* (H) interlobar pleural branch, (J) anterior branch, (K) lateral branch, (L) posterior branch, (M) apical branch.

C. Standard pattern of right bronchial arteries seen in a lateral view of a right lung (Case 7). (Hilum faces x-ray tube.)

Upper lobe: (A) apical pleural branch, (B) apical branch, (C) posterior branch, (D) anterior branch. *Middle lobe:* (E) lateral branch, (F) medial branch, (G) interlobar pleural branch, (H) annulus. *Lower lobe:* (I) anterior branch, (K) cardiac (medial) branch, (L) lateral branch, (M) posterior branch, (N) apical branch.

D. Lateral view (Case 3) of right bronchial tree superimposed on right bronchial arterial pattern. (1) Apical pleural branch. Some alveolar fogging has occurred. The hilum faces away from x-ray tube. About one-third of normal size. (*B, C,* and *D* from Cudkowicz, L., and Armstrong, J. B.: Thorax, 6:342–358, 1951.)

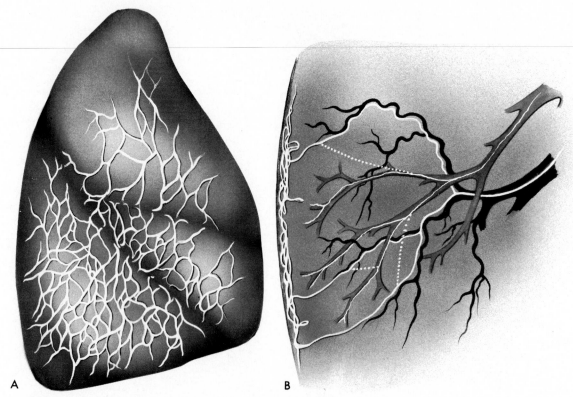

A   B

Figure 10–34. The lymphatic drainage of the pleura and lungs. *A.* A drawing of the lateral aspect of the right lung shows the pleural lymphatics to be much more numerous over the lower half of the lung than over the upper. *B.* In a coronal section through the midportion of the lung, lymphatic channels from the pleura enter the lung at the interlobular septa and extend medially to the hilum along venous radicals (dark shaded vessels); lymphatic channels originating in the peripheral parenchyma extend medially in the bronchovascular bundles (light shaded vessels). Communicating lymphatics (dotted lines) extend between the peribronchial and perivenous lymphatics. (From Fraser, R. G., and Paré, J. A. P.: Diagnosis of Diseases of the Chest. Philadelphia, W. B. Saunders Co., 1970.)

the smaller bronchi have only a single plexus of lymphatics which terminates at the alveolar ductules. Here they join the lymphatics accompanying the pulmonary veins that form at this point.

There are no lymphatics in the walls of the air spaces distal to the alveolar ductules.

Lymphatics of the Pulmonary Artery. The larger branches of the pulmonary artery are accompanied by two lymph channels, one of which is situated between the artery and its accompanying bronchus. These intercommunicate freely by means of a rich plexus. The smaller arterial branches are accompanied by only single lymph channels. Communications between the periarterial and peribronchial lymphatics occur in many places but predominantly in the region of bifurcations and at the distal end of the alveolar ductules.

Lymphatics of the Pulmonary Veins. As in the case of the

arteries and bronchi, lymph channels accompany all of the veins, except in the region of the alveolar sacs.

Lymphatics of the Pleura. There is only a single plexus of lymphatics in the pleura, arranged in polyhedral rings. There are smaller rings within these larger ones, with smaller lymph channels.

Direction of Lymph Flow. The valves situated in the hilus, pleura, and at the junction of the deep and superficial systems permit flow in one direction only. *The flow in the peribronchial, periarterial, and perivenous lymphatics is toward the interior of the lung* or hilus.

The *valves situated just beneath the pleura permit flow of lymph toward the pleura.* In the subpleural region, the pleural lymphatics occasionally dip into the lung and then return to the surface to become pleural again (Trapnell, 1963).

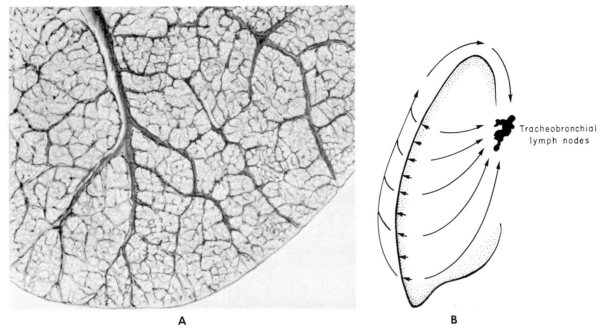

Figure 10–35. *A.* Drawing of lower surface of middle lobe showing lymphatic vessels outlining the lobules and acini of the lung parenchyma. (From Twining, E. W.: A Textbook of X-Ray Diagnosis. H. K. Lewis & Co., Publishers, *B.* Diagrammatic illustration of the drainage of the lymphatics of the lungs. The superficial lymphatics are situated in the pleura and drain into the pleural space and around to the hili thereby. The deep lymphatics follow along the pulmonary arterial branches, veins, and bronchi and drain toward the hilus. The two sets of lymphatics communicate with one another immediately adjoining the pleura and in the region of the hilus, but are otherwise separate.

The valves situated in the pleura allow free circulation of the lymph within this space. The pleural lymphatics together with the lymphatics from the interior of the lung all enter the tracheobronchial lymph nodes.

In the presence of an obstructed lymph channel, a reversal of lymph flow can occur. These obstructed and distended lymphatics appear linear and stellate in relation to hilar lymph nodes.

Lymphoid Tissue. Lymphoid tissue may occur in the form of lymph nodes, lymph follicles, or small masses of lymphoid tissue. Lymph nodes in the normal lung are associated with the larger divisions of the bronchi, and are situated at the places where branching takes place (Fig. 10–36). There is in old age a definite increase in the lymphoid tissue independent of that produced by disease, but dependent to a great extent on the amount of irritating particles inhaled (such as carbon). In the normal lung, lymph nodes are not present in the pleura.

The following groups of lymph nodes occur (Fig. 10–36): (1) the paratracheal group; (2) the tracheobronchial group, the right being more constant than the left, but those on the left are in close proximity to the recurrent nerve (they are connected with the anterior and posterior mediastinal nodes, and also with the inferior deep cervical nodes); (3) the bifurcation group, which are likewise in communication with the posterior mediastinal nodes; (4) the bronchopulmonary group, lying in the hilus of the corresponding lung, in the angles between the branches of the bronchi;

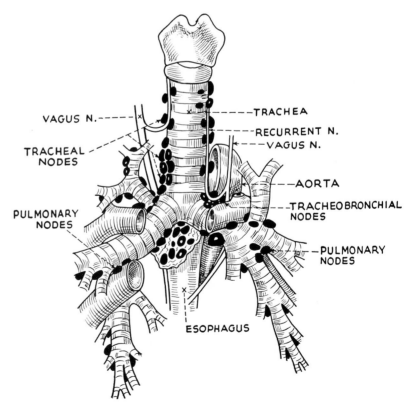

Figure 10–36. Lymph nodes of the tracheobronchial tree. (After Sukienikow.)

(5) the pulmonary groups, lying in the lung substance, usually in the angles of the branching bronchi up to the third branching. The nodes in the left upper lobe may lie in the anterior mediastinum in close proximity with the aorta and ductus arteriosus.

The hilar nodes receive lymph not only from the more peripheral lymphatics of the lung but also from the pleura, by lymph channels which drain along the interlobar fissures and over the anterior and posterior lung surfaces toward the hilus. This accounts for the great frequency with which these fissures are visible in both pleural and pulmonary disease.

Lymphatic Pathways of the Mediastinum. Fraser and Paré have divided the lymphatic pathways of the mediastinum according to the three conventional compartments of the mediastinum (see Chapter 11), although usually the intrathoracic lymph nodes are considered to be divided into a parietal group and a visceral group. The parietal lymph nodes drain the thoracic wall and certain extrathoracic tissues, whereas the visceral group are involved mostly with intrathoracic structures.

Group 1: Lymph Nodes of the Anterior Mediastinal Compartment

(1) *The sternal, anterior parietal, or internal mammary group.* This group of nodes is distributed along the internal mammary arteries behind the anterior costochondral cartilages bilaterally. They drain the upper anterior abdominal wall, the anterior thoracic wall, the anterior portion of the diaphragm, and the medial portions of the breast. They communicate with a visceral group of anterior mediastinal lymph nodes and cervical nodes.

(2) *The anterior mediastinal lymph node group.* These are visceral nodes, lying posterior to the sternum in the lower thorax, along the superior vena cava and innominate vein on the right and in front of the aorta and carotid artery on the left. Some of these nodes are situated anterior to the thymus.

Group 2: The Posterior Mediastinal Lymph Nodes (Fig. 10–38)

This group of lymph nodes lies posteriorly in the intercostal spaces and in paravertebral areas. They drain the parietal pleura and vertebral column. This group consists of parietal nodes and mediastinal visceral nodes, which communicate with each other. The posterior mediastinal group of visceral nodes lie along the lower esophagus and descending aorta, and drain the posterior portion of the diaphragm, the pericardium, the esophagus, and the lower lobes of the lungs.

Group 3: The Middle Mediastinal Lymph Nodes (Fig. 10–39)

The parietal group of lymph nodes in this chain are located mainly around the pericardial attachment to the diaphragm,

whereas the visceral group consists mainly of the tracheobronchial and bifurcation nodes and bronchopulmonary nodes (see also Figure 10–36).

The lymph from the anterior mediastinal nodes flows into the right lymphatic duct or bronchomediastinal duct, and the thoracic duct on the left. The posterior mediastinal lymph nodes drain into the thoracic duct and the cisterna chyli from the lower thoracic region. They also communicate with the visceral mediastinal lymph nodes draining mainly via the thoracic duct.

The middle mediastinal lymph nodes communicate with anterior mediastinal and posterior nodes, and also drain into the bronchomediastinal trunk on the right and the thoracic duct on the left (Rouviere). The bronchomediastinal trunk receives the lymph from the right lung and empties via the right lymphatic duct into the beginning of the innominate vein. Near their terminations, both thoracic ducts lie close to the lower deep cervical lymph nodes.

THE LUNG HILI

The hilus of the lung (Fig. 10–40) is a wedge-shaped depressed area on the mediastinal surface of the lung above and behind the pericardial impression on the lung, within which the blood vessels, lymph vessels, nerves, and bronchi enter and leave the lung. Bronchial lymph nodes are located among those structures. The hilus is surrounded by the reflection of the pleura from the surface of the lung on to the pulmonary root. The mediastinal surface of the lung presents the pericardial impression produced by structures in the posterior mediastinum and the superior mediastinum in addition to the hili.

The term "root of the lung" is, strictly speaking, applied to a number of structures that enter and leave the lung on its mediastinal surface. It constitutes a pedicle that attaches the lung to the mediastinal wall of the pleural cavity. The large structures forming the pulmonary root are: (1) the two pulmonary veins, (2) the pulmonary artery, (3) the bronchus, (4) bronchial arteries and veins, (5) pulmonary nerves, and (6) lymph vessels and some lymph nodes (bronchial).

In the case of the left lung, the major arteries and veins and their branches are arranged in the form of a triangle, with the pulmonary veins forming the anterior and inferior apices of the triangle and the left pulmonary artery forming the superior apex; the bronchus is in the center of the triangle. The pulmonary artery lies higher in the left root than in the right, and crosses the bronchus on the left before it divides into its branches.

These root structures can be moderately well distinguished on radiographs in the posteroanterior and oblique projections. By common usage, the terms "hilus" and "root" are used interchangeably.

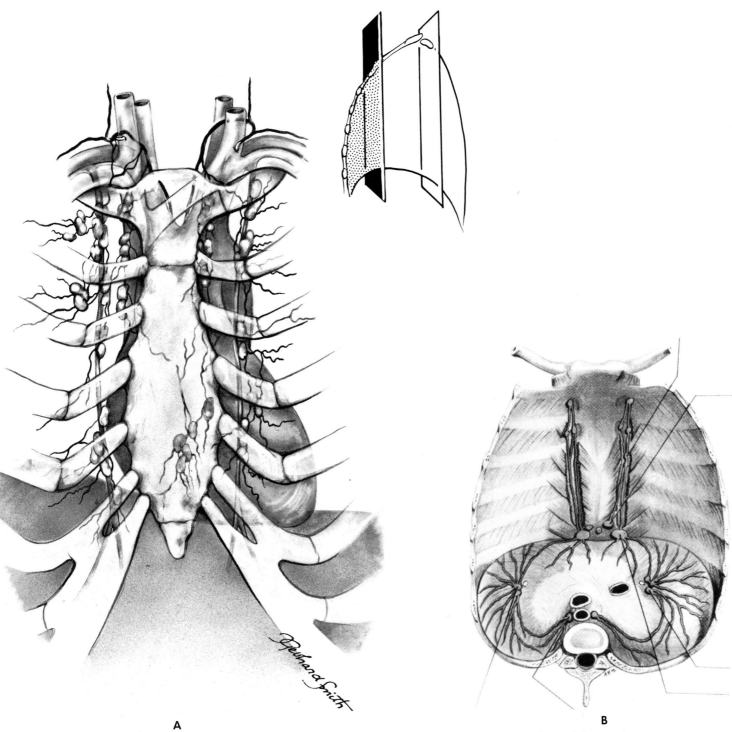

A   **B**

Figure 10–37. *A.* Anterior Mediastinal Lymph Nodes. The nodes illustrated are chiefly those of the anterior parietal group scattered along the internal mammary arteries and behind the anterior intercostal spaces and costal cartilages bilaterally. The prevascular (visceral) group relate to the superior vena cava and innominate vein on the right and to the aorta and carotid artery on the left. (From Fraser, R. G., and Paré, J. A. P.: Diagnosis of Diseases of the Chest. Philadelphia, W. B. Saunders Co., 1970.) *B.* The anatomy of the internal mammary lymph nodes. From Cunningham's Textbook of Anatomy, 10th ed. London, Oxford University Press, 1964.)

Figure 10–37 continued on the following page.

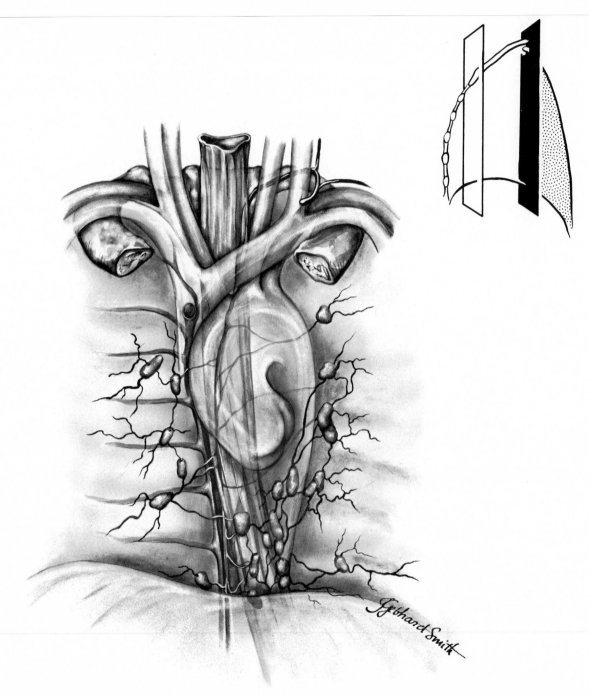

Figure 10-38.   Posterior Mediastinal Lymph Nodes. The intercostal (posterior parietal) group lies laterally, in the intercostal spaces, and medially, in the paravertebral areas adjacent to the heads of the ribs. The visceral group of posterior mediastinal nodes is situated along the lower esophagus and descending aorta. (From Fraser, R. G., and Paré, J. A. P.: Diagnosis of Diseases of the Chest. Philadelphia, W. B. Saunders Co., 1970.)

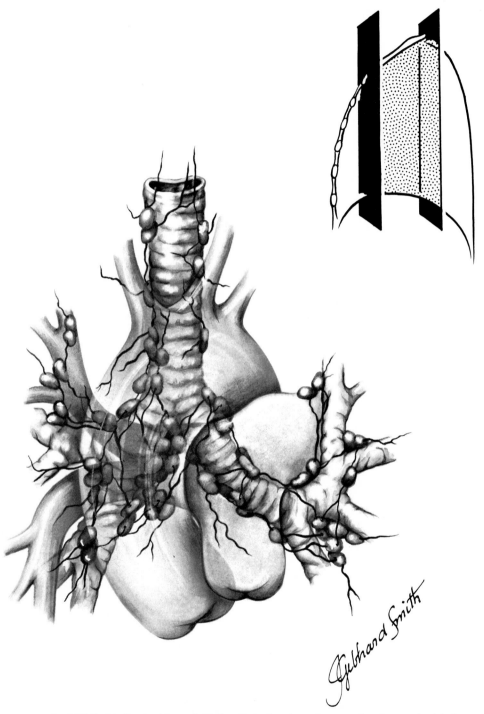

Figure 10–39. The Middle Mediastinal Lymph Nodes. Only the visceral group of nodes are depicted, consisting of the tracheobronchial, carinal, and bronchopulmonary nodes. See text for description. (From Fraser, R. G., and Paré, J. A. P.: Diagnosis of Diseases of the Chest. Philadelphia, W. B. Saunders Co., 1970.)

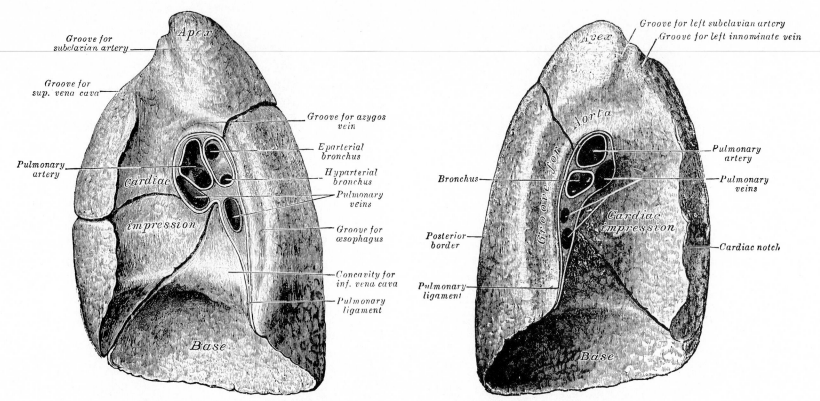

Figure 10-40. Structures in the lung hili. (From Gray's Anatomy of the Human Body, 29th edition. Goss, C. M. (ed.) Philadelphia, Lea & Febiger, 1973.)

THE THORACIC CAGE, PLEURA, AND DIAPHRAGM

There are several important component parts of the thoracic cage, all of which may be visualized to some extent radiographically. These are: (1) the soft tissue structures of the thoracic wall, such as the skin, breasts, and muscular tissues; (2) the bony structures of the thoracic cage, consisting chiefly of ribs, costal cartilage, sternum, and thoracic spine; (3) the pleura, both visceral and parietal; and (4) the diaphragm.

Soft Tissue Structures of the Thoracic Wall

Skin and Subcutaneous Tissues. The skin and subcutaneous tissues of the thoracic cage cannot be entirely ignored in the consideration of the radiographic anatomy of the chest. Normally, these tegmental layers are seen only over the clavicle (Fig. 10–41), and as outlining shadows of the thoracic cage; abnormally,

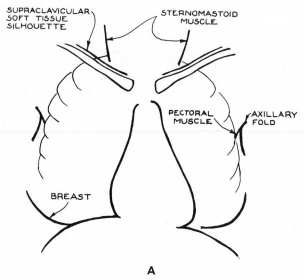

Figure 10-41. A. Soft tissues of the thoracic cage as seen radiographically.

Figure 10-41 continued on the opposite page.

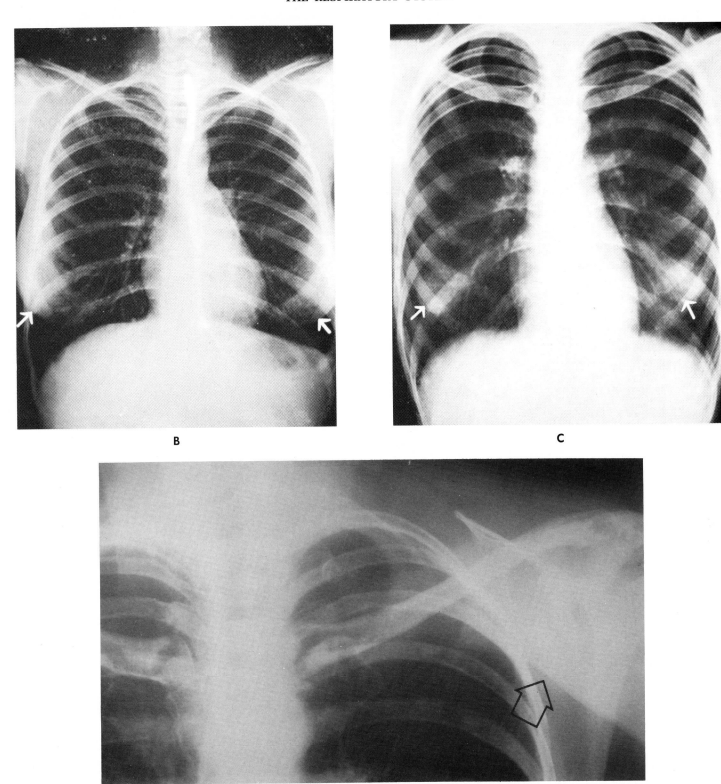

Figure 10–41 *Continued.*   *B.* Projection of female breast shadows over the lung substance. *C.* Radiograph showing areola and nipple shadows. *D.* Close-up view of the axilla in a patient following radical mastectomy. There is complete absence of the pectoral muscles.

shadows contained within the skin and subcutaneous tissues can produce very dense shadows that must be differentiated from pulmonary constituents. Free air in the skin and subcutaneous tissues also produces its individual appearance. The fact that structures contained within the skin have radiographic significance must not be overlooked.

The Breasts. The breasts are situated in the superficial fascia covering the anterior aspect of the thoracic cage, and in the female usually extend from the level of the second or third rib to the level of the sixth. The hemispherical shadow of the female breast is cast over that of the pectoralis major muscle (Fig. 10–41 B), and together they form a notable haziness that may obscure to a great extent the lung substance proper. At the level of the fourth or fifth rib, the nipple, in turn, may cast an even denser shadow than that of the breast (Fig. 10–41 C), and has the ap-

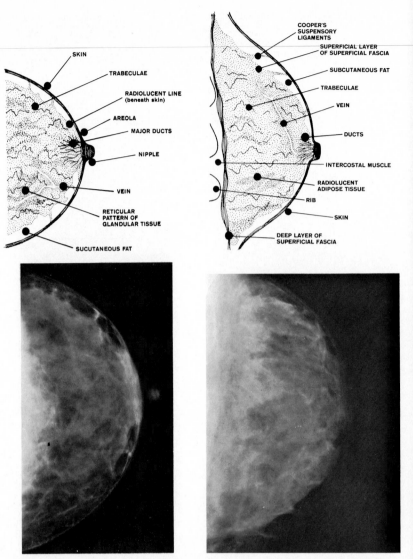

Figure 10–43. Representative mammograms in the craniocaudad (*left*) and mediolateral (*right*) projections and labeled line drawings of each. (From Egan, R. L.: Mammography, 1964. Courtesy of Charles C Thomas, Publisher, Springfield, Illinois.)

Figure 10–43 continued on the opposite page.

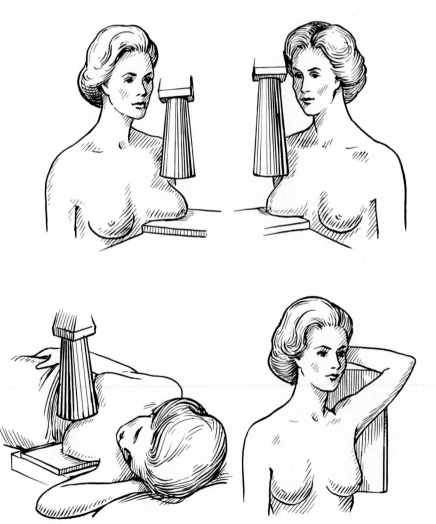

Figure 10–42. Diagrams illustrating position of patient for soft tissue mammography.

pearance of a rather dense nodule. Occasionally the areola around the nipple may also be distinguished. Of course, the size and shape of the breasts vary considerably among both women and men, and will vary in the same woman according to the physiologic state of the breast.

The breast may be investigated radiographically in several ways: (1) soft tissue study tangential to the breast (Figs. 10–42 and 10–43); (2) study of the breast following injection of CO_2 into tissues around the breast (Fig. 10–44); and (3) injection of opaque media into the lactiferous ducts (Fig. 10–45).

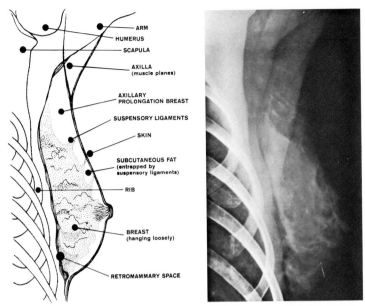

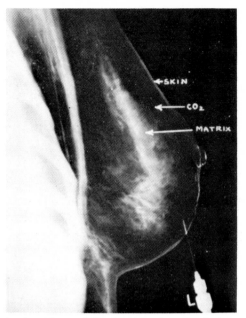

Figure 10–43 *Continued.* Representative mammogram in the axillary projection with labeled line drawing. (From Egan, R. L.: Mammography. 1964. Courtesy of Charles C Thomas, Publisher, Springfield, Illinois.)

Figure 10–44. Study of breast following injection of soft tissues with air. (From N. F. Hicken et al., Amer. J. Roentgenol., *39*, 1938.)

The main purpose of these studies is to demonstrate abnormal mass lesions within the breast.

Muscular Tissues. The following muscles of the thoracic cage may produce a shadow upon the radiograph: (1) the pectoralis major and minor; (2) the sternocleidomastoid; (3) the serratus anterior; and (4) the intercostal muscles (may be seen on oblique views of the ribs and chest). Their importance lies chiefly in the fact that they must be differentiated from abnormal shadows in the chest. By the injection of air, these muscle shadows can be delineated more clearly.

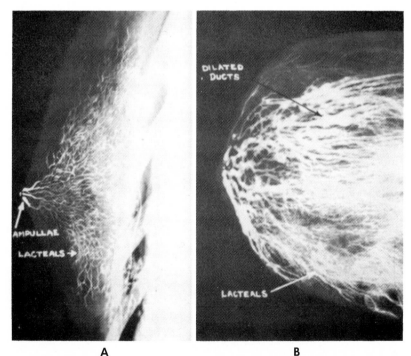

A   B

Figure 10–45. Radiographs of breast after injection of the ducts with lipiodol. *A.* Virginal breast. *B.* Multiparous breast.

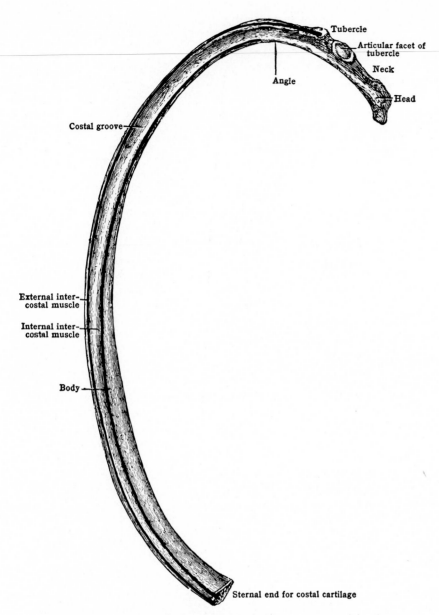

Tubercle

Articular facet of tubercle

Neck

Angle

Head

Costal groove

External inter-costal muscle

Internal inter-costal muscle

Body

Sternal end for costal cartilage

Figure 10–46. Anatomic drawing of a typical rib. (From Anson, B. J. (ed.): Morris' Human Anatomy, 12th ed. Copyright © 1966 by McGraw-Hill, Inc. Used by permission of McGraw-Hill Book Company.)

When it is desired to differentiate any of these soft tissue structures, it is well to mark or delineate the structures with wire, and compare a radiograph so obtained with one obtained without the delineation. This permits the radiologist to distinguish at a glance the cause of the shadow.

The Ribs

Gross Anatomy Related to Radiographic Anatomy. The typical rib (Fig. 10–46) consists of a head, neck, tubercle, body or shaft, and costal cartilage. The body has an angle and a costal groove. The heads of the upper nine ribs articulate with two thoracic vertebrae—the one with which each rib is in numerical correspondence, and the one above. Each rib has two articular facets for this purpose. The tenth, eleventh, and twelfth ribs have only one articulation, and articulate with only one vertebral body.

Anatomic Features of Radiographic Significance. The inferior aspect of the neck may have a notched appearance (Fig. 10–47), and this notching must not be confused with the abnormal notching and undulation that occur more peripherally in association with dilated intercostal arteries (as in coarctation of the aorta) (Fig. 10–48 A, B, C, D).

The inferior margin of the rib where the costal groove is identified may have a somewhat irregular appearance, particularly at the angle of the rib. This irregularity at the angle is due to the fact that the bone is slightly thickened in this location (Fig. 10–49).

There is usually a slight widening of the rib as it joins the costal cartilage, and a ring-like shadow may be seen in this location (see Fig. 10–50 A and B). This slight flare of the ribs must not be confused with the abnormal rosary which occurs in vitamin D deficiency in children (Fig. 10–50 C).

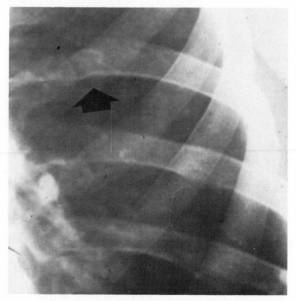

Figure 10–47. Magnified view of neck of rib to show normal concavity.

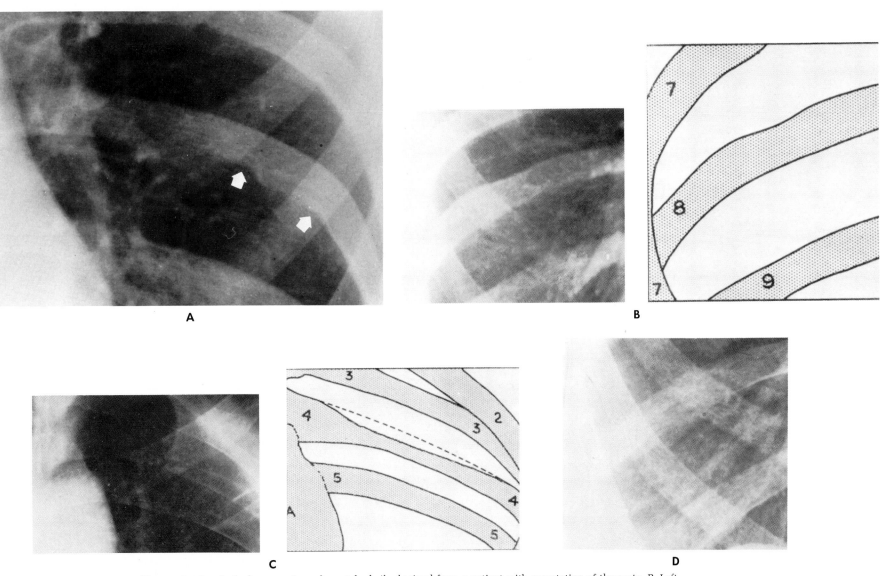

Figure 10–48. *A.* A close-up view of a notched rib obtained from a patient with coarctation of the aorta. *B. Left,* Shallow indentation of posterior aspect of eighth rib as often seen in healthy individuals. Note sharp cortical margin. *Right,* Diagram of left radiograph. *C.* Varying extent of erosion of the upper cortical rib margin. Note fuzzy outline of lesions. *Left,* Shallow, long erosion of left fourth rib. *Right,* Diagram of radiograph. *D.* Short, shallow erosions of right ninth rib. (*B, C,* and *D* from Noetzl, M., and Steinbach, H. L.: Amer. J. Roentgenol., *87:* 1058, 1962.)

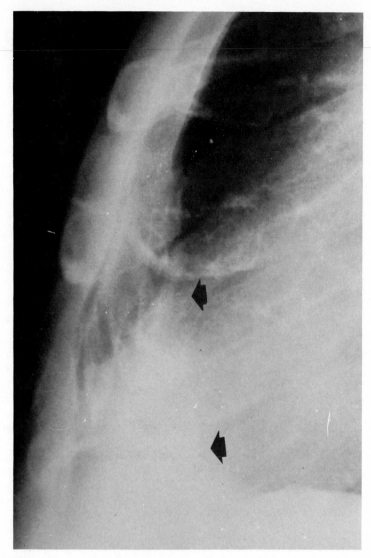

Figure 10–49.   Radiograph of a rib, demonstrating the normal slight irregularity and thickening at its angle.

The gas shadows over ribs are very disturbing at times, and make a study of bony detail extremely difficult. These gas shadows must not be confused with areas of true bone absorption or replacement.

The last rib may simulate a transverse process of the lumbar spine, but can be identified frequently by its articulation with the twelfth thoracic vertebra. This transition between the ribs and the transverse processes of the lumbar vertebrae is usually a gradual one, and is exemplified in the anatomic changes visible in the last three thoracic ribs.

Mode of Radiographic Examination of the Ribs.   Ribs may be studied in any of the routine radiographs of the chest. Ordinarily, however, for greatest accuracy, special studies of the ribs are desirable. These are obtained by placing the ribs in question in various degrees of obliquity (essentially the same as that shown in Fig. 10–53), centering over the area of maximum suspicion and obtaining movable grid films. Usually at least three such views are obtained. *It is not unusual to find that routine radiographs of the chest are inadequate for rib detail, and that the study is considerably better when done as a special or separate procedure*

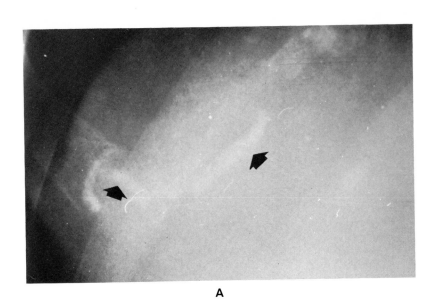

A

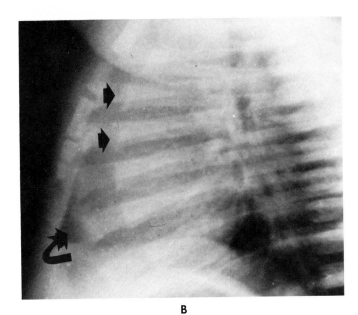

B

C

Figure 10–50.   A. Calcified costal cartilage, lower chest. B. Costochondral junctions in a newborn infant as seen in lateral view. The curvilinear area is the costochondral junction farthest from the film, whereas the straight areas are those closest to the film. C. Calcified costochondral cartilage in the upper chest adjoining the manubrium.

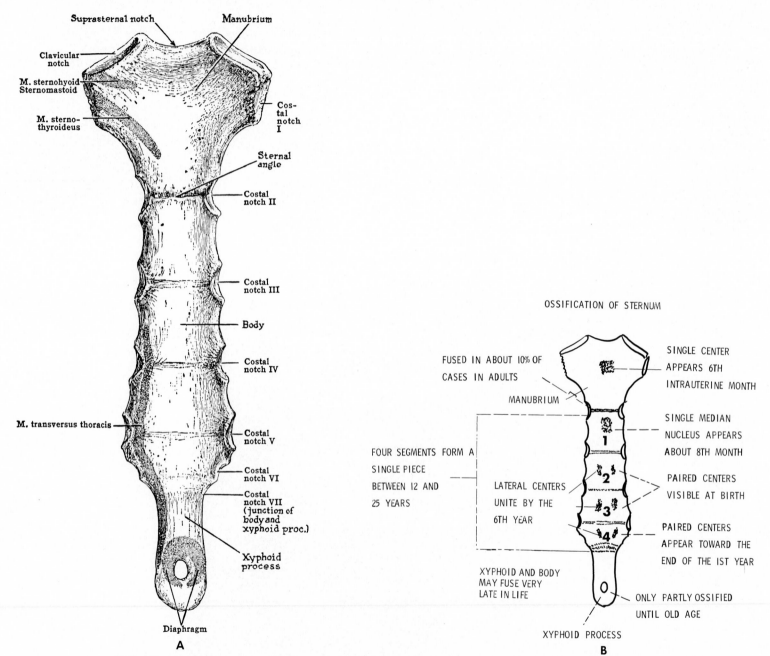

Figure 10–51. A. Gross anatomy of the sternum. (Adapted from Anson, B. J. (ed.): Morris' Human Anatomy, 12th ed. Copyright © 1966 by McGraw-Hill, Inc. Used by permission of McGraw-Hill Book Company.) B. Ossification of sternum.

The Sternum

Gross Anatomy and Correlated Radiographic Anatomy. The sternum consists of the manubrium, body, and xiphoid process. The body in youth consists of four segments. The manubrium ordinarily is united with the sternal body by a cartilaginous union only, until old age. The manubrium has a suprasternal notch (Fig. 10–51), a clavicular articular surface on either side for articulation with the clavicle, and a rough portion just below the clavicular articulation where the cartilage of the first rib is implanted.

The angle between the body of the sternum and the manubrium is called the sternal angle, and the cartilage of the second rib joins the sternum at this point.

The body of the sternum is composed of four segments that fuse in adolescence, leaving a transverse ridge at each site of fusion. There are small protuberances on either side of the sternum at these junction lines, and the rib cartilages for the third, fourth, and fifth ribs join the sternum at these protuberances.

The seventh rib cartilages join the sternum at the junction of the body and xiphoid process, and the sixth rib cartilages join the sternum slightly above this level.

The upper margin of the manubrium is at the level of the lower border of the body of the second thoracic vertebra; the sternal angle, with the upper border of the body of the fifth thoracic vertebra; and the xiphoid process, with the eighth or ninth thoracic vertebra (Fig. 10–52).

With the exception of the manubrium, the sternum will ordinarily not be visible on straight posteroanterior views of the chest, and requires special projections for the demonstration of its radiographic anatomy (Fig. 10–53).

Variations with Growth and Development (Figs. 10–51 *B*, 10–54). Ordinarily, there are one or two centers of ossification already present and ossified at birth for four of the segments of the sternum. The paired centers of the fourth segment of the body of the sternum appear toward the end of the first year of life, but the center of ossification for the xiphoid process usually does not appear until about 3 years of age.

The segments of the body of the sternum unite from below upward. First the paired lateral centers unite with one another by the sixth year. Then the four segments of the body form a single bony piece between 12 and 25 years. The manubrium and body fuse in about 10 per cent of adults, and the body and xiphoid process fuse late in life in about 30 per cent of adults. The xiphoid process may remain only partly ossified until old age (Anson; Gabrielsen and Ladyman).

Generally, the enchondral ossification of the sternum is very slow and irregular.

These normal lines of fusion of the various segments must not be confused with fractures.

Modes of Radiographic Examination. *1. Oblique View of the Sternum* (Fig. 10–53). Since the sternum overlies the heart and mediastinal structures, it must be projected away from these structures to be visualized radiographically. Either oblique projection may be employed as illustrated. In either case, the lung structures are projected over the sternum, so that bony texture is very difficult to evaluate accurately. Gross abnormalities are readily manifest, but minute changes in the sternum can escape detection.

The manner in which the film is obtained, and the associated anatomy are shown in Figure 10–53.

2. Lateral View of the Sternum (Fig. 10–55). This view is particularly helpful since it shows the structure of the sternum

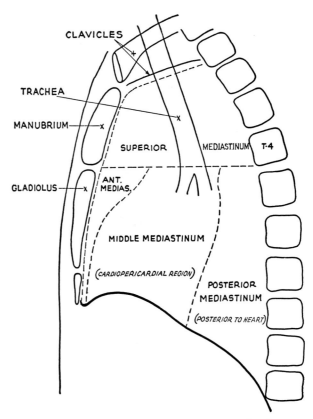

Figure 10–52. The compartments of the mediastinum, also demonstrating the usual topographic relationship of the sternum to the spine.

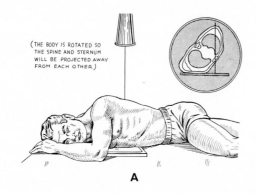

(THE BODY IS ROTATED SO THE SPINE AND STERNUM WILL BE PROJECTED AWAY FROM EACH OTHER.)

A

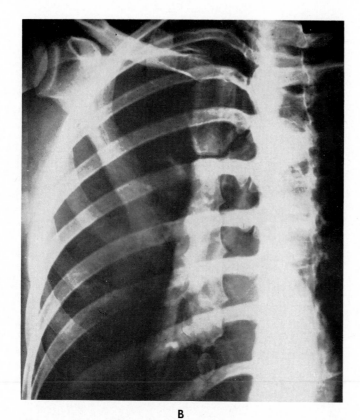

B

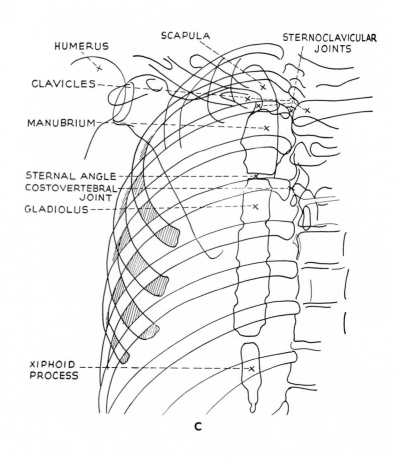

C

Figure 10–53. Oblique view of sternum and sternoclavicular joints (also ribs). *A.* Position of patient similar in both. *B.* Radiograph of sternum. *C.* Labeled tracing of *B.*

Figure 10–53 continued on the opposite page.

Points of Practical Interest With Reference to Figure 10–53, and Comments Relating to Body Section Radiography of the Sternum

1. Sometimes the sternum is difficult to visualize with sufficient clarity in this view. Under these circumstances, body section radiography is recommended. The best technique for this is as follows:
   (a) A mobile cart is placed at right angles to the x-ray table, and the patient lies prone on the cart, with his chest overlapping the table, so that he is as nearly as possible *perpendicular to the x-ray table.*
   (b) *The long axis of the sternum is therefore in contact with the surface of the x-ray table but at right angles to the long axis of this table.*
   (c) The cassette is placed in the tray so that its long axis corresponds to that of the sternum.
   (d) The body section study is thereafter made in the usual manner, and two or three "cuts" may be made.

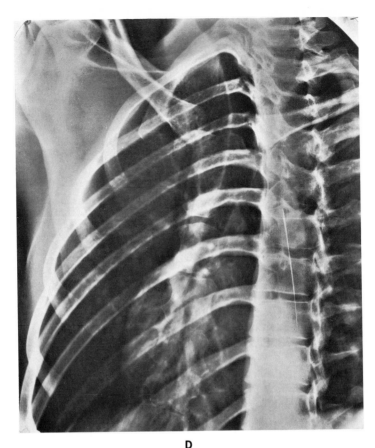

D

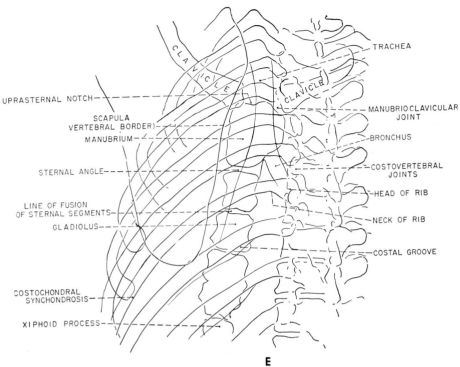

TRACHEA

UPRASTERNAL NOTCH

SCAPULA
VERTEBRAL BORDER)

MANUBRIUM

STERNAL ANGLE

LINE OF FUSION
OF STERNAL SEGMENTS

GLADIOLUS

COSTOCHONDRAL
SYNCHONDROSIS

XIPHOID PROCESS

MANUBRIOCLAVICULAR
JOINT

BRONCHUS

COSTOVERTEBRAL
JOINTS

HEAD OF RIB

NECK OF RIB

COSTAL GROOVE

E

Figure 10–53 *Continued.* D. Radiograph of sternoclavicular joints. E. Labeled tracing of D.

without the interference of overlying structures. This is only one perspective, however, and one cannot ordinarily obtain a clear anatomic concept from one projection alone. Moreover, in certain people, the sternum is somewhat depressed and the ribs overlie the sternum in considerable part. It is most difficult to obtain a clear idea of the structure of the sternum in such people.

This view is also valuable since it shows the relationship of the sternum to the underlying structures.

The method by which this view is obtained, along with film and tracing, are illustrated in Figure 10–55.

3. Body Section Radiographs of the Sternum (Fig. 10–56). Body section radiographs must frequently be employed to obtain an unobstructed view of the sternum. A much more detailed visualization of the bony texture and structure can thus be obtained. Several sections are necessary, and caution must be used in interpretation since the entire sternum is not visualized at one level.

A study of the bony texture of the sternum is of particular interest and importance since the sternal marrow is one of the important hematopoietic organs, and as such can be readily affected by diseases of the blood-forming apparatus, lymphoid structures, or any of the cellular components of the marrow.

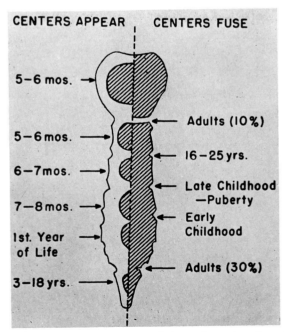

CENTERS APPEAR   CENTERS FUSE

5–6 mos.

5–6 mos.

6–7 mos.

7–8 mos.

1st. Year
of Life

3–18 yrs.

Adults (10%)

16–25 yrs.

Late Childhood
—Puberty

Early
Childhood

Adults (30%)

Figure 10–54. Ossification and fusion of the various sternebrae (infant and adult sternum) (Also see Fig. 10–51 *A*). (From Currarino, G., and Silverman, F. N.: Radiology, 70:532–540, 1958.)

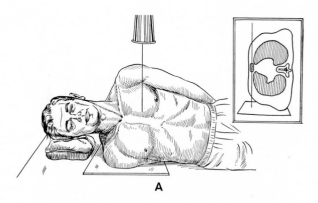

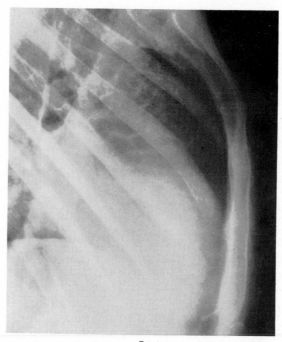

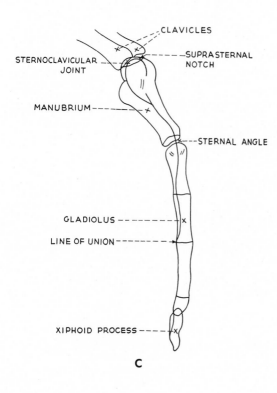

Figure 10–55. Lateral view of sternum. *A.* Position of patient. *B.* Radiograph. *C.* Labeled tracing of *B.*

Points of Practical Interest With Reference to Figure 10–55

1. This view of the sternum gives us maximum clarity of the sternum, but unfortunately has the following disadvantages:
   (a) When the sternum is depressed at all, it is concealed behind the costal cartilages and some lung in this projection. This is especially true of the condition called "pectus excavatum."
   (b) Abnormalities which do not affect the entire width of the sternum may be obscured by the unaffected portion. Body section radiographs are helpful when this is suspected.
   (c) The various segments of the sternum must be recognized and differentiated from other abnormalities which may be stimulated at the costosternal junctions.
2. The retrosternal mediastinal and pleural shadows should always be examined very carefully. This is also true of the shadows which are superficial to the sternum. The clue to abnormality is often found here where it may escape detection by inspection of the sternal shadow only.

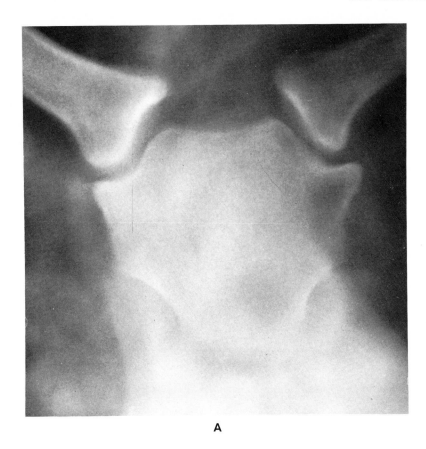

A

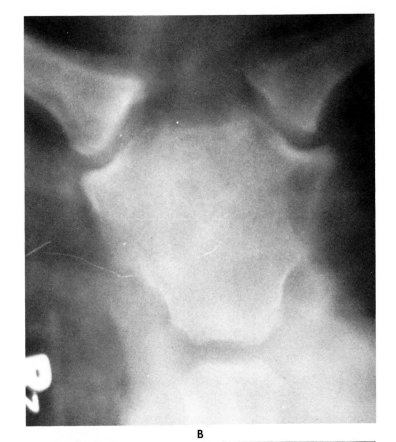

B

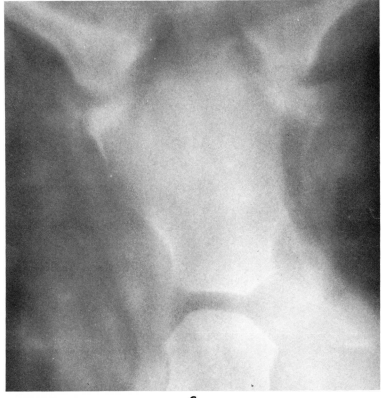

C

Figure 10–56. *A* and *B.* Tomographs of manubrium. *C.* Tomograph of sterno-manubrial junction.

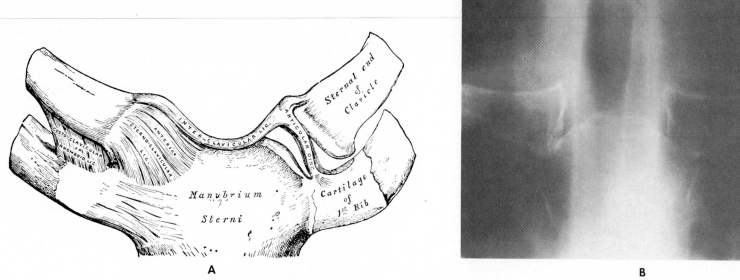

Figure 10–57. *A.* Gross anatomy of sternoclavicular joint. (From Gray's Anatomy of the Human Body, 29th ed. Goss, C. M. (ed.) Philadelphia, Lea & Febiger, 1973.) *B.* Body section radiograph of the sternoclavicular joints. This is obtained in the prone position, centering over the sternoclavicular joints.

Sternoclavicular Joints (Fig. 10–57). The sternoclavicular joint is a two-chambered synovial or diarthrodial joint with an articular disk between the two chambers. Each chamber is usually distinct and separate from the others, unless the articular disk happens to be unusually thin (as in the case of the temporomandibular joint).

These joints are usually demonstrated on oblique projections such as those employed for the sternum proper (Fig. 10–53), except that the tube is centered over the joint. *A comparison film of the opposite side is always obtained so that the two sternoclavicular joints can be compared in the same patient.*

The Pleura

Gross Anatomic Features as Applied to Radiographic Anatomy. The pleura lines the entire thoracic cavity and invests the entire lung, and invaginations of the pleura form the interlobar fissures. That portion lining the thoracic cavity is called the *parietal pleura,* and that investing the lung is called the *visceral pleura.* The interlobar fissures are formed by invagination into the lung of two closely approximated layers of visceral pleura.

The lines of pleural reflection do not accurately correspond on the two sides of the thorax. These lines of reflection also vary in different subjects, depending upon body habitus.

The pleura is composed of a layer of endothelial cells resting on a membrane of connective tissue, within which are situated blood vessels, lymphatics, and nerves.

There is a thin layer of serous fluid between the two opposing layers of pleura ordinarily, with a slow and steady filtration and absorption occurring normally. The visceral pleural blood supply is obtained from the bronchial arteries as previously indicated, whereas the parietal pleura is supplied by systemic arteries that are branches of the subclavian artery and thoracic aorta. Also, the reader is referred to the previous discussion of the lymphatics in connection with the lung. The superficial lymphatics drain the visceral pleura outward, and communicate by means of short tributaries with the deep lymphatics that drain in the opposite direction toward the lung hilus. The parietal lymphatics do not drain directly into the hilar lymph nodes but rather into the lymph trunks at the junction of the internal jugular and subclavian veins.

Ordinarily, the pleura does not cast a significant radiographic shadow, except perhaps minimally in the costophrenic angles. When the pleural shadow can be identified, it is usually indicative of an abnormality.

There are usually small blebs or ruptured alveoli at the lung apices (Cunningham) which cast a shadow on the chest radiograph (Fig. 10–58). This may simulate pleural disease and must not be confused with an abnormal appearance of the pleura or lungs in this location.

Ordinarily, the costophrenic angles are sharply delineated, and any significant degree of blunting is indicative of previous

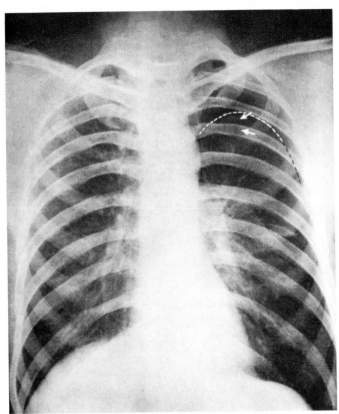

Figure 10–58. Chest film to demonstrate small blebs or ruptured alveoli at lung apices: chest film of patient with spontaneous rupture into the pleural space of one of these blebs on the left. There are similar blebs in the right apex.

pleural disease; since these areas represent the most dependent portions of the pleura, disease is readily seen in these locations.

The cardiophrenic angles, however, vary considerably in appearance, and although the reflection of the pleura is normally sharp in this location also, a greater variability exists in the appearance of the pleural shadow here. An increased acuity of the appearance of this angle is of significance in detecting excessive fluid within the pericardial space, and thus an accurate conception of these angles must be constantly borne in mind.

The Diaphragm

Composition and Normal Attachments of the Diaphragm. The diaphragm consists of a peripheral muscular portion that completely surrounds an aponeurotic membrane and arches over the abdominal contents, separating the abdomen from the chest. There is extensive peripheral attachment to the xiphoid process, the lower six costal cartilages, the ribs, the first three lumbar vertebrae on the right side, and the first two on the left side. With varying degrees of curvature, the fibers arch centrally

and end in the central tendon. This latter tendon is more anterior than posterior and thus is not truly central. It is incompletely divided into three lobes or leaflets. The middle one is anterior and intermediate in size, whereas the right lateral one is the largest and the left lateral the smallest. The crura of the diaphragm are two elongated musculotendinous bundles that arise on each side of the aorta and are partly separated from the lumbar vertebrae by the upper lumbar arteries, but are firmly attached to the upper three vertebrae on the right and the upper two on the left. There is a tendency for the cupola of the diaphragm to descend with age (Fig. 10–59).

Normal Openings in the Diaphragm (Fig. 10–60). The diaphragm is pierced by numerous structures: the superior epigastric artery, the musculophrenic artery, the splanchnic nerves, and the sympathetic trunks behind; the aorta, azygos vein, and thoracic duct passing between the crura; the inferior vena cava,

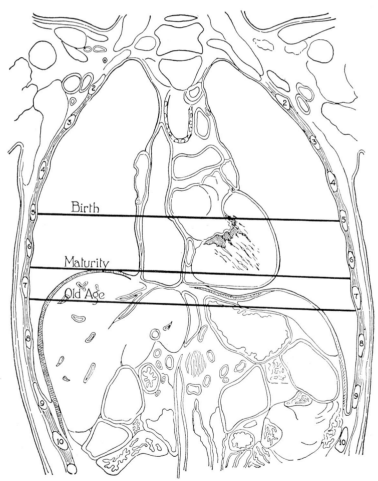

Figure 10–59. Diaphragm at various ages. (From Scamon, in Meyers and McKinlay, The Chest and the Heart, Charles C Thomas, Publishers.)

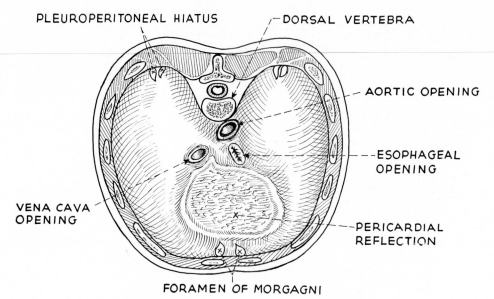

PLEUROPERITONEAL HIATUS   DORSAL VERTEBRA

AORTIC OPENING

ESOPHAGEAL OPENING

VENA CAVA OPENING

PERICARDIAL REFLECTION

FORAMEN OF MORGAGNI

Figure 10–60.   Normal openings of the diaphragm.

and small branches of the right phrenic nerve passing through the foramen venae cavae; and the esophageal opening, transmitting the esophagus and two vagus nerves.

Three-Dimensional Concept of the Diaphragm (Fig. 10–61). The posterior attachment of the diaphragm is considerably lower than the anterior, and there is much lung substance and diaphragm which cannot be seen from the posteroanterior projection.

Moreover, much of the pleural space is likewise obscured from view by virtue of the attachments of the diaphragm. For that reason, it is important to attempt to visualize the structures behind it and frequently to obtain lateral and oblique projections.

Occasionally, the diaphragm may have a slightly irregular appearance, and by projection, a structure which actually lies beneath the diaphragm will be projected above a portion of it. Every effort must be made to obviate such projection phenomena and understand them when they occur.

Tenting and Scalloping of the Diaphragm.   Occasionally, the contour of the diaphragm is broken into two or more arches, the outlines appearing as a scalloped margin (Fig. 10–62). This is usually caused by an irregular contraction of the diaphragmatic musculature, and usually these irregularities become less evident in expiration.

Occasionally, several peaks are present on the diaphragmatic surface that are likewise due to the rib attachments of the diaphragm. Occasionally, these are due to abnormal pleurodiaphragmatic adhesions, and the two processes must not be confused. This is spoken of as "tenting" of the diaphragm.

Overlapping Shadows Due to Diaphragm, Liver, and Heart Anteriorly (Fig. 10–63).   The anteromedian part of the diaphragmatic dome, the heart shadow, and the anterior margin of the

liver overlap one another in the lateral projection, producing a triangular shadow that may be confused with an interlobar effusion or consolidation of the inferior portion of the right middle lobe. Care must be exercised not to make this error of interpretation.

Roentgen Significance of the Transverse Thoracis Muscle (Shopfner et al.).   The transverse thoracis muscle is the plane of muscular and tendinous fibers and muscle situated on the front wall of the thoracic cage (Fig. 10–63 *B*). It originates on either side from the lower third of the posterior surface of the sternal body xiphoid process and medial ends of the costal cartilages of the lower three or four true ribs. It is inserted by slips into the lower borders and inner surface of the costal cartilages of the second, third, fourth, fifth, and sixth ribs. Usually, it is directed obliquely downward, producing a density of varying size and contour in the lateral chest roentgenogram that may cause difficulty in differential diagnosis since it may resemble a retrosternal mass (Fig. 10–63 *C* and *D*).

The thickness of the muscle varies, depending upon the size of the patient, between 2 and 4 mm. Its appearance varies somewhat, depending upon the degree of rotation of the patient from the true lateral. It is ordinarily not visualized in oblique projections of 45 to 60 degrees. Actually, perfectly positioned lateral roentgenograms likewise do not show this shadow, which is apparent only when there is a slight rotation from the true lateral position which throws this muscle into relief. It is not important except that it should be recognized as a normal anatomic structure not to be confused with possible pathologic entities. Generally, a true lateral view with expiration can prevent its visualization since it blends imperceptibly with the

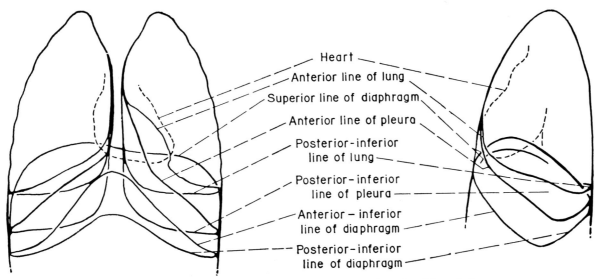

Figure 10–61.   Isometric concept of the diaphragm on frontal and lateral views.

shadow of the sternum. Slight obliquity and deep inspiration allow the lower portion of the muscle to appear on one side as a linear density. Differentiation can thereby be achieved with reasonable accuracy.

Diaphragmatic Movements.   On quiet breathing, the range of motion of the diaphragm is about 1 to 2 cm. On deep breathing it will increase to 3 to 5 cm., or even somewhat more. There is usually an accompanying flare of the ribs upward and outward (Fig 10–64). Occasionally, half of the diaphragm will move somewhat more than the other, or in slightly different sequence, but marked differences in any area of the diaphragm or inequalities between the two sides are of definite pathologic significance.

The diaphragmatic position at rest is also of considerable im-

portance, whether it be elevated or depressed, and localized elevations are likewise noteworthy, since they may be related to masses underlying the diaphragm.

ROUTINE POSITIONS IN THE RADIOGRAPHY OF THE CHEST

Chest Fluoroscopy.   Fluoroscopy offers the first mode of examination of the chest. However, for consistent demonstration of fine detail, for avoidance of considerable magnification, and for the sake of permanent record and future comparison, radiography has no substitute.

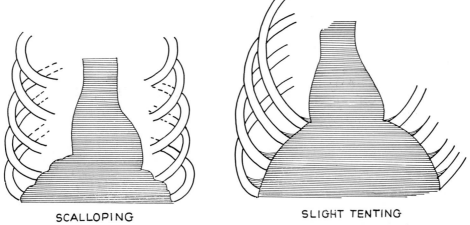

SCALLOPING   SLIGHT TENTING

Figure 10–62.   Diagrammatic illustration of tenting and scalloping of the diaphragm.

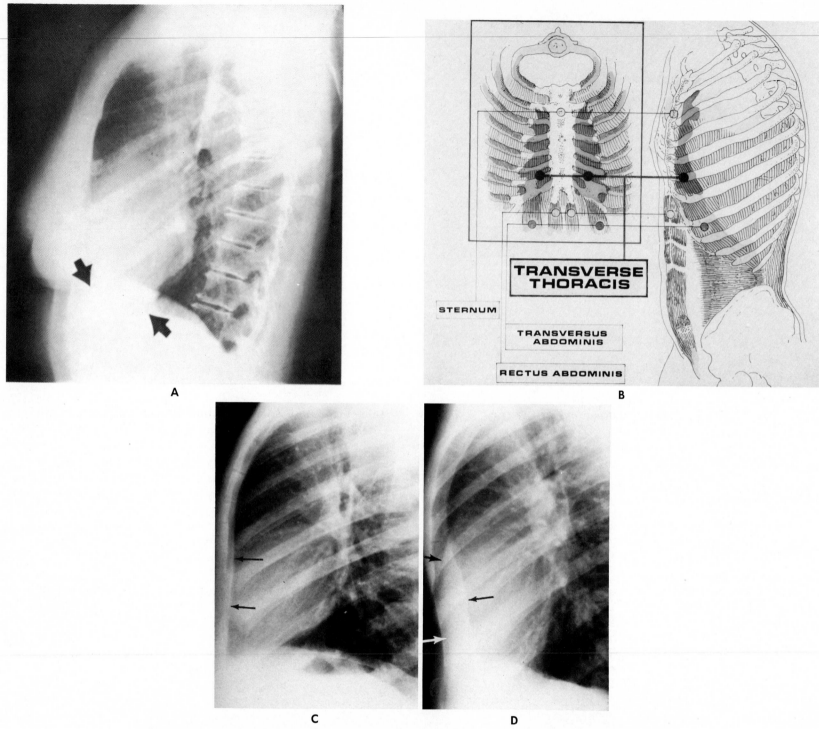

Figure 10–63. *A.* Lateral view of the chest, demonstrating a rather dense ovoid area produced by overlapping shadows of the heart, liver, and diaphragm anteroinferiorly. This must not be confused with an interlobar effusion. *B.* Artist's sketch of transverse thoracis muscle showing its relationship to other anatomic structures in the antero-posterior and lateral views. *C.* True lateral chest roentgenogram of 7-year-old female. The transverse thoracis muscle shows a thin strip of density (arrows) contiguous to the sternum. *D.* Same patient as in *C.* Slight rotation from the true lateral position causes the origin and lowest inserting fibers of the muscle to cast a triangular density (arrows). Only slight rotation from the true lateral is necessary to produce the density because of the sternal width being interposed between the muscle of the two sides. (*B, C,* and *D* from Shopfner, C. E., Jansen, C., and O'Kell, R. J.: Amer. J. Roentgenol., *103*:140–148, 1968.)

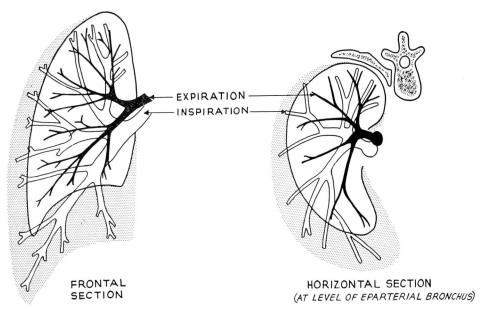

Figure 10–64. Longitudinal and transverse sections through thorax, showing mode of expansion of lungs with respiration. (After Caffey, J.: Pediatric X-ray Diagnosis, 6th ed. Springfield, Illinois, Charles C Thomas, 1972.)

A very useful routine to follow in fluoroscopy of the chest is as follows:

1. Notation of the position and contour of the trachea and ιarynx, in phonation and at rest.
2. Detection of the movement and symmetry of the two halves of the diaphragm.
3. Notation of the clarity of the costophrenic and cardiophrenic angles.
4. Examination of the lung fields, bilaterally, for notation of any differences in clarity of the two sides.
5. Examination of the lung apices, requesting the patient to move his scapula forward so as to improve the visibility of the lung apices.
6. Notation of the type of rib movement and flare with respiration.
7. Simultaneously, the heart and mediastinum must also be studied, as well as the esophagus in its entirety. (These structures will be described subsequently.)

Fluoroscopy has the great advantage of offering the immediate opportunity of turning the patient in any degree of obliquity, or into the erect or recumbent positions. Spatial relationships as well as physiologic function are thus elucidated.

It has the disadvantage of requiring the exposure of the radiologist as well as the patient to considerably greater x-ray exposure than would be necessary by the film studies alone. Even though we may be well below presently considered tolerance levels for exposure to x-ray irradiation, any exposure must be regarded as potentially dangerous.

Posteroanterior View of the Chest (Fig. 10–65). This view is ordinarily obtained with a 6-foot film-target distance so that it can be utilized for study of cardiac size and contour as well. The patient's shoulders are rotated forward so that the scapulas are projected away from the lung fields, and the patient is asked to stop respiration after full inspiration and hold his breath for the film in inspiration, and similarly to stop respiration after forced exhalation for the film in expiration. Both of these studies have definite characteristics. The film in inspiration will show the aerated lung to best advantage, and if there are any unaerated portions, they can be demonstrated by contrast. The film in expiration, on the other hand, will demonstrate any areas that are unusually well aerated. In either case, the mediastinum will normally remain stationary, but abnormally it will shift to one side or the other if unfixed by disease. The excursion of the diaphragm in the two phases of respiration may also be studied in this manner.

Films in both inspiration and expiration (exhalation) are particularly valuable in children. Needless to say, it is not always possible to time the exposure in a child or infant exactly as one would desire it. The value of these views in children is as follows: (1) the history in relation to a child's chest abnormality is notoriously poor, since often it is obtained from the parent who may be unaware of the fact that the child may have inhaled a foreign body; (2) the two frontal views of the chest, even though they may not be perfectly timed in relation to inspiration or expiration, usually supplement one another in any case in an area of difficult diagnosis. Sometimes one of the films is

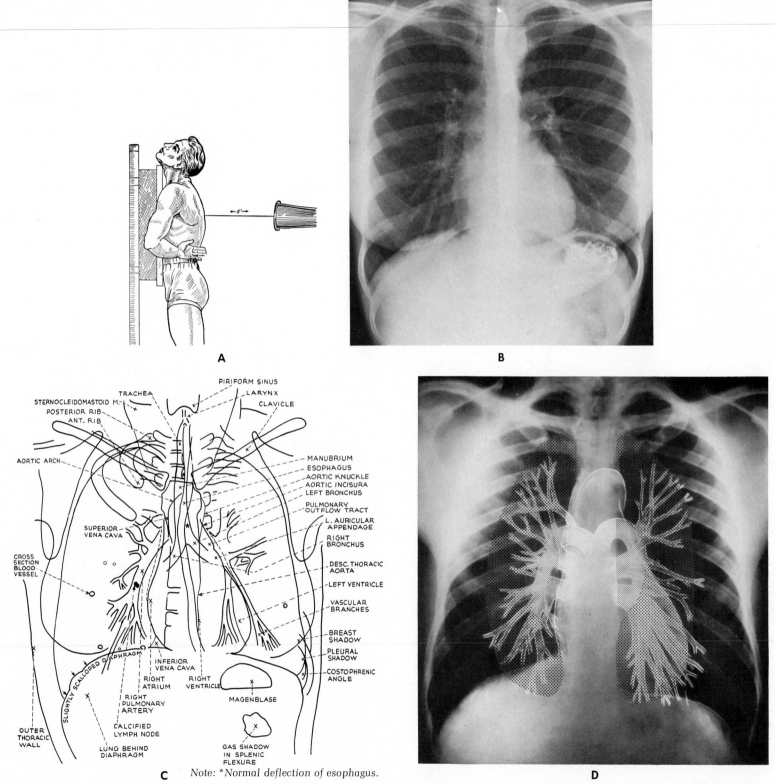

A

B

PIRIFORM SINUS
LARYNX
CLAVICLE
TRACHEA
STERNOCLEIDOMASTOID M.
POSTERIOR RIB
ANT. RIB
AORTIC ARCH
MANUBRIUM
ESOPHAGUS
AORTIC KNUCKLE
AORTIC INCISURA
LEFT BRONCHUS
PULMONARY OUTFLOW TRACT
L. AURICULAR APPENDAGE
SUPERIOR VENA CAVA
RIGHT BRONCHUS
CROSS SECTION BLOOD VESSEL
DESC. THORACIC AORTA
LEFT VENTRICLE
VASCULAR BRANCHES
BREAST SHADOW
PLEURAL SHADOW
COSTOPHRENIC ANGLE
SLIGHTLY SCALLOPED DIAPHRAGM
INFERIOR VENA CAVA
RIGHT ATRIUM
RIGHT VENTRICLE
MAGENBLASE
OUTER THORACIC WALL
RIGHT PULMONARY ARTERY
CALCIFIED LYMPH NODE
GAS SHADOW IN SPLENIC FLEXURE
LUNG BEHIND DIAPHRAGM

C   *Note: *Normal deflection of esophagus.*   D

Figure 10–65.   Posteroanterior view of chest. *A.* Position of patient. *B.* Radiograph (female). *C.* Labeled tracing of *B. D.* Normal radiograph of chest showing three zones of study in the parenchyma.

faulty because of motion on the film or some other feature in the roentgen technique difficult to control in an infant or child. We are then particularly happy to have the two films for comparison. Actually, in infants at least eight ribs should appear above the level of the diaphragm when counted posteriorly in inspiration (White). On the other hand, when nine or more ribs are visible, overinflation, such as may occur with air trapping in bronchiolitis, is to be suspected.

Gross Subdivisions of the Lung Fields (Fig. 10–65). Arbitrarily one can subdivide the lung fields into three zones, depending on the size of the vascular radicles. The vascular branches gradually assume a smaller caliber proceeding from the hilus to the lung periphery. The inner one-third zone contains the largest channels; the middle one-third zone contains vessels of intermediate size; and the peripheral one-third zone usually has vessels that are 1 mm. or less in diameter. This arbitrary subdivision permits the radiologist to attribute definite significance to shadows that are inordinately large in diameter or size, particularly in the middle and outer zones. (See final section in this chapter: Methods of Studying Radiographs of the Chest.)

Lateral Views of the Chest (Fig. 10–66). When a lateral view of one lung is desired, that side of the patient is placed closest to the film, and the arms are raised out of the projection as much as possible. A relatively close film-to-target distance (36 to 48 inches) is desired in this instance to "blur out" the lung that is farthest from the film.

The anatomic parts are illustrated in Figure 10–67. A detailed discussion of the anatomy will be deferred until after the entire thorax and its contents have been reviewed from the correlated gross anatomic standpoint.

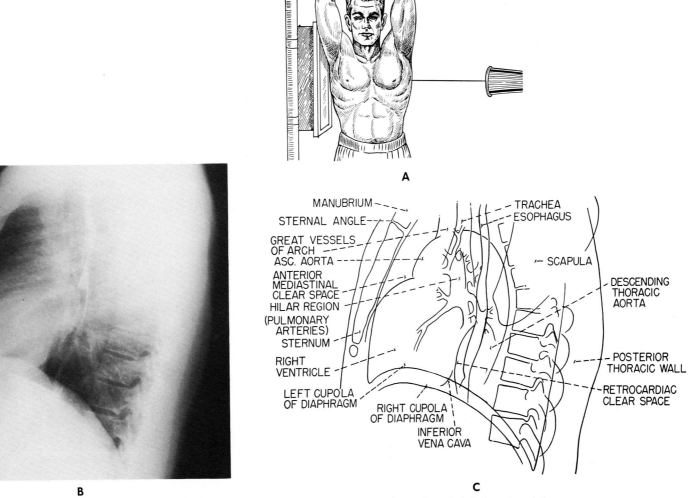

Figure 10–66. Lateral view of chest. *A.* Position of patient. *B.* Radiograph. *C.* Labeled tracing of *B.*

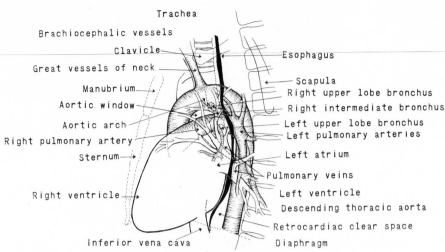

Figure 10–67. Lateral view of the chest showing anatomic relationships.

Oblique Views of the Chest (Figs. 10–68 to 10–71). These projections are obtained by rotating the thorax 45 degrees, with the side in question closest to the film. In posteroanterior oblique views the anterior aspect of the patient is closest to the film. On the other hand, in anteroposterior oblique views the posterior aspect of the patient is closest to the film.

The left posteroanterior oblique view (Fig. 10–69) (or right anteroposterior oblique) is ordinarily best for visualization of the trachea and its bifurcation. A portion of the left lung is obscured by the spine, but other portions of the left lung are seen in better detail. The right posteroanterior (or left anteroposterior) oblique (Figs. 10–70 and 10–71), on the other hand, gives the clearest visualization of the right retrocardiac space and right lung.

Anteroposterior View of the Chest (Fig. 10–72). This projection has the disadvantage of not permitting the scapulas to be projected out of the lung fields as readily as in the posteroanterior

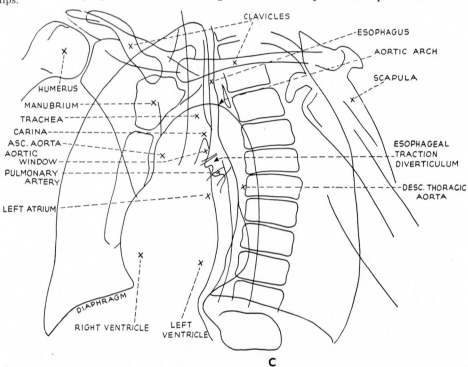

Points of Practical Interest With Reference to Figure 10–68

1. The 45-degree obliquity may be increased to 50 or 55 degrees on occasion, to obtain maximum clearance of the spine.
2. Ordinarily the left ventricle clears the spine, and the right ventricle forms a smooth uninterrupted convexity with the ascending portion of the arch of the aorta.
3. This view gives maximum clarity of the bifurcation of the trachea, the arch of the aorta, and the posterior basilar portion of the left ventricle. Pulsations are ordinarily of maximum amplitude in this portion of the cardiac silhouette.
4. Although the right ventricle is seen very adequately in most instances in this view, the straight lateral is preferable, since the relationship of the right ventricle to the retrosternal space is more informative. Likewise, the left ventricle is more accurately evaluated in the straight lateral view by noting its relationship to the shadow of the inferior vena cava. It should not normally project more than 5 or 6 mm. beyond this shadow in the lateral projection.

Figure 10–68. Left posteroanterior oblique view of chest. *A*. Position of patient. *B*. Radiograph. *C*. Labeled tracing of *B*.

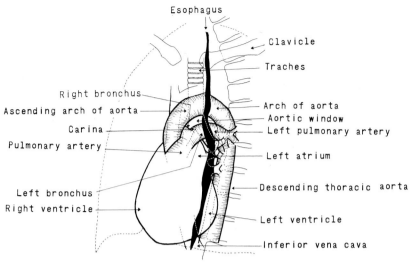

CHEST, LEFT ANTERIOR OBLIQUE
VIEW

Esophagus

Clavicle

Traches

Right bronchus

Ascending arch of aorta

Carina

Pulmonary artery

Arch of aorta

Aortic window

Left pulmonary artery

Left atrium

Left bronchus

Right ventricle

Descending thoracic aorta

Left ventricle

Inferior vena cava

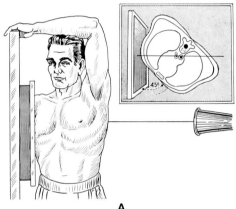

A

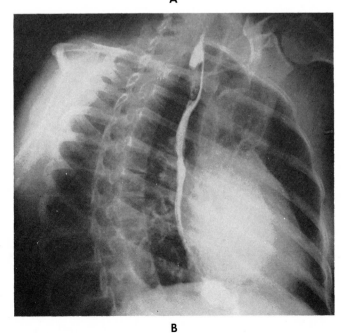

B

Figure 10-69. Left anterior oblique view of the chest showing anatomic relationships.

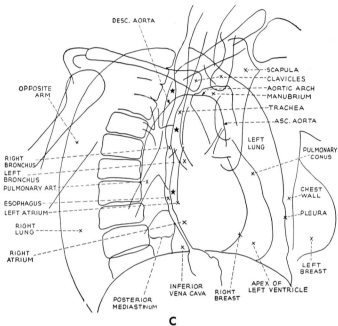

C

DESC. AORTA

OPPOSITE ARM

SCAPULA
CLAVICLES
AORTIC ARCH
MANUBRIUM
TRACHEA
ASC. AORTA

LEFT LUNG

PULMONARY CONUS

RIGHT BRONCHUS
LEFT BRONCHUS
PULMONARY ART.

ESOPHAGUS
LEFT ATRIUM

RIGHT LUNG

RIGHT ATRIUM

CHEST WALL

PLEURA

LEFT BREAST

POSTERIOR MEDIASTINUM

INFERIOR VENA CAVA

RIGHT BREAST

APEX OF LEFT VENTRICLE

*Note: *Undulation of esophagus in regions of . . .*
    1. Above arch of aorta
    2. At arch of aorta and pulmonary art.
    3. Left atrium (slightly prominent in
       this case)

Figure 10-70. Right posteroanterior oblique view of chest. *A.* Position of patient. *B.* Radiograph. (The left atrium is enlarged slightly but is shown for demonstration of its indentation upon the esophagus.) *C.* Labeled tracing of *B.*

Points of Practical Interest with Reference to Figure 10-70

1. The patient's right shoulder is placed against the film and the body turned approximately 45 degrees from the film, with the left arm resting in a convenient position, away from the body.
2. The central ray is directed just medial to the scapula nearest the x-ray tube at approximately the level of the sixth or seventh thoracic vertebra.
3. The patient is placed in proper position and then barium paste is administered. He is instructed to swallow and then take a deep breath and hold it while the x-ray exposure is made.
4. The maximum area of the right lung field is demonstrated in this view, but it is partially obscured by the shadow of the spinal column.
5. This view is most advantageous for demonstration of the left atrium and its possible enlargement, since any slight enlargement will cause a significant impression upon the esophagus, as indicated.
6. This view is also valuable for demonstration of the anterior apical portion of the left ventricle, which is most significantly involved in anterior apical myocardial infarction, a rather common disease entity.

647

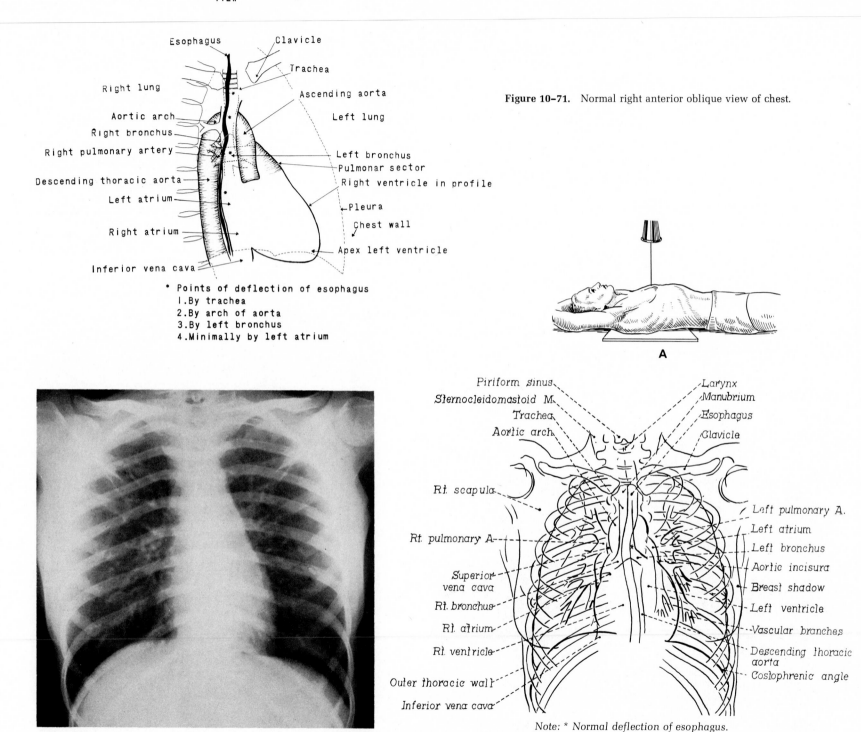

CHEST,RIGHT ANTERIOR OBLIQUE
VIEW

Esophagus · Clavicle · Trachea · Right lung · Ascending aorta · Aortic arch · Left lung · Right bronchus · Right pulmonary artery · Left bronchus · Pulmonar sector · Right ventricle in profile · Descending thoracic aorta · Left atrium · Pleura · Chest wall · Right atrium · Apex left ventricle · Inferior vena cava

* Points of deflection of esophagus
1. By trachea
2. By arch of aorta
3. By left bronchus
4. Minimally by left atrium

Figure 10–71. Normal right anterior oblique view of chest.

A

Piriform sinus · Larynx · Sternocleidomastoid M. · Manubrium · Trachea · Esophagus · Aortic arch · Clavicle · Rt. scapula · Left pulmonary A. · Left atrium · Rt. pulmonary A. · Left bronchus · Aortic incisura · Superior vena cava · Breast shadow · Rt. bronchus · Left ventricle · Rt. atrium · Vascular branches · Rt. ventricle · Descending thoracic aorta · Outer thoracic wall · Costophrenic angle · Inferior vena cava

Note: * Normal deflection of esophagus.

B   **C**

Figure 10–72. Anteroposterior view of chest. *A.* Position of patient. *B.* Radiograph. The main differences between Figures 10–65 and 10–72 are: (1) the projection of the clavicles; (2) the scapulas are projected over the lung fields in the anteroposterior view; (3) the superior mediastinal structures appear somewhat fuller in the anteroposterior view; (4) the obliquity of the ribs is different. *C.* Labeled tracing of *B.*

projection The clavicle, however, is projected out of the subapical portion of the lung fields, and thus this view has this slight advantage. This projection is usually the only one possible in a very sick patient who cannot sit or stand up, and who cannot be rolled over onto his abdomen readily.

It will be noted that the rib structures have a different appearance in this projection compared with that in the posteroanterior view.

Apical Lordotic View (Fig. 10–73).   This projection is particularly useful for clear demonstration of the lung apices and subapical areas. It also has its application in demonstrating the anterior mediastinum tangentially. Distortion of the lower chest areas is maximum in this view.

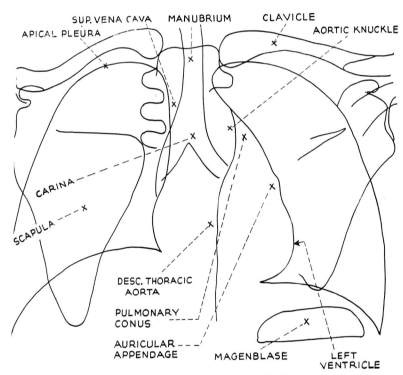

Note: *Apical portion of lung is completely clear*

C

Points of Practical Interest with Reference to Figure 10–73

1. By standing the patient approximately 1 foot in front of the vertical cassette stand and then having him lean directly backward, a proper obliquity of the chest is obtained.
2. The top of the cassette is adjusted so that the upper border of the film is about 1 inch above the shoulders.
3. The central ray passes through the region of the manubrium. Occasionally a slight angle of 5 degrees toward the head may prove to be of advantage in demonstrating the apices more clearly.
4. This view gives a very distorted picture of the lung fields and mediastinum, but is particularly valuable in showing more clearly: (1) the apices; (2) the interlobar areas of the lungs; and (3) the region of the pulmonary sector of the cardiac shadow.

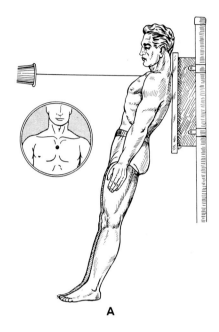

A

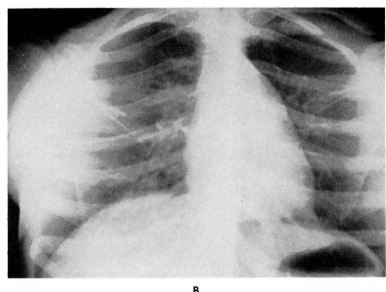

B

Figure 10–73.   Apical lordotic view of chest. *A.* Position of patient. *B.* Radiograph. *C.* Labeled tracing of *B.*

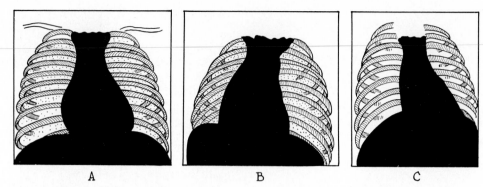

Figure 10–74. Diagram illustrating changes in appearance of mediastinum with position of patient. *A.* Upright. *B.* Lying on right side. *C.* Lying on left side.

Lateral Decubitus Film Studies. By placing the patient on one side or the other and utilizing a horizontal x-ray beam, a posteroanterior projection can be obtained. By gravity, the mediastinal structures will shift downward, and thus show the paramediastinal lung areas to better advantage (Fig. 10–74). If there is any free fluid in the chest, it will shift away from the side of the chest which is uppermost, and thus it is possible to obtain a clearer concept of a portion of lung or pleura that would otherwise be obscured. Also, this method offers an accurate means of estimating small amounts of free pleural fluid that might otherwise escape detection.

It is possible to detect amounts of fluid in excess of (but not less than) 100 cc in this manner, whereas on other conventional views of the chest one cannot ordinarily detect fluid unless it exceeds about 300 cc. in volume.

Air Gap Technique. The air gap technique provides a positioning frame that displaces the patient's chest 6 to 10 inches from the cassette (Fig. 10–75). This has two advantages: (1) The air gap of 6 to 10 inches acts as a filter for secondary radiation, making this procedure a "gridless technique." There are no grid lines to interfere with the interpretation of the film (Watson; Jackson). The air gap roentgenogram is considered by some to be of greater value than the over-penetrated grid roentgenogram on this basis. The kilovoltage is raised to 120 Kv., since lower values are found to give inadequate penetration. Also, the use of these higher voltages reduces the patient's dose (Trout et al.). (2) The air gap roentgenogram may be considered a midchest laminagram since the structures in the midchest are seen in greatest detail, whereas the anterior and posterior chest regions are perhaps diminished in sharpness. Ideally, the distance of the tube-target from the film should be 10 feet for optimum results (3.05 meters).

Most adults require an exposure of 1000 Ma., 120 Kv., and one-40th of a second. Infants and children require an exposure of at least 300 Ma., 110 Kv., and one-60th of a second.

The disadvantage of this technique is that soft pulmonary infiltrates and small densities tend to be obscured. Moreover, a patient with a wide chest is most difficult to fit on the frame, unless the cassette is placed crosswise to the beam. If the anteroposterior position is utilized, it is important to move the scapulae out of the way by special positioning of the patient.

Positive Pressure Radiography. The Valsalva maneuver may be utilized in radiologic diagnosis to increase intrathoracic pressure and lower the effective filling pressure of both cardiac ventricles. This maneuver, originally described by Valsalva in 1704 for use in patients with middle ear disease and tympanic membrane perforation, requires the patient to blow against the closed mouth and nose to aid in diagnosis and therapy. Weber in 1951 emphasized a similar pressure against a closed glottis with its associated alteration in heart sound and pulse. More recently, Whitley and Martin have utilized this procedure as a diagnostic tool in chest disease. A mercury column is positioned so that it is superimposed over the edge of the posteroanterior film of the chest (Fig 10–77), and thus an instantaneous record of the pressure at the moment the film is made is obtained. The exposure is made approximately 5 to 6 seconds after initiation of the patient's positive pressure effort. This timing is important because after 8 to 10 seconds there is a return to normal pressures and cardiac output. The miminum level of intrabronchial pressure to assume a consistent response has been estimated to be between 30 and 40 mm of mercury. A precise level in any individual is determined by his lung compliance, venous pressure, and vasomotor tone. In the overshoot or post-Valsalva maneuver phase following the release of the pressure, the visualization of the enlarged left atrial appendage is improved, as might occur in mitral stenosis. The overshoot phenomenon is best determined approximately 8 to 10 seconds after the cessation of the Valsalva maneuver. During the maneuver, there is a diminution in cardiac size and intrapulmonary vasculature, since cardiac output has been lowered temporarily and visualization of the pulmonary vascular bed and the aorta and its principal branches has been improved by increased aeration of surrounding lung and diminished size of vasculature.

The Valsalva maneuver, as utilized above, has been found useful in the following circumstances: (1) differentiation of en-

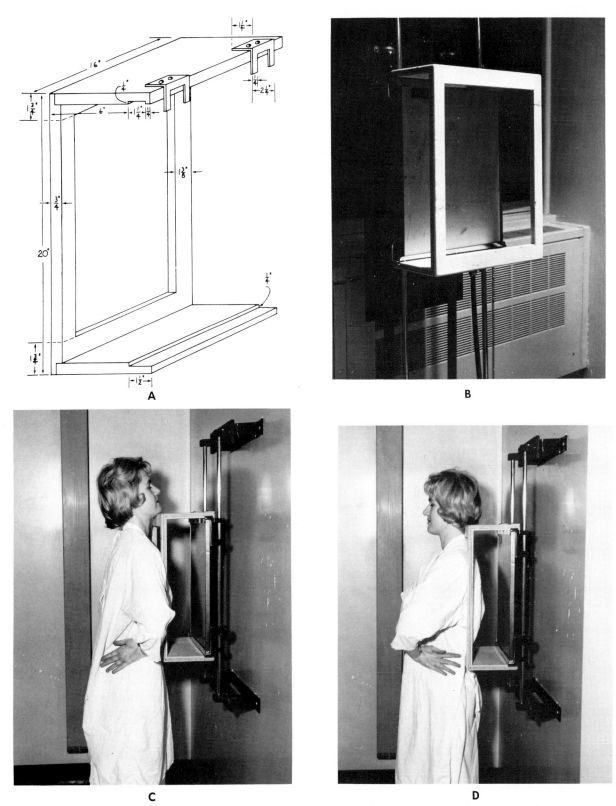

Figure 10–75.   *A.* A drawing of the frame, indicating its dimensions. *B.* The frame is ready for use. *C.* The patient is positioned against the frame for a posteroanterior roentgenographic study. *D.* The patient is positioned for an anteroposterior study. (From Jackson, F. I.: Amer. J. Roentgenol., *92*:688–691, 1964.)

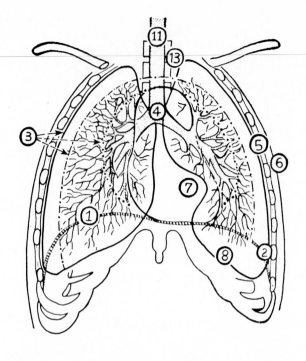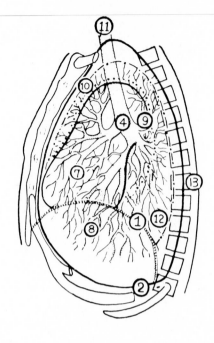

1. DIAPHRAGM
2. COSTOPHRENIC SINUSES
3. ZONES OF LUNG FIELDS
4. TRACHEA IN THORAX
   AND HILI
5. RIBS AND PLEURA
6. THORACIC WALL
7. HEART
8. UNDER DIAPHRAGM
9. HILI ON LATERAL VIEW
10. ANT. MEDIASTINUM
11. TRACHEA IN NECK
12. POST. MEDIASTINUM
13. VERTEBRA

Figure 10–76. A suggested routine to be followed in examining radiographs of the chest.

larged hilar vessels from hilar lymphadenopathy; (2) differentiation of hyperemia, both isolated and associated with other abnormalities, from infiltration and fibrosis of the lung; (3) differentiation of pulmonary arteriovenous fistula from solid tumors; (4) visualization of the miliary and small nodular pulmonary densities; (5) differentiation of focal nodular areas of hyperemia and infiltration from ill-defined tumor nodules.

METHOD OF STUDYING RADIOGRAPHS OF THE CHEST (Fig. 10–76)

1. Localize the abnormal shadow with respect to the chest wall, pleura, lung parenchyma, or mediastinum. If localized in the lung, determine the exact lobe or segment involved if possible

2 Study the level of the diaphragm on each side, noting its general contour and position and any abnormalities contiguous with it.

3 Study the costophrenic and cardiophrenic sinuses in relation to their clarity and sharpness for indication of pleural disease

4. Survey the lung fields. First compare the two sides in relation to one another. Second, divide the lung fields into three zones as shown in Figure 10–65 D. The innermost zone contains hilar blood vessels of large caliber, the intermediate or middle zone contains the medium-sized blood vessels, and the outer zone contains the very small blood vessels, usually so small that only minimal detection is obtained in the usual radiographs. When any shadows that are extraordinary in any respect appear, therefore, in any of these zones, they are immediately suspicious of abnormality.

5. Note the lung apices particularly, and take care to look

tion is noted? Is there an accentuation of the interstitial pattern? Is there arterial distention?

7. Study the thoracic cage, tracing each rib carefully. The widths and symmetry of the intercostal spaces are evaluated simultaneously. The clavicle, scapulae, and visible bony structures of the neck should be noted. Although the skeletal structures of the dorsal spine are not seen adequately enough for careful diagnosis, it can be noted whether or not there is a scoliosis or other significant spine deformity which may affect the radiographic diagnosis of chest lesions. Is there a sternal depression or deformity, pectus excavatum, or pectus carinatum?

8. Study the soft tissue structures of the thoracic cage (Fig. 10–41 *A*). Identify the breasts, nipples, areoli, muscular shadows, particularly the pectoralis major and minor, and the sternocleidomastoids, which very often cast a significant soft tissue shadow across the medial aspect of the lung apices. A tegmental shadow, ordinarily seen above the superior border of the clavicle, must be identified and distinguished from the abnormal.

9. Any unusual pleural shadows are identified. The pleura does not ordinarily cast a significant visible shadow, except occasionally the posterior mediastinal (paraesophageal) stripe to a minimal degree in the costophrenic sinuses (Fig. 10–78) and

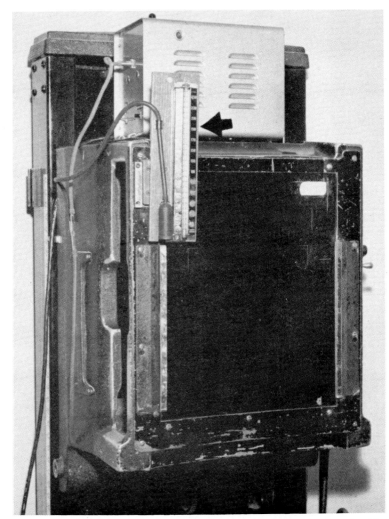

Figure 10–77. Stereoscopic 14 × 17 inch cassette changer equipped with a manometer (arrow) which will register the extent of positive pressure obtained during positive pressure film studies. The film exposure is triggered after maximum pressure is achieved by the electronic device in the box above the cassette holder. (From Whitley, J. E., and Martin, J. F.: Amer. J. Roentgenol., 91:297–306, 1964.)

"under the bones" so that no actual pulmonary markings of unusual character are overlooked.

6. Study the hilar blood vessels and mediastinum. The position of the trachea and its major ramifications should be noted. The trachea is ordinarily located near the midline. A further analysis of the mediastinum will follow in later chapters; here, it is enough to say that a study of the mediastinum cannot be separated from a study of the respiratory system.

The major hilar blood vessels should be traced so that arteries and veins are distinguished, especially in the lung apices and the lung bases. Is there a "deflection" or "cephalization-of-flow" phenomenon in the upright position so that venous disten-

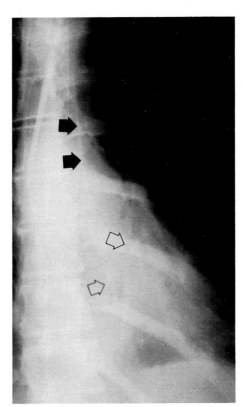

Figure 10–78. Posterior mediastinal (paraesophageal) pleural stripe. Air bronchogram (open arrows) with atelectasis of the left lower lobe and deflection of the posterior mediastinal stripe to the left (closed black arrows).

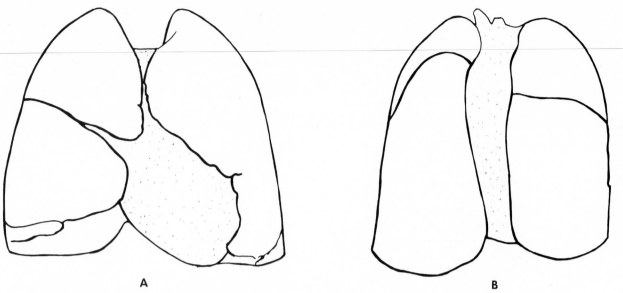

Figure 10–79. Line diagrams illustrating the pleural demarcation zones anteriorly and posteriorly. (Also see the fissures and lobes of the lungs.) *A* and *B*. Frontal and posterior views of lungs.

overlying the lung apices. In the region of the lung apices small blebs may occur normally. They are without pathologic significance and must be identified and distinguished from a pathologic process.

10. Identify structures underlying the diaphragm. A posteroanterior erect chest film offers a very good opportunity for visualizing free air under the diaphragm. Dense areas of calcification such as calcified cysts of the liver are also identified. The distance of the stomach (fundal air bubble or Magenglase) from the left hemidiaphragm should be noted. Is there a filling defect in the fundus? Is the spleen enlarged?

11. In the lateral projection of the chest it is particularly important to identify the *mediastinal shadow* and to form in the mind's eye a concept of the normal in this regard. Identify the left and right pulmonary artery, the trachea, and the bifurcations. We find the lateral projection extremely valuable in detecting abnormal lymphadenopathy or tumor masses in the central mediastinum.

12. In the lateral view identify the *anterior mediastinal clear space* which is just anterior to the cardiac silhouette and underlies the sternal shadow. On occasion the lateral view is the only projection in which the clear space is obliterated in the presence of a space-occupying lesion in the anterior superior mediastinum.

13. In the lateral projection, *the pleural reflection over the internal mammary vessels should be studied.* Metastases will at times produce detectable masses in this location.

14. In the oblique projections, further care must be exercised to identify the trachea and bronchial structures which can be seen to excellent advantage. The oblique views are also particu-

larly valuable in analysis of the cardiac silhouette, especially when barium delineates the esophagus (this will be described in Chapters 11 and 12).

15. Study the clear pneumonic space in the posterior mediastinum and identify the relationship it has with the posterior margin of the left ventricle and the reflection of the inferior vena cava especially.

16. Study the dorsal spine.

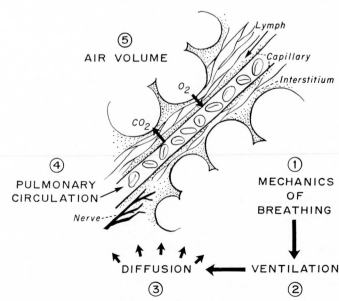

Figure 10–80. Diagrammatic basis for various pulmonary function tests.

Appendix 1

PULMONARY PHYSIOLOGY—ITS PLACE IN PULMONARY ROENTGEN DIAGNOSIS
(Tables 10–1, 10–2)

The morphology of the chest provides:

1. An adequate delivery of oxygen to the alveolus.

2. An adequate permeation of oxygen from the alveolus to a capillary and its red cell content and plasma.

3. A reverse passage of carbon dioxide from the capillary and its contents to the alveolus.

4. An efficient delivery of blood to and from the primary lobule of the lung.

5. Adequate compliance of the chest in overcoming frictional resistance and other forces resistant to exchange of gases and flow of blood (Fig. 10–80).

Thus, in evaluating the chest film we must think of the chest as a model of a gaseous volume and a blood circulatory space. Both of the compartments in this model must be analyzed.

The physiologic tests of pulmonary function indicate how the disease has altered this function. An anatomic, bacteriologic, or pathologic concept such as may be obtained radiographically is usually not rendered.

The radiologist may supplement the tests of pulmonary function that measure pressure, blood flow, vascular resistance, and the distribution of blood in the pulmonary circulation by defining the size of veins and arteries, the presence of venous arterial shunts, the presence or absence of vascular occlusion, pulmonary venous or arterial hypertension, and diminution in pulmonary capillary volume. In some instances it is possible to locate specific areas which may be so involved.

Apart from these considerations, the interstitium of the lung must also occupy the attention of the radiologist. In certain patients, a tentative diagnosis of "alveolar-capillary block" or impairment of diffusion is justified on the basis of the classical clinical picture. Physiologic tests can confirm this diagnosis. Only microscopic examination of the pulmonary tissues can actually establish the exact cause of the alteration. Such may occur in patients with Boeck's sarcoid of the lung, granulomatoses, pulmonary scleroderma, alveolar cell carcinoma, diffuse metastatic lesions in the lungs, and occasional cases of chemical poisonings of the lungs when the diffusion apparatus is disturbed.

With regard to evaluation of pulmonary disability, there may be gross roentgen changes in the lungs of patients with completely normal function, as in some cases of silicosis. Minor anatomic roentgen lesions in the lungs of patients may be associated with severe disturbances of pulmonary function, as in chronic obstructive pulmonary emphysema. In evaluation of pulmonary disability, tests of *function* of the lungs should replace tests that

evaluate only anatomic alterations in the lungs. In general, compensation cases should be settled by such objective tests as airway resistance, pulmonary compliance, arterial blood studies, thoracic mass volume, and diffusing capacity; these do not require the claimant's cooperation. Neither the physician nor the physiologist can ever conclude that the dyspneic patient does not in fact have dyspnea. It is possible that the patient's complaint may be caused by rather elusive factors such as chronic irritation of nerve endings somewhere in the respiratory tract, or the existence of some alveoli with decreased compliance and consequent under-inflation. Every effort should be made to determine (1) the presence or absence of functional impairment; (2) the nature of the impairment; (3) the severity of the disturbance; and (4) whether the degree of abnormality is compatible with the claim of disability.

TABLE 10–1 ROLES OF THE PULMONARY PHYSIOLOGIST AND RADIOLOGIST IN CHEST DISEASE EVALUATION

	Pulmonary Physiologist Evaluates	Radiologist Evaluates
Mechanical factors in ventilation	Yes	To some extent
Lung volume	Yes	To a limited extent
Distribution of air ventilating alveoli	Yes	No
O_2 and CO_2 diffusion	Yes	Qualitatively
Pulmonary capillary blood flow	Yes	To some extent
Lung compliance on resiliency	Yes	To some extent
How disease has altered function	Yes	
Anatomic, bacteriologic, or pathologic diagnosis	No	Yes, well
Differentiation of types of edema or alveolar infiltrate	No	To a considerable extent
Presence of small regional impairments	No	Yes, well
Arterial pressure	Not by usual studies	Yes
Venous pressure	Not by usual studies	Yes
Interstitial pressure	Not by usual studies	Yes
Asymmetry of vascularity	Not by usual studies	Yes

TABLE 10–2 ROLE OF THE RADIOLOGIST IN THE STUDY OF VASCULARIZATION OF THE LUNGS

I. Distribution of vascularization: is it normal?
II. Size of pulmonary arteries and veins.
   A. Rapid tapering of pulmonary arteries, resulting in pulmonary artery hypertension greater than 25 to 35 mm. Hg.
     1. Interstitial edema with loss of compliance.
     2. Intra-alveolar edema.
   B. Pulmonary venous hypertension.
     1. Venous distention.
     2. Upper lobe veins more distended than others.
III. Septal lines of interstitium: capillary pressure 18 mm. or greater and pulmonary artery diastolic pressure of greater than 25 mm. Hg.

REFERENCES

Alavi, S. M., Keats, T. E., and O'Brien, W. M.: The angle of tracheal bifurcation: its normal mensuration. Amer. J. Roentgenol., *108*:546–549, 1970.

Amplatz, K., and Haut, G.: Lateral decubitus bronchography with a single bolus. Radiology, *95*:439–440, 1970.

Anson, B. J. (ed.): Morris' Human Anatomy. 12th edition. New York, McGraw Hill, 1966.

Bean, W. J., Graham, W. L., and Jordon, R. B.: Diagnosis of lung cancer by transbronchial brush biopsy technique. J.A.M.A., *206*:1070–1072, 1968.

Bean, W. J., Jordan, B., Gentry, H., and Nice, C. M.: Fissure lines in the pediatric roentgenogram. Amer. J. Roentgenol., *106*:109–113, 1969.

Bjork, L., and Lodin, H.: Pulmonary changes following bronchography with Dionosil oily (animal experiment). Acta Radiol., *47*:177, 1957.

Burko, H., Carwell, G., and Newman, E.: Size, location and gravitational changes of normal upper lobe pulmonary veins. Amer. J. Roentgenol., *111*:687–689, 1971.

Cauldwell, E. W., Siekert, R. G., Lininger, R. E., and Anson, B. J.: The bronchial arteries; an anatomic study of 150 human cadavers. Surg. Gyn. Obst., *86*:395–412, 1948.

Chang, L. W. M., Lee, F. A., and Gwinn, J. L.: Normal lateral deviation of the trachea in infants and children. Amer. J. Roentgenol., *109*:247–251, 1971.

Cudkowicz, L., and Armstrong, J. B.: Observations on the normal anatomy of the bronchial arteries. Thorax, *6*:342–358, 1951.

Cunningham, D. J.: Manual of Practical Anatomy. 12th edition. London, Oxford University Press, 1958.

Davies, C. N.: Inhaled particles and vapours. A formalized anatomy of the human respiratory tract. Elmsford, New York, Pergamon Press, 1961.

Davies, L. G., Goodwin, J. F., Steiner, R. E., and Van Leuven, B. D.: Clinical and radiological assessment of pulmonary arterial pressure in mitral stenosis. Brit. Heart J., *15*:393–400, 1953.

Doppman, J. L., and Lavender, J. P.: The hilum and the large left ventricle. Radiology, *80*:931–936, 1963.

Eller, J. L., Roberts, J. F., and Ziter, F. M. H., Jr.: Normal nasopharyngeal soft tissue in adults: a statistical study. Amer. J. Roentgenol., *112*:537–541, 1971.

Faber, L. P., Monson, D., Amato, J. J., and Jensik, R. J.: Flexible fiberoptic bronchoscopy (Abstract). Presented at Ninth Annual Meeting of Society of Thoracic Surgeons, Jan. 22–24, 1973.

Felson, B.: Lobes and interlobar pleura. Fundamental roentgen considerations. Amer. J. Med. Sci., *230*:572–584, 1955.

Fennessy, J. J.: Bronchial brushing in the diagnosis of peripheral lung lesions; preliminary report. Amer. J. Roentgenol., *98*:474–481, 1968.

Fennessy, J. J.: Transbronchial biopsy of peripheral lung lesions. Radiology, *88*:878–882, 1967.

Fischer, F. K.: The bronchial tree: technique of bronchography. *In* Schinz, H. C., et al.: Roentgen Diagnostics, Vol. 3. First American edition. London, Heinemann, 1953, p. 2023.

Fischer, H. W., and Balug, S. M.: Aerosol bronchography. Radiology, *92*:150–154, 1969.

Fleischner, F., Hampton, A. O., and Castleman, B.: Linear shadows in lung: interlobar pleuritis, atelectasis and healed infarction. Amer. J. Roentgenol., *46*:610–618, 1941.

Fraser, R. G., and Paré, J. A. P.: Diagnosis of Diseases of the Chest. Philadelphia, W. B. Saunders Company, 1970.

Gabrielsen, T. O., and Ladyman, G. H.: Early closure of sternal sutures. Amer. J. Roentgenol., *89*:975–983, 1963.

Heitzman, E. R., Markarian, B., Berger, I., and Dailey, E.: Secondary pulmonary lobule: A practical concept for interpretation of chest radiographs. Radiology, *93*:507–519, 1969.

Holden, W. S., and Cowdell, R. H.: Late results of bronchography using Dionosil oily. Acta Radiol., *49*:105–112, 1958.

Ikeda, S., Yanai, N., Ishikawa, S.: Flexible bronchofiberscope. Keio J. Med., *17*:1–16, 1968.

Jackson, F. I.: The air gap technique: An improvement by anteroposterior positioning for chest roentgenography. Amer. J. Roentgenol., *92*:688–691, 1964.

Jacobson, G., Schwartz, L. H., and Sussman, M. L.: Radiographic estimation of pulmonary artery pressure in mitral valvular disease. Radiology, *68*:15–24, 1957.

Johannesson, S.: Roentgenologic investigation of nasopharyngeal tonsil in children of different ages. Acta Radiol. (Diag.), *7*:299–304, 1968.

Kahn, B. S.: Bronchofiberoscopy. J. Wadsworth Hospital, Los Angeles, Calif., Aug. 1933.

Lambert, M., and Waugh, W.: Accessory bronchiole-alveolar communications. J. Path. Bact., *70*:311–314, 1955.

Lehmann, Q. H., and Fletcher, G. H.: Contribution of the laryngogram to the management of malignant laryngeal tumors. Radiology, *83*:486–500, 1964.

L'Heureux, P. R., and Baltaxe, H. A.: Emulsified Ethiodol as bronchographic contrast agent. Radiology, *95*:273–275, 1970.

MacLean, K. S.: Bronchial abrasion microbiopsy instrument. J.A.M.A., *166*:2160–2161, 1958a.

McLean, K. H.: Pathogenesis of pulmonary emphysema. Amer. J. Med., 25:62–74, 1958b.

Macklin, C. C.: Alveolar pores and their significance in the human lung. Arch. Path., 21:202–216, 1936.

Milne, E. N.: Physiological interpretation of plain radiographs in mitral stenosis, including review of criteria for radiological estimation of pulmonary arterial and venous pressures. Brit. J. Radiol., 36:902–913, 1963.

Miller, W. S.: The Lung. Second edition. Springfield, Ill., Charles C Thomas, 1950.

Nadel, J. A., Wolfe, W. G., Graf, P. D., Youker, J. E., Samel, H., Austin, J. H., Hinchcliffe, W. A., Greenspan, R. H., and Wright, R. R.: Powdered tantalum. New Eng. J. Med., 283:281–286, 1970.

Newton, T. H., and Preger, L.: Selective bronchial arteriography. Radiology, 84:1043–1051, 1965.

Noetzl, M., and Steinbach, H. L.: Subperiosteal erosion of the ribs in hyperparathyroidism. Amer. J. Roentgenol., 87:1058, 1962.

Owsley, W. C., Jr.: Palate and pharynx. Amer. J. Roentgenol., 87:811–821, 1962.

Pump, K. K.: Morphology of finer branches of bronchial tree of human lung. Disease Chest, 46:370–398, 1963.

Reid, L.: Secondary lobule in adult human lung, with special reference to its appearance in bronchograms. Thorax, 13:110–115, 1958.

Reich, S. B., and Abouav, J.: Interalveolar air drift. Radiology, 85:80–86, 1965.

Reich, S. B.: Production of pulmonary edema by aspiration of water soluble non-absorbable contrast media. Radiology, 92:367–370, 1969.

Reid, L. M.: Selection of tissue for microscopic study from lung injected with radiopaque material. Thorax, 10:197–198, 1955.

Reid, L. M., and Simon, G.: Peripheral pattern in normal bronchogram and its relation to peripheral pulmonary anatomy. Thorax, 13:103–109, 1958.

Rizutti, R. J., and Whalen, J. P.: The nasopharynx: Roentgen anatomy and its alteration in the base view. Radiology, 104:537–540, 1972.

Robbins, L. L., and Hale, C. H.: Roentgen appearance of lobar and segmental collapse of lung: Preliminary report. Radiology, 44:107–114, 1945a.

Robbins, L. L., and Hale, C. H.: Roentgen appearance of lobar and segmental collapse of lung. IV. Collapse of lower lobes. Radiology, 45:120–127, 1945b.

Rouviere, H.: Anatomy of the Human Lymphatic System. Tobias, M. J., Trans. Edwards, Ann Arbor, Michigan, 1938.

Rubin, P., Bunyagidj, S., and Poulter, C.: Internal mammary lymph node metastases in breast cancer: detection and management. Amer. J. Roentgenol., 111:588, 1971.

Sargent, E. N., and Sherwin, R.: Selective wedge bronchography: Pilot studies in animals for development of a proper technique. Amer. J. Roentgenol., 113:660–679, 1971 (29 ref.).

Schoenbaum, S. W., Pinsker, K. L., Rakoff, S. J., Peavey, H. H., and Koerner, S. K.: Fiberoptic bronchoscopy: complete evaluation of the tracheobronchial tree in the radiology department. Radiology, 109:571–575, 1973. (Also several personal communications.)

Shopfner, C. E., Jansen, C., and O'Kell, R. T.: Roentgen significance of the transverse thoracis muscle. Amer. J. Roentgenol., 103:140–148, 1968.

Simon, M.: Pulmonary veins in mitral stenosis. J. Fac. Radiol., 9:25–32, 1958.

Simon, M.: Pulmonary vessels: their hemodynamic evaluation using routine radiographs. Radiol. Clin. N. Amer., 1:363–376, 1963.

Smiddy, J. F., Ruth, W. E., Kerby, G. R., Renz, L. E., and Raucher, C.: Flexible fiberoptic bronchoscope [Letter]. Ann. Intern. Med., 75:971, 1971.

Sovak, M.: Bronchography with a directable double catheter. Radiology, 90:152, 1968.

Steiner, R. E.: Radiology of pulmonary circulation: Chamberlain lecture. Amer. J. Roentgenol., 91:249–264, 1964.

Trapnell, D. H.: Recognition and incidence of intrapulmonary lymph nodes. Thorax, 19:44–50, 1964.

Trapnell, D. H.: The peripheral lymphatics of the lung. Brit. J. Radiol., 36:660–672, 1963.

Trout, E. D., Graves, D. E., and Slauson, D. B.: High kilovoltage radiography. Radiology, 52:669–683, 1949.

Turner, A. F., Law, F. Y. K., and Jacobson, G.: A method for the estimation of pulmonary venous and arterial pressures from the routine chest roentgenogram. Amer. J. Roentgenol., 116:97–106, 1972.

Upham, T., Graham, L. S., and Stecke, R. J.: Determination of in vivo persistence of tantalum dust following bronchography, using reactor activated tantalum and total body counting. Amer. J. Roentgenol., 111:690–694, 1971.

Viamonte, M., Parks, R. E., and Smoak, W. N. III: Guided catheterization of the bronchial arteries. Part I. Technical considerations. Radiology, 85:205–230, 1965.

Von Hayek, H.: The Human Lung. New York, Hafner Publishing Co., Inc., 1970.

Wanner, A., Zighelboim, A., and Sackner, M. A.: Nasopharyngeal airway: a facilitated access to the trachea. For nasotracheal suction bedside bronchofiberoscopy and selective bronchography. Ann. Intern. Med., 75:593–595, 1971.

Watson, W.: Gridless radiography at high voltage with air gap technique. X-ray Focus (Ilford), *2*:12, 1958.

Weibel, E. R.: Morphometry of the Human Lung. New York, Academic Press, 1963.

Werthemann and Vischer, quoted in Holden, W. S., and Cowdell, R. H.: Late results of bronchography using Dionosil oily. Acta Radiol., *49*:105–112, 1958.

White, H.: Respiratory disease in later infancy. Sem. Roentgenol., 7:85–121, 1972.

Whitley, J. E., and Martin, J. F.: The Valsalva maneuver in roentgenologic diagnosis. Amer. J. Roentgenol., *91*:287–306, 1964.

Willson, J. K. V., and Eskridge, M.: Bronchial brush biopsy with a controllable brush. Amer. J. Roentgenol., *109*:471–477, 1971.

Xerox Corporation: Progress report: Xeroradiography. No. 3, September, 1972. Xerox Corp., P.O. Box 5786, Pasadena, California 91107.

Zamel, N., Austin, J. H. M., Graf, P. D., Dedo, H. H., Jones, M. D., and Nadel, J. A.: Powdered tantalum as a medium for human laryngography. Radiology, *94*:547–553, 1970.

11

The Mediastinum, Excluding the Heart

BASIC ANATOMY

Mediastinal Boundaries

The mediastinum is that compartment of the thoracic cage that is bounded laterally by the parietal pleural reflections along the medial aspects of both lungs, superiorly by the thoracic inlet, inferiorly by the diaphragm, anteriorly by the sternum, and posteriorly by the anterior surfaces of the thoracic vertebral bodies.

Arbitrary Compartments of the Mediastinum

For descriptive purposes the mediastinum is divided into four compartments (Fig. 11–1): (1) the *superior mediastinum,* bounded superiorly by the thoracic inlet and inferiorly by a line drawn from the manubriosternal angle to the intervertebral disk between the T4 and T5 vertebrae. Below this imaginary line the *inferior mediastinum* has three compartments or subdivisions; (2) an *anterior mediastinum* bounded anteriorly by the sternum and other tissues beneath the sternum, and posteriorly by the pericardium covering the heart and major vessels anteriorly; (3) a *middle mediastinum,* which contains the heart, the aorta, the origin of the great vessels to the upper extremities and neck, the pulmonary arteries, superior and inferior venae cavae, and the vessels of the root of the lung; and (4) the *posterior mediastinum,* which is bounded anteriorly by the heart and posteriorly by the thoracic spine.

Major Anatomic Structures Contained in the Mediastinum

When the mediastinum is viewed from its *right side* with the mediastinal and costal parts of the pleura removed and the pericardium open (Fig. 11–2 *A*), the major structures visualized are (from top to bottom): esophagus, trachea, right vagus nerve, right phrenic nerve, azygos vein, superior vena cava, right atrium of the heart, inferior vena cava, greater splanchnic nerve, and a number of intercostal veins, arteries, and nerves. In cross section the superior and middle right pulmonary arteries, the superior and inferior pulmonary veins, and the right bronchus may be visualized.

Similarly, when the *left side* of the mediastinal septum is viewed (Fig. 11–2 *B*) with the mediastinal and costal parts of the pleura removed, the pericardium opened, and the structures exposed and partly dissected, the following structures can be seen (from top to bottom): esophagus, major vessels arising from the

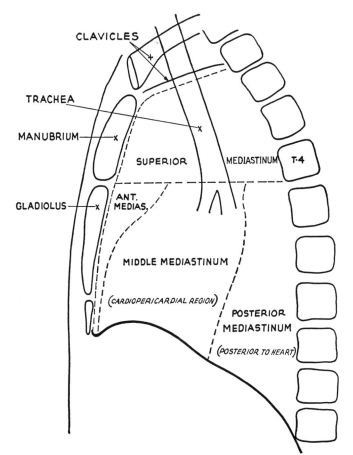

Figure 11–1. Compartments of the mediastinum.

659

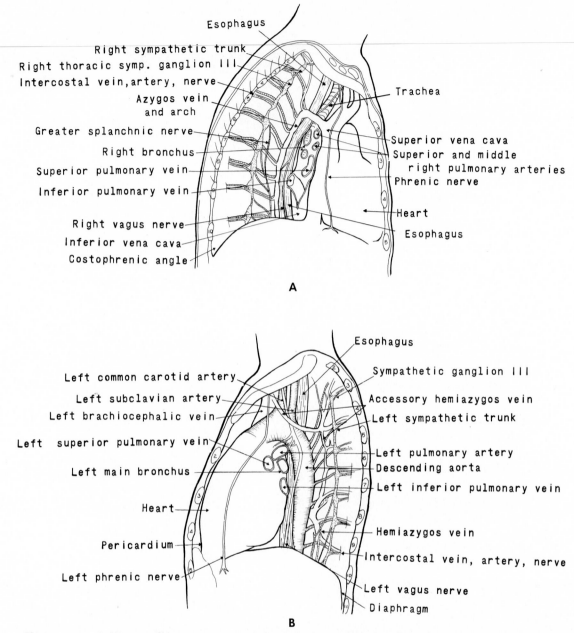

Esophagus
Right sympathetic trunk
Right thoracic symp. ganglion III
Intercostal vein, artery, nerve
Azygos vein and arch
Greater splanchnic nerve
Right bronchus
Superior pulmonary vein
Inferior pulmonary vein
Right vagus nerve
Inferior vena cava
Costophrenic angle

Trachea
Superior vena cava
Superior and middle right pulmonary arteries
Phrenic nerve
Heart
Esophagus

A

Esophagus
Left common carotid artery
Left subclavian artery
Left brachiocephalic vein
Left superior pulmonary vein
Left main bronchus
Heart
Pericardium
Left phrenic nerve

Sympathetic ganglion III
Accessory hemiazygos vein
Left sympathetic trunk
Left pulmonary artery
Descending aorta
Left inferior pulmonary vein
Hemiazygos vein
Intercostal vein, artery, nerve
Left vagus nerve
Diaphragm

B

Figure 11–2. *A.* Diagram illustrating a view of the mediastinum from its right aspect (left lung removed). *B.* Diagram illustrating a view of the mediastinum from its left aspect (right lung removed). (After Pernkopf, E.: Atlas of Topographical and Applied Human Anatomy, Vol. 2. Philadelphia, W. B. Saunders Co., 1964.)

arch of the aorta (including the left common carotid artery and the left subclavian artery), left brachiocephalic vein, the entire arch and descending aorta, hemiazygos vein, left vagus nerve, left phrenic nerve, left ventricle of the heart, and, in cross section, the left pulmonary artery, left inferior pulmonary vein, left superior pulmonary vein, and left main bronchus. There are, in addition,

the segmental intercostal veins, arteries, and nerves, as well as the left sympathetic trunk, and some of the sympathetic ganglia.

In *sagittal section,* along the line of the superior and inferior venae cavae, passing through the right aspect of the cavity of the left atrium, one may visualize: the right innominate vein and the opening of the left innominate vein, a small portion of the ascending aorta, the auricle of the right atrium, the right ventricle, left atrium, superior vena cava, right pulmonary artery in cross section, and the right bronchus with the azygos vein above it (Fig. 11–3).

Figure 11–3 is also useful as a supplement to cross-sectional diagrams of the chest, which help greatly in further understanding the structures of the mediastinum.

In *frontal perspective,* a diagram of a radiograph is very helpful in revealing the structures of the mediastinum (Fig. 11–4). Thus, the following structures can be identified: the trachea with its left and right main bronchi, the pulmonary arteries and veins, the azygos knob adjoining the inferior margin of the superior vena cava and producing an ovoid shadow in the right tracheobronchial angle, the arch of the aorta and descending thoracic aorta, the thoracic spine with its paraspinal lines, and the pleural contours of the mediastinum medially. These will be identified more clearly as the radiographs of the mediastinum are shown in greater detail.

A line drawing showing the *boundaries of the anterior and posterior mediastinal pleura* as they adjoin the mediastinum is shown in Figure 11–5. Anteriorly, the lower left mediastinal pleura diverges from the midline to accommodate the heart and pericardium. Beneath the sternum, the soft tissue space is identifiable where the costal and mediastinal pleurae meet. The pleura at the level of the manubrium passes backward over the superior mediastinum from the sternum to the vertebral column and is reflected over the apex of lung; it protrudes slightly above the first rib laterally but no higher than the first rib posteriorly. The anterior margins of the two pleurae converge behind the sternoclavicular joints and come into apposition with each other at the lower border of the manubrium, remaining in apposition to approximately the fourth costal cartilage. The left pleura at this level turns away from the median plane as much as 2 to 3 cm. and finally reconverges with the right pleura at the level of the xiphoid process.

The fat and remains of the *thymus* (in the adult) lie beneath the manubrium and anterior to the innominate veins. Somewhat laterally, beneath the costal cartilages, the internal mammary vessels descend deeply to the pectoralis muscles. The thymus in the adult cannot be identified unless it is enlarged or unless it is the site of tumor formation.

A study of the *caudal cross section* of the superior medias-

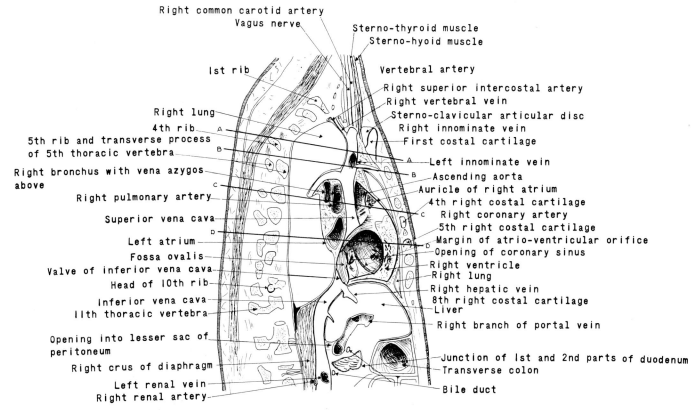

Figure 11–3. Line drawing illustrating the sagittal anatomy of the chest along the line of the superior and inferior venae cavae. (After Cunningham's Textbook of Anatomy, 6th ed. London, Oxford University Press, 1931.)

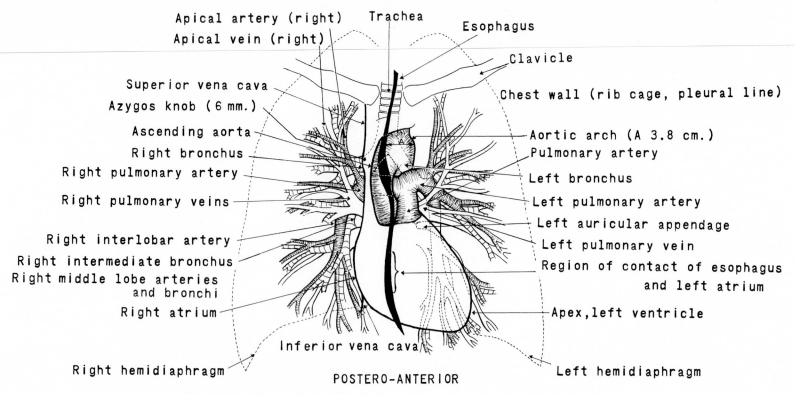

Apical artery (right)   Trachea   Esophagus
Apical vein (right)

Superior vena cava
Azygos knob (6 mm.)
Ascending aorta
Right bronchus
Right pulmonary artery
Right pulmonary veins

Right interlobar artery
Right intermediate bronchus
Right middle lobe arteries and bronchi
Right atrium

Clavicle
Chest wall (rib cage, pleural line)
Aortic arch (A 3.8 cm.)
Pulmonary artery
Left bronchus
Left pulmonary artery
Left auricular appendage
Left pulmonary vein
Region of contact of esophagus and left atrium
Apex, left ventricle

Inferior vena cava

Right hemidiaphragm

POSTERO-ANTERIOR

Left hemidiaphragm

Figure 11–4.   Diagram of chest film showing arteries, veins, and relationships to bronchi.

tinum (Fig. 11–6) reveals the structures that descend from the neck into the inferior mediastinum. Thus, anteriorly the fat and remains of the thymus can be identified, as well as the left and right innominate veins, the trachea, esophagus, left subclavian

and left common carotid arteries and innominate artery, and nerves such as the right and left phrenic, right and left vagus, and laryngeal (cross section at the level of the third thoracic vertebra).

The *innominate veins and innominate artery* lie anterior to the trachea. At the level of the trachea the left common carotid artery can be identified. The left subclavian artery and the esophagus lie posterior to the level of the trachea. The trachea lies just to the right of the midline, while the esophagus, more posteriorly, lies in the midline closely applied to the thoracic vertebrae.

Descending into the *inferior mediastinum,* the cross-sectional diagrams allow us to detect more accurately the contents of the anterior, middle, and posterior compartments. At the inferior margin of the superior mediastinum, fourth thoracic level, the pericardium comes into intimate contact with the substernal connective tissue and fat, separating the right and left pleural sacs (Fig. 11–7). The internal mammary vessels lie immediately anterior to the pericardium at this level, just anterior to the pleural margins. These are important anatomic landmarks, since enlargement of the internal mammary vessels (as in coarctation of the aorta), or enlargement of the lymph nodes and lymphatics that course along the internal mammary vessels, or infiltration

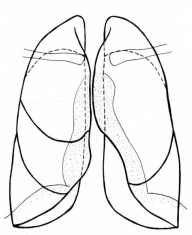

Figure 11–5.   Line diagram showing the boundaries of the anterior and posterior mediastinal pleura.

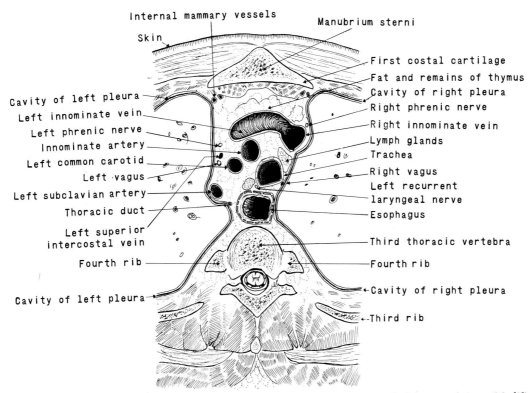

Figure 11–6.   Line drawing of the cross-sectional anatomy of the chest at the level of the manubrium. (Modified from Cunningham's Textbook of Anatomy, 6th ed. London, Oxford University Press, 1931.)

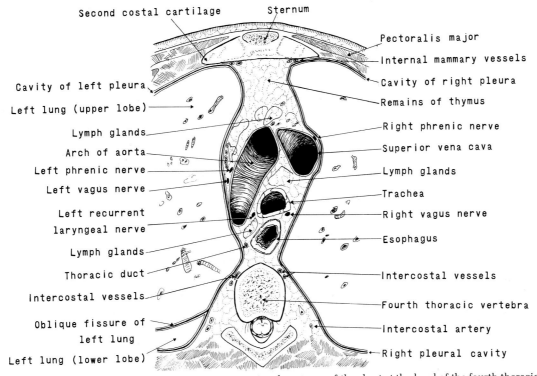

Figure 11–7.   Line drawing illustrating the cross-sectional anatomy of the chest at the level of the fourth thoracic vertebra. (Modified from Cunningham's Textbook of Anatomy, 6th ed. London, Oxford University Press, 1931.)

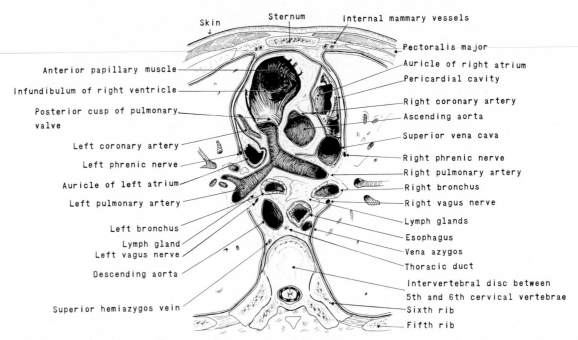

Figure 11–8. Line drawing illustrating the cross-sectional anatomy of the chest at T5 level, just below the inferior boundary of the superior mediastinum. (Modified from Cunningham's Textbook of Anatomy, 6th ed. London, Oxford University Press, 1931.)

by any neoplasia or fluid, may be recognized beneath the sternum in a lateral view of the chest at this level.

The remains of the thymus, fat, and areolar tissue, as well as lymph nodes, compose the rest of the anterior mediastinum at this level. In the midmediastinum, the major vessels such as the arch of the aorta, the superior vena cava, and adjoining lymph nodes come into view. The phrenic nerves, vagus nerves, and trachea with the left recurrent laryngeal nerve adjoining may be identified here as well. In the posterior mediastinum, the main structures are the esophagus, thoracic duct, and lymph nodes. The thoracic duct is situated to the left of the esophagus. Occasionally the esophagus can be seen on radiographs when it contains air in sufficient quantities, but otherwise it requires barium esophagrams for delineation.

In infancy and early childhood, the thymus gland extends into the anterior mediastinum, producing a distinct shadow in lateral and frontal projections. Farther down in the mediastinum the following structures can be seen (Figs. 11–8, 11–9). *At the level of the intervertebral disk between the fifth and sixth thoracic vertebrae*, the heart and pericardium are in contact with the internal aspect of the covering structures of the sternum. At this level the infundibulum of the right ventricle is shown anteriorly, and the pulmonary arteries are shown posteriorly in the cardiac cross section. The left and right bronchi are also shown in cross section,

the left being closer to the midline. In the posterior compartment, the esophagus and the azygos vein are shown to the right of the midline and the descending aorta to the left. The azygos vein lies slightly posterior and lateral to the esophagus, and very close to it. All of these structures are in close proximity with the soft tissues covering the spine. The superior hemiazygos vein and the thoracic duct also lie in this posterior compartment, with the thoracic duct lying between the descending thoracic aorta and esophagus, and the superior hemiazygos vein lying posterior to the descending thoracic aorta.

Descending the mediastinum farther still (Fig. 11–9) to the interspace between the seventh and eighth thoracic vertebrae, the heart can be seen occupying most of the mediastinum at this level. The left atrium and pulmonary veins are seen in the posterior aspect of the cardiac silhouette. The esophagus and descending thoracic aorta are closely applied against the left atrium, which explains why a slight enlargement of this cardiac chamber causes a significant displacement of the esophagus. The descending thoracic aorta lies just to the left of and almost in the same sheath as the esophagus. It can be readily understood why the esophageal displacement is a "tug of war" between the left atrium on the one hand and the descending thoracic aorta on the other. This is an important concept in understanding the radiographic pathology of this region. The azygos vein and superior hemia-

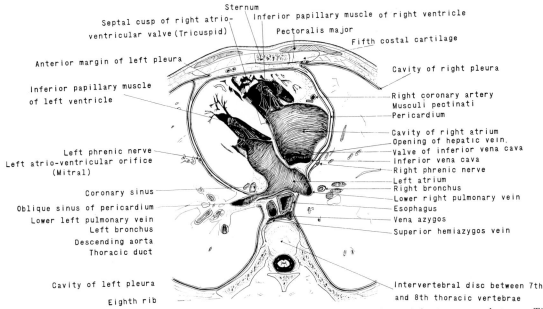

Figure 11–9. Line drawing illustrating the cross-sectional anatomy of the chest at the interspace between T7 and T8 levels. (Modified from Cunningham's Textbook of Anatomy, 6th ed. London, Oxford University Press, 1931.)

zygos vein lie to the right of the esophagus, posteriorly on the one hand (azygos vein), and directly posterior to the descending thoracic aorta (superior hemiazygos vein), on the other.

Thoracic Gutters. The posterior mediastinum is a very narrow structure at this level, narrower than the width of the spine. Note also how far the lung extends posterior to the posterior mediastinum in Figures 11–8 and 11–9. These concavities compose the so-called *thoracic gutters.* The space between the right and left pleurae is approximately 2 cm. or less in the posterior mediastinum at this level, just enough to allow easy visibility for the paraspinous ligamentous silhouette (Fig. 11–10). The vagus nerves are closely applied to the esophagus on each side. There are also numerous paravertebral lymph nodes in this region that can be particularly important when enlarged and detectable.

In a line diagram of the *left lateral roentgenogram* of the chest with barium in the esophagus, the following important indentations in the esophagus can be seen (Fig. 11–11): (1) indentation to the left and slightly posteriorly at the level of the aortic arch, (2) slight indentation anteriorly by the left main bronchus close to the bifurcation of the trachea, and (3) a minimal impression at the level of the left atrium, unless the left atrium is significantly enlarged.

The trachea, on the other hand, is slightly indented on its left side by the arch of the aorta.

In the *lateral view,* the relationship of the sternum to the thoracic vertebral column varies somewhat, depending on body build, the presence of kyphosis, the shape of the sternum, and the presence or absence of air-trapping in the anterior lung fields. In

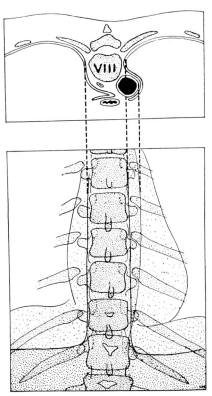

Figure 11–10. *Upper,* cross section through the posterior mediastinum at the level of the eighth thoracic vertebra. *Lower,* diagram taken from a roentgenogram depicting the posterior portions of the visceral or parietal pleura as lines along the vertebral column. Dotted lines indicate anatomic substrates of pleural lines and aortic lines in cross section. (From Lachman, E.: Anat. Rec., 83:521, 1942.)

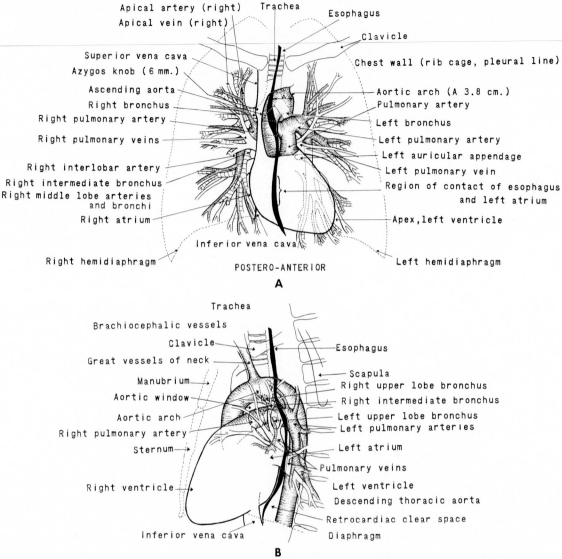

Figure 11–11. *A.* Line diagram of chest showing a frontal view of the mediastinum. *B.* Line diagram of chest showing a left lateral view.

general, however, in a young man of average build the following relationships are demonstrated:

Upper border of manubrium	Opposite interspace between T2 and T3
Sternal angle (junction of manubrium and sternum)	Lower border of T4
Xiphisternal joint	T9

Azygos and Hemiazygos Veins.   Line drawings illustrating the anatomy of the azygos and hemiazygos veins and their tributaries are shown in Figure 11–12 *A* and *B*. The azygos and as-

cending lumbar veins constitute a continuous channel for venous drainage of the posterior body wall. In the abdomen the ascending lumbar veins receive the intercostal lumbar veins; in the thorax the azygos veins receive the thoracic posterior intercostal veins. In the thorax also the azygos ultimately terminates in the superior vena cava, forming a small knob at this point which can be identified on most roentgenograms of the chest (posteroanterior view) and measured. The size of the azygos knob becomes significant when interpreting distention of the azygos system such as occurs in certain decompensated states. Together with the lumbar veins, the azygos system constitutes a bypass between the superior and inferior venae cavae.

Azygos Venous System.   The azygos venous system of the

thorax is composed of three primary channels: (1) the azygos vein and right superior intercostal vein on the right, (2) the hemiazygos, and (3) the accessory hemiazygos veins forming a continuous channel on the left. Other thoracic channels drain into the azygos system, including the left intercostal, esophageal, bronchial, pericardiac, mediastinal, and phrenic veins.

Thus, the azygos vein has its origin in the thorax at the level of the twelfth thoracic vertebra. It first lies ventral to the fifth to

the twelfth right intercostal arteries and to the right of the thoracic duct and thoracic aorta. Near the sternal angle it bends forward, arching cranially over the root of the right lung, and then empties into the superior vena cava just before the latter pierces the pericardium.

On its left margin the azygos receives the hemiazygos vein as a single or double communication at the eighth or ninth vertebral level. A little higher, at the sixth or seventh thoracic level, it re-

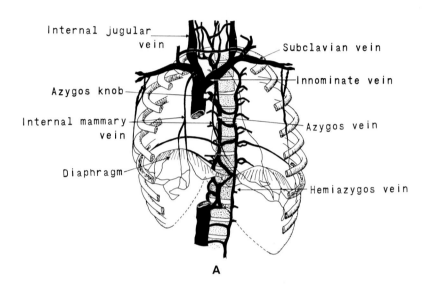

A

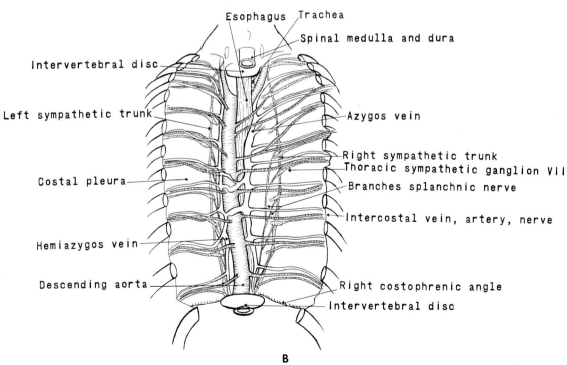

B

Figure 11–12. Line drawings illustrating the anatomy of azygos and hemiazygos venous systems.

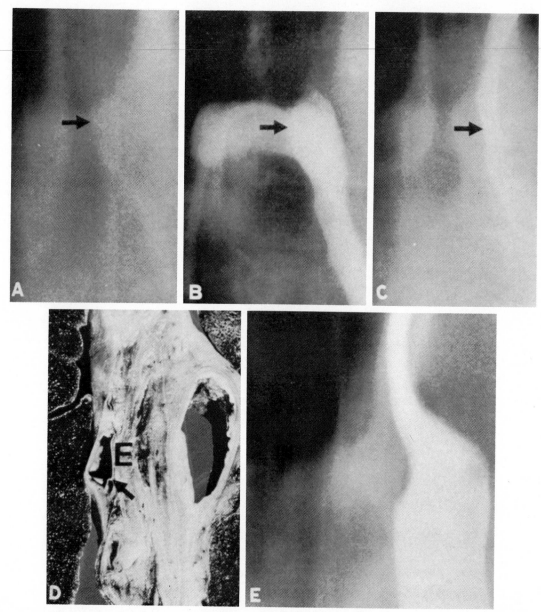

Figure 11–13. *A.* An anteroposterior laminagram shows an elliptical shadow outlined by lung on its right side at the level of T5 (arrow). *B.* An anteroposterior azygogram (same patient) shows this shadow to represent the posterior portion of the azygos arch, the "azygos knob" (arrow). *C.* An anteroposterior laminagram with barium in the esophagus demonstrates the imprint of the posterior azygos arch on the esophagus (arrow). *D.* A coronal section of the thorax through the level of the posterior azygos arch shows the intimate relationship of this structure (arrow) to the esophagus (*E*). *E.* Left posterior oblique esophagram shows the azygos "imprint" on the esophagus. (From Heitzman, E. R., Scrivani, J. V., Martino, J., and Moro, J.: Radiology, *101*:249–258, 1971.)

ceives the accessory azygos vein. In about 15 per cent of individuals the intercostal veins of the left side of the thorax drain directly into the azygos vein and the hemiazygos and accessory hemiazygos veins are incompletely formed.

The *hemiazygos vein*, formed from a number of venous roots, perforates the diaphragm just lateral to the left crus and courses along the left margin of the thoracic vertebral bodies, receiving intercostal veins along its left side. It lies just dorsal to the esophagus and to the left of the aorta. Throughout its entire course it lies in contact with the left mediastinal pleura. At the level of the ninth vertebra the hemiazygos vein turns to the right, passes behind the aorta and joins the azygos vein. In about 40 per cent of people, the hemiazygos vein is continuous above with the accessory hemiazygos vein (Anson).

The *accessory hemiazygos vein* is a longitudinal vein lying on the left margin of the fifth through the seventh thoracic vertebral bodies, and receiving posterior intercostal veins. It empties into the azygos veins through a trunk that crosses to the right behind the aorta, usually at the level of the seventh thoracic vertebra. There are usually valves in this venous system at the junctions of the azygos and intercostal veins, the hemiazygos and accessory hemiazygos veins with the azygos trunk, and, especially, the azygos and the superior vena cava.

The Azygos Knob. The azygos "knob" is that portion of the azygos vein that turns at a sharp angle from a prespinal location to join the superior vena cava. The knob is very close to the esophagus, which lies to the left and slightly anterior to it.

Knowledge of the normal dimension of the azygos knob has proved to be useful in the differentiation of a number of chest conditions, particularly inflammatory and neoplastic pulmonary infiltration from acute congestive pulmonary interstitial edema. In congestive pulmonary interstitial edema, the azygos knob measurement is increased, whereas in inflammatory or neoplastic pulmonary infiltrative diseases (which may resemble interstitial edema), the azygos knob is normal in size (Keats et al.). However, once the acute phase of interstitial pulmonary edema gives way to actual pleural effusion, the azygos arch dilatation may disappear. The azygos knob is also slightly dilated in pregnancy. In contrast with the normal measurement in women (3 to 7 mm.), in pregnant women the azygos knob ranges from 3 to 15 mm., with an average of 7.14 mm. Azygos measurement may be erroneous in the presence of lymph node enlargement in the area of the azygos arch. Differentiation, however, is possible, since the azygos arch enlarges in the supine position while an azygos lymph node in this immediate location will not.

The method of measurement of the azygos knob proposed by Keats et al. is shown in Figure 11–14. This measurement is obtained on *erect* teleroentgenograms of the chest, and is possible in 56 per cent of the normal patients surveyed.

Others have indicated other maximum dimensions: Felson, 10 mm.; Fleischner and Udis, 6 mm. Doyle et al. and Wishart used tomography to obtain comparable measurements. In the *supine* position on tomography, Doyle's maximum was 14.2 ± 2.6 mm. Felson's technique was apparently comparable to that of Keats et al. (Table 11–1).

The normal vein width in children was studied by Wishart in 762 chest radiographs of patients from birth to 14 years of age with the results shown in Table 11–1. The azygos vein does not increase uniformly in size with age. Respiratory activity, posture,

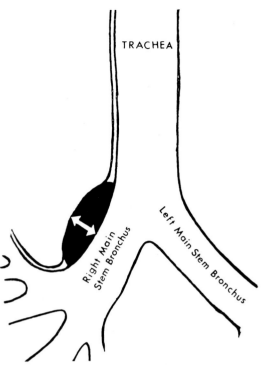

Figure 11–14. Method of measurement of azygos "knob" proposed by Keats et al. (From Keats, T. E., Lipscomb, G. E., and Betts, C. S., III: Radiology, 90:990–994, 1968.)

and anatomic arrangement may cause changes in its width from subject to subject and from time to time in the same subject, making clinico-radiologic correlation somewhat uncertain. It was pointed out by Preger et al. that when the width of an azygos vein

TABLE 11–1 AVERAGE VALUES FOR AZYGOS VEIN SHADOW WIDTH*

Investigator	Conditions of Measurement	Normal Range
Fleischner and Udis, 1952	Upright posteroanterior teleroentgenogram	Up to 6 mm.
Doyle et al., 1961	Supine anteroposterior tomograms	14.2 ± 2.6 mm.
Felson, 1967	Upright anteroposterior teleroentgenograms	Up to 10 mm.
Keats et al., 1968	Erect teleroentgenogram	3–7 mm.
	Age	Mean ± 1 Standard Deviation
Wishart, 1972	Birth to 6 months	3.5 ± 1.3 mm.
	6 to 24 months	4.1 ± 1.0 mm.
	2 to 7 years	4.8 ± 1.2 mm.
	8 to 14 years	5.1 ± 1.6 mm.

*Modified from: Wishart, D. L.: Normal azygos vein width in children. Radiology, *104*:115–118, 1972.

is greater than 15 mm. as measured on a *supine* adult chest roentgenogram, it is associated with a raised central venous pressure above 10 cm. of water. The formula proposed as the result of this study was: the central venous pressure in centimeters of water equals the azygos vein width in millimeters × 1.4 minus 3, but the 95 per cent confidence limits for central venous pressure were ± 7 cm. from this predicted value. The tabular relationship of the width of the azygos vein in millimeters to the predicted central venous pressure is shown in Table 11–2.

An excellent drawing showing in cross section the arch of the azygos vein as it joins the superior vena cava forming the visualized knob is shown in Figure 11–15 (Tori and Garusi).

Failure of the superior part of the inferior vena cava to develop normally, with consequent continuation of the inferior vena cava as the azygos vein, is a diagnosis that can be rendered accurately with present methods of cardiac catheterization and angiocardiography. Its importance lies in the fact that half of the cases of azygos-cava anomaly also have an abnormality of abdominal situs that includes foregut, midgut, and colon malrotation. There is also a high order of association of this azygos-cava anomaly with asplenism-cyanotic and lethal heart disease, symmetry of organs, and other anomalies such as bilateral superior vena cava (Pacofsky and Wolfel).

Changes in Size and Configuration of the Mediastinum Normally. Ordinarily, the mediastinum is quite mobile, changing inspiration and expiration (Fig. 11–16). The mediastinum varies in the thoracic cage. Also, the mediastinum changes its shape in inspiration and expiration (Fig. 11–16). The mediastinum varies in size and configuration with body build, being long and thin in the asthenic individual, and short and stocky in the sthenic per-

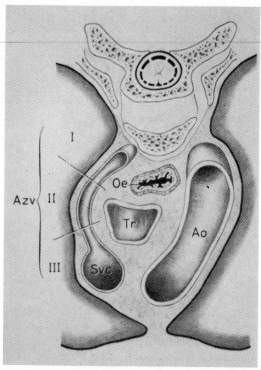

Figure 11–15. Drawing (modified from Andreassi) of a transverse section of thorax at the level of the fourth dorsal vertebra illustrates how the arch describes a medially concave curve, first passing laterally from the point of origin (I, posterior segment), then in a forward direction (II, intermediate segment), and, finally, turning inward and downward (III, terminal segment). (Ao, aorta; Azv, azygos vein; Oe, oesophagus; Svc, superior vena cava; Tr, trachea.) (From Tori, G., and Garusi, G. F.: Amer. J. Roentgenol., 87:238, 1962.)

TABLE 11–2   PREDICTED CENTRAL VENOUS PRESSURE*

Width of Azygos Vein (mm.)	Estimated Central Venous Pressure (to nearest cm.)	95 Per Cent Confidence Limits (to nearest cm.)
4	3	0–10
6	5	0–12
8	8	1–15
10	11	4–18
12	14	7–21
14	17	10–24
16	19	12–26
18	22	15–29
20	25	18–32
22	28	21–35
24	31	24–38
26	33	26–40
28	36	29–43

*From Preger, L., Hooper, T. I., Steinbach, H. L., and Hoffman, J. I. E.: Width of azygos vein related to central venous pressure. Radiology, *93*:521–523, 1969.

son. The mediastinum also changes as the individual grows, as is illustrated in Figure 11–16.

Paramediastinal Recesses. There are several so-called weak spots of the mediastinum, where protrusion may more readily occur from one side of the chest to the other. There is one situated anteriorly in the region of the shrunken thymus gland. Another weak spot exists where the esophagus and aorta are slightly separated in the lower posterior mediastinum; herniation of lung almost invariably occurs from right to left in this situation. The third is situated in the upper posterior mediastinum where the two pleural surfaces are in almost complete contact (between T3 and T5 and the esophagus in this area).

A detailed knowledge of the pleural reflections, especially around the azygos vein, is useful in the evaluation of many abnormalities of the cardiovascular system and also the right side of the mediastinum posterior to the hilus (Heitzman et al.) (Fig. 11–13). A deep inspiratory effort or a Valsalva maneuver will force lung into the mediastinal recesses and against pathologic pro-

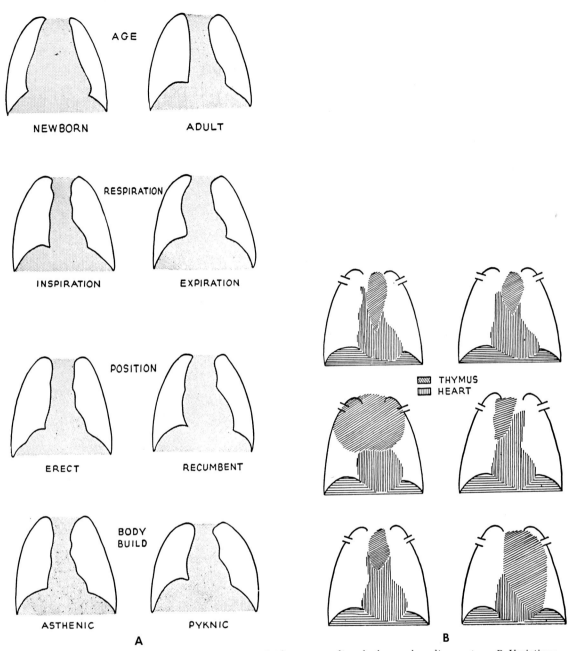

Figure 11-16. A. Normal factors causing variation in the supracardiac shadow and cardiac contour. B. Variations in size and position of supracardiac thymic shadow in the infant.

cesses that may distort these recesses. If the mediastinum is mobile, which it usually is normally, these recesses can be accentuated by placing the patient on his side, or minimized by placing the patient supine. Thus, evaluation of enlarged mediastinal lymph nodes, left atrial enlargement, posterior mediastinal masses, herniation of lung, or massive right pleural effusions may be significantly aided with this knowledge.

Thoracic Duct. The relationships of the thoracic duct are illustrated in Figure 11-17. It arises in the abdomen from the cisterna chyli on the first and second lumbar vertebrae, enters the

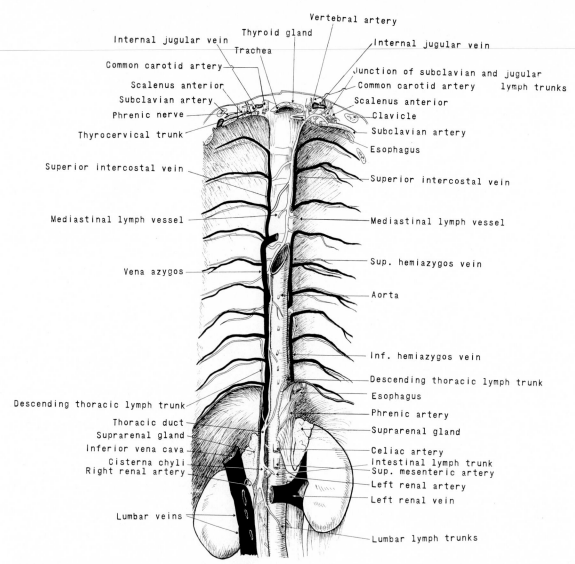

Figure 11–17.   Line drawing illustrating the anatomic relationships of the thoracic duct. (Modified from Cunningham's Textbook of Anatomy, 6th ed. London, Oxford University Press, 1931.)

posterior mediastinum along with the aorta on its right, and continues upward in the posterior mediastinum between the descending aorta and azygos vein, posterior to the esophagus. At T5 level, it crosses to the left of the median plane and extends through the superior mediastinum, along the left border of the esophagus. In the root of the neck it arches behind the left carotid sheath, travels downward and in front of the subclavian artery, and terminates in the upper end of the left innominate vein. It has numerous valves and many tributaries, and varies considerably in course and termination. The thoracic duct can be visualized radiographically.

Mediastinal Lymph Nodes. The numerous mediastinal lymph nodes are liberally distributed along the internal mammary vessels, in juxtavertebral loci, and in foci adjoining the diaphragm anteriorly and lateral to the pericardial sac (Fig. 11–18). As shown in Chapter 10, they are nestled among the large vessels, both arteries and veins, and are found adjacent to the lower esophagus and descending aorta, and at bifurcations of the trachea and bronchi in both hili and lungs. Although normally not visible, they have great significance in inflammatory and neoplastic disease.

The right paratracheal lymph node chain represents a prin-

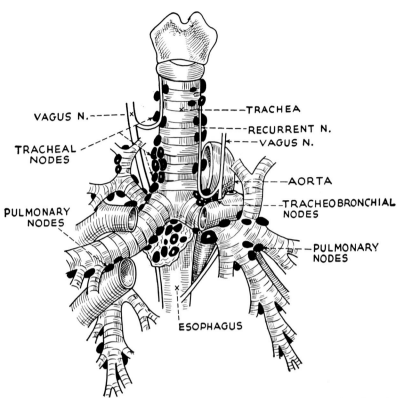

VAGUS N.

TRACHEA

RECURRENT N.

VAGUS N.

TRACHEAL NODES

AORTA

TRACHEOBRONCHIAL NODES

PULMONARY NODES

PULMONARY NODES

ESOPHAGUS

Figure 11–18.   Lymph nodes of the tracheobronchial tree. (After Sukienikow.)

cipal drainage area for the entire right lung and a major portion of the left (Rouviere and Valette; McCort and Robbins). Thus, the careful analysis and identification of each shadow of this region on the chest radiograph is imperative.

The *lymphatic drainage of the esophagus* also has great significance, since usually it occurs in longitudinal pathways in submucous and muscular lymphatic networks, extending from the internal jugular chain through the paratracheal nodal group and the posterior mediastinal nodes into the nodes of the cardia and lesser curvatures of the stomach. Careful observation of metastases from neoplasms of the esophagus corroborates the early spread of these lesions to subdiaphragmatic sites.

The Thymus

Basic Anatomy.   The thymus is a bilobed structure, largest in the child and regressing after puberty so that in the aged adult it becomes so intermingled with adjoining mediastinal parenchyma that it is difficult to ascertain its true shape or boundary. Its largest absolute size occurs during adolescence (Anson).

In the newborn it ranges in size from 4 to 6 cm. in length, 1.2 to 4.0 cm. in thickness. The gland lies mainly between the two anterior mediastinal pleural margins, but may extend superiorly into the neck as far as the lower pole of the thyroid gland. It is situated beneath the manubrium and upper part of the body of the sternum and their adjoining costal cartilages, approximately to the level of the fourth cartilage.

In the infant it is found in the superior and anterior mediastinum, and although it is largest in young adolescents, being almost three times its birth weight at that time, it is not as apparent on roentgenograms of the chest as it is in the infant, in view of the relative size and position of adjoining structures.

Thymic Patterns in the Newborn (Tausend and Stern).   The pattern of the thymus in the newborn is extremely variable. In a study involving some 1020 frontal chest roentgenograms obtained from infants born consecutively, no prominence was found on either side in 517, or approximately 50 per cent. In 276, the prominence was on the right side, and in 75 it occurred on the left side.

The frequently described "sail sign," a triangular prominence of the superior mediastinal image (Fig. 11–19 *a* and *d*), was encountered in less than 5 per cent of the thymic prominences.

An undulating contour of the lateral margin of the thymus, presumably caused by indentations by the anterior rib segments, was found rather frequently (Fig. 11–19 *d, e,* and *f*). Figure 11–19 *d* shows the scalloped margin as well as the sail sign. Even a cervical thymus gland may be encountered on occasion (Moseley and Som). Apparently the lumen of the trachea is seldom if ever compressed or displaced by a prominent thymus, regardless of its size or situation. On rare occasions there are radiolucent areas within the prominent thymus, suggesting the presence of fatty tissue (Fig. 11–19 *g*). The thymus gland decreases in size under stress and with the administration of steroid hormones (Tausend and Stern).

Thymic Angiography.   The arteries supplying the thymus are derived from the internal mammary and from the superior and inferior thyroid arteries. Technically, selective internal mammary arteriography is involved, and this requires bilateral selective catheterization.

On the other hand, normal thymic venography is apparently more feasible; two of the normal thymic venous patterns are illustrated in Figure 11–20. As shown in these diagrams, drainage occurs from the thymic region into the superior vena cava and the left innominate vein, and indirect drainage of the inferior thyroidal vein flows into the thymus and thereafter into thymic venous tributaries. The main thymic vein, the vein of Keynes, drains into the left innominate vein, 1 to 2 cm. from its junction with the superior vena cava (Yune and Klatte). Arteriography of the thymus gland has been accomplished by both selective subclavian and internal mammary angiography (Boijsen and Reuther).

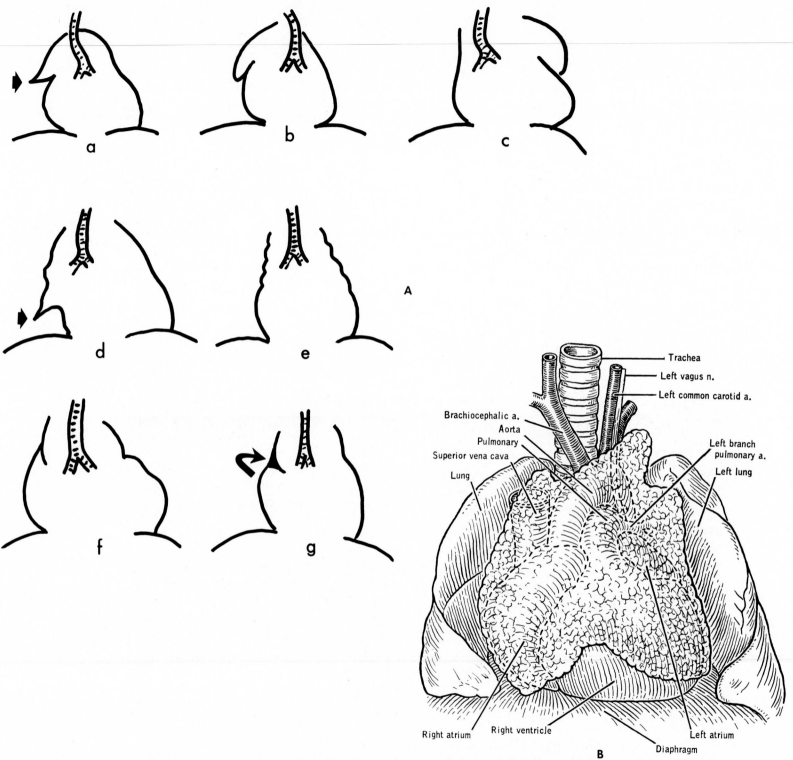

Figure 11–19. *A.* Variations in shape of the thymus gland in the newborn infant. (Modified from Tausend, M. E., and Stern, W. Z.: Amer. J. Roentgenol., 95:125–130, 1965.) *B.* Thymus of a full-term stillborn infant to show its relation to subjacent structures in the superior and anterior mediastinum prior to inflation of the lungs. Right and left lungs have been retracted laterally. (From Anson, B. J. (ed.): Morris' Human Anatomy, 12th ed. Copyright © 1966 by McGraw-Hill, Inc. Used by permission of McGraw-Hill Book Company.)

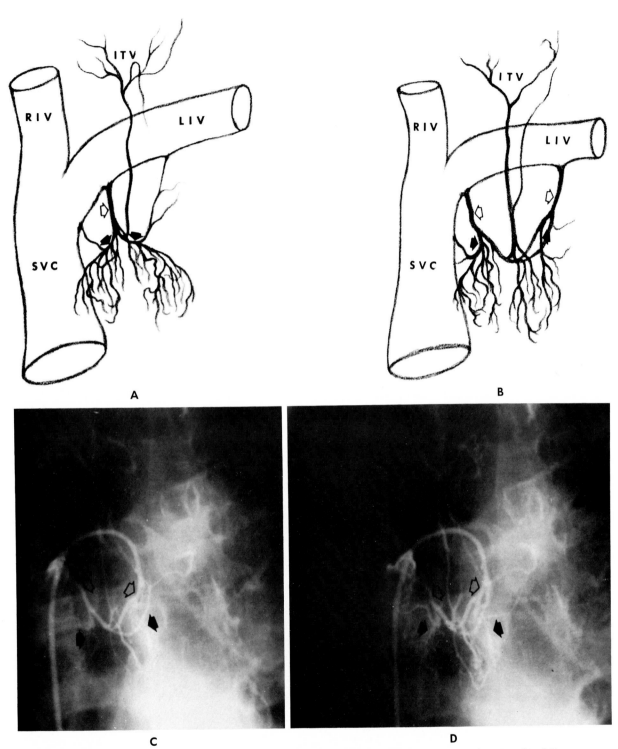

Figure 11–20. *A.* Normal thymic venous pattern as described by Kreel, showing main thymic vein of Keynes (open arrow) and lateral thymic veins (solid arrows). (LIV) left innominate vein; (ITV) inferior thyroidal vein; (RIV) right innominate vein; (SVC) superior vena cava. *B.* Variations of the normal thymic venous pattern. Diagram shows right and left limbs of the main thymic vein arcade (open arrows) and lateral thymic veins (solid arrows). (LIV) left innominate vein; (ITV) inferior thyroidal vein; (RIV) right innominate vein; (SVC) superior vena cava. *C.* Normal thymic venogram (early phase). *D.* Normal thymic venogram (late phase). The catheter tip is in the left side limb of the arcade. (From Yune, H. Y., and Klatte, E. C.: *Radiology, 96:*521–526, 1970.)

Mediastinal "Stripes": The Pulmonary Ligament

Inferior Pulmonary Ligament.   The inferior pulmonary ligament (Fig. 11–21) is a fibrous sheath connecting the visceral pleura on the medial surface of the lower lobe of each lung to the parietal pleura covering the mediastinum. It is actually composed of a double layer of pleura extending in a sheetlike manner from the inferior margin of the pulmonary hilus to the diaphragm, and loosely attaching the medial surface of the lung to the mediastinum. It tends to divide the anterior and posterior parts of the mediastinum below the root of the lung into compartments (Rabinowitz and Wolf). It assumes a triangular shape when the lung is displaced away from the mediastinum from any cause, and hence, has been referred to as the "triangular ligament." The apex of this triangle is situated inferior to the root of the lung, below the inferior pulmonary veins, and extends to the diaphragm with a bare area on the diaphragm between the two leaves of the ligament. Occasionally, the ligament does not reach the diaphragm and terminates in a free falciform border (Rabinowitz and Wolf) (Fig. 11–21 B). In normal subjects it is not visualized roentgenographically, but it does influence the radio-logic appearance of a number of pathologic entities such as pneumothorax, mediastinal pleural effusions, and pulmonary atelectasis. It also must be considered in surgery of this portion of the chest.

Patterns of Pleural Reflections of the Left Superior Mediastinum (Blank and Castellino).   A chain of anterior mediastinal lymph nodes lies along the distribution of the phrenic and vagus nerves called the "left prevascular nodes" (Fig. 11–22 A). These nodes lie along the anterior and superior convexities of the aortic arch and continue anterior to the left carotid artery. They are somewhat lateral to the left paratracheal lymph nodes, and hence are important from the standpoint of potential distortion of the mediastinal silhouette when they become enlarged. The five basic contours for the pleural reflection of the left superior mediastinum in this location are shown in Figure 11–22 B (from Blank and Castellino). Two reflections of the pleura are identifiable: reflection A is apparently due to the pleural reflection "over the undivided portion of the pulmonary artery and is separated from this vessel by connective tissue." The relationships of the main pulmonary artery to the left cardiac margin are basic to the appearance of reflection A, although this reflection also covers fat and lymph nodes in the mediastinum.

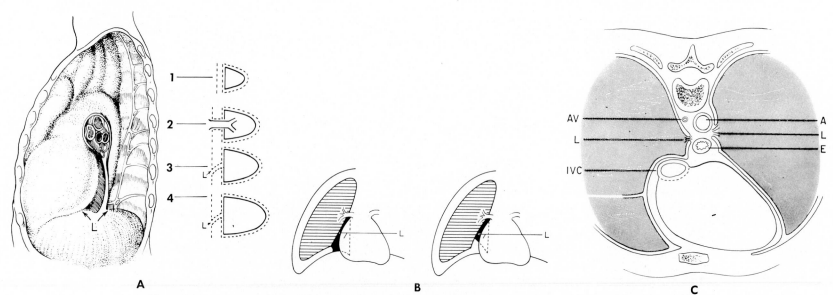

A   B   C

Figure 11–21.   *A.* Diagrammatic view of the left side of the mediastinum. The pulmonary ligament (*L*) extends downward and backward from the hilus to the dome of the diaphragm. It has been cut along its attachment to the lung.

The side drawings are cross sections through various levels of the hemithorax to demonstrate the relationship of the visceral and mediastinal pleurae (dotted lines) to the lung and the pulmonary ligament at several levels. Above the hilus (1), the visceral and mediastinal pleurae are completely separated and the lung lies free within the thorax. The pleura that surrounds the hilus (2) is connected to both the visceral and mediastinal portions. The pulmonary ligament (3, 4) is composed of a double layer of pleura that bridges the visceral and mediastinal pleurae and attaches the lung to the mediastinum.

B. Schematic drawings to demonstrate the triangular configuration of the pulmonary ligament (*L*). The lung is shown retracted away from the mediastinum so that the ligament is stretched out as a sheet. The dotted lines represent the retrocardiac extension of the ligament. In the first drawing, the ligament is fully developed and its inferior margin is attached to the diaphragm. In the second drawing, the ligament fails to reach the diaphragm and ends inferiorly in a free falciform border.

C. Schematic cross section of the chest shows the relationship of the pulmonary ligaments to the mediastinal structures. Pulmonary ligament (*L*); aorta (*A*); esophagus (*E*); inferior vena cava (*IVC*); azygos vein (*AV*). (From Rabinowitz, J. G., and Wolf, B. S.: Radiology, 87:1013–1020, 1966.)

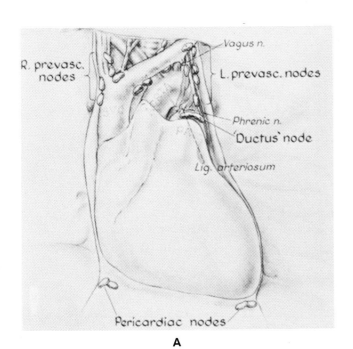

A

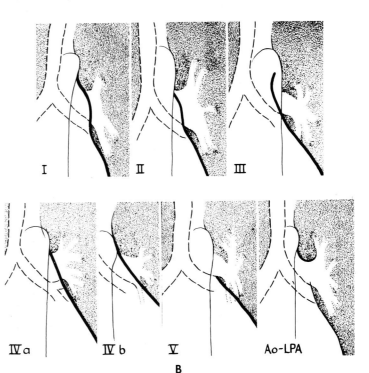

B

Figure 11–22. *A.* Diagrammatic representation of left and right prevascular chains of the anterior mediastinal lymph nodes. *B.* Diagrammatic representation of "reflections A and B." The heavy line in panels I–IVb represents the appearance of the pleural reflections between the aortic arch and "left heart border." "Reflection A" represents that portion extending from the aortic arch to the level of the left main bronchus. Five variations are shown.

Type I. A double curve with the lower portion convex, and the cephalad portion concave to the left (23%).

Type II. A single curve convex to the left (8%).

Type III. A line with the lower portion straight and the cephalad portion concave to the left (5%).

Type IV. A straight or slightly concave line which either intersects with (IVa — 14%) or forms a tangent passing slightly lateral to (IVb — 2%) the aortic arch.

Type V. No continuous border seen (48%).

Panel labeled Ao-LPA represents the appearance of "reflection B," indicated by heavy line extending from aortic arch and merging with the upper border of the left pulmonary artery. This reflection is present in only 38% of cases. When present, it may coexist with "reflection A" (36%) or be seen alone (64%).

In older persons the uncoiled descending thoracic aorta projects lateral to the mediastinal pleural reflections and must not be mistaken for them. Portions of transverse processes or posterior rib ends should not be confused with these reflections. Other abnormalities such as congenital cardiovascular anomalies, abnormal accumulations of fat, and primary mediastinal tumors will also produce changes in the mediastinal pleural reflections and must be considered in formulating a differential diagnosis. Finally, it must be emphasized that only the predominant recurring patterns have been presented here. (From Blank, N., and Castellino, R. A.: Radiology, *102*:585–589, 1972.)

Reflection B is "probably due to projection of a segment of mediastinal pleura where it is not inseparably applied to the adventitia of the aorta and left pulmonary artery." It is usually concave to the left but may be straight in whole or in part. At times it is obscured by overlying ribs and transverse processes.

Posterior Mediastinal Line. The posterior mediastinal line between the right and left lungs probably has various component parts: (1) the esophageal-pleural stripe, which represents the pleural contact with the esophagus, and (2) the approximation of the right and left lung posterior to the collapsed esophagus between the esophagus and the spine.

At times the anterior mediastinal line, which represents the interface between the right and left lungs anterior to the heart and great vessels, is also superimposed on a teleroentgenogram. These lines may be identified, particularly in the high kilovoltage chest roentgenogram, and may be deflected in the event of a shift of lung from one side to the other (Fig. 11–23) (Cimmino and Snead).

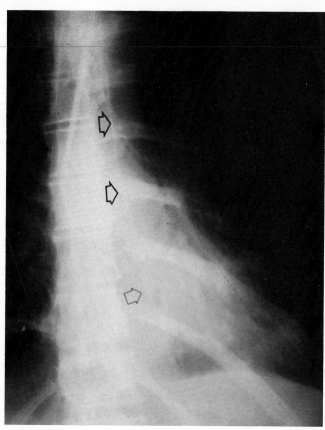

Figure 11–23. Arrows point to "posterior mediastinal stripe" shifted to left with atelectasis of left lower lobe.

RADIOLOGIC EXAMINATION OF THE MEDIASTINUM

The radiologic techniques of examination of the mediastinum include the following:

1. Posteroanterior and lateral chest roentgenograms may be made with maximal inspiration, moderate overpenetration, and barium in the esophagus (using high kilovoltage, short exposure time, and a Bucky grid).
2. Fluoroscopic examination may be used to evaluate the following parameters, especially:
   a. Pulsation—intrinsic or by impact.
   b. Abnormal response to positive intrathoracic pressure.
   c. Relationship of the movement of the mass lesion to structures within the chest: diaphragm, tracheobronchial tree, esophagus, heart, and major vessels.
   d. The relationship of the cardio-pericardial shadow to the epicardial fat (especially to exclude pericardial effusions).

3. Body section radiography. This is especially useful in:
   a. Determining the relationship of the abnormality to a specific anatomic structure.
   b. Studying the relationship of the abnormality to the vascular structures of the mediastinum.
   c. Studying the nature of calcification in the lesion, if it is present.
   d. Studying the nature of fat within the lesion, if it is present.
4. Angiography. This is especially useful in:
   a. Determining the relationship of the abnormality to opacified vascular structures such as the heart, aorta, major vessels arising from the aorta including the internal mammary (Boijsen and Reuter), and pulmonary arteries and veins.
   b. Studying the great veins leading into the heart (venacavography).
   c. Studying the azygos venous system (azygography). This may be done by intraosseous injection of the contrast agent or by selective catheterization.
5. Bronchography may indicate widening, narrowness, or filling defects in the air passages.
6. Myelograms may demonstrate the status of the subarachnoid space and indicate whether the mediastinal lesion is related to the spine or spinal cord.
7. Pneumomediastinography (Sumerling and Irvine). In this technique, the gas is introduced into the fascial planes of the mediastinum by a number of different routes. Tomography coupled with this technique is especially helpful in certain cases. This method is useful for:
   a. Ascertaining the exact relationship of a lesion to the adjoining structures.
   b. Helping to determine resectability of a lesion in the mediastinum, or of bronchogenic carcinoma.
8. Diagnostic pneumothorax and pneumoperitoneum may be used to localize the suspected lesion in relation to these potential spaces; they are especially helpful in studying herniation from the abdomen into the thoracic cage. These procedures must be performed with great care, in order to avoid a tension pneumothorax and its deleterious symptoms.
9. Radioisotopic techniques:
   a. Blood pool scans.
   b. Radioisotopic angiograms.
   c. Study of pericardial effusions.
   d. Localization of some tumors: thymoma, thyroid, and occasionally, lymph node enlargements.

Fluoroscopy and Routine Film Studies of the Chest. These have already been considered in Chapter 10. It should be emphasized that the examination of the mediastinum requires good delineation of the esophagus with barium contrast, which may be accomplished with either thick or thin barium. Air contrast has at times been used for a similar purpose. Because the mediastinum includes the esophagus, heart, and major blood vessels, it is difficult to separate the anatomic investigation of the mediastinum from these other entities. This is arbitrarily being done here for ease of description. The anatomy of the esophagus proper will be described with the anatomy of the alimentary tract (Chapter 13), and anatomy of the heart will be described in Chapter 12 in conjunction with the cardiovascular system. Other modes of investigation are distributed as follows: *angiography,* see Chapter 12; *bronchography,* see Chapter 10; *myelography,* see Chapter 9.

Pneumomediastinography. Pneumomediastinography has been utilized as a diagnostic tool since 1936 (Condorelli). Various methods for inducing pneumomediastinum have been described: (1) the retro- or transsternal method (Condorelli); (2) the suprasternal notch method (Hare and Mackay); and (3) the presacral technique utilized for retroperitoneal air insufflation (Palubinskas and Hodson).

For a more complete bibliography and details regarding pneumomediastinography the student is referred to Oliva's review of this subject. A large number of approaches have been suggested but in actual practice only five are frequently employed:

1. *Retrosternal access* (Fig. 11–24 *A*) was originally suggested by Condorelli in 1934. In this procedure a needle is advanced through the suprasternal notch and then along the posterior wall of the sternum for a distance of 4 centimeters, making certain continuously that the needle is not situated in a vessel. During the continued insufflation, the pressure varies between minus 5 and plus 5 cc. of water. Ordinarily one utilizes 300 to 400 milliliters of gas.

2. *Transtracheal access* (Fig. 11–24 *B*) was also suggested by Condorelli et al. in 1949. This approach allows better visualization of the posterior mediastinum; the anterior mediastinum is seen only after a large amount of gas has been utilized.

3. *Retroperitoneal access* was first suggested by Ruiz-Rivas in 1950. It is accomplished by a simultaneous injection into both the anterior and posterior mediastina, using the technique of pneumoretroperitoneography by the precoccygeal route into the retroperitoneal spaces and from there into the mediastina.

4. Other *direct pathways* are employed, either through the sternum, next to the sternum, or beneath the xiphoid. A pretracheal pathway may also be used.

5. *Indirect approaches* through the back have also been utilized. These have the advantages of more constant visualization of both the anterior and posterior mediastina.

Tomography is essential to success. Tomograms which have been supplied to us by Sumerling are reproduced with the further advantage of Logetronic printing. It is readily apparent that large anatomic structures may be seen, including the thoracic aorta, trachea, superior vena cava, thymus, pulmonary artery, chambers of the heart such as the right ventricle and left

atrium in margin, azygos vein, left innominate vein, right innominate vein, left carotid artery, left subclavian artery, thyroid (particularly when enlarged), right and left bronchi, pulmonary vein, and paramediastinal pleura. The gas apparently surrounds the organs, which are otherwise without contrast of their own, rendering them visible through the delineation of their margins. Unfortunately, superimposition of shadows makes the tomographic technique essential in both frontal and lateral views as shown.

With special equipment, axiotransverse tomography may also be employed, but relatively little experience with this technique has been reported (Oliva).

The procedure is generally well tolerated by the patient, although too large amounts of gas can induce a feeling of retrosternal pressure and produce pain similar to angina, but this disappears in a very short time. The appearance of subcutaneous emphysema in the supraclavicular and neck area and even dysphagia is not of significant concern. In the presence of cardiac failure, the retrosternal approach can lead to the perforation of an enlarged blood vessel, but this can be detected by good technique. The transtracheal approach can lead to the perforation of the esophagus, but ordinarily this is not followed by any serious sequelae. The precoccygeal approach is practically without danger, although significant subcutaneous emphysema, scrotal emphysema, and even perforation of the rectum may occur. It is probable that pneumomediastinography is closely akin to surgical mediastinoscopy and is an alternative method for the observation and demonstration of vessels, bronchi, lymph nodes, and tumors of the mediastinum (Fig. 11–24).

It must be emphasized further, however, that with a completely obstructed mediastinum the capacity of this area of the anatomy is virtually zero and hence, the technique can be used to distinguish a benign noninfiltrating tumor from a severely infiltrating one. Needless to say also, the transtracheal technique is contraindicated in the presence of an acute infectious process of the respiratory organs.

The transsternal technique has been utilized either directly through the bone or through the manubriosternal junction. The procedure is best done under fluoroscopic control; carbon dioxide, air, or nitrous oxide is usually employed. Because nitrous oxide and carbon dioxide are absorbed very rapidly, the first injection may be made with these gases to determine whether or not the injection is proceeding well, and thereafter air may be utilized. Image amplifier fluoroscopic control is extremely helpful.

If dissection of the gas into the mediastinum proceeds normally, 300 to 500 cc. of the gas may be employed.

Stringent precautions must be taken against the possibility of gas embolism. The examination is contraindicated in patients with a bleeding diathesis.

In the *anteroposterior view* the gas outlines the following anatomic structures in different tomographic levels: the left innominate vein, superior vena cava, azygos vein in the right tracheobronchial angle, aorta, innominate artery, left carotid artery, and left subclavian artery. Ordinarily, dissection of the gas occurs around the main pulmonary artery and aortic arch, outlining the aortic window. The outer walls of the trachea and bronchi are often outlined as far as the primary divisions. In some cases, the ligamentum arteriosum can be identified. With appropriate tomography the thymus in the adult may also be seen in the anteroposterior projection as two thin shadows on either side of the midline. The right lobe of the thymus is closely related to the superior vena cava (Fig. 11–24).

Lateral tomograms are particularly useful for outlining the thymus. The external surface of the heart and the esophagus may also be demonstrated. In the adult, the gas diffuses into the neck, and anteroposterior tomograms will clearly delineate the lobes of the thyroid gland (Fig. 11–24).

The *potential spaces of the mediastinum in the newborn* are indicated in Figure 11–25 *A* and *B*. The anterior mediastinum extends to the left of the midline adjacent to the anterior chest wall, and separation of the anterior mediastinum from the middle mediastinum occurs at its posterolateral borders by the apposition of pericardium to mediastinal pleura. Air in the anterior mediastinum is limited superiorly by the superior sternopericardial ligament. This forms the superior attachment of pericardium to the upper sternum, and the thymus is said to lie above this ligament. If the air does not rise above this ligament the typical sail sign on the chest roentgenogram with pneumomediastinum is not obtained in the newborn (Franken). A pneumomediastinum may dissect along the fibrous layer of prevertebral fascia, perivisceral fascia, esophageal fascia, and even parietal and visceral pericardial fascia, as shown in Figure 11–26 *A* and *B*. Under these cir-

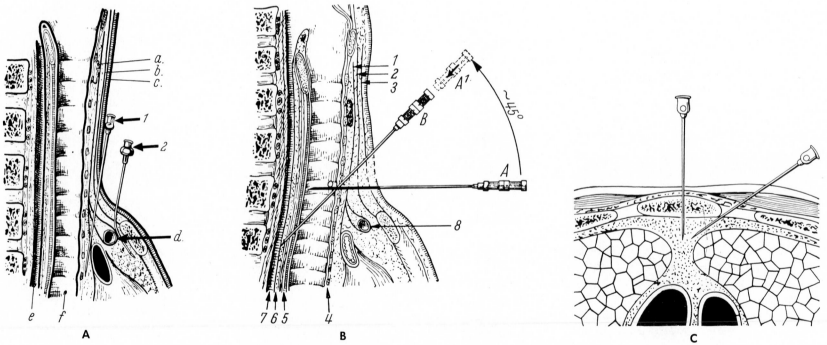

Figure 11–24. *A.* Direct approach for the introduction of the gas according to Condorelli: (1) Pretracheal access (posterior mediastinum); (2) Retrosternal access (anterior mediastinum): *a.* deep part of the middle cervical fascia, *b.* superficial part of the middle cervical fascia, *c.* superficial cervical fascia, *d.* left brachiocervical venous trunk, *e.* esophagus, *f.* trachea. (From Condorelli, L., Truchetti, A., and Pidone, G.: Ann. Radiol. Diag., 23:33, 1951.) *B.* Transtracheal approach for the introduction of air into the posterior mediastinum according to Condorelli: (A) Position of the needle for the perforation of the skin and the anterior tracheal wall. (B) Position of the needle for the perforation of the posterior tracheal wall. (1) Deep part of the middle cervical fascia; (2) superficial part of the middle cervical fascia; (3) superficial cervical fascia; (4) anterior wall of the trachea; (5) posterior wall of the trachea; (6) areolar, loose connective tissue between trachea and esophagus; (7) esophagus; (8) left brachiocervical venous trunk. (From Cocchi, U.: Pneumoretroperitoneum and Pneumomediastinum. Georg Thieme Verlag, Stuttgart, 1957.) *C.* Schematic drawing of the transsternal and parasternal approaches according to Sansone (anterior pneumomediastinum). (From Sansone, G.: Minerva Pediat., 3:293, 1951.)

Figure 11–24 continued on the opposite page.

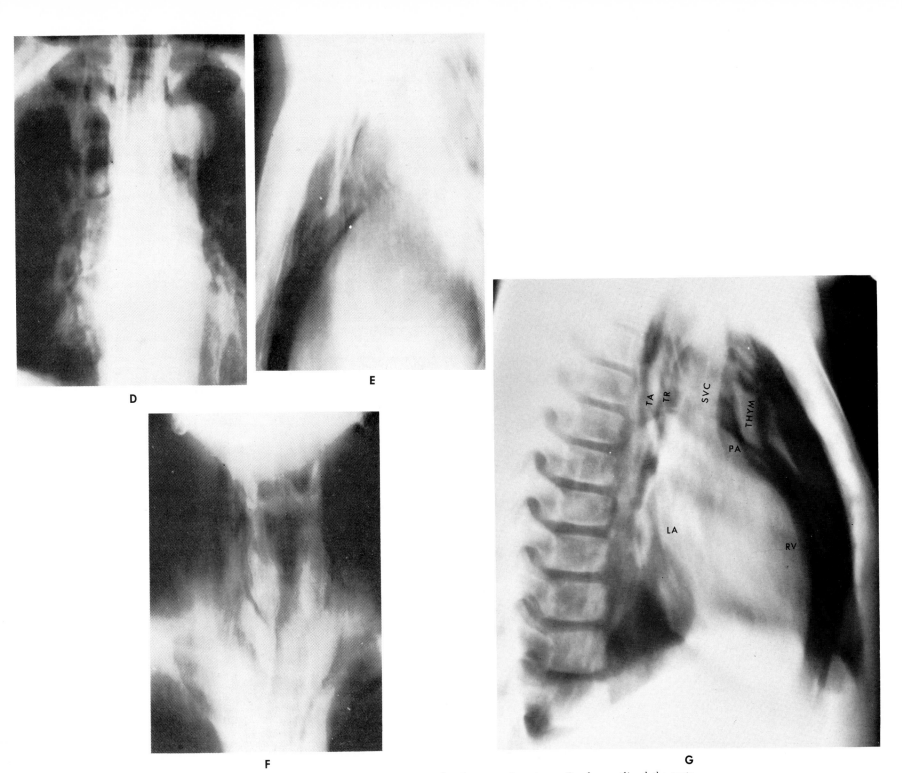

Figure 11–24 *Continued.* D. Anteroposterior tomogram showing normal anatomy. Gas has outlined the aorta, main pulmonary artery, ligamentum arteriosum, azygos vein, left subclavian artery and superior vena cava. Gas also diffused around the trachea and main bronchi, outlining their walls. E. Lateral tomogram showing the two lobes of the thymus outlined by gas in the anterior mediastinum. The trachea, esophagus, left innominate vein, and superior vena cava are also seen. Gas has diffused between the right ventricular outflow tract and the aorta. F. Anteroposterior tomogram of the cervical region shows the two lobes of the thyroid gland outlined by gas immediately below the larynx. (From Sumerling, M. D., and Irvine, W. J.: Amer. J. Roentgenol., 98:451–460, 1966.) G. Lateral view of pneumomediastinum in a child, demonstrating the thymus (THYM); superior vena cava (SVC); trachea (TR); thoracic aorta (TA); left atrium (LA); right ventricle (RV); and pulmonary artery (PA). (Courtesy of Dr. M. D. Sumerling.)

Figure 11–24 continued on the following page.

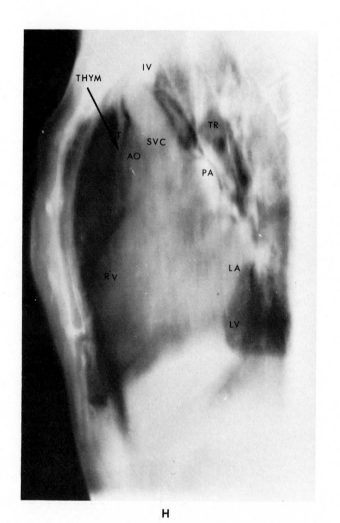

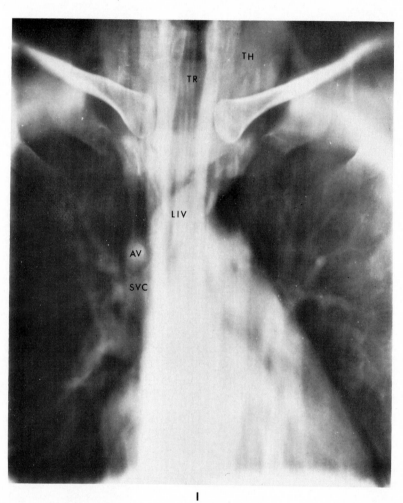

H

I

Figure 11–24 *Continued.   H.* Lateral view of pneumomediastinum in an adult, showing the thymus (THYM) to be much smaller and the anterior mediastinal clear space much more noticeable than it is in a child. Other structures visualized in this study are the aorta (AO); superior vena cava (SVC); innominate vein (IV); pulmonary artery (PA); and, as previously, the trachea, left atrium, left ventricle, and right ventricle. *I.* Representative frontal view which shows the thyroid (TH); trachea (TR); left innominate vein (LIV); azygos vein or knob (AV); and superior vena cava (SVC). (Courtesy of Dr. M. D. Sumerling.)

Figure 11–24 continued on the opposite page.

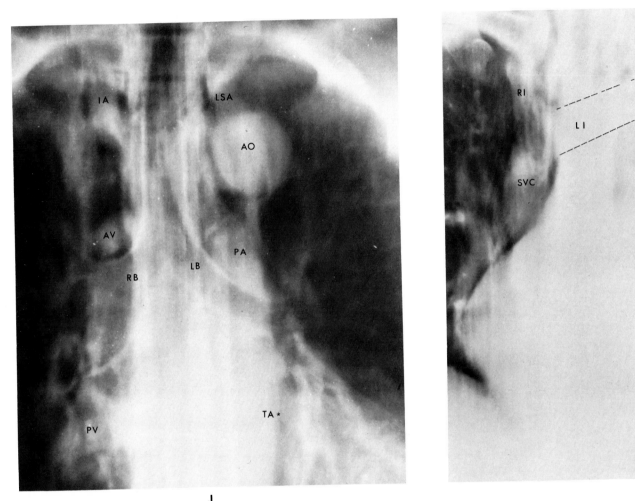

Figure 11-24 *Continued.* *J.* Frontal view of an older individual showing a much more prominent aorta (AO); left subclavian artery (LSA); thoracic aorta (TA); pulmonary vein (PV); right and left bronchi (RB and LB); and right innominate artery (IA). *K.* A left innominate vein (LI) draining into the superior vena cava (SVC). A right innominate vein (RI) is also present. The paramediastinal pleura (PP) is also shown quite clearly, particularly along the left cardiac margin. (Courtesy of Dr. M. D. Sumerling.)

Figure 11-24 continued on the *following page.*

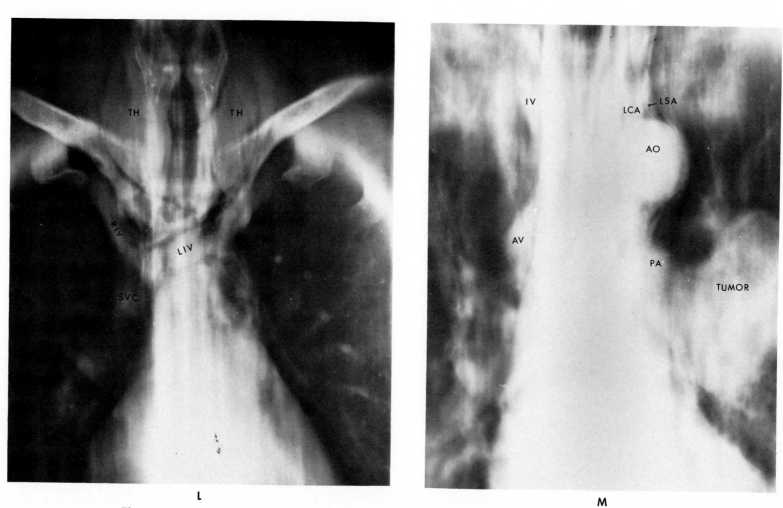

Figure 11-24 *Continued.* *L.* Somewhat similar structures are shown but the thyroid (TH) is shown to be significantly enlarged. *M.* A tumor is noted in the left lung, but additionally one can see a separation between the left subclavian artery (LSA) and the left common carotid artery (LCA). Other structures are much the same as those previously shown. (Courtesy of Dr. M. D. Sumerling.)

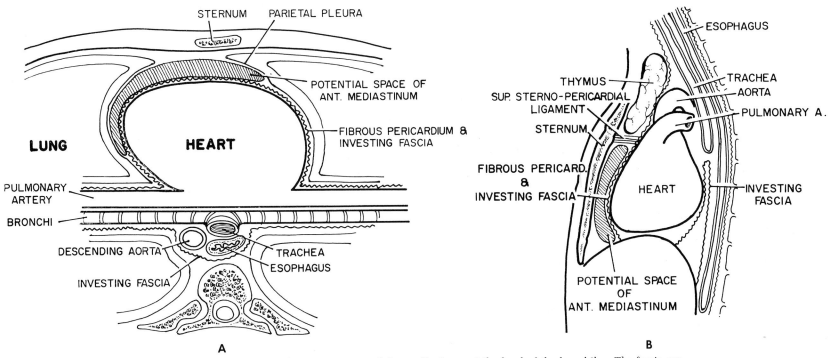

Figure 11-25. *A.* Diagrammatic cross section of the mediastinum at the level of the lung hilus. The fascia surrounding the pulmonary vessels is continuous with the fibrous pericardium and the investing fascia of the trachea and great vessels. The anterior mediastinum is anterior to this fascia. Because of the levoposition of the heart, more potential space is available to the left of midline. Air collecting in this region could therefore displace the heart posteriorly and to the right. *B.* Diagrammatic sagittal section of the mediastinum in the midline. The superior sterno-pericardial ligament limits the superior extent of the anterior mediastinum, and the thymus lies above this ligament. (From Franken, E. A., Jr.: Amer. J. Roentgenol., *109*:252–260, 1970.)

cumstances, air may be shown to dissect into peribronchial tissues from the hilar region. These mediastinal fascial planes constitute a "highway connecting the lung to the mediastinum" (Marchand).

Venography of the Azygos and Vertebral Veins. Opacification of the vertebral and azygos veins has been accomplished by femoral vein injection with simultaneous inferior caval compression (Anderson). Thirty to 35 cubic centimeters of a suitable contrast agent such as Hypaque or Renografin are injected simultaneously into both femoral veins after pressure has been applied tightly against the patient's abdomen with a plastic plate and a "football air bladder."

The vertebral veins and azygos system may also be demonstrated by intraosseous venography (Fischgold et al.). This is accomplished by injecting the contrast agent directly into a spinous process of the thoracic vertebrae or the posterior segment of the last rib. Three to four films are obtained during and after the injection. It is also possible to opacify the azygos system by retrograde injection through a catheter inserted through the superior vena cava (Ranniger; Stauffer et al.).

Abrams has studied the lumbar and azygos system by ciné

techniques. In this instance a catheter is passed from the femoral vein into the inferior vena cava and then into a third, fourth, or fifth lumbar vein. Thirty cc. of 76 per cent Renografin are then injected in 5 seconds if both this vein and an ascending lumbar vein reached from a left common iliac vein are injected. A diagrammatic representation of the azygos venous system so visualized and examples of its appearance at the upper thoracic level and via osseous vertebral venography are shown in Figure 11-27. Numerous variations, implications, and applications may be shown, and the reader is referred to Abrams and a comprehensive reference for this purpose.

Investigation of the Thoracic Duct (Rosenberger and Abrams). Various techniques have been devised for study of the thoracic duct in the living. Retrograde injection of contrast agent has been used in patients with advanced neoplastic disease (Bierman et al.; Brzek et al.). Operative injection of the thoracic duct at the time of surgery has also been tried. Lymphangiography affords an excellent opportunity for study of the thoracic duct. The technique for this procedure has already been described in relation to the lymphatics of the lower extremity, and it will be referred to again in the study of the lymphatics and lymph nodes

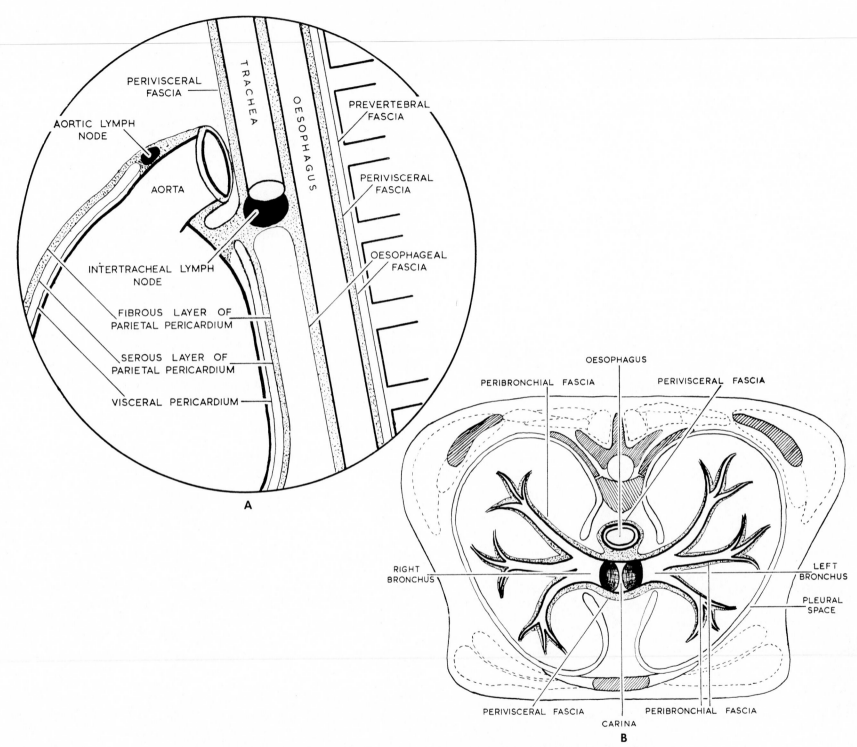

Figure 11–26. *A.* Diagram showing the distribution of the perivisceral fascia at the bifurcation of the trachea and the relation of the intertracheal and aortic glands to the serous layers of the pericardium. The stippled area represents the subfascial connective tissue plane. *B.* Transverse section through the thorax. Diagram showing the manner in which the perivisceral fascia is prolonged around the right and left bronchi into the lung substance to form the peribronchial fascia. The stippled area represents the subfascial plane, occupied by connective tissue and in which lie the bronchial vessels and the pulmonary lymphatics. (From Marchand, P.: Thorax, 6:359–368, 1951.)

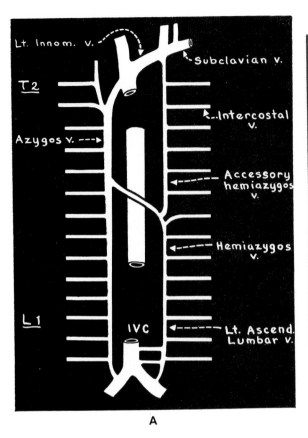

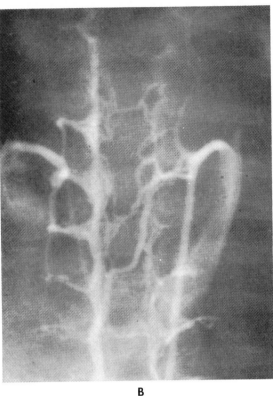

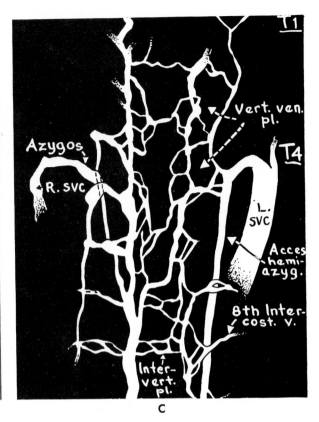

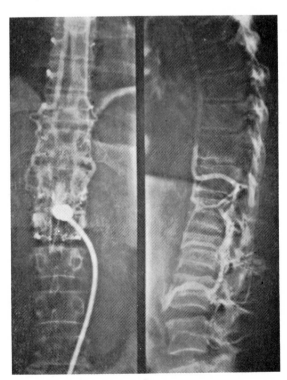

Figure 11-27. *A.* Diagrammatic representation of the azygos venous system. The segmental lumbar veins are joined to each other by a longitudinal vessel, the ascending lumbar vein. The right ascending lumbar vein as it enters the thorax becomes the azygos vein, and the left ascending lumbar vein is continuous with the hemiazygos vein. The hemiazygos vein crosses in front of the vertebral column at the level of the eighth or ninth thoracic vertebra to join the azygos vein. The accessory hemiazygos vein is continuous with the hemiazygos, receives the upper thoracic veins on the left, and joins the left superior intercostal vein above.

B and *C.* The vertebral veins at the upper thoracic level. The vertebral venous plexuses are opacified following the injection of the opaque medium into the left saphenous vein. The primitive paired arrangement of both the azygos and the superior vena cava veins is preserved, the accessory hemiazygos emptying into the left superior vena cava and the azygos emptying into the right superior vena cava. The medial portions of the intercostal veins are opacified. (R.SVC, right superior vena cava; L.SVC, left superior vena cava.)

D. Osseous vertebral venography. The opaque medium is injected into the spinous process and rapidly fills the paravertebral plexuses and the azygos system. (Courtesy of Dr. Franz P. Lessman, Roswell Park Memorial Institute, Buffalo, N.Y.) (Reproduced from Abrams, H. L.: Angiography, 2d ed. Boston, Little, Brown & Co., 1971.)

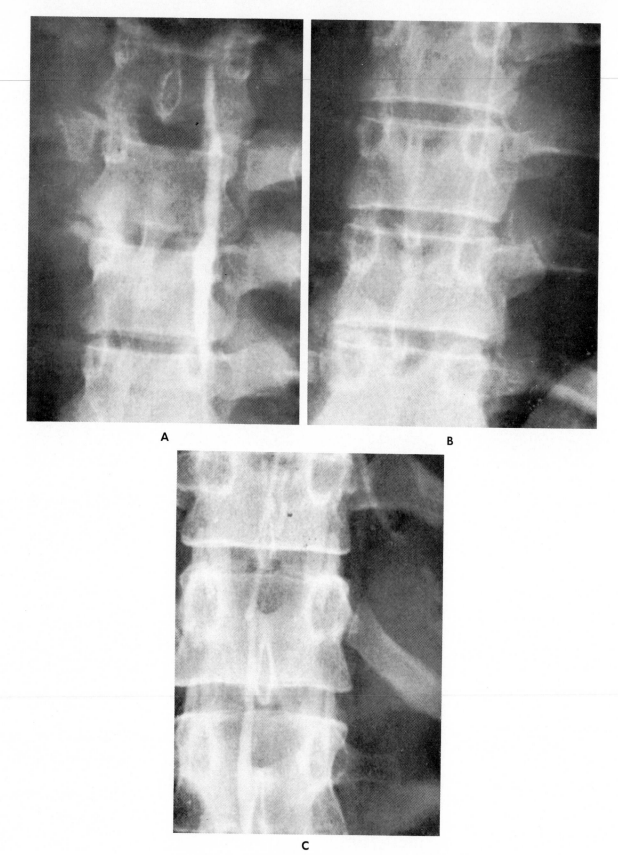

A

B

C

Figure 11–28. *See opposite page for legend.*

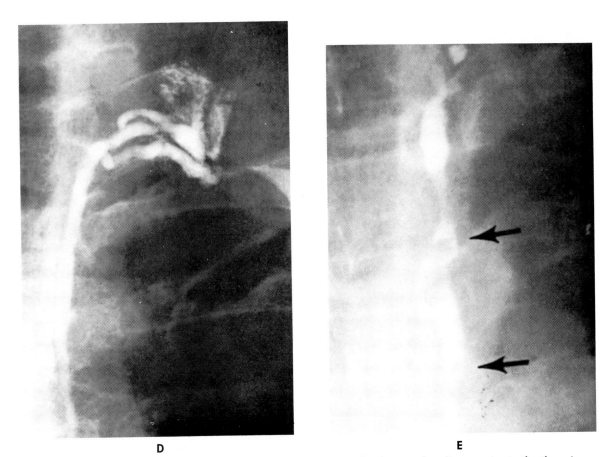

D   **E**

Figure 11–28. The thoracic duct. *A.* Upper thoracic segment. The thoracic duct lies anterior to the thoracic spine on its left side, immediately adjacent to the descending aorta. Above the left main-stem bronchus it parallels the course of the trachea. *B.* Mid-thoracic portion. The duct in its lower portion moves toward the midline, again following the course of the aorta. *C.* Caudal segment of the thoracic duct. The lowest portion of the duct overlies the first lumbar vertebra. It is now to the right of the midline. Its most caudal segment is continuous with the cisterna chyli. As it extends cephalad over the eleventh and twelfth thoracic vertebrae, it begins to move to the left and reaches the left of the midline at the interspace between the tenth and eleventh thoracic vertebrae. *D.* The thoracic duct, cephalic segment. The upper one-third of the duct resembles an inverted J. Notice that it becomes three separate channels just prior to its entry into the junction of the internal jugular and left subclavian veins. A few supraclavicular lymph nodes are filled with contrast agent. *E.* Valves in the thoracic duct. Valves can usually be visualized in the thoracic duct and may vary in number from two to thirteen. They are bicuspid and quite variable in size. The maximum observed diameter of a valve was 6 mm. (From Abrams, H. L.: Angiography, 2d ed. Boston, Little, Brown & Co., 1971.)

of the abdominal region. In brief review, this procedure involves the injection of a vital stain into the web space between the great toe and the second toe, surgical dissection of the subcutaneous lymphatic in this region, and insertion of a very fine catheter tip into the lymphatic. Next, a contrast agent such as Ethiodol in 3 to 5 cc. quantities is injected, and films of the lower extremities, the abdomen, and the chest are routinely taken 1 to 2 hours after the injection. Films are obtained as required in anteroposterior, lateral, and oblique projections (for a comprehensive review of this technique see Fuchs).

As noted previously, the thoracic duct is a continuation of the cisterna chyli from its abdominal segment into the thorax, enter-ing the thorax through the aortic hiatus of the diaphragm. A representative illustration is shown in Figure 11–28. As visualized by Rosenberger and Abrams, the maximum diameter of the thoracic duct varied between 1 and 7 mm., and no difference in distribution of size was detected by them with or without mediastinal masses. Valves in the thoracic duct were noted in most cases (Fig. 11–28 *E*), and the maximum observed diameter of a valve was 6 mm. Multiple thoracic channels were observed in a number of cases, and variations of normal were not unusual. The roentgen signs of normality and abnormality were carefully documented by Rosenberger and Abrams.

REFERENCES

Abrams, H. L.: The vertebral and azygos veins. *In* Abrams, H. L. (ed.): Angiography. Second edition. Vol. 1. Boston, Little, Brown & Co., 1971.

Anderson, R. K.: Diodrast studies of the vertebral and cranial venous systems. J. Neurosurg., *8*:411, 1951.

Anson, B. (ed.): Morris' Human Anatomy. 12th edition. New York, McGraw-Hill, 1966.

Bierman, H. R., Byron, R. L., Jr., Kelly, K. H., Gilfillan, R. S., White, L. P., Freeman, N. E., and Petrakis, N. L.: The characteristics of thoracic duct lymph in man. J. Clin. Invest., *32*:637, 1953.

Blank, N., and Castellino, R. A.: Patterns of pleural reflections of the left superior mediastinum. Radiology, *102*:585–589, 1972.

Boijsen, E., and Reuter, S. R.: Subclavian and internal mammary angiography in the evaluation of anterior mediastinal masses. Amer. J. Roentgenol., *98*:447–450, 1966.

Brzek, V., Kren, V., and Bartos, V.: Retrograde lymphographie des ductus thoracicus. Fortschr. Roentgenstr., *102*:125–131, 1965.

Cimmino, C. V., and Snead, L. O.: The posterior mediastinal line on chest roentgenograms. Radiology, *84*:516–518, 1965.

Condorelli, L.: Il pneumo-mediastino artificiale; ricerche anatomiche preliminari. Tecnica delle iniezioni nelle loggie mediastiniche anteriore e posteriore. Minerva Medica, *1*:81–86, 1936.

Doyle, F. H., Read, A. E., and Evans, K. T.: The mediastinum in portal hypertension. Clin. Radiol., *12*:114–129, 1961.

Felson, B.: Letter from the editor. Sem. in Roentgenol., *2*:323, 1967.

Fischgold, H., Adam, H., Ecoiffier, J., and Piequet, J.: Opacification des plexus rachidiens et des veines azygos voie osseusse. J. Radiol. et Électrol., *33*:37, 1952.

Fleischner, F. G., and Udis, S. W.: Dilatation of the azygos vein: a roentgen sign of venous engorgement. Amer. J. Roentgenol., *67*:509, 1952.

Franken, E. A., Jr.: Pneumomediastinum in the newborn. Amer. J. Roentgenol., *109*:252–260, 1970.

Fuchs, W. A.: Technique in complications of lymphangiography. *In* Abrams, H. L. (ed.): Angiography. Second edition. Boston, Little, Brown & Co., 1971.

Hare, W. S. C., and Mackay, I. R.: Radiological assessment of the thymic size in myasthenia gravis and systemic lupus erythematosus. Lancet, *1*:746–748, 1963.

Heitzman, E. R., Scrivani, J. V., Martino, J., and Moro, J.: The azygos vein and its pleural reflections. II. Applications in the radiological diagnosis of mediastinal abnormalities. Radiology, *101*:259–266, 1971.

Hughes, D. L., Hanafee, W. N., and O'Loughlin, B. J.: Diagnostic pneumomediastinum. Radiology, *12*: 1962.

Issard, H. J., Bergelson, V. D., and Foreman, J.: Mediastinal pneumography. Amer. J. Roentgenol., *75*:771–778, 1956.

Keats, T. E., Lipscomb, G. E., and Betts, C. S., III: Mensuration of the arch of the azygos vein and its application to the study of cardiopulmonary disease. Radiology, *90*:990–994, 1968.

Knutsson, F.: The mediastinal pleura. Acta Radiol., *43*:265–275, 1955.

Kreel, L., Blendis, L. M., and Piercy, J. C.: Pneumomediastinography by trans-sternal method. Clin. Radiol., *15*:219–223, 1964.

McCort, J. J., and Robbins, L. L.: Roentgen diagnosis of intrathoracic lymph-node metastases in carcinoma of the lung. Radiology, *57*:339–359, 1951.

Marchand, P.: The anatomy and applied anatomy of the mediastinal fascia. Thorax, *6*:359–368, 1951.

Moseley, J. E., and Som, M.: Cervical thymus gland. J. Mt. Sinai Hospital, *21*:289–295, 1954–55.

Oliva, L. E.: Pneumomediastinography. *In* Rigler, L. G. (ed.): Roentgen Diagnosis. Vol. 1, General Principles and Methods. Second American edition. New York and London, Grune & Stratton, 1968.

Pacofsky, K. B., and Wolfel, D. A.: Azygos continuation of the inferior vena cava. Amer. J. Roentgenol., *113*:362–365, 1971.

Palubinskas, A. J., and Hodson, C. J.: Transintervertebral retroperitoneal gas insufflation. Radiology, *70*:851–854, 1958.

Preger, L., Hooper, T. I., Steinbach, H. L., and Hoffman, J. I. E.: Width of azygos vein related to central venous pressure. Radiology, *93*:521–523, 1969.

Rabinowitz, J. G., and Wolf, B. S.: Roentgen significance of the pulmonary ligament. Radiology, *87*:1013–1020, 1966.

Ranniger, K.: Retrograde azygography. Radiology, *90*:1097, 1968.

Rosenberger, A., and Abrams, H. L.: The thoracic duct. *In* Abrams, H. L. (ed.): Angiography. Second edition. Boston, Little, Brown & Co., 1971.

Rouviere, H., and Valette, G.: Physiologie du Systeme Lymphatique. Paris, Masson et Cie, 1937.

Ruiz-Rivas, M.: Generalized subserous emphysema with a single puncture. Amer. J. Roentgenol., *64*:723–739, 1950.

Stauffer, H. M., LaBree, J. W., and Adams, F. H.: Normally situated arch of azygos vein; roentgenologic identification and catheterization. Amer. J. Roentgenol., *66*:353, 1951.

Stranahan, A., Alley, R. D., Kousel, H. W., and Reeve, T. S.: Operative thoracic ductography. J. Thoracic Surg., *31*:183, 1956.

Sumerling, M. D., and Irvine, W. J.: Pneumomediastinography. Amer. J. Roentgenol., *98*:451–460, 1966.

Swart, B.: The width of the azygos vein as a roentgen diagnostic criterion of pathological collateral circulation. Fortschr. Roentgenstrahl., *91*:415–444, 1959.

Tausend, M. E., and Stern, W. Z.: Thymic patterns in the newborn. Amer. J. Roentgenol., *95*:125–130, 1965.

Tori, G., and Garusi, G. F.: The azygos vein. Amer. J. Roentgenol., *87*:235–247, 1962.

Vallebona, A.: Transverse stratigraphy of the mediastinum. Stratigrafia, *2*:73–89, 1957.

Wishart, D. L.: Normal azygos vein width in children. Radiology, *104*:115–118, 1972.

Yune, H. Y., and Klatte, E. C.: Thymic venography. Radiology, *96*:521–526, 1970.

12

The Heart and Major Blood Vessels

BASIC ANATOMY OF THE CARDIOVASCULAR SYSTEM

Introduction. The heart, its major blood vessels, and the blood contained within these structures are all of the same order of density, and hence any studies of the heart without contrast media in the blood must necessarily be contour studies.

These studies, therefore, presuppose a knowledge of the normal positions of the various cardiac chambers, so that they can be placed in proper position for study; they also are based upon a knowledge of the normal contours of these chambers when in these various degrees of obliquity.

The Heart. The heart is enclosed within the pericardium, and normally there is only a thin layer of fluid between the inner layer of pericardium and the epicardium of the heart. The heart is obliquely situated in the chest so that about one-third of it is situated on the right and about two-thirds on the left of the median plane (Fig. 12–1).

The heart contains four chambers—two atria and two ventricles. The atria are separated from the ventricles by the *coronary sulcus*. The groove which separates the two atria is barely visible on the posterior surface, and is hidden from view on the anterior surface by the pulmonary artery and the aorta. There are two grooves separating the ventricles—the *anterior longitudinal sulcus* near the left border of the heart, and the *posterior longitudinal sulcus* on the diaphragmatic surface of the heart. The base of the heart is the upper posterior and right aspect of the heart, while the apex is rounded and extends inferiorly and to the left (Fig. 12–2).

The right atrium is slightly larger than the left and forms the upper right margin of the heart (Fig. 12–3). It has a principal cavity and a smaller anterior pouch called the auricle. The superior and inferior venae cavae open into the right atrium, as does also the coronary sinus (Fig. 12–4). These channels return the blood from the upper and lower parts of the body and the heart musculature respectively.

Situated in the lower part of the septum between the right and left atria is the fossa ovalis, an oval depression that corresponds with the foramen ovale of the fetus.

692

The left atrium, like the right, contains a principal cavity and an auricle. There are four pulmonary veins (Fig. 12–5) that open into the upper part of the posterior surface of the left atrium. The left atrium forms the greater part of the posterior surface of the heart and the base of the heart. It is in close proximity with the esophagus in this sector, and any enlargement of the left atrium must necessarily displace the esophagus posteriorly, and usually to the right (Figs. 12–6, 12–7). (Also see cross-section diagrams of mediastinum in Chapter 11.).

The right ventricle forms the larger part of the anterior (or sternocostal) surface of the heart, and it also forms a small portion of the diaphragmatic surface. Its upper and left portion forms

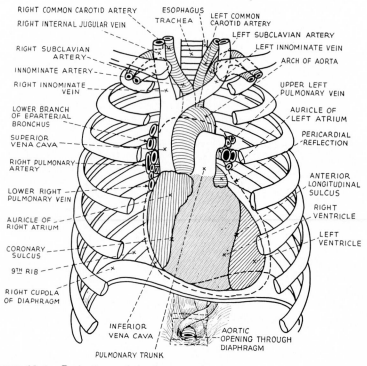

Figure 12–1. Projections of the heart in the thoracic cage with lung and rib structures removed. Frontal projection.

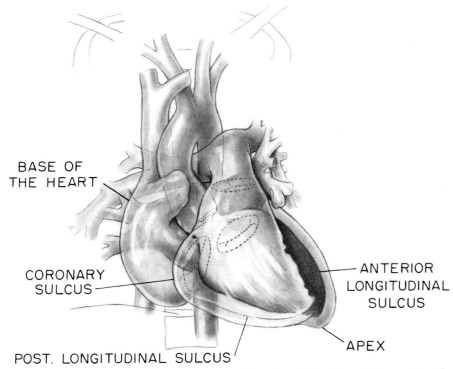

Figure 12-2. Frontal view of a normal heart (transparent) showing relationships of inflow and outflow tracts to chambers. (After Schad, N., et al.: Differential Diagnosis of Congenital Heart Disease. New York, Grune & Stratton, 1966.)

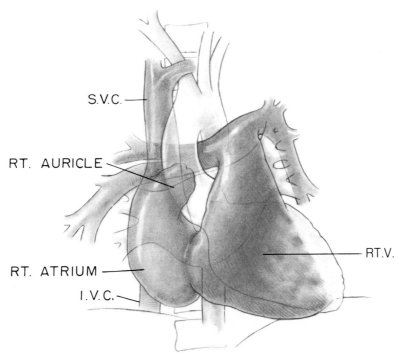

Figure 12-3. Frontal view of the heart showing the relationship of inflow and outflow tracts to the right cardiac chambers. (I.V.C.) inferior vena cava, (S.V.C.) superior vena cava, (RT.V.) right ventricle. (After Schad, N., et al.: Differential Diagnosis of Congenital Heart Disease. New York, Grune & Stratton, 1966.)

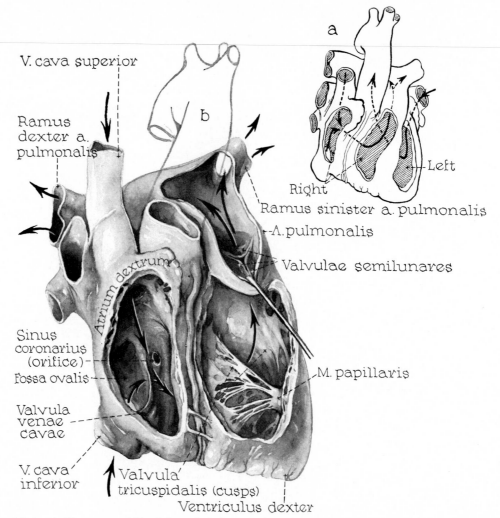

Figure 12–4. *A.* The course of blood through the chambers of the heart. *B.* The right atrium and right ventricle opened up for view, along with the outflow tract from the right ventricle to the pulmonary artery. (From Anson, B. J.: An Atlas of Human Anatomy. Philadelphia, W. B. Saunders Co., 1968.)

a conical pouch called the conus arteriosus or pulmonary conus. The wall of the right ventricle is thinner than that of the left, bearing a ratio of about 1 to 3 to the latter. The opening of the pulmonary artery is situated at the uppermost part of the conus arteriosus, above and to the left of the right atrioventricular opening (Figs. 12–4, 12–8, 12–9).

The left ventricle forms much of the left cardiac border below the coronary sulcus, and a considerable part of the diaphragmatic surface of the heart. The left atrioventricular orifice is below and to the left of the orifice connecting with the aorta (Fig. 12–10).

There are four series of valves regulating blood flow between the chambers of the heart and great vessels, situated between left atrium and left ventricle (mitral valves), left ventricle and aorta (aortic valves), right atrium and right ventricle (tricuspid valves), and right ventricle and pulmonary artery (pulmonary valves) (Fig. 12–11). There are three cusps (Fig. 12–12) to each of the above valves, with the exception of the mitral valve, which has only two. The tricuspid and mitral valves are attached by means of narrow bands (chordae tendineae) to the papillary muscles of the ventricular walls.

The Cardiac Cycle (Fig. 12–12). The heart normally pulsates regularly by contraction at a rate of approximately 60 to 80 times per minute. Its wave of contraction is known as systole and its period of rest as diastole. The atrial systole normally precedes

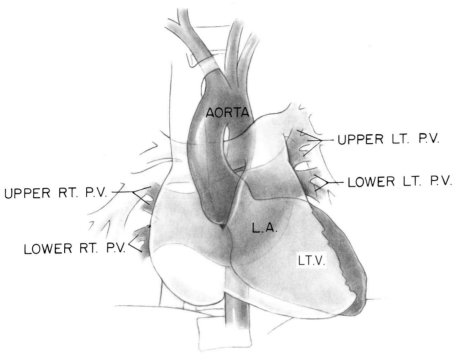

Figure 12–5. Frontal view of the heart showing the relationship of inflow and outflow tracts to the left cardiac chambers. (RT. P.V.) right pulmonary veins, (L.A.) left atrium, (LT.V.) left ventricle (shaded), (LT. P.V.) (left pulmonary veins). (After Schad, N., et al.: Differential Diagnosis of Congenital Heart Disease. New York, Grune & Stratton, 1966.)

the ventricular. When the ventricles contract, the bicuspid and tricuspid valves close, preventing the regress of the blood from the ventricles back to the atria, and as the pressure rises, the pulmonary and aortic valves open and allow the flow of the blood into the pulmonary artery and the aorta. When the ventricular con-

traction ceases, these latter valves close. During the period of rest, the blood from the systemic and pulmonary veins flows into the atria.

The technique of cardiac catheterization and selective angio-cardiography will be reviewed subsequently. The diagnostic pro-

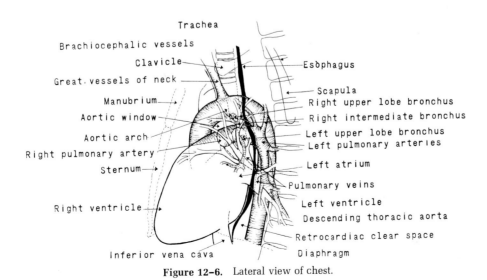

Figure 12–6. Lateral view of chest.

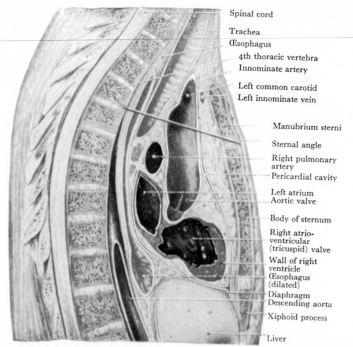

Spinal cord
Trachea
Œsophagus
4th thoracic vertebra
Innominate artery
Left common carotid
Left innominate vein

Manubrium sterni
Sternal angle
Right pulmonary artery
Pericardial cavity
Left atrium
Aortic valve
Body of sternum
Right atrioventricular (tricuspid) valve
Wall of right ventricle
Œsophagus (dilated)
Diaphragm
Descending aorta
Xiphoid process
Liver

Figure 12–7. Sagittal section of thorax of an old man. The upper border of manubrium sterni and the bifurcation of trachea are lower than in a young adult. The thick black line is the artificial boundary that separates the superior mediastinum from the other three. (From Cunningham's Manual of Practical Anatomy, 12th ed., Vol. 2. London, Oxford University Press, 1958.)

outside the scope of this text (see Kory et al. for a brief interpretive summary).

Fluoroscopically, the pulsations in the various portions of the heart vary somewhat in their appearance and sequence, the contractions being most forceful in the region of the left ventricular apex posteriorly (best seen in the left anterior oblique projection). The sequence and character of the pulsations, as well as the rhythm, require close study, since variations from the normal pattern are of considerable significance.

The Aorta. The aorta arises from within the cardiac silhouette in a sheath shared with the pulmonary artery. The *ascending* aorta begins on a level with the third intercostal space along the left sternal margin and ascends posterior to the sternum as far as the superior border of the right costosternal articulation or sternal angle. This segment is 5 to 5.5 cm. in length usually and 28 to 30 mm. in diameter. There is a dilatation of the aorta near its point of origin caused by the three *aortic sinuses,* one to the right and one to the left, and a third posteriorly (Fig. 12–13). The *right and left coronary arteries* arise from the superior borders of the right and left aortic sinuses.

The *arch of the aorta* lies in the superior mediastinum posterior to the manubrium, covered by an attachment of fibrous pericardium. It begins at the second right costal cartilage and curves superiorly, dorsally, and to the left and then caudally

cedures performed under radiologic control permit sampling of blood and pressure measurements in the various chambers of the heart, aorta, and pulmonary arteries proximally and distally. These measurements permit the estimation of valvular abnormalities as well as cardiac output determinations.

Figure 12–12 presents graphically the normal percentage of oxygen saturation and oxygen volume, and pressure ranges in heart chambers and great vessels. Pressure tracings are shown in relation to the electrocardiogram both in the right and left heart, with inclusion also of aortic and pulmonary pressure determinations.

In the pulmonary wedge position, 97 to 99 per cent saturated blood can be withdrawn from the wedged catheter, approximating the values of pulmonary venous blood. Note that the phasic pressures in the right atrium, left atrium, and pulmonary artery wedge position have the same overall characteristics. There are small differences in amplitude and timing of the various phases.

The level of peak systolic pressure of the left ventricle is approximately five times that in the right, but the phasic pressures in the right and left ventricles are very similar in contour. A detailed discussion of these curves, phases, and interpretation is

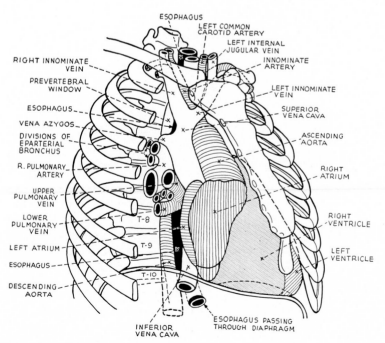

ESOPHAGUS
LEFT COMMON CAROTID ARTERY
LEFT INTERNAL JUGULAR VEIN
RIGHT INNOMINATE VEIN
INNOMINATE ARTERY
PREVERTEBRAL WINDOW
LEFT INNOMINATE VEIN
ESOPHAGUS
SUPERIOR VENA CAVA
VENA AZYGOS
DIVISIONS OF EPARTERIAL BRONCHUS
ASCENDING AORTA
R. PULMONARY ARTERY
RIGHT ATRIUM
UPPER PULMONARY VEIN
LOWER PULMONARY VEIN
RIGHT VENTRICLE
T-8
LEFT ATRIUM
T-9
LEFT VENTRICLE
ESOPHAGUS
DESCENDING AORTA
T-10
INFERIOR VENA CAVA
ESOPHAGUS PASSING THROUGH DIAPHRAGM

Figure 12–8. Projections of the heart in the thoracic cage with lung and rib structures removed. Right anterior oblique projection.

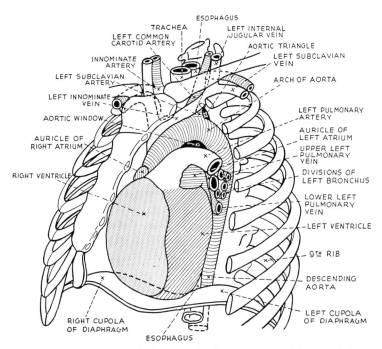

Figure 12–9. Projections of the heart in the thoracic cage with lung and rib structures removed. Left anterior oblique projection.

Variations in the main branches of the arch of the aorta, along with their statistical incidence, are indicated in Figures 12–14 and 12–15.

Anomalously, the right aortic arch may persist, resulting in a complete reversal of the branches and structures of the aortic arch. This may occur with or without a situs inversus of all of the viscera, and occurs in approximately 20 per cent of those individuals who have a tetralogy of Fallot. Also, the distal portion of the right aortic arch may persist, an anomaly that is associated with the disappearance of some or all of the proximal part. This abnormality may result in the right subclavian artery appearing to originate from the descending thoracic aorta. In these instances, the right subclavian artery passes to the right, dorsal to the trachea and esophagus, and making an esophageal impression. Other abnormalities are described with congenital anomalies in roentgenologic texts dealing with the abnormal.

The usual branches of the aortic arch are: the *brachiocephalic*, the *left common carotid*, and the *left subclavian arteries*. These supply the head and neck, superior limbs, and part of the thoracic wall (Fig. 12–16). A *thyroidea ima artery* may arise from the arch between the brachiocephalic and left common carotid arteries. (The brachiocephalic trunk and subclavian vessels have been described in relation to the upper extremity.)

along the left side of the vertebral column to a level between the fourth and fifth thoracic vertebrae, where it continues as the *descending thoracic aorta*. It arches across the right pulmonary artery and left bronchus. The aortic arch lies to the left of the trachea and esophagus.

Just beyond the origin of the left subclavian artery, the aorta narrows somewhat and is called the *isthmus*, this segment extending to the point of origin of the *ligamentum arteriosum*. The latter structure is attached to the concavity of the arch approximately opposite the third thoracic vertebra. The proximal arch of the aorta usually has a diameter of approximately 28 mm., but it diminishes in size beyond the subclavian to an average of 23 mm. When this measurement exceeds 37 mm., the aorta can be considered dilated or aneurysmal. The thymus overlies the arch of the aorta between the pleural cavities anteriorly.

Within the concavity of the arch of the aorta are the following structures: the *right pulmonary artery*, the *bifurcation of the pulmonary trunk*, the *left bronchus*, the *ligamentum arteriosum*, the *left recurrent laryngeal nerves*, the *superficial cardiac plexus*, and several *bronchial lymph nodes*.

Dorsal to the arch of the aorta are the following structures: the *superior vena cava, trachea, esophagus, thoracic duct, deep cardiac plexus*, and *left retrolaryngeal nerve*. The *left brachiocephalic vein* is superior and somewhat ventral. The chief three branches of the arch of the aorta arise along its cephalic border.

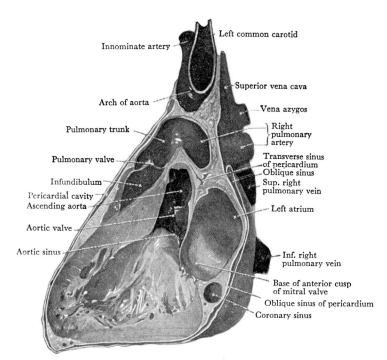

Figure 12–10. Sagittal section of heart and pericardium. (From Cunningham's Manual of Practical Anatomy, 12th ed., Vol. 2., London, Oxford University Press, 1958.)

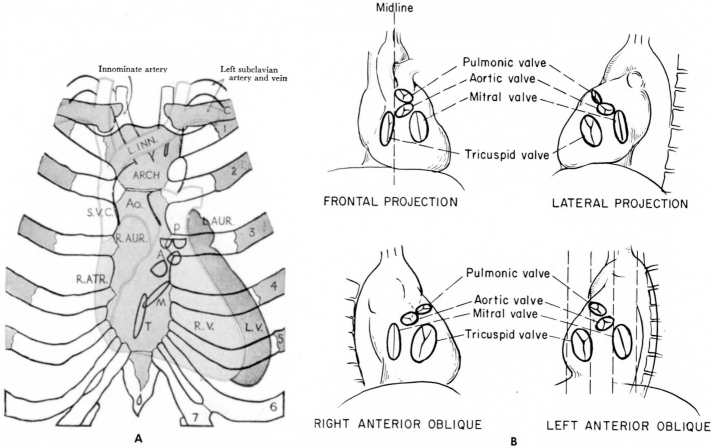

PROJECTION OF CARDIAC VALVES
IN ROUTINE POSITIONS IN RADIOGRAPHY

Figure 12–11. A. Relation of heart and great vessels to anterior wall of thorax. (1 to 7) Ribs and costal cartilages, (A) aortic orifice, (Ao) ascending aorta, (C) clavicle, (L.V.) left ventricle, (M) mitral orifice, (P) pulmonary orifice, (R.V.) right ventricle, (S.V.C.) superior vena cava, (T) tricuspid orifice. (From Cunningham's Manual of Practical Anatomy, 12th ed., Vol. 2. London, Oxford University Press, 1958.) B. Cardiac valves in routine radiographic projections.

The *common carotid arteries* ascend into the neck and are different on each side. They are 8 to 12 cm. long, extending from the sternoclavicular articulation to the superior border of the thyroid cartilage (Fig. 12–16). At the level of the fourth cervical vertebra they divide into internal and external carotid arteries. The common carotid arteries are contained in a common sheath with *the internal jugular vein* and the *vagus nerve* on each side. At the sternoclavicular joint the jugular vein lies ventrolateral to the artery, but as it ascends it becomes dorsolateral. The common carotid artery is unbranched except at its termination and does not diminish in size as it ascends in the neck, but there is a slight

dilatation for approximately 1 cm. at its bifurcation which provides for the *carotid sinus*, part of a mechanism that regulates blood pressure.

The collateral circulation of the common carotid and subclavian arteries is shown diagrammatically in Figure 12–17.

The *external carotid artery* is distributed to the anterior part of the neck, the pharynx, the tongue, oral cavity, face, temporal and infratemporal fossae, nasal cavity, and the greater part of the scalp and cranial meninges (Fig. 12–16 *B*).

There is some variability in the point of origin of the external carotid artery, but it arises at the superior border of the thyroid cartilage or the fourth cervical level in about two-thirds of the cases. It may, however, arise at the third cervical level or at the superior margin of the fifth cervical vertebra. It generally terminates posterior to the neck of the mandible, dividing into two main branches: the *maxillary* and *superficial temporal arteries*. Eight independent branches arising from the external carotid may usually be counted, given off in the following order: *superior thyroid, ascending pharyngeal, lingual, facial, occipital, posterior auricular, superficial temporal*, and *maxillary*. The *sternocleido-mastoid artery* is also an independent branch. These major branches are indicated in Figure 12–16 *B*.

Returning to the distal portion of the arch of the aorta at the point of origin of the ligamentum arteriosum, a very slight dilatation of the aorta may occur, sometimes referred to as the *"ductus diverticulum"* (Fig. 12–18). Beyond this there may be in infants, a further slight fusiform dilatation, which His has called the *aortic spindle*. This structure may persist into adult life. In the adult, the site of insertion of the ligamentum arteriosum may appear on aortography as a very slight irregularity.

The *descending aorta* follows a downward course to the left of the vertebral column giving off numerous small branches, most of them intercostal arteries. The small *bronchial arteries* and

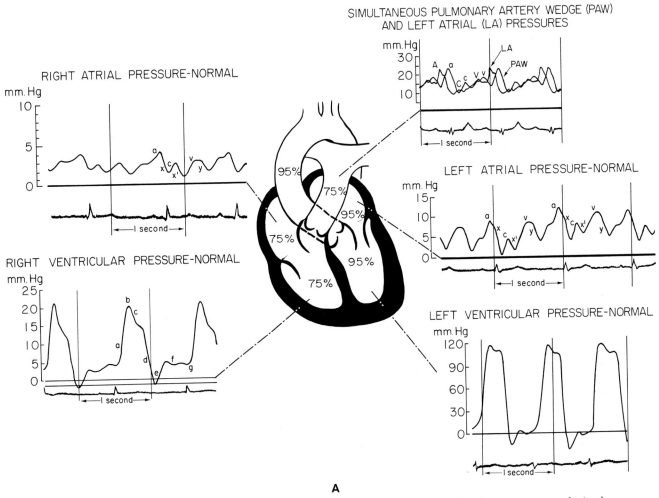

A

Figure 12–12. *A.* Diagram of the heart and its major blood vessels indicating the related pressure curves obtained from the right atrium, the right ventricle, and simultaneously from the pulmonary artery and left atrium, as well as normal pressure curves for the left atrium and left ventricle. The average oxygen saturation in the right atrium, right ventricle, pulmonary artery, left atrium, left ventricle, and aorta are also indicated.

Figure 12–12 continued on the following page.

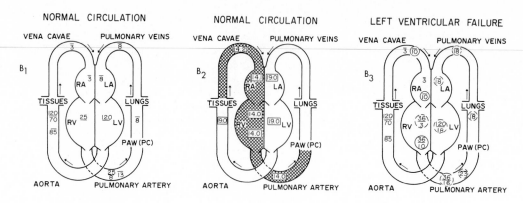

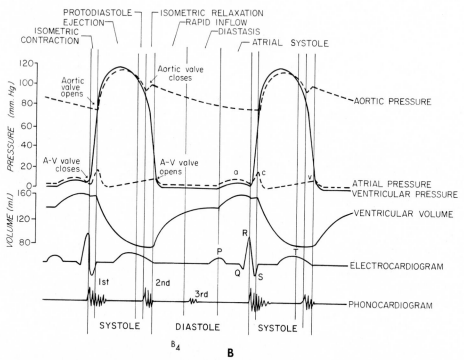

Figure 12–12 *Continued.* B1. Schematic diagram of the normal circulation showing representative mean pressures in millimeters of mercury in the various heart chambers, great vessels and pulmonary artery wedge (PAW). (RA) Right atrium, (RV) right ventricle, (LA) left atrium, (LV) left ventricle, (PC) pulmonary capillary.

B2. Diagram of the normal circulation showing representative values for oxygen content of the blood expressed in volumes per cent in the various heart chambers and major vessels. The cross-hatched area represents venous blood. (Abbreviations as previously indicated.)

B3. The figures encircled by interrupted lines are representative pressure values which may be recorded in the presence of left ventricular failure. Those figures encircled by solid lines are representative pressure values for right ventricular failure. (B1, B2, and B3 redrawn from: Kory, R. C., Tsagaris, T. J., and Bustamante, R. A.: A Primer of Cardiac Catheterization. 1965. Courtesy of Charles C Thomas, Publisher, Springfield, Ill.)

B4. Correlation of the dynamic acoustic and electrical events of the cardiac cycle: this figure provides simultaneous recording of left atrial, left ventricular, and aortic pressures together with the electrocardiogram and phonocardiogram. (LV) left ventricle, (LA) left atrium. The numbers 1, 2, and 3 refer to the first, second, and third heart sounds respectively. (Redrawn from Guyton, A. C.: Textbook of Medical Physiology, 4th ed. Philadelphia, W. B. Saunders Co., 1971.)

Figure 12–12 continued on the opposite page.

Figure 12–12 *Continued.* C. Calculations of mitral and aortic valve areas, intracardiac pressures, oxygen content variation between right heart vessels and chambers, average oxygen contents and saturations in various heart chambers and vessels, and representative oxygen content evaluation in left to right shunts. (From Kory, R. C., Tsagaris, T. J., and Bustamante, R. A.: A Primer of Cardiac Catheterization, 1965. Courtesy of Charles C Thomas, Publisher, Springfield, Illinois.)

SHUNT FLOW

A CENTRAL CIRCULATORY shunt is defined as an abnormal communication between the pulmonary and systemic circulations connecting either of the two pairs of cardiac chambers or the great vessels.[50] Shunting of blood may occur from left to right, right to left, or may be bidirectional.

A. OXYGEN METHOD FOR DETECTION OF SHUNTS

The determination of O_2 content in blood samples drawn at different levels within the heart and great vessels aids in determining the presence, direction, and volume of central circulatory shunts.

The average normal values for the O_2 content and saturation in the various chambers of the heart and great vessels are shown in Table 12C.

TABLE 12C

AVERAGE O_2 CONTENTS AND SATURATIONS IN VARIOUS HEART CHAMBERS AND VESSELS

	O_2 Content vol. %	O_2 Saturation
SUPERIOR VENA CAVA (SVC)	14 (± 1)	70%
INFERIOR VENA CAVA (IVC)	16 (± 1)	80%
RIGHT ATRIUM (RA)	15 (± 1)	75%
PULMONARY ARTERY (PA)	15.2 (± 1)	75%
RIGHT VENTRICLE (RV)	15.2 (± 1)	75%
BRACHIAL ARTERY (BA)	19.0 (± 1)	95%+

There is moderate variation in venous oxygen content from chamber to chamber even in patients without shunts. The limits of this variation which may occur normally are indicated in Table 12B (Gorlin).

A. CALCULATION OF MITRAL VALVE AREA

The formula in general use for calculation of mitral valve area[47] is:

$$\text{MITRAL VALVE AREA, cm.}^2 = \frac{\text{Mitral valve flow (ml./sec.)}}{31\sqrt{\text{Diastolic gradient across the mitral valve}}}$$

$$\text{where: Mitral valve flow} = \frac{\text{Cardiac output (ml./min.)}}{\text{Diastolic filling period (sec./min.)}}$$

$$\begin{array}{l}\text{Diastolic filling} \\ \text{period} \\ \text{(sec./min.)}\end{array} = \begin{array}{l}\text{diastolic period} \\ \text{per beat} \\ \text{(sec./beat)}\end{array} X \begin{array}{l}\text{heart rate} \\ \text{(beats/min.)}\end{array}$$

$$\begin{array}{l}\text{Diastolic gradient} \\ \text{across the mitral} \\ \text{valve (mm. Hg)}\end{array} = \begin{array}{l}\text{left atrial} \\ \text{mean pressure} \\ \text{(mm. Hg)}\end{array} \text{minus} \begin{array}{l}\text{left ventricular} \\ \text{mean diastolic} \\ \text{pressure (mm. Hg.)}\end{array}$$

$$\text{and} \quad 31 \quad = \quad \text{empirical constant}$$

The *normal mitral valve area* is 4.5 cm.² Clinical disability is present with mitral valve areas of 1.0 cm.² or less (Lewis et al.).

B. CALCULATION OF AORTIC VALVE AREA

The formula in general use for calculation of aortic valve area is:

$$\begin{array}{l}\text{AORTIC VALVE} \\ \text{AREA, cm.}^2\end{array} = \frac{\text{Aortic valve flow (ml./sec.)}}{44.5\sqrt{\text{Systolic pressure gradient across the aortic valve}}}$$

$$\begin{array}{l}\text{where: Aortic valve flow} \\ \text{(ml./sec.)}\end{array} = \frac{\text{Cardiac output (ml./min.)}}{\text{Systolic ejection period (sec./min.)}}$$

$$\begin{array}{l}\text{Systolic ejection period} \\ \text{(sec./min.)}\end{array} = \begin{array}{l}\text{Systolic ejection period} \\ \text{per beat} \\ \text{(sec./beat)}\end{array} X \begin{array}{l}\text{Heart rate} \\ \text{(beats/min.)}\end{array}$$

$$\begin{array}{l}\text{Systolic pressure} \\ \text{gradient across} \\ \text{the aortic valve} \\ \text{(mm. Hg)}\end{array} = \begin{array}{l}\text{left ventricular} \\ \text{mean systolic} \\ \text{pressure} \\ \text{(mm. Hg)}\end{array} \text{minus} \begin{array}{l}\text{aortic} \\ \text{mean systolic} \\ \text{pressure} \\ \text{(mm. Hg)}\end{array}$$

$$\text{and} \quad 44.5 \quad = \quad \text{gravity acceleration factor}$$

The *normal aortic valve* area is 3-4 cm.² Clinical disability is generally present when the valve area is 0.75 cm.² or less (Wood) and is always present with a valve area of 0.5 cm.² or less (Gorlin et al.).

The formulas for calculation of the tricuspid and pulmonary valve areas are similar to the formulas for calculating the mitral and aortic valve areas, respectively, but are rarely used clinically.

Similar formulas can be used for estimating the size of a patent ductus arteriosus or the size of defects in the atrial or ventricular septa.

TABLE 12A

INTRACARDIAC PRESSURES — NORMAL RESTING VALUES

	Pressure in mm. Hg.		
Site of Measurement	Systolic	Diastolic	Mean
Right atrium (RA)	°	°	< 5
Right ventricle (RV)	< 30	< 5 (End-diastolic)	°°
Pulmonary Artery (PA)	< 30	< 10	< 20
°°°Pulmonary Artery Wedge (PAW)	°	°	< 12
Left atrium (LA)	°	°	< 12
Left ventricle (LV)	120	< 10 (End-diastolic)	°°
Aorta (Ao)	120	70	95

°Since the pressures in the right and left atria are comparatively low and since the systolic and diastolic levels are subject to wide respiratory fluctuation, only the mean atrial pressures are commonly reported in cardiac catheterization studies.

°°Since systolic pressures in the ventricles are related to ventricular ejection and diastolic pressures to ventricular filling, *mean* ventricular pressure values have no physiologic meaning and are not reported.

°°°The pulmonary artery wedge (PAW) pressure, also termed the pulmonary "capillary" pressure, is obtained by "wedging" the catheter into a small branch of the pulmonary artery. This pressure is essentially the same as the pressure in the left atrium (LA).

TABLE 12B

MAXIMAL NORMAL LIMIT OF O_2 CONTENT VARIATION BETWEEN RIGHT HEART CHAMBERS AND VESSELS

	Maximal Increase in O_2 Content Over the Proximal Chamber
PA (between PA and RV)	0.5 vol. %
RV (between RV and RA)	0.9 vol. %
RA (between RA and SVC)	1.9 vol. %

If the increase in oxygen content of blood in a particular chamber exceeds that of the more proximal chamber by more than the value listed, a left-to-right shunt at that chamber or great vessel level is probably present. Thus, if the O_2 content of the right ventricle exceeds the O_2 content of the right atrium by more than 0.9 vol. %, a ventricular septal defect with a left-to-right shunt is likely. However, when the shunt is small (less than 25% of the systemic flow), this method may not be sensitive enough to detect the presence of such a shunt.

Examples of commonly encountered left-to-right shunts with representative O_2 content values are shown in Table 12D.

TABLE 12D

REPRESENTATIVE O_2 CONTENT VALUES IN LEFT-TO-RIGHT SHUNTS

	O_2 Content (vol. %)		
	Atrial Septal Defect (ASD)	Ventricular Septal Defect (VSD)	Patent Ductus Arteriosus (PDA)
BRACHIAL ARTERY (BA)	20	20	20
PULMONARY ARTERY (PA)	17	17	17
RIGHT VENTRICLE (RV)	17	17	14
RIGHT ATRIUM (RA)	17	14	14
SUPERIOR VENA CAVA (SVC)	14	14	14

C

Figure 12-12 Continued. *See opposite page for legend.*

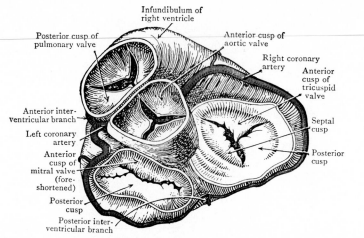

Figure 12–13. Base of ventricular part of the heart, showing arterial orifices and their valves, aortic sinuses and origin of the coronary arteries. (From Cunningham's Manual of Practical Anatomy, 12th ed., Vol. 2. London, Oxford University Press, 1958.)

esophageal branches also arise from this segment of the aorta (the bronchial arteries are described in Chapter 11 and the esophageal blood vessels will be described in conjunction with the alimentary tract in Chapter 13).

The descending thoracic aorta passes from the left side of the vertebral column, becoming more medial in its descent, and finally lies immediately in front of the vertebral column at the level of the diaphragm. It is related anteriorly to the root of the left lung, pericardium, esophagus, and diaphragm. On its right side lie the azygos vein and thoracic duct and on the left are situated the left pleura and lung. It ends at the lower border of the twelfth thoracic vertebra, where it pierces the diaphragm and continues as the abdominal aorta.

Pulmonary Artery (Fig. 12–19 *A, B, C*). The pulmonary artery is a short, wide artery about 5 cm. in length, extending from the conus arteriosus upward and backward and passing in front of and then to the left of the ascending aorta. Under the aortic arch it divides into right and left branches.

The entire artery is contained within the pericardium. On each side of its origin is the auricle of the corresponding side and a coronary artery.

The right branch of the pulmonary artery is longer than the left and passes horizontally to the right under and posterior to the ascending aorta and superior vena cava, and anterior to the right bronchus, to the root of the right lung where it divides into two branches. These follow the course of the right main stem bronchus rather closely as indicated in Chapter 10.

The left branch of the pulmonary artery passes horizontally in front of the descending aorta and left bronchus to the root of the left lung, where it likewise divides into two main branches, one for each lobe of the lung. It is connected with the distal concavity of the arch of the aorta by the ligamentum arteriosum. On the left of the latter structure is the left recurrent nerve. The other branches of the left pulmonary artery have been previously described in connection with the blood supply of the lungs (Chapter 10).

In frontal perspective, the pulmonary artery and occasionally its left branch constitute part of the left cardiac-pericardial silhouette (Fig. 12–19 *A*). In the right anterior oblique projection it is the right pulmonary artery that is seen almost in its entirety and the left pulmonary artery appears considerably foreshortened. The left pulmonary artery is seen to best advantage in the left anterior oblique projection (Fig. 12–19 *B*). The lateral view provides an excellent study of the pulmonary outflow tract, including the infundibulum and pulmonary conus. These form a considerable portion of the superior part of the anterior cardiac border (Fig. 12–19 *C*).

The branches of the pulmonary artery conform closely to the bronchial ramifications in both lungs. To identify the bronchi is to identify the normal pulmonary arterial distribution.

Pulmonary Veins (Fig. 12–20). There are usually two pulmonary veins on each side, each about 15 mm. long; occasionally there may be three on the right. Each vein enters the left atrium of the heart. The *right superior pulmonary vein* lies dorsal to the superior vena cava; the *left pulmonary veins* lie ventral to the thoracic aorta. Pulmonary veins within the lung lie in segmental septae, unlike the arteries, and therefore drain adjacent bronchopulmonary segments (see Chapter 10).

The two pulmonary veins on the right side drain areas as follows: the *right superior pulmonary vein* drains the right upper and middle lobe; the lower lobe is drained by the *right inferior pulmonary vein*. The *left pulmonary veins* are paired, one for each lobe. The left veins enter the left atrium ventral to those of the right.

Right Pulmonary Artery Measurements (Chang). The normal upper limits for the inspiratory measurement of the right descending pulmonary artery of normal male adults was shown to have a maximum measurement of 16 mm. Measurements of 17 mm. or more may be regarded as abnormal. In the adult female, the comparable measurement was 15 mm., with an indication that 16 mm. or more is abnormal.

During inspiration, when the intra-alveolar pressure falls, the size of the right descending pulmonary artery increases, and during expiration the vessel's size decreases owing to compression. There is a 1 to 2 mm. difference between inspiratory and expiratory measurements (2 mm. difference was noted in 69 per cent of cases).

Other measurements are shown in Figure 12–21. The 16.3 mm. measurement indicates the sum of the diameters of the apical vein of the right upper lobe at the level of the right upper

(Text continued on p. 708.)

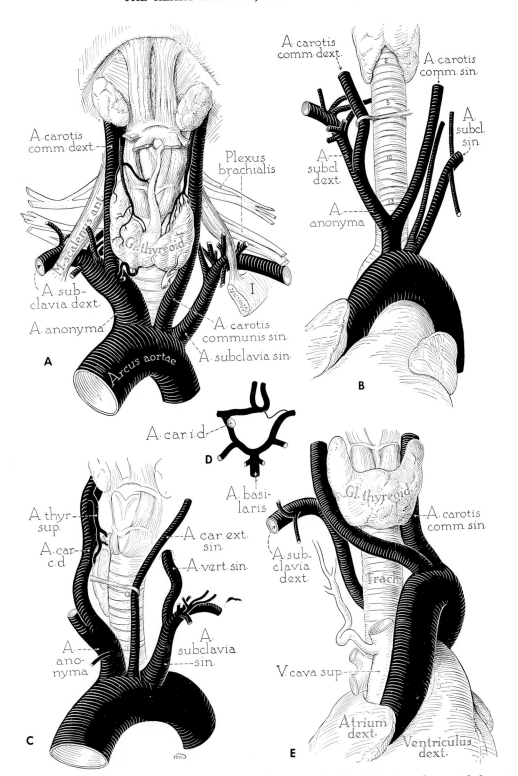

Figure 12–14. Branches of the aortic arch. Variation in the pattern of origin. *A.* Regular schema. *B.* Left common carotid from the innominate. *C.* Absence of left internal carotid artery. *D.* Form of the arterial circle (of Willis) in the same specimen. *E.* Retroesophageal right subclavian artery. (From Anson, B. J.: An Atlas of Human Anatomy. Philadelphia, W. B. Saunders Co., 1963.)

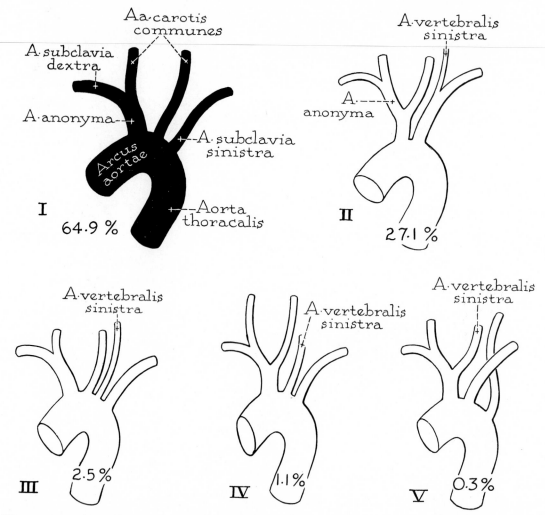

Figure 12–15. Types of branching of the aortic arch encountered in 1000 adult cadavers. I. The arrangement regarded as "normal" for man is actually encountered more frequently than all other types combined. In specimens of this variety, three branches leave the arch in the following succession, from the specimen's right to left: innominate (with right common carotid and right subclavian as derivatives); left common carotid; left subclavian. II. An arrangement distinguished by reduction in the number of stems to two, both common carotid arteries arising from the innominate. III. Here the distinguishing feature is increase, not reduction, in the number of derived branches. The left vertebral artery (usually arising from the subclavian) is the additional vessel. IV. Differing from the preceding variety, the feature is replacement, the left vertebral artery (not the left common carotid, as in Type I) being the second stem in right-to-left succession. Both common carotid arteries arise from a common stem, as they do in examples of Type II. V. In this departure from the anatomic norm, the left vertebral artery arises from the innominate, and the order of the left common carotid and left subclavian arteries is reversed.

VI to VIII (facing page). Three patterns similar in respect to the position of origin of the right subclavian artery; the latter vessel arises as the last branch of the aortic arch, reaching the right upper extremity by passing dorsal to the esophagus. In respect to the origin of the other branches, the types differ. IX. A bi-innominate sequence, in which paired vessels (in turn having matching main branches) are the only derivatives of the aortic arch. X and XI. In both these varieties the left vertebral artery arises from an aortic trunk from which the left subclavian is also derived. However, in Type X a regular innominate artery is present (as in Type I), whereas in Type XI the "innominate" (with regular branches) arises from an aortic trunk shared with the common carotid. XII. Here, as in Type III, an extra vessel arises from the arch between the innominate and the left subclavian, but the added derivative is the *a. thyreoidea ima* instead of the *a. vertebralis*. XIII. Unification is the distinguishing feature of this departure from the typical scheme of branching; the usual branches (see Type I) take origin from the aortic arch through a single trunk as an intermediary vessel. XIV. An infrequent variety with all branches derived from a common stem (as in

(Legend is continued on the opposite page.)

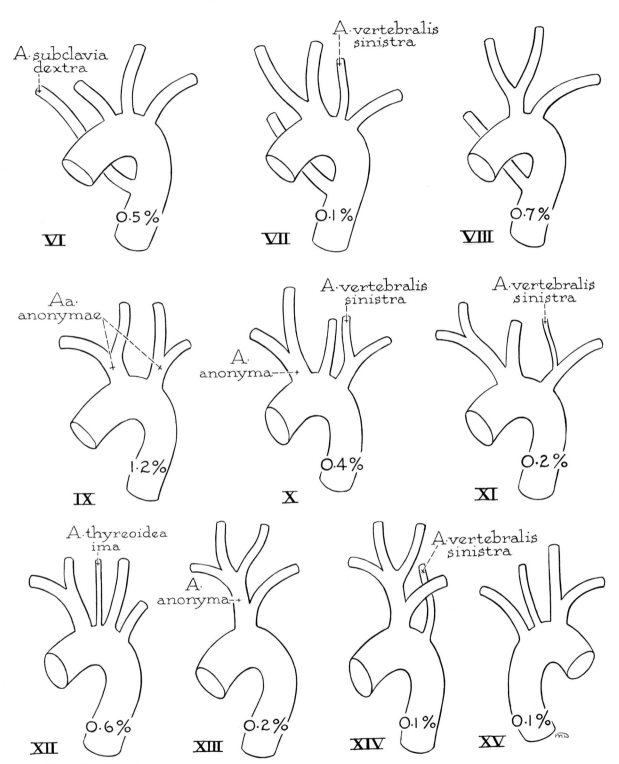

Figure 12–15 *Continued.*
Type XIII) with the exception of the left vertebral, which arises from the arch to the right of the common stem.
XV. In this rare variety, in which the arch passes in a reversed direction from heart to thoracic aorta, the branches maintain a normal succession in relation to the body itself; however, their position on the aortic arch itself is as a mirror-image of the "standard" scheme of derivation. (From Anson, B. J.: An Atlas of Human Anatomy. Philadelphia, W. B. Saunders Co., 1963.)

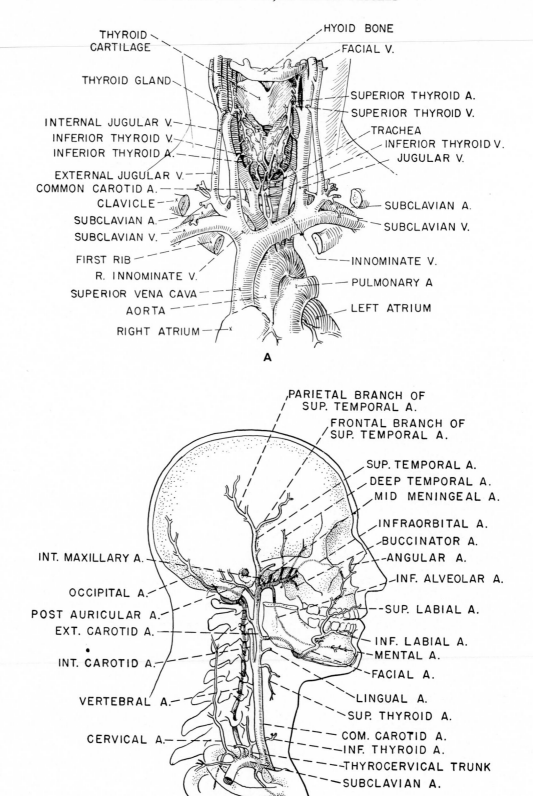

Figure 12–16.   *A.* Diagram of major circulation in the neck. *B.* Major deep arteries of head and neck, lateral view.

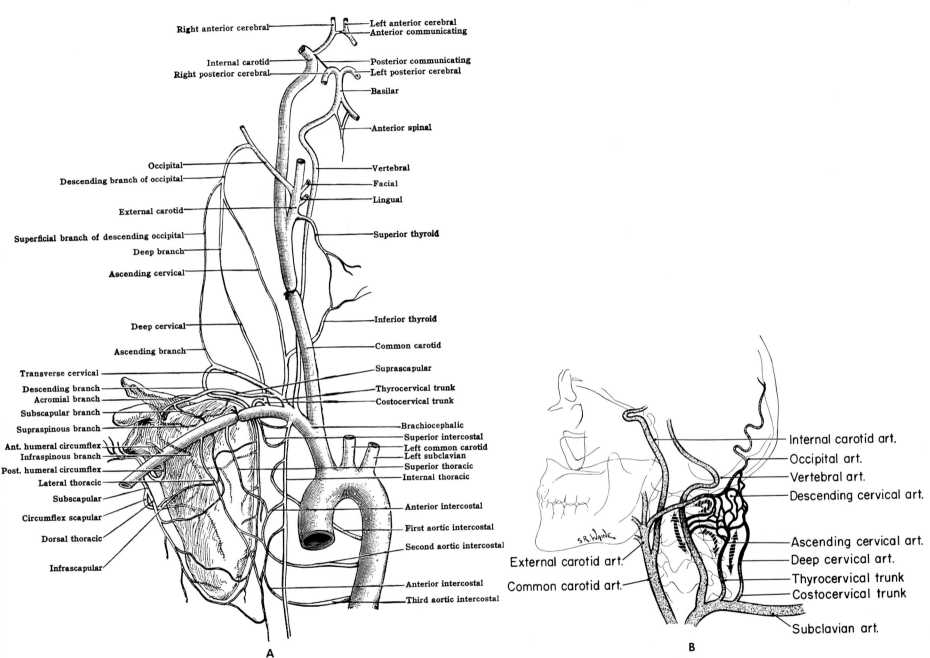

Figure 12–17. Semischematic diagram showing the potential collateral circulation of the common carotid and subclavian arteries. (From Anson, B. J. (ed.): Morris' Human Anatomy, 12th ed. Copyright © 1966 by McGraw-Hill, Inc. Used by permission of McGraw-Hill Book Company.) *B.* The "cervical arterial collateral network" which joins the carotid, subclavian, and vertebral arteries. (From Bosniak, M. A.: Amer. J. Roentgenol., 91:1222, 1964.)

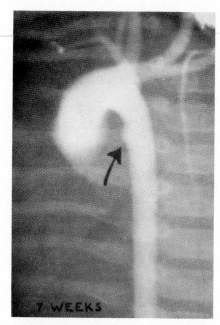

Figure 12–18. Normal aorta. Seven weeks. The aortic arch and its great branches are clearly defined. The silhouette of the arch and the descending aorta resembles an inverted J. A localized bulge at the site of the ligamentum arteriosum (*arrow*) is present. This corresponds to the "ductus diverticulum," or "infundibulum" of the ductus. (From Abrams, H. L.: Angiography, 2nd ed., Vol. 1. Boston, Little, Brown & Co., 1971.)

lobe bronchus and the posterior segmental vein of the right upper lobe at the point at which it is crossed by the anterior segmental artery. The 18.1 mm. measurement is the sum of the diameters of the superior and inferior basal veins of the right lower lobe measured 1 cm. from their junction (Lavendar et al.).

Mean measurements of arterial diameters with standard deviations as related to age and body area in children are given in the adjoining figure (Fig. 12–22).

Various Factors Influencing Cardiac Contour
(Fig. 12–23)

Constitutional Features. The general contour of the chest cavity is closely related to the contours of the organs contained therein. Thus, it has been demonstrated in anatomic sections that the outline of the circumference of the heart is closely related to the form of the circumference of the chest. In a circular chest, the cardiac contour tends to be circular also; in an ovoid chest, it tends to be ovoid.

If one arbitrarily divides the population into three groups—the asthenic or long, slender type, the pyknic or short, stocky type, and the athletic or muscular, well-proportioned group—the following cardiac contours will be characteristic:

In the asthenic group, the mediastinum as a whole is long and narrow, the diaphragm is low, and the cardiac silhouette

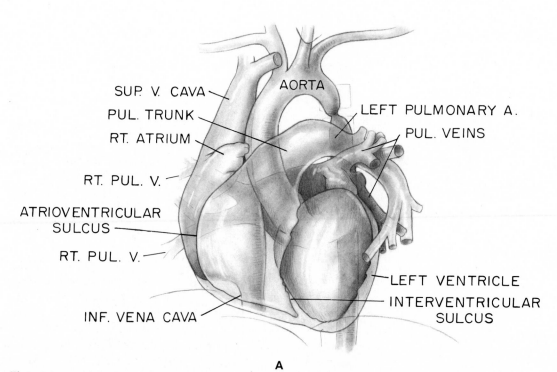

A

Figure 12–19. A. Heart in left anterior oblique projection, rotation 30°, showing the relative positions of the major vessels and the inflow and outflow tracts by translucency of overlying chambers. There is a coarctation of the aorta in its most frequent location.

Figure 12–19 continued on the opposite page.

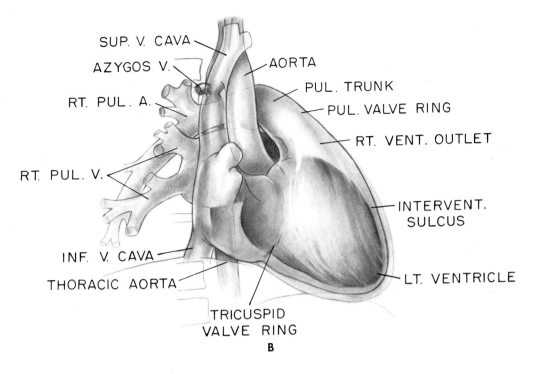

SUP. V. CAVA

AZYGOS V.

RT. PUL. A.

RT. PUL. V.

INF. V. CAVA

THORACIC AORTA

TRICUSPID VALVE RING

AORTA

PUL. TRUNK

PUL. VALVE RING

RT. VENT. OUTLET

INTERVENT. SULCUS

LT. VENTRICLE

B

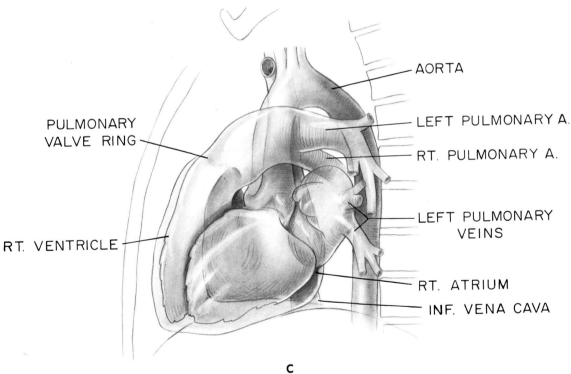

PULMONARY VALVE RING

RT. VENTRICLE

AORTA

LEFT PULMONARY A.

RT. PULMONARY A.

LEFT PULMONARY VEINS

RT. ATRIUM

INF. VENA CAVA

C

Figure 12–19 *Continued.* *B.* Normal heart in right anterior oblique projection, rotation 60°, showing the relationship of inflow and outflow tracts to the chambers of the heart by translucency of the chambers. *C.* Lateral view of a normal heart showing inflow and outflow tracts to the ventricles and atria. (*A–C* modified from Schad, N., et al.: Differential Diagnosis of Congenital Heart Disease. New York, Grune & Stratton, 1966.)

Figure 12–19 continued on the following page.

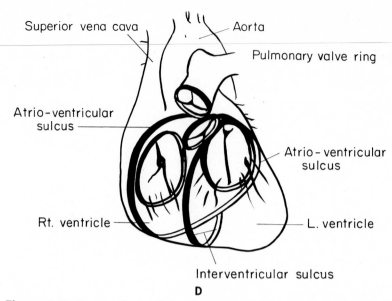

Superior vena cava

Aorta

Pulmonary valve ring

Atrio-ventricular sulcus

Atrio-ventricular sulcus

Rt. ventricle

L. ventricle

Interventricular sulcus

D

Figure 12–19 *Continued. D.* Slight normal left anterior oblique radiograph of the heart showing the relative positions of the pulmonary valve ring, the aortic valve ring, the tricuspid valve ring, and the mitral valve ring, with respect to the aorta, pulmonary artery, and left and right ventricles.

tends to be long, narrow, and rather straight up and down. Only the pulmonic shadow tends to be prominent. Extreme examples of this group are called "pendulous hearts," which indeed is most descriptive.

In the pyknic individual, the mediastinal shadow as a whole tends to be short and wide. The diaphragm is high, and the convexity of all the cardiac contours is marked. The heart appears diminished in height and somewhat boot-shaped, and is pushed upward and transversely by the high diaphragm. This type is indicated as horizontal or transverse.

In the athletic and sthenic individual, heart size tends to be at the upper limits of normal, and cardiac contour approaches the median group type.

Age (Fig. 12–24). Age is an important factor conditioning the relative size and shape of the heart and contiguous mediastinal structures. In younger individuals the cardiac shadow tends to be more globular and to reveal less differentiation than in the adult. In the newborn, the transverse diameter is very long in comparison with the diameter of the chest. The right side of the heart is larger than the left, and the atria and auricular appendages are large in comparison with the ventricles. The right border of the heart is therefore curved and the aortic knob cannot be differentiated.

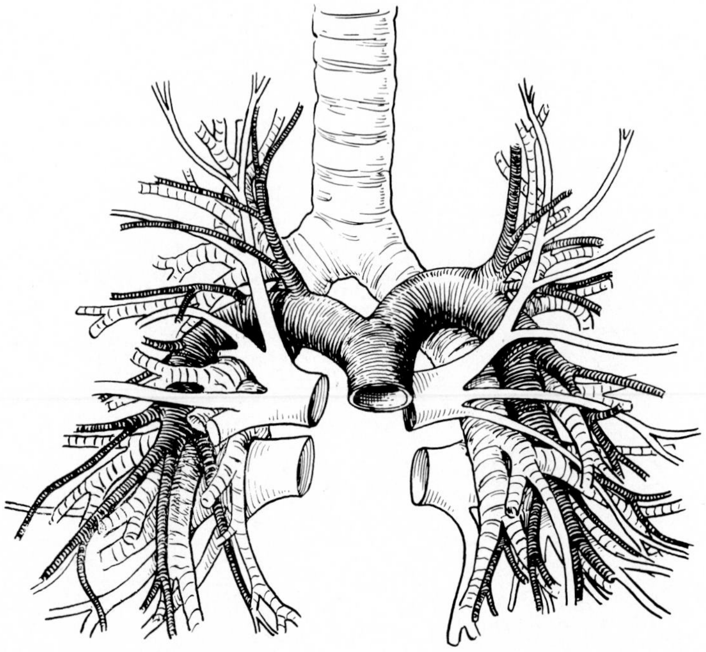

Figure 12–20. Line diagram showing the relationship of the major ramifications of the tracheobronchial tree, pulmonary artery, and pulmonary veins to one another.

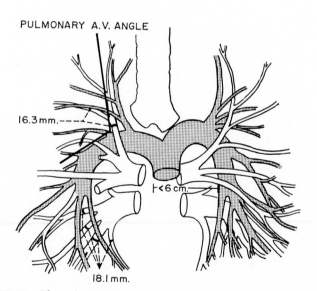

PULMONARY A.V. ANGLE

16.3 mm.

|<6 cm.

18.1 mm.

Figure 12–21. The pulmonary arteriovenous angle, which becomes more obtuse with passive hyperemia of the lungs. Also shown are several measurements which are occasionally quoted in the literature (after Logue et al.). The measurement 16.3 mm. indicates the sum of the diameters of the apical vein of the right upper lobe at the level of the right upper lobe bronchus, and the posterior segmental vein of the right upper lobe at the point at which it is crossed by the anterior segmental artery. The 18.1 mm. is the sum of the diameters of the superior and inferior basal veins of the right lower lobe measured 1 cm. from their junction. (From Lavender, J. P., and Doppman, J.: Brit. J. Radiol., 35:303–313, 1962.)

MEAN MEASUREMENTS OF ARTERIAL DIAMETERS WITH STANDARD DEVIATIONS AS RELATED TO AGE AND BODY AREA

Age (yr.)	Primary Branch			Secondary Branch			Tertiary Branch		
	No.	Mean (mm.)	Standard Deviation (mm.)	No.	Mean (mm.)	Standard Deviation (mm.)	No.	Mean (mm.)	Standard Deviation (mm.)
0– 2	25*	6.1	1.2	25*	2.7	0.9	25	1.5	0.5
2– 4	16	7.3	1.0	16	4.0	0.6	16	2.2	0.4
4– 6	25	8.4	1.0	25	4.3	0.7	25	2.4	0.6
6– 8	49	9.1	1.1	49	4.5	0.7	49	2.5	0.4
8–10	26	9.1	0.7	26	4.7	0.7	26	2.8	0.5
10–12	39	10.0	1.1	39	5.0	1.1	39	3.0	0.5
12–14	28	10.6	1.0	28	5.6	1.1	28	3.0	0.6
Total	208								
Area (m²)									
0.21–0.4	11	5.8	1.0	9	3.1	1.6	11	1.4	0.4
0.41–0.6	9	6.5	1.4	8	3.5	1.1	9	1.8	0.6
0.61–0.8	18	8.3	0.8	18	4.0	0.7	18	2.3	0.5
0.81–1.00	23	9.6	1.2	23	4.8	0.7	23	2.5	0.5
1.01–1.20	17	10.0	1.1	17	5.1	0.7	17	2.8	0.6
1.21–1.40	14	10.3	1.3	14	5.1	0.4	14	3.0	0.7
Total	92								

* Out of 60 normal infant chest roentgenograms only 25 could be measured.

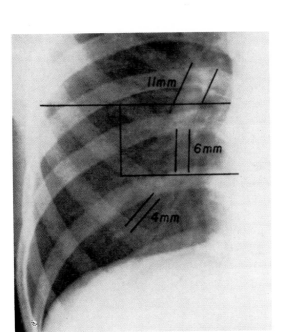

Figure 12–22. Division of the right lower lobe into three areas with the arterial diameters shown in each area. (From Leinbach, L. B.: Amer. J. Roentgenol., 89:996, 1963.)

During the last half of the first year, the long axis of the heart tends to rotate and descend slightly in the thorax, and the thymic shadow begins to regress. A rather definitive cardiac shadow is established between the sixth and the eighth year, but there is a relative prominence of the pulmonary artery (and conus) on the left in the frontal projection that persists in a variable degree throughout adolescence, and does not completely disappear until the early twenties.

As age increases, there is a gradual diminution of the size of the base of the heart and a tendency to increasing prominence of the aortic knob and superior vena cava shadows. The cardiac and retrocardiac structures change their relationships slightly, as shown in Figure 12–25. When arteriosclerosis of the aorta is present, there is usually a tendency toward elongation and redundancy of the entire thoracic aorta, but particularly of the aortic arch.

Cardiac Cycle. The size and shape of the cardiac silhouette varies in accordance with systole and diastole. Cardiac measure-

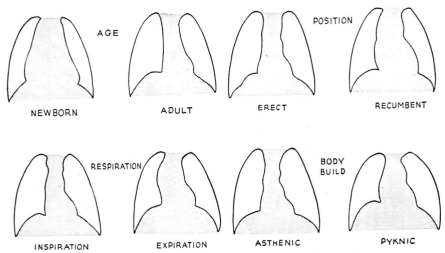

Figure 12–23. Normal factors causing variation in the supracardiac shadow and cardiac contour.

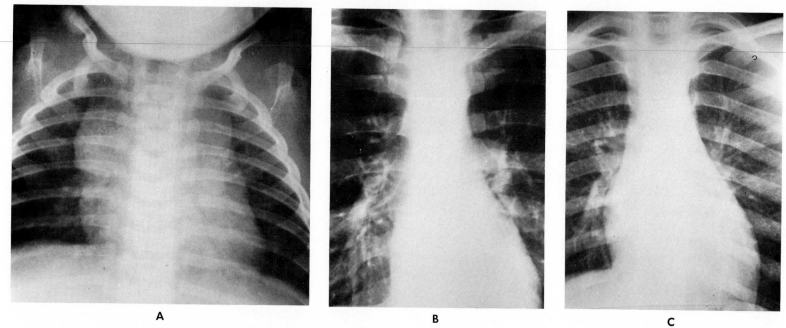

A   B   C

Figure 12–24. Heart and mediastinum in respect to age. *A.* Infant 4 months of age. *B.* Child 6 years of age. *C.* Normal adult, erect inspiration performing a Valsalva maneuver. *D.* Heart, mediastinum, and chest in a patient of asthenic build, showing the heart to be rather pendulous in contour.

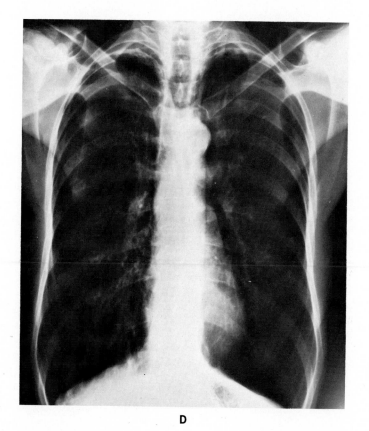

D

ments in systole and diastole were carefully made by Gammill et al., who postulated that maximum and minimum sizes of the heart with respect to the cardiac cycle would be more useful in evaluating cardiac size than the single chest roentgenogram exposed at random during the cardiac cycle. However, 52 per cent of their patients showed changes of 0.3 cm. or less and 41 per cent showed alterations of 0.4 to 0.9 cm. in the two phases of the cardiac cycle. In 7 per cent, the variation was between 1.0 cm. and 1.7 cm. Their patients also showed changes in frontal area as well as in other measurements proposed.

This difference in cardiac size and shape tends to be greater with contraction rates below 60 per minute.

For a most accurate assay, the cardiac configuration and size must be studied in identical phases of the cardiac cycle; when such accuracy is lacking, due allowance must be made for this variable factor.

Body Position (Fig. 12–25). There are quite definite changes in the cardiovascular silhouette in the different positions of the body. The change from the erect to the recumbent position causes a broadening of the cardiac silhouette, particularly at its base. The area of the cardiac shadow increases in proportion to increase in diameter and the broad diameter. These changes are probably secondary to the changes in position of the sternum, ribs, and diaphragm.

In the lateral prone position, the mediastinal structures tend to shift toward the lowermost side with the force of gravity. The lower leaf of the diaphragm ascends and increases its respiratory

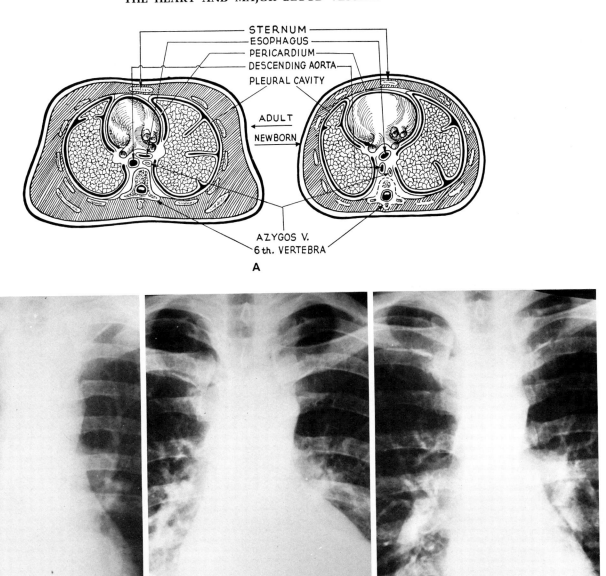

Figure 12–25.   *A.* Differences in infantile and adult posterior mediastinal relationships. (Modified from Caffey.)
B. Heart and mediastinum in a patient supine in full inspiration. *C.* Heart and mediastinum in same patient, erect
during expiration. *D.* Heart and mediastinum in same patient erect in full inspiration and Valsalva maneuver.

excursions, while the uppermost leaf descends. The mediastinal
shadow tends to return to the midline on deep inspiration against
the forces of gravity. This movement with deep inspiration is
greatest in asthenic persons.

Respiration.   During ordinary quiet or tidal respiration, no
significant changes in the cardiac silhouette are noted. However,
with forced inspiration, changes are produced depending upon
whether breathing is predominantly costal or diaphragmatic. In

the diaphragmatic type, there is a slight caudal shift of the heart
that is ordinarily not observed in the costal type of forced inspiration. There is a tendency for the left heart border to move
medially, and the left contour is less curved. The vascular basilar
shadows are elongated. The retrosternal and retrocardiac shadows are increased in radiolucency.

In forced expiration, the cardiac shadow rises and is somewhat displaced to the left. The cardiac base appears wider and

shortened, and the retrosternal and retrocardiac shadows are diminished in radiolucency. When the Valsalva experiment is performed by closing the glottis at the end of full inspiration and forcing expiration, there is a slow decrease in the size of the entire cardiac silhouette, probably related to the increased intrathoracic pressure. A slowing of the heart rate occurs in some, while in others the rate increases.

The position of the diaphragm will affect cardiac size and contour significantly, not only with respect to respiration but also with regard to: (1) abdominal distention or other intraabdominal or subdiaphragmatic disease, (2) unilateral elevation from any cause, and (3) the presence or absence of increased intrathoracic tension.

Valsalva Maneuver. If the glottis is closed after deep inspiration and positive pressure is maintained against the closed glottis, cardiac size gradually diminishes for several cardiac cycles. This is called a "positive pressure study" and has been suggested as a means of differentiating compressible vascular structures from noncompressible mass lesions in the chest (Whitley and Martin; see Chapter 10).

Thoracic Deformities. Thoracic deformities alter the position of the heart as well as its size and contour. For example, dorsal lordosis, funnel chest, or pectus excavatum may produce a rotation of the heart toward the left or a flattened appearance with displacement posteriorly; kyphoscoliosis produces a rotation of the heart toward the side opposite the scoliosis.

Intrathoracic Pulmonary or Pleural Pathologic Processes. These very often affect cardiac size and contour.

Pregnancy (Fig. 12–26). In pregnancy the diaphragm is elevated and hypervolemia occurs, with a tendency toward increased cardiac size. The lungs show an increased vascularity, caused by engorgement of the breasts that imparts an increased haziness to both lung bases.

Microcardia. The heart may be small (microcardia) in association with malnutrition from any cause. A "microcardia" has been reported in patients with widespread carcinomatosis, lymphoma, ulcerative colitis, scleroderma, hepatoma, and anorexia nervosa (Altemus).

BASIC RADIOLOGIC METHODS OF CARDIAC STUDY

Role of Radiologic Examination of the Heart. It is important first to consider the part that the radiologic examination plays in the total clinical examination of the heart. Our basic physical diagnostic armamentarium consists of *inspection* to determine normal and abnormal pulsations, vascular distention, and cyanosis; *percussion* to determine mediastinal size; *palpation* to verify further facts noted above as well as the detection of palpable thrills; and *auscultation* for study of cardiac and mediastinal sounds.

The radiographic examination of the heart gives more accu-

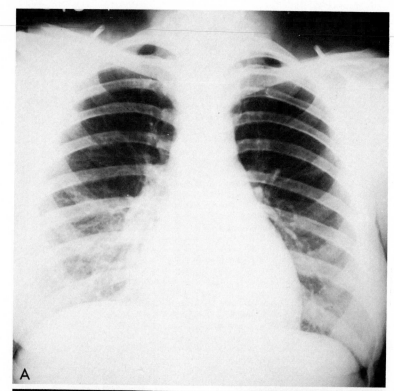

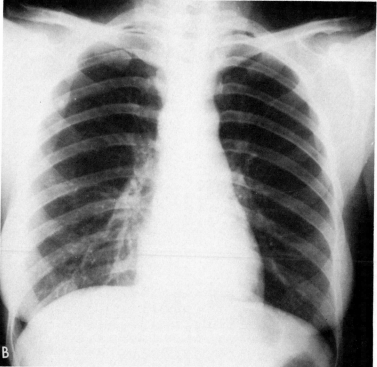

Figure 12–26. Posteroanterior views of the chest showing changes in heart size and lung appearance as the result of pregnancy. *A*. Near term pregnancy. *B*. Approximately 1 year after delivery.

rate data regarding cardiac size, contour, and pulsations than any of the above methods, *but it can never be a substitute for auscultation, for the determination of palpable thrills, and for the detection of cyanosis.* Thus the cardiac roentgenologic examination is a very useful adjunct in the total examination but it must not be regarded as independent of all other means of study.

Radiologic Methods Used in the Roentgen Cardiac Examination

1. **The Posteroanterior (PA) Teleroentgenograms of the Chest** (6 foot target-to-film distance), preferably with barium outlining the esophagus (Fig. 12–27).

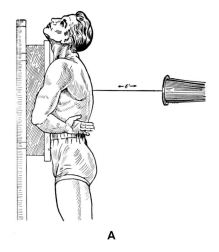

A

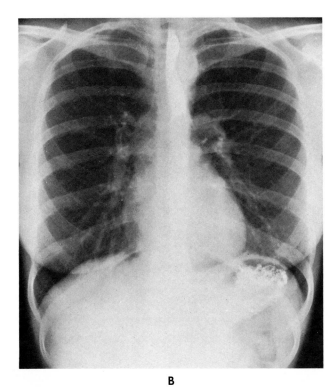

B

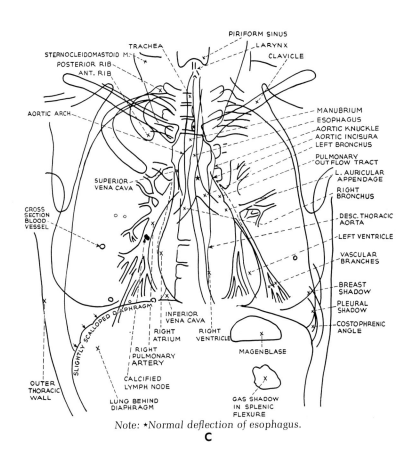

Note: *Normal deflection of esophagus.

C

Figure 12–27 Cardiac esophagram, posteroanterior projection. *A.* Position of patient. *B.* Radiograph (female). *C.* Labeled tracing of *B.*

Points of Practical Interest With Reference to Figure 12–27

1. The exact course of the esophagus in this projection is noteworthy. At the base of the neck there is a slight deflection toward the left so that the esophageal projection falls behind the left sternoclavicular joint in a perfectly centered film. Thereafter it courses to the right at the level of the transverse portion of the arch of the aorta. From this position, there is a slight gradual deflection toward the left so that the diaphragm is penetrated to the left of the midline. An enlargement in any of the contiguous structures will alter this course perceptibly.
2. It is also important to trace the aortic shadow as it courses to the left of the middle, with its left margin ordinarily separate and distinct from the paraspinous shadow. This is a straight line normally below the level of the arch of the aorta; abnormally, it becomes convex, or S-shaped with elongation of the aorta.
3. The position of the "left" ventricular apex with reference to the left hemidiaphragm is important. This portion of the cardiac silhouette is not always due to the left ventricle, but may be related to the right ventricle, particularly in congenital heart disease.

2. **The Left and Right Anterior Oblique Films of the Chest,** also with barium outlining the esophagus, and usually following fluoroscopy (Figs. 12–28 and 12–29).

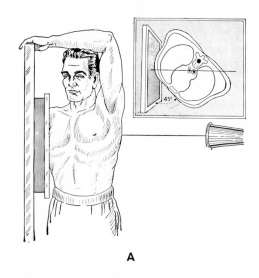

A

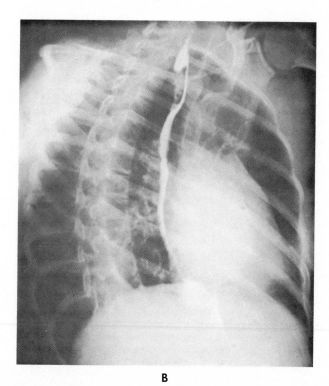

B

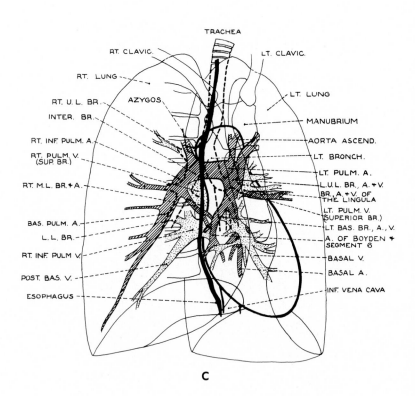

C

Figure 12–28.   Cardiac esophagram, right anterior oblique projection. (There is a minimal enlargement of the left atrium in this case, purposely chosen to show its position.) *A.* Position of patient. *B.* Radiograph. *C.* Labeled tracing of *B.*

Points of Practical Interest With Reference to Figure 12–28

1. The relative convexity of the pulmonary sector is noteworthy. This area becomes concave in many (but not all) cases of pulmonic or infundibular stenosis; or it may increase in prominence with dilatation of the pulmonary artery.

2. When the heart enlarges diffusely, the esophagus is often displaced posteriorly —but this type of displacement is not sharply localized to the region of the left atrium. For this reason, the region of the left atrium as it impinges on the esophagus must be known accurately by the student. Once this is established, the differential diagnosis becomes less difficult.

3. Air shadows in the esophagus may produce some confusion in interpretation. These are frequent and normal, except possibly when excessive.

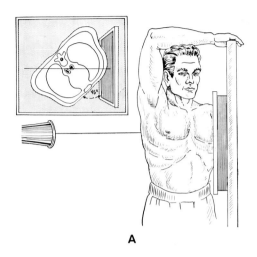

A

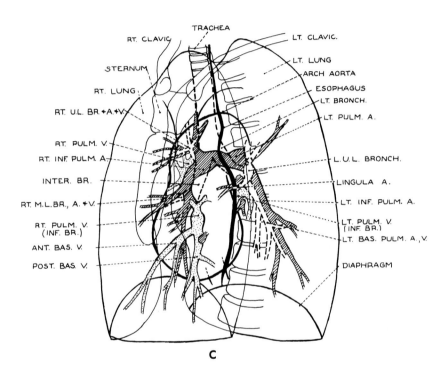

C

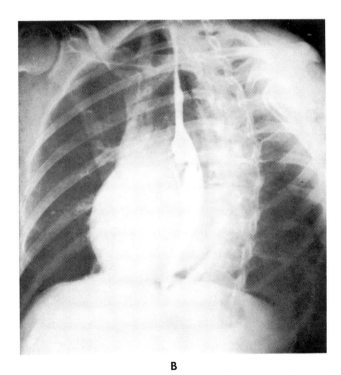

B

Figure 12-29. Cardiac esophagram, left anterior oblique projection. *A.* Position of patient. *B.* Radiograph. *C.* Labeled tracing of *B.*

Points of Practical Interest With Reference to Figure 12-29

1. The student should learn to identify the following anatomic areas of the cardiac silhouette particularly, in this view: right and left ventricle; arch of aorta; left atrium; and the position of the aortic and mitral valves. The relative prominence of each of these areas should be noted.

2. The trachea and its bifurcation can be clearly identified in this projection. Position and contour description will help detect such abnormalities as narrowness, deflection, compression, and filling defects.

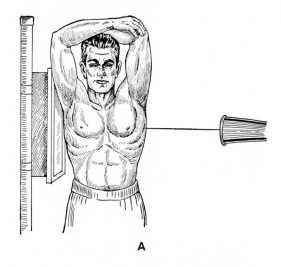

A

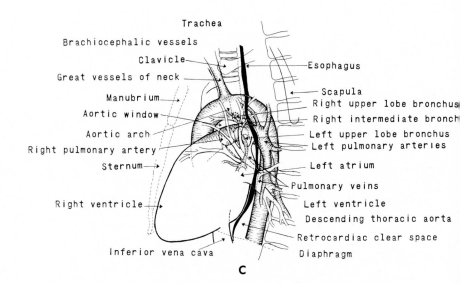

Trachea
Brachiocephalic vessels
Clavicle
Great vessels of neck
Manubrium
Aortic window
Aortic arch
Right pulmonary artery
Sternum
Right ventricle
Inferior vena cava

Esophagus
Scapula
Right upper lobe bronchus
Right intermediate bronch
Left upper lobe bronchus
Left pulmonary arteries
Left atrium
Pulmonary veins
Left ventricle
Descending thoracic aorta
Retrocardiac clear space
Diaphragm

C

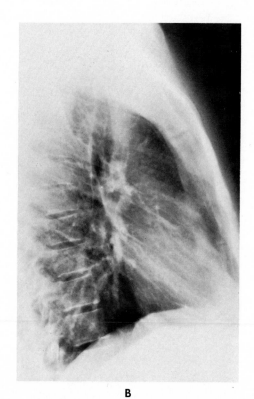

B

Figure 12–30. Lateral view of the chest with barium in the esophagus. *A.* Position of patient. *B.* Radiograph. *C.* Labeled tracing of *B.*

Points of Practical Interest With Reference to Figure 12–30

1. The following areas are of particular interest and value for identification:
   (a) The relationship of the right ventricle to the posterior margin of the sternum. With enlargement of the right ventricle, its shadow "rises" higher on the sternum.
   (b) The degree of clarity of the anterior mediastinal clear space.
   (c) The relationship of the left ventricle posteriorly to the shadow of the inferior vena cava. This will allow early and accurate detection of enlargement of the left ventricle.
   (d) The relationship of the esophagus to the left atrium.
   (e) The relative prominence of the pulmonary arteries. This requires considerable experience, but is very valuable from the standpoint of detecting abnormalities of lymph node origin, or tumor masses.

3. **A Lateral Film of the Chest with Esophagram** (Fig. 12–30).

4. **A PA or AP Teleroentgenogram of the Chest in the Recumbent Position** for comparison with the erect film, if pericardial fluid is suspected (Fig. 12–31). Other special procedures such as kymography, angiocardiography, cardiac catheterization, orthodiagraphy, and retrograde aortography are considered outside the scope of this text.

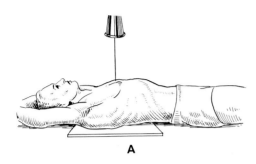

A

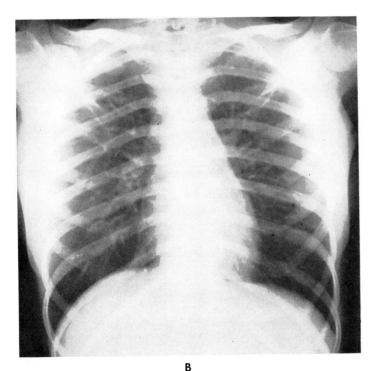

B

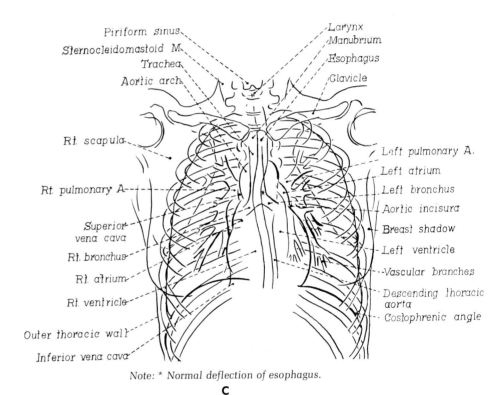

*Note: * Normal deflection of esophagus.*

C

Figure 12–31. Anteroposterior recumbent study of chest. *A.* Position of patient. *B.* Radiograph. *C.* Labeled tracing of *B.*

Points of Practical Interest With Reference to Figure 12–31

1. Although it is difficult to obtain a view of the upper lung fields in this projection because of the shadows of the scapulae, considerable improvement will result if the patient crosses his arms above his head, thus rotating the scapulae outward.

2. The clavicles, on the other hand, are projected above the lung apices sufficiently so that this area of the lungs may be more clearly shown.

3. The analysis of the cardiac silhouette is not as favorable in this projection in the adult, because of the straightening of the left margin and broadening of the base.

5. **Fluoroscopy.** Fluoroscopy with image amplification should precede the film studies. The following outline is recommended.

The Heart and Mediastinal Structures are Studied in the Frontal Projection. (1) The pulsations along the left cardiac border are investigated and the radiologist proceeds around the periphery of the mediastinum, studying carefully the pulsations of the pulmonary arteries, aorta, and right atrium. (2) The cardiac position is carefully noted, both in inspiration and expiration, and changes with respiration are detected.

The Patient is Thereafter Turned in the Right Anterior Oblique Position. (1) Once again the cardiac contour and pulsations are carefully noted. The pulsations in the apex of the left ventricle are particularly important, since this area is prone to suffer from coronary vascular impairment. (2) The pulmonary outflow tract is observed, since this projection is particularly suited for this purpose. (3) The anterior margin of the ascending aorta is then studied. (4) Thereafter the posterior mediastinal space is viewed. Normally this space is clear, because it is occupied by structures of lesser opacity such as the esophagus, aorta, and veins. The prominence of the left atrium in relation to the posterior mediastinum is particularly noteworthy. Its relationship to the esophagus (barium-filled) is particularly important.

The Patient is Then Turned in the Left Anterior Oblique Position. (1) In this position the posterior basilar portion of the left ventricle is studied. The pulsations here are usually of greater amplitude than elsewhere. Some concept of left ventricular size can be obtained from the fact that in the 45 degree obliquity the left ventricle normally clears the spine. (2) The anterior margin of the heart in this projection is formed by the right ventricle usually. A fairly straight line is formed by the anterior margin of the right ventricle and the ascending aorta in this projection. Any unusual convexities, either in the right ventricle or in the ascending aorta, are of pathologic significance. (3) This position affords the most accurate means of studying the arch of the aorta in relation to the left pulmonary artery, which lies beneath it. There is ordinarily a clear space known as the "aortic window" between the aortic arch and the pulmonary artery. Any enlargement of a contiguous structure will cause its obliteration.

Size of Fluoroscopic Field. By carefully restricting the size of the fluoroscopic field, the cardiac shadow is surveyed for any areas of calcification and hyperlucency. (1) Care must be exercised to insure that the calcification is projected within the heart in every view and pulsates synchronously with the heart, since calcified mediastinal lymph nodes can cause occasional confusion. (2) The heart normally does not contain calcification, but the following cardiopericardial structures may contain calcium abnormally (Fig. 12–32): (a) the pericardium, (b) the coronary vessels, (c) the myocardium, (d) the endocardium, (e) the papil-

lary muscles, (f) the cardiac valves (Fig. 12–33), and (g) the rings at the base of the cardiac valves and the aortic sinus of Valsalva.

The position of the cardiac valves in various projections is indicated in Figure 12–33. Calcified valves may be differentiated by their characteristic "dance," which is synchronous with the cardiac pulsations. The motion is jerky and steplike.

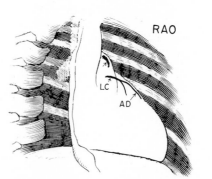

CALCIFIED LEFT CORONARY A.   CALCIFIED LEFT CORONARY A.

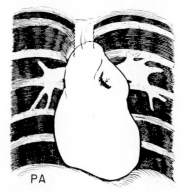

CALCIFIED PATENT DUCTUS

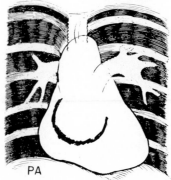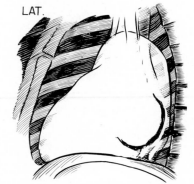

CALCIFIED LEFT ATRIUM   CALCIFIED LEFT ATRIUM

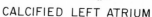

A

Figure 12–32. *A, B,* and *C.* Cardiopericardial structures which may contain calcium as depicted radiographically.

Figure 12–32 continued on the opposite page.

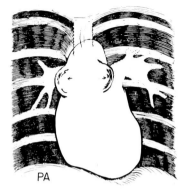

CALCIFIED SINUS OF VALSALVA
ANEURYSM

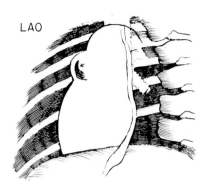

CALCIFIED SINUS OF VALSALVA

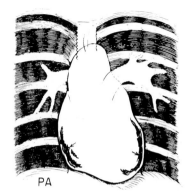

CALCIFIED PERICARDIUM

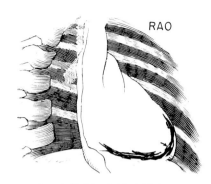

CALCIFIED PERICARDIUM
WITH CONSTRICTIVE PERICARDITIS

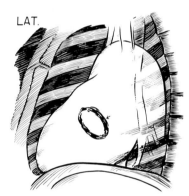

CALCIFIED MITRAL RING

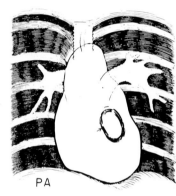

CALCIFIED MITRAL RING

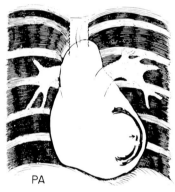

CALCIFIED
MYOCARDIAL INFARCT

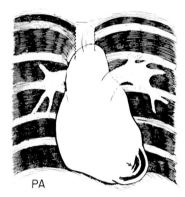

CALCIFIED
LEFT VENTRICULAR ANEURYSM

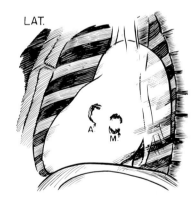

CALCIFIED MITRAL VALVE
CALCIFIED AORTIC VALVE

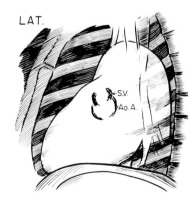

CALCIFIED SINUS OF VALSALVA
CALCIFIED AORTIC ANNULUS

B

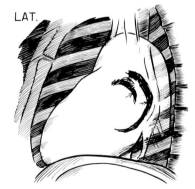

CALCIFIED LEFT ATRIUM
WITH CALCIFIED THROMBUS

C

Figure 12–32 Continued.

PROJECTION OF CARDIAC VALVES
IN ROUTINE POSITIONS IN RADIOGRAPHY

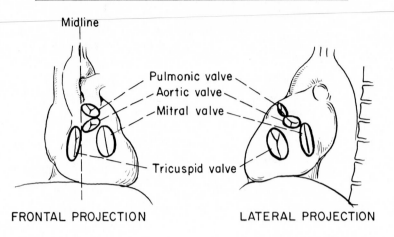

Midline

Pulmonic valve
Aortic valve
Mitral valve

Tricuspid valve

FRONTAL PROJECTION   LATERAL PROJECTION

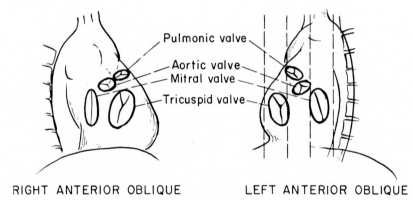

Pulmonic valve

Aortic valve
Mitral valve
Tricuspid valve

RIGHT ANTERIOR OBLIQUE   LEFT ANTERIOR OBLIQUE

Figure 12–33.

Aortic sinus of Valsalva calcification is best seen in the lateral view. It is identified by its calcified origin near the left coronary artery and is projected near the anterior wall of the ascending aorta into the base of the heart. The appearance resembles a parentheses when there are two portions calcified, or a comma when only one is calcified.

The motion as visualized cinefluoroscopically conforms to the pulsation of the ascending aorta, and the calcification is contiguous with the ascending aorta in all projections (Levitan and Reilly).

Fluoroscopy with image amplification and cineradiography has proved to be of great value in the detection of cardiac or intracardiac calcifications, even when the more conventional procedures fail.

(3) *Under image amplification, the epicardial fat can often be seen. Pericardial effusion* outside this fat layer may thereby

often be differentiated from other causes of cardiopericardial enlargement.

A barium swallow should always be part of the fluoroscopic and radiographic study of the heart, with good delineation of the esophagus in all projections. Since the esophagus is so closely applied to the descending aorta on the one hand and the posterior cardiac structures on the other, changes in the course of the esophagus are of considerable value in the interpretation of cardiovascular and aortic anatomy.

The patient is then lowered into a recumbent position and a study of the mediastinum is repeated as described earlier in the frontal and oblique projections, noting carefully the changes that occur with change in body position.

The cardiac valves in the living person are farther to the right and nearer to the midline than might be expected from anatomic textbooks which are based upon cadaver studies. Moreover, since calcified valves are themselves pathologic and are frequently associated with cardiac hypertrophy and dilatation, a study of cardiac valves in such subjects can hardly be compared with normal studies on human cadavers.

The demonstration on roentgenograms requires a very small focal spot, extremely rapid exposure, and coning down over the valve area in the proper degree of obliquity as determined fluoroscopically.

PLAIN FILM ROUTINE STUDIES OF HEART (USING BARIUM IN THE ESOPHAGUS)

1. **The 6 Foot Posteroanterior View of the Heart with Barium in the Esophagus.** The various parts demonstrated in silhouette along the right margin of the central mediastinal shadow are as follows (Fig. 12–27): the inferior vena cava, in the right cardiophrenic angle; the right atrium, forming the major portion of the right cardiac shadow; the ascending portion of the arch of the aorta; and the superior vena cava, extending above and to the right of the latter. The anatomic parts contributing to the left side of the shadow are as follows (from above downward): the aortic knob, which forms a knucklelike shadow superiorly; the aortic incisura, which is the notch between the aortic knob and the pulmonary artery below it; the left auricular appendage, which may protrude very slightly below the pulmonary artery; and the large sweeping convex shadow below this, which extends down to the diaphragm. There is frequently a less dense shadow in the vicinity of the left ventricular apex caused by the pericardial fat pad, which has a triangular appearance and should not enter into the computation of the cardiac size.

The esophagus after it descends into the thorax lies in close proximity with the aorta. It has various impressions upon it, and the uppermost indentation is that produced by the arch of the aorta, which displaces the esophagus to the right and posteriorly.

Normally, in this projection, the esophagus descends straight downward, and any deviation is significant from the standpoint of cardiac chamber enlargement. A study of the esophagus in this view is therefore of value in detection of such abnormalities as rightsided aorta, left atrial enlargement, and abnormalities of the descending thoracic aorta.

This 6 foot film of the heart is also called a teleroentgenogram and is obtained for evaluation of cardiac size and contour in the posteroanterior projection. Actually, this is usually the routine chest film obtained in most clinics. As indicated in Chapter 1, distortion and magnification are two major problems in radiography that to a great extent can be obviated if a long film-to-target distance is utilized. The degree of magnification and distortion will vary in accordance with the relative distances of the anatomic part and the tube target from the film. A 6 foot film-to-target distance has been found to be practicable, and for all ordinary adult chests the magnification is no greater than 5 to 10 per cent. Since this study is usually combined with a study of the lung fields, an extremely short exposure is employed, about one-tenth to one-twentieth of a second (or even less). A short exposure of this type will usually portray the heart in some phase between systole and diastole, and hence allowance must be made for such differences as may occur in the various phases of the cardiac cycle, which may be 1 cm. or more. The cardiac size will also vary somewhat in the different phases of respiration, being smallest in deep sustained inspiration.

The pericardium, which invests the entire heart and is attached to the diaphragm below and the base of the major vessels above, ordinarily does not cast a shadow of its own, and is normally not distinguishable.

2. **The Right Anterior Oblique View with Esophagram.** In this position the patient is rotated so that his right side is in contact with the cassette, and he is rotated away from the cassette approximately 45 degrees (Fig. 12–28). The esophagus occupies the space between the descending aorta and the posterior margin of the cardiac shadow, and there is a slight undulation of the esophagus produced by the impression of certain structures upon it. We depend upon the esophagus to delineate most accurately the retrocardiac structures. The uppermost impression upon the esophagus after it enters the thorax is that produced by the arch of the aorta as it displaces the esophagus to the right and posteriorly. Just below this indentation, another slight posterior impression is frequently produced by the left atrium. This impression is virtually absent normally, and an impression beyond a minimal degree (such as is illustrated in Fig. 12–28) is indicative of left atrial enlargement, a most significant finding. The right atrium forms the lowermost slight convexity in the cardiac outline posteriorly in this projection.

The retrocardiac space is ordinarily fairly large, and when encroached upon is likewise an indication of abnormality.

The descending thoracic aorta overlaps the anterior margin

of the thoracic spine in its descent, and, significantly, the esophagus descends in practically the same sheath as the aorta. Elongation and tortuosity of the aorta therefore have a definite bearing on the appearance of the esophagus.

The trachea and left bronchus can be identified as a straight air shadow above the shadow of the left atrium, and just above the left atrium, the pulmonary artery can usually be seen as a circular opaque shadow (seen end-on).

Between the left atrial impression and that of the aorta, there is frequently a lesser impression produced by the bronchial bifurcation.

The anterior border of this central mediastinal shadow permits delineation of the following structures: the ascending portion of the arch of the aorta seen superiorly; usually a small notch between this shadow and that of the pulmonary conus, which has a slight anterior convexity; seen below this shadow is that of the left ventricle or right ventricle depending upon the degree of rotation of the patient. This view forms a valuable one for visualization of the anterior apical area of the left ventricle (frequently involved by infarction) and the main pulmonary artery (frequently involved in congenital heart disease).

3. **The Left Anterior Oblique View with Barium in the Esophagus.** In this position, the patient is rotated 45 degrees with the left anterior shoulder against the cassette (Fig. 12–29). When sufficiently rotated, the left ventricle just barely clears the anterior margin of the thoracic spine. This is the posterior basilar portion of the left ventricle. Above this lies the left atrium. The arch of the aorta is seen in its entirety. The anterior margin of the silhouette is formed inferiorly by the right ventricle (this is the only view in which the right ventricle is adequately and definitely seen), and above this by the right atrium. The tracheal bifurcation is seen very clearly in this projection. The left pulmonary artery is seen in the clear space above the left atrium, and that portion beneath the arch of the aorta is known as the aortic window.

The aortic triangle is frequently identified above the arch of the aorta, bounded by the arch of the aorta below, the dorsal spine posteriorly, and the left subclavian artery anteriorly. The latter can be faintly identified branching from the aortic arch.

In this projection, the esophagus is normally not diverted from a relatively straight course. Deviations, if they occur, are of pathologic significance.

4. **The Anteroposterior Recumbent Study of the Cardiopericardial Shadow** (Fig. 12–31). There is a normal change in shape of the cardiopericardial shadow that accompanies a change in posture from the erect to the recumbent position. This has been previously described and is due to the upward shift of the diaphragm. In the presence of fluid in the pericardial space in excess of about 300 cc., this change in shape becomes most pronounced when the pericardial fluid shifts from the lower portion of the space to the base of the heart. This produces a marked widening of the base of the heart.

These recumbent studies are also sometimes necessary if the patient cannot stand erect.

In any case, the film-target distance should be carefully stated so that adjustment can be made for distortion and magnification. (The method of determination of magnification will be described in conjunction with pelvicephalometry in Chapter 17.)

5. **The Lateral View of the Chest with Barium in the Esophagus** (Fig. 12–30). The lateral view of the chest with barium in the esophagus is a valuable adjunct in the study of the heart, particularly in the following circumstances:

(a) It allows the radiologist another perspective for study of the relationship of the esophagus to the left atrium. The course of the esophagus is normally straight. Indentation in the region of the left atrium is usually an indication of enlargement of this chamber.

(b) The right ventricle is seen in silhouette anteriorly, and when enlarged encroaches upon the anterior mediastinal clear space. The right ventricle in this perspective usually forms a smooth convexity anteriorly from its junction with the shadow of the aorta, gradually meeting the anterior chest wall in the vicinity of the xiphoid process of the sternum inferiorly. Its junction

with the chest wall above this level is usually an indication of chamber enlargement. This is particularly true in congenital heart disease.

(c) The pulmonary arteries form an ovoid structure identifiable below the arch of the aorta. These can be evaluated for size and differentiated from other mediastinal structures that may on occasion be enlarged, such as mediastinal lymph nodes.

(d) The ascending portion of the aorta and arch of the aorta can be fully evaluated as to size and contour.

(e) The relationship of the left ventricle posteriorly projected over the shadow of the inferior vena cava shadow is of importance in evaluating the size of the left ventricle (Fig. 12–34). Ordinarily the shadow of the inferior vena cava is seen about 5 to 18 mm. behind that of the adjoining left ventricular shadow. With enlargement of the latter chamber, particularly in association with mitral insufficiency, the left ventricle protrudes beyond 18 mm. posteriorly. Such enlargement of the left ventricle is not apt to occur with relatively pure mitral stenosis.

(f) In attempting differentiation of diffuse cardiac enlargement from pericardial effusion, a careful study of the pulsations of the heart *posteriorly* in this projection may be very helpful. These

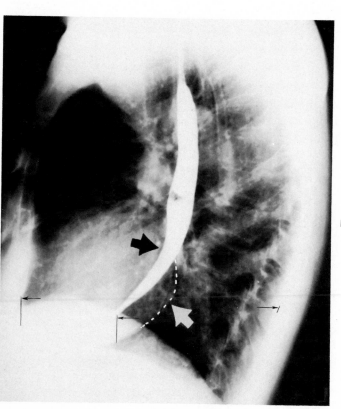

LV   Left ventricle
IVC   Inferior vena cava
LD   Left hemidiaphragm
RD   Right hemidiaphragm

A

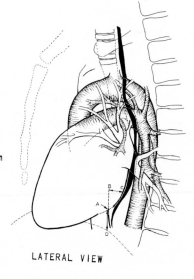

LATERAL VIEW

Eyler et al.:Radiology 73:56,1959.
   Mitral insuff. A > 15 mm.
   Mitral stenosis A < 15 mm.
Keats and Rudhe:Radiology 83:616,
               1964.
   Atrial secundum defect
     IVC partially
       free of heart shadow.
   Ventricular septal defect
     IVC is over mass of
       heart with large shunt.

Point A = crossing of inferior
        vena cava & left ventricle.

Point B is 2 cm.cephalad to A.
Line BC parallels plane of
     dorsal vertebrae.
Line AD is vertical distance to
     left hemidiaphragm.
Left ventricular enlargement
     Present when BC >18 mm.
Left ventricular hypertrophy
     Suspect when AD < 0.75 cm.

B

Figure 12–34. A and B. Important measurements on lateral view of the heart.

may be more accurately ascertained with the aid of kymograms. With pericardial effusion, pulsations in this area are usually completely lacking, whereas with diffuse cardiac enlargement some degree of pulsation is usually manifest here.

DETERMINATION OF CARDIAC ENLARGEMENT (Fig. 12–35)

Definition of the "Normal" Sized Heart. It can be assumed that the majority of a large population is normal, and the problem of determining the "normal" sized heart on a radiograph becomes one of correlating various cardiac measurements with any other bodily factors that allow a high statistical correlation in the majority of the population. In statistical terms, this is called a "high correlation coefficient." It is thus possible to determine how many chances (per hundred) the individual heart has of being within normal limits. In the individual case, this statistical approach

may cause inaccuracy, but in the consideration of a large group it is a satisfactory means of assay. *We must be cognizant of the fact that the boundary between the normal and the abnormal is an arbitrary one, based upon statistical correlation alone.*

Introduction. Increase in cardiac size is the most consistent indication of cardiac disease. Cardiac mensuration is an accurate method for determination of cardiac enlargement; correlation with actual cardiac weight, however, is not very satisfactory, since the element of dilatation in respect to enlargement cannot be accurately evaluated separately from cardiac hypertrophy.

Greatest accuracy and best correlation is obtained by the determination of relative cardiac volume. Ungerleider and Gubner's frontal area method is also included for reference.

Measurements are made directly on teleroentgenograms of the chest obtained in suspended respiration at a 6 foot target-to-film distance. The cardiac image is magnified to approximately 5 per cent. The most frequent and useful measurements obtained from the teleroentgenograms are (Fig. 12–36):

(Text continued on page 729.)

CARDIAC MENSURATION

1. UNGERLEIDER AND GUBNER NOMOGRAM METHOD
(FOR INDIVIDUALS 56–80" HT; 95–300# WT.)

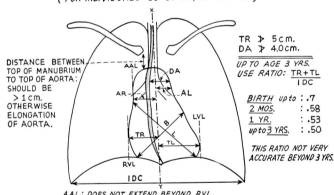

DISTANCE BETWEEN TOP OF MANUBRIUM TO TOP OF AORTA: SHOULD BE >1 cm. OTHERWISE ELONGATION OF AORTA.

TR ≯ 5 cm.
DA ≯ 4.0 cm.

UP TO AGE 3 YRS.
USE RATIO: $\dfrac{TR+TL}{IDC}$

BIRTH up to	: .7
2 MOS.	: .58
1 YR.	: .53
up to 3 YRS.	: .50

THIS RATIO NOT VERY ACCURATE BEYOND 3 YRS.

A AL : DOES NOT EXTEND BEYOND RVL.
RVL : DOES NOT EXTEND BEYOND MEDIAL 1/3 of DIAPHRAGM.
LVL : DOES NOT EXTEND BEYOND MEDIAL 1/2 of DIAPHRAGM.

1. $A = \frac{\pi}{4} L \times B = .7854 \times L \times B$
2. GREATEST TRANSVERSE DIAMETER (GTD) OF HEART: TR + TL
3. COMPARE MEASURED AND CALCULATED VALUES FOR A and GTD WITH VALUES ANTICIPATED FROM BODY HEIGHT AND WEIGHT. NORMAL RANGE IS VALUE ANTICIPATED ± 10%
4. MEASURED AORTIC VALUE : AR + AL
   ANTICIPATED AORTIC VALUE :

CHART VALUE	
−1 mm. For each 3 YRS. < 43 YRS.	+ 1 mm. For each 3 YRS. > 43 YRS.

2. USE SIMILAR MEYER'S TABLES FOR CHILDREN 3–16 YRS. OF AGE EXCEPT A = .68 × L × B.

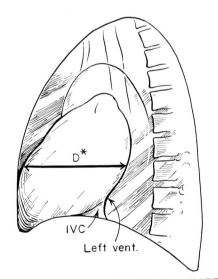

LATERAL VIEW OF NORMAL HEART

*D = Greatest anterior-posterior measurement of heart

A

Figure 12–35. *A. Left,* Cardiac mensuration by the Ungerleider and Gubner technique. *Right,* lateral view of the normal heart showing the method of obtaining D, the greatest anteroposterior measurement of the heart in calculation of cardiac volume.

Figure 12–35 continued on the following page.

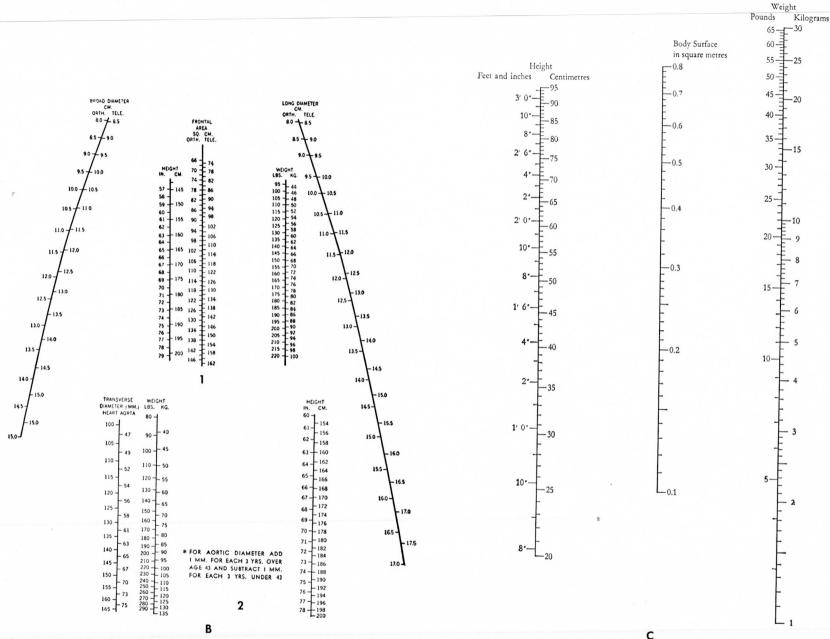

Figure 12-35 *Continued. B.* (1) Nomogram showing the frontal area of the heart predicted from height and weight, and actual area obtained from the measured long and broad diameters (for both orthodiagrams and tele-rentgenograms). Values exceeding 10 per cent above predicted values are abnormal. (2) Nomogram showing the predicted transverse diameter from height and weight, and diameter of the aorta. For the aortic diameter add 1 mm. for each 3 years over age 43 and subtract 1 mm. for each 3 years under 43.

Figure 12-35 continued on the opposite page.

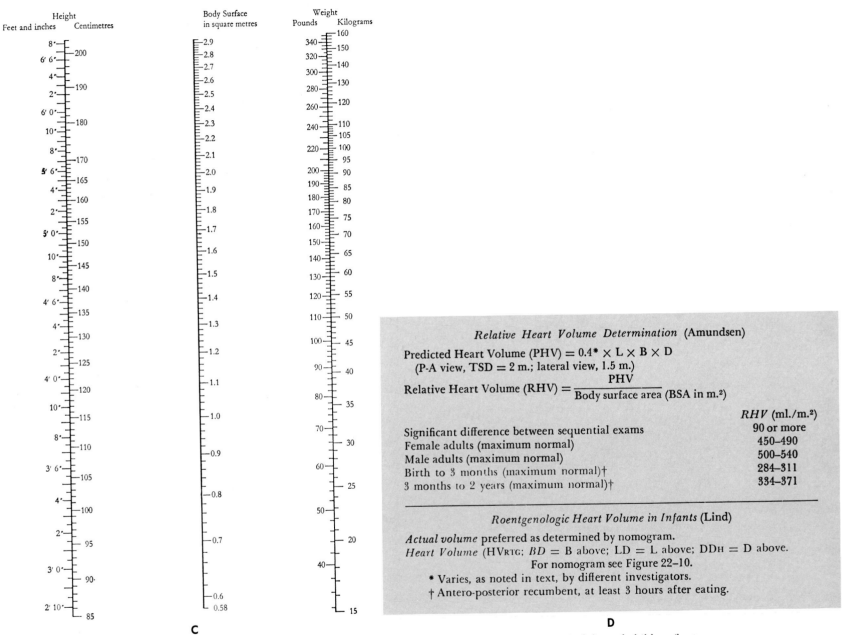

Height
Feet and inches   Centimetres

Body Surface
in square metres

Weight
Pounds   Kilograms

Relative Heart Volume Determination (Amundsen)

Predicted Heart Volume (PHV) = 0.4* × L × B × D
(P-A view, TSD = 2 m.; lateral view, 1.5 m.)

$$\text{Relative Heart Volume (RHV)} = \frac{\text{PHV}}{\text{Body surface area (BSA in m.}^2)}$$

	RHV (ml./m.²)
Significant difference between sequential exams	90 or more
Female adults (maximum normal)	450–490
Male adults (maximum normal)	500–540
Birth to 3 months (maximum normal)†	284–311
3 months to 2 years (maximum normal)†	334–371

Roentgenologic Heart Volume in Infants (Lind)

Actual volume preferred as determined by nomogram.
Heart Volume (HVRTG; *BD* = B above; LD = L above; DDH = D above.
For nomogram see Figure 22–10.
* Varies, as noted in text, by different investigators.
† Antero-posterior recumbent, at least 3 hours after eating.

C   D

Figure 12–35 *Continued.* C. Nomogram for the determination of body surface area of adults and children (by Du Bois). *Key:* The body surface area is given by the point of intersection with the middle scale of a straight line joining height and weight. *D.* Summary of concepts of relative heart volume determination and roentgenologic heart volume in infants according to Amundsen and Lind respectively. Mannheimer's values for children are presented in Table 12–1.

Figure 12–35 continued on the following page.

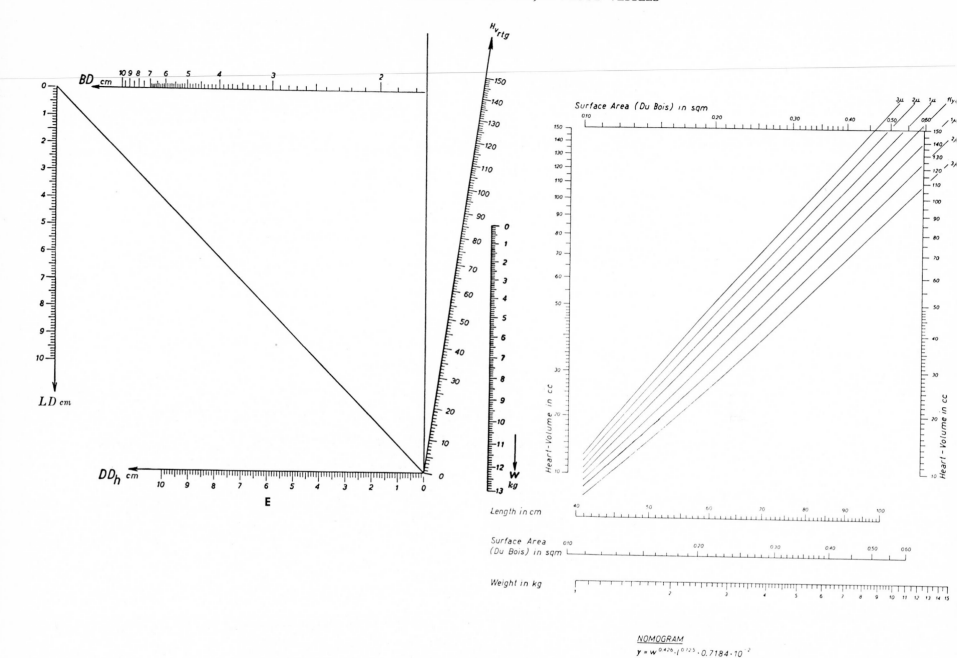

$$\underline{NOMOGRAM}$$

$$y = w^{0.426} \cdot l^{0.725} \cdot 0.7184 \cdot 10^{-2}$$

$$H_v = 289.42 \, y - 19.06 \qquad \textbf{F}$$

Figure 12–35 *Continued.*   E. Nomogram for roentgenologic heart volume in infants. *Key to nomogram:* A line is drawn connecting DD_h and BD. A second line is drawn from LD to the point of intersection of the line between DD_h and BD with the diagonal; this is continued until it cuts the vertical line with no scale. This latter point is joined by a straight line to the weight scale (in kilograms). The point of intersection of this line with the Hv_{rtg} scale indicates the roentgenologic heart volume. F. Nomogram for predicted heart volume and comparison with the roentgenologic heart volume in infants. *Key to nomogram:* The surface area is read at the point at which a straight line connecting weight and length intersects the surface-area scale. From this point of intersection a line is drawn to the same point on the opposite surface-area scale. The intersection of the vertical line and the regression line [F(Y)] represents the predicted heart volume read on the heart-volume scale. A line is drawn from the point on the heart-volume scale representing the roentgenologic heart volume to the same point on the opposite scale. The intersection of this line with the vertical line from the surface-area scale indicates the position of the roentgenologic heart volume, within the standard deviation limits (mμ), that is, the relationship between the roentgenologic and predicted heart volume.

Figure 12–35 continued on the opposite page.

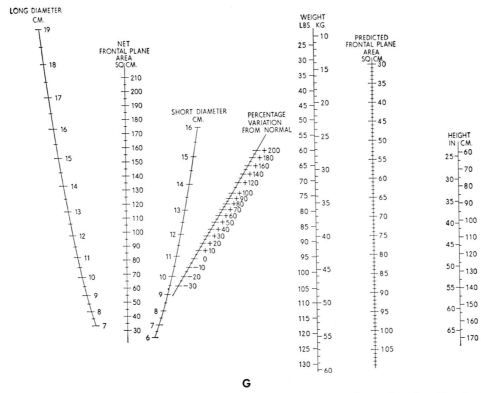

G

Figure 12–35 *Continued.* G. Nomograms showing the frontal area of the hearts from 6-foot chest films in children between the ages of 3 and 16 years inclusive. (From Meyer, R. R., in Radiology, 53:363–370, 1949.) The long and short diameters are obtained as previously described and the net frontal plane area is obtained from the nomogram portion reading "net frontal plane area." Next, the predicted frontal plane area is obtained from the nomogram by placing a straight edge between the appropriate body weight and height. When the ruler is placed so that it connects the values for "net" and "predicted frontal plane area," the "percentage variation from normal" is read off the sloping center scale at the point intersected by the ruler.

Transverse Diameter (TR + TL). This is the sum of the maximum projections of the right and left borders of the heart from the midline.

Long Diameter (L). This is the distance between the left ventricular apex and the small notch on the right border of the heart between the right atrium and the superior vena cava.

Broad Diameter (B). This is the greatest diameter of the cardiac shadow perpendicular to the long diameter. Occasionally, it is necessary to extend the right cardiac margin inferiorly in its natural curvature to delineate the lower margin of this diameter.

Anteroposterior Diameter (D). This is the greatest anteroposterior dimension of the cardiac silhouette on the lateral view.

Aortic Arch Diameter (AR + AL). This is the sum of the maximum extensions to the right and to the left of the aortic shadow from the midline as projected above the base of the heart. When the esophagus is also delineated, the maximum extension to the left of the aortic shadow in relation to the lateral margin of the esophagus is a measure of the diameter of the descending limb of the arch of the aorta. Normally, this measurement may vary between 1.8 and 3.8 cm.; a measurement greater than 4 cm. is abnormal. These measurements have no correction for magnification, and do not take into account the 3 mm. thickness of tissue between the lumen of the esophagus and the aorta.

DETERMINATION OF RELATIVE CARDIAC VOLUME (Amundsen)

The physical factors employed are (1) a target-to-film distance on frontal view of 2 meters, and (2) a target-to-film distance on lateral view of 1.5 meters.

Basic Formula. Volume = K × L × B × D (Fig. 12–35), where K = 0.42 (standard deviation 7.4 per cent) based on 45 cases, comparing calculated value with autopsy-determined value.

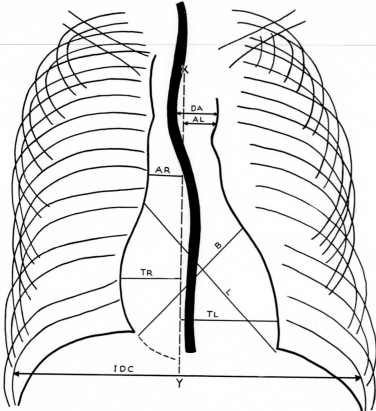

Figure 12–36. Diagram of teleroentgenograms of heart showing most frequent and useful cardiac measurements obtained therefrom: (*TR*) Maximum projection of the right cardiac border from the midline, (*TL*) maximum projection of the left cardiac border from the midline, (*TR plus TL*) the greatest transverse diameter of the heart, (*L*) the long diameter of the heart which extends from the junction of the cardiac silhouette and vascular pedicle on the right to the apex on the left, omitting consideration of the fat pad frequently seen in this location, (*B*) the broad diameter of the heart, which is the greatest diameter of the cardiac shadow perpendicular to the long diameter. It may be necessary to extend the lower right heart border in its natural curve, (*XY*) the midline in a perfectly straight PA projection (falls over spinous processes of dorsal spine), (*AR*) the maximum extension to the right of the vascular pedicle from the midline. (Note: The vascular pedicle shadow usually includes superior vena cava as well as aorta.) (*AL*) The maximum extension to the left of the vascular pedicle from the midline, (*AR plus AL*) the aortic arch diameter, (*DA*) the measurement of the descending aorta which represents the distance from the left margin of the esophagus to the outermost left margin of the aortic knob, (*IDC*) the greatest internal diameter of the chest.

Relative heart volume is defined as the volume per square meter of surface area using the DuBois nomograms for calculation of surface area from body height and weight. Thus, the formula for *relative heart volume* is:

$$\frac{0.42 \times L \times B \times D}{\text{Body surface area in square meters}}$$

A difference of 90 ml. per square meter or more between two successive examinations of the same patient indicates a significant change in relative heart volume.

The mean volume per square meter for adult males is 420 ± 40 cc., and for adult females it is 370 ± 40 cc. The second or third standard deviation indicates a suspicion of cardiomegaly, and above this limit there is only a 3 per cent chance of a normal heart size.

The second to third standard deviation above the mean is:

Female adults	450–490 ml. per sq. m.
Male adults	500–540 ml. per sq. m.
Birth to 3 months	284–311 ml. per sq. m.
3 months to 2 years	334–371 ml. per sq. m.

In infants, Lind's technique calls for carefully centered anteroposterior *supine* films.

Nomograms for the determination of body surface area of children and adults are appended for use.

Transverse Diameter of the Aorta. Measurements AR and AL are added together (Fig. 12–35 *E*). Ungerleider and Gubner's nomogram for predicting aortic diameter is used, corrected as follows: (1) 1 mm. is added for each 3 years over the age of 43, and (2) 1 mm. is subtracted for each 3 years under the age of 43.

Since the *relative heart volume* is more accurate than the frontal area of the heart, we no longer employ the nomogram for *cardiac frontal area.*

Normal Heart Volumes in Children (Table 12–1; Fig. 12–35 *C*). These values may be utilized along with those of Amundsen and Lind.

Relative heart volume calculation is now considered the method of choice for daily practice for both children and adults.

TABLE 12–1 NORMAL HEART VOLUMES IN CHILDREN*

Age	Volume per Square Meter of Body Surface (Relative Heart Volume)	Standard Error of the Mean
0–30 days	196	22.6
30–90 days	217.8	33.9
90–360 days	282	35.8
1–2 years	295	30.4
2–4 years	304	41.5
4–7 years	310	36.2
7–9 years	324	28.6
9–12 years	348	33.6
12–14 years	369	53.8
14–16 years	398	61.9

*Adapted from Mannheimer, in Keats, T. E., and Enge, I. P.: Radiology, 85:850, 1965.

Frontal Cardiac Area. This may be determined with a fair degree of accuracy in accordance with the formula:

$$A = \pi/4 \; L \times B$$

where A is the frontal area, and L and B are the long and broad diameters respectively. The frontal area of the heart provides a reasonably accurate concept of cardiac size, although relative heart volume is considered more accurate.

The frontal cardiac area may be determined by utilization of nomograms as shown in Figure 12–35 *B*-1 for adults, and Figure 12–35 *B* for children.

The bodily factors most frequently employed for correlation are body height, weight, surface area, age, and sex. Weight is a better criterion than height but fails in the presence of obesity. Height is therefore a valuable criterion to compensate for this failure. Height groups are also found to be better criteria than age groups in children.

The correlation coefficient of body surface area with cardiac frontal area has been found to be as high as 0.84 to 0.92 (1.0 being perfect). Since the surface area equals 0.425 W × 0.725 H × 71.84 (where W and H are the weight and height respectively), there is a sufficiently high correlation between surface area and the product of height and weight to use the latter as a substitute for surface area.

The greatest internal diameter of the chest has a poor correlation with cardiac frontal area.

The right and left cardiac margins must be delineated as separate and distinct from the pericardial fat pads in the cardiophrenic angles (Fig. 12–37).

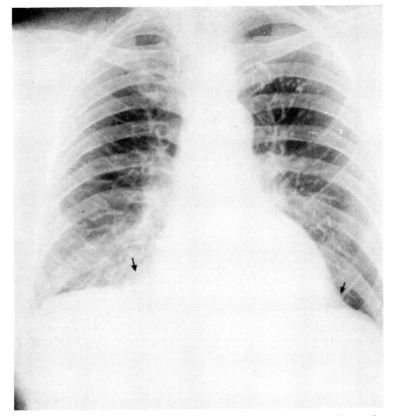

Figure 12–37. Pericardial fat pads. These are distinguished from the cardiac margins in both the right and left cardiophrenic angles.

RADIOGRAPHIC CARDIAC CONTOUR CHANGES IN RELATION TO SPECIFIC CHAMBER ENLARGEMENT

Introduction. As a matter of principle we have not included abnormalities of anatomy, but, in this region we shall demonstrate cardiac contour changes when specific chambers are enlarged to emphasize some of the normal roentgenographic anatomy.

Left Ventricle. Contour changes with left ventricular enlargement are indicated in Fig. 12–38. The left ventricular contour is rounded, extends farther laterally, and in the left lateral view is displaced posterior to the reflection of the inferior vena cava by a distance of 18 mm. or more, when measurements are made as demonstrated in the illustration. In the left anterior oblique view, the left ventricle usually overlaps the spine more than 1 cm. in the 45 degree obliquity. *Patients with a giant left atrium, a deformity of the left hemidiaphragm, a markedly enlarged right ventricle, or depression of the sternum (pectus excava-*

tum) cannot be evaluated by this method (Dinsmore et al.; Hoffman and Rigler).

Right Ventricle (Fig. 12–39). In infants, when the right ventricle is enlarged, it is projected above the left ventricular apex, imparting a squared appearance to this left margin near the diaphragm—the so-called "coeur en sabot" (wooden shoe) shape. In frontal view either no changes may be detected, or the right atrium may be displaced somewhat toward the right. The best view for detection of right ventricular enlargement is the straight lateral, in which an encroachment can be noted on the anterior and superior mediastinal clear space as the enlarged right ventricle "climbs the sternum" on its internal aspect.

Left Atrial Enlargement (Fig. 12–40). In the frontal projection, the right cardiac border assumes a double-contoured appearance because of the projection of the right margin of the left atrium toward it. The esophagus is usually displaced toward the right but occasionally toward the left, depending upon any associated aortic elongation that may be present and affecting the esophagus. There is a prominence of the left auricular appendage,

HYPERTROPHY AND DILATATION
LEFT VENTRICLE

POSTERO-ANTERIOR

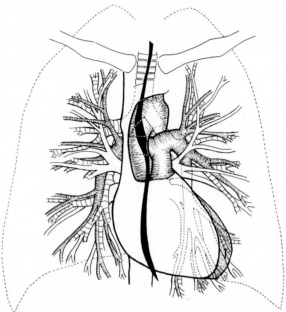

LEFT ANTERIOR OBLIQUE

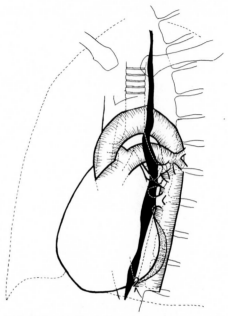

1. Left ventricular contour is rounded, extends farther laterally, and left diaphragm is depressed; <u>rounding</u> due to hypertrophy, <u>distension</u> to left due to dilatation.

A

2. Left ventricle extends beyond retrocardiac space and cannot "clear the spine" readily; is rounded.

B

Figure 12-38. Diagrams showing changes in appearance of cardiac contour with left ventricular hypertrophy and dilatation.

Figure 12–38 continued on the opposite page.

producing an extra "hump" beneath the pulmonary sector, and it contributes to the convexity of the left cardiac margin. The left bronchus may be slightly displaced upward.

In the right anterior oblique as well as the right or left lateral views, the esophagus is displaced posteriorly in the region of the left atrium. A notch may be detected in the contour at the interatrial groove along the posterior margin of the heart. In the left anterior oblique view, the aortic window is usually obliterated by the enlarged left atrium or its appendage.

Also in the lateral view, the trachea, the right bronchus, and the left bronchus are normally in line with one another. The major bronchi appear tapered.

If, in the lateral view, the left upper lobe bronchus is displaced posteriorly, it is a good indication of left atrial enlargement and is sometimes a more sensitive indicator than displacement of the esophagus posteriorly (Lane and Whalen).

Right Atrial Enlargement (Fig. 12–41). Isolated right atrial enlargement is rare. It usually accompanies a diffuse or right ventricular enlargement. In the frontal view, the right cardiac margin may extend toward the right, but this is not a reliable sign (Klatte et al.). The most reliable indicators are revealed by the following methods:

1. Study of the heart fluoroscopically in the left anterior oblique view, in at least 45 degrees obliquity. Right atrial pulsations can be readily distinguished from those of the right ventricle on the right border of the heart. If the right atrium occupies 50 per cent or more of this border, right atrial enlargement is almost certainly present.

2. On film studies, the left anterior oblique and lateral views are most accurate. Here, when the right atrium is enlarged, the right auricular appendage produces a squared appearance of the right cardiac border.

LATERAL

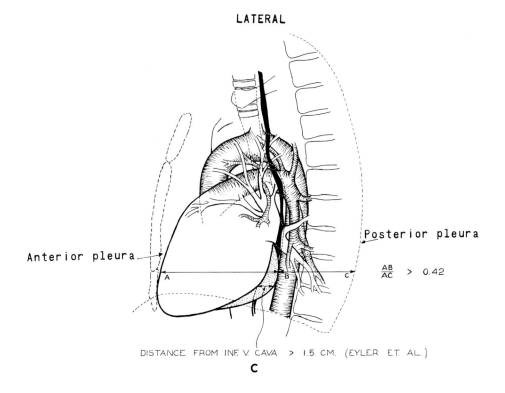

Anterior pleura

Posterior pleura

$$\frac{AB}{AC} > 0.42$$

DISTANCE FROM INF. V. CAVA > 1.5 CM. (EYLER ET. AL.)

C

RIGHT ANTERIOR OBLIQUE

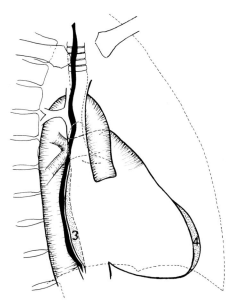

4. Anterior apical portion of heart extends farther anteriorly.

Heart intersects left leaf of diaphragm.

3. Heart as a whole is displaced posteriorly and comes close to spine.

LEFT VENTRICULAR HYPERTROPHY

D

Figure 12-38 Continued.

RIGHT VENTRICLE HYPERTROPHY AND DILATATION.

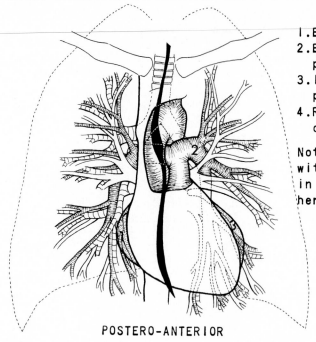

1. Enlarged right atrium.
2. Enlargement and dilatation of pulmonary arteries.
3. Increased convexity in left pulmonary sector.
4. Right ventricle bulges convexly on anterior aspect.

Note: "Wooden shoe" shape associated with right ventricular hypertrophy in tetralogy of Fallot not included here.

POSTERO-ANTERIOR

A

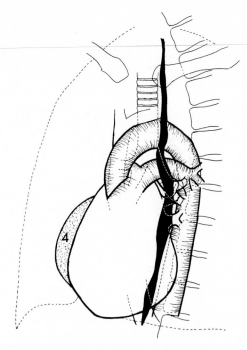

LEFT ANTERIOR OBLIQUE

B

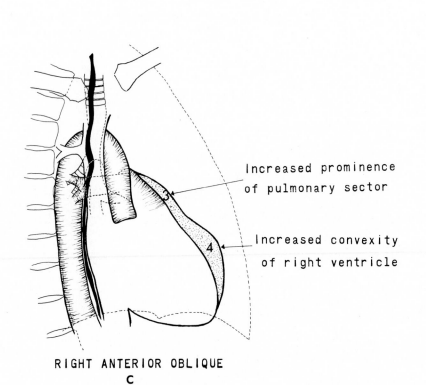

Increased prominence of pulmonary sector

Increased convexity of right ventricle

RIGHT ANTERIOR OBLIQUE

C

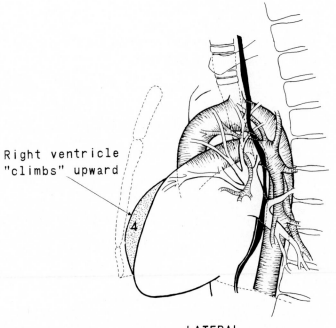

Right ventricle "climbs" upward

LATERAL

Right ventricle enlargement and encroachment on mediastinal clear space

D

Figure 12–39. Diagrams showing cardiac contour changes with right ventricular hypertrophy and dilatation in the various conventional views.

In the lateral view, the right atrium, when markedly enlarged, protrudes posterior to the esophagus. This, however, is not a reliable sign by itself and is valid only when the right atrium is judged to be enlarged in the left anterior oblique view. (The left ventricle, when enlarged, also protrudes behind the esophageal shadow in the lateral projection, and the left anterior oblique view is necessary to distinguish this possibility.)

The right hemidiaphragm may be elevated, with right-sided cardiac dilatation and failure because of an engorged liver.

Aorta. In the frontal projection, there is no convexity to the right of the vascular pedicle at the base of the heart. The aortic knob falls 1 to 2 cm. below the clavicles, and the measurement of the descending limb of the arch of the aorta does not exceed 3.8 cm., or 4 cm. in markedly sthenic individuals. In the left anterior oblique projection, the anterior margin of the ascending limb of the arch of the aorta forms a smooth continuous convexity with the anterior border of the right ventricle. The aortic window is well preserved.

Main Pulmonary Artery. The pulmonary artery is best visualized in the right anterior oblique projection, and normally is not visualized in the other projections to good advantage. It forms a continuous straight line, or a slightly convex curve anteriorly above the left ventricular margin when the patient is rotated 45 degrees. Abnormality of the conus is also best reflected in this segment but may also be demonstrated by secondary enlargement or distortion and increased pulsations of the pulmonary arteries. For a more complete description and illustration of aortic and pulmonary artery abnormalities, the reader is referred to our companion texts, Analysis of Roentgen Signs and Roentgen Signs in Clinical Practice.

SPECIAL STUDIES OF THE HEART AND MAJOR BLOOD VESSELS

Newer advances in surgery of the heart and peripheral vascular system have necessitated great accuracy in depiction of cardiac abnormalities in diagnostic studies. Special techniques in cardiac radiology, and the greater collaborative efforts of radiologist, cardiologist, and physiologist, have helped greatly in the achievement of this aim. The most important of these special cardioradiologic techniques are: (1) venous angiocardiography, (2) selective angiocardiography, (3) aortography, (4) peripheral arteriography, (5) azygography, (6) venography, and (7) lymphangiography.

However, before delving into these special contrast studies, a few comments in relation to orthodiagraphy and kymography are in order.

Orthodiagraphy. An orthodiagram is an outline drawing of the heart made on a celluloid cover or transparent paper placed over the fluoroscopic screen while moving the screen and x-ray tube independently, so that only the central ray is employed to record every point on the cardiac border. Since only the central ray is employed, the complete absence of divergent beams eliminates the element of magnification. Also, it is possible to plot the points in a given phase of the cardiac cycle and in a given respiratory phase also, eliminating these variables as well. It is very time-consuming and requires a specially constructed independently moving fluoroscopic screen and x-ray tube; *the advantages gained are not usually sufficiently great to warrant the performance of this procedure or the hazards of radiation exposure to patient and physician.*

Magnification of Teleroentgenograms and the Fallacy of Comparison of Orthodiagrams with Teleroentgenograms. In orthodiagraphy the central ray is employed in a designated phase of respiration and cardiac cycle. Teleroentgenography, on the other hand, is a 6 foot projection of the heart in suspended inspiration in no definite phase of the cardiac cycle. Even at 6 feet a certain amount of magnification (approximately 5 per cent) is inevitable, depending upon the distance of the heart from the film on the one hand, and the distance of the heart from the tube-target on the other. Differences of cardiac measurements in systole and diastole will impose an additional 5 to 10 per cent variation. Differences produced by body habitus and phase of respiration, as well as body position, impose additional necessary corrections. (Apparatus is available, however, by means of which a roentgenogram of the heart in any phase of the cardiac cycle can be obtained by triggering the x-ray exposure during any desired phase of the electrocardiogram.)

The complexity of this comparison can be seen immediately, and it is readily apparent that no actual constant arithmetical factor can be given between orthodiagraphy and teleroentgenography.

Kymography (Boone et al.) (Fig. 12–42). The conventional multiple-slit kymograph consists of a sheet of lead in which multiple parallel slits about 1 mm. wide have been cut about 1 cm. apart. This is placed over a cassette, and the lead sheet is made to move the distance between the slits (1 cm.) during three to five cardiac systoles. As the slits descend, an outline of the pulsations of each portion of the cardiac outline is obtained. The peaks represent diastole and the valleys systole. The configuration of the contractions can be studied, and abnormalities in pulsations recorded for future reference and comparison. However, respiratory changes, the changes in contour with the rotary movement of the heart, and the neutralization effects of one chamber on another all make this method of recording pulsations rather inaccurate. A more accurate method has been advocated (Boone et al.) which employs the current in a photoelectric cell as the recording medium of the pulsation. The cardiac pulsations at a given point will interrupt the passage of a fine x-ray beam through the chest at

LEFT ATRIAL ENLARGEMENT

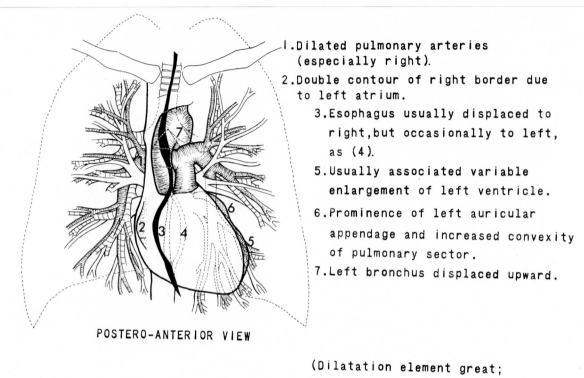

1. Dilated pulmonary arteries (especially right).
2. Double contour of right border due to left atrium.
   3. Esophagus usually displaced to right, but occasionally to left, as (4).
5. Usually associated variable enlargement of left ventricle.
6. Prominence of left auricular appendage and increased convexity of pulmonary sector.
7. Left bronchus displaced upward.

POSTERO-ANTERIOR VIEW

(Dilatation element great; hypertrophy minimal; seldom unassociated with other pathology.)

A

Figure 12-40. Diagrams illustrating cardiac contour changes with left atrial enlargement in the conventional projections.

Figure 12-40 continued on the opposite page.

this point, and this variation in the intensity of the x-ray beam after it has passed through the body is recorded by means of a photoelectric cell. Records can be obtained which are indicative of abnormality at given points in the cardiac outline, but here, too, the torsion of the heart with pulsations and the respiratory effect will modify the curve obtained, and thus produce inaccuracies.

Application of Special Contrast Studies to a Study of the Heart and Major Blood Vessels (Venous Angiocardiograms). In 1938, Robb and Steinberg described a method for visualization of the cardiac chambers and major blood vessels leading from the heart, by means of the rapid injection of a relatively large quantity (50 cc.) of double concentration (70 per cent) Diodrast into a vein of the arm or leg. This method of examination was called "cardioangiography."

Originally, their method required timing the films in accordance with the major and lesser circulation times which were ob-

tained prior to the Diodrast injection. More recently, apparatus has been devised which permits obtaining films at very rapid intervals, up to 12 per second with 16 or 35 mm. movie films with very high frame frequencies per second (24 to 60 being most frequently employed). This allows the production of sequential films for twelve or more seconds after the injection depending on the "program selection." With the aid of such apparatus, it is unnecessary to time the exposures with great accuracy, so long as a sufficient number of exposures is obtained while the dye is passing through the right side of the heart, and then the left side of the heart and aorta. Simultaneous or near simultaneous films may be obtained in two planes perpendicular to one another.

It is essential in this method of examination that a large bulk of the dye (up to 50 cc.) be injected very rapidly (in 2 seconds or less), so that the concentration of the dye in the blood will be sufficiently high to produce a good contrast not only in the right side

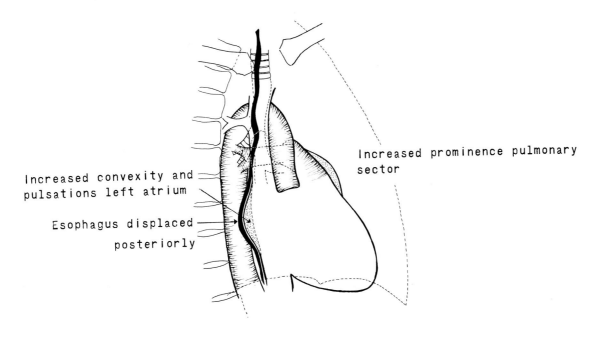

Increased convexity and
pulsations left atrium

Esophagus displaced
posteriorly

Increased prominence pulmonary
sector

RIGHT ANTERIOR OBLIQUE

B

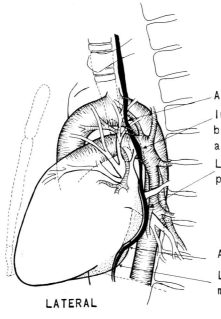

Aortic impression on esophagus

Impression by tracheobronchial
bifurcation displaced by pulmonary
arteries

Left atrium displacing esophagus
posteriorly

Atrioventricular groove

Left ventricular hypertrophy
may be associated

LATERAL

C

Figure 12–40 *Continued.*

RIGHT ATRIAL ENLARGEMENT

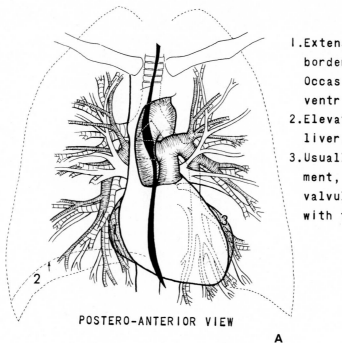

1. Extension to right of right atrial border, with increased convexity. Occasionally enlarged right ventricle does this.
2. Elevated diaphragm from enlarged liver.
3. Usually left-sided heart enlargement, since mitral and aortic valvular disease are associated with tricuspid.

POSTERO-ANTERIOR VIEW

A

"Squaring off" of right atrial appendage

Right atrial margin comprises 50% or more of entire right cardiac margin, judged by studying pulsations

LEFT ANTERIOR OBLIQUE

B

Figure 12–41. Diagrams showing cardiac contour changes which may be present with right atrial enlargement.

Figure 12–41 continued on the opposite page.

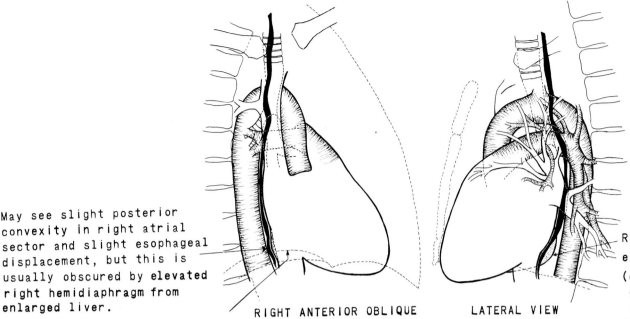

May see slight posterior convexity in right atrial sector and slight esophageal displacement, but this is usually obscured by elevated right hemidiaphragm from enlarged liver.

RIGHT ANTERIOR OBLIQUE

C

Right atrium protrudes behind esophagus –
(compare with right anterior oblique view to exclude left ventricle)

LATERAL VIEW

D

Figure 12–41 *Continued.*

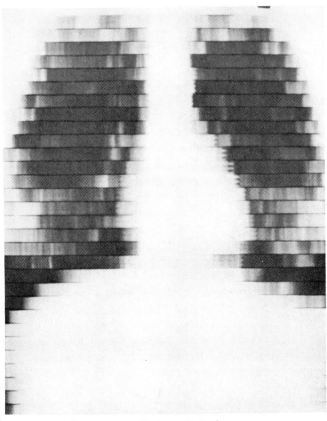

Figure 12–42. Posteroanterior kymogram.

of the heart, but also in the left. For this reason a special syringe with a large bore and a large bore needle (12 gauge) must be employed. It is sometimes advisable in children to expose a vein in the ankle and insert the needle under direct visualization. Special automatic pressure injectors have also been devised for this purpose. At best, the concentration of the dye in the left side of the heart under normal conditions allows only a moderate intensification and visualization of the anatomy.

In normal individuals, the superior vena cava and the right atrium are visualized in 1 to 1½ seconds; the right ventricle and pulmonary arteries in 3 to 5 seconds (Fig. 12–43); and the left atrium, left ventricle, and aorta in 6 to 10 seconds following the beginning of the injection period.

On the right side (Fig. 12–43 *A*), the following structures can be identified: the *superior vena cava and its tributaries* (which may be referred to as the inflow tract); *the right atrial and ventricular cavities and walls;* the *auricular appendage;* the *tricuspid valve;* the *trabeculae;* the *ventricular septum;* the *pulmonic valve;* and the *pulmonary artery with its subdivisions.*

The space between the right border of the contrast-filled atrium and the right border of the cardiac silhouette represents the free wall of the right atrium, which normally measures 2 to 3 mm. in diameter. When this space is increased, pericardial effusion is indicated.

The right atrial appendage or auricle extends cephalad and medially from the upper portion of the right atrium, overlapping to some extent the inflow tract. The *tricuspid valve* is in an

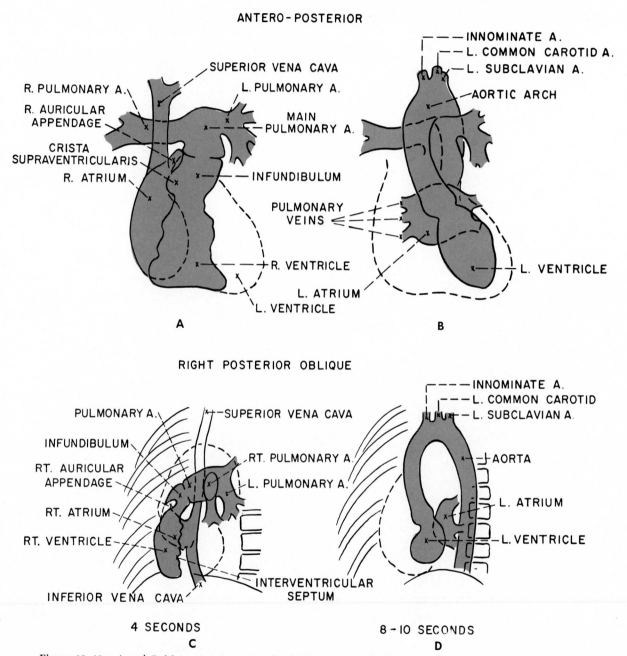

Figure 12-43. A and B. Major structures visualized in venous angiocardiograms in the anteroposterior projection. A. Lesser circulation phase. B. Greater circulation phase. C and D. Major structures visualized in venous angiocardiograms in the right posterior oblique projection. C. Lesser circulation phase. D. Greater circulation phase.

Figure 12-43 continued on the opposite page.

LEFT POSTERIOR OBLIQUE

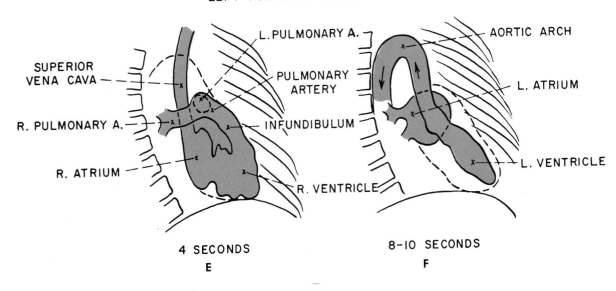

4 SECONDS
E

8-10 SECONDS
F

RIGHT LATERAL

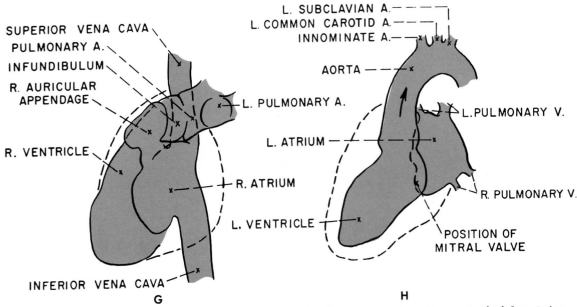

G

H

Figure 12–43 *Continued.* E and F. Major structures visualized in venous angiocardiograms in the left posterior oblique projection. E. Lesser circulation phase. F. Greater circulation phase. G and H. Major structures visualized in venous angiocardiograms in the right lateral projection. G. Lesser circulation phase. H. Greater circulation phase.

oblique plane between the right atrium and right ventricle and may be represented as an ellipse (Fig. 12–44). The inferior margin of the *tricuspid annulus* is adjacent to the junction of the *inferior vena cava* and *right atrium*. The *coronary sinus* is situated in this same region. (This similarity in position may give rise to confusion in catheterization, because the catheter may enter the coronary sinus and advance into the great cardiac vein rather than upward into the outflow tract of the right ventricle.) The atrium and ventricle tend to lie over one another in the immediate vicinity of the tricuspid annulus.

The *right ventricle* is a chamber roughly triangular in shape, divided into two component parts: (1) a large trabeculated inflow

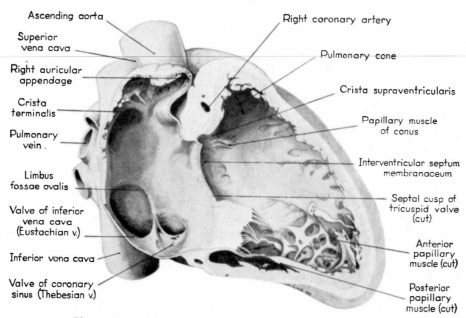

Ascending aorta

Superior
vena cava

Right auricular
appendage

Crista
terminalis

Pulmonary
vein

Limbus
fossae ovalis

Valve of inferior
vena cava
(Eustachian v.)

Inferior vena cava

Valve of coronary
sinus (Thebesian v.)

Right coronary artery

Pulmonary cone

Crista supraventricularis

Papillary muscle
of conus

Interventricular septum
membranaceum

Septal cusp of
tricuspid valve
(cut)

Anterior
papillary
muscle (cut)

Posterior
papillary
muscle (cut)

Figure 12–44 Right side of the heart opened in a plane approximately parallel to the septa, to show the interior of the right atrium and the right ventricle. A segment of the septal leaflet of the tricuspid valve has been cut away to expose more fully the region of the membranous portion of the interventricular septum. (From Gould, S. E. 1959. Pathology of the Heart, 2d ed. Courtesy of Charles C Thomas, Publisher, Springfield, Illinois.)

portion communicating with the right atrium, and (2) a tubular upper portion representing the *outflow tract.* The right border of the inflow portion is formed by the *tricuspid valve,* whereas the left border is formed by the *interventricular septum.* The right border of the outflow tract is formed by a sheet of muscle extending from the tricuspid to the pulmonic valve lying in front of the aorta; it is a localized prominence in this muscle that is called the *crista supraventricularis.* The *pulmonic valve,* when normal, is not easily identified in the frontal view and is best seen in oblique or lateral projections. The *pulmonary trunk* is visualized cephalad to the pulmonic valve and branches almost immediately into *right and left pulmonary arteries.* The right pulmonary artery courses in a direct horizontal direction to the right and is clearly identified in this projection; the left pulmonary artery is directed posteriorly and is foreshortened. It is best demonstrated in a left lateral or steep left anterior oblique view. Contrast agent may remain in the superior vena cava or in the right atrium, obscuring the right pulmonary artery.

In the *lateral projection* (Fig. 12–44) the right atrium is projected posterior to the right ventricle, and the posterior margin of the right atrium is clearly identified. The anterior margin of the right atrium is formed by the tricuspid valve and

annulus of this valve that forms a boundary between the right atrium and the right ventricle. The atrial appendage rises cephalad to the tricuspid valve, extending anteriorly and superiorly and overlapping the pulmonic valve very slightly. The ostium of the coronary sinus lies in the inferior portion of the atrium just in front of the entrance of the inferior vena cava. It curves posteriorly from the superior vena cava and can be recognized in this way.

Because of the interference by the right atrial appendage, the *right ventricle* is best studied by selective angiocardiography. The inflow portion of the right ventricle lies in front of the tricuspid valve, with the crista supraventricularis situated just superior and anterior to the tricuspid annulus. It marks the inferior margin of the infundibulum—the outflow portion of the right ventricle. The outflow portion is readily identified as a tubular sector leading directly to the pulmonic valve. The valve cusps are readily identified in the lateral view. This view is also best for identifying an *infundibular stenosis,* a common congenital anomaly. The left pulmonary artery is clearly identified in the lateral view as it courses posteriorly, but the right pulmonary artery is too foreshortened in this view to be accurately seen.

On the left side (Fig. 12–43 *B*), the following components may be seen: the *pulmonary veins;* the *left atrial and ventricular cavities and walls;* the *auricular appendage;* the *aortic valve;* and the *entire thoracic aorta* with its main branches.

In *frontal projection,* the left heart is first identified by detecting the left atrium, which lies just above and to the right of the left ventricle. The two superior pulmonary veins enter the uppermost portion of the left atrium, whereas the inferior pulmonary veins can be identified below them forming a horizontal V-shaped structure that extends on each side of the circular left atrium. The left atrial appendage has a hooklike contour extending upward and to the left and overlying the left superior pulmonary vein. The left ventricle, for the most part, can be identified below the level of the mitral valve as well as the aortic valve. It is oval in shape with its apex pointing downward and to the left. Generally, the *trabeculation of the left ventricular cavity is much finer than that of the right ventricle* and hence, one can identify right and left ventricles by the trabecular architecture—an important differentiation in certain congenital heart conditions. The superior margin of the annulus of the mitral valve is continuous with that of the aortic ring and is usually not well identified in frontal view. The membranous portion of the interventricular septum cannot be delineated on angiocardiograms, but it lies beneath the anterior portion of the posterior cusp of the aortic valve, a small part of the adjacent right cusp, and the commissure between the two. In frontal projection the right cusp is seen *en face;* the left cusp forms the left border of the aortic valve, whereas the noncoronary cusp forms the right border. The right coronary artery can often be identified faintly in angiocardiograms but it is best identified by selective angiography (to be discussed subsequently). It arises from the midportion of the aortic valve, whereas the left coronary artery originates from the left border of the aortic valve. The entire right border of the left ventricle is formed by the interventricular septum, the upper part being membranous and the remainder being muscular.

In some anomalous conditions it is important to recall that the tricuspid valve attachment reaches almost to the aortic valve and actually crosses the membranous septum.

In the *lateral view* (Fig. 12–45) the left atrium is projected posterior to the left ventricle. The anterior margin of this chamber is formed by the mitral valve. The left atrial appendage arises above the mitral valve and extends anteriorly and cephalad to the sinuses of Valsalva. The posterior border of the atrial cavity is a free wall of the atrium, and the pulmonary veins enter its superior and middle portions. The mitral valve forms the posterior boundary of the left ventricle and its upper margin extends to the aortic valve in the region of the commissure between the left (coronary) and posterior (noncoronary) cusps. The left ventricular cavity extends inferiorly and anteriorly from the mitral valve and aortic sinuses; its entire anterior margin is formed by the interventricular septum. In lateral view, the right coronary cusp of the aortic valve forms the anterior border of the valve; the left and posterior cusps are projected obliquely, posteriorly, with the posterior noncoronary cusp lower than the left cusp (coronary). The membranous portion of the interventricular septum lies directly below the commissure between the right and noncoronary cusp.

The right coronary artery may occasionally be identified on angiocardiograms but is best visualized in selective angiocardiography or selective coronary arteriograms. The right coronary artery arises from the upper portion of the right sinus of Valsalva; the left coronary artery is foreshortened in this lateral view.

When the right ventricle is enlarged, the sulcus between the ventricle and right atrium is displaced anteriorly. This in turn will displace the position of the coronary artery.

The tricuspid valve lies anterior to the mitral valve.

The supraventricular crest lies directly in front of the right sinus of Valsalva.

The wall thickness of the right ventricle may at times be measurable—2 to 3 mm. The left ventricular wall, *smoother than that of the right,* usually measures between 7 and 10 mm. in thickness.

The *arch of the aorta* is demonstrable as it extends anteriorly and upward, and then arches posteriorly and to the left. It descends down the left side of the thoracic spine and in the posterior mediastinal space as a tubular structure approximately 3.5 cm. in diameter. The wall thickness of the aorta is usually in the order of 3 mm.

The *innominate, left common carotid, and left subclavian arteries* can occasionally be distinguished as they branch from the arch of the aorta along its anterior aspect.

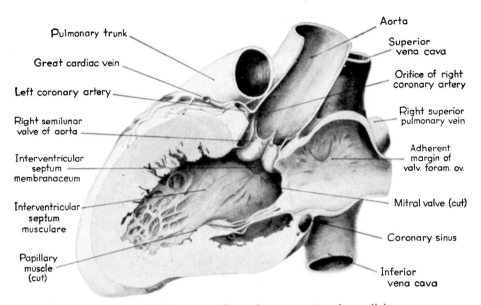

Figure 12–45. Left side of the heart opened in a plane approximately parallel to the septa, to show the interior of the left atrium and left ventricle. A segment of the anterior leaflet of the mitral valve has been cut away to expose more fully the region of the membranous portion of the interventricular septum and the aortic orifice. (From Gould, S. E. 1959. Pathology of the Heart, 2d ed. Courtesy of Charles C Thomas, Publisher, Springfield, Illinois.)

The *aortic triangle* is likewise delineated. It is bounded anteriorly by the left subclavian artery, posteriorly by the spine, and inferiorly by the arch of the aorta.

CATHETERIZATION OF THE HEART

Cardiac Catheterization. In view of the great technical advances made by cardiac surgeons in relation to open heart surgery and repair of defects, the roentgen examination of the heart and its inflow and outflow tracts has become much more exacting. The surgeon must know the answers to many questions, such as the size and extent of a defect or stenosis, the degree of overriding of the aorta, and the appearance of the pulmonary arteries, veins, and systemic arteries.

In recent years, the technique of cardiac catheterization has been increasingly applied and developed in this direction. Passing a catheter into the right heart and then sequentially into the pulmonary artery provides the physician with the following opportunities: (1) blood samples may be obtained from any of these areas or all of them, and *gas analysis* may be performed on the samples to determine the site of shunt formation; (2) the *volume of blood shunting* may be calculated; (3) *pulmonary blood flow* may be readily calculated; (4) *pressures* in the various chambers may be recorded and evaluated in relation to the dynamics of the cardiac circulation (see Chapter 11); (5) if the catheter takes an *abnormal route,* a defect may be recognized directly—for example, a patent interatrial septum; (6) at the end of these procedures, one may selectively inject into any region a quantity of opaque media under sufficient pressure to visualize carefully a given area without too much interference from adjoining areas. This latter technique is called "selective angiocardiography," in contrast to the previously described venous angiocardiography.

Selective Angiocardiography.   There are different types of catheters used for this purpose, each with its own advocates. A mechanical pressure device for the injection must usually be employed to provide a satisfactory jet of contrast media within ½ to 1 second. A number of these are available commercially, varying in complexity and cost from several hundred dollars to several thousand. Injection directly into the right ventricle is by far the most common procedure, and the injection is followed by serial films taken as rapidly as 12 per second (simultaneously in two planes), or by 16 or 35 mm. cineradiographs for cinema depiction. Care must be exercised to locate the catheter tip accurately, lest the injection be made into a coronary vein.

The projection planes most frequently employed are the straight frontal (anteroposterior), right posterior oblique, and lateral. Usually, a simultaneous biplane technique is desirable.

Most of the catheters now used by angiographers, with the exception of expensive preshaped molded varieties, are supplied in long rolls and are custom-made for a particular use, being discarded after one use. Usually they are radiopaque in order to facilitate manipulation and guidance under fluoroscopic control, with image amplification. Generally, polyethylene catheters seem to change the least when made radiopaque; the lead oxide incorporated into polyethylene in Kifa tubing was one of the earliest materials used for this purpose. (Lead is now prohibited from such use.) Radiopaque polyethylene catheters are available from many manufacturers and are supplied in rolls of 10 to 20 feet, color-coded according to their size.

Most catheters are inserted percutaneously by the Seldinger technique. As shown in Figure 12–46, this involves the initial insertion of a special type of needle through both walls of the artery and gradual retraction of the tip of the cannula into the arterial lumen after withdrawal of the needle insert. A guidewire is then passed through the cannula into the artery, and the cannula is removed over the guidewire. A catheter is then gently rotated over the guidewire into the lumen of the artery. To accomplish this, the catheter must be carefully tapered by heating it with the guidewire still in place. With the guidewire in place the catheter is then bent into its desired curve and immersed in hot water (over 140 degrees F.), after which it is immediately plunged into cold water so that the shaping is permanent. Side holes are usually provided in the catheter, as close to the end hole as possible to concentrate the bolus, yet to avoid a jet stream. The side holes, appropriately placed, help prevent recoil of the catheter out of the vessel during injection of the contrast material.

The proximal end of the catheter is usually equipped with a special adapter attached to a Luer-lock stopcock. Catheters, of course, must be thoroughly tested to avoid leakage around the stopcock or connector. Various catheter-manipulating devices that allow for ease of insertion into the desired blood vessels are also commercially available.

Some catheters used for angiocardiography are inserted directly into surgically exposed arteries or veins, making end holes unnecessary. Absence of the end hole decreases the chance of intramural injection into a cardiac chamber. One such commer-

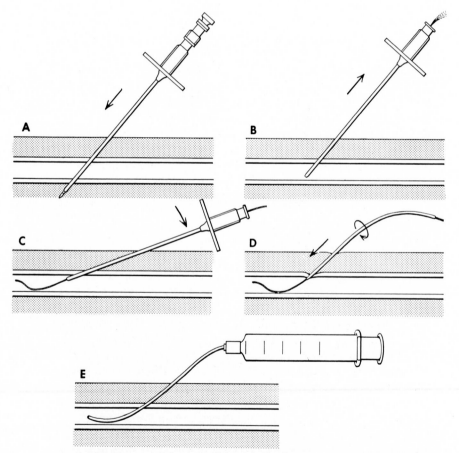

Figure 12–46.   Application of Seldinger technique of arterial puncture. *A.* Puncture of both walls of the vessel. *B.* Retraction of tip of cannula into arterial lumen after withdrawal of needle insert. *C.* Passage of guidewire through cannula into artery. *D.* Passage of smoothly tapered catheter tip over guidewire into artery; gentle rotation of the catheter facilitates the entry. *E.* Catheter in lumen of artery after withdrawal of guidewire. (From Curry, J. L., and Howland, W. J.: Arteriography. Philadelphia, W. B. Saunders Co., 1966.)

cially available device is the Lehman ventriculography catheter, made of woven Dacron (or Teflon) with thin walls and a closed distal tip, and four side holes 4 cm. from the tip. The Rodriquez-Alvarez catheter has thin walls of smooth nylon reinforced with woven Dacron, and six openings arranged in three opposing pairs within the first centimeter of the tip. (For a more detailed discussion of catheters see Bierman.)

Injection rates in various portions of the heart or major blood vessels vary in order to obtain most satisfactory visualization. For example, selective coronary arteriography is performed at injection rates of 4 cc. per second approximately, with hand injections. Aortography or angiocardiography requires larger injection volumes in short periods of time. Whereas 8 to 10 cc. per second is adequate within a cardiac chamber, aortography requires injection rates of up to 40 or 50 cc. per second. These high rates require mechanical injectors, which are now commercially available so that the desired rate of injection and timing can be very accurately controlled.

Much has been written concerning other aspects of this highly specialized technique, for example, the advantages of large film studies as opposed to ciné film studies. With the ciné technique, it is now possible to expose several hundred frames in 1 second, if desired. Each has its proponents, and its advantages and disadvantages. A radiology study group under the aegis of an intersociety commission for heart disease resources formulated guidelines for optimal equipment for a catheterization-angiocardiography laboratory, and the reader is referred to their preliminary report for greater detail regarding the organization and space required for the laboratory, and specific equipment, electrical power, and physiologic monitors necessary (Abrams). (Detailed chapters devoted to this equipment as well as to catheters, injectors, and other aspects of angiography are also available in this text.)

Various contrast media have been suggested for selective angiocardiography; the agents usually used are Renografin (meglumine diatrizoate), Hypaque (sodium diatrizoate), and iothalamate (Jacobson and Paulin).

Apart from coronary arteriography (which will be discussed subsequently), selective angiocardiography in relation to the heart and major vessels at this writing includes the passage of a catheter into the right atrium, right ventricle, pulmonary artery, right and left pulmonary artery branches, through the foramen ovale into the left atrium, and through the mitral valve into the left ventricle. Catheters are also passed backward from the arm or leg into the ascending aorta, the sinuses of Valsalva, and through the aortic valve into the left ventricle.

In view of the complexity of this procedure, radiation exposure must be kept to an absolute minimum. An accurate record of fluoroscopic time, physical factors employed, and films made during all procedures should allow the radiologist to estimate the approximate radiation dosage to the patient. The gonads and all other body areas not required for diagnosis should be carefully protected from the primary beam and, as far as possible, from external scatter as well.

Several other techniques for catheterization of the left chambers of the heart are also available: (1) retrograde catheterization of the left ventricle from a peripheral artery; (2) direct puncture of the left chambers of the heart by a transthoracic needle; (3) transbronchial needle puncture of the left atrium; and (4) catheterization of the left atrium and ventricle by a transseptal needle and overlying catheter. Transbronchial and direct transthoracic cardiac puncture are seldom employed because the placement of a large-bore catheter into the left heart is difficult and risky with these techniques, and they do not allow easy positioning of the patient for repeated injections of the contrast agent. Generally, for left ventricular catheterization, retro-aortic catheterization via the femoral artery using a Seldinger technique is preferred. However, complications of transseptal puncture for left heart catheterization are few (Bell). This technique is diagrammatically illustrated in Figure 12-47.

Representative Angiocardiograms. Representative angiocardiograms are shown in Figure 12-48. With *right heart visualization*, there is rapid sequential filling of the superior vena cava, right atrium, and right auricular appendage. The tricuspid valve region is identified between the right atrium and right ventricle, and thereafter filling of the infundibulum and pulmonary artery and its major branches is shown. In the *lateral view* (Fig. 12-48 G-K), the right auricular appendage overlaps the pulmonary artery, although usually the pulmonary valve can be identified as an umbrella-shaped structure just above the projection of the right atrial appendage. Note that during atrial systole, the atrial ventricular border shifts dorsally. The crista terminalis presses into the lumen, resembling a membrane.

On *left heart visualization,* the left ventricle, mitral valve (Fig. 12-49), and left atrium appear as shown. The superior and inferior right pulmonary veins are clearly in evidence, whereas those on the left are somewhat obscured. The left auricular appendage is seen projected just above the left ventricle to the left of the midline. The aorta may thereafter be visualized. The aortic sinuses and valves as well as the coronary arteries may also be visualized following selective catheterization of the left ventricle.

In *lateral view* these structures may once again be identified and the thickness of the left ventricle readily measured.

Gross differences between the normal child and adult are shown in Figure 12-50. In frontal perspective in the adult the cardiac chambers are more horizontally disposed, with a much tighter U-shaped curve of the right heart. In the left heart, the axes of both the inflow and outflow tracts lie in a more horizontal plane in infants and children than in adults.

In venous angiography when injection is made in both arms, the entire venous inflow tract to the heart is excellently visualized (Fig. 12-51).

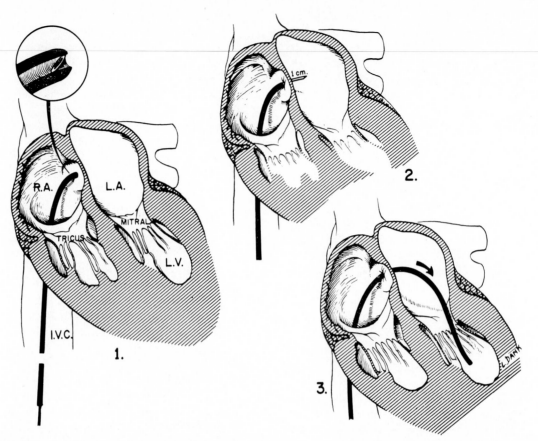

Figure 12–47. Diagrammatic representation of transseptal puncture with catherization of left atrium and left ventricle by the overlying catheter. (1) Proper positioning of needle and catheter for septal puncture, (2) septal puncture by the needle, and (3) catheterization of left ventricle by the overlying catheter. (From Schobinger, R. A., and Ruzicka, F. F., Jr.: Vascular Roentgenology. New York, The Macmillan Company, 1964.)

CORONARY ARTERIOGRAPHY AND VENOGRAPHY

Basic Anatomy. Two coronary arteries supply the heart. The *left coronary* originates from the left aortic sinus at the level of the free edge of the valve cusp. Its short common stem bifurcates or trifurcates about 0.5 to 2 cm. from its origin (Fig. 12–52). The *anterior interventricular or descending branch* courses downward in the anterior interventricular groove just to the right of the apex of the heart, and may ascend a short distance up the posterior interventricular groove. There are branches to the adjacent anterior right ventricular wall and septal branches, supplying the anterior two-thirds of the apical portion of the septum. The

anteroapical portions of the left ventricle ordinarily have several branches. The second branch of the left coronary artery, the *circumflex,* runs in the left atrioventricular sulcus, giving off branches to the upper lateral left ventricular wall and left atrium. When there is a third branch of the left coronary artery, it originates between the anterior interventricular and circumflex branches and supplies the left ventricle.

The *right coronary artery* arises from the right anterior sinus of Valsalva (aortic sinus) and courses along the right atrioventricular sulcus. It rounds the acute margin of the right ventricle to reach the crux (junction of the posterior interventricular sulcus and the posterior atrioventricular groove). It gives off branches to the anterior right ventricular wall; the branch along the acute

(Text continued on page 750.)

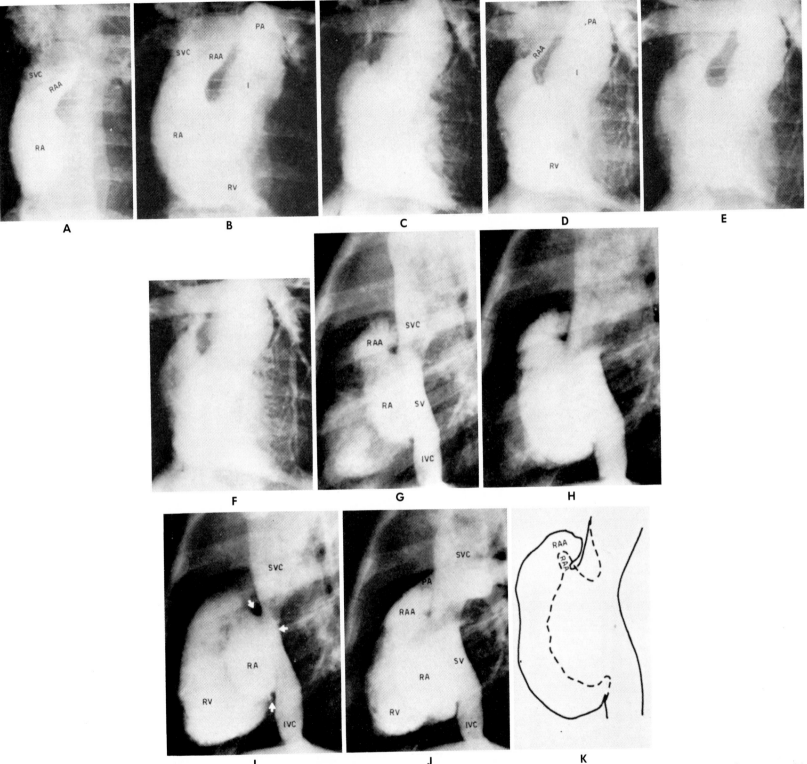

Figure 12–48. Representative angiocardiograms. *A–F.* Lesser circulation phase, frontal projection. Right auricular appendage lies directly to the right of the infundibulum and the right ventricle and lower part of the pulmonary artery which, consequently, in lateral projection, are overlapped by the appendage. (AO) Aorta, (I) infundibulum, (IVC) inferior vena cava, (LA) left atrium, (LV) left ventricle, (PA) pulmonary artery, (RA) right atrium, (RAA) right auricular appendage, (RV) right ventricle, (SV) sinus venosus, (SVC) superior vena cava. *G–K.* Lesser circulation phase, lateral projection. During atrial systole, the atrioventricular border is shifted dorsally, while the dorsal wall of the atrium remains in the same position. The crista terminalis presses into the lumen like a membrane (*I,* lower arrow). Sphincter mechanism of the venae cavae is clearly visible. *K.* Collective picture of appearance of atrium in late diastole (solid line) and late systole (broken line). (From Diagnosis of Congenital Heart Disease, 2d ed., by Kjellberg, Sven R., et al. Copyright © 1959 by Year Book Medical Publishers, Inc., Chicago. Used by permission.)

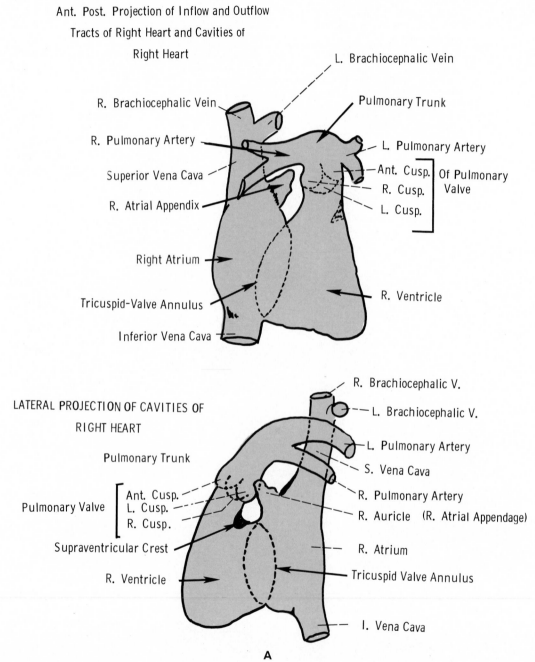

Ant. Post. Projection of Inflow and Outflow
Tracts of Right Heart and Cavities of
Right Heart

L. Brachiocephalic Vein

R. Brachiocephalic Vein

Pulmonary Trunk

R. Pulmonary Artery

L. Pulmonary Artery

Superior Vena Cava

Ant. Cusp. ─┐ Of Pulmonary
R. Cusp. ──┤ Valve
L. Cusp. ───┘

R. Atrial Appendix

Right Atrium

R. Ventricle

Tricuspid-Valve Annulus

Inferior Vena Cava

LATERAL PROJECTION OF CAVITIES OF
RIGHT HEART

R. Brachiocephalic V.

L. Brachiocephalic V.

Pulmonary Trunk

L. Pulmonary Artery

S. Vena Cava

Pulmonary Valve ─┤ Ant. Cusp.
L. Cusp.
R. Cusp.

R. Pulmonary Artery

R. Auricle   (R. Atrial Appendage)

Supraventricular Crest

R. Atrium

R. Ventricle

Tricuspid Valve Annulus

I. Vena Cava

A

Figure 12–49.   A. Anteroposterior and lateral projections of inflow and outflow tracts of the right heart and the cavities of the right heart, also showing the relative positions of the cusps of the pulmonary valve.

Figure 12–49 continued on the opposite page.

Ant. Post. Projection Left Heart and Aorta
as seen in Angiography

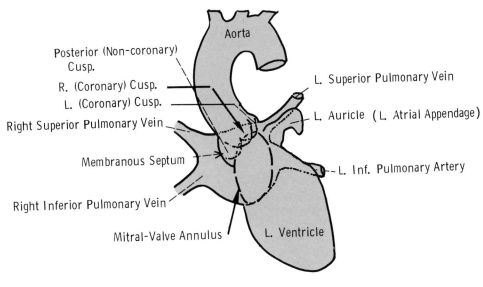

Posterior (Non-coronary)
Cusp.
R. (Coronary) Cusp.
L. (Coronary) Cusp.
Right Superior Pulmonary Vein
Membranous Septum
Right Inferior Pulmonary Vein
Mitral-Valve Annulus

Aorta
L. Superior Pulmonary Vein
L. Auricle (L. Atrial Appendage)
L. Inf. Pulmonary Artery
L. Ventricle

Lateral Projection of Cavities of Left Heart

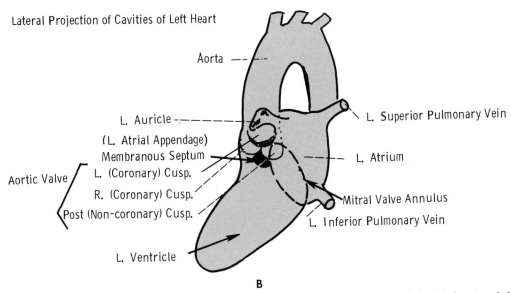

Aorta
L. Auricle
(L. Atrial Appendage)
Membranous Septum
Aortic Valve
L. (Coronary) Cusp.
R. (Coronary) Cusp.
Post (Non-coronary) Cusp.
L. Ventricle

L. Superior Pulmonary Vein
L. Atrium
Mitral Valve Annulus
L. Inferior Pulmonary Vein

B

Figure 12–49 *Continued.* B. Anteroposterior and lateral projections of the cavities of the left heart and the outflow tracts, also showing the relative positions of the cusps of the aortic valves.

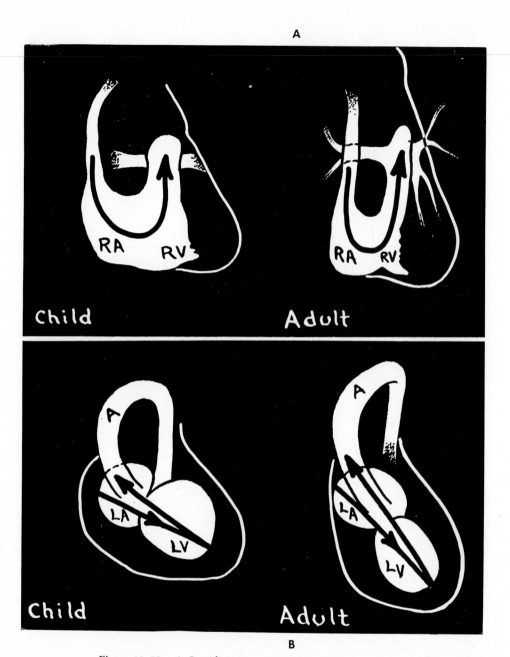

Figure 12–50. *A.* Semidiagrammatic tracings of the normal right heart as seen in representative frontal angiocardiograms of children and adults. Note the more horizontal relationships of the cardiac chambers in the child, and the much tighter "U"-shaped curve of the right heart in the adult. This difference reflects the change from a relatively transverse position of the heart in infancy and childhood to a more vertical position in adult life, and parallels the changing configuration of the thoracic cage. *B.* Semidiagrammatic tracings from angiocardiograms of the normal left heart and aorta in children and adults. Frontal projection. The axes of both the inflow and outflow tracts of the left ventricle lie in a more horizontal position in infants and children than in adults. This reflects the transverse position of the heart and the relatively greater horizontal diameter of the chest in the early years. (From Abrams and Kaplan: Angiocardiographic Interpretation in Congenital Heart Disease, Charles C Thomas.)

margin of the heart and another supplying the posterior interventricular branch are usually well developed. The posterior papillary muscle of the left ventricle usually has a dual supply from both the left and the right coronary arteries. One branch, which originates from the right coronary artery, ascends along the anteromedial wall of the right atrium and supplies the *superior vena caval branch or nodal artery,* posterior and to the left of the superior vena caval ostium. It then rounds this ostium to the sinoatrial node.

Variations in the branching pattern of the coronary artery are frequent. In about two-thirds of the cases, the right coronary artery is dominant, crossing the crux and supplying part of the left ventricular wall and the ventricular septum. In 15 per cent of cases the left coronary artery is dominant and its circumflex branch crosses the crux, supplying the posterior interventricular branch and all of the left ventricle, the ventricular septum, and part of the right ventricle. In 18 per cent of cases both coronary arteries reach the crux and this is the so-called "balanced coronary arterial pattern" (Netter). In about 40 per cent of cases, a large anterior atrial branch of the left coronary artery courses toward the superior vena cava rather than the anterior atrial branch of the right coronary artery. It is also quite common for the first, second, and even third branches of the right coronary artery to originate independently from the right aortic sinus rather than from the right coronary artery proper.

Oblique projections of the right and left coronary arteries are shown diagrammatically in Figure 12–53.

The two largest veins are the *great cardiac vein* in the anterior interventricular groove along with the left coronary artery, and the *middle cardiac vein* in the posterior interventricular groove, along with the posterior interventricular branch of the right coronary artery. There may also be a large *posterior left ventricular vein* as well. Small valves may be present in each of these larger veins. The oblique vein of the left atrium enters the coronary sinus near its junction with the great cardiac vein and it does not have a valve. The small cardiac vein may enter the coronary sinus as shown (Fig. 12–54), or it may enter the right atrium independently. There are anterior cardiac veins that do almost always enter the right atrium independently. As shown in the illustration, there are veins in the inferior interventricular groove and the atrioventricular groove along the right border that appear to flow into the small cardiac vein and thence into the coronary sinus. Small veins situated in the atrial septum and ventricular walls that enter the cardiac chambers directly are called the *Thebesian* veins.

Coronary Arteriography

Brief Review of Technique. (For greater detail see Abrams and Adams, and Judkins.) This procedure requires the skilled

(Text continued on page 754.)

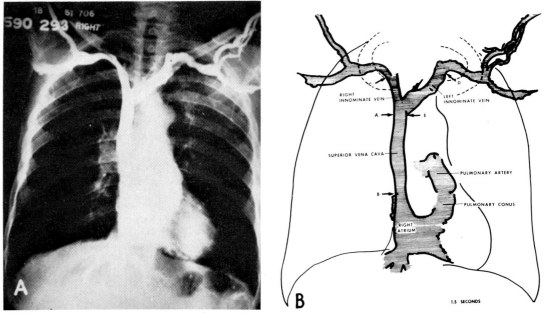

Figure 12–51. The superior vena cava and innominate veins as visualized by venous angiocardiography. (From Roberts, D. J., Jr., Dotter, C. T., and Steinberg, I.: Am. J. Roentgenol., 66:341–352, 1951.)

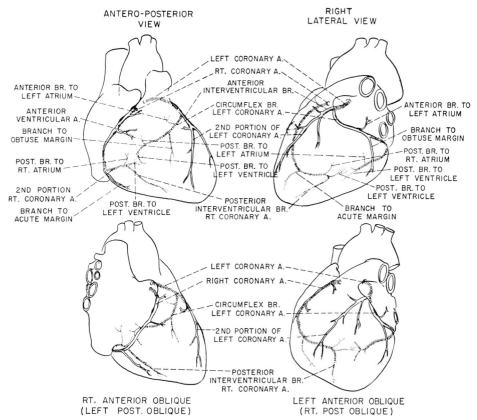

Figure 12–52. Diagram of coronary circulation as might be seen in frontal, lateral and oblique projections. (Modified from Guglielmo and Guttadauro: Acta Radiol., Supp. 97, 1952.)

RIGHT CORONARY ARTERY LEFT ANTERIOR OBLIQUE

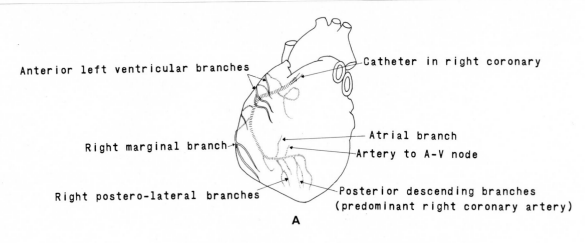

Anterior left ventricular branches

Catheter in right coronary

Right marginal branch

Atrial branch

Artery to A-V node

Right postero-lateral branches

Posterior descending branches
(predominant right coronary artery)

A

RIGHT CORONARY ARTERY — RIGHT ANTERIOR OBLIQUE

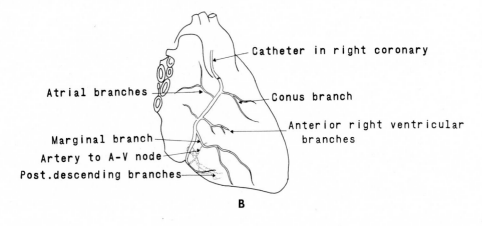

Catheter in right coronary

Atrial branches

Conus branch

Anterior right ventricular
branches

Marginal branch

Artery to A-V node

Post. descending branches

B

LEFT CORONARY ARTERY   LEFT ANTERIOR OBLIQUE

Catheter

Left atrial branch

Artery to sinus node

Left coronary artery

Posterior division

Anterior descending branch

Left marginal branch

Septal branches

Diagonal branch

Anterior interventricular branch

Antero-lateral branch

Postero-lateral branch

Posterior circumflex branch

Posterior descending branches

C

Figure 12–53.   Oblique projections of the coronary arteries.

Figure 12–53 continued on the opposite page.

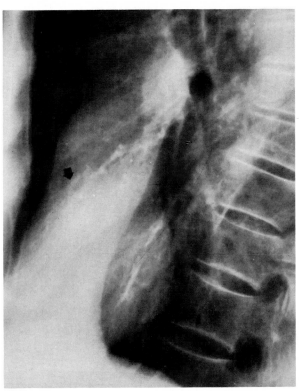

LEFT CORONARY ARTERY   RIGHT ANTERIOR OBLIQUE

Catheter

Superior left atrial branch

Septal branches

Posterior circumflex

Inferior left atrial branch

A-V node branch

Posterior descending branches

Postero-lateral branches

Left marginal branch

Left coronary artery

Posterior division

Anterior division

Diagonal branch

Antero-lateral branch

Anterior descending branch

D

E

Figure 12–53 *Continued.* D. Right anterior oblique projection of left coronary artery. E. Calcification in coronary arteries seen on plain film.

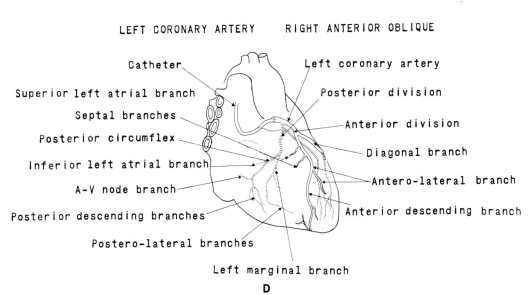

Oblique vein over posterior wall of left atrium

Small valve may occur here

Coronary sinus

Small valve may occur here

Great cardiac vein in anterior inter-ventricular groove with left coronary artery

Small cardiac vein

Veins from left ventricle

Atrioventricular groove along right border

Middle cardiac vein

Inferior interventricular groove

Figure 12–54. Lateral erect view of the veins of the heart.

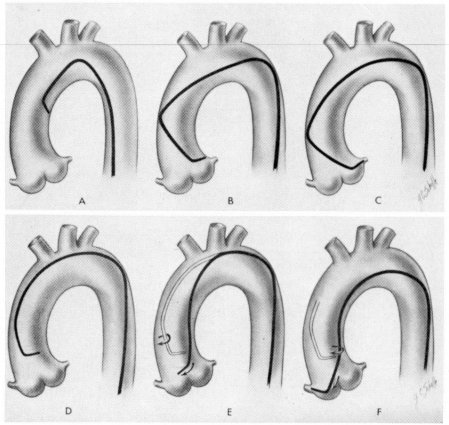

Figure 12–55. *A, B,* and *C.* Diagrammatic illustrations of left coronary catheterization. *D, E,* and *F.* Diagrammatic illustrations of right coronary catheterization (see text). (From Judkins, M. P.: Radiol. Clin. N. Amer., 6:467–492, December, 1968.)

collaboration of radiologists and cardiologists, each with a thorough knowledge of the cardiac pharmacology. The two basic techniques for coronary artery visualization involve: (1) the introduction of a catheter into a supravalvular site with a forceful injection, which allows visualization of the coronary arteries as they leave the aortic sinuses; and (2) selective coronary arteriography whereby a catheter is inserted into the ostium of each coronary artery in sequence for injection. There are a number of modifications of the selective approach: (a) by a cutdown technique over the brachial artery and the insertion of a single catheter into each coronary artery sequentially; or (b) a percutaneous femoral approach involving insertion of a specially shaped catheter into each coronary ostium separately. In this latter approach usually the catheter is separately shaped for each of the two insertions. Each technique has its proponents, but some would prefer a technique that obviates the need for performing a

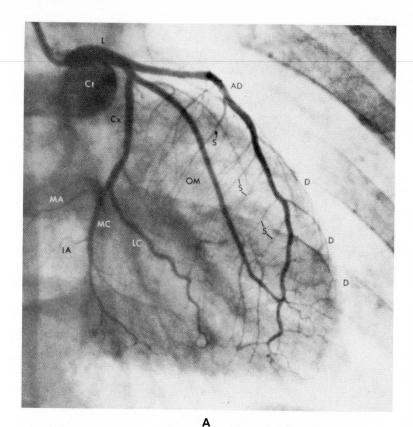

A

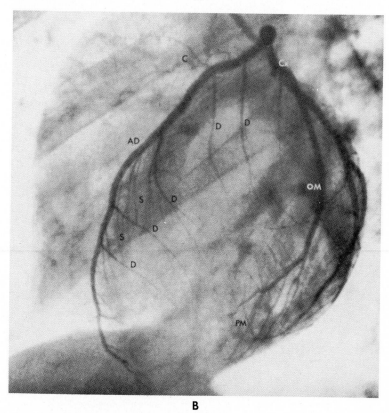

B

Figure 12–56. *See opposite page for legend.*

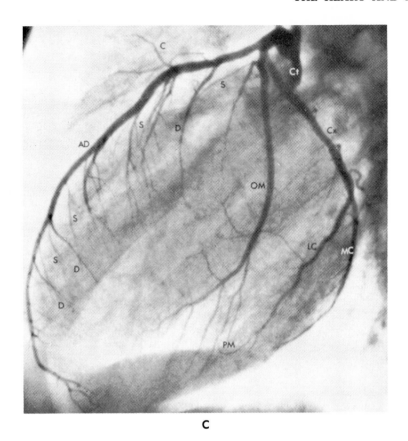

C

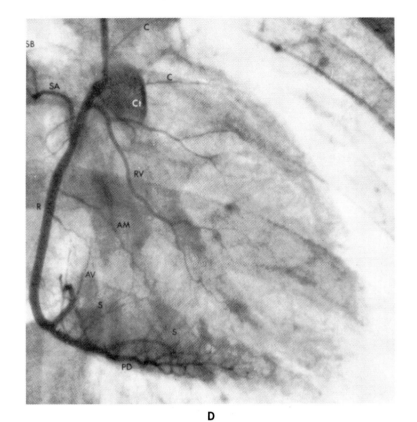

D

Figure 12–56. *A–C.* High-resolution normal left selective coronary arteriography. *A.* Right anterior oblique 20°. *B.* Left anterior oblique 70°. *C.* Lateral. Contrast agent injections of each coronary artery are filmed in three projections by both cinéfluorography and high-resolution serial techniques. These three projections were selected because they uncover and give dimension to all parts of the coronary tree. In each, the heart is projected free of the spine.

Legend: L, Left main; AD, anterior descending; D, diagonal; S, septal; C, conus branches; Cx, circumflex; OM, obtuse marginal; LC, lateral circumflex; MC, medial circumflex; AC, atrial circumflex; MA, middle arterial; IA, inferior atrial; PM, papillary muscle artery; Ct, contrast material in the sinus of Valsalva.

D–F. High-resolution normal right selective coronary arteriography. *D.* Right anterior oblique 20°. *E.* Left anterior oblique 70°.

Legend: R, Right main; C, conus branch; RV, right ventricular artery; SA, sinus node artery; SB, sinus node branch; PA, posterior atrial branch; AS, atrial septal branch; AM, acute marginal; PD, posterior descending; AV, atrioventricular node artery; PL, posterior lateral arteries; MA, middle atrial; IA, inferior atrial; S, septal; Ct, contrast material in the sinus of Valsalva. (*A–F* from Judkins, M. P.: Radiol. Clin. N. Amer., 6:467–492, December, 1968.)

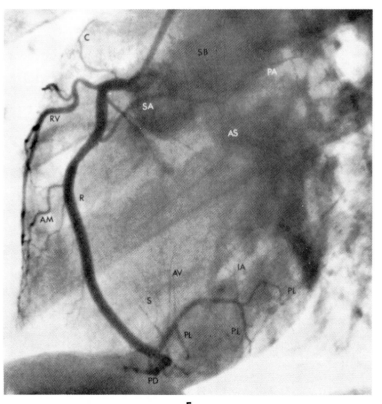

E

Figure 12–56 continued on the following page.

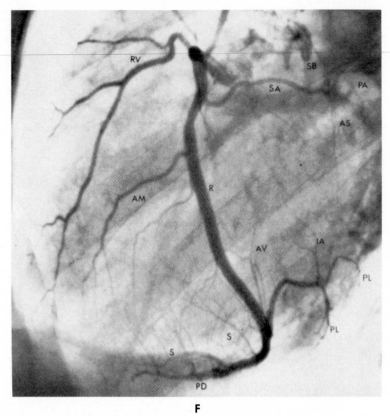

F

Figure 12–56 *Continued.* *F.* Lateral film in high-resolution normal right selective coronary arteriography. See full legend on page 755.

cutdown over any artery, particulary the small caliber brachial artery with its associated difficulties of catheter manipulation. Many different injection devices have been described for use with selective coronary arteriography. Many, however, require a manual injection of small volumes (4 to 8 ml.) of contrast agent into each coronary artery.

Serialographic rapid film technique or coronary cinéangiography may be employed. Left ventricular cinéangiography should probably be an integral part of coronary arteriography so that ventricular contractility may be assessed prior to the visualization of the coronary arteries. It should be emphasized that experienced personnel, careful monitoring of cardiac rhythm, and "adequate facilities for immediate resuscitation and cardioversion, and prompt surgical intervention in the event of vascular occlusion or hemorrhage are mandatory to keep a low incidence of complications. Under ideal conditions the risk should be no greater than that of thoracic aortography or other intracardiovascular diagnostic procedures" (Abrams and Adams) (Fig. 12–55).

Select Coronary Arteriograms for Demonstation of Anatomy. Normal left and right selective coronary arteriograms, with important branches labeled, are indicated in Figure 12–56. Some variations of normal are illustrated in Figure 12–57. Numerous other variations could be described (Levin and Baltaxe). Also, numerous anastomoses of the coronary arteries are described, with preferential pathways of collateral flow. These are illustrated in Figures 12–58 and 12–59.

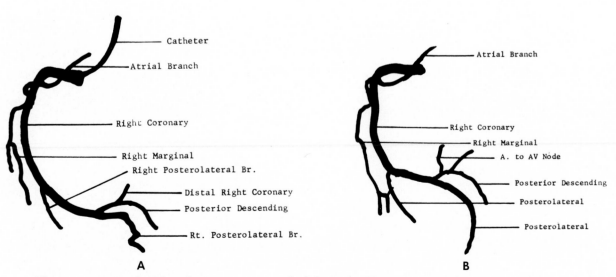

A

B

Figure 12–57. *A* and *B.* The right coronary artery in the left anterior oblique in two different phases of respiration.

Figure 12–57 continued on the opposite page.

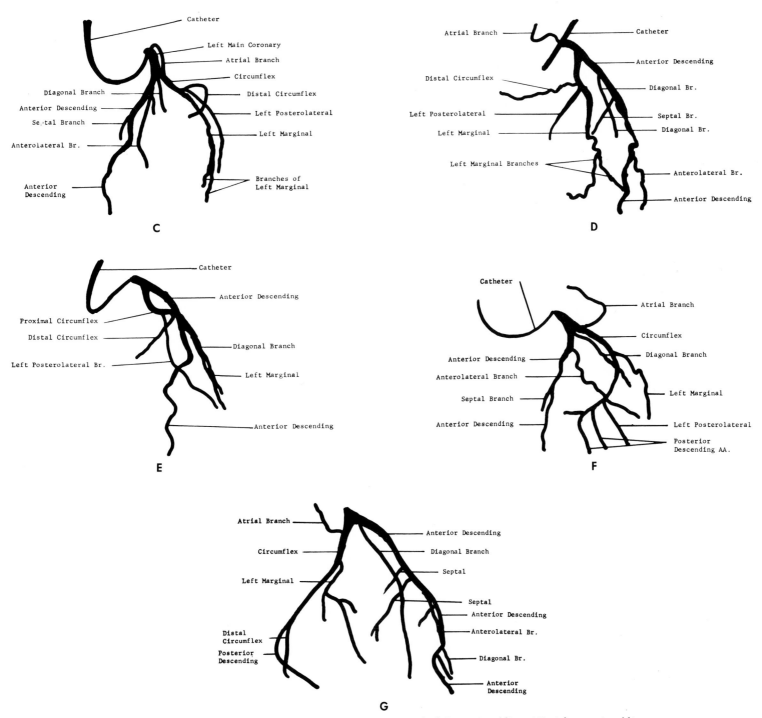

Figure 12–57 *Continued.* *C, D,* and *E.* A left coronary artery in the left anterior oblique (*C*), right anterior oblique (*D*), and posteroanterior projections (*E*).

F and *G.* A left coronary artery in the left (*F*) and right (*G*) anterior oblique projections. (From Sewell, W. H.: Amer. J. Roentgenol., 97:359–368, 1966.)

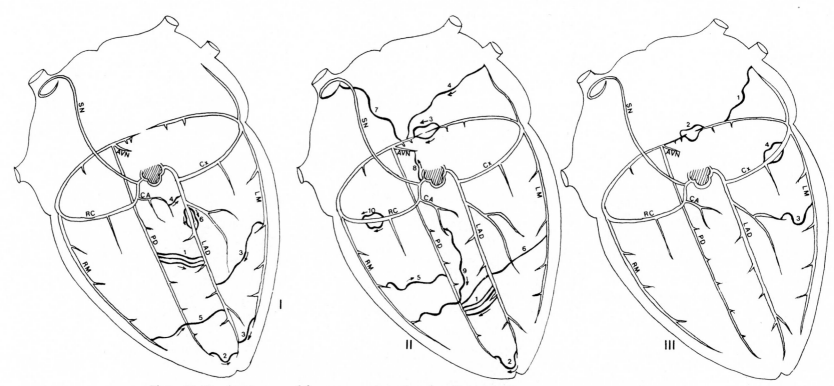

Figure 12–58. Anastomoses of the coronary arteries in order of frequency.

I. Left Anterior Descending Artery: (1) septal anastomoses, (2) anastomoses over the apex, (3) left marginal anastomoses to the LAD, (4) Vieussen's circle, (5) right marginal anastomoses to the LAD, (6) intracoronary anastomoses.

II. Right Coronary Artery: (1) septal anastomoses, (2) apical anastomoses, (3) left circumflex anastomoses with distal RC, (4) atrial circumflex anastomoses with distal RC, (5) right marginal anastomoses with posterior descending, (6) left marginal anastomoses with posterior descending, (7) sinus node artery anastomoses with distal RC, (8) Kugel's artery, (9) conus artery anastomoses with the right marginal branches, (10) intracoronary anastomoses across occlusion.

III. Left Circumflex Artery: (1) anastomoses from the left atrial circumflex to the circumflex, (2) anastomoses from the right coronary artery to the left circumflex, (3) diagonals over left margins to the left circumflex, (4) intracoronary anastomoses bridging the occlusion.

(LC) left main coronary artery; (Cx) left circumflex artery; (RC) right coronary artery; (AVN) atrioventricular node artery; (LAD) left anterior descending artery; (LM) left marginal artery of the obtuse angle; (RM) right marginal artery of the acute angle; (SN) sinus node artery; (CA) conus artery. (From Jochem, et al.: Amer. J. Roentgenol., *116*:60, 1972.)

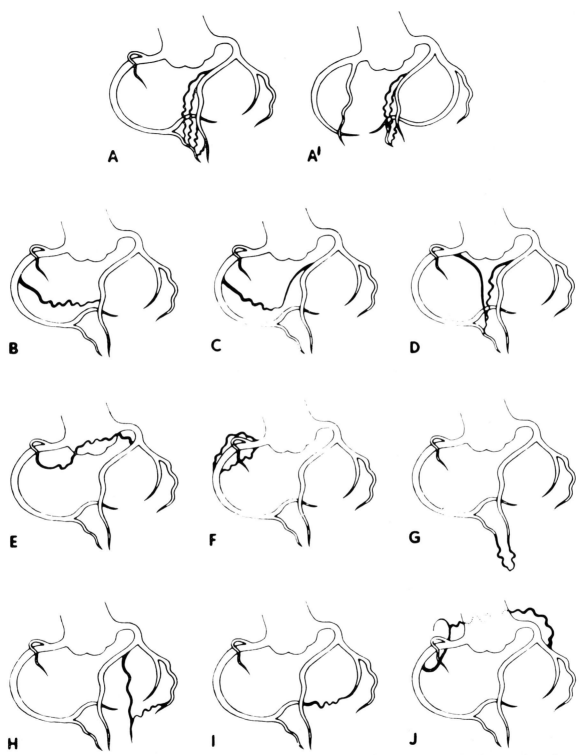

Figure 12–59. Coronary collaterial pathways. Schematic presentation of different interarterial connections. *A.* Septal collaterals. *A'.* Same collaterals as in *A* with a more prominent left circumflex artery. *B.* Epicardial collaterals of right ventricular wall. *C.* Collateral in moderator band. *D.* Collateral in crista supraventricularis. *E.* Epicardial collateral of the pulmonary conus. *F.* Direct by-passing collateral. *G.* Epicardial collateral at apex. *H.* Collateral in left ventricular wall. *I.* Collateral in atrioventricular sulcus. *J.* Collateral in atrial wall. (From Paulin, S.: Investigative Radiol., 2:147–159, 1967.)

REFERENCES

Abrams, H. L.: Angiography, Vol. 1. Second edition. Boston, Little, Brown & Co., pp. 119–122, 1971.

Abrams, H. L., and Adams, D. F.: Coronary arteriography. *In* Abrams, H. L. (ed.): Angiography. Second edition. Boston, Little, Brown & Co., 1971.

Altemus, L. R.: Malnutrition with microcardia. Amer. J. Roentgenol., *99*:674–680, 1967.

Amundsen, P.: The diagnostic value of conventional radiological examination of the heart in adults. Acta Radiol. (Suppl.), *181*:1–87, 1959.

Anson, B. J.: Atlas of Human Anatomy. Philadelphia, W. B. Saunders Co., 1963.

Bell, A. L. L.: Catheterization of the left heart by transseptal needle and overlying catheter. *In* Schobinger, R. A., and Ruzicka, F. F. (eds.): Vascular Roentgenology. New York, Macmillan, 1964.

Bierman, H. R.: Selective Arterial Catheterization, Springfield, Ill., Charles C Thomas, 1969.

Boone, B. R., Chamberlain, W. E., Gilbeck, F. G., and Henny, G. C.: Interpreting the electrokymogram of heart and great vessel motion. Amer. Heart. J., *34*:560–681, 1947.

Bosniak, M. A.: An analysis of some anatomic-roentgenologic aspects of the brachiocephalic vessels. Amer. J. Roentgenol., *91*:1222–1231, 1964.

Boyden, E. A.: Segmental Anatomy of the Lungs: A Study of the Patterns of the Segmental Bronchi and Related Pulmonary Vessels. New York, McGraw Hill Book Co., 1955.

Chang, C. H. J.: Right pulmonary artery measurements. Amer. J. Roentgenol., 87:929–935, 1962.

Cunningham, D. J.: Manual of Practical Anatomy, Vol. 2. 12th edition. London, Oxford University Press, 1958.

Dinsmore, R. E., Goodman, D. J., and Sanders, C. A.: Some pitfalls in evaluation of cardiac chamber enlargement on chest roentgenograms. Radiology, 87:267–273, 1966.

Gammill, S. L., Krebs, C., Meyers, P. et al.: Cardiac measurements in systole and diastole. Radiology, 94:115–119, 1970.

Gorlin, R.: Normal variations in venous oxygen content. *In* Warren, V. J. (ed.): Methods in Medical Research. Vol. 7. Chicago, Year Book Medical Publishers, 1958.

Gorlin, R., McMillan, I. K. R., Medd, W. E., Matthews, M. D., and Daley, R.: Dynamics of the circulation in aortic valvular disease. Amer. J. Med., *18*:855, 1955.

His, quoted in Abrams, H. L.: Angiography. Second edition. Boston, Little, Brown & Co., 1971.

Hoffman, R. B., and Rigler, L. G.: Evaluation of left ventricular enlargement in the lateral projection of the chest. Radiology, 85:93–100, 1965.

Jacobson, B., and Paulin, S.: Experience with different contrast media in coronary angiography. Acta Radiol. (Suppl.), *270*:103, 1967.

James, T. N.: Anatomy of the Coronary Arteries. New York, Paul B. Hoeber, Inc., 1961.

Jochem, W., Soto, B., Karp, R. B., et al.: Radiographic anatomy of the coronary collateral circulation. Amer. J. Roentgenol., *116*:50–61, 1972. fig. 9.

Judkins, M. P.: Percutaneous transfemoral selective coronary arteriography. Radiol. Clin. N. Amer., *6*:467–492, December, 1968.

Klatte, E. C., Tampas, J. P., and Campbell, J. A.: Evaluation of right atrial size. Radiology, *81*:48–55, 1963.

Lane, E. J., Jr., and Whalen, J. P.: A new sign of left atrial enlargement: posterior displacement of the left bronchial tree. Radiology, 93:279–284, 1969.

Lavender, J. P., and Doppman, J.: The hilum in pulmonary venous hypertension. Brit. J. Radiol., *35*:303–313, 1962.

Leinbach, L. B.: Normal pulmonary arteries in children. Amer. J. Roentgenol., 89:995–998, 1963.

Levin, D. C., and Baltaxe, H. A.: Posterior descending coronary artery. Amer. J. Roentgenol., *116*:41–49, 1972.

Levitan, L. H., and Reilly, H. F., Jr.: Aortic sinus of Valsalva calcification: a roentgen sign on the lateral chest film. Radiology, 87:1074–1075, 1966.

Lewis, B. M., Gorlin, R., Haussay, H. E. J., Haynes, F. W., and Dexter, L.: Clinical and physiological correlation in patients with mitral stenosis. Amer. Heart J., *43*:2, 1952.

Lind, J.: Heart volume in normal infants. Acta Radiol., (Suppl.), *82*:3–127, 1950.

Meschan, I.: Analysis of Roentgen Signs. Philadelphia, W. B. Saunders Co., 1973.

Michelson, E., and Salik, J. O.: The vascular pattern of the lung as seen on routine and tomographic studies. Radiology, 73:511–526, 1959.

Netter, F. H.: Ciba Collection of Medical Illustrations, Vol. 5. Ciba Pharmaceutical Company, Division of Ciba-Geigy Corporation, 1969.

Paulin, S.: Coronary angiography: technical, anatomic and clinical studies. Acta Radiol. (Suppl.), *233*:5–215, 1964.

Paulin, S.: Interarterial coronary anastomoses in relation to arterial obstruction demonstrated in coronary arteriography. Invest. Radiol., *2*:147–159, 1967.

Robb, G. P., and Steinberg, I.: Practical method of visualization of chambers of the heart, the pulmonary circulation, and the great blood vessels in man. J. Clin. Invest., *17*:507, 1938; Amer. J. Roentgenol., *41*:1–17, 1939.

Sewell, W. H.: Roentgenologic anatomy of human coronary arteries. Amer. J. Roentgenol., *97*:359–366, 1966.

Ungerleider, H. E., and Gubner, R.: Evaluation of heart size measurements. Amer. Heart J., *24*:494–510, 1942.

VonHayek, H.: The Human Lung. New York, Hafner Publishing Co., Inc., 1960.

Wilson, W. J., Lee, G. B., and Amplatz, K.: Selective coronary arteriography. Amer. J. Roentgenol., *100*:332–340, 1967.

Wood, P.: Aortic stenosis. Amer. J. Cardiol., *1*:553, 1958.

13

The Upper Alimentary Tract

PRINCIPLES INVOLVED IN STUDY OF THE ALIMENTARY TRACT

The walls of the alimentary tract are intermediate in radiographic density, and hence require some type of contrast material for detection by means of x-rays. Normally, there is a variable amount of gas in the stomach and colon that permits a relatively gross and inadequate visualization of these structures. In the normal adult, gas in the small intestine is considered abnormal and the introduction of contrast material into the small intestine is therefore essential.

Although negative contrast may be employed in the visualization of the gastrointestinal tract, it is usually supplementary to the more significant positive contrast with radiopaque media.

Since the physiology and function of the gastrointestinal tract are readily altered by so many factors such as hypotonicity or hypertonicity, alkalinity, acidity, proteins, fats, carbohydrates, amino acids, and any slight mechanical irritation, it is essential for any opaque contrast medium to be physiologically inert.

The most commonly used medium thus employed in present-day radiography of the gastrointestinal tract is barium sulfate in water suspension, although bismuth salts, radioactive Umbrathor and barium sulfate in isotonic saline, "buttermilk," or other commercial suspensions are also employed by some, or used on special occasions. In certain patients, in whom obstruction by barium mixtures may occur, organic soluble iodides are utilized by intubation techniques. In infants or other patients in whom aspiration is a potential danger, small quantities of iodized oil are helpful, at least until it is certain that aspiration is not taking place. Iodized oil is a poor contrast agent beyond the esophagus because it distorts the normal physiologic pattern.

On certain occasions, it is advantageous to use so-called double contrast in which gas is introduced after administering the barium suspension. The gas and barium suspension are thus mixed and are helpful in outlining polyps and small tumors. The gas employed may be air, carbon dioxide, or a mixture of both, as when ginger ale, carbonated water or Seidlitz powder are introduced into the stomach.

The usual radiologic methods include: (1) fluoroscopy, (2) spotfilm radiography, (3) routine radiography in certain positions; any or all of the usual erect, recumbent, supine, prone, lateral or oblique positions are employed.

Other methods of radiologic study of the upper alimentary tract include *hypotonic duodenography, angiography,* and *endoscopic pancreatocholangiography,* as well as other pararadiologic procedures not included in this text, such as ultrasonography and radioisotopic scanning procedures.

Parietography—the demonstration of the walls of the gastrointestinal tract by filling the peritoneal cavity and the lumen of the studied organ simultaneously with air or gas—is a further refinement of the air contrast technique. This may be especially helpful when combined with tomography.

In many of these methods, *pharmacoradiography,* or the injection of drugs in order to influence the radiologic examination, may be employed.

There are two major principles involved in the radiologic anatomy of the gastrointestinal tract:

1. We are examining a dynamic, moving, functioning system of organs. They are not static. Their structure must at all times be considered along with their function, and the two aspects are inseparable.

2. When the lumen of a hollow organ is filled with contrast substance, we can visualize the inner lining with accuracy, but the wall of the organ outside the innermost lining can be studied only indirectly as it affects the lumen or the mucosa. It is conceivable that considerable abnormality may exist outside the lumen within the wall of the organ, which may not be reflected in the mucosal pattern.

(Parietography, does, however, permit visualization of the outer walls of the gastrointestinal tract simultaneously with the lumen of the studied organ, particularly when combined with tomography.)

THE MOUTH AND OROPHARYNX

The mouth and oropharynx are so readily examined by direct inspection and palpation that it is not usual to employ the radiograph except for demonstration of hidden structures.

In a direct lateral view (Fig. 13–1), the air within the mouth and pharynx permits a contrast visualization of the tongue surface, the hard and soft palate, and the nasopharynx and oropharynx.

Special views of the salivary glands may be obtained after the injection of iodized water soluble contrast agents into the ducts. Soft tissue studies of the floor of the mouth or the cheek are also feasible.

Brief mention of the radiography of the teeth has already been made (see Chapter 6), and will not be further discussed in this text.

Soft Tissue Study of the Mouth and Pharynx by Lateral Projection. This projection is identical with that employed for a lateral view of the cervical spine, except that technical factors are varied slightly to emphasize the soft tissues rather than the skeletal structure (see Chapters 9 and 10).

The structures demonstrated in profile are: the tongue and floor of the mouth, the hard and soft palate and uvula, the vallecula at the base of the tongue and the pyriform sinuses on either side, the nasopharynx above the palate with turbinates and eustachian orifice, the lymphoid structures in the nasopharynx, and the epiglottis. The laryngeal structures seen in this projection have been previously described (Chapter 10).

The width of the soft tissues projected under the sphenoid is considerably narrower in the adult than in the child, owing to the markedly enlarged lymphoid apparatus in the child after 3 to 6 months of age. This view affords a ready means of investigating these lymphoid and adenoid structures (Chapter 10).

The width of the retro-oropharyngeal soft tissues in the child is also considerably greater than it is in the adult when these structures are compared with the retrolaryngeal soft tissues between the larynx and the cervical spine. Thus in the newborn and infant, the ratio of the retro-oropharyngeal soft tissues to the retrolaryngeal soft tissues is approximately 1 to 1, while in the adult it is usually in the order of 1 to 3. These measurements are of value in the detection of space-occupying lesions such as inflammations and tumors in these locations, which by direct inspection are difficult to evaluate because they may be posterior to the visible mucosa, or because the patient may be unable to open his mouth. (See Chapter 10.)

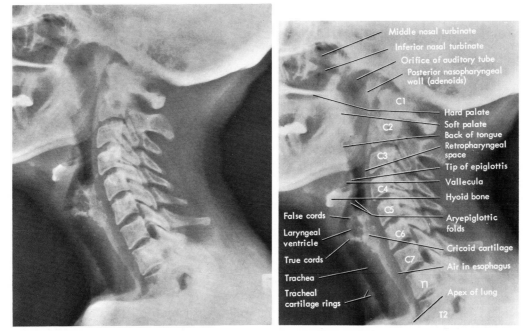

Figure 13–1. Lateral soft tissue film of neck.

Soft Tissue Radiography of the Floor of the Mouth with the Aid of the Occlusal Type Dental Film. By placing an occlusal type dental film in the mouth (Fig. 13–2) and directing the x-ray beam perpendicular to it, the soft tissues of the submandibular area are penetrated, as well as the mandible. These soft tissues are not visualized in sufficient detail to distinguish the various anatomic structures such as the salivary glands and ducts, lymph nodes, and tongue, but this method of examination does afford a ready means of investigating abnormal calcareous deposits in these structures. Hence an understanding of the normal appearance of this projection is essential.

Soft Tissue Radiography of the Cheek. This can be performed in a similar manner by placing an occlusal film on the inside of the cheek. Care must be exercised to place the film sufficiently posterior to obtain a visualization of as much of Stenson's duct as possible, since occasionally calcareous deposits in this location may lead to obstructive inflammation and symptoms.

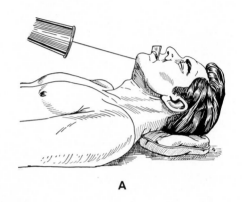

A

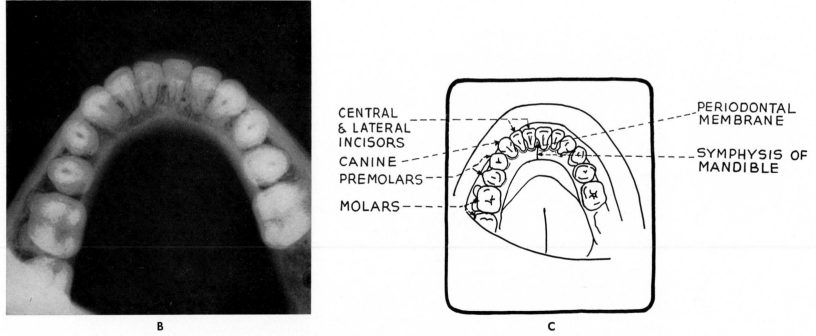

B   C

Figure 13–2. Occlusal type dental film of floor of mouth. *A.* Position of patient. *B.* Radiograph. *C.* Labeled tracing of *B.*

Radiography of the Hard Palate. Apart from the lateral projection previously described, the hard palate may be visualized by means of an occlusal film in the mouth as illustrated in Figure 13–3. There are considerable differences in density in the various portions of the hard palate owing to the presence of the aerated sinuses, the alveolar process, and the bony nasal septum, all of which overlie the palate. This variation in density is important in interpretation of the osseous structure of the hard palate.

The incisive foramen and the major palatine foramen can usually be identified. Frequently, the midline suture as well as the transverse palatine suture can also be noted.

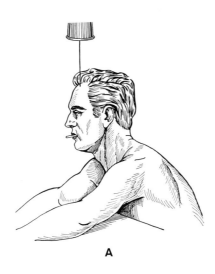

A

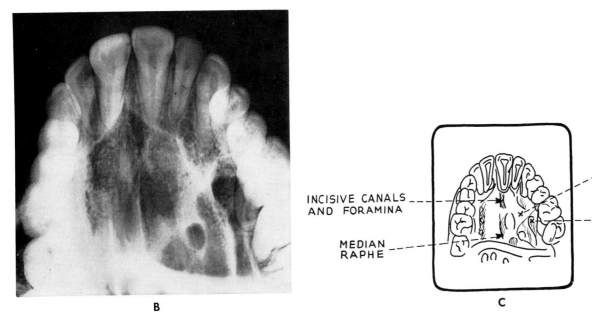

B   C

INCISIVE CANALS AND FORAMINA

MEDIAN RAPHE

PALATINE PROCESS OF MAXILLA

MAXILLARY SINUS

Figure 13–3. Method of radiography of hard palate with occlusal type dental film. A. Position of patient. B. Radiograph. C. Labeled tracing of B.

THE SALIVARY GLANDS

Normal Anatomy. There are three salivary glands, each with a separate duct or ducts opening into the mouth: the parotid, the submaxillary, and the sublingual.

The parotid gland is the largest of these and lies on the side of the face, below and in front of the ear, bounded by the zygoma above, the sternomastoid muscle behind, and the ramus of the mandible in front. Approximately one-quarter or one-third of the gland is usually deep to the posterior margin of the mandible and extends almost to the pharyngeal wall, being separated from the latter by the branches of the carotid artery, several veins and nerves, and small muscles. Actually, the anterior surface of the gland is wrapped around the posterior margin of the ramus of the mandible. The parotid duct (or Stensen's duct) runs across the masseter muscle superficially, accompanied by branches of the facial nerve. At the anterior margin of the masseter muscle, it turns sharply inward, pierces the buccinator muscle, and opens into the vestibule of the oral cavity on a small papilla opposite the second upper molar tooth. It is approximately 6 cm. in length.

The submaxillary gland lies in the submaxillary triangle on either side of the neck. This gland lies under cover of the body of the mandible for the most part, in its submaxillary fossa. There are a few small lymph nodes embedded in the substance of the gland, and the external maxillary artery runs through its superior and posterior portion. The submaxillary duct (Wharton's duct) runs forward, inward, and upward to open into the floor of the mouth, in a papilla on the plica sublingualis close to the frenulum of the tongue. This duct is about 5 cm. in length.

The sublingual gland is the smallest of the salivary glands, and is more deeply situated. It lies under the mucosa of the floor of the mouth, just posterior to the symphysis and in the sublingual fossa of the medial surface of the mandible. It has approximately 12 separate excretory ducts which open on the plica sublingualis, for the most part, but one or two of them may open into the submaxillary duct. This latter point is important from the standpoint of sialography, since one of the ducts opening into the submaxillary duct may be injected by error, and the submaxillary gland visualized instead of the sublingual.

Radiographic Technique of Examination. The salivary glands may be examined by means of plain radiographs, or after the injection of contrast media into the salivary duct. Plain radiographs are of value only when a calculus is suspected. In other instances, contrast studies are necessary.

With regard to *plain radiographs,* the following studies may be performed:

1. For parotid calculi, a lateral view (in stereoscopic projection preferably) is taken, centering over the gland, with the neck extended and the mouth open.

2. For submaxillary and sublingual calculi, a stereoscopic lateral view is obtained with the mouth closed, and usually it is best to incline the x-ray tube slightly cephalad to prevent superimposition of the two rami of the mandible. Also a view of the floor of the mouth is obtained with the aid of an occlusal type dental film as previously described.

Sialograms are defined as the radiographic demonstration of the salivary ducts and alveoli by the injection of contrast media. The technique is as follows (Chisholm et al.; Park and Mason):

The duct may be dilated with olive-tipped lacrimal probes. A sterile polyethylene catheter is thereafter inserted with a wire stylus for rigidity for a distance of 3 to 4 cm.

The contrast medium usually employed is a diatrizoate such as Hypaque or Renografin. It may be injected directly or by means of a glass reservoir positioned 70 cm. above the patient's head. If direct injection is employed, the injection is continued until definite pain is experienced by the patient. In the second technique (Park and Mason, 1966), underfilling seldom occurs because the film is taken while the contrast medium is still flowing and the pressure is therefore maintained. Moreover, overfilling rarely occurs because of the almost constant pressure. Usually 1 to 2 cc. of the contrast agent is adequate.

Films are obtained in the anteroposterior, lateral, or lateral-oblique positions (Fig. 13–4) at the completion of the filling phase. The polyethylene catheter may be plugged while the films are checked for adequacy. These films are then followed by a secretory film taken 5 minutes after the completion of the filling phase. To insure rapid expulsion of the contrast medium, salivary flow is stimulated by a few drops of lemon juice or by sucking on a lemon for 1 minute, after which the patient rinses his mouth. Normally, the gland should be empty within 5 minutes, although a faint "acinar" cloud may persist for up to 24 hours.

The emptying phase is considered as important as the "filling phase" to be described.

The Normal Filling Phase Sialogram. The appearance of the normal sialogram simulates the skeletal structure of a leaf (Fig. 13–4).

The parotid duct is somewhat narrower than the submaxillary, angulating sharply as it leaves the masseter muscle and passing obliquely through the buccinator muscle. There is usually a large forked branch from the parotid duct directed superiorly, called the "socia parotidis," but otherwise the branching ducts tend to join the main duct almost at right angles.

The secondary ductules of the submaxillary duct are less regular than those of the parotid, but are otherwise very similar.

The sublingual gland has numerous excretory ducts, and ordinarily only a small segment of the gland is visualized by a single injection. Occasionally, as mentioned earlier, a portion of the sublingual gland may be visualized after injecting the submaxillary duct, since the sublingual excretory duct may empty into the submaxillary duct rather than into the mouth.

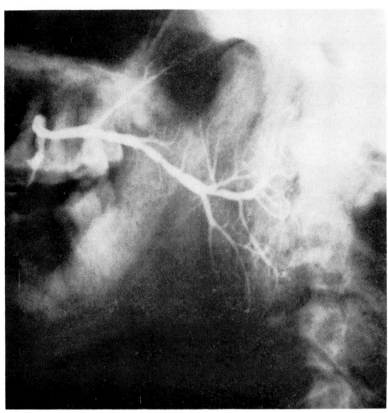

Figure 13–4. Normal sialogram of the parotid gland. (Courtesy Dr. L. B. Morettin, Galveston, Texas.)

ROENTGENOLOGIC CONSIDERATIONS OF THE HYOID APPARATUS

Basic Anatomy (Porrath). The hyoid bone is suspended in the anterior portion of the neck above the larynx, beneath the mandible, and anterior to the epiglottis. It is connected inferiorly by broad membranous bands to the thyroid cartilages of the larynx, and by other broad ligamentous sheaths to the epiglottis. It is suspended from the styloid processes by two ligaments, the stylohyoid ligaments, which may be variably ossified. The stylohyoid ligaments attach to the lesser horns of the hyoid bone, which consists of a body and two pairs of processes, the greater and lesser horns (Fig. 13–5).

There is a synovial articulation between the lesser and greater horns of the hyoid bone, and a synchondrosis of the greater horn with the body of the hyoid bone. The synovial articulations are subject to all diseases of synovia, such as rheumatoid arthritis.

Roentgen Appearance. In the lateral view (Fig. 13–6), the

body of the hyoid bone is parallel to the body of the mandible and to the thyroid cartilages.

The stylohyoid ligaments extending from the free tips of the styloid process to the lesser horns vary considerably in degree of ossification as well as in length and width.

The paired lesser horns of the hyoid are small and conical and are united to the body of the hyoid by fibrous tissue and occasionally a synovial joint. As pointed out previously, the lesser horns articulate with the greater horns by means of a synovial joint.

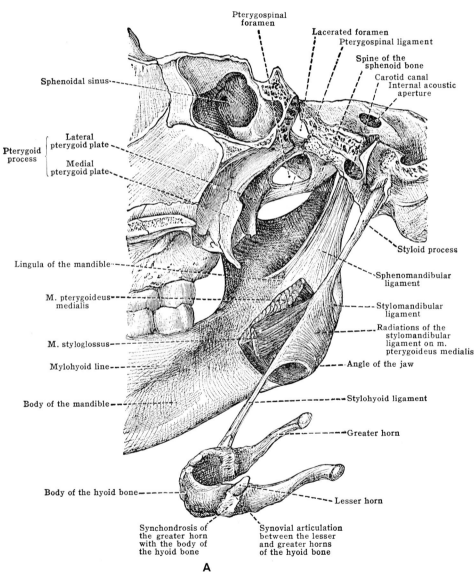

Figure 13–5. A. Ligaments of the temporomandibular articulation and of the hyoid bone; medial view. (After Toldt.) (From Anson, B. J. (ed.): Morris' Human Anatomy, 12th ed. Copyright © 1966 by McGraw-Hill, Inc. Used by permission of McGraw-Hill Book Company.)

Figure 13–5 continued on the following page.

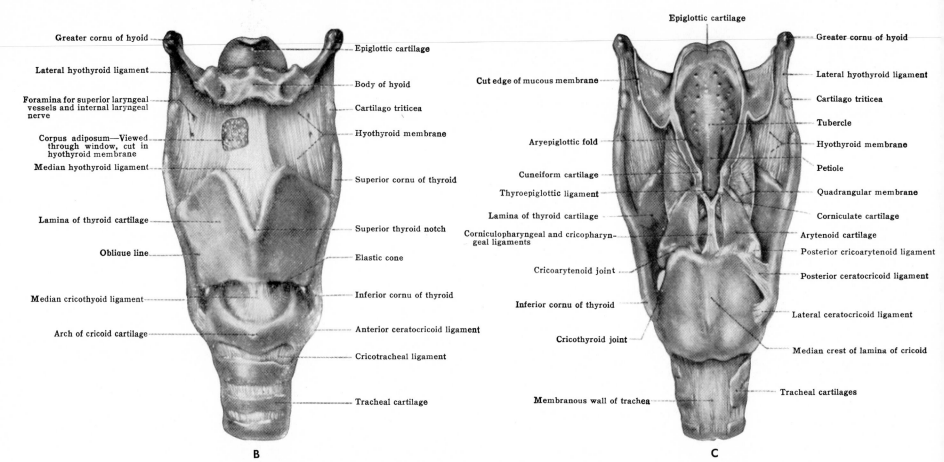

Figure 13–5 *Continued.* B. Laryngeal skeleton, as viewed from the ventral aspect. C. Laryngeal skeleton, as viewed from the dorsal aspect. (From Anson, B. J. (ed.): Morris' Human Anatomy, 12th ed. Copyright © 1966 by McGraw-Hill, Inc. Used by permission of McGraw-Hill Book Company.)

Figure 13–5 continued on the opposite page.

The posterior surface of the hyoid is parallel to the epiglottis and is separated from it by the hyothyroid membrane and loose areolar tissue. Several bursae may be interposed between the membrane and the bone in these regions.

The recognition of hyoid fractures as well as anomalies of this bone require a good appreciation of the normal roentgen anatomy (Porrath).

THE ESOPHAGUS

Gross Anatomy and Relationships of the Esophagus. The esophagus extends from the pharynx at the inferior border of the cricoid cartilage to the cardiac orifice of the stomach opposite the eleventh thoracic vertebra. Its course is in the midline anterior to the vertebral column, but it deviates to the left at the base of the neck for a short distance. At about the level of the seventh thoracic vertebra it passes slowly to the left and anteriorly to reach the esophageal orifice of the diaphragm, and it maintains this direction until it reaches the stomach.

Its length varies between 25 and 30 cm., and its breadth between 12 mm. and 30 or more mm. in its distended state.

In cross section it usually appears as a flattened tube, or a tube with a stellate lumen.

There are certain anatomic relationships of the esophagus (Fig. 13–7) which are of definite importance:

In the neck it is loosely connected by areolar tissue with the posterior aspect of the trachea. It is possible, however, for an abnormal structure such as aberrant thyroid tissue to lie between the trachea and esophagus, and hence it is important to obtain a lateral visualization of the base of the neck with barium in the esophagus when studying the thyroid gland.

In the thorax, the trachea lies anterior to the esophagus as far as the fifth thoracic vertebra near which the trachea bifurcates.

The *arch of the aorta,* passing back to reach the vertebral column, crosses to the left side of the esophagus, causing a *slight deviation of the esophagus to the right.*

The *thoracic aorta* lies first to the left of the esophagus, then posterior to it, and finally, both posterior and to the right of it.

Immediately *below the level of the bifurcation of the trachea,* the esophagus is *crossed by the left bronchus,* and in the rest of its

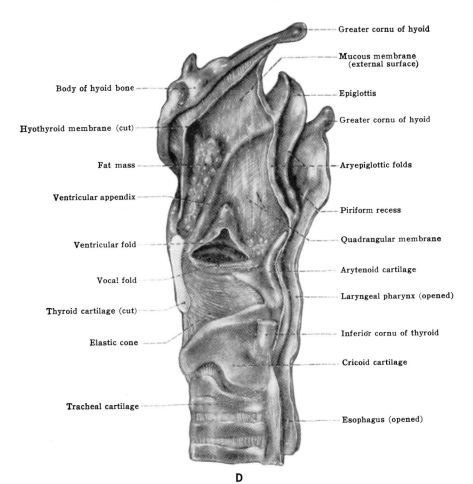

D

Figure 13–5 *Continued.* D. Larynx and certain related structures as viewed from the left. The left lamina of the thyroid cartilage has been removed and the laryngeal ventricle opened. All muscles have been removed and the hyothyroid membrane partially cut away. (Anson, B. J. (ed.): Morris' Human Anatomy, 12th ed. Copyright © 1966 by McGraw-Hill, Inc. Used by permission of McGraw-Hill Book Company.)

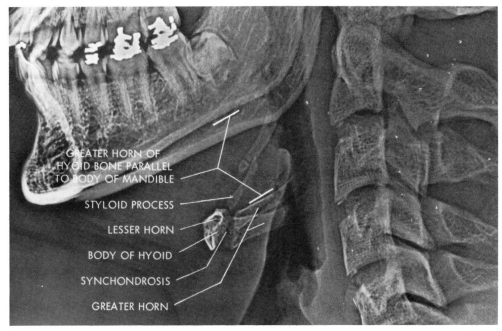

Figure 13–6. Xeroradiograph of the hyoid bone in the lateral view, with parts labeled.

769

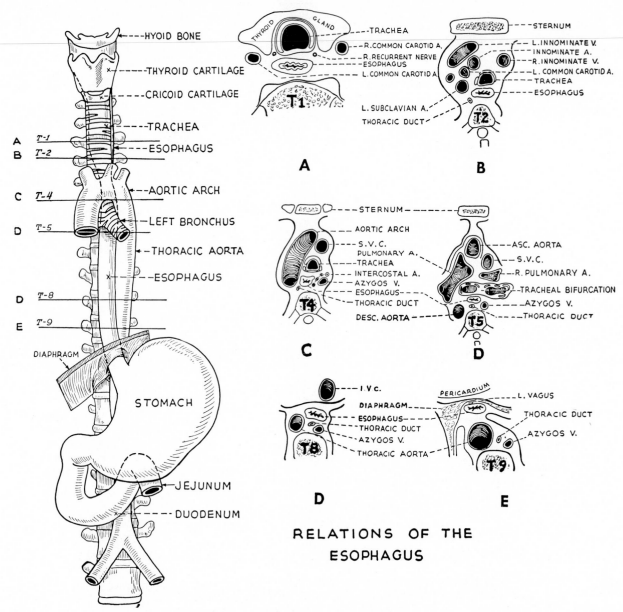

Figure 13–7. Relationship of esophagus to contiguous structures at various levels.

thoracic course it *lies close to the posterior surface of the pericardium.*

In this location it is situated in the posterior mediastinum, and is *separated from the vertebral column by the azygos vein, thoracic duct, and lower thoracic aorta.* It is in *close proximity with the left atrium,* and any enlargement of the latter structure is reflected in displacement of the esophagus posteriorly and to the right (Fig. 13–8).

The two *vagus nerves* descend to the esophagus after forming the anterior and posterior pulmonary plexuses, and unite with the sympathetic branches to form the anterior and posterior esophageal plexuses. The left vagus then winds anteriorly and the right posteriorly, and the two vagi descend in the esophageal sheath through the diaphragm to reach the stomach.

The esophagus is connected with the *esophageal orifice of the diaphragm* by strong fibrous tissue throughout its circumference,

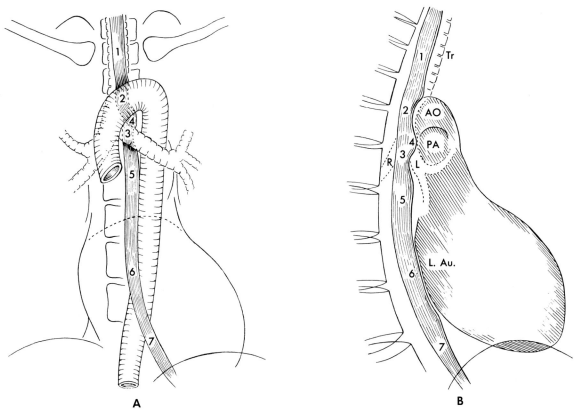

Figure 13–8. Segments of the esophagus. *A.* The segments of the thoracic esophagus (anteroposterior view):
(1) paratracheal segment, (2) aortic segment, (3) bronchial segment, (4) interaorticobronchial triangle, (5) interbronchial segment, (6) retrocardiac segment, (7) epiphrenic segment.

    B. The segments of the esophagus (right anterior oblique view). Shown are: trachea (Tr), right (R) and left (L)
main bronchi, pulmonary artery (PA), left auricle (L. Au), and the different segments of the paratracheal (1), aortic
(2), bronchic (3), interaorticobronchial (4), interbronchial (5), retrocardiac (6), and epiphrenic (7) esophagus. (From
Brombart, M.: Roentgenology of the esophagus. *In* Margulis, A. R., and Burhenne, H. J., (eds.): Alimentary Tract
Roentgenology, 2nd ed. St. Louis, C. V. Mosby Co., 1973.)

but any defects in this supportive tissue may cause hiatal protrusion of the stomach.

    The *abdominal portion of the esophagus* is approximately 1 to
3 cm. in length and runs in the esophageal groove on the posterior
surface of the liver.

    The *phrenic ampulla* is that portion of the esophagus that lies
just above the esophageal orifice of the diaphragm (Fig. 13–9). It is
rather bulbous, varies in size, and causes confusion radiographically with a hiatal hernia of the stomach through the diaphragm. The esophageal ampulla appears as a segmented ovoid
structure 3 to 5 cm. in length and 2 to 4 cm. in diameter, and it is
separable from the stomach pattern below. The hiatal herniation
of the fundus through the diaphragm has considerably more variation in size, and its rugal pattern can usually be more closely
identified with that of the contiguous portion of the stomach

    The esophageal vestibule is another name for the intra-ab-
dominal portion of the esophagus. The vestibule is often situated
above the diaphragm, producing a sliding hernia. The inferior
esophageal sphincter and mucosal junction between esophagus
and stomach are, under these circumstances, situated between
the vestibule and the ampulla.

    The diaphragm and its ligamentous esophageal attachments
(phrenicoesophageal membrane) at the esophageal hiatus produce a valve like action called a constrictor cardiae.

    Normal Points of Narrowness in the Esophagus. There are
four definite constrictions in the normal esophagus (Fig. 13–8):
one at its cricoid beginning, a second at the level of the aortic
knob, a third opposite the crossing of the left bronchus, and the
fourth at the place where it passes through the diaphragm. The
lumen at the site of the upper constrictions is smaller than the

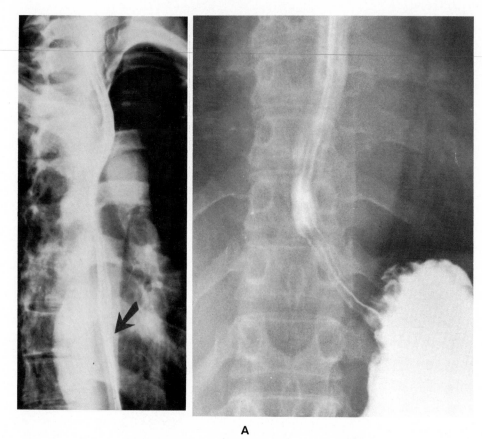

A

Figure 13–9. *A. Rugal pattern of the esophagus.*

Figure 13–9 continued on the opposite page.

fourth, and ordinarily, when a foreign body fails to pass down the esophagus, the site of obstruction occurs at one of the upper points of narrowness.

Esophageal Lip (Fig. 13–10). The esophageal lip is an indentation on the posterior aspect of the esophagus at its junction with the hypopharynx. It is postulated that this is caused by the cricopharyngeal muscle. Differential diagnosis of this formation from a foreign body or other abnormality may cause some problems. It is probable that the esophageal lip is not associated with dysphagia and is of no definite pathologic significance (Siebert et al.).

The Normal Rugal Pattern of the Esophagus. The mucous coat of the esophagus is very loosely connected with the muscular coat by the areolar tissue of the submucous layer. When the esophagus is empty, the mucous coat is thrown into a series of longitudinal folds (Fig. 13–9); otherwise it is very smooth in contrast with the mammillated gastric mucous membrane.

The longitudinal folds of the empty or partially empty esophagus impart to the radiographic picture the typical rugal pattern attributed to this organ. These consist of parallel lines throughout the esophagus which become more closely approximated as

the distal funnel end of the esophagus is reached just above the cardia (Fig. 13–11).

Abnormalities in the esophageal wall are reflected to a great extent in alteration of this normal rugal pattern, either by the appearance of abnormal folds or by the lack of folds.

The Normal Swallowing Function. The process of deglutition has been thoroughly studied by cineradiography in recent times. Briefly, the sequence of events is as follows:

1. There is a forward and upward movement of the tongue which displaces the contents of the mouth backward.

2. The soft palate is raised and the palatoglossal and palatopharyngeal muscles relax.

3. The hyoid and the lateral walls of the pharynx then rise abruptly.

4. The epiglottis deflects the food bolus into the lateral food channels and then reverts back and inferiorly to cover the laryngeal vestibule. The role of the epiglottis is secondary to the sphincteric action of the supraglottic laryngeal musculature.

5. The cricopharyngeus relaxes ahead of the advancing bolus.

6. There is a continued contraction of the muscles around the

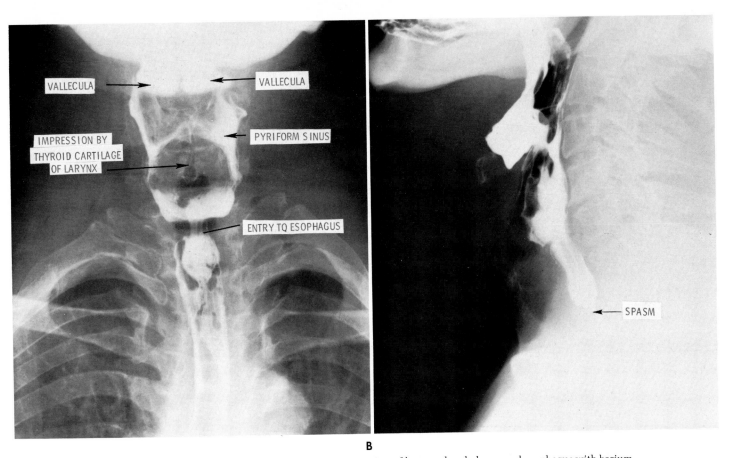

B

Figure 13–9. *Continued.* *B.Left,* Normal anteroposterior view of laryngeal and pharyngeal esophagus with barium.
Right, Lateral view of a patient with cricopharyngeal spasm and barium accumulating in the vallecula.

Figure 13–9 continued on the following page.

mouth, and the supraglottic muscles and epiglottis prevent the food from entering the larynx. The elevation of the soft palate simultaneously approximates it to the posterior pharyngeal wall, preventing the return of the material into the mouth or nasopharynx.

7. Intrapharyngeal pressure rises with the entry of the bolus into the pharynx, but in the region of the cricopharyngeus, the high resting pressure falls abruptly on swallowing, with an equally abrupt return to high pressure after the passage of the bolus into the esophagus. Thus, the cricopharyngeus acts as a true sphincter, preventing egress of material back into the hypopharynx.

8. The tubular portion of the esophagus, by means of a peristaltic wave, transports the food bolus toward the stomach. The peristalsis begins in the posterior pharynx and is shallow in type and nonocclusive.

9. The function of the gastroesophageal segment is quite complex. There is a small pouch formed just above the esophageal hiatus, depending upon the quantity of fluid swallowed, the consistency of the fluid, the caliber of the submerged segment as defined by Wolf, and the height of intra-abdominal pressure. Pressure in the submerged segment as well as in the ampulla remains somewhat elevated, and as the peristaltic wave descends to it, the combined pressures of peristaltic and submerged pressure force the food bolus into the stomach. When the food bolus has left the ampullary region and submerged segment, the elevated pressure zone in the esophagogastric region persists so that no significant reflux is thereby permitted. These pressure relationships are illustrated in Figure 13–12.

Basic Anatomic Concepts Regarding the Lower Esophagus. Great interest and considerable confusion have arisen in relation to that segment of the esophagus just above the diaphragm and

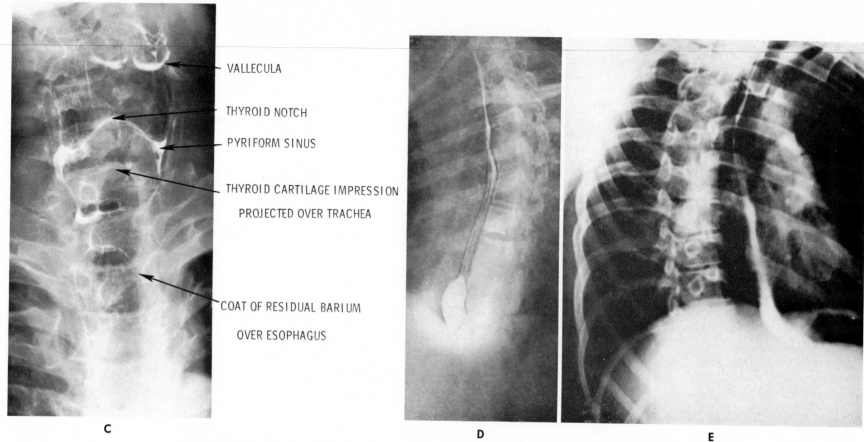

Figure 13–9 *Continued.* *C.* Pharyngeal region and upper esophagus coated with a thin coat of barium. *D* and *E.* Radiograph of esophagus. *D.* Demonstrating the esophageal phrenic ampulla (intensified). *E.* Showing rugal pattern of esophagus.

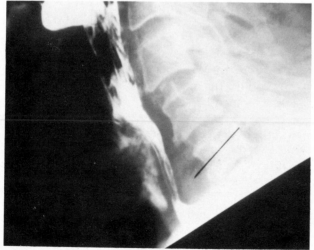

Figure 13–10. Lateral view of the pharyngeal and upper esophagus, demonstrating an esophageal lip.

extending to the stomach (Lerche; Johnstone; Berridge; Wolf, 1973). A dynamic functional concept of the gastroesophageal junction is necessary. Fluoroscopy has shown that the junctional area between the esophagus and stomach is mobile and undergoes changes in position, shape, and architecture according to changes in body position, intra-abdominal pressure, and swallowing movements of the patient (Adler, 1962) (Fig. 13–13).

Although there is no morphologically discernible sphincter in the distal esophagus, newer manometric recording devices have made it possible to demonstrate a long-suspected sphincterlike action inherent in the function of the distal esophagus in a segment about 4 cm. in length that straddles the diaphragm at the esophageal hiatus. The resting intraluminal pressure within this segment is higher than that within the stomach. The sphincterlike action of this segment appears to be completely separate from the behavior of the diaphragm.

In an effort to clarify the terminology in respect to this area, Wolf (1970) has called the long narrow segment that is sometimes

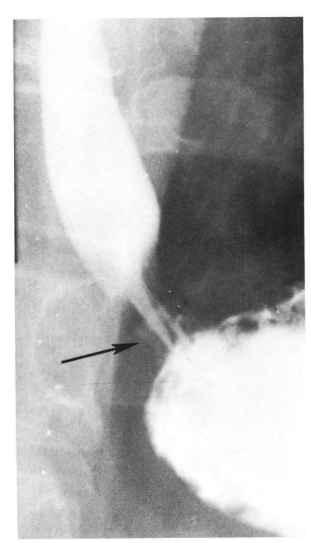

Figure 13-11. Radiograph showing normal rugal pattern of the lower esophagus.

lishing a high pressure zone to prevent reflux from the stomach to the esophagus. It is when the fundus slides above the diaphgram through a patulous hiatus to create a hiatal hernia that the function of this segment is most vulnerable and the barrier furnished by it to regurgitation and reflux may be inadequate to protect the lower esophagus from the refluxing digestive enzymes of the stomach.

The junction of the vestibule and fundus of the stomach is often demarcated by an epithelial ring which can be identified radiographically (Fig. 13-14).

With a hiatal hernia, a ring is often identified between the esophagus and herniated portion of stomach; it is called a

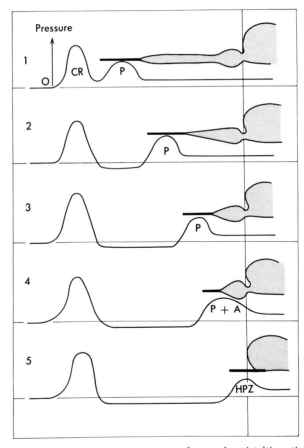

Figure 13-12. Diagrammatic representation of normal peristaltic activity of the esophagus during the act of swallowing. (1) The reconstituted resting cricopharyngeal sphincter (CR) returns to a state of elevated pressure as the stripping wave (P) enters the proximal esophagus. (2 to 5) The peristaltic stripping wave continues distally without change in the tubular configuration of the body of the esophagus. The size of the pouch formed above the hiatus depends on the quantity of fluid swallowed, the consistency of the fluid, the caliber of the submerged segment, and the height of intra-abdominal pressure. Note that in contrast to pressure in the body of the esophagus, pressure in the ampulla may rise while it still contains barium so that an elongated pressure curve (P + A) is obtained (4). With complete emptying, elevated pressure in the esophagogastric region persists, that is, the esophagogastric composite sphincter is reconstituted. (From Wolf, B. S.: Roentgenology of the esophagogastric region. In Margulis, A. R. and Burhenne, H. J., (eds.): Alimentary Tract Roentgenology, 2nd ed. St. Louis, C. V. Mosby Co., 1973.)

referred to as the esophageal vestibule when beneath the diaphragm the "submerged segment," and he further names "A," "B," and "C" rings (Fig. 13-13). In this terminology, the cardia (CO) is the orifice at the junction between the esophagus and the diaphragm; it is normally situated beneath the diaphragm. The A ring, originally referred to by Lerché as the inferior esophageal sphincter, is an inconstant constriction at the superior margin of the esophageal ampulla. The B ring refers to the true mucosal junction between the esophagus and the stomach when there is a hernia of the stomach above the diaphragm. The submerged segment, or C ring, is defined by the constrictor cardiae or phrenicoesophageal membrane of the diaphragm.

The submerged segment functions most effectively when a portion of the esophagus lies beneath the diaphragm (esophageal vestibule), where the diaphragmatic contraction assists in estab-

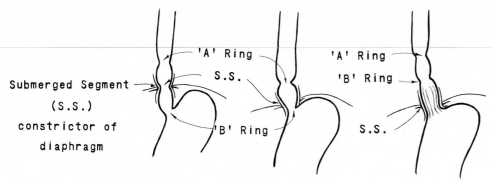

Figure 13-13. Anatomic concept of lower esophagus, modified from Wolf et al.

"Schatzki ring" or a "Templeton ring"). This is in fact a B ring. It is probably of clinical significance when its transverse measurement is less than 13 mm. (Fig. 13-15) and when there is an associated reflux to the level of the tracheal bifurcation.

Figure 13-16 illustrates what Wolf considers a variety of

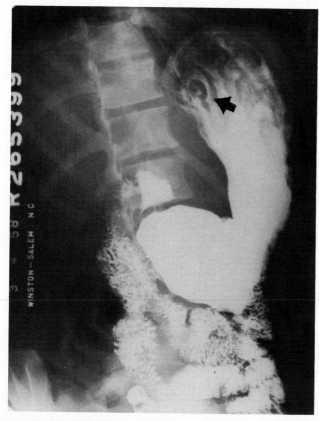

Figure 13-14. "Epithelial ring" at the cardioesophageal junction.

pressure profiles in patients with sliding hernias; they are significant only in so far as they contribute to a knowledge of the normal anatomic landmarks at this junction. One or another of the A or B rings or the submerged segment itself may act as a barrier to reflux from the stomach and as a high pressure zone. It is when no high pressure zone is functioning that symptoms of "epigastric burning" (pyrosis) are probable.

Barrett's epithelium is a *columnar epithelium* which may be found in the upper and lowermost portions of the esophagus and may represent an embryonic type of epithelium. This may, at times, be situated between the squamous epithelium and the normal simple columnar epithelium of the esophagus.

The phrenic esophageal ampulla is a physiologic dilatation of the lower esophagus which can be identified particularly when this region is distended by a bolus of food or barium. It may be seen most clearly in full inspiration. The ampulla is accentuated by a contraction or constriction of the esophagus just proximal to it.

The anatomic presence of the inferior esophageal sphincter has been demonstrated by Lerché. The narrowing produced in the esophageal appearance in this area is due in part to the contraction of the sphincter and in part to the downward pull of the phrenoesophageal membrane, the upper end of which is attached at this point.

The phrenicoesophageal membrane is the anchoring apparatus for the lower esophagus to the diaphragm. This membrane divides into an ascending portion that is attached at the level of the inferior esophageal sphincter and a descending portion that is attached to the muscular coat of the cardia of the stomach in the region of the gastroesophageal junction. The phrenicoesophageal membrane ordinarily serves as a channel for the esophagus, resisting excessive shortening or lengthening of the organ during the act of respiration. On the other hand, in deep inspiration the diaphragm constricts the lower end of the esophagus (constrictor diaphragmatis) and in expiration the area expands fully. With changes in position, there is a sliding movement of the esophagus in this area so that the relationship of the esophagus to the diaphragm actually changes with respiration.

The gastroesophageal vestibule corresponds with the abdominal portion of the esophagus or submerged segment. This has been referred to as the gastric antrum or antechamber of the stomach. When the phrenic ampulla is full, the vestibule is ordinarily empty. It is essential that the gastroesophageal vestibule be recognized so that it is not mistaken for a sliding hiatal hernia. When the vestibule is empty the longitudinal rugae are thin and parallel and resemble closely the rugal pattern of the esophagus above this level. When the vestibule is full, however, the rugae are effaced and closely resemble the rugae of the gastric fundus. Hence, serial film studies are necessary to differentiate this area accurately.

HERNIATIONS

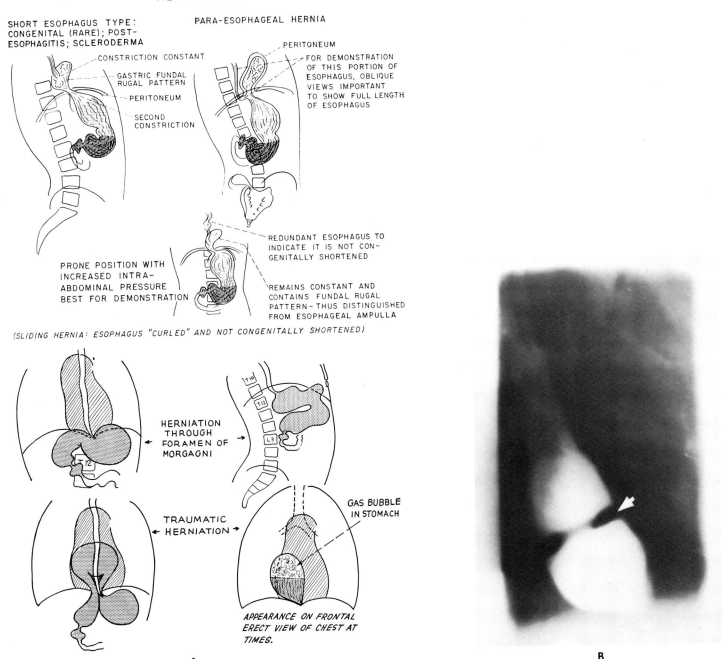

SHORT ESOPHAGUS TYPE:
CONGENITAL (RARE); POST-
ESOPHAGITIS; SCLERODERMA

PARA-ESOPHAGEAL HERNIA

CONSTRICTION CONSTANT

GASTRIC FUNDAL
RUGAL PATTERN

PERITONEUM

SECOND
CONSTRICTION

PERITONEUM

FOR DEMONSTRATION
OF THIS PORTION OF
ESOPHAGUS, OBLIQUE
VIEWS IMPORTANT
TO SHOW FULL LENGTH
OF ESOPHAGUS

PRONE POSITION WITH
INCREASED INTRA-
ABDOMINAL PRESSURE
BEST FOR DEMONSTRATION

REDUNDANT ESOPHAGUS TO
INDICATE IT IS NOT CON-
GENITALLY SHORTENED

REMAINS CONSTANT AND
CONTAINS FUNDAL RUGAL
PATTERN—THUS DISTINGUISHED
FROM ESOPHAGEAL AMPULLA

(SLIDING HERNIA: ESOPHAGUS "CURLED" AND NOT CONGENITALLY SHORTENED)

HERNIATION
THROUGH
FORAMEN OF
MORGAGNI

TRAUMATIC
HERNIATION

GAS BUBBLE
IN STOMACH

APPEARANCE ON FRONTAL
ERECT VIEW OF CHEST AT
TIMES.

A

B

Figure 13–15. *A.* Summary diagram illustrating herniations of the stomach through the diaphragm. *B.* Radiograph demonstrating Schatzki's ring.

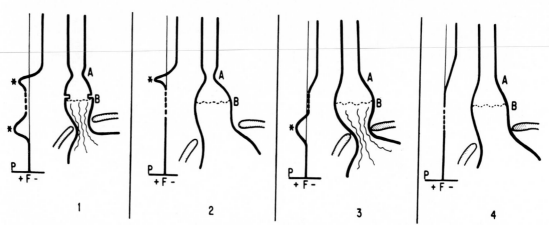

Figure 13–16. Diagram illustrating a variety of pressure profiles in patients with sliding hernias. Panels *1–4*. A and B levels are indicated in each panel. F indicates fundic pressure; pressure (P) higher than F is on the plus (+) side, lower than F on the minus (—) side. Peak pressures are indicated by asterisks (*) on the pressure curves. The length of plateau region varies (dashes) depending on the size of the hernia. Panel *1* shows two peaks of resting pressure, one in the region of the A ring and another at the level of the hiatus. Panel *2* shows one peak related to the A level and a wide barium column traversing the hiatus. Panel *3* shows a single peak in the region of the hiatus with a relatively narrowed gastric channel or collar within the hiatus. Panel *4* shows no peak and a continuous wide barium channel extending from the tubular esophagus into the stomach below the diaphragm. A "B" ring is shown in Panel *1* but may or may not be present in any of these configurations. The Z line, although indicated, is not evident roentgenologically. (From Wolf, B. S.: Amer. J. Roentgenol., *110*:274, 1970.)

The constrictor cardia is at the gastroesophageal junction and ordinarily is located beneath the diaphragm at the junction of the esophageal and gastric mucosa. There is an abrupt change from the squamous epithelium of the esophagus to the columnar epithelium of the stomach at this site. At times, this epithelial line appears as an epithelial ring (Fig. 13–14) as previously illustrated.

Blood Supply of the Esophagus

Venous Drainage of the Lower Esophagus and Its Importance. The veins of the esophagus form a plexus exteriorly (Fig. 13–17). The venous drainage of the lower esophagus passes to the coronary vein of the stomach, and the latter vein empties into the portal vein. Higher up, the veins of the esophagus empty into the azygos system and thyroid veins. (See Chapter 12.)

Thus, the esophagus forms a communicating link between the portal circulation on the one hand and the systemic veins on the other, since the azygos vein empties into the superior vena cava.

Obstruction of the portal vein from any cause may, in turn, cause considerable distention of the lower esophageal veins and other tributaries of the coronary vein of the stomach. These irreg-

ular distentions are spoken of as "varices," and have the appearance and the same physiologic significance as hemorrhoids in the case of the anal canal (Fig. 13–18). These veins may rupture and cause considerable embarrassment from bleeding. They produce a marked irregularity of the rugal pattern of the lower esophagus, especially when the venous pressure is increased as in the case of forced expiration. Indeed, the relative disappearance of the irregularity in deep inspiration, and reappearance with forced expiration is pathognomonic of esophageal varices.

Arterial Supply of the Esophagus. The arterial supply of the esophagus is derived from esophageal branches of the aorta (Fig. 13–19), bronchial arteries, the inferior phrenic artery, and left gastric arteries. Veins accompany these arteries, which usually number three at the most. At times, esophageal branches are received from the bronchial arteries. Ascending branches of esophageal arteries from an abnormal level are also shown.

The veins form a plexus on the outer surface of the esophagus opening into the left gastric, azygos, and thyroid veins cranially, as previously described, thus establishing a communication between portal and systemic veins.

Lymphatics in the Esophagus. The lymphatics in the esophagus arise chiefly in the mucosa and drain into the inferior deep cervical, posterior mediastinal, and superior gastric lymph nodes.

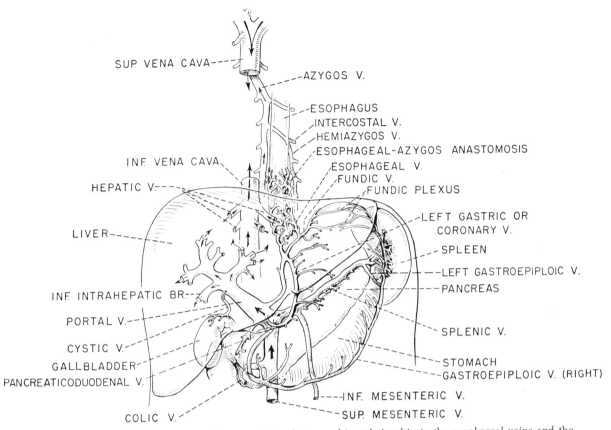

Figure 13-17. Anatomic diagram of the portal circulation and its relationship to the esophageal veins and the azygos venous system.

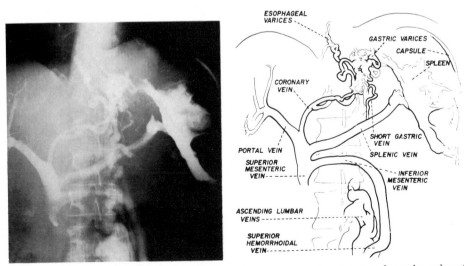

Figure 13-18. Roentgenogram at 12 seconds demonstrates coronary vein, gastric and esophageal varices. The anastomosis between the inferior mesenteric vein and superior hemorrhoid plexus is demonstrated. The latter is also seen to drain into the vertebral venous plexus. Tracing at right. (From Evans, J. A., and O'Sullivan, W. D.: Amer. J. Roentgenol. *77,* 1957.)

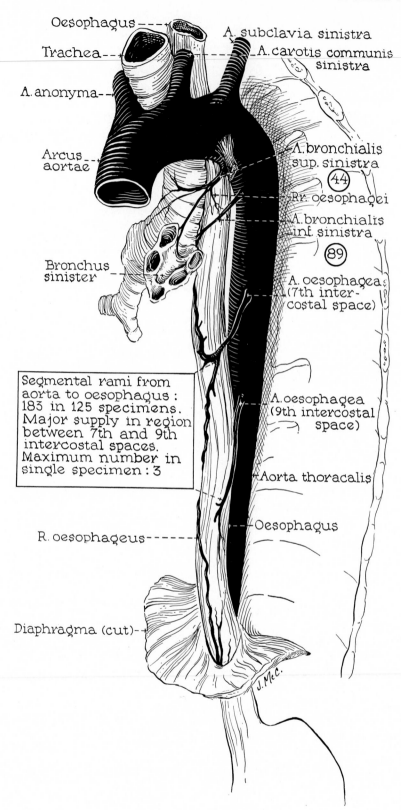

Oesophagus

Trachea

A. anonyma

Arcus aortae

Bronchus sinister

Segmental rami from aorta to oesophagus : 183 in 125 specimens. Major supply in region between 7th and 9th intercostal spaces. Maximum number in single specimen : 3

R. oesophageus

Diaphragma (cut)

A. subclavia sinistra

A. carotis communis sinistra

A. bronchialis sup. sinistra

(44)

Rr. oesophagei

A. bronchialis inf. sinistra

(89)

A. oesophagea (7th intercostal space)

A. oesophagea (9th intercostal space)

Aorta thoracalis

Oesophagus

J. McC.

Technique of Examination of the Esophagus

Fluoroscopy. The proper examination of the esophagus involves a combination of fluoroscopy and radiography, with spot film radiography in selected areas. We now consider cinefluoroscopy and radiography to be an essential part of this examination with respect to the swallowing function.

The sequence is as follows: (1) survey fluoroscopy of chest; (2) survey fluoroscopy of abdomen; (3) the swallowing of a single mouthful of thin barium is studied in frontal and oblique perspective; (4) for mucosal detail, the swallowing of thick barium paste is thereafter viewed in frontal and oblique perspectives; (5) the patient is then placed in the supine position and the study is repeated. When the patient is in the left posterior oblique, regurgitation is assayed by gravity and positive pressure (Valsalva maneuver). The water test is done in this position also.

The Trendelenburg position is utilized when a hiatal hernia is suspected.

The prone position for demonstration of a hiatal hernia with the patient straining is particularly useful and is repeated with both thick and thin barium with the patient in the right anterior oblique position. Spot films are obtained in at least two separate sequences.

Technique of the Water Test (Linsman; Crummy). The patient is supine and turned obliquely on his left side. After the fundus of the stomach is filled with barium, he is asked to drink a mouthful of water through a straw. He is asked to swallow this while his esophagogastric junction is carefully studied fluoroscopically. The bolus of water is identified by the air swallowed with the water, and the water is detected as it enters the stomach. Normally, very little of the barium is observed to reflux into the esophagus at this juncture. With a positive water test a large amount of barium is seen to reflux up the esophagus, usually above the level of the hilar vessels and frequently above the aortic arch. At such times, clearing of the esophagus is slow and several peristaltic waves are required to empty the esophagus of the regurgitated barium.

Figure 13–19. Thoracic sources of esophageal arteries, diagrammatic. The encircled numbers represent the frequency with which esophageal rami arose from the particular bronchial artery in 125 dissections. Ascending branches of esophageal arteries from abdominal level and descending branches of the segmental esophageal arteries of thoracic level are also shown. (From Anson, B. J.: An Atlas of Human Anatomy. Philadelphia, W. B. Saunders Co., 1963.)

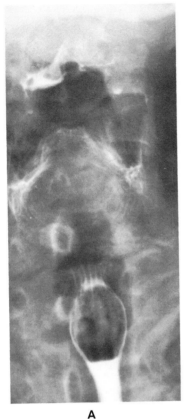

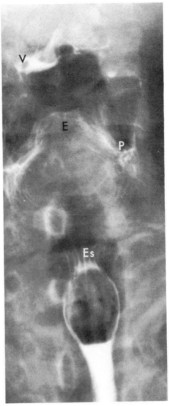

A   **B**

Figure 13–20.   *A.* Anteroposterior view of neck with barium in the esophagus. *B.* Same view labeled: (V) vallecula, (E) epiglottis, (P) pyriform sinus, (Es) upper esophagus.

In studies correlating reflux of barium into the esophagus as demonstrated by the water-siphonage test of de Carvalho (Crummy), in 650 routine upper gastrointestinal studies in patients with pyrosis ("heartburn"), the following statistics were reported:

- *a.* 10.3 per cent of the patients had reflux, and 68.6 per cent of these complained of pyrosis.
- *b.* 89.7 per cent did not have reflux, and 3.4 per cent of these complained of pyrosis.
- *c.* 10.1 per cent of the total group complained of pyrosis, and 69.6 per cent of these had a positive water test.
- *d.* 30.4 per cent of those with pyrosis as a complaint showed no reflux when tested.
- *e.* 46 of these 650 patients had hiatal herniae.
- *f.* Of 48 per cent with pyrosis, 91 per cent had a positive water test.
- *g.* Of 52 per cent who were asymptomatic, 91.7 per cent had a negative water test.
- *h.* In only 14 cases did reflux occur with change of position

only. All 14 had a positive water test, but only half of these had pyrosis.

Thus the water test is highly satisfactory for detection of gastroesophageal reflux, and reflux occurring under these circumstances correlates well with pyrosis, especially in patients with hiatal hernia.

Spot Film Radiography.   Spot films are obtained whenever a suggestion of abnormality is seen. (Water test films and films of the lower esophagus are routine.)

Cineradiography.   We now consider cineradiography (or video tape recording) an essential part of a study of the swallowing function and use it routinely, usually in the erect, supine, and prone positions.

Films Obtained.   (1) Anteroposterior film study of the esophagus, including neck to diaphragm (Figs. 13–20, 13–21). (2) Right anterior oblique projection (Fig. 13–22). (3) Left anterior oblique projection (Fig. 13–23). (4) A lateral view of the neck with barium in the esophagus (Fig. 13–24).

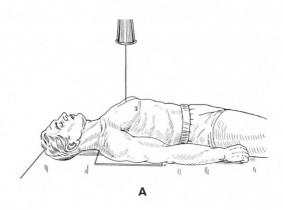

A

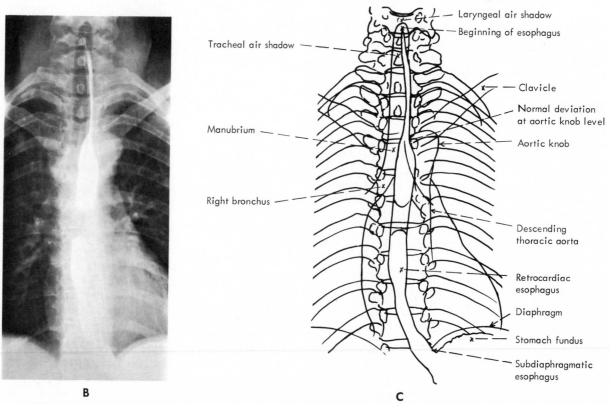

B   C

Figure 13–21.   Anteroposterior film study of esophagus. *A.* Position of patient. *B.* Radiograph. *C.* Labeled tracing of *B.*

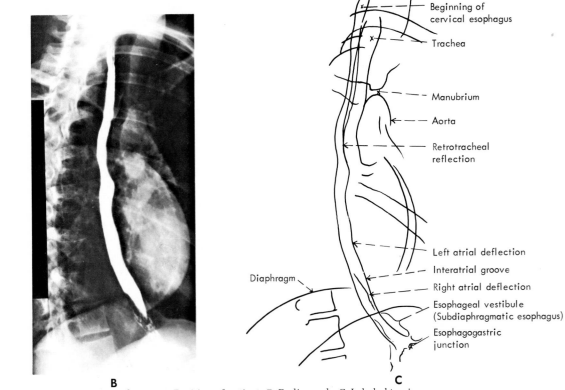

Figure 13-22. Right anterior oblique view of esophagus. *A.* Position of patient. *B.* Radiograph. *C.* Labeled tracing. (This same view is frequently taken in the recumbent position as well.)

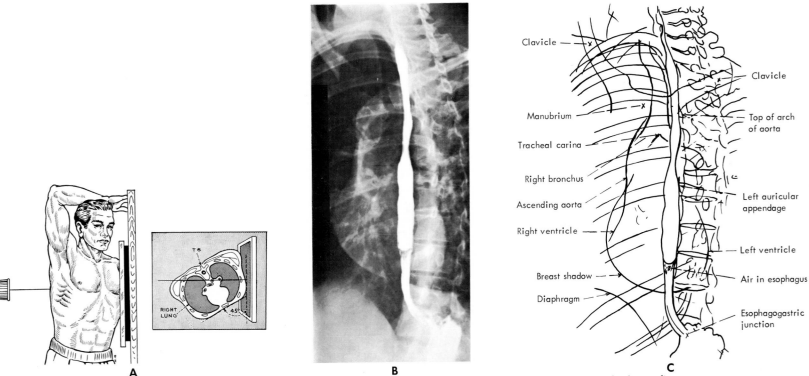

Figure 13-23. Left anterior oblique projection of esophagus. *A.* Position of patient (recumbent may also be used). *B.* Radiograph (intensified). *C.* Labeled tracing.

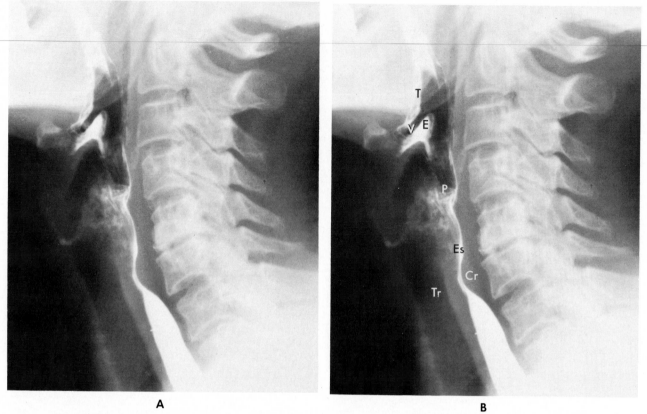

Figure 13-24. *A.* Lateral roentgenogram of the neck with barium in the esophagus. *B.* Same radiograph labeled: (T) back of tongue, (V) vallecula, (E) tip of epiglottis, (P) pyriform sinus, (Es) upper esophagus above (Cr) cricopharyngeus muscle impression, (Tr) trachea.

Special Procedure for Suspected Swallowing of Foreign Body. (1) Lateral films of the neck and chest without contrast media. (2) Lateral film of the neck during deglutition, so that the calcified, cartilaginous structures will be elevated, bringing into clear relief any postcricoid foreign body. (3) Routine fluoroscopy of the esophagus as outlined above.

It has been recommended by some that the swallowing of a small cotton ball soaked with barium or a barium-filled gelatin capsule be employed. If this is done, interpretation must be carried forward with great caution since either of these may be delayed in transit and false conclusions drawn.

A plain survey film of the abdomen prior to the introduction of barium is advisable, as is an AP or PA film of the chest to determine whether or not the suspected foreign body has been aspirated into the chest or swallowed into the gastrointestinal tract below the level of the esophagus.

Routine Film Studies of the Esophagus

Anteroposterior Film Study of the Neck (Fig. 13–20). The cervical portion of the esophagus begins at the lower border of the

cricoid cartilage approximately at the level of the sixth cervical vertebra. The pharyngoesophageal junction is usually closed and the esophagus collapsed. Occasionally, however, air may be detected in this sector. Although the esophageal inlet relaxes during swallowing, it immediately contracts and tapers again afterwards. A peristaltic wave passing downward in unbroken succession may be visualized in the pharynx. The esophagus is in the midline at its origin and deviates slightly to the left in the caudal part of the neck and cranial part of the thorax. Its rugal pattern is longitudinal, cephalocaudad. At the base of the neck the esophagus protrudes slightly beyond the left margin of the trachea. The tracheal air shadow may be clearly identified in relation to the barium-containing cervical esophagus.

Since the esophagus is relatively longer in a newborn infant than in the adult, the cervical esophagus is farther cranial in children, corresponding to the more cranial vertebral level of the larynx.

In **lateral projection** (Fig. 13–24) the esophagus is immediately posterior to the trachea and separated from it by a thin fascial plane.

The Anteroposterior Film Study Below the Neck (Fig. 13–21). In this projection, the esophagus is tapered superiorly and inferiorly immediately above the diaphragm, and is largely a midline structure, except where it deviates to the right by the left bronchus impression in the upper part of its course, and slightly to the left and anteriorly in the region of the diaphragm in the lower part of its course. There may be a very slight impression by the left auricular appendage, displacing the esophagus slightly to the right also. If this displacement is more than extremely slight, it is usually indicative of enlargement of the left atrium.

Right Anterior Oblique Projection (Fig. 13–25). In this

projection the esophagus is rather closely applied to the spine in the neck and to the posterior margin of the pericardium in the thorax. The previously described "aortic" indentation in the region of the left bronchus is also seen to displace the esophagus slightly posteriorly. There is a slight indentation of the esophagus in the region of the left atrium, which is in a posterior position. The clear space behind the esophagus increases above the diaphragm, in view of the gradually increasing anterior course of the esophagus.

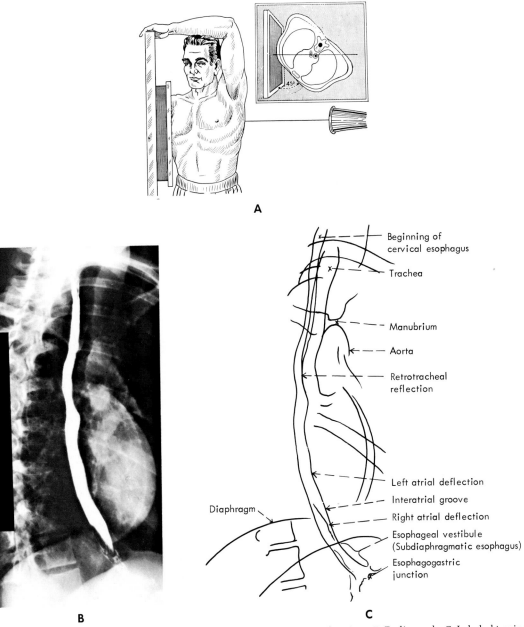

Figure 13–25. Right anterior oblique view of esophagus. *A.* Position of patient. *B.* Radiograph. *C.* Labeled tracing. (This same view is frequently taken in the recumbent position as well.)

Left Anterior Oblique Projection (Fig. 13–26). In this view, the slight posterior impression produced by the left bronchus is once again seen, but otherwise, the esophagus courses directly down to the diaphragm on the anterior aspect of the thoracic spine.

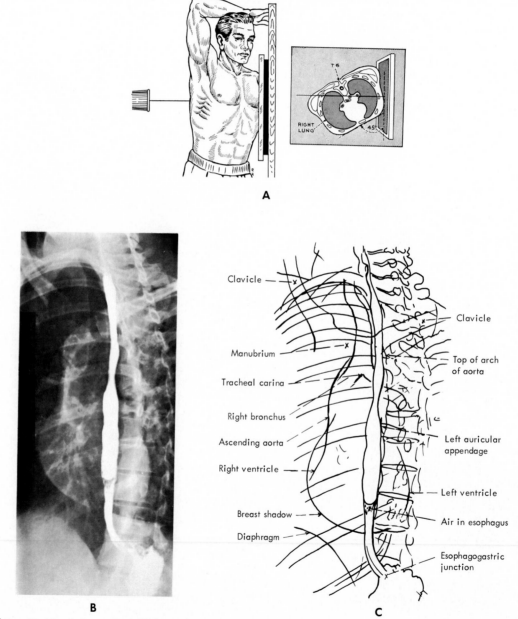

A

B

C

Clavicle

Clavicle

Manubrium

Top of arch of aorta

Tracheal carina

Right bronchus

Ascending aorta

Left auricular appendage

Right ventricle

Left ventricle

Breast shadow

Air in esophagus

Diaphragm

Esophagogastric junction

Figure 13–26. Left anterior oblique projection of esophagus. *A.* Positioning of patient (recumbent may also be used). *B.* Radiograph (intensified). *C.* Labeled tracing.

Iodized Oil Study. Iodized oil is possibly somewhat less irritating when inhaled into the trachea or bronchial tree than is the barium sulfate suspension. On the other hand, it is more expensive and somewhat more irritating to gastric mucosa.

When a patient gives a history of extreme difficulty in swallowing, followed by considerable coughing, it usually indicates that he inhales the swallowed bolus, at least in part. In such instances, an iodized oil such as Dionosil (oily) may be injected by syringe onto the back of the tongue and swallowed. The barium sulfate suspension may be used thereafter if inhalation of the Dionosil has not occurred.

This is particularly true in cases of pharyngeal palsies, pseudopharyngeal palsies, and such congenital anomalies as esophageal atresias, where there is usually a communication between the esophagus and the trachea or bronchial tree. Barium sulfate suspension may be used initially, however, if desired,

since it has been tolerated as a bronchographic agent also (Fig. 13–27).

THE STOMACH AND DUODENUM

Subdivisions of the Stomach. The stomach is arbitrarily divided into three parts: the fundus, the body, and the pyloric portion (Fig. 13–28).

The fundus is that portion of the stomach that lies above a horizontal plane through the junction of the stomach and esophagus (this latter being called the "cardiac orifice" or "cardia"), and the pyloric portion is that part that falls between the incisura angularis and the pylorus. The body is represented by the intervening portion.

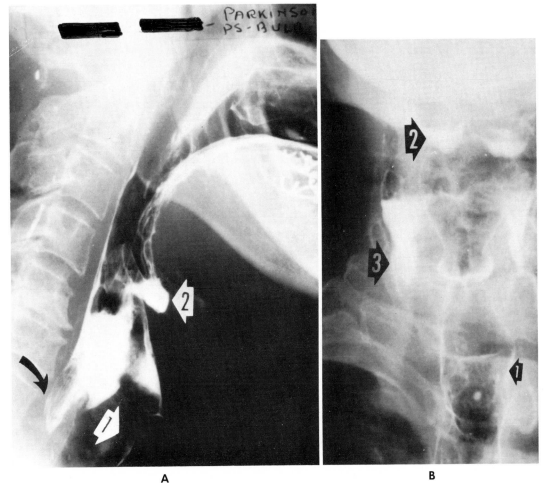

A   **B**

Figure 13–27. *A* and *B*. Pseudobulbar palsy in a patient with Parkinson's disease. (1) Trachea, (2) vallecula, (3) pyriform sinuses.

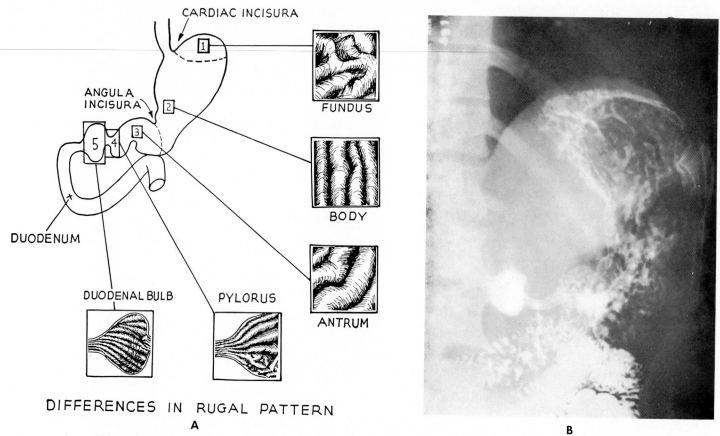

Figure 13–28. Stomach. *A.* Subdivisions and rugal pattern. *B.* Radiograph showing rugal pattern. (The distal portion of the pyloric antrum is in a contracted state and its rugal pattern merges imperceptibly with the pattern of the pyloric canal.)

The right wall of the cardia merges into the lesser curvature of the stomach, while the left wall is deeply notched by the cardiac incisura.

A pyloric constriction marks the junction between the stomach and duodenum. The pyloric sphincter is sharply demarcated from the duodenum, but blends imperceptibly with the thickened masculature of the pyloric antrum. The pyloric canal traverses the pyloric sphincter and is approximately 5 mm. in length. The gastric mucous membrane is continued into the duodenum without any alteration visible to the naked eye.

The greater curvature corresponds in its greater part with the attachment of the gastrosplenic and gastrocolic ligaments.

Stomach Contour Variations in Accordance with Body Build (Fig. 13–29). Gastric tone and contour normally follow the habitus of the individual closely. In the individual who is short and stocky, the stomach is usually high in position and "steerhorn" in shape, its lumen being largest above and tapering toward the pylorus. It extends more quickly toward the right. At

times, it is even horizontal in position. The incisura angularis is difficult to identify, and occasionally the pylorus is the lowermost part of the stomach.

In the sthenic individual, the eutonic stomach is J-shaped, and the body of the stomach tends to be vertical in the frontal projection and uniform in size. The lowermost part of the stomach in the erect position tends to be at the level of the iliac crests.

In asthenic individuals, the stomach tends to be hypotonic, and shaped rather like a fishhook. The greater curvature tends to sag down into the pelvis, with the greatest diameter between the incisura angularis and the adjoining greater curvature.

Each of the stomach types may occur in individuals of any body build, but in general the hypotonic stomach tends to occur more frequently in underweight individuals, whereas the steerhorn type tends to occur more frequently in the overweight. Indeed, according to a study which we have conducted, when the hypotonic stomach occurs in an overweight individual, it is almost invariably symptomatic. Likewise, a cascade stomach tends

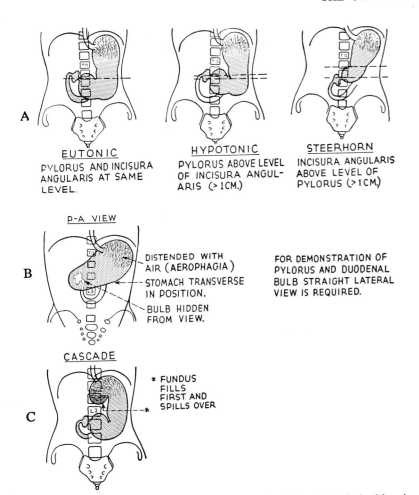

EUTONIC
PYLORUS AND INCISURA
ANGULARIS AT SAME
LEVEL.

HYPOTONIC
PYLORUS ABOVE LEVEL
OF INCISURA ANGUL-
ARIS (>1 CM.)

STEERHORN
INCISURA ANGULARIS
ABOVE LEVEL OF
PYLORUS (>1 CM.)

P-A VIEW

B

DISTENDED WITH
AIR (AEROPHAGIA)
STOMACH TRANSVERSE
IN POSITION.
BULB HIDDEN
FROM VIEW.

FOR DEMONSTRATION OF
PYLORUS AND DUODENAL
BULB STRAIGHT LATERAL
VIEW IS REQUIRED.

CASCADE

C

* FUNDUS
FILLS
FIRST AND
SPILLS OVER

Figure 13–29. Variations in stomach contour. A. In relation to body build and general stomach type. B. The infantile stomach. C. The cascade stomach.

to be symptomatic in an overweight person, whereas in normal or underweight individuals the cascade stomach is relatively asymptomatic. The symptoms are vague abdominal distress, sometimes suggestive of peptic ulcer.

The normal relationships of each type of stomach to each type of body build have been carefully worked out and tabulated as shown in Figure 13–11. Measurements can be taken as indicated and should fall within the normal range; if they are outside this normal range, the physician should be strongly suspicious of displacement of the stomach by some extrinsic lesion (see Table 13–1). A more accurate method of measurement in the left lateral erect with compression is illustrated in Figure 13–30 B.

Variations of the Stomach in Different Positions (Fig. 13–30). Gravity will influence the position of the gastric contents and the position and contour of the stomach. Thus, in the supine recumbent position, there is a tendency for the stomach to move up-

ward. At the same time, gastric contents will flow into the fundus, and the air in the stomach, which in the erect position is found in the fundus, will move anteriorly to occupy the anterior portion of the body of the stomach. Some of the air is invariably trapped in the pyloric portion also, but if there is sufficient barium suspension in the stomach, the pyloric portion and duodenal bulb will fill with it as well as with trapped air, producing a double contrast effect.

In the prone recumbent position, gravity tends to reverse these positional relationships. The barium mixture usually flows into the pyloric portion while the gas moves into the fundus. At the same time, there is a tendency for the stomach itself to move downward slightly, more closely resembling the appearance in the erect position.

In order to separate the shadows of the pyloric antrum and the duodenal bulb, it is usually necessary to place the patient in a slight right anterior oblique position. Otherwise, these structures usually overlie one another.

The lateral projection also finds wide usefulness, in that one can demonstrate positional relationships of the stomach to the pancreas and the omental bursa with greatest accuracy in this projection. The *left* lateral *standing* view is most valuable for this purpose since the relationship of the stomach to retrogastric structures is most accurately depicted thereby, particularly with compression. On the other hand, in the *right* lateral *recumbent* position, the stomach swings forward on its two areas of fixation (diaphragm and postbulbar duodenum), changing its relationship to the retrogastric structures. In this latter view, however, the pyloric antrum and body of the stomach fall anteriorly away from the level of the duodenum, producing a clearer depiction of the pylorobulbar area.

When the patient is supine, the stomach does not necessarily fall closely toward the retrogastric structures. This relationship is sometimes altered by the fact that the gas content of the stomach causes it to rise anteriorly. In our experience, therefore, a left lateral study of the stomach, obtained with a horizontal x-ray beam and the patient lying supine, is *less* valuable for study of stomach relationships to retrogastric structures than is the left lateral erection position, especially with compression.

Other Factors Which Influence Gastric Contour. Vagal stimulation increases gastric tone, whereas sympathetic stimulation decreases it. Thus, when an individual is frightened or otherwise emotionally disturbed, the stomach tends to be hypotonic. These psychic effects are usually temporary. Pathologic processes in the gastrointestinal and biliary tracts will also cause changes in gastric contour, but these are outside the scope of the present text.

The Duodenum. The duodenum is ordinarily examined simultaneously with the stomach, and it is discussed separately here for the sake of convenience only. The first part of the duodenum—the duodenal bulb—is integrated both structurally

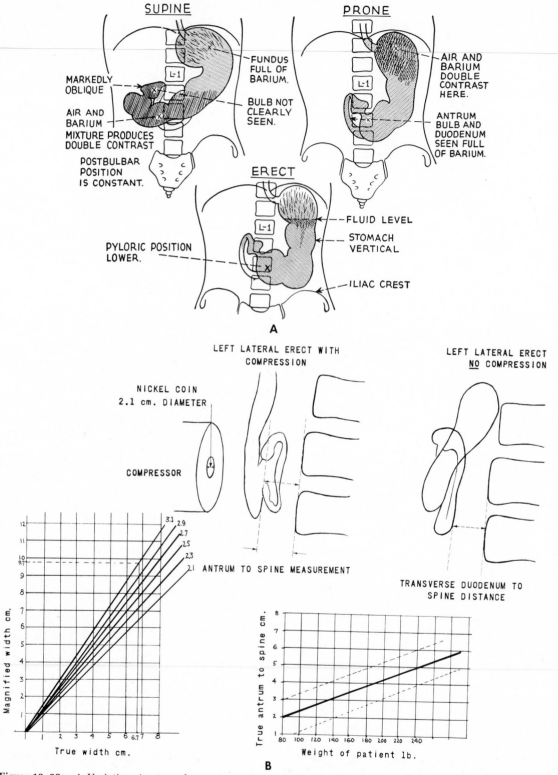

Figure 13–30.   *A.* Variations in stomach contour in relation to body position. *B.* Method of measuring "retroantral" and "retroduodenal" space. The coin on the compressor allows correction for magnification (graph, lower left). The normal standards for antrum to spine are shown in the graph, lower right. (From Poole, G. J.: Radiology, *97:71–81, 1970.)

and functionally with the pyloric antrum. The structure of the remainder of the duodenum resembles that of the small intestine.

The duodenum differs from the rest of the small intestine in several important respects:

1. It has no mesentery, and is fixed to the posterior abdominal wall for the most part.
2. The ducts of the liver, gallbladder, and pancreas open into it (at the duodenal papilla, or ampulla of Vater) in the descending part of the duodenum.
3. The duodenum contains some distinctive glands of its own, the duodenal glands of Brunner.
4. It is the shortest, widest, and most fixed portion of the small intestine.

Subdivisions. The duodenum is variably described as consisting of three or four parts (Fig. 13–31):

1. The superior portion, or duodenal bulb, which runs superiorly backward and to the right, is in direct continuity with the pylorus of the stomach. This portion has a mesentery of its own for a short distance.
2. The descending portion, which begins at the neck of the gallbladder, runs down on the posterior abdominal wall and usually ends approximately opposite the upper border of the fourth lumbar vertebra on the right of the vertebral column.
3. The inferior part is variably described as having one or two separate parts. It consists of a transverse portion, which crosses to the left of the midline, across the vena cava, aorta, and vertebral column; and an ascending portion, which ascends on the left of the vertebral column to the inferior surface of the pancreas. There it bends abruptly forward, forming the duodenojejunal flexure.

The duodenum is in the form of a U, with the superior portion more anterior than the descending part, the transverse portion coming directly forward and to the left, and the ascending portion in the same plane as the superior portion but to the left of the midline.

Gross Anatomy and Relationships of Each Subdivision of the Duodenum

THE SUPERIOR PORTION, DUODENAL BULB OR CAP. SITES OF NORMAL "FLECK" FORMATION. This first part of the duodenum is rather conical in shape, approximately 3.5 to 5 cm. in length, and

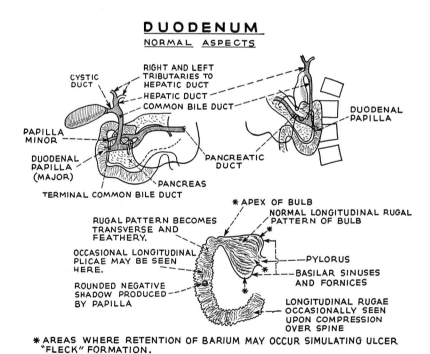

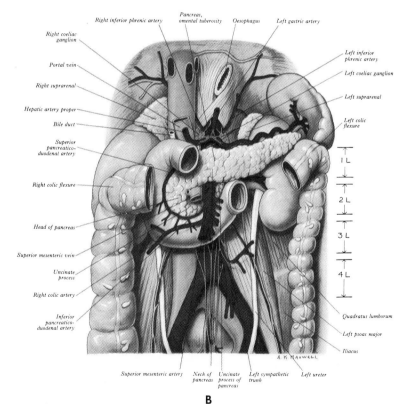

A

B

Figure 13–31. *A.* Normal relationships of the bile ducts to the duodenum, and the narrow mucosal patterns of the duodenum proper. *B.* A dissection to show the duodenum and pancreas. The right and left hepatic veins have been cut away at their points of entry into the inferior vena cava. The superior hypogastric plexus is shown in front of the sacral promontory and the sympathetic nerves which form it are seen descending across the bifurcation of the aorta, the left common iliac vein and the body of the fifth lumbar vertebra. (In this specimen the left renal artery is situated anterior to the left renal vein at the hilus of the kidney.)

3 cm. in diameter. It is described as having a base and an apex, the base forming a "stem-and-leaf" relationship with the pyloric canal (Fig. 13–32 A and B.)

As previously indicated, the rugal pattern of the bulb more closely resembles that of the pyloric antrum than the remainder of the duodenum, tending to be rather parallel, or parallel in spiral fashion from the base to apex. The contraction pattern and motor physiology of the bulb form a transition between that of the antrum and the distal duodenum.

Radiologically, a "fleck" (from the German meaning "spot") is a loculation of barium of any size from a few millimeters to 2 or more centimeters which strongly suggests a break in the normal mucosal structure and ulceration. In view of the great frequency of ulceration in this area, the detection of a fleck in this location is of extreme importance.

There are certain locations in the duodenal bulb, however, where fleck formation may be a normal variant, and these must be differentiated from the pathologic variety: (1) when the pylorus closes, there may be a dimple of mucosa at the base of the bulb in which the barium may accumulate, giving rise to the appearance of a fleck (Fig. 13–32 C); (2) the outer periphery of the base of the bulb occasionally acts as a groove, or sinus, in which barium may accumulate, and when seen in profile, gives the appearance of fleck formation at the base of the bulb; (3) the concentration of rugae at the apex of the bulb may simulate fleck formation on occasion also; (4) flecks of an inconstant variety may be simulated by peristaltic waves passing over the duodenal bulb.

The anatomic relationships of the bulb which are important are as follows (Fig. 13–33): the duodenal bulb forms the inferior boundary of the foramen epiploicum (foramen of Winslow), and hence a pathologic penetration of the bulb finds ready access into the lesser omental bursa. The hepatic artery is also in contact for a short distance with the superior margin of the bulb. Below, the bulb rests on the head and neck of the pancreas. There are several large blood vessels which come into close contact with this area (Fig. 13–33 B), and are of considerable importance from the standpoint of possible erosion of an ulcer. On the left side lie the portal vein, gastroduodenal artery (and bile duct); close to the posterior aspect is the right side of the inferior vena cava; and adjoining the inferior margin are the superior pancreaticoduodenal and the right gastroepiploic vessels (Fig. 13–34).

The common bile duct may occasionally indent the bulb, giving rise to an apparent deformity, and the gallbladder lies in close apposition with the superior and right margins of the first part of the duodenum, occasionally producing an indentation of the duodenum.

THE SECOND, OR DESCENDING PART OF THE DUODENUM. DESCRIPTION OF VILLI AND PLICAE CIRCULARES. This part of the duodenum is retroperitoneal in position with the root of the transverse mesocolon, crossing it at its middle. The head of the pancreas is in contact with its left margin (Fig. 13–35) and occasionally overlaps it both anteriorly and posteriorly, and along this margin run the branches of the pancreaticoduodenal arteries. The bile duct, after descending behind the duodenal blub, passes between the head of the pancreas and this part of the duodenum, where it joins with the pancreatic duct. The two together pierce the duodenal wall obliquely, and open by a common orifice on its inner aspect at the apex of the duodenal papilla (ampulla of Vater) medially (Fig. 13–36).

The mucous membrane of this part of the duodenum, as well

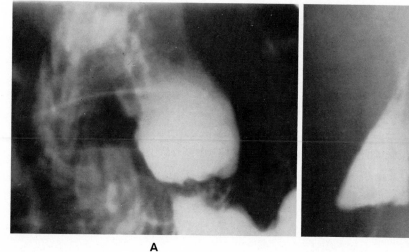
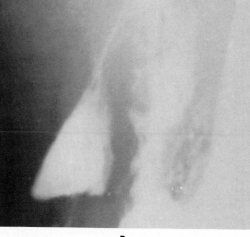
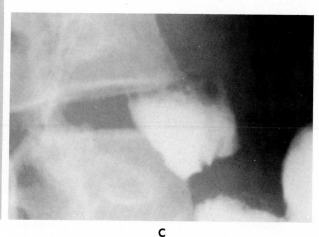

A   B   C

Figure 13–32. Spot film radiographs of the duodenal bulb in the right anterior (A) and left anterior oblique (B) position. C. There is a "dimple" at the base of the duodenal bulb when the pylorus closes normally. The dimple simulates an ulcer niche.

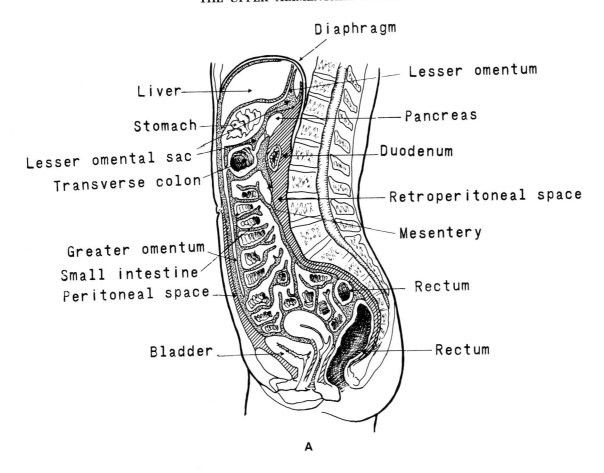

A

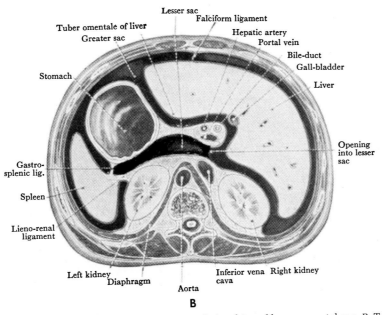

B

Figure 13–33. *A.* Sagittal diagram of abdomen showing relationships of lesser omental sac. *B.* Transverse section of abdomen to show the arrangement of peritoneum at the level of the opening into lesser sac. (From Cunningham's Manual of Practical Anatomy, 12th ed., Vol. 2. London, Oxford University Press, 1958.)

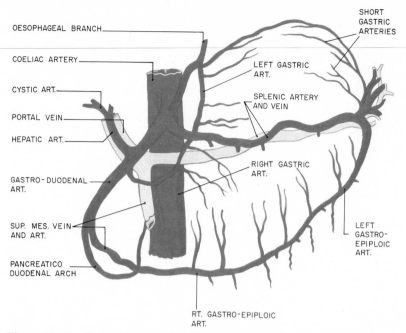

Figure 13–34. Coeliac artery and its branches. (Redrawn from Cunningham's Manual of Practical Anatomy, 12th ed., Vol. 2. London, Oxford University Press, 1958.)

as all parts of the small intestine, presents a soft, velvety internal surface which is caused by the presence of the minute mucosal processes known as villi. These begin at the edge of the pyloric valve where they are quite broad, but they become narrower as they proceed down the small intestine. The only place they are not found is immediately over the solitary lymph nodules. These villi play an important part in the absorption function of the small intestine (Figs. 13–31 A and 13–38).

The mucous membrane of the small intestine is thrown into numerous folds which may to a great extent disappear upon distention, but there are permanent folds known as the plicae circulares (Fig. 13–37) or valvulae conniventes. They are crescentic folds running around the small intestine in circular fashion. They may bifurcate, and they usually project about 8 mm. into the lumen of the small intestine. *They begin in the second part of the duodenum* (Fig. 13–38), and gradually become more prominent, so that in the region of the duodenal papilla, they are very distinct and remain prominent in the rest of the duodenum. The combination of the plicae circulares and the villi imparts a feathery pattern to the duodenum and jejunum when viewed radiographically in the absence of distention, and this is the typical rugal pattern not only of the duodenum but also of the

jejunum. The absence of plicae circulares in the duodenal bulb accounts for its closer resemblance radiographically to the pyloric antrum (Fig. 13–39).

THE HORIZONTAL PORTION OF THE INFERIOR PART OF THE DUODENUM (THIRD PART). This part is somewhat concave upward, is retroperitoneal, and is crossed by the superior mesenteric vessels and the root of the mesentery near the midline. It crosses the inferior vena cava, and is closely applied to the inferior aspect of the head of the pancreas.

THE ASCENDING PORTION OF THE INFERIOR PART OF THE DUODENUM (FOURTH PART). This part lies on the aorta, the left renal vein, and occasionally also the left renal artery (Fig. 13–40 A). As previously indicated, it extends obliquely anteriorly and to the left, and its left side lies in contact with some coils of small intestine. In addition to being clothed by peritoneum anteriorly (as is the case of the second and third parts), it is also covered by peritoneum on its left side.

The duodenojejunal flexure is fixed by the musculus suspensorius (suspensory ligament) of Treitz, opposite the left side of the first or second lumbar vertebrae. This latter suspensory muscle blends with the muscular coat of the duodenum, passes upward behind the pancreas to blend partially with the celiac artery, and then is attached to the right crus of the diaphragm.

In the neighborhood of the ascending part of the duodenum, three peritoneal fossae may frequently be present (Fig. 13–40 B). Two of these, the superior and inferior duodenal fossae, are formed by slips of fibrous tissue covered by peritoneum extending from the left side of the duodenum to the peritoneal surface adjoining it, and form very small pouches directed caudad and cephalad respectively. The third, however, which is called the paraduodenal fossa, is produced by a fold of peritoneum formed by the inferior mesenteric vein as it courses along the left lateral side of the ascending part of the duodenum. The inferior mesenteric vein is accompanied in part of its course by the left colic artery. This fossa is capable of forming a hernial sac, and therefore may be of some clinical significance.

IMPORTANCE OF A STUDY OF THE DUODENAL CONTOUR. The duodenum is in a fixed position for the most part, and hence variations from its normal position become significant in the detection of space-occupying lesions in adjoining structures, such as the pancreas, lesser omental bursa, colon, gallbladder, and biliary ducts.

There is, however, a considerable variation in different individuals in the normal contour of the duodenum. To a great extent, this is correlated with body habitus. Thus in pyknic individuals with high steer-horn stomachs (Fig. 13–41 and Table 13–1) the duodenal loop appears widened; and in asthenic individuals, portions of the duodenal loop will appear to be very close to one another, and sometimes overlapping. Occasionally, there is a redundancy of the first part of the duodenum (Fig. 13–42) with a greater segment peritonealized than is ordinarily seen. In some

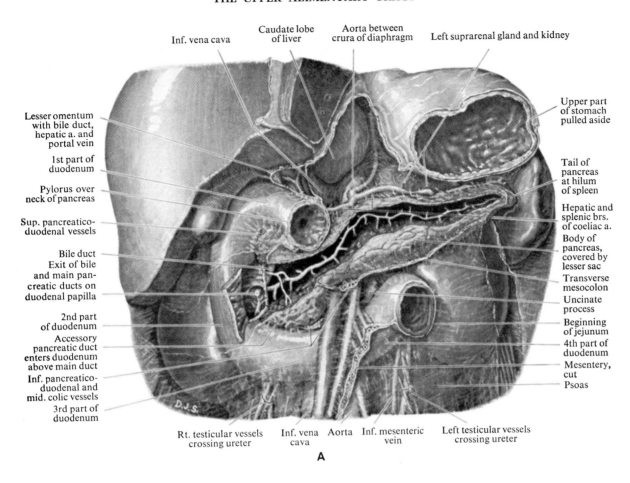

Inf. vena cava

Caudate lobe of liver

Aorta between crura of diaphragm

Left suprarenal gland and kidney

Upper part of stomach pulled aside

Lesser omentum with bile duct, hepatic a. and portal vein

1st part of duodenum

Pylorus over neck of pancreas

Sup. pancreatico-duodenal vessels

Bile duct
Exit of bile and main pancreatic ducts on duodenal papilla

2nd part of duodenum

Accessory pancreatic duct enters duodenum above main duct

Inf. pancreatico-duodenal and mid. colic vessels

3rd part of duodenum

Tail of pancreas at hilum of spleen

Hepatic and splenic brs. of coeliac a.

Body of pancreas, covered by lesser sac

Transverse mesocolon

Uncinate process

Beginning of jejunum

4th part of duodenum

Mesentery, cut

Psoas

Rt. testicular vessels crossing ureter

Inf. vena cava

Aorta

Inf. mesenteric vein

Left testicular vessels crossing ureter

A

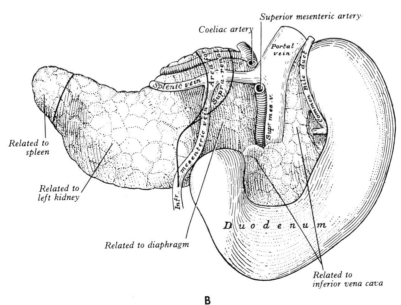

Coeliac artery

Superior mesenteric artery

Portal vein

Splenic vein

Related to spleen

Related to left kidney

Related to diaphragm

Duodenum

Related to inferior vena cava

B

Figure 13–35. *A.* Dissection of duodenum and pancreas. Transverse colon and part of stomach removed. (Reprinted by permission of Faber and Faber, Ltd., from Anatomy of the Human Body, by Lockhart, Hamilton, and Fyfer: Faber and Faber, London; J. B. Lippincott Company, Philadelphia.) *B.* Posterior aspect of the pancreas and duodenum from behind. (From Warwick, R., and Williams, P. L.: Gray's Anatomy, 35th British ed. Longman, London (for Churchill Livingstone), 1973.)

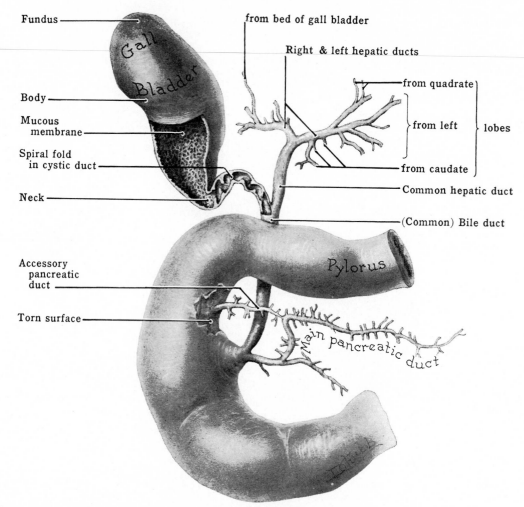

Figure 13–36. Extrahepatic bile passages and the pancreatic ducts. (Reproduced by permission from J. C. B. Grant: An Atlas of Anatomy, 5th ed. Copyright © 1962 by The Williams and Wilkins Company.)

individuals, the second part of the duodenum may be virtually lacking, and it would appear that the superior part of the duodenum connects almost directly with the horizontal part of the inferior portion of the duodenum.

These normal variations and anomalies must be constantly borne in mind when radiography of the duodenum is attempted.

Variations in the appearance of the duodenal bulb (Fig. 13–43). This is by far the most important part of the duodenum from the standpoint of incidence of abnormality. The normal bulb is usually very regular. It tends to be conical or triangular in shape, and variations from this configuration are usually of considerable significance. The apex of the bulb is usually surrounded by the feathery mucosa of the duodenum which contains plicae circulares, but the mucosal pattern of the bulb proper usually consists of fairly parallel rugae, or rugae arranged in the form of a spiral (Figs. 13–28 and 13–38).

The body habitus of the individual will to some extent cause some variation in the appearance of the bulb. In the short, squat person, the bulb tends to be small and posterior, hiding as it were behind the pyloric antrum. Occasionally also, in such people, the bulb will extend obliquely downward, especially if the stomach is high and steer-horn in type (Fig. 13–44 *A* and *B*).

Occasionally, the bulb is large and patulous in type, and tends to remain filled for a considerable period of time.

The normal rugae are ordinarily quite flexible and elastic, and can be quite readily obliterated by pressure, in contrast to the abnormal "fleck" which has already been mentioned (Fig. 13–45 *A* and *B*).

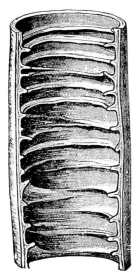

Figure 13–37. Anatomic presentation of the plicae circulares of the small intestine (jejunum). (From Cunningham's Textbook of Anatomy, 6th ed. London, Oxford University Press, 1931.)

The duodenum distal to the duodenal bulb. The second, third, and fourth portions of the duodenum have the normal feathery mucosal pattern already described. They appear as a single loop, with peristaltic waves carrying the barium around this loop.

Occasionally the duodenal papilla in the middle of the descending part of the duodenum will fill with barium or produce a small filling defect in the contour of the duodenum. This must not be interpreted as abnormal (Fig. 13–46).

There may be a slight hesitation when the barium passes the duodenojejunal junction, and usually an angulation can be detected in this region. This angle tends to be more obtuse in pyknic individuals.

Important Anatomic Relationships of the Stomach. The position of the stomach varies in different individuals, and in the same individual depending upon posture and emotional factors, as well as upon the digestive state (Figs. 13–29 and 13–30). The

The posture of the patient will also affect the appearance of the bulb. The duodenal bulb is best seen and most copiously filled when the patient is lying obliquely prone on his right side. It is least filled in the supine position.

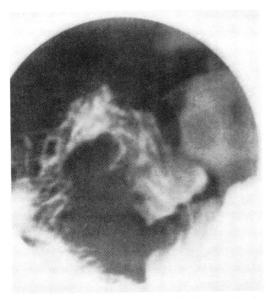

Figure 13–38. Mucosal pattern of the duodenal bulb and the change in pattern which occurs at the beginning of the second part of the duodenum.

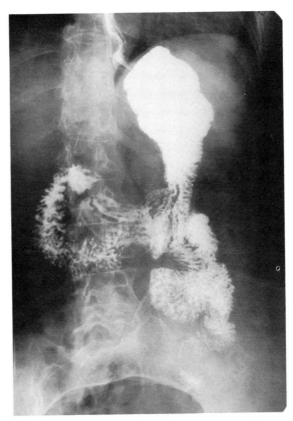

Figure 13–39. Anteroposterior view of stomach in slight left posterior oblique. Note the excellent double contrast of the distal stomach while the fundus is completely filled with barium. Note also the changes in mucosal pattern which occur more distally in the bulb and duodenum as well as in the jejunum.

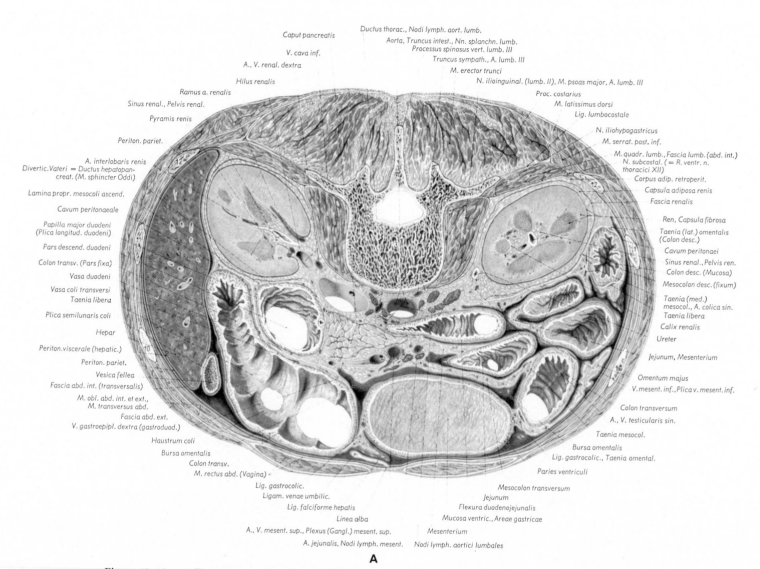

Caput pancreatis
Ductus thorac., Nodi lymph. aort. lumb.
Aorta, Truncus intest., Nn. splanchn. lumb.
V. cava inf.
Processus spinosus vert. lumb. III
A., V. renal. dextra
Truncus sympath., A. lumb. III
Hilus renalis
M. erector trunci
N. ilioinguinal. (lumb. II), M. psoas major, A. lumb. III
Ramus a. renalis
Proc. costarius
Sinus renal., Pelvis renal.
M. latissimus dorsi
Pyramis renis
Lig. lumbocostale
Periton. pariet.
N. iliohypogastricus
M. serrat. post. inf.
A. interlobaris renis
M. quadr. lumb., Fascia lumb. (abd. int.)
Divertic.Vateri = Ductus hepatopan-
N. subcostal. (= R. ventr. n.
creat. (M. sphincter Oddi)
thoracici XII)
Lamina propr. mesocoli ascend.
Corpus adip. retroperit.
Cavum peritonaeale
Capsula adiposa renis
Fascia renalis
Papilla major duodeni
(Plica longitud. duodeni)
Ren, Capsula fibrosa
Pars descend. duodeni
Taenia (lat.) omentalis
(Colon desc.)
Colon transv. (Pars fixa)
Cavum peritonaei
Vasa duodeni
Sinus renal., Pelvis ren.
Vasa coli transversi
Colon desc. (Mucosa)
Taenia libera
Mesocolon desc. (fixum)
Plica semilunaris coli
Taenia (med.)
mesocol., A. colica sin.
Hepar
Taenia libera
Periton.viscerale (hepatic.)
Calix renalis
Periton. pariet.
Ureter
Vesica fellea
Jejunum, Mesenterium
Fascia abd. int. (transversalis)
M. obl. abd. int. et ext.,
Omentum majus
M. transversus abd.
V.mesent. inf.,Plica v. mesent. inf.
Fascia abd. ext.
V. gastroepipl. dextra (gastroduod.)
Colon transversum
Haustrum coli
A., V. testicularis sin.
Bursa omentalis
Taenia mesocol.
Colon transv.
Bursa omentalis
M. rectus abd. (Vagina)
Lig. gastrocolic., Taenia omental.
Lig. gastrocolic.
Paries ventriculi
Ligam. venae umbilic.
Mesocolon transversum
Lig. falciforme hepatis
Jejunum
Linea alba
Flexura duodenojejunalis
A., V. mesent. sup., Plexus (Gangl.) mesent. sup.
Mucosa ventric., Areae gastricae
A. jejunalis, Nodi lymph. mesent.
Mesenterium
Nodi lymph. aortici lumbales

A

Figure 13–40.   *A.* Transverse section through abdomen at the level of the third lumbar vertebra. Section through spatium hepatorenale (compartment for liver, colon, duodenum, and kidneys) and spatium retrogastricum (cavum bursae oment.) of cavum peritonaei. (From Pernkopf, E.: Atlas of Topographical and Applied Human Anatomy. Vol. 2, Thorax, Abdomen, and Extremities. Philadelphia, W. B. Saunders Co., 1964.)

Figure 13–40 continued on the opposite page.

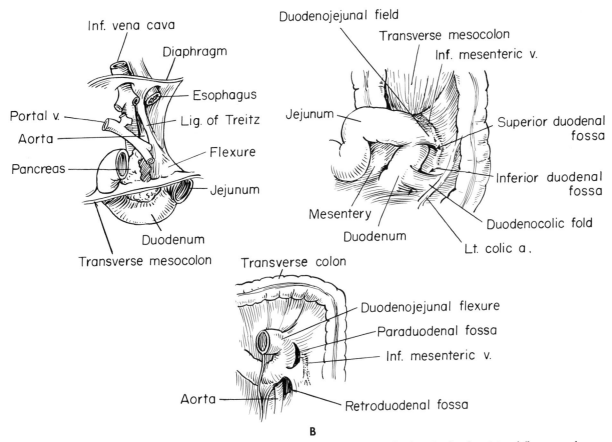

Figure 13–40 *Continued.* B. Line drawing indicating the structures involved at the duodenojejunal flexure and the duodenal fossae and folds. Note the superior duodenal fossa, the inferior duodenal fossa, and the paraduodenal fossa, and the relationship to the duodenojejunal flexure.

pylorus may lie as high as the twelfth thoracic vertebra, or as low as the upper sacrum. It may lie in the midline, or to the right or left of it. Associated with these different positions of the pylorus, there is a difference in the position of the first part of the duodenum, and its relation to the head of the pancreas. Likewise, the stomach may be high and the liver low, and vice versa, indicating no definite relation between their relative positions (Fig. 13–47).

Ordinarily, the stomach is obliquely placed in the left upper abdominal cavity (Fig. 13–48), with the fundus somewhat more lateral than the pylorus. In the lateral projection, the fundus is posterior to the liver, in apposition with the diaphragm above and behind. The body of the stomach is anterior, lying immediately under the anterior abdominal wall. The pyloric antrum extends obliquely posteriorly, superiorly, and to the right. Usually the pylorus is situated just above the head of the pancreas (Fig. 13–

48) in the posterior part of the abdomen, in a plane just anterior (1 to 2 cm.) to the plane of the second part (retroperitoneal portion) of the duodenum.

The hepatogastric and hepatoduodenal ligaments constitute the lesser omentum which is attached to the lesser curvature of the stomach and forms a part of the omental bursa—an anatomic relationship of considerable practical significance (Fig. 13–49).

The spleen lies posterior and somewhat lateral to the body of the stomach, with the gastrosplenic ligament attaching it to the greater curvature of the stomach (Fig. 13–50).

The head of the pancreas lies in the duodenal loop (Fig. 13–48), whereas the body of the pancreas lies posterior to the pyloric portion of the stomach. The tail of the pancreas usually lies just posterior to the body of the stomach, and comes into contact with the medial surface of the spleen. The pancreas forms a large part

(Text continued on page 804.)

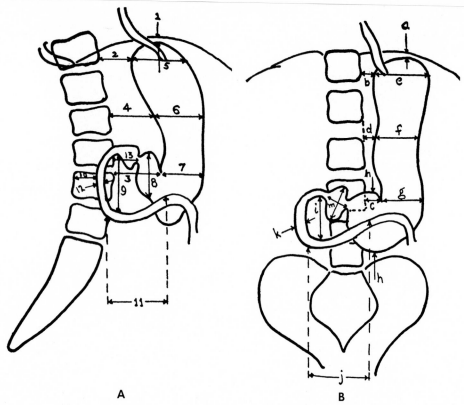

A   **B**

Figure 13–41. Lateral *(A)* and frontal *(B)* views of the stomach showing the various measurements which can be taken in an effort to associate the normal stomach with body build. (From Meschan, I., et al.: South. Med. J., *46,* 1953.)

1, Distance between top of fundus and diaphragm.
2, Cardia of stomach to anterior spine.
3, Stomach to anterior spine at level of cardia.
4, Stomach to anterior spine midway between cardia and incisura angularis.
5, Horizontal measurement of fundus at level of cardia.
6, Horizontal midway measurement of body of stomach at level of measurement 4.
7, Horizontal measurement of stomach at level of incisura angularis.
8, Maximal vertical measurement of pyloric antrum.
9, Maximal vertical internal diameter of duodenal loop.
10, Minimal measurement of outer margin of second portion of duodenum to posterior margin of vertebral bodies.
11, Maximal horizontal internal diameter of duodenal loop.
12, Maximal outer diameter of second part of duodenum.
13, Distance between pylorus and anterior margin of spine.

a, Measurement between diaphragm and top of fundus.
b, Distance between cardia and lateral margin of spine.
c, Distance between incisura angularis and lateral margin of spine.
d, Distance between stomach and lateral margin of spine midway between b and c.
e, Maximal horizontal measurement of fundus at level of cardia.
f, Midway measurement of body of stomach at level of measurement d.
g, Horizontal measurement of body of stomach at level of incisura angularis.
h, Maximal vertical measurement of pyloric antrum.
i, Maximal vertical internal diameter of duodenal loop.
j, Maximal horizontal internal diameter of duodenal loop.
k, Diameter of second part of duodenum.
m, Ratio of the measurement of base of the bulb over its height from apex to pylorus.

TABLE 13–1 RELATIONSHIPS OF STOMACH AND DUODENUM TO THE SPINE IN DIFFERENT WEIGHT AND STOMACH TYPE GROUPS (BOTH ASYMPTOMATIC AND SYMPTOMATIC SUMMATED)*

Weight Group	Stomach Type	No. of Cases	4 Rt. Lat.[a]		4 Lt. Lat.[a]		9 Rt. Lat.[a]		10 Rt. Lat.[a]		11 Rt. Lat.[a]		13 Rt. Lat.[a]	
			Avg. of Medians	Range	Avg. of Medians	Range	Avg. of Medians	Range	Avg. of Medians	Range	Avg. of Medians	Range	Avg. of Medians	Range
Normal	J-shape	58	5.5	1—8.5	4	0—8	6.5	4—9.5	3	—1—9	3	0—12.5	4	—0.5—8
	Fish-hook	10	4	1.5—6	3	0.5—6.5	6	4—8	3	2.5—4	5.6	3.5—8	4.5	2.5—9
	Cascade[b]	13	6	1—13	5.5	1.5—13	6	4.5—6	4.3	2—9.5	6.6	1—11	6	2.5—9
	Steer-horn	9	5	0—11	4	1—13	6.5	5.5—8	3.5	—0.5—5	5.5	1.5—9	5	2.5—10
Underwt	J-shape	56	4.5	1.5—7	2	0.5—8	5.5	2—11	3	—0.5—7	4	0—9	3	0.5—6.5
	Fish-hook	21	4	0—7.5	2.6	—1.5—4.5	5.5	3.5—8	2.5	0—5	3	1.5—5	2.5	1—4
	Cascade[b]	5	5	2—8	2.6	0—5	6	5.5—6.5	2.5	2—3.5	4.5	4—5	3	2—5
	Steer-horn	3	5	4.5—6	6.5	0.5—7.5	8	8	4.5	2—6	7	6.5—8	4	1.5—5
Overwt	J-shape	13	5.5	1.5—10	4	1.5—8.5	6.5	4—9	3.3	2—7	4.5	3.5—9	3.5	1.5—9.5
	Fish-hook	5	5	3—7.5	4	0—5.5	5	3—7.5	2.5	0—4	4.5	2—9.5	4.6	3—6.5
	Cascade[b]	10	5	2—11	5.5	0—9	7	4—9	4	1—7.5	5	1.5—10	5.6	3—12
	Steer-horn	8	6	2.5—9.5	4.6	2.5—8	6	5.5—8	4	3.5—5.5	5	3—7.5	4.5	3—7.5
	Total	**211**												

*From Meschan, I. et al.: The normal radiographic adult stomach and duodenum. South. Med. J., *46*:878, 1953.
[a]Measurements are defined in Figure 13–41.
[b]Asymptomatic cascade is farther from spine than symptomatic.

DUODENAL ANOMALIES

DEFECTIVE ATTACHMENT OF DUODENAL MESENTERY

MOBILE DUODENUM

DUODENUM APPEARS INVERTED

RECUMBENT

DUODENUM HAS NORMAL APPEARANCE

ERECT

NONROTATION OF DUODENUM

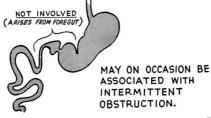

NOT INVOLVED
(ARISES FROM FOREGUT)

LOWER DUODENUM CURVES TO RIGHT INSTEAD OF LEFT AND JOINS JEJUNUM IN RIGHT UPPER QUADRANT
(USUALLY NONROTATION OF JEJUNUM ALSO.)

MAY ON OCCASION BE ASSOCIATED WITH INTERMITTENT OBSTRUCTION.

REDUNDANCY – FIRST PART

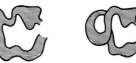

REDUNDANCY – 3rd PART

INVERTED DUODENUM

MAY PREDISPOSE TO PANCREATITIS DUE TO TWIST OF BILE DUCT AND REFLUX INTO PANCREAS.

INVERSION BEGINS IN 2nd PART USUALLY.

Figure 13–42.

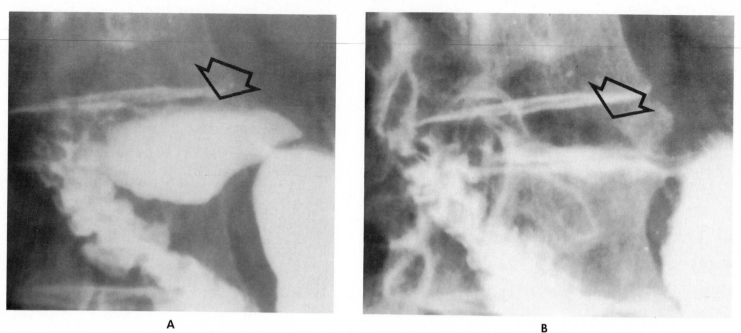

Figure 13-43. *A* and *B*. Normal duodenal bulb in two stages of contraction, *B* simulating an elongated pyloric canal.

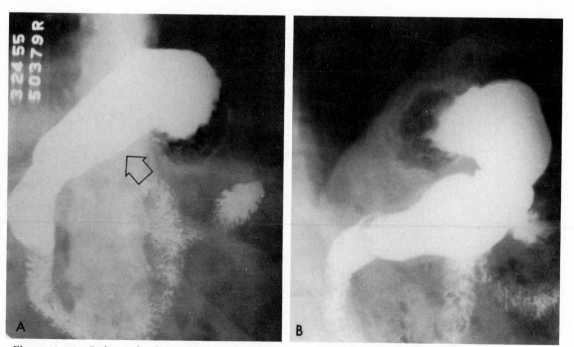

Figure 13-44. Radiographs demonstrating an intermittent type of organoaxial rotation of the stomach. In *A* the inferior margin of the stomach is concave and the stomach is situated high under the diaphragm. In *B* the stomach is in a relatively normal position. This type of rotation has also been referred to as incomplete volvulus.

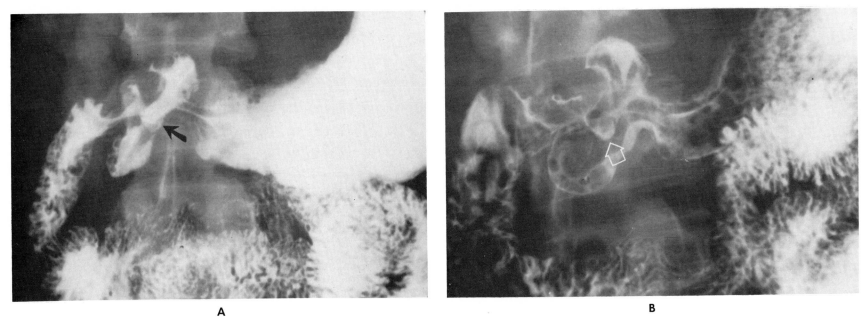

Figure 13-45. *A* and *B.* Duodenal ulcer showing the advantages of double contrast with barium and air, (*A*) erect, and (*B*) supine. Both views show the ulcer.

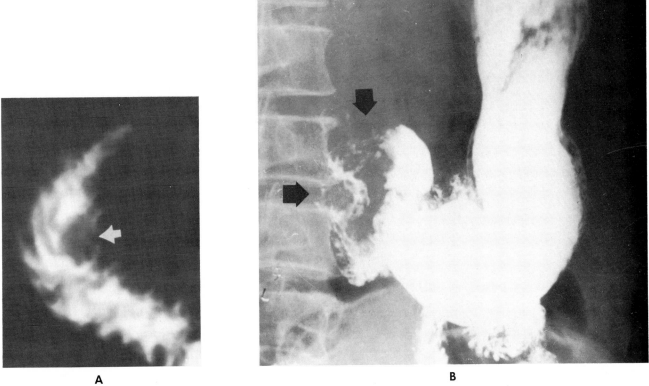

Figure 13-46. *A.* Occasional normal appearance of the major papilla indenting the second part of the duodenum. *B.* Abnormal indentations on the second part of the duodenum (for comparison with *A*). (Carcinoma of the pancreas with matted lymph nodes and a dilated common duct.)

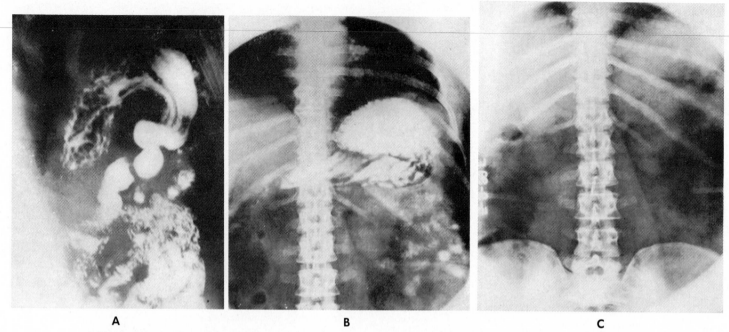

Figure 13–47. "Cascade" stomach. *A.* Radiograph in the right anterior oblique position. *B.* Slight cascade stomach in anteroposterior projection. *C.* Same as *B* without the barium, showing how the fundus of such a stomach may simulate a mass in the left upper quadrant. (*B* and *C* courtesy of Drs. H. L. Friedell and C. C. Dundon, University Hospitals, Cleveland, Ohio.)

of the posterior wall of the lesser omental bursa, whereas the posterior wall of the stomach forms the greater part of the anterior wall of this important "sac." Abnormalities of this bursa and the pancreas are therefore frequently reflected in pressure upon the stomach, with alteration of the normal gastric contour (Fig. 13–51).

The transverse colon is loosely connected with the greater curvature of the stomach via the greater omentum, which hangs like an apron over the entire intestinal tract. The splenic flexure of the colon is lateral to the lower greater curvature of the stomach and closely applied to the undersurface of the spleen.

In most texts dealing with gross anatomy, there is reference to the "stomach chamber" or "bed" in which the stomach is said to lie. Radiographically, the stomach usually extends more inferiorly than is indicated by the dissection of the cadavers.

When the patient lies down, the stomach moves freely about its two points of fixation, the diaphragm superiorly and the postbulbar duodenum inferiorly. In the right lateral projection, it swings anteriorly like a hammock, and is no longer closely applied to the retrogastric structures. In the right lateral position with the patient lying down, the relationship of fundus-to-body-to-antrum will vary from one patient to another, depending upon

adjoining pressure phenomena. When the patient lies on his left side, the stomach is concave toward the left, with the fundus and duodenal bulb being uppermost. Any food or barium in the stomach under these circumstances will tend to gravitate to the body of the stomach and air will rise to the fundus and duodenal bulb. Thus, the left posterior oblique, approximately 45 degrees with the patient lying supine on his left side, is particularly valuable for obtaining double contrast visualization of the fundus, antrum, and duodenal bulb (and sometimes the remainder of the duodenum as well). When the patient is in the prone position, in the right anterior oblique, the fundus of the stomach continues to retain some air, but barium contained within the stomach will gravitate to the body and antrum as well as to the duodenal bulb. When the patient is lying directly prone, there is some pressure of the spine upon the adjoining portion of the pyloric antrum and duodenal bulb. The right anterior oblique view frees the stomach from pressure against the spine and hence, is ordinarily the desired view for optimum visualization of peristalsis. The left lateral erect film offers the best opportunity to study the stomach in relation to the structures posterior to it.

To demonstrate gastroesophageal reflux, the optimum positions are as follows: first, the patient lies supine on the left side in

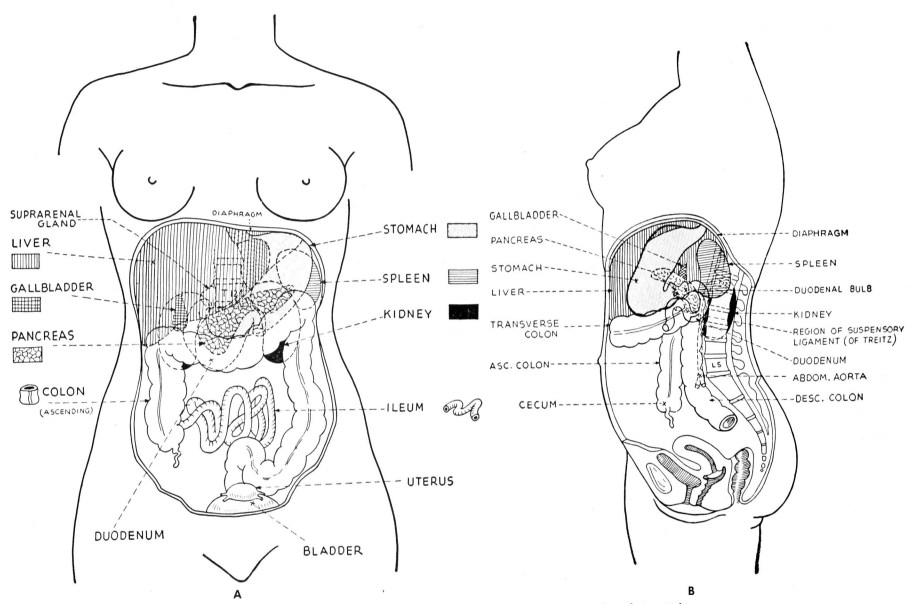

Figure 13–48. Important anatomic relationships of the stomach. *A.* Anteroposterior view. *B.* Lateral view (right, recumbent).

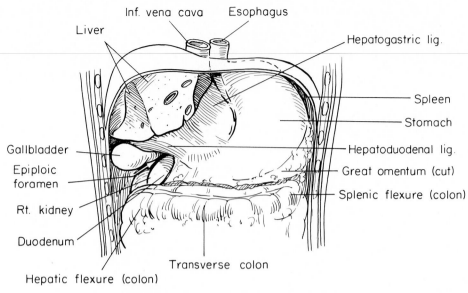

Figure 13–49. Stomach *in situ*, with hepatic ligaments, greater omentum cut.

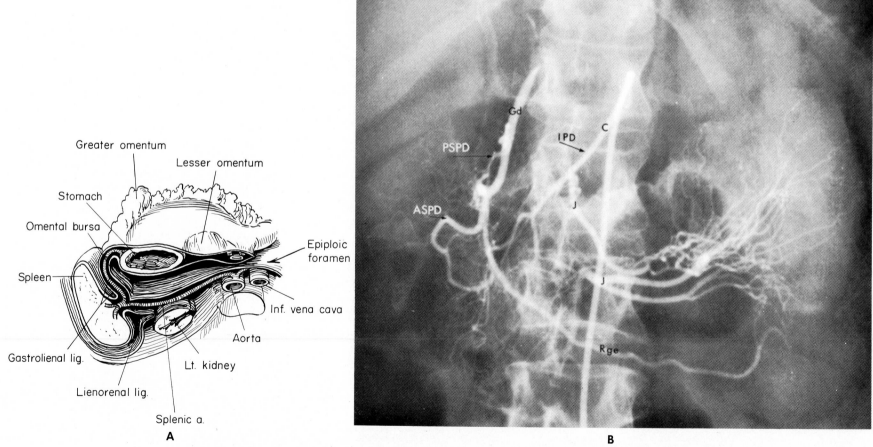

Figure 13–50. *A.* Cross-section showing relation of stomach, spleen, and adjoining structures to lesser omental bursa and epiploic foramen. *B.* Celiac arterial axis as related to the stomach, spleen, and greater omentum. (J) Catheter *in situ*, (Rge) right gastroepiploic artery, (C) celiac artery, (IPD) inferior anterior pancreaticoduodenal artery, (PSPD) posterior superior pancreaticoduodenal artery, (ASPD) anterior superior pancreaticoduodenal artery, the latter two making an arcade. (From Ruzicka, F. F., and Rossi, P.: Radiol. Clin. N. Amer., 8:3–29, 1970.)

Figure 13–50 continued on the opposite page.

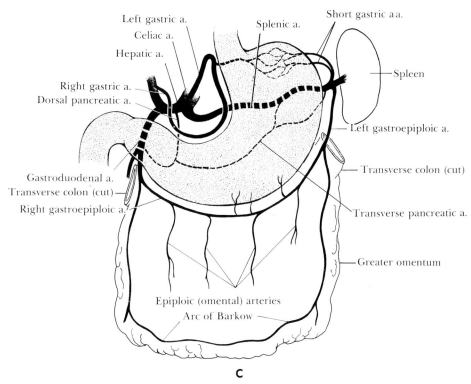

Left gastric a.

Celiac a.

Hepatic a.

Splenic a.

Short gastric a.a.

Spleen

Right gastric a.

Dorsal pancreatic a.

Left gastroepiploic a.

Transverse colon (cut)

Gastroduodenal a.

Transverse colon (cut)

Right gastroepiploic a.

Transverse pancreatic a.

Greater omentum

Epiploic (omental) arteries

Arc of Barkow

C

Figure 13–50 *Continued.* *C.* Line drawing representative of celiac arterial axis as related to stomach and greater omentum. (Modified from Ruzicka, F. F., and Rossi, P.: Radiol. Clin. N. Amer., 8:3–29, 1970.)

a moderate Trendelenburg position; second, the patient bends forward so that the esophagus lies below the level of the fundus of the stomach. Both methods demonstrate a gastroesophageal reflux in the presence of an incompetent gastroesophageal junction.

The Rugal Pattern of Each Subdivision of the Stomach (Fig. 13–28). When the stomach is wholly or partially empty, the muscular layers contract and throw the mucosa into numerous folds or rugae which project into the interior of the stomach. The rugae of the fundus tend to be arranged in a mosaic, which gradually becomes more regular in the body of the stomach. The mosaic appearance is more marked along the greater curvature and this pattern gradually diminishes toward the pylorus.

The rugae tend to remain parallel in a narrow segment on the lesser curvature of the stomach throughout the entire length of the stomach from the cardia to the pylorus. These longitudinal rugae form the "magenstrasse," which seems to consitute a channel for the usual descent of the food, although not invariably so.

The rugae in the pylorus are thin parallel folds. These parallel folds continue into the duodenal cap or bulb, where they either remain parallel or spiral toward the apex of the duodenal bulb.

Between the rugae, there are minute depressions caused by the openings of the small gastric glands, and minute ridges around them, giving the stomach mucosa the so-called mammillated appearance. These minute mammillae are not recognizable radiographically.

The rugal pattern of the stomach must not be thought of as completely static—it can vary in the same individual under different physiologic conditions. Thus, it will vary in accordance with the degree of vascularity of the mucosa and submucosa and also with the degree of distention of the stomach. Cold tends to make the rugae smaller and more numerous, and certain chemicals such as pilocarpine and physostigmine have the same effect, whereas atropine has the opposite effect.

However, the rugal pattern will change in certain pathologic states such as inflammation, ulceration, and neoplastic infiltration, as well as from extrinsic pressure, and the rugae thus become one of the most accurate indices which the radiologic examination of the stomach furnishes. Examination for rugal pattern constitutes one of the most important aspects of the gastrointestinal examination, if not the most important.

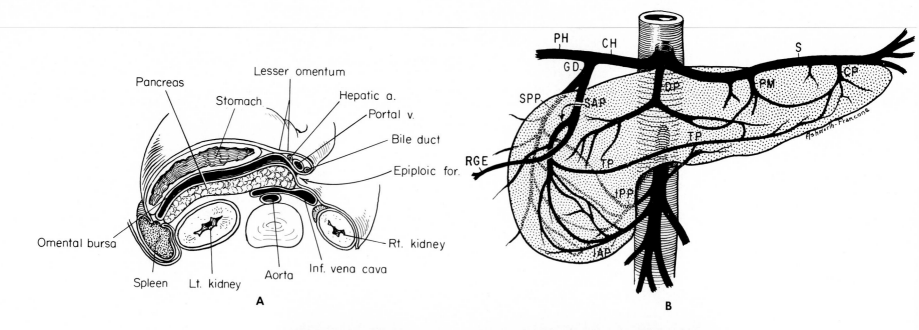

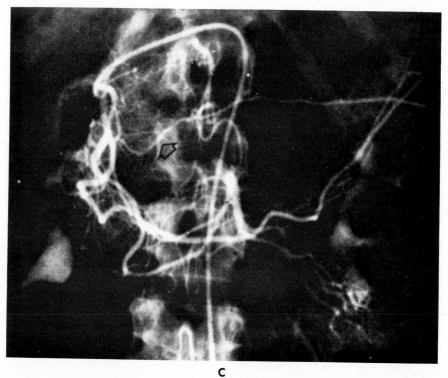

Figure 13–51. *A.* Transverse section relations of pancreas and stomach to lesser omental sac. *B.* Schematic drawing of the arterial supply to the pancreas. (CH) common hepatic, (PH) proper hepatic, (GD) gastroduodenal, (RGE) right gastroepiploic, (SAP) superior anterior pancreaticoduodenal, (SPP) superior posterior pancreaticoduodenal, (IAP) inferior anterior pancreaticoduodenal, (IPP) inferior posterior pancreaticoduodenal, (S) splenic, (DP) dorsal pancreatic, (PM) pancreatic magna, (CP) caudal pancreatic, (TP) transverse pancreatic. *C.* Superselective arteriography of the normal gastroduodenal artery with visualization of its pancreaticoduodenal branches. The transverse pancreatic (unfilled arrow), dorsal pancreatic (filled arrow), and branches of the superior mesenteric artery are filled through anastomotic vessels. (*B* and *C* from Rösch, J., and Judkins, M. P.: Seminars in Roentgenol., *3:*296–309, 1968.)

Physiologic Considerations Concerning the Stomach

Gastric Glandular Secretions (Figs. 13–52 and 13–53). Gastric glandular secretions arise from (1) cardiac glands, situated in a 5 mm. zone (approximately) around the esophagogastric junction or cardia; (2) fundic glands situated for the most part throughout the remainder of the fundus and body of the stomach; and (3) pyloric glands, situated in the region of the antrum. There is no sharply demarcated boundary line in the stomach in respect to these glandular secretions. The fundic glands contain chief cells which are responsible for pepsinogen secretion; parietal cells are responsible for the secretion of hydrochloric acid as well as intrinsic factors. There are scattered argentaffin cells throughout the body and antrum, and occasionally parietal cells are also found in the antrum. In addition, the hormone gastrin is secreted by the antrum. This apparently is responsible for stimulating the activity of parietal cells.

Although mucus is found predominantly surrounding the cardiac orifice, where it is secreted by cardiac glands, and in the antrum, secreted by pyloric cells, mucous secretions are found throughout the entire stomach and arise from fundic glands as well.

In subtotal gastric resection in the treatment of persistent peptic ulcer, it is important to extirpate those portions of the stomach that are predominantly responsible for acid secretion and also the portion responsible for gastrin secretion that, if allowed to remain, will stimulate the remaining parietal cells to hyperactivity. Subtotal resections of the stomach, therefore, must include for the greatest efficiency the entire body and antrum of the stomach and possibly portions of the fundus.

Gastric and Duodenal Evacuation, Tone, and Peristalsis. Usually, from two to five simultaneous peristaltic waves are observed in the stomach, with the greatest activity occurring in the distal half. The stomach will empty its contents when the pressure in the stomach exceeds the pressure in the duodenum;

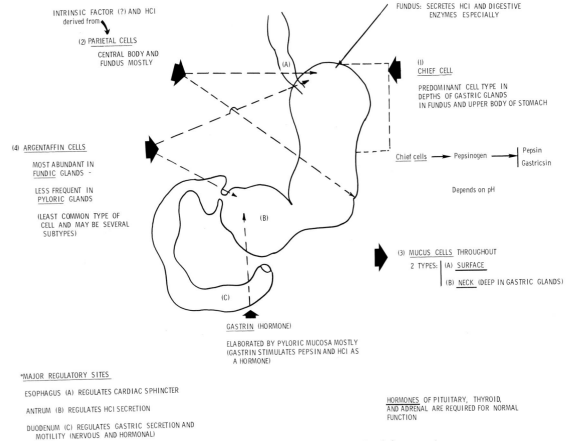

Figure 13–52. The sites of origin of the gastric glandular secretions.

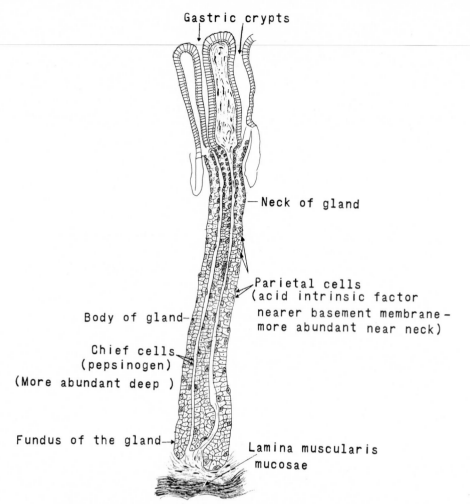

Figure 13-53. Histology of a fundic gland. (Modified from Jordan, H. E.: A Textbook of Histology. New York, D. Appleton-Century, 1934.)

regurgitation from the duodenum will occur when there is a reversal of this pressure relationship. The pyloric antrum, pylorus, and duodenal bulb tend to act as a single unit in response to various food stimuli.

After the introduction of barium into the stomach, emptying begins almost immediately, and the main bulk of the barium meal will have left the stomach in 1 to 2 hours, with no residual trace after 3 hours. Hyperacidity in the stomach will permit the retention of a coating of barium on the gastric mucosa that in itself is not an indication of abnormality. Six hour retention to any significant degree is pathologic, and it is customary to obtain a film 3 to 6 hours later for this purpose. On the other hand, retention in infants may be normal up to 8 hours after a barium meal, but anything beyond 8 hours may be interpreted as pathologic.

The main function of the pyloric sphincter normally is to prevent regurgitation from the duodenum into the stomach (Quigley and Meschan). The entire process of gastric evacuation is very aptly described by Quigley and Louckes as follows: "The stomach is a tolerant organ and accepts with relative indifference substances which are very hot, cold, hypertonic, or distinctly irritant. . . , and the volume which may be ingested without gastric rebellion may stretch the very elastic gastric wall almost to the point of rupture."

"The duodenum, in contrast, will only accept chyme in small quantities and after the chyme is prepared to meet rigid requirements. If chyme enters the duodenum too rapidly or is too hot or cold or contains excessive concentrations of fats, alcohol, condiments, etc., the duodenum revolts by producing nausea or vomiting or signals by a 'feed-back' mechanism to the stomach that evacuation should be retarded and the material retained by the stomach until it is made more acceptable to the duodenum. This 'feed-back' mechanism operates in a more moderate form to depress the antral peristalsis and insure the chyme of being delivered to the duodenum in moderate quantities and in a form which will be readily tolerated."

"In brief, it is the purpose of the stomach to accept almost anything that is presented to it in almost any volume, and, by bringing this material to body temperature and proper isotonicity and dilution (fats, condiments, etc.) to make it acceptable to the relatively 'intolerant' duodenum and then deliver it to the duodenum at a moderate rate."[1]

In the presence of gastric retention it must not be assumed that the obstruction is necessarily pyloric in origin. At times, inadequacy of the evacuation mechanism may result from a hypotonicity of the stomach from some undetermined cause (that is, vagotomy). It would be folly to treat such dysfunction with atropine-like drugs (Fig. 13-54).

Gastric Tone. Vagal stimulation increases gastric tone, whereas sympathetic stimulation decreases it. Thus, when a person is frightened or otherwise emotionally disturbed, the stomach tends to be hypotonic. Pathologic processes in the gastrointestinal tract elsewhere or the biliary tract may also cause changes in the stomach.

Factors Influencing Rate of Gastric Evacuation. Of practical importance are the following normal considerations:

The type of meal will alter the rate of gastric evacuation considerably. The presence of any food will depress gastrobulbar peristalsis and prolong the emptying time by about three times. This function is caused by a reflex or hormone (enterogastrone) operating from the duodenum. The presence of alkali such as sodium bicarbonate in the stomach will increase the rate of gastric evacuation. Only isotonicity, with no food substances contained in the meal, will not alter the rate of evacuation. Normally, with

[1]Quigley, J. P., and Louckes, H. S.: Amer. J. Digest. Dis., 7:672–676, 1962.

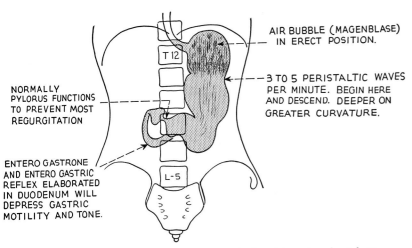

NORMALLY
PYLORUS FUNCTIONS
TO PREVENT MOST
REGURGITATION

ENTERO GASTRONE
AND ENTERO GASTRIC
REFLEX ELABORATED
IN DUODENUM WILL
DEPRESS GASTRIC
MOTILITY AND TONE.

T 12

L-5

AIR BUBBLE (MAGENBLASE)
IN ERECT POSITION.

3 TO 5 PERISTALTIC WAVES
PER MINUTE. BEGIN HERE
AND DESCEND. DEEPER ON
GREATER CURVATURE.

Figure 13–54. Diagram illustrating résumé of gastric motor physiology.

food-free barium suspension, emptying will begin almost immediately after the introduction of the barium into the stomach, and the main bulk of the meal will have left the stomach in 1 hour, with no residual trace in 2 or 3 hours. Hypoacidity in the stomach will permit the retention of a coating of barium on the gastric mucosa, which in itself is not an indication of abnormality. Six hour retention of any significant degree in the adult, or 8 hour retention in the infant is pathologic, and it is customary to obtain a film in 6 or 8 hours for this purpose.

Cascade Stomach (Fig. 13–47).   Occasionally, the posterior portion of the fundus of the stomach will fill first, and the remainder of the stomach will fill by overflow from the fundus. This is called a cascade stomach. It may be related to overdistention of the splenic flexure of the colon or to localized muscular hypertonus. Occasionally it is related to adhesions between the stomach and the diaphragm, but it cannot be properly called a normal variation under these circumstances.

Methods of Roentgenologic Study of the Stomach and Duodenum

Technique of Fluoroscopy and Spot Film Compression Radiography (Figs. 13–55, 13–56, and 13–57)

1. With the patient standing, after the initial survey of the chest and abdomen, the patient is given a cup of barium suspension containing 100 grams of barium sulfate suspended in a glassful (8 oz.) of water.

2. The manner in which the barium enters the stomach is carefully studied. Ordinarily, this first swallow of barium follows

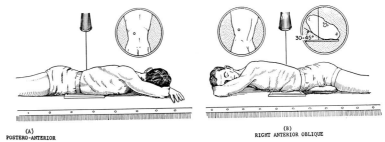

(A)
POSTERO-ANTERIOR

(B)
RIGHT ANTERIOR OBLIQUE

Figure 13–55.   Radiographic examination of the esophagus, stomach, and duodenum.

along the "magenstrasse" on the lesser curvature of the stomach. In the presence of excessive fluid in the stomach the barium drops into the fluid like pellets in a glass of water. The lesser curvature is normally smooth below the level of the cardia and any variation is of definite significance. Spot films of the rugal pattern of the stomach are obtained at this time, particularly in the right anterior oblique, using compression if desirable (Fig. 13–57 A, B, C).

If the barium fills the duodenal bulb and spills over into the second part of the duodenum at this point, an additional spot film of the duodenal bulb is obtained (Fig. 13–57 D).

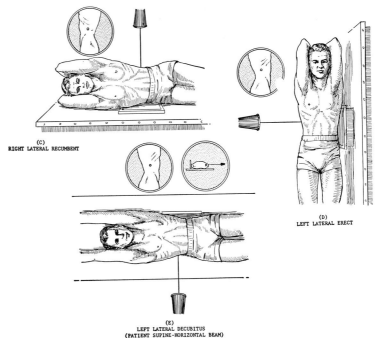

(C)
RIGHT LATERAL RECUMBENT

(D)
LEFT LATERAL ERECT

(E)
LEFT LATERAL DECUBITUS
(PATIENT SUPINE-HORIZONTAL BEAM)

Figure 13–56.   Diagrams illustrating the routine positioning technique for examination of the stomach radiographically, apart from fluoroscopy.

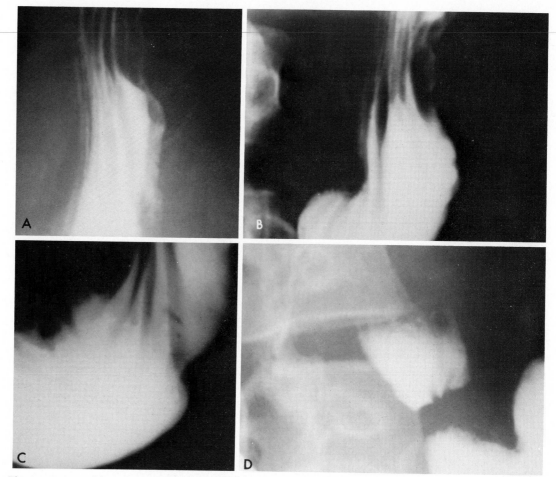

Figure 13–57. Films ordinarily obtained during fluoroscopy and routine study of the stomach and duodenum. *A.* Initial spot film of gastric rugae (body of stomach) immediately following the first swallow of barium. *B.* Second spot film showing the rugal pattern of the body and antrum. *C.* Third spot film demonstrates the lower half of the body and antrum of the stomach. *D.* Spot film showing the distal antrum, pyloric canal, and initial filling of the duodenal bulb.

Figure 13–57 continued on the opposite page.

3. Otherwise, the patient, still in the right anterior oblique, is given additional swallows of barium, and the swallowing function as well as the stomach are studied. The gastroesophageal junction and the action of the constrictor diaphragmae are particularly noted. The patient is in frontal and right anterior oblique projections at this point, and additional spot film studies of the duodenal bulb are obtained in these projections (Fig. 13–57 *E*).

4. The patient then swallows the remainder of the barium, and peristalsis and contour of the stomach and duodenum are studied in all projections. An additional spot film of the stomach or duodenal bulb in the left anterior oblique projection is obtained if necessary (Fig. 13–57 *F*).

This provides a profile study of the duodenal bulb on its anterior and posterior aspect as well as the stomach on its lesser and greater curvature.

5. The patient is then turned with his right side toward the table, arms above his head, leaning slightly in the right anterior oblique, and the tilt table is turned into the horizontal so that the patient is lying somewhat prone on his right side.

6. The gastroesophageal junction, peristalsis of the stomach, and the duodenum are then studied in this right lateral relationship. A spot film of the entire duodenal loop is obtained at this juncture (Fig. 13–57 *G*), and, if desired, an additional film of the gastroesophageal junction.

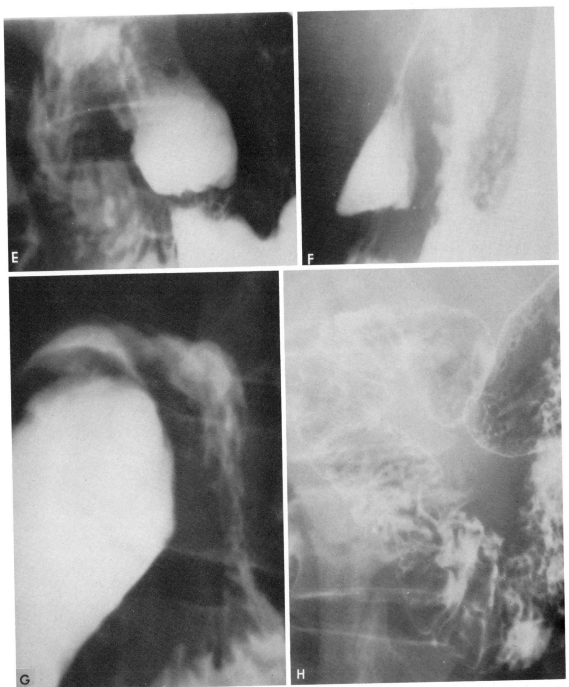

Figure 13–57 *Continued.* E. Somewhat later spot film study of the duodenal bulb after the barium has emptied from it into the second part of the duodenum (patient still in the erect position). F. Spot film study in the left anterior oblique, demonstrating the full duodenal bulb, especially in relation to its anterior and posterior margins. The apex of the bulb and second part of the duodenum are also well demonstrated. G. This film study, with the patient lying on his right side, slightly oblique toward prone, demonstrates the relationship of the stomach, the duodenum, and the duodenal bulb. H. Patient supine with right side elevated, left side down. The air rises into the duodenal bulb and second part of the duodenum, imparting to these structures a double contrast. A spot film is then obtained.

Figure 13–57 continued on the following page.

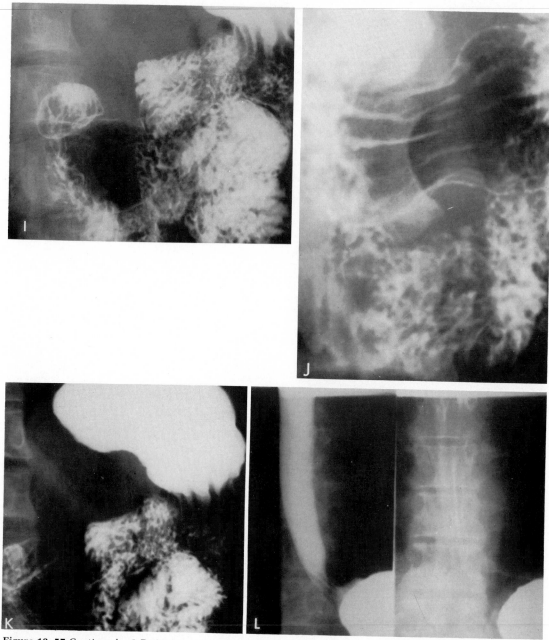

Figure 13–57 *Continued.*   *I.* Patient supine on his left side with the air rising into the antrum and duodenal bulb. A full film of the stomach is then obtained. *J.* Patient supine with air occupying the body of the stomach for demonstration of double contrast visualization of the rugae of the body of the stomach. *K.* Patient supine with the barium moving by gravity into the fundus of the stomach. The full contour of the fundus of the stomach is thereby studied. *L.* Patient supine on left side. Additional swallows of barium are given and the esophagus studied both morphologically and physiologically. The patient is asked to strain with the Valsalva maneuver immediately after swallowing and then after the esophagus is emptied. The esophagus is studied for possible gastroesophageal reflux. This may be followed by a "water test" in all cases where hiatal hernia is demonstrated and where esophageal reflux is suspected.

Figure 13–57 continued on the opposite page.

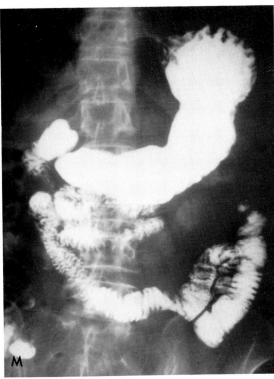

Figure 13–57 *Continued.* M. The full 14 × 17 posteroanterior film of the stomach and proximal small intestine obtained with routine Bucky technique, immediately following the fluoroscopy.

swallows of barium, the patient is encouraged to empty the contents of his mouth, and attempt an additional straining maneuver to see whether or not gastroesophageal reflux is obtained in this projection (Fig. 13–57 *M*).

10. Further tests for gastroesophageal reflux may be made by turning the patient into the Trendelenburg position at this time and studying regurgitation with a swallow of water. The barium normally will reflux back somewhat into the esophagus, but abnormally a considerable admixture of water with the barium rises from the stomach back into the esophagus.

11. If a hiatal hernia is noted or if esophageal varices are suspected, thick barium is then administered in order to study the rugal pattern of the lower esophagus with and without the Valsalva maneuver. Varices will impart a wormlike pattern to the lower esophageal rugae which is accentuated by the Valsalva maneuver. This accentuation is virtually pathognomonic of esophageal varices in contrast with other irregularities such as esophagitis, which produce a somewhat similar appearance.

This routine of examination of the esophagus, stomach, and duodenum is the one we have followed satisfactorily for a considerable period of time. Other routines in current use may be found in the study reported by Burhenne of 15 different institutions in the United States and Europe.

The pyloric canal is ordinarily no greater than 5 mm. in length and 5 to 8 mm. in diameter. The direction of the long axis of the pylorus, like that of the stomach, will depend upon those factors discussed under variation in gastric contour. Tone, body habitus, and emotional influences all play a part, as previously indicated. The pylorus is ordinarily centrally placed with respect to the base of the duodenal bulb; eccentricity is of pathological significance. Its appearance in relation to the duodenal bulb resembles that of a basal stem to its leaf. The rugae of the pyloric canal are quite narrow and parallel in contrast with the slightly wider rugal pattern of the antrum on the one side and the spiral pattern of the duodenal bulb on the other.

Attention is paid throughout this examination to the position, contour, pliability, and peristalsis of the stomach, and points of tenderness and masses nearby. If pancreatic disease is suspected from the clinical history, it is particularly important to study the patient in the left lateral erect position.

The importance of spot film compression radiography can hardly be overemphasized in the radiographic study of the gastrointestinal tract. Film visualization of an anatomic part is far more accurate and detailed than is fluoroscopy, and this method of film radiography has the additional advantage of compression, the patient being turned so that the desired anatomy is demonstrated. The permanent recording of a part under fluoroscopic control is possible. It has been repeatedly demonstrated that compression may bring out a defect which otherwise might escape detection.

7. The patient is next turned to the prone or the 45 degree oblique position, and peristalsis of the entire stomach and duodenum is carefully studied and spot films obtained as necessary.

8. Next, the patient is turned onto his left side at an obliquity of 45 degrees. Gas in the stomach will then rise to the pyloric antrum, duodenal bulb, and duodenum. One or two spot films of the entire duodenal loop are taken with the double contrast provided by the air entering the antrum and the duodenum (Fig. 13–57 *H*). Additional spot films of the stomach are obtained with this double contrast evaluation (Fig. 13–57 *I* and *J*). With the patient lying somewhat flatter on his back, the entire fundus is carefully studied since it is now filled with barium (Fig. 13–57 *K*).

9. In the same position (45 degrees oblique, supine, left side down), the patient is given an additional half cup of barium to swallow. The entire esophagus is then studied and spot films are obtained of the esophagogastric junction with the patient performing the Valsalva maneuver (Fig. 13–57 *L*). After several

Routine Films Obtained Following Fluoroscopic Study

In addition, the *routine radiographs usually obtained are:* (1) recumbent posteroanterior (prone), straight frontal projection (Fig. 13-58); (2) right anterior oblique prone (Fig. 13-59); (3) right lateral recumbent (Fig. 13-60); (4) posteroanterior full abdominal view in 4 or 6 hours for study of the extent of gastric evacuation (Fig. 13-61).

These are demonstrated in the accompanying illustrations, and the various anatomic portions labeled.

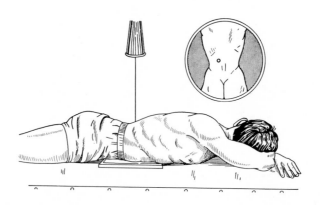

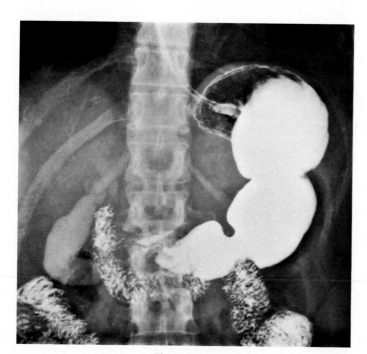

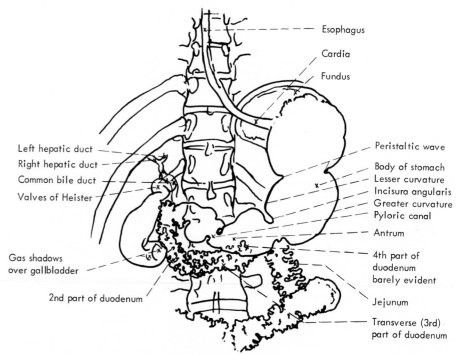

Figure 13-58. Recumbent posteroanterior projection of stomach and duodenum. (An oral cholecystogram was also obtained at this time in the film illustrated.)

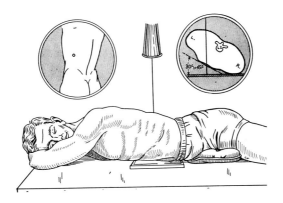

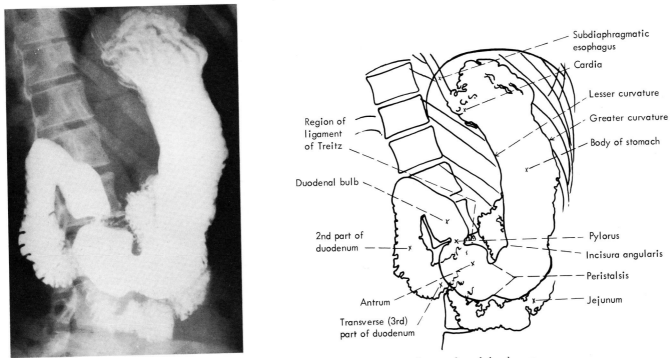

Figure 13–59. Right anterior oblique prone projection of stomach and duodenum.

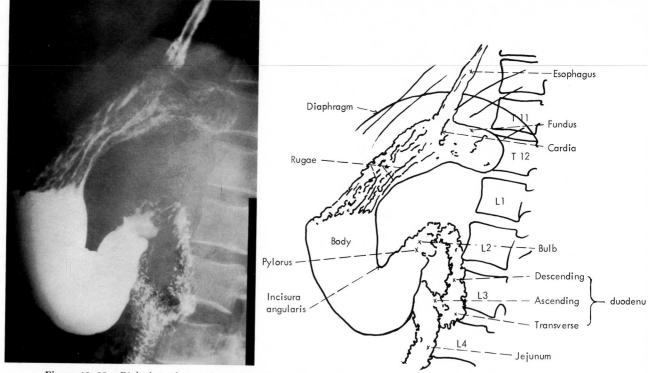

Figure 13–60. Right lateral recumbent view of stomach and duodenum.

Labels on diagram: Esophagus, Diaphragm, T 11, Fundus, Cardia, Rugae, T 12, Body, L1, Pylorus, L2, Bulb, Incisura angularis, Descending, L3, Ascending, Transverse, L4, Jejunum, duodenum

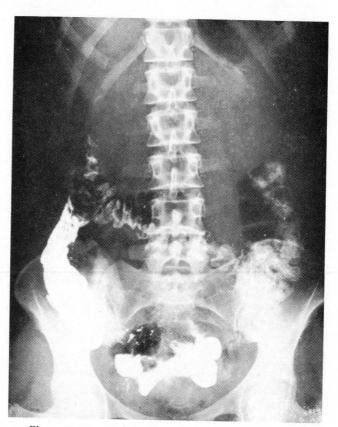

Figure 13–61. Six-hour film study of gastric evacuation.

Additional studies of the stomach and duodenum may be carried out as follows:

Left Lateral Erect Film of Stomach and Duodenum (Fig. 13–62). The left lateral erect view of the stomach and duodenum is most useful to demonstrate the exact relationship of the stomach to retrogastric structures. Anatomic detail is obscured, and hence this film study is obtained when especially indicated by clinical history suggesting pancreatic or retrogastric disease.

Anteroposterior View of Stomach in Slight Left Posterior Oblique (Fig. 13–57 *J*). In this position, the air in the stomach rises and when admixed with the barium furnishes a double contrast visualization of the body, antrum, and bulb, and a com-

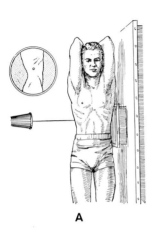

A

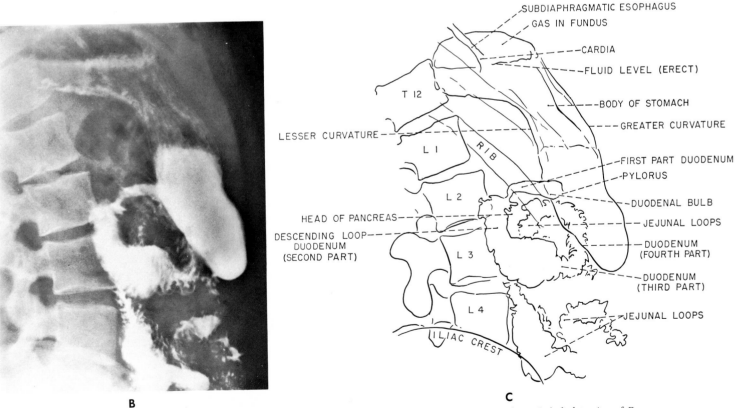

B

C

Figure 13–62. Left lateral erect film of stomach. A. Position of patient. B. Radiograph. C. Labeled tracing of B.

pletely barium-filled fundus. Filling defects and mucosal disturbances are thereby sometimes intensified in these areas.

Air Insufflation of the Stomach.   Air may be introduced into the stomach as a special examination either by stomach tube, or indirectly by Seidlitz powders or a carbonated drink. The stomach should be empty for this examination. The direct introduction of air has the advantage of permitting the examination of the dry gastric mucosa, following which the addition of a small amount of barium mixture permits double contrast. The carbonated drink method has the disadvantage of diluting the barium which interferes with its coating property.

In either case the patient is first examined fluoroscopically in all projections, and films in any desired position are obtained.

Special Studies of the Stomach and Duodenum

Hypotonic Duodenography. Hypotonic duodenography refers to a barium and gas study of the duodenum after the administration of a gas-producing medication or intubation, followed immediately by an atropinelike drug. Double contrast visualization of the duodenum has proved to be of considerable value in studying both intraluminal and extraluminal disorders of this area. Thirty to 60 mg. of Pro-banthine is administered intramuscularly (or 30 mg. intravenously, adult dose) for this purpose. The barium may be injected by tube also if a duodenal tube is used for the introduction of the air. At times, it may be satisfactory to allow air to enter the duodenum from the stomach at the time the antivagal drug is administered. The patient should be in the supine left posterior oblique position. *Probanthine is contraindicated in patients with heart abnormalities or glaucoma. Two to five mg. of glucagon may be used instead in nondiabetic patients.*

Some advantages of double contrast in the duodenum and hypotonic duodenography are shown in Figure 13–63.

Duodenal atony occurs about 5 minutes after the intramuscular introduction of 60 mg. of Pro-banthine and lasts about 20 minutes. The subtle alteration in the pancreaticoduodenal interface has been carefully studied by this method in the normal (Ferruci et al.). The method allows: (1) differentiation of duodenal mucosal fold effacement, (2) differentiation of pathologic papillary defects from normal papilla, and (3) straightening of the contour of the duodenum. Lesions of the tail of the pancreas cannot be studied in this way (Fig. 13–64).

Utilization of Water Soluble Contrast Media for Gastrointestinal Study.   Water soluble contrast media have been recommended by some (Rea; Jacobson et al.), when barium is contraindicated. This is best administered by gastric tube since it is bitter to taste. A flavoring agent may be added to make it more palatable but this may alter normal physiologic responses.

Sixty cc. of 60 per cent Hypaque or Gastrografin or 50 grams of powdered Hypaque dissolved in 75 cc. of sterile water, to which 10 drops of a wetting agent (Tween–80) have been added, are utilized as the contrast agent.

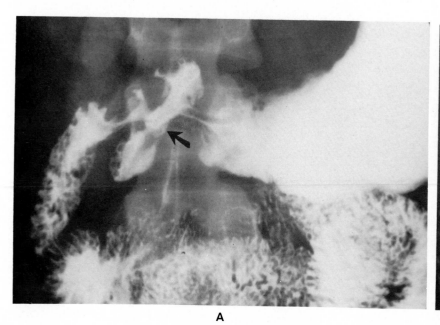

A

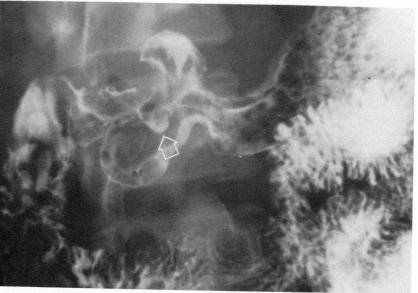

B

Figure 13–63.   *A* and *B.* Duodenal ulcer showing the advantages of double contrast with barium and air, (*A*) erect, and (*B*) supine. Both views show the ulcer.

Figure 13–63 continued on the opposite page.

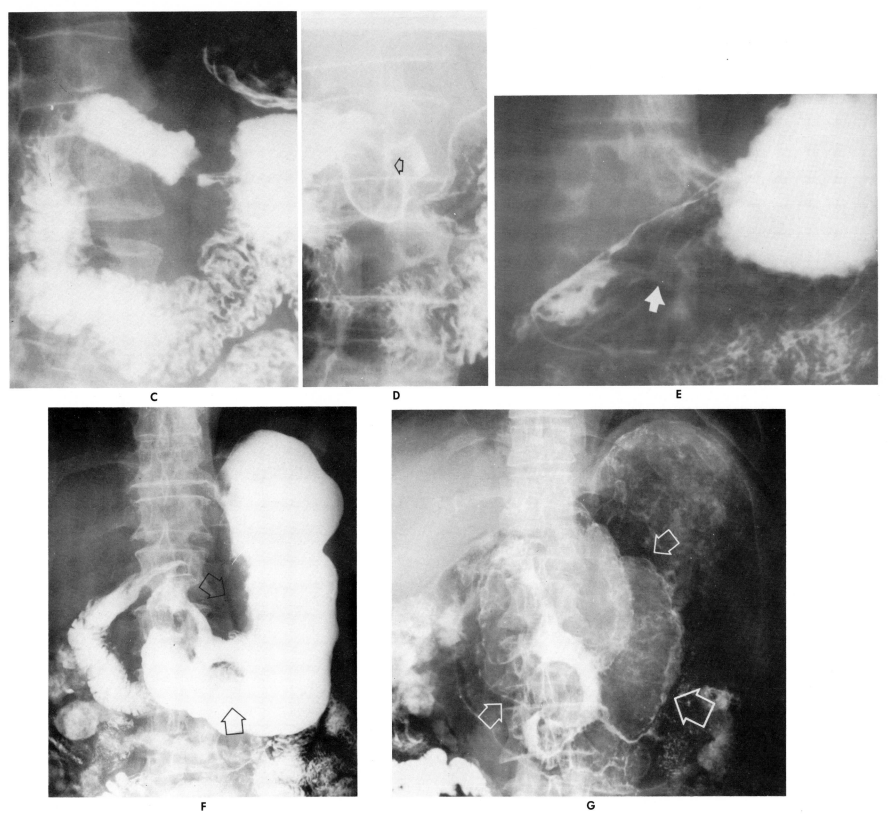

C

D

E

F

G

Figure 13–63 *Continued.* *C* and *D.* Once again a demonstration of the advantages of the left oblique supine study and double contrast demonstration of the ulcer on the posterior wall of the duodenum, not otherwise readily demonstrable. *E.* Double contrast barium-air representation of a healed gastric ulcer seen en face. The stellate radiation of the rugal pattern with a tendency to puckering of the mucosa with outright fleck formation is characteristic. *F.* Radiograph demonstrating large irregular carcinomatous filling defects of the stomach. *G.* Double contrast barium and air study of the stomach showing a large irregular polypoid carcinoma partly filling the stomach, in association with a markedly dilated stomach.

Figure 13–63 continued on the following page.

821

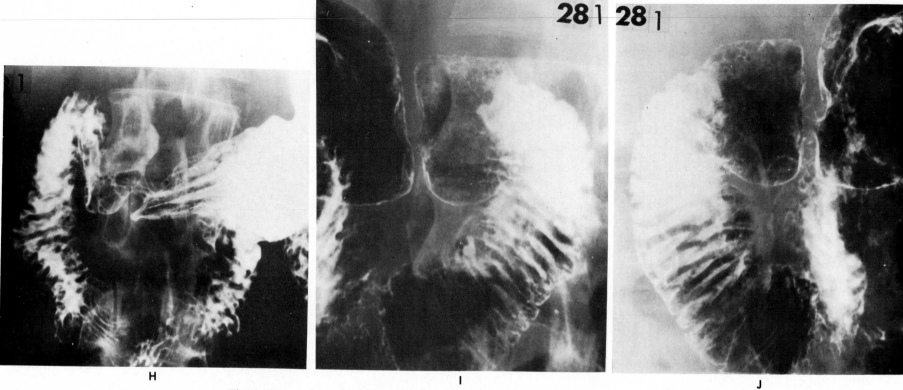

Figure 13–63 *Continued.*   Hypotonic duodenography. *H.* Routine film of the duodenum. *I* and *J.* Duodenum following hypotonic duodenography demonstrating the marked double contrast obtained in the duodenal bulb and duodenum.

For examination of the lower gastrointestinal tract, or in dehydrated patients, the use of these water soluble media is probably contraindicated since they are hyperosmotic and cause further water imbalance. They are also probably contraindicated in infants, in whom dehydration by the hyperosmotic medium may be disturbing unless intravenous fluids are administered simultaneously. However, in general, these agents (Hypaque or Gastrografin) may be used whenever barium mixtures can be used, with the proviso that small quantities be employed (Sidaway; Neuhauser).

Emergency Study of the Upper Gastrointestinal Tract for Bleeding. When patients are unable to stand for any reason, we have modified our technique for fluoroscopy as follows:

1. The patient lies obliquely on his right side, prone, facing the examiner. He drinks one or two swallows of barium from a straw.

2. The swallowing function and esophagus are studied as the barium is swallowed and moves into the stomach.

3. The stomach is then studied with small and large quantities of barium, first in this position (right oblique, prone), then with the patient on his left side, and finally rotating the patient onto his back.

4. When the patient is supine, he is turned toward his left and lies obliquely on his left side, permitting a double contrast visualization of the antrum and duodenum.

5. Thick barium may be administered, particularly if esophageal varices are suspected. The patient may be asked to carry out, with caution, the Valsalva maneuver.

6. Spot films are taken as necessary throughout the procedure. There is a greater tendency in this examination to make "full spot" films of the entire stomach and duodenum rather than the smaller, more confined views.

7. Routine posteroanterior, right anterior oblique, right lateral, and left posterior oblique views are obtained. A left lateral decubitus view may also be obtained if desired.

This procedure is not intended to replace the routine gastrointestinal examination, which is repeated at a suitable interval after cessation of the emergency (Knowles et al.; Hampton).

Pharmacoradiology in Evaluation of Gastrointestinal Disease. Smooth muscle stimulation by means of pharmacodynamic agents has long been recommended for evaluation of stomach and duodenum (Pancoast; Ritvo; Adler et al.; Bachrach; Rasmussen; Silbiger and Donner). Such agents as insulin, morphine, Dilaudid, atropine, Prostigmin, pethidine, Pro-banthine, opium derivatives, Mecholyl, physostigmine, Benzedrine, and Pantopon have found their proponents.

Morphine has been considered by some as the most reliable stimulant of gastric peristalsis (Silbiger and Donner). Eight milligrams of morphine were employed by the latter investigators. Within 2 to 10 minutes following intravenous administration, there was an increase in peristalsis which lasted 20 to 45 minutes. There was a second phase of prolonged depression of intestinal propulsion and diminution of tone. Neoplastic infiltrates of the gastric wall invariably resulted in disordered peristaltic patterns. Gastric ulcers, the postoperative stomach, and various infiltrating lesions may be studied to good advantage this way. Active intestinal bleeding and hypersensitivity to the drug are considered contraindications.

Parietography. In this examination, the gastric wall is isolated between two layers of air by gastric inflation and pneumoperitoneum. Body section radiography is also employed. This procedure permits definition of wall thickness of the suspected region and defines the extent of a tumor if present. Approximately 800 to 1200 ml. of air are introduced in the peritoneal cavity on the evening prior to the examination. The gas in the stomach is derived from tartaric acid which becomes mixed with a succeeding dose of sodium bicarbonate (250 to 300 ml. of gas estimated). Body section radiographs are obtained at 1 cm. intervals ordinarily, at 11 to 19 cm. from the posterior skin surface (Porcher and Buffard).

Celiac Angiography for Visualization of the Stomach, Duo-

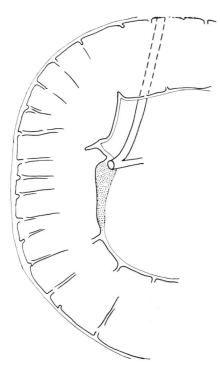

Figure 13–64. Anatomic diagram of normal features of duodenal hypotonic study. (From Ferrucci, J. T., Jr., Benedict, K. T., Page, D. C., Fleischli, D. J., and Eaton, S. B.: Radiology, 96:401–408, 1970.)

denum and Pancreas. See No. 11 in the following section on techniques of examination of the pancreas.

THE PANCREAS

Introduction. The radiologic diagnosis of pancreatic disease leaves much to be desired. The examination of the pancreas must be performed largely by indirect methods, such as careful study of the stomach and duodenum, as well as angiology. It is possible, however, that with greater expertise and refinement of technique our diagnostic accuracy will be considerably enhanced in the future.

Basic Anatomy. The pancreas is both an endocrine and an exocrine gland, its endocrine function being carried forward by the islets of Langerhans. The two hormones secreted are insulin and glucagon. These hormones help regulate glucose, lipid, and protein metabolism. The acini of the pancreas secrete digestive juices into the duodenum.

The pancreas is arbitrarily divided into four parts: *head, neck, body* and *tail.*

Head. The head of the pancreas lies within the curvature of the duodenum (Fig. 13–40 *B*). The prolongation of the left and caudal border of the head of the pancreas is called the "uncinate process" (Fig. 13–65). As shown in the posterior view of the pancreas and duodenum, the superior mesenteric artery and vein cross the uncinate process on its right aspect. The posterior surface of the pancreas is without peritoneum and is in contact with the aorta, inferior vena cava, common bile duct, renal veins, and right crus of the diaphragm (Fig. 13–51). The anterior surface is, in its lower part, below the level of the transverse colon, and is covered by peritoneum and separated from the transverse colon by areolar tissue.

The *neck* of the pancreas is that constricted portion just to the left of the head (Fig. 13–65). Superiorly it adjoins the pylorus. It is proximal to the origin of the portal vein and the gastroduodenal artery.

The *body* of the pancreas is separated anteriorly from the stomach by the omental bursa. The posterior surface of the body of the pancreas is closely related to the aorta, splenic vein, left kidney and its vessels, left suprarenal, the origin of the superior mesenteric artery, and the crura of the diaphragm. The inferior surface of the body is coated by peritoneum and is in close proximity to the duodenojejunal flexure, the coils of the jejunum, and the left flexure of the colon. Along its anterior aspect, the layers of the transverse mesocolon diverge. The superior border of the body of the pancreas is close to the celiac artery, with the hepatic artery to the right and the splenic artery to the left (Fig. 13–65).

The *tail* of the pancreas extends laterally toward the left to the surface of the spleen and is situated in the phrenicolienal ligament.

The exocrine secretions of the pancreas empty into the duo-

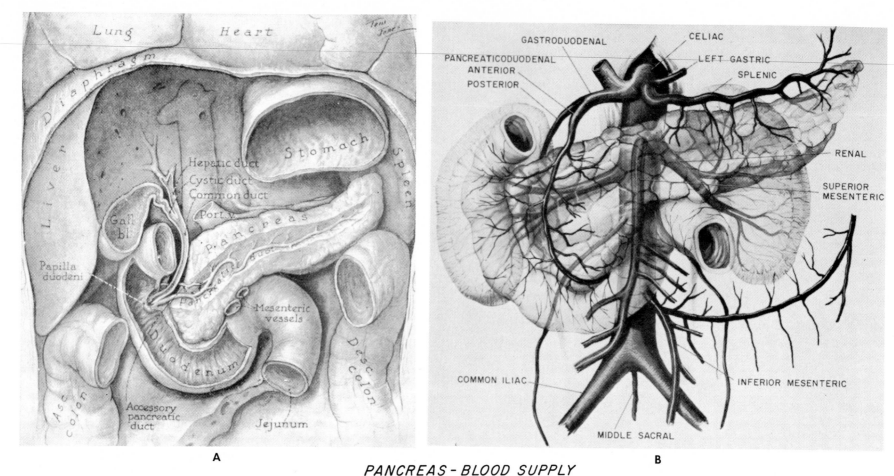

PANCREAS-BLOOD SUPPLY

Figure 13–65. *A.* The gross anatomy of the biliary system. (From Jones, T.: Anatomical Studies. Jackson, Michigan, S. H. Camp and Co., 1943.) *B.* Arterial circulation of the pancreas (isometric diagram). *C.* Pancreatic blood supply in simple diagram to demonstrate the anterior and posterior pancreaticoduodenal arcade in conjunction with the celiac axis and the superior mesenteric arteries and veins. The transverse pancreatic artery is also shown, in its relationship to the splenic artery and the pancreatica magna artery. (*B* and *C* from Bierman, H. R.: Selective Arterial Catheterization, 1969. Courtesy of Charles C Thomas, Publisher, Springfield, Illinois.)

denum through two ductal systems: first, a *major duct* (of Wirsung), which extends the full length of the pancreas toward the right, opening into the descending duodenum at a common orifice with the common bile duct, the *major papilla* (ampulla of Vater). Second, the *minor pancreatic duct* (of Santorini) drains

part of the head of the pancreas and enters the duodenum just above the duct of Wirsung by a separate opening in the duodenum.

The arterial blood supply of the pancreas (Fig. 13–66 *A*) is derived from *four* main sources: (1) numerous small branches

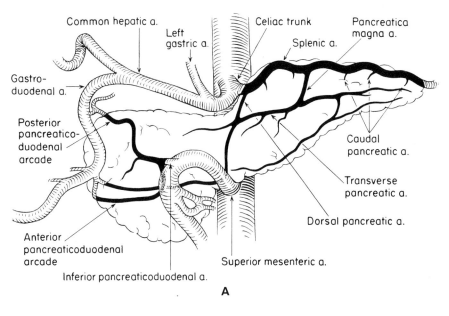

A

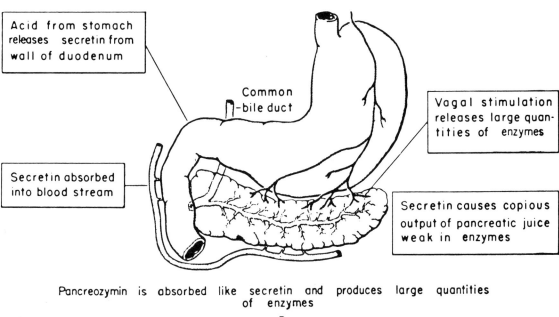

B

Figure 13–66. *A.* Line drawing of arterial supply of the pancreas. The pancreatic branches are enlarged for emphasis. In this example, the dorsal pancreatic artery arises from the splenic artery and gives off the transverse pancreatic artery. It receives an anastomotic branch from the anterior pancreaticoduodenal arcade. The relationships of the pancreatic arteries are variable and must be evaluated in each patient. (From Reuter, S. R., and Redman, H. C.: Gastrointestinal Angiography. Philadelphia, W. B. Saunders Co., 1972.) *B.* Regulation of pancreatic secretion. (From Guyton, A. C.: Textbook of Medical Physiology, 4th ed. Philadelphia, W. B. Saunders Co., 1971.)

from the *splenic* artery; (2) the retroduodenal branch of the *gastroduodenal* artery; (3) the *superior pancreaticoduodenal* arising from the gastroduodenal artery; and (4) the *inferior pancreaticoduodenal* which arises from the superior mesenteric artery and anastomoses with the superior pancreaticoduodenal in the head of the pancreas.

A *dorsal pancreatic artery* may give rise from the celiac artery just distal to the origin of the splenic artery and opposite the point of origin of the left gastric. This supplies the body of the pancreas centrally with branches extending toward the head and tail. This artery, called by some the superior, instead of arising from the celiac trunk may originate from the superior mesenteric artery.

The *superior pancreaticoduodenal* artery may divide into two main segments, one anterior and one posterior, surrounding the head of the pancreas and its uncinate process. The arcade formed around the head of the pancreas also supplies the duodenum its ventral aspect.

The pancreas also receives branches directly from the *common hepatic artery.*

One of the branches from the splenic artery is often sufficiently large to be identified as a single branch called the *pancreatica magna artery.* It is distributed along the pancreatic duct.

The pancreatic veins drain directly into the portal vein by means of the *splenic and superior mesenteric veins.*

The *lymphatics* terminate in numerous lymph nodes near the root of the superior mesenteric artery, following the course of blood vessels and terminating in the pancreaticolienal, pancreaticoduodenal, and preaortic lymph nodes.

Pancreatic Exocrine Secretions. Pancreatic juice contains enzymes for digesting all three major types of food: proteins, carbohydrates, and fat. There are a number of proteolytic enzymes which, as synthesized in the pancreas, are inactive but become active after they are secreted into the intestinal tract by enzymes released from the intestinal mucosa whenever chyme comes in contact with the mucosa. If this were not the case, the pancreatic juice might digest the pancreas itself. There is additionally, however, another substance called trypsin inhibitor stored in the cells of the pancreas which prevents the activation of pancreatic proteolytic enzymes.

Pancreatic secretion, like gastric secretion, is regulated by both nervous and hormonal mechanisms. The most important hormone in this regard is *secretin.* A second hormone is *pancreozymin.* When chyme enters the intestine it causes the release and activation of secretin, which is absorbed into the blood and in turn causes the pancreas to secrete large quantities of fluid containing a high concentration of bicarbonate ion and a low concentration of chloride ion. Hydrochloric acid, particularly in the chyme, is capable of causing a great release of secretin, although almost any type of food will cause at least some release.

The secretin response is particularly important in the prevention of too great acidity in the small intestine, since the small intestine cannot withstand the intense digestive properties of gastric juice. Moreover, the tendency toward alkaline environment assists the action of the pancreatic enzymes per se.

Pancreozymin is largely responsible for secretion of the digestive enzymes from the pancreas and is somewhat similar to the effect of vagal stimulation. The type of secretion of the pancreas in response to secretin is called "hydrelatic" secretion and the secretion in response to pancreozymin is called "ecbolic" secretion (Fig. 13–66 B).

Technique of Examination of the Pancreas

1. **Plain Films of the Abdomen.** Anteroposterior and lateral views of the abdomen centered over the pancreas (with oblique views taken as necessary) are helpful from the standpoint of revealing (a) pancreatic calcification (Fig. 13–67); (b) an abnormal gas distribution, such as free air in the immediate vicinity of the pancreas or lesser omental bursa; or (c) displacement of adjoining organs such as the stomach, duodenum, kidney, or spleen.

2. **Air Contrast Studies of the Stomach and Duodenum.** Air contrast may be used in the stomach and duodenum to accentuate the pancreatic region, particularly when calcareous masses are noted therein. Air contrast ordinarily does not obscure the areas of calcification, whereas barium contrast introduced into the stomach and duodenum might do so. Body section radiography may be used in conjunction with the air contrast to enhance its efficacy.

3. **Endo- and Perigastric Gas with Selective Celiac Arteriography During the Phase of Maximal Secretion** (stimulation by pharmacologic agents) (Taylor, et al.). This combination of an angiographic identification of the pancreas, plus the visualization of the stomach and duodenum by gas intraluminally, permits the identification of the pancreas in conjunction with the gastric mucosa and thickness of the gastric wall.

Selective celiac arteriography in itself is very helpful in identifying certain lesions of the pancreas (Fig. 13–68). However, the interpretation of angiograms of the pancreas offers some difficulty and the efficacy of this technique for identification of carcinoma in the pancreas, for example, is somewhat controversial.

4. **Intubation of the Stomach and Duodenum with Opaque Tube.** The main purpose of this examination is to delineate the region of the pancreas for better visualization of any suspicious oblique or negative shadows in this area (Weens and Walker). A discussion of pancreatic calculi or calcified cysts of the pancreas is outside the scope of this text and the student is referred to special reports of these disorders for further information (Stein et al.; Poppel; Becker et al.; Meschan: *Analysis of Roentgen Signs,* Chapter 28).

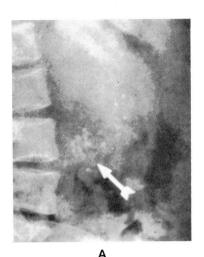
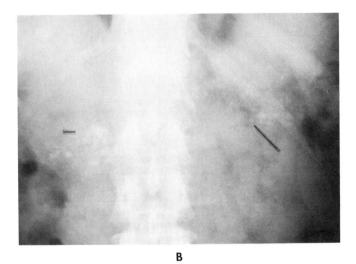

A   **B**

Figure 13–67. Pancreatic calculi. *A.* Lateral projection. The calcific shadows lie anteriorly to the second and third lumbar vertebrae. *B.* After the administration of an opaque meal. The calcific shadows are visualized within the loop of the duodenum (black marker). (From Ritvo, M., and Shauffer, I. A.: Gastrointestinal X-ray Diagnosis. Philadelphia, Lea & Febiger, 1952.)

5. **Opaque Meal in Stomach and Duodenum.** The close relationship of the pancreas to the stomach and duodenum has already been described. Impressions upon the stomach and alterations of the detailed mucosal pattern of the duodenum may be the only evidence of pancreatic abnormality. Cinefluorography and cineradiography are particularly useful for detailed analysis of areas of pliability or incipient rigidity in the second part of the duodenum (Salik). Greater variability in appearance, less rigidity and induration, and the absence of fixed corrugations favor a diagnosis of pancreatitis over carcinoma. Hypotonic duodenography is particularly helpful with opaque studies of the stomach and duodenum in revealing minute abnormalities related to the pancreas (Fig. 13–69).

6. **Barium Enema** (Chapter 14). The peritoneal reflection of the transverse mesocolon lies in very close proximity to the pancreas; and hence, lesions of the pancreas may extend to and involve the colon, especially its transverse portion. The barium enema may corroborate plain films of the abdomen that reveal inordinate shadows in the immediate vicinity of the transverse colon (Salik; Eyler et al.).

7. **Excretory Urogram** (Chapter 16). The tail of the pancreas may lie just anterior to the left kidney and extends to the hilum of the spleen. Abnormal enlargement of the pancreas, especially involving the lesser omental bursa, may displace or distort the left kidney, ureter, or spleen (Marshall et al.).

8. **Cholecystograms and Cholangiograms** (Chapter 15). Cholecystograms and cholangiograms may at times reveal evidence of an obstructed or a displaced common duct. The max-

imum diameter of the common duct in chronic pancreatitis for example, seldom if ever exceeds 25 mm. Obstruction of the common duct due to carcinoma may cause an enlargement of over 30 mm. Unfortunately, intravenous cholangiography fails in about one-third of the cases of acute inflammations of the pancreas (Schultz). Conspicuous dilatation of the pancreatic duct and its tributaries coupled with narrowness of the transduodenal portion of the common duct may also indicate inflammations of the pancreas (Sachs and Partington).

9. **Percutaneous Cholangiography** (Chapter 15). When complete obstruction of the common bile duct occurs at its site of entry into the pancreas, considerable dilatation of the more proximal regions in the biliary tree results. Direct percutaneous injection of a contrast agent through the liver into one of the dilated constituent branches will not only demonstrate severe dilatation, but also the more characteristic appearances of the common bile duct. At the site of obstruction, there may be a jagged, notched appearance and a reversal of the usual convexity of the common bile duct toward the left (Flemma et al.; Evans; Darke and Beal).

10. **Further Comments About Selective Pancreatic Angiography.** As indicated earlier, the arterial supply of the pancreas is somewhat variable, with the major supply coming from the splenic, celiac, gastroduodenal, and superior mesenteric arteries. Selective study of the pancreas is probably best accomplished by celiac or superior mesenteric angiograms. Inflation of the stomach in conjunction with this study is helpful (Lunderquist). Superselective catheterization of the hepatic, splenic, gastroduodenal, dorsal pancreatic, inferior pancreatic, or duodenal arteries

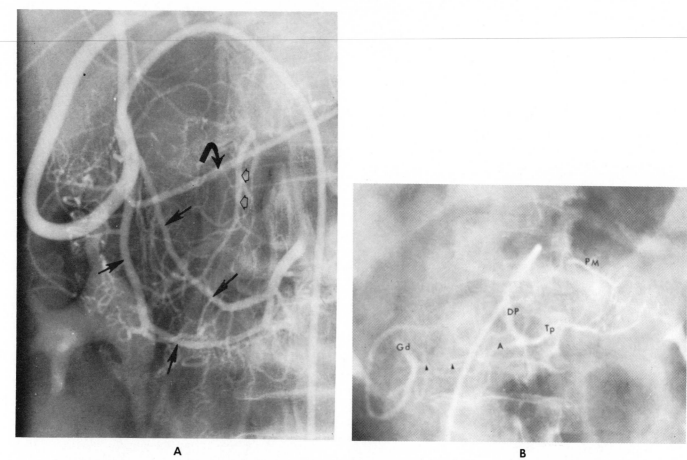

A   **B**

Figure 13–68. *A.* Normal pancreatic arcades. Direct serial magnification angiography during a gastroduodenal artery injection clearly demonstrates the pancreatic arcades (*straight arrows*), the transverse pancreatic artery (*curved arrow*) and the dorsal pancreatic artery (*open arrow*). (From Baum, S., and Athanasoulis, C. A.: Angiography. *In* Eaton, S. B., and Ferrucci, J. T. (ed.): Radiology of the Pancreas and Duodenum. Philadelphia, W. B. Saunders Co., 1973.) *B.* Selective dorsal pancreatic injection. Catheter passed via celiac artery. (*DP*). Dorsal pancreatic artery, (*A* and arrowheads), anastomotic branch from dorsal pancreatic artery to pancreaticoduodenal arcade, (*Gd*) gastroduodenal artery, (*Pm*) pancreatica magna, (*Tp*) transverse pancreatic. (From Ruzicka, F. F., Jr., and Rossi, P.: Radiol. Clin. N. Amer., 8:3–28, 1970.)

has been attempted, and it has been noted that injections must be made at least into both gastroduodenal and splenic arteries for adequate demonstration of the entire pancreas. It is probable that pharmacologic agents will serve to enhance these techniques (Bierman). (See also Fig. 13–68.)

11. **Splenoportography.** The splenic vein and tail of the pancreas are in close contiguity with one another. Splenic vein occlusion and distortion have been described in association with pancreatic tumors or large masses (pseudocysts) of the pancreas (Bookstein and Whitehouse; Rösch and Herfort; Varriale et al.).

12. **Retropneumoperitoneum with Body Section Radiography.** This method involves a combination of the retroperitoneal insufflation of a gas, gaseous distention of the stomach, and body section radiography in both the sagittal and coronal planes. Simultaneous pneumoperitoneum, introduction of con-

trast agent in the stomach, urinary tract, or biliary tree, and other expedients have also been utilized in conjunction with this method. These methods are still in the process of evaluation and it is questionable whether the discomfort and perhaps even the dangers of the procedure are justified when compared with other possible methods that might be employed in identical cases (Mosely).

13. **Direct Pancreatography.** This method involves direct insertion of a needle or catheter into the pancreatic duct at surgery (Doubilet et al., 1959). The original method involved transduodenal sphincterotomy and direct injection of a suitable contrast agent (from 2 to 5 ml. of 50 per cent sodium diatrizoate is recommended). This injection is made slowly during a 5 minute period, with the last 2 ml. introduced during the x-ray exposure. The tube may be left in place for drainage. Corrosion prepara-

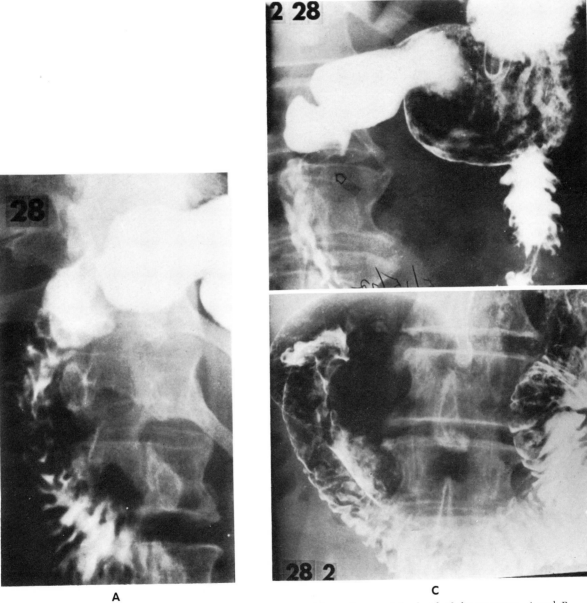

Figure 13–69. Hypotonic duodenography in a patient with carcinoma of the head of the pancreas. *A* and *B*. Prior to the hypotonic study. *C*. The hypotonic study. Although the rigid impression upon the duodenum is visible in *A* and *B*, it is better shown following the gaseous distention of the duodenal loop.

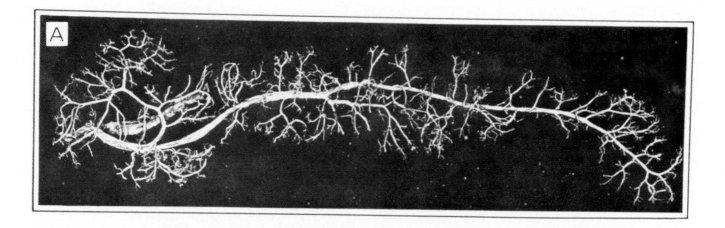

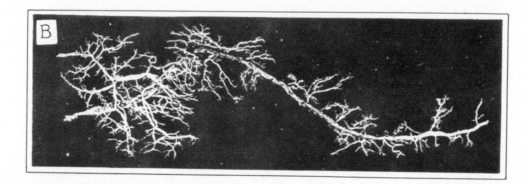

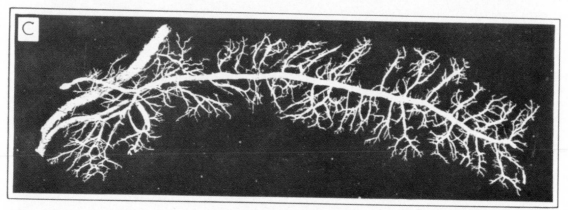

Figure 13–70.   Corrosion preparations of the pancreatic ducts. *Dimensions:* total length 8.2 inches (average). The main duct begins 1 inch from the tail, and has a diameter of 0.5 mm., which gradually increases to 3.5 mm. in diameter in the head of the pancreas. (Reproduced by permission from J. C. B. Grant: An Atlas of Anatomy, 5th ed. Copyright © 1962, The Williams and Wilkins Company.)

tions of the pancreatic duct are shown in Figure 13–70. Normal pancreatograms reveal only the main ducts of the pancreas. With acute inflammation the radiopaque solution permeates the acinar tissue, showing not only the smaller ramifications as shown in Figure 13–70 but even some of the parenchymal tissue. Serial pancreatograms will depict resolution of such inflammation.

14. **Endoscopic Pancreatocholangiography** (peroral pancreaticobiliary ductography). Cannulation of the ampulla of Vater through a fiberoptic duodenoscope may be performed with the aid of x-ray television (Ogoshi et al.; Oi; Tagaki et al.; Gotton et al.; Kusagai et al.; Robbins et al.; Okuda et al.). The technique of the examination is described as follows: A fiberduodenoscope, Model JF-B of the Olympus Company, Tokyo, has been used. This instrument, 10 mm. in diameter and 1250 mm. long, is inserted perorally into the stomach and thereafter into the duodenum. Its tip is equipped with a rigid lens system that can be bent at will 120 degrees up and down, and 90 degrees right and left. It contains lenses and holes for illumination, fixed focus for visualization and photography, a small hole for injecting air and washing fluid, and a larger hole for passing a forceps and cannula. A Teflon cannula 1.7 mm. in external diameter is passed through the duodenoscope into the ampulla of Vater and sodium meglumine diatrizoate is then injected into the cannulated duct system. Usually only 2 to 3 cc. are required. The injection is terminated and left lateral and posteroanterior (sometimes left oblique) roentgenograms are taken. The cannula and scope are withdrawn and several more roentgenograms are taken in various projections, including the right oblique view and erect positions. The speed of disappearance or excretion of the contrast medium into the duodenum is checked on the television screen. If too great a volume of contrast agent is used, a pancreatitis may ensue and this should be avoided. After the procedure an antibiotic is used to prevent acute pancreatitis and infection.

After successful pancreatography the common duct may be visualized with a cannula withdrawn halfway and contrast medium reinjected (Fig. 13–71). The accessory pancreatic duct may be visualized as communicating with the duct of Wirsung. Usually, barium swallow study and hypotonic duodenography are carried out prior to the duodenoscopy. Representative ductograms are shown in Figure 13–71.

Okuda et al. note that the length of the normal pancreatic duct by this technique is usually 15.8 mm. on the average, and slightly longer in the presence of inflammation. The maximum duct diameter of the head of the normal pancreas is 3.9 mm., but this measurement is considerably larger in the presence of chronic pancreatitis. (There is no indication in this report of magnification in relation to these measurements.) Normally, the ductal system clears in an average of 4 minutes and 6 seconds, but considerably longer retention occurs in abnormal states.

15. **Measurement of the Retrogastric and Retroduodenal Spaces: an Index of Pancreatic or Lesser Omental Bursal In-**volvement. Various methods have been proposed for measurement of the retrogastric space (Poppel et al.; Scheinmel and Mednick; Meschan et al.; Poole). The normal range of distances in centimeters between the stomach and duodenum and the spine on left lateral roentgenograms of the abdomen according to body habitus has been proposed by a number of investigators. The limits of normal vary considerably according to the gross judgment of body habitus. Such great variations of normal make the validity of measurement difficult to interpret except in the presence of "extrinsic tumor impression on the visceral [which was] ... the single most important statistical factor in evaluating the presence of a retroperitoneal mass" (Herbert and Margulis). Poole, in studying this issue, noted that "the only variable measurements in the midline cross-section at the level of the stomach are the thicknesses of the prepancreatic fat, and the width of the pancreatic neck, which is 1 to 1.5 cm. thick normally in the midline. Many other structures, however, are present such as the lesser sac, fat, aortic lymph nodes, and the aorta itself." Poole devised an anterior abdominal wall compression device which contained a nickel coin (measuring 2.1 cm. in diameter) on its flat surface. He used this device to press the midline stomach against the retroperitoneal structures. After the barium was swallowed, the fluoroscopic pressure cone was applied to the midline puddle of barium with sufficient force to splay the mucosal folds and flatten the column of barium. Adequate compression was noted by displacement of the central midbarium column to both sides of the midline. A lateral spot film was taken. The midline antrum-to-spine distance was measured from the posterior pressure defect to the anterior vertebral body. After the antrum-to-spine measurement, the patient was placed in the right lateral decubitus position to allow barium to enter the horizontal duodenum, and then he was brought upright and placed in the posteroanterior position. When the midline duodenum was identified in the posteroanterior projection, the patient was then turned laterally and a spot film taken without pressure (Fig. 13–72). The duodenum-to-spine distance was measured from the posterior aspect of the midline horizontal duodenum to the spine. The measurements obtained from spot films were corrected for magnification by the magnification of the coin marker on the compressor device. A nomogram is provided to correct for such magnification (Fig. 13–72). A direct linear correlation exists between the weight of the normal individual and his true antrum-to-spine measurement. For an average weight of 148 pounds the average corrected antrum-to-spine distance was 3.14 cm. The 95 per cent confidence limits are shown in the accompanying graph. The duodenum-to-spine normal measurement exhibited no relationship to body weight. The mean value was 1.3 cm., with a standard deviation of 5 mm. The upper limit of normal was 2.3 cm. (two standard deviations). This method obviates many of the variables previously noted by compressing the barium-containing midline viscus against the retroperitoneum, thus accurately defining its anterior margin.

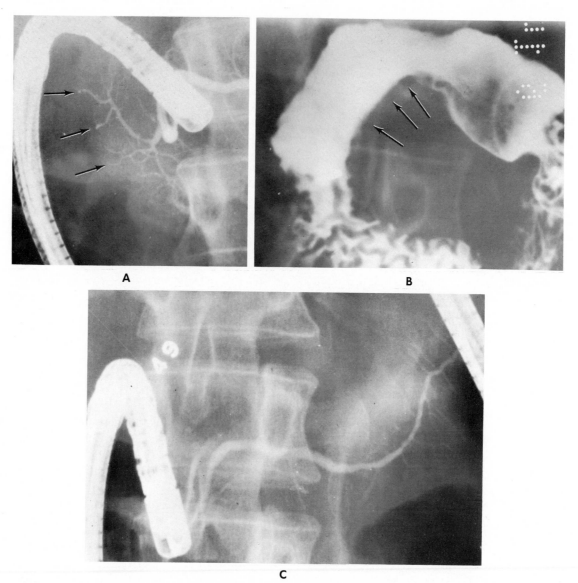

Figure 13-71. Detection of malignant disease by peroral retrograde pancreaticobiliary ductography. (From Robbins, A. H., et al.: Amer. J. Roentgenol., *117*:432–436, 1973.)

A. Barium studies suggest pressure defect on second part of duodenum. *B.* Ductogram reveals normal tributary ducts in same region. *C.* Main pancreatic duct is normal and other branches are normal as well. (Patient had chronic pancreatitis.)

Figure 13-71 continued on the opposite page.

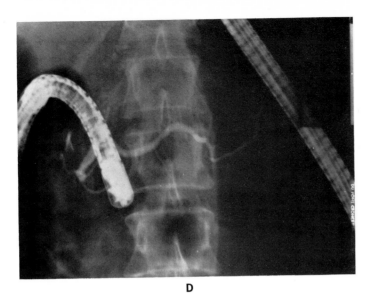

D

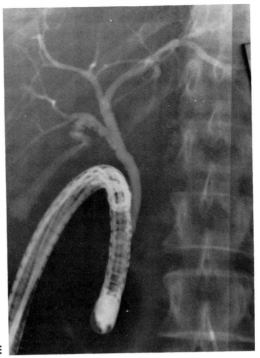

E

Figure 13-71 *Continued.* D. Another normal pancreatic ductogram. E. A normal cholangiogram.

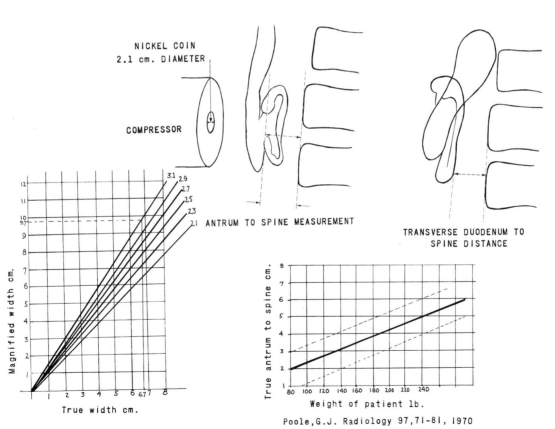

Figure 13-72. Method of measuring "retroantral" and "retroduodenal" space. The coin on the compressor allows correction for magnification (graph, lower left). The normal standards for antrum to spine are shown in the graph, lower right. The transverse duodenum-to-spine distance plus 2 standard deviations was 2.3 cm. (From Poole, G. J.: Radiology 97:71–81, 1970.)

GASTRIC AND DUODENAL ANGIOGRAPHY

Blood Supply of the Stomach

The Celiac Trunk. The celiac trunk or axis is the first unpaired branch of the abdominal aorta (Fig. 13–73). It arises from the ventral side, usually at about the upper margin of the first lumbar vertebra. It may vary in its origin, however, between the lower margin of T12 and the lower margin of L1. It is a very short branch and it lies ordinarily about an average of 1 cm. above the origin of the superior mesenteric artery, although this measurement may range between 1 and 2.2 cm. Usually the celiac artery terminates in three branches but occasionally in four. The three typical branches are the *left gastric, common hepatic,* and *splenic* (Fig. 13–73). Additional branches may occasionally go to the dorsal pancreatic, the left or right phrenic, and a middle or accessory middle colic.

The classical pattern of branching of the celiac artery is found in 93 per cent of cases (Ruzicka and Rossi) (Fig. 13–75). A representative simultaneous selective celiac and superior mesenteric artery angiogram of the type I pattern is shown in Figure 13–76.

The *left gastric artery* courses upward toward the cardiac end of the stomach and passes between the layers of the gastrohepatic ligament, following the lesser curvature of the stomach closely. After reaching the region of the cardia of the stomach it descends from left to right downward toward the pylorus, ultimately anastomosing with the right gastric artery (Fig. 13–74). It thus forms an arterial arch or arcade on the lesser curvature of the stomach with the right gastric artery. The main branches of the left gastric artery are the *esophageal* and the *hepatic.* One to three esophageal branches ascend along the right anterior and posterior surfaces of the esophagus, supplying the cardiac and distal portions of the esophagus. These branches anastomose with other esophageal arteries from the aorta, bronchial branches, posterior intercostal, and phrenic arteries as described in the section on the esophagus.

The hepatic branch of the left gastric artery occurs in about 25 per cent of individuals.

The *common hepatic artery* arises along the right aspect of the celiac trunk and to the right of the superior margin of the head of the pancreas (Fig. 13–73). In the region of the first part of the duodenum it gives off the *gastroduodenal artery,* and then turns forward into the hepatoduodenal ligament, where it continues toward the liver as the hepatic artery proper. In the hepatoduodenal ligament, the hepatic artery is situated on the ventral side of the portal vein to the left of the common bile duct. As it reaches the porta hepatis it divides into two main branches, a *right* and *left hepatic branches.* Some of the variations of normal branching of the hepatic arteries are shown in Figure 13–77.

The *right gastric artery* is ordinarily a branch of the hepatic artery proper. It usually arises distal to the origin of the gastroduodenal, but it may arise from other arteries, such as the left hepatic (40 per cent); right hepatic (5 per cent); middle hepatic (5 per cent); gastroduodenal (8 per cent); and common hepatic. The right gastric artery descends from its origin, giving off branches to the pylorus and stomach, and reaches the lesser curvature where it turns to the left and ascends along the lesser curvature, ultimately anastomosing with the left gastric artery in the arcade described previously.

The *right hepatic branch* of the hepatic artery passes between the portal vein and the common hepatic duct to enter the right lobe of the liver. It usually lies to the right of the right hepatic duct. Aberrant right hepatic arteries from other sources in the celiac trunk occur in about 18 per cent of individuals, usually as a branch of the superior mesenteric artery (Fig. 13–77). Outside the liver the right hepatic artery gives off the *cystic artery* to the gallbladder and it may also provide a *middle hepatic artery.* The intrahepatic distribution of the hepatic artery will be described subsequently in conjunction with the anatomy of the liver.

The *left hepatic artery* supplies the left lobe of the liver and is

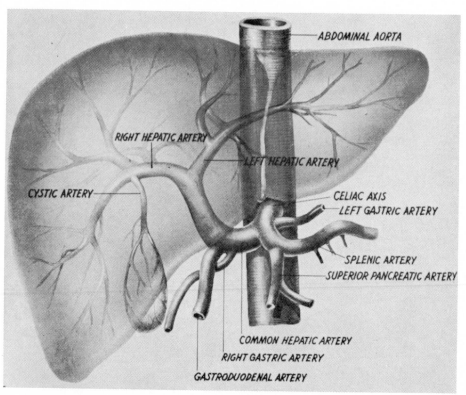

Figure 13–73. Classic arterial circulation of the liver. (From Bierman, H. R.: Selective Arterial Catheterization, 1969. Courtesy of Charles C Thomas, Publisher, Springfield, Illinois.)

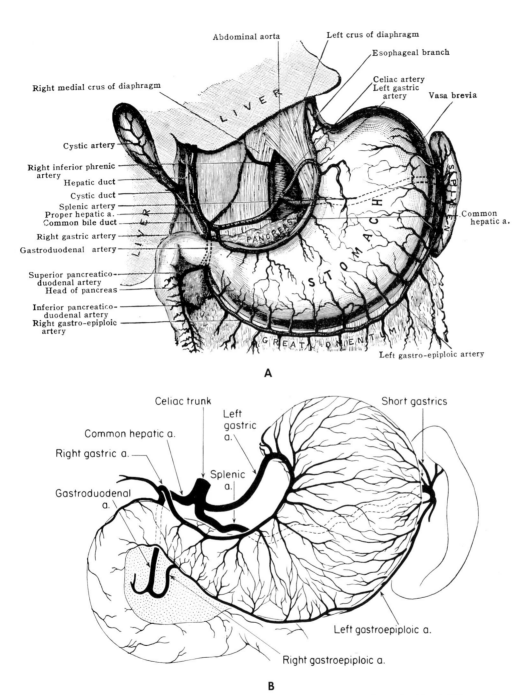

Figure 13-74. *A.* Celiac artery and its usual main branches. (From Anson, B. J. (ed.): Morris' Human Anatomy, 12th ed. Copyright © 1966 by McGraw-Hill, Inc. Used by permission of McGraw-Hill Book Company.) *B.* Line drawing of arterial supply of the stomach. The arteries to the stomach are enlarged for emphasis. The left gastroepiploic and right gastric arteries are frequently not identified at angiography unless they are serving as a collateral pathway. (From Reuter, S. R., and Redman, H. C.: Gastrointestinal Angiography. Philadelphia, W. B. Saunders Co., 1972.)

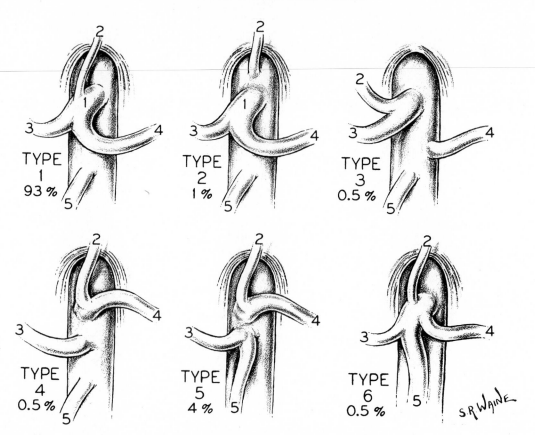

Figure 13–75. (1) Celiac trunk, (2) left gastric artery, (3) common hepatic artery, (4) splenic artery, (5) superior mesenteric artery, (6) right hepatic artery, (7) left hepatic artery, (8) gastroduodenal artery, (9) proper hepatic artery. (From Ruzicka, F. F., and Rossi, P.: N.Y. State J. Med., 23:3032–3033, 1968, reproduced with permission.)

usually considerably smaller than the right. An aberrant left hepatic artery occurs in about 25 per cent of individuals.

A *middle hepatic artery* supplies the quadrate lobe of the liver. It may arise from either the right or left hepatic artery and it gives off branches to the left side of the quadrate lobe and in some instances sends a branch to the left lobe. In rare instances, it gives rise to the cystic artery, to be described later.

The *gastroduodenal artery* descends dorsal to the first part of the duodenum to the lower margin of the pylorus, where it divides into a *right gastroepiploic artery* and an *anterior superior pancreaticoduodenal artery.* The gastroduodenal artery lies to the left of the common bile duct at its origin and terminally lies on the ventral aspect of the head of the pancreas, as described in the section on the pancreas. It has three main branches — a *posterior superior pancreaticoduodenal,* an *anterior superior pancreaticoduodenal,* and the *right gastroepiploic.* There may be other small duodenal branches. The pancreaticoduodenal branches form the arcade previously described in the section on the pancreas. The right

gastroepiploic artery courses along the greater curvature of the stomach, ultimately to anastomose with the left gastroepiploic artery, which arises from the splenic artery. The right gastroepiploic artery thereafter passes in the gastrocolic ligament or in the greater omentum. It is ordinarily larger than the left and passes much farther to the left than the midline. The right and left gastroepiploic arteries form an arcade supplying the anterior and superior surfaces of the stomach along its greater curvature.

The *splenic artery* is the largest branch arising from the celiac trunk and is generally the first branch of the celiac. It arises to the right of the midline and crosses the aorta to reach the spleen on the left, varying in length from 8 to 32 cm. It is often very tortuous, particularly in elderly persons. Its diameter varies from 4 to 11 mm. Generally, it embeds itself in the superior border of the pancreas and reaches the tail of the pancreas, where it divides into its *two main terminals* (Fig. 13–78), the *superior* and *inferior,* and occasionally, even a third branch called the middle terminal. Throughout its pancreatic course, it lies ceph-

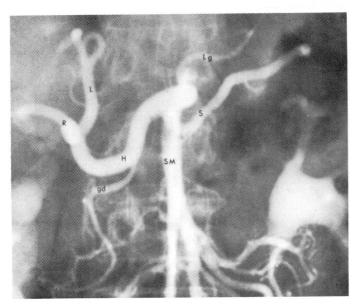

Figure 13–76. Simultaneous selective celiac and superior mesenteric artery injections show type I pattern (see Figs. 13–75 and 13–77 also). Anteroposterior view. (S) Splenic artery, (SM) superior mesenteric, (gd) gastroduodenal, (H) proper hepatic, (R) right hepatic, (L) left hepatic, (Lg) left gastric. (From Ruzicka, F. F., and Rossi, P.: Radiol. Clin. N. Amer., 8:3–29, 1970.)

alad to the splenic vein. Its most constant branches are the *pancreatic, left gastroepiploic, short gastric, superior and inferior terminal, and splenic branches.*

The pancreatic branches arising from the splenic artery are usually small, as previously indicated, but occasionally some may be very large. The largest of these is the *dorsal pancreatic,* which in turn forms the *inferior pancreatic artery* (supplying the inferior edge of the pancreas) and anastomoses with the caudal pancreatic branches of the *pancreatica magna.* The dorsal pancreatic may communicate with the superior mesenteric artery or its branches. The *pancreatica magna artery* is the largest pancreatic branch and enters the pancreas at the junction of its middle and left third. It represents the main blood supply of the tail of the pancreas. Caudal pancreatic branches arise from the splenic before its terminal division and penetrate the tail of the pancreas, anastomosing with the inferior pancreatic and pancreatica magna radicals.

The *left gastroepiploic artery* reaches the stomach below the fundus and descends along the left side of the greater curvature in the anterior layer of the greater omentum. As previously mentioned, it anastomoses with the right gastroepiploic artery and provides an arcade on the greater curvature of the stomach. It

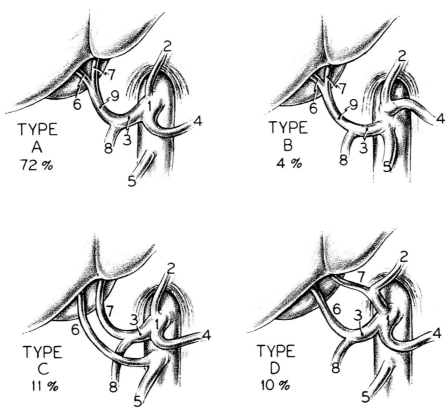

Figure 13–77. (1) Celiac trunk, (2) left gastric artery, (3) common hepatic artery, (4) splenic artery, (5) superior mesenteric artery, (6) right hepatic artery, (7) left hepatic artery, (8) gastroduodenal artery, (9) proper hepatic artery. (From Ruzicka, F. F., and Rossi, P.: N.Y. State J. Med., 23:3032–3033, 1968, reproduced with permission.)

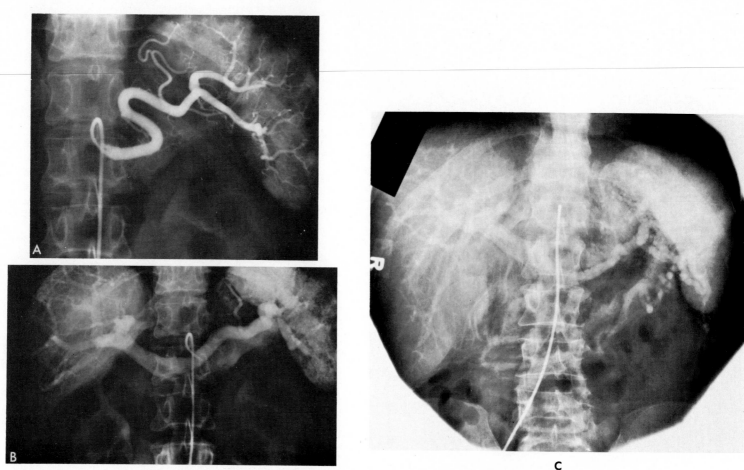

Figure 13-78.   Normal splenic arteriogram in the evaluation of the pancreatic body and tail.

    A. Arterial phase of a selective splenic arteriogram demonstrates the pancreatica magna and short pancreatic arteries supplying the body and tail of the pancreas.

    B. During the venous phase of the same injection, the splenic vein and portal vein are optimally visualized. The close association of the splenic vein with the opacified normal pancreatic body and tail is apparent. (From Eaton, S. B. and Ferrucci, J. T., Jr., Radiology of the Pancreas and Duodenum, W. B. Saunders Co., 1973.)

    C. Portal or splenoportal venogram following celiac arteriogram.

Figure 13-78 continued on the opposite page.

gives off various gastric, pancreatic, and splenic arterial branches. The *short gastric arteries* are small branches from the splenic artery which pass to the greater curvature of the stomach in its cardiac or fundic region.

The *terminal arteries* of the splenic send from two to twelve small splenic branches into the substance of the spleen.

Venous Drainage.   The *veins of the stomach* drain directly or indirectly into the portal vein which will be described in more detail in Chapter 14. However, short gastric veins from the greater curvatures and fundus may drain into the splenic vein (Fig. 13-78 *C, D*), and the left gastroepiploic vein also drains into the splenic from the greater curvature of the stomach. The right gastroepiploic from the right end of the greater curvature drains into the superior mesenteric vein. *A coronary vein* runs the length of the lesser curvature from the cardia to the portal vein in the same distribution as the left and right gastric arteries. There are additional pyloric veins along the pyloric part of the lesser curvature which join directly into the portal vein.

Lymphatic Drainage.   The *lymphatic drainage of the stomach* and its zones of flow are illustrated in Figure 13-79. The visceral nodes consist of gastric, hepatic, and pancreaticolienal. The gastric nodes are situated along the left gastric artery and the right half of the greater curvature. The hepatic nodes are situated along the hepatic artery, near the neck of the gallbladder and in

Cunningham, D. J.: Manual of Practical Anatomy. 12th edition. London, Oxford University Press, 1958.

Darke, C. T., and Beal, J. M.: Percutaneous cholangiography. Arch. Surg., *91*:558–563, 1965.

Doubilet, H., Poppel, M. H., and Mulholland, J. H.: Pancreatography. Ann. N.Y. Acad. Sci., *78*:829–851, 1959.

Doubilet, H., Poppel, M. H., and Mulholland, J. H.: Pancreatography. Radiology, *64*:325–339, 1955.

Evans, J. A.: Specialized roentgen diagnostic techniques in the investigation of abdominal disease. Radiology, *82*:579–594, 1964.

Eyler, W. R., Clark, M. D., and Rian, R. L.: An evaluation of roentgen signs of pancreatic enlargement. J.A.M.A., *181*:967–971, 1962.

Ferrucci, J. T., Jr., Benedict, K. T., Jr., Page, D. L., Fleischli, D. J., and Eaton, S. B.: Radiographic features of normal hypotonic duodenogram. Radiology, *96*:401–408, 1970.

Flemma, R. J., Schauble, J. F., Gardner, C. E., Anlyan, W. G., and Capp, M. P.: Percutaneous transhepatic cholangiography in the differential diagnosis of jaundice. Surg. Gynec. Obstet., *116*:559–568, 1963.

Gotton, P. B., Salmon, P. R., and Blumgart, L. H.: Cannulation of papilla of Vater via fiber duodenoscope: assessment of retrograde cholangiopancreatography in 60 patients. Lancet, *1*:53–58, 1972.

Grant, J. C. B.: Atlas of Anatomy. Fifth edition. Baltimore, Williams and Wilkins Co., 1962.

Guyton, A. C.: Textbook of Medical Physiology. Fourth edition. Philadelphia, W. B. Saunders Co., 1971.

Hampton, A. O.: A safe method for the roentgen demonstration of bleeding ulcers. Amer. J. Roentgenol., *38*:565–570, 1937.

Herbert, W. W., and Margulis, A. R.: Diagnosis of retroperitoneal masses by gastrointestinal roentgenographic measurements: a computer study. Radiology, *84*:52–57, 1965.

Jacobson, G., Berne, C. J., Meyers, H. I., and Rosoff, L.: The examination of patients with suspected perforated ulcer using a water soluble contrast medium. Amer. J. Roentgenol., *86*:37–49, 1961.

Johnstone, A. S.: Observations on the radiological anatomy of the esophagogastric junction. Radiology, *73*:501–510, 1959.

Knowles, H. C., Felson, B., Shapiro, N., and Schiff, L.: Emergency diagnosis of upper digestive tract bleeding by roentgen examination without palpation. ("Hampton" technique.) Radiology, *58*:536–541, 1952.

Kusagai, T., Kuno, N., and Aoki, I.: Fibroduodenoscopy: analysis of 353 examinations. Gastrointestinal Endoscopy, *18*:9–16, 1971.

Lerche, W.: The esophagus and pharynx in action: a study of structure in relation to function. Springfield, Illinois, Charles C Thomas, 1950.

Lowman, R. M.: Retroperitoneal tumors: a survey and assessment of roentgen techniques. Radiol. Clin. N. Amer., *3*:543–566, 1965.

Lunderquist, A.: Angiography in carcinoma of the pancreas. Acta Radiol. (Diag.), Suppl. *235*:1, 1965.

Marshall, S., Lapp, M., and Schulte, J. W.: Lesions of the pancreas mimicking renal disease. J. Urol., *93*:41–45, 1965.

Morettin, L. B.: Normal and abnormal sialograms of the parotid gland. Personal communication.

Meschan, I., Landsman, H., Regnier, G., et al.: The normal radiographic adult stomach and duodenum. A study of their contour and size and their critical relationships to spine in both symptomatic and asymptomatic individuals. South Med. J., *46*:878–887, 1953.

Mosely, R. D., Jr.: Roentgen diagnosis of pancreatic disease. Arch. Intern. Med., *107*:31–36, 1961.

Neuhauser, E. D. B.: quoted in Sidaway, M. E.: The use of water soluble contrast medium in pediatric radiology. Clin. Radiol., *15*:132–138, 1964.

Ogoshi, K., Tobita, Y., and Hara, Y.: Endoscopic observation of duodenum and pancreato-choledochography using duodenal fibroscope under direct vision. Gastroenterology, *12*:83–96, 1970.

Oi, I.: Fibroduodenoscopy and endoscopic pancreato-cholangiography. Gastrointestinal Endoscopy, *17*:59–62, 1970.

Okuda, K., Someya, N., Goto, A., Tadahiko, K., Emura, T., Yasumoto, M., and Shimokawa, Y.: Endoscopic pancreato-cholangiography. Amer. J. Roentgenol., *117*:437–445, 1973.

Pancoast, H. K.: Possible effects of morphine on intestinal motility. Amer. J. Roentgenol., *2*:549–551, 1914.

Pansky, B., and House, E. L.: Review of Gross Anatomy. New York, MacMillan Co., 1964.

Park, W. M., and Mason, D. K.: Hydrostatic sialography. Radiology, *86*:116, 1966.

Pernkopf, E.: Atlas of Topographical and Applied Human Anatomy. Volumes 1 and 2. Philadelphia, W. B. Saunders Co., 1963.

Poole, G. J.: A new roentgenographic method of measuring the retrogastric and retroduodenal spaces: statistical evaluation of reliability and diagnostic utility. Radiology, *97*:71–81, 1970.

Poppel, M. H.: Roentgen Manifestations of Pancreatic Disease. Springfield, Illinois, Charles C Thomas, 1951.

Poppel, M. H., Sheinmel, A., and Mednick, E.: The procurement and critical appraisal of the width diameter of the midline retrogastric soft tissues. Amer. J. Roentgenol., *61*:56–60, 1949.

Porcher, P., and Buffard, P.: Malignancy of the stomach. *In* Margulis, A. R., and Burhenne, H. J. (eds.): Alimentary Tract Roentgenology. St. Louis, C. V. Mosby Co., 1967.

Porrath, S.: Roentgenologic considerations of the hyoid apparatus. Amer. J. Roentgenol., *105*:63–73, 1969.

Quigley, J. P., and Louckes, H. S.: Gastric emptying. Amer. J. Digest. Dis., *7*:672–676, 1962.

Quigley, J. P., and Meschan, I.: The gastric evacuation of fat with special reference to pyloric sphincter activity. Gastroenterol., *4*:272–275, 1937.

Rasmussen, T.: Pharmacoradiography of the stomach. Nord. Med., *44*:1563–1566, 1950.

Rea, C. E.: Conservative versus operative treatment of perforated peptic ulcer. Surgery, *32*:654–657, 1952.

Ritvo, M.: Drugs as an aid in roentgen examination of the gastrointestinal tract: the use of Mecholyl, physostigmine, and Benzedrine in overcoming atonicity, sluggishness of peristalsis, and spasm. Amer. J. Roentgenol., *36*:868–874, 1936.

Robbins, A. H., Paul, R. E., Jr., Norton, R. A., Schimmel, E. M., Tomas, J. G., and Sugarman, H. J.: Detection of malignant disease by peroral retrograde pancreatico-biliary ductography. Amer. J. Roentgenol., *117*:432–436, 1973.

Rösch, J.: Roentgenology of the Spleen and Pancreas. Springfield, Illinois, Charles C Thomas, 1967.

Rösch, J., and Herfort, K.: Contribution of splenoportography to the diagnosis of diseases of the pancreas. Acta Med. Scand., *171*:263–272, 1962.

Ruzicka, F. F., and Rossi, P.: Normal vascular anatomy of the abdominal viscera. Radiol. Clin. N. Amer., *8*:3–29, 1970.

Sachs, M. D., and Partington, P. F.: Cholangiographic diagnosis of pancreatitis. Amer. J. Roentgenol., *76*:32–38, 1956.

Salik, J. O.: Pancreatic carcinoma and its early roentgenologic recognition. Amer. J. Roentgenol., *86*:1–28, 1961.

Schultz, E. H.: Aid to diagnosis of acute pancreatitis by roentgenologic study. Amer. J. Roentgenol., *89*:825–836, 1963.

Schultz, E. H.: Cervical disk disease simulating intramedullary neoplasms by myelography. Radiology, *84*:389, 1965.

Sheinmel, A., and Mednick, E. A.: The roentgen diagnosis of upper abdominal retroperitoneal space-occupying lesions. Amer. J. Roentgenol., *65*:77–92, 1951.

Sidaway, M. E.: The use of water soluble contrast medium in pediatric radiology. Clin. Radiol., *15*:132–138, 1964.

Siebert, T. L., Stein, J., and Poppel, M. H.: Variations in the roentgen appearance of the "esophageal lip." Amer. J. Roentgenol., *81*:570–575, 1959.

Silbiger, M. L., and Donner, M. W.: Morphine in the evaluation of gastrointestinal disease: a cineradiographic study. Radiology, *90*:1090–1096, 1968.

Stein, G. N., Kalser, M. H., Sarian, N. N., and Finkelstein, A.: An evaluation of the roentgen changes in acute pancreatitis: correlation with clinical findings. Gastroenterology, *36*:354–361, 1959.

Tagaki, K., Ikeda, S., and Nakagawa, Y.: Retrograde pancreatography and cholangiography by fibroduodenoscope. Gastroenterology, *59*:445–452, 1970.

Taylor, D. A., Macken, K. L., Fiore, A. S., Colcher, H., Bachman, A. L., and Seaman, W. B.: New method of visualizing gastric wall. Further studies. Radiology, *86*:711–717, 1966.

Varriale, P., Bonanno, C. A., and Grace, W. J.: Portal hypertension secondary to pancreatic pseudocysts. Arch. Intern. Med. (Chicago), *112*:191–198, 1963.

Weens, H. S., and Walker, L. A.: Radiologic diagnosis of acute cholecystitis and pancreatitis. Radiol. Clin. N. Amer., *2*:89–106, 1964.

Wolf, B. S.: Roentgen features of normal and herniated esophagogastric region. Amer. J. Digest. Dis., *5*:751–769, 1960.

Wolf, B. S.: Roentgen features of the normal and herniated esophagogastric region; clinical correlations. *In* Glass, G. B. J. (ed.): Progress in Gastroenterology. Vol. 2, New York, Grune and Stratton, 1970, pp. 288–315.

Wolf, B. S.: Sliding hiatal hernia: the need for re-definition. Amer. J. Roentgenol., *117*:231–247, 1973.

Small Intestine, Colon, and Biliary Tract

THE SMALL INTESTINE

Gross Anatomy. The small intestine during life varies considerably in length. It is well known, for example, that the entire small intestine can be traversed by a Miller-Abbott tube several feet in length, whereas its length at autopsy is usually 20 to 22 feet; probably with good muscle tone during life it varies between 15 and 17 feet. In formalin-hardened bodies, it rarely measures longer than 12 or 13 feet in length. There is a gradual diminution in diameter from the pylorus to the ileocecal valve (valvula coli).

The jejunum and ileum are completely covered with peritoneum and therefore vary considerably in position, except at the two ends where relative fixation occurs. However, the small intestine is usually distributed in the abdomen according to a fairly regular pattern (Fig. 14–1). Thus, the proximal jejunum usually lies in the left half of the abdomen between the level of the pancreas and the intercrestal line. The distal ileum usually lies deep in the pelvis posteriorly, with the terminal ileum arising out of the pelvis to meet the cecum in the right lower quadrant anteriorly. The distal jejunum and proximal ileum are distributed in the right half of the abdomen for the most part.

The root of the mesentery, about 15 cm. long, is attached to the posterior abdominal wall along a line running obliquely from the left side of the body of the L2 vertebra to the right sacroiliac joint, crossing the third part of the duodenum, the aorta, the inferior vena cava, the right gonadal vessels, the right ureter, and the right psoas muscle (Fig. 14–2). It is approximately 20 cm. broad, on the average, tending to become narrower as it reaches the lower end of the ileum. The mesentery contains blood vessels, lymphatics, lymph nodes, and nerves of the small intestine, as well as fat.

The mucous membrane of the small intestine is enormously increased in surface area by the formation of circular folds (valvulae conniventes), upon which are mounted intestinal villi (Figs. 14–3 and 14–4). The circular folds give a characteristic coiled-spring appearance to the inner aspect of the small intestine. These folds reach their maximum development in the distal half of the duodenum and proximal part of the jejunum, where

they may be as much as 8 mm. in height and extend around two-thirds of the circumference of the bowel, branching in the course of their extension. Thereafter they gradually become smaller and less numerous so that they are virtually absent in the lower ileum (Fig. 14–3). Although they extend through the wall of the bowel and involve the whole thickness of the mucous membrane and a core of submucosa, they do not involve the serosa, unlike the valvulae semilunares of the colon.

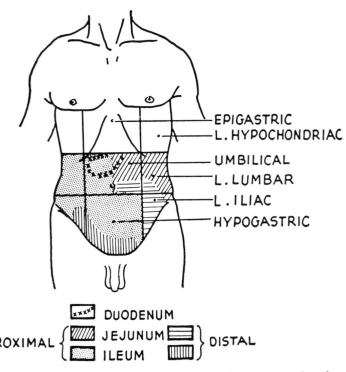

SCHEME OF NORMAL POSITION OF SMALL INTESTINE

EPIGASTRIC
L. HYPOCHONDRIAC
UMBILICAL
L. LUMBAR
L. ILIAC
HYPOGASTRIC

DUODENUM
PROXIMAL { JEJUNUM / ILEUM } DISTAL

Figure 14–1. Approximate distribution of the small intestine within the abdomen.

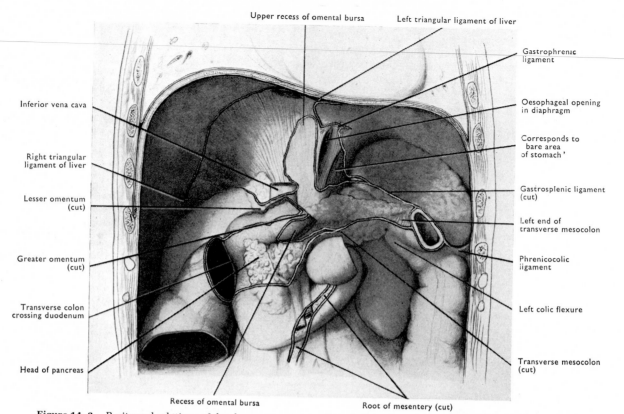

Figure 14-2. Peritoneal relations of duodenum, pancreas, spleen, kidneys, etc. From a body hardened by injection of formalin. When the liver, stomach, and intestines were removed the lines of the peritoneal reflections were carefully preserved. (From Cunningham's Textbook of Anatomy, 10th ed. London, Oxford University Press, 1964.)

The intestinal villi are mounted on these folds and measure less than half a millimeter in height. They begin at the pyloric orifice where they are broad and short, becoming longer and narrower as they approach the ileocecal valve. These villi are actu-

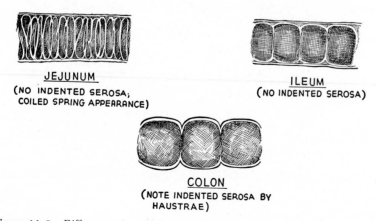

Figure 14-3. Differences in roentgen appearance of distended small and large intestines.

ally present on and between the circular folds but never over solitary lymph nodules. In the center of each villus there is a lymph channel—a central lacteal—which joins the submucous lymph plexuses and a vascular capillary network that drains into a vein at the base of the villus.

Major Differences Between Jejunum and Ileum. The main differences between the jejunum and ileum from the radiographic standpoint can be summarized as follows:

1. There is a gradual diminution in diameter as the cecum is approached, and thus the lumen of the ileum is smaller than that of the jejunum. The average diameter of the jejunum measures 3 to 3.5 cm.; that of the ileum, 2.5 cm. or less.

2. The plicae circulares commence in the second part of the duodenum (see the description in the preceding chapter). The maximum number and size of plicae circulares are found in the midjejunum, and they diminish toward the ileum, practically ceasing a little below the middle of this portion. This fact is important because the mucosal pattern of the ileum differs from that of the proximal jejunum by being considerably smoother and less feathery (Fig. 14-5). Barium tends to have a more clumped appearance in the ileum than in the jejunum as a result of this fundamental difference. In the ileocecal region, the rugae tend to be

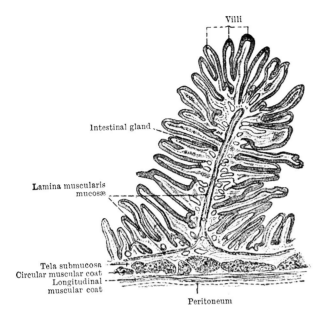

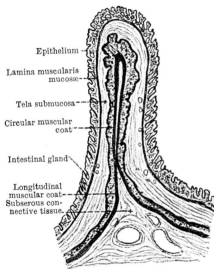

Figure 14–4. Diagrammatic presentation of the differences in transverse section between the plicae circulares of the small intestine and plicae semilunares of the large intestine. (From Cunningham's Textbook of Anatomy, 6th ed. London, Oxford University Press, 1931.)

parallel in type approaching the appearance of the rugae in the pylorus.

3. The aggregate lymphatic nodules, or Peyer's patches, are most numerous in the ileum and considerably fewer in number in the jejunum. They are more prominent in young people and tend to atrophy as age advances. They are not ordinarily distinguishable radiographically and normally do not play a significant role in radiographic diagnosis.

4. In the adult, because the mesentery of the ileum contains

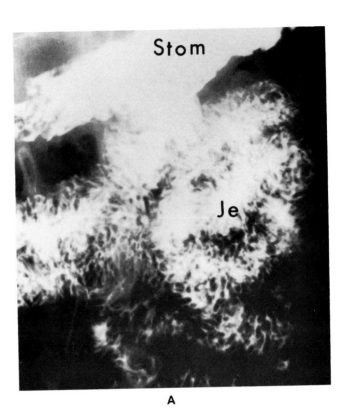

A

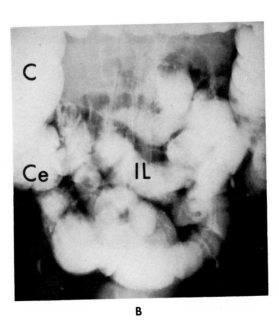

B

Figure 14–5. A. Radiograph of jejunal mucosal pattern. B. Radiograph of ileal mucosal pattern.

considerably more fatty tissue than that of the jejunum, it appears to be considerably thicker than the latter structure.

Intestinal Glands. The crypts between the villi contain one or two tubular structures connected with intestinal glands or "crypts of Lieberkühn." The villi are otherwise covered by a single layer of cylindrical epithelial cells with glandular cells of three types occasionally interspersed: (1) goblet cells, (2) oxyphilic granular cells of Paneth, and (3) argentaffine cells.

The goblet cells secrete mucous fluid. Generally, they are found low in the crypts along the lower part of the villi, but occasionally they are located in the upper regions of the villi as well. The oxyphilic granular cells of Paneth are characteristically situated in the floor of the crypts; they participate in enzyme production. Argentaffine or yellow cells have a high affinity for silver and chromium, and their characteristic site is in the fundi of the crypts of Lieberkühn. They are associated with the production of serotonin, and they are found with particular frequency in the duodenum and the appendix.

The secretions from these glands are rapidly reabsorbed by the villi so that there is a constant circulation of fluid from the crypts to the villi, thus supplying a watery vehicle for absorption of food substances from the small intestine. The epithelial cells of the mucosa of the small intestine contain large quantities of digestive enzymes, enabling them presumably to digest food substances during absorption through the epithelium (Guyton).

There is a constant reproductive cycle of these epithelial cells from deep within the crypts of Lieberkühn toward the surface of the mucosa. The life cycle of an intestinal epithelial cell is approximately 48 hours. Thus, excoriation of the small intestine is rapidly repaired. One of the chief effects of radiation on the small intestine, however, is significant impairment of the reproductive capacity of the crypts of Lieberkühn.

Motility Study of the Small Intestine. It has been well established that many systemic diseases (such as vitamin deficiency, protein deficiency, certain anemias, allergic states, and so on) are capable of producing considerable changes in the motility pattern of the small intestine, and for that reason, a close study of the normal small intestinal motility is imperative.

Cannon was one of the first investigators to demonstrate intestinal motility, both by direct inspection of the exposed intestine in anesthetized animals and also by radiographic studies in the intact animal. He described *rhythmic segmentation, pendulum movements* and *peristaltic waves.*

The movements of rhythmic segmentation occur at a rate of 8 to 9 per minute in the duodenum, becoming progressively slower farther down the small intestine. These contractions appear to divide the small intestine into segments, imparting to it the appearance of a "chain of sausages." Such chopping movements of the intestinal chyme tend to mix the chyme with intestinal secretions and promote absorption.

The pendular movements consist of small constrictive waves that sweep forward and then backward, up and down a few centimeters of the gut. By moving the contents back and forth within the intestinal lumen these movements further keep the intestinal contents thoroughly mixed.

Peristaltic waves propel the intestinal contents toward the anus at a velocity of approximately 1 to 2 cm. per second. Usually, the contents travel visibly only a few centimeters at a time. Peristaltic activity generally increases immediately after a meal and is produced by the so-called "gastroenteric reflex." Intense irritation of the intestinal mucosa may produce a rapid peristaltic movement, the so-called "peristaltic rush," which may pass over large lengths of intestine in a few minutes, sweeping the contents into the colon.

A significant delay of the intestinal contents may occur in the region of the ileocecal valve, often relieved by a gastroileal or gastroenteric reflex at the time of another meal.

Actually, our present-day concept is not quite so clear-cut as Cannon's description might indicate. Barium usually passes quite rapidly into the jejunum for approximately 30 or 40 cm., and thereafter the movement of the barium column proceeds quite slowly. The lumen of the jejunum is usually sufficiently collapsed to permit a ready and accurate visualization of the rugal pattern. Peristaltic waves are the most common type of motility, but occasionally an overall circular movement of a whole segment of small bowel is superimposed. The barium column gradually moves on into the ileum, where there is a smoother and less fluffy pattern, and where the barium tends to remain longer in continuous cylinders. Ordinarily, the barium remains clumped in the distal ileum for a considerable period of time, and periodically a peristaltic wave will be seen to carry a small portion of the barium into the terminal ileum, which rises out of the pelvis to meet the cecum. Peristaltic waves are intermittent over the terminal ileum. In the distal ileum, there is virtually no rugal pattern visible, and all movement is difficult to observe fluoroscopically, since the ileal loops are conglomerated and difficult to palpate in view of their posterior position.

The average time for the head of the barium column to reach the ileocecal region is $1\frac{1}{2}$ to 2 hours, but it is not unusual for a period of 4 hours to elapse before barium appears in the cecum. Abnormality, either primary or secondary, in the emptying of the stomach will of course affect the emptying time of the small intestine, and any abnormality of the terminal ileum may be reflected in a delayed emptying of the stomach.

Special Anatomy of the Ileocecal Valve (Valvula Coli). The terminal ileum projects into the cecum at its termination, producing folds or a papillary protrusion that function as a sphincter. The serosa of the ileum does not participate in this protrusion and helps to prevent abnormal invagination of the terminal ileum into the ascending colon (called "intussusception"). The filling defect produced by this anatomic structure is readily visualized radiographically (Figs. 14–6, 14–7).

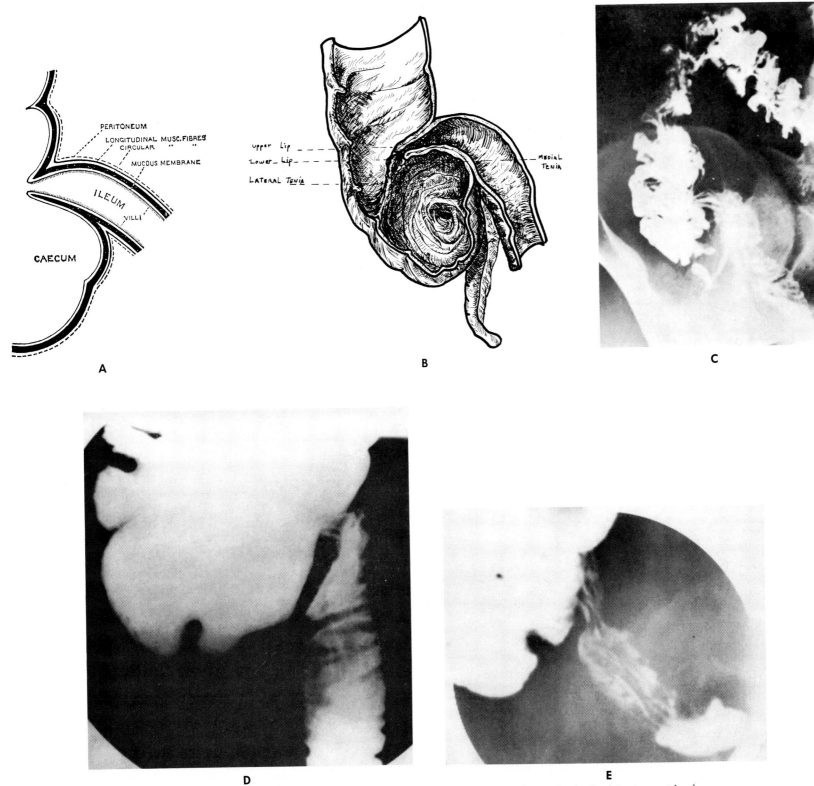

Figure 14–6. Ileocecal junction. A. Diagrammatic section. (From Cunningham's Textbook of Anatomy, 6th ed. London, Oxford University Press, 1931.) B. Line drawing of the ileocecal valve. (From Rubin, S., Dann, D. S., Ezekial, C., and Vincent, J.: Amer. J. Roentgenol., 87:708, 1962). C, D, E. Ileocecal junction; spot film studies.

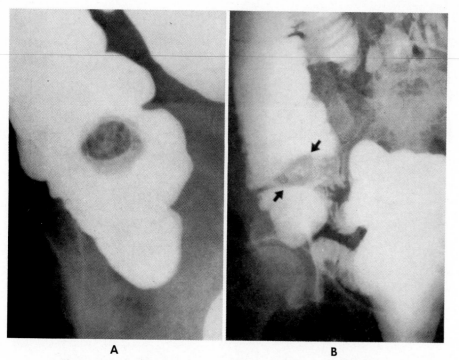

A   **B**

Figure 14–7. Difference between prolapse (*A*) and prominent ileocecal valves (*B*). In the former the central slitlike valve orifice is not filled with barium, whereas in the latter it stands out clearly. This is a posteriorly situated valve. (From Hinkel, C. L.: Amer. J. Roentgenol., *68*, 1952.)

The function of this valve is sphincteric—much like that of the pyloric valve—but it is unknown if its main function is to prevent regurgitation as is the case with the pyloric sphincter. In performing barium enema examinations, it is possible to force barium from the colon into the terminal ileum in at least half of the cases, and this incompetency is probably of no pathologic significance. Ordinarily, however, in gaseous distention of the colon from any mechanical obstructive cause at a lower level in the colon, the ileocecal valve will prevent passage of the gas back up into the small intestine for a considerable period of time.

THE LARGE INTESTINE

Gross Anatomy. The large intestine is approximately 5 to 5½ feet in length and varies in diameter from 1½ to 3 inches. Commencing at the cecum, it is further subdivided into ascending colon, transverse colon, descending and iliac colon, sigmoid or pelvic colon, and rectum.

The cecum is found in the right lower quadrant of the abdomen ordinarily, but its position is most variable. It is usually situated anteriorly, with only the omentum and abdominal wall lying over it. The terminal ileum joins the cecum usually on its

medial or posterior aspect, and the vermiform appendix springs from the cecum on the same side as the ileocecal junction. The upper end of the cecum is continuous with the ascending colon. There is considerable variation, however, in the position of the cecum, both in respect to its posterior peritoneal attachment and to its relationship to the pelvic rim or the abdomen. Some variations in attachment of the posterior peritoneum to the cecum are shown in Figure 14–8. Variations in the contour of the cecum, terminal ileum, and appendix, when on the right side of the abdomen, are shown in Figure 14–9. Variations in position of the appendix and cecum are shown in Figure 14–10.

The vermiform appendix is part of the cecum. It arises from the point where the three taeniae of the large intestine merge into one uniform coat of longitudinal muscle. It varies considerably in length from 2.5 to 25 cm., averaging 6 to 9 cm. Unless inflamed, it varies in position freely in the same individual in relation to its attachment to the cecum. Its movement depends considerably on the length and width of the peritoneal fold that represents its mesentery. At times it points upward toward the liver and sometimes it is "retrocolic" rather than retrocecal, lying behind or to the right of the ascending colon. It contains masses of

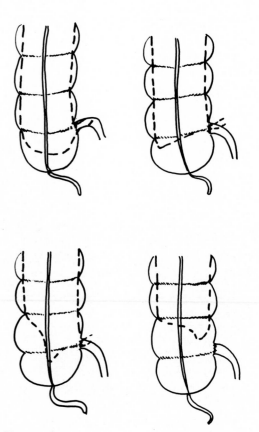

Figure 14–8. Diagram showing variations in position of the posterior peritoneal attachment of the cecum.

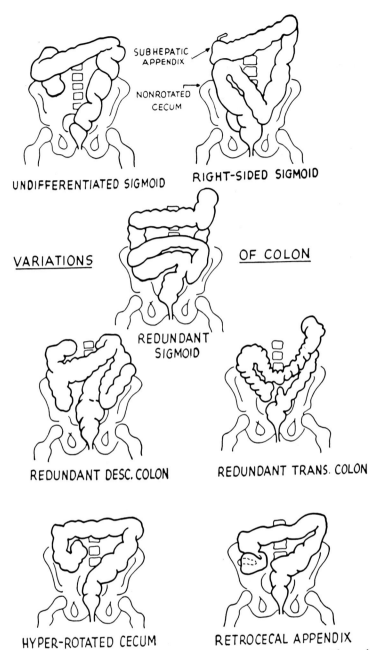

UNDIFFERENTIATED SIGMOID   RIGHT-SIDED SIGMOID

SUBHEPATIC APPENDIX

NONROTATED CECUM

VARIATIONS   OF COLON

REDUNDANT SIGMOID

REDUNDANT DESC. COLON   REDUNDANT TRANS. COLON

HYPER-ROTATED CECUM   RETROCECAL APPENDIX

Figure 14–9. Variations in contour and position of the cecum. The redundancy of various parts of the colon is also illustrated.

The lower portion of the ascending colon may be on a partial mesentery, and, like the cecum, rather anterior in position, but very soon it proceeds posteriorly in most instances, assuming a partially covered retroperitoneal position. When it reaches the inferior surface of the liver, it turns forward and to the left (forming the hepatic flexure). It lies between the quadratus lumborum laterally, and the psoas major muscle medially. Its posterior surface is ordinarily not peritonealized, thus giving it a relatively fixed position, but it is surprisingly mobile radiographically despite these anatomic limitations.

The hepatic flexure is ordinarily situated lateral and anterior to the descending portion of the duodenum, and posterior to the thin anterior margin of the liver. Its peritoneal relations are similar to those of the ascending colon.

The transverse colon has a long mesentery, and as a result is subject to wide variation in length and position. It usually hangs down in front of the small intestine, at a considerable distance from the posterior abdominal wall, with only the greater omentum and anterior abdominal wall lying over it. *Along its first few centimeters, however, it is usually firmly attached to the anterior surface of the second part of the duodenum and the head of the pancreas*—a factor of considerable importance when these structures are distended by a space-occupying lesion, since there is in such cases a secondary displacement of this portion of the colon. Toward the left, the mesentery shortens, bringing this segment close to the tail of the pancreas, with the stomach lying anterior and to the right. At the inferior surface of the spleen, it passes into the splenic flexure, which is again retroperitoneal *but at a higher level than the hepatic flexure.*

The posterior surface of the greater omentum adheres to the upper surface of the transverse mesocolon and to the serosal coating on the anterior side of the transverse colon. The omentum droops down from the greater curvature of the stomach, forming a double fold over the middle part of the transverse colon.

The splenic flexure is perhaps the most constant part of the colon, being held in position by the phrenicocolic ligament, which is attached laterally to the diaphragm opposite the ninth to the eleventh rib posteriorly.

The descending and iliac portions of the colon are the narrowest parts. The descending colon first lies in contact with the lateral margin of the left kidney, and then in a comparable position with the ascending colon on the right. The posterior surface is not peritonealized and the descending colon is less mobile ordinarily than the ascending.

The iliac colon lies in the iliac fossa and, like the descending colon, is not peritonealized on its posterior surface.

The pelvic or sigmoid colon has a mesentery of its own, which accounts for the mobility of this portion of the colon, and is somewhat variable in width. It usually lies for the most part in the pelvis minor, but occasionally with marked redundancy it may escape above into the abdominal cavity. In the child at birth,

lymphoepithelial tissue and some glandular elements such as argentaffine cells, the latter of which give rise to carcinoid tumors, the appendix being a frequent site of these neoplasms. Since the lumen of the vermiform appendix is often patent, it may be visualized radiographically at the time of a barium enema or following the ingestion of oral barium.

THE COLON

ANOMALIES OF THE CECUM, ABNORMALITIES OF POSITION

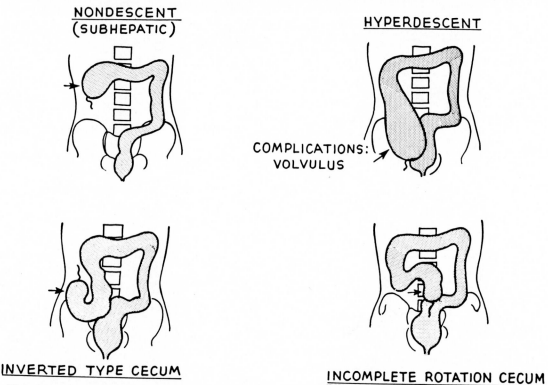

Figure 14–10. Variations of the contour of the ascending colon in particular, demonstrating abnormalities of contour as well as position of the cecum.

owing to the small size of the pelvis minor, only the terminal part of the pelvic colon lies in this area. In the child, the pelvic colon usually arches over to the right side, and lies in great part in the right iliac fossa. At the termination of the pelvic colon, it arches backward and downward to form the rectosigmoid junction.

The rectosigmoid junction is usually the narrowest point in the colon, and this narrowness may extend for 1 to 1.5 cm. *This narrowness sometimes is difficult to distinguish from an abnormal constriction,* and the radiologist must be thoroughly familiar with the normal variations of this region (Fig. 14–20D). Ordinarily, the rectosigmoid junction is found at the level of the third sacral vertebra. The peritoneal coat continues down from the sigmoid but only over the anterior and lateral rectal walls for about 1 to 2 cm.

The rectum is a true retroperitoneal organ. The peritoneal reflection between the rectum and the bladder in the male, or between the rectum and the uterus in the female forms the *rectovesical* or *rectouterine recess or pouch.*

Rectum and Anal Canal. The rectum and anal canal are more accurately examined by the proctoscope and sigmoidoscope and by digital palpation than by radiographic methods, and for that reason less radiographic emphasis is placed upon these regions. The rectum has only a partial covering of peritoneum, and no sacculations; it is very distensible, particularly in its midportion, and this area is therefore called the rectal ampulla. The rectum first follows the hollow of the sacrum and coccyx, and then turns gently forward and finally abruptly downward to join the anal canal. There are three (and sometimes as many as five) crescentic folds, called the plicae transversales (plicae of Houston), which project into the lumen of the rectum. These pass around two-thirds of the rectal circumference and produce indentations on the radiograph of the rectum. They are variable in position and occasionally are poorly developed or virtually absent. It is probable that these are similar in origin to the plicae semilunares of the rest of the colon, but in the absence of the taeniae coli they take on a somewhat different appearance. There are creases in addition, however, that involve the entire wall of the rectum in their structure.

Some of the distinguishing features of the anal canal and rectum in relation to the sigmoid are shown in Figure 14–11. The superior and inferior plicae of Houston or rectal valves (also called the plica transversalis of Kohlrausch) are located on the left side, between 2 and 4 cm. from the rectosigmoid junction. The middle rectal valve lies just inferior to the peritoneal cul-de-sac, usually on the right side at or slightly above the level of the peritoneal reflection, approximately the distance that a probing finger can reach in rectal digital examination. This is usually the largest of the three valves, but their size varies individually, as does their number. These rectal valves occupy one-third to one-half the circumference of the rectum. The superior rectal valve is below the level of the rectosigmoid junction, which has also been called the

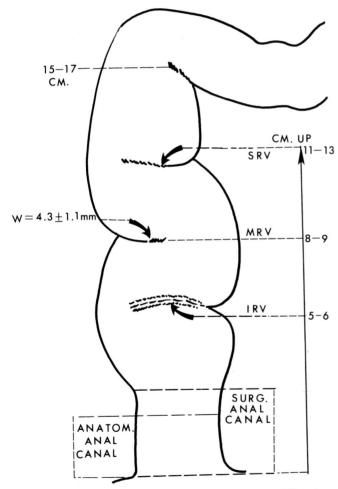

Figure 14–11. Diagram illustrating the rectum, the valves of Houston, and the position of the rectosigmoid junction. (W) Width, (SRV) superior rectal valve, (MRV) middle rectal valve, (IRV) inferior rectal valve.

"third sphincter" (Cohen). Although there is considerable variability in the rectal valves, some identification of them is possible roentgenographically (in 83 per cent of cases in the lateral projection, according to Cohen).

The sphincteric portion of the rectum is actually the upper third of the surgical anal canal, usually about 4 to 6 cm. above the anal verge.

The lower two-thirds of the surgical anal canal is identical with the *anatomic anal canal*, and extends to the margin where the anal tube opens outward, approximately where hair stops growing in the margin of the anal skin.

The axis of the anal canal is, in adults, directed anteriorly toward the umbilicus, in contrast to that of the rectum, which is directed posteriorly along the margin of the sacrum. *However, in infants, both the rectal and anal axes take the same direction because the child still lacks the adult rectal curves. This may predispose to anal and rectal prolapse in childhood.*

The average width of the prominent rectal fold is 4.3 mm. ± 1.1 mm., with a range of 2 to 7 mm. The 95 per cent limit is therefore approximately 6.5 mm.

The fascia of Waldeyer is a thin layer of fatty areolar tissue which lies anterior to the sacrum between it and the rectal wall. This layer is continuous with the extraperitoneal layer of areolar tissue. When the rectum is filled with barium, it balloons out to fill the hollow of the sacrum so that the presacral space normally becomes very small. Examples of normal and abnormal appearances are shown in Figure 14–12. When the rectum is empty the space is rather large because the rectum falls away from the sacral concavity. The retrosacral distance in randomly selected normal patients is usually less than 1 cm. in width, with a mean value of 0.7 cm. and a range of 0.2 to 1.6 cm. It is thought that any measurement above 2 cm. can be interpreted as abnormal (Chrispin and Fry). Others have measured this distance more conservatively (Edling and Eklof), but in our experience the measurements of Chrispin and Fry apparently are more applicable. When this space was measured in a large series of children without signs of inflammatory large bowel disease, it was found to range between 1 and 5 mm., with over half of the measurements falling at 3 mm. (Eklof and Gierup). These measurements are 2 mm. below those given by Rudhe.

Normal Anatomic Relationships and Variations of Position in the Colon

1. Although in most patients the ascending colon is "retroperitoneal," usually to the point where it passes over the inferior portion of the right kidney, there is a mesentery, albeit short, of the ascending colon in 26 per cent of persons (Treves).

2. It will be recalled that the transverse mesocolon is attached to the midportion of the head of the pancreas and to the inferior surface of the body and tail of the pancreas. It passes above the duodenojejunal junction and over the upper portion of the an-

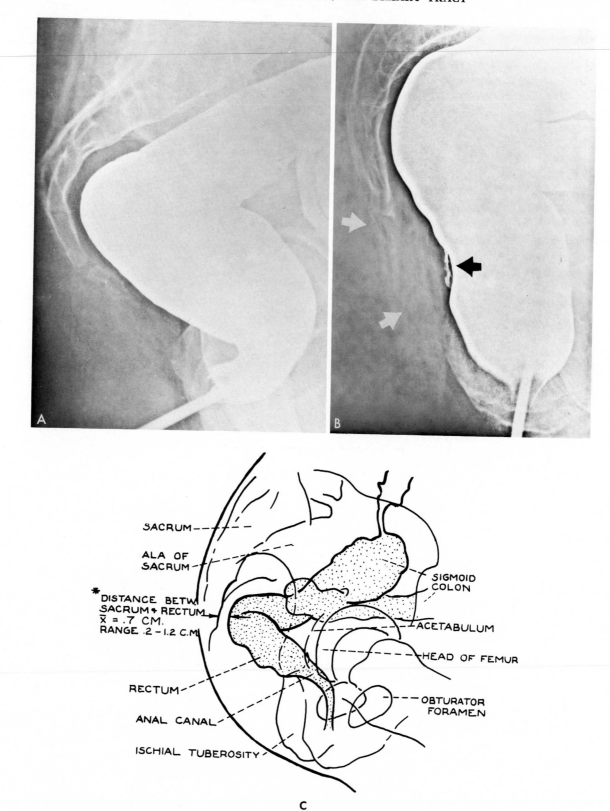

Figure 14–12. Lateral view of sacrum, coccyx, and barium-filled rectum, demonstrating (*A*) normal close application of rectum to sacrum and coccyx even with sharp angulation of the sacrum, and (*B*) displacement of barium-filled rectum by a chordoma which has partially destroyed the tip of the sacrum and adjoining coccyx. C. Diagram showing rectosacral distance and its measurement.

terior surface of the left kidney, and then descends abruptly. It is fixed at this level by the phrenicocolic ligament.

3. The colon in this region is related closely to the inferior and posterior portions of the tip of the spleen—this relationship is illustrated in Figure 14–13. This ligament is a strong peritoneal fold, extending from the splenic flexure of the colon to the parietal peritoneum overlying the posterolateral aspect of the diaphragm at the level of the eleventh rib. This is the most posterior portion in position of the entire colon. The splenic angle, radiographically visualized because of contrast afforded by extraperitoneal fat (see Chapter 15), marks the site of the phrenicocolic ligament on a plain radiograph. At this site the colon becomes retroperitoneal and starts to descend. This ligament also bridges the limit of the left paracolonic gutter and is related to some of the roentgen signs of abnormality, thus assuming considerable significance at times (Meyers) (for more detail on the colon "cutoff sign" see *Analysis of Roentgen Signs*).

4. The descending segment of the colon is without a mesen-

tery in 64 per cent of the cases, while 36 per cent do have a mesocolon (Treves).

5. The relationship of frontal and lateral perspectives of the colon has been very carefully documented by Whalen and Riemenschneider, and is shown in Figure 14–14. In this correlation they point out that the splenic flexure as visualized roentgenographically may not actually represent the point of anatomic splenic flexure. Thus, in their diagram, all of the area from points 4 to 5 (Fig. 14–14) is mesenteric, since although point 4 is that portion of the colon which has been called the splenic flexure roentgenographically, it is point 5 that is actually fixed retroperitoneally, is in constant relation to the inferior tip of the spleen, and hence, is the point of attachment of the phrenicocolic ligament. The area of attachment of the phrenicocolic ligament is indeed a constant one to look for.

6. Such close analysis of the relationship of the colon to contiguous organs is important in predicting causes of displacement of the colon, such as: (a) enlargement of the liver will depress

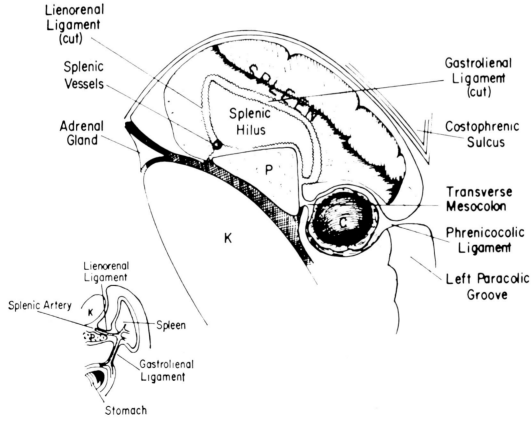

Figure 14–13. The phrenicocolic ligament is continuous with the transverse mesocolon and the gastrolienal ligament and indirectly with the lienorenal and gastrocolic ligaments. Posteriorly and laterally, it reflects to the parietal peritoneum. The small horizontal diagram shows the tail of the pancreas ensheathed intraperitoneally by the leaves of the lienorenal ligament. (From Meyers, M. A.: Radiology, 95:539–545, 1970.)

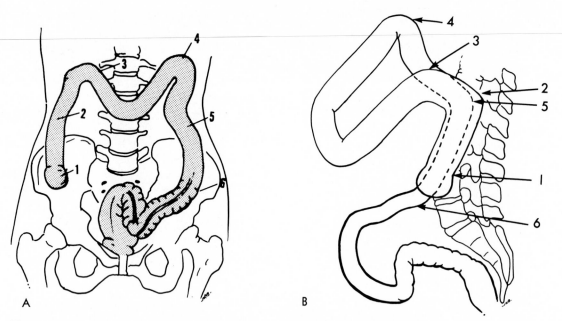

Figure 14–14. Diagrammatic drawings of the entire colon in frontal (A) and lateral (B) projections. The known anatomic portions of the colon are labeled from 1 to 6. (1) Ileocecal area; (2) the most distal portion of the fixed retroperitoneal right colon, the most posterior portion of the right flexure; (3) the area of the colon as it passes over the second portion of the duodenum, where the mesentery begins to lengthen; (4) the roentgenographic splenic flexure; (5) the anatomic splenic flexure; (6) that portion of colon which again becomes mesenteric, the beginning of the sigmoid colon. (From Whalen, J. P., and Riemenschneider, P. A.: Amer. J. Roentgenol., 99:55–61, 1967.)

point 2 of the colon (Fig. 14–14) and push to the left the area between points 2 and 3; (b) enlargement of the gallbladder will depress point 3, but will not affect the area from points 2 to 3; (c) right kidney masses will displace anteriorly the area from points 2 to 3 and will depress this segment (with the exception of lesions of the inferior pole of the right kidney which lie beneath the mesocolon, and which would thus elevate the segment from points 2 to 3); (d) right adrenal masses will displace the colon in the same way as would masses affecting the upper pole of the right kidney.

(e) Lesions of the pancreas will depress the area of the colon between points 3 and 4, at the point of insertion of the mesocolon.

(f) Lesions of the left kidney will elevate the distal portion of the segment from point 3 to point 4, and will laterally displace the portion of the colon from point 4 to point 5. Most of the kidney tissue on the left side is below the insertion of the mesocolon, and the fixed portions of the left colon are lateral to the kidney (exception: a mass arising in the superior pole of the left kidney).

(g) Left adrenal masses will displace the colon in the same way as a mass situated in the superior portion of the left kidney, depressing the segment between points 4 and 5.

(h) Enlargement of the spleen will depress point 5 of the colon and displace to the right and anteriorly the portion from point 4 to point 5. An enlargement in the region of the tail of the pancreas could displace the colon in the same way as masses in or enlargements of the spleen.

(i) Retroperitoneal tumors will displace the colon anteriorly from points 1 to 3 and points 5 to 6.

Distinguishing Features between the Large and Small Intestines. Those features which distinguish the large from the small intestine are: (1) the *taeniae coli,* which are longitudinal bands of muscle running along the outer surface of the large intestine and symmetrically placed around its circumference; (2) the *appendices epiploicae,* which are small peritoneal processes projecting from the serous coat of the large intestine; and (3) the *haustral sacculations* of the large intestine (Fig. 14–15).

The taeniae coli are the three longitudinal muscle bands into which the longitudinal musculature of the large intestine is principally concentrated; they pass from the cecum to the rectum, where they disappear in a fan-shaped process to form a more continuous layer of muscle around the rectum.

The appendices epiploicae usually contain fat and project from the serous coat of the entire large intestine, with the exception of the rectum. Their importance radiologically lies in the fact that occasionally they undergo calcification.

The haustral sacculations are produced by crescentic folds of the entire wall of the large bowel that result in a segmented appearance, each haustral segment measuring 3 to 5 cm. in length.

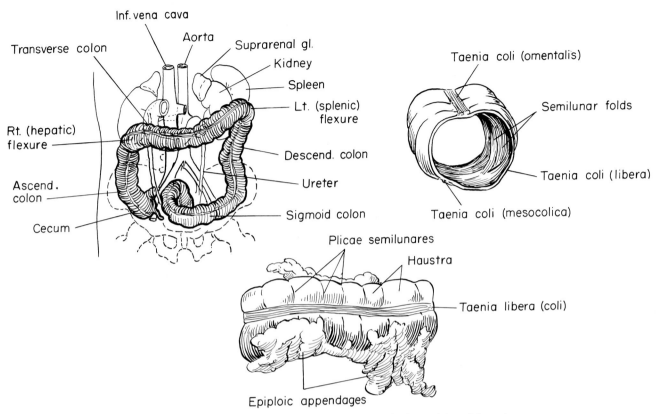

Figure 14–15. Distinguishing anatomic features and relationships of the colon.

There are creases or folds on the interior of the large intestine that correspond with the external folds, which are called the plicae semilunares of the colon. These plicae differ from those of the small intestine in that: (1) they contain not only the mucosal fold, but the submucosal layer and also a portion of the muscular layer as well; and (2) they are much more widely separated—each of these folds extends around one-third the circumference of the wall of the large intestine between two taeniae coli.

The radiographic representation of these differences (Fig. 14–3 and 4) between the plicae circulares of the small intestine and the plicae semilunares of the colon is of considerable practical significance in attempting to differentiate the gas-distended small and large intestine. The plicae circulares are very closely placed with respect to one another, and are most conspicuous in the jejunum and least conspicuous in the ileum. Occasionally, they are completely effaced in the ileum. They form a sharp margin with the outer wall of the small bowel, since they are purely mucosal folds, and have no contribution from the outer layers of the wall of the small bowel. The plicae semilunares of the colon, on the other hand, are usually 3 to 5 cm. apart, are most conspicuous in the transverse colon, and have rounded margins, in which there is a contribution from the entire wall of the large intestine.

The widest parts of the colon are the cecum and the full rectum. There is a gradual diminution in the caliber of the colon from the cecum to the rectosigmoid junction.

Mucosal Pattern of the Large Intestine. When the colon is full (Fig. 14–16) only the normal haustral pattern of the colon is visible. This is slightly more irregular in the ascending colon than in the transverse, and *may be virtually absent in the descending colon and sigmoid* when the latter portions of the colon are examined radiographically. The haustral appearance of the descending and pelvic colons is therefore variable.

When the colon is empty (Fig. 14–17), its mucosa is thrown into numerous irregular folds. These folds, however, are coarser than those of the small intestine because of the lack of the plicae circulares and villi. The pattern, however, is an irregular mosaic throughout the colon, except in the iliac and pelvic colons where these folds assume a more regular and parallel appearance. The pattern of the cecum (Fig. 14–18) differs also slightly from that of the rest of the colon, in that there is a greater tendency toward a spiral arrangement of the rugal pattern.

An examination of the rugal pattern of the colon is a very important part of the colonic examination, and for that reason a film after evacuation of a barium enema is never omitted.

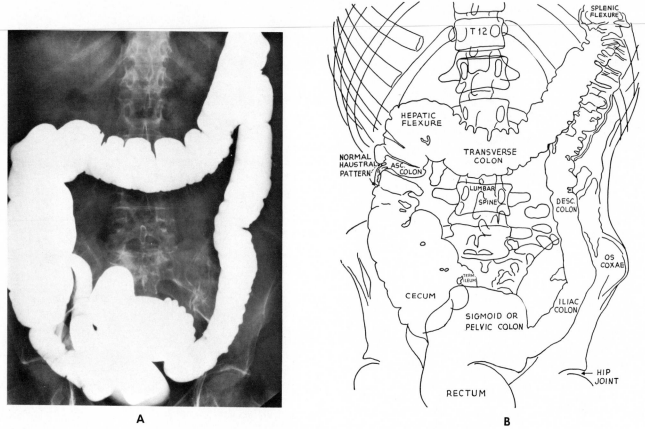

Figure 14–16. Colon distended with barium. *A.* Radiograph. *B.* Tracing.

Special Anatomy of the Vermiform Appendix. The appendix usually arises from the cecum on its medial or posterior aspects, about 2.5 to 4 cm. from the ileocecal valve. It is extremely variable in size and position (Figs. 14–9; 14–10). There is a "valve" at its orifice in the cecum that probably does not function in life, although occasionally the appendix even with a patent lumen will not fill immediately at the time of a barium enema and will be seen to contain barium 24 or more hours later.

At postmortem examination total occlusion of the lumen of the appendix is found in 3 or 4 per cent of cases, whereas almost total or partial obliteration of the lumen is found in an additional 25 per cent (Cunningham). In persons past the age of 60, the lumen is obliterated in more than 50 per cent of the cases, and may represent a retrogressive normal change with age.

In disease of the appendix, its lumen is obliterated in practically all (but not all) instances, but since obliteration of the appendix in the adult is such a frequent finding without definite disease, the mere lack of visualization of the appendix radiographically is not indicative of abnormality. However, when the appendix is visualized, it can be taken as good evidence, though not conclusive, of a normal appendix.

Fecal concretions and calculi (called "coproliths") are found in the appendix under many circumstances, and may permit a partial visualization of this structure, despite their presence. In infants and children a coprolith of the appendix usually is indicative of associated appendicitis.

Variation in Size and Position of the Subdivisions of the Colon. The dividing line between anatomic variations and congenital malformations is not a sharp one. Marked redundancies of the sigmoid colon and transverse colon are found so frequently that they can be considered anatomic variants. These various types of redundancies are illustrated in Figure 14–19.

Failures of rotation, however, are congenital aberrations which have considerable practical significance. These are outside the scope of the present text, but the most frequent of these are illustrated (Fig. 14–19). In nonrotation of the cecum, the cecum lies lateral to the ascending colon, and the appendix ascends toward the liver, giving rise to the so-called subhepatic appendix (Fig. 14–9). In hyper-rotation of the colon, the cecum appears to acquire an extra twist which places it medial to the ascending colon, pointing medially or upward (Figs. 14–9, 14–19). The appendix is in a variable position in these cases, but is not found

half of the colon. The hindgut consists of the distal half of the colon beyond the midtransverse colon to the rectum. These areas correspond closely to major blood supply.

Anomalies of intestinal rotation are principally limited to

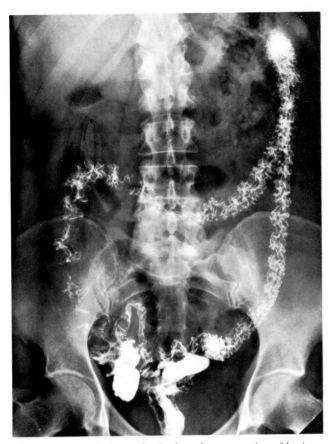

Figure 14–17. Radiograph of colon after evacuation of barium.

in its usual location. A schematic representation of the normal fetal rotation of the midgut in successive stages is shown in Figure 14–19 C. The foregut consists of the stomach and superior portion of the duodenum down to approximately the major papilla of the duodenum. The midgut consists of the remaining portion of the duodenum, the whole of the small intestine, and the proximal

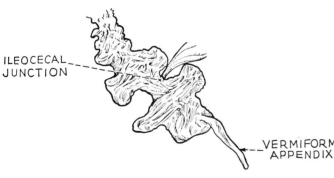

Figure 14–18. Representative mucosal pattern of cecum.

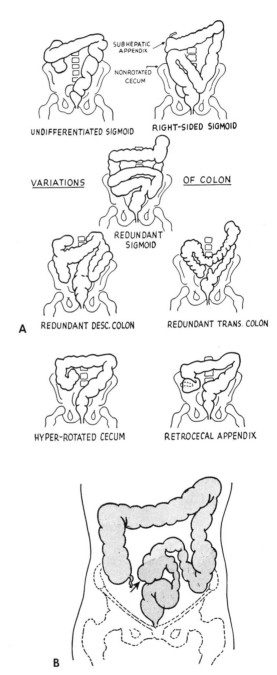

Figure 14–19. *A.* Variations in contour of the normal colon. *B.* Tracing of a colon with marked redundancy of the sigmoid region.

Figure 14–19 continued on the following page.

THE COLON
ANOMALIES OF THE CECUM, ABNORMALITIES OF POSITION

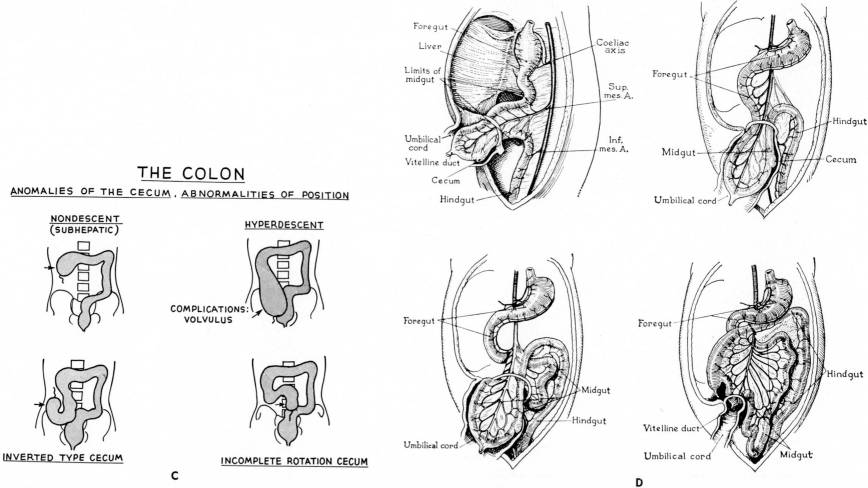

NONDESCENT (SUBHEPATIC)

HYPERDESCENT

COMPLICATIONS: VOLVULUS

INVERTED TYPE CECUM

INCOMPLETE ROTATION CECUM

C

D

Figure 14–19 *Continued.* *C.* Variations of the contour of the ascending colon in particular, demonstrating abnormalities of contour as well as position of the cecum. *D.* Schematic representation of normal fetal rotation of the midgut in successive stages. *Upper left,* Lateral view at the fifth fetal week. The foregut, hindgut, and midgut are suspended from the posterior wall in the common dorsal mesentery. Part of the midgut and superior mesenteric artery protrudes out into the umbilical cord and forms a physiologic umbilical hernia. The foregut derives its blood supply from the celiac axis, the midgut from the superior mesenteric artery, and the hindgut from the inferior mesenteric artery. *Upper right,* Frontal view at the eighth fetal week. The midgut has rotated 90 degrees counterclockwise so that the prearterial segment now lies on the right and the postarterial segment on the left. External rotation is complete. *Lower left,* Frontal view at the tenth fetal week. The midgut is returning to the abdominal cavity and is undergoing internal rotation. *It is noteworthy that the proximal end of the midgut returns first and that it passes to the right and behind the superior mesenteric artery.* Succeeding loops are then packed into the left upper abdominal quadrant and later in the right side and lower portions of the abdomen. *Lower right,* At approximately the eleventh fetal week all of the midgut has returned to the abdominal cavity and has rotated an additional 180 degrees counterclockwise from its position as shown at upper right and a total of 270 degrees from its original position as shown at upper left. The process of rotation is now complete and the mesenteries are then fixed onto the posterior wall of the abdomen in the areas which are indicated in stipple.

In the case of failure of rotation or incomplete rotation the cecum and small intestine remain in their early fetal patterns and, more important, the stage of fixation is missed. Without its anchorage to the posterior abdominal wall, the malplaced midgut is prone to twist around the superior mesenteric artery on a narrow mesenteric pedicle to form a volvulus. The volvulus usually impinges on the third portion of the duodenum and causes complete or incomplete obstruction at this level. (Modified from Golden, Radiologic Examination of the Small Intestine, *in* Caffey, J.: Pediatric X-Ray Diagnosis, 4th ed. Chicago, Year Book Medical Publishers, 1961.)

Figure 14–19 continued on the opposite page.

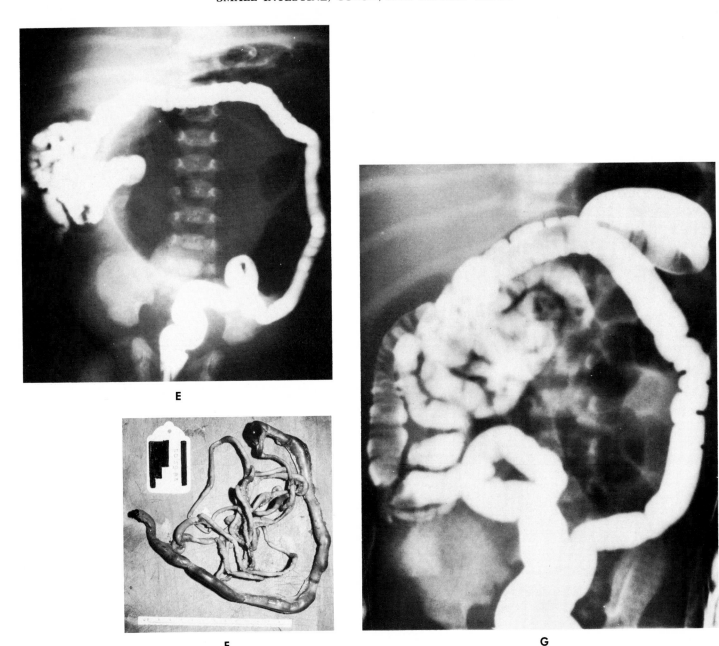

Figure 14–19 *Continued.*   E. Barium enema in an "unused colon" in a neonate with a large peritoneal abscess. F. Photograph of a neonatal "unused colon." G. Barium enema in a neonate with jejunal atresia, but with meconium in the colon.

the midgut. The most common problem is incomplete rotation—the cecum fails to migrate completely from the left lower quadrant to its normal position in the right lower quadrant. The midgut hangs on the superior mesenteric artery. The cecum and terminal ileum are either free or attached in the subhepatic region by peritoneal bands. If the entire midgut is unattached, a

twisting (volvulus) may occur, usually in a clockwise direction. This not only occludes the blood supply to the midgut but also increases the pressure on the duodenum.

Variations in Appearance of the Normal Colon.   Apart from the marked redundancy of the descending colon or sigmoid, or increased mobility of the cecum on its long mesentery with

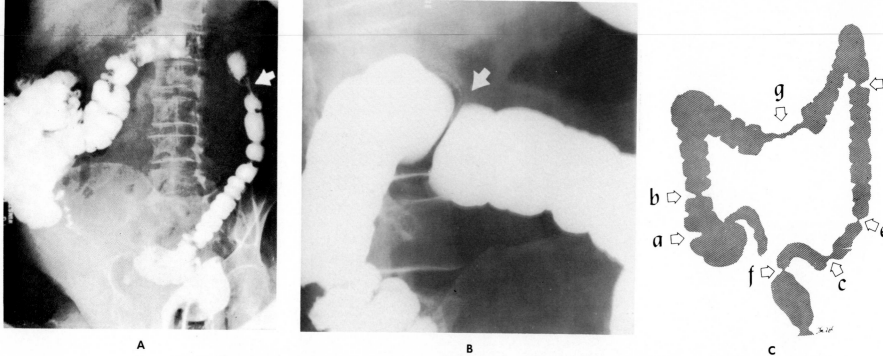

A   **B**   **C**

Figure 14–20. A. Annular constriction in the distal portion of the splenic flexure representing a segmental contraction simulating an area of abnormal narrowness. This is the so-called Payr-Strauss focal contraction. B. Radiograph demonstrating an area of segmental contraction in the transverse colon just beyond the hepatic flexure at
Cannon's ring point. C. The approximate locations of inconstant segmental contractions which may simulate disease in the barium-filled colon. They are designated by the names of their describers; *a*, Busi; *b*, Hirsch; *c*, Moultier;
d, Payr-Strauss; *e*, Balli; *f*, Rossi; *g*, Cannon's ring. (Part *C* after Templeton, *in* Bockus, H. L.: Gastroenterology.
Vol. 2, 2nd ed. Philadelphia, W. B. Saunders Co., 1964.)

Figure 14–20 continued on the opposite page.

various rotational abnormalities, there are other variations of
normal as follows:

1. *Variations in the Appearance of the Haustral Pattern.*
There are seven areas of normal narrowness or focal contraction
of the colon that are inconstantly seen radiographically and that
are not found at autopsy. These must be carefully differentiated
from organic or neoplastic defects. The most common of these is
Cannon's ring, which is located approximately in the middle of
the transverse colon and represents the junction of the primitive
midgut and hindgut. The other areas of narrowness producing
somewhat similar appearances are shown in Figure 14–20 *A, B,
C,* and *D.*

2. *Innocuous Filling of Intestinal Glands or Innominate
Grooves* (Williams; Sasson; Dassel). The major secretion obtained from the colon is mucus from small cryptlike glands—the
glands of Lieberkühn. Ordinarily, mucus is not grossly discernible in the feces unless excretion is excessive. When barium sulfate enters the colonic glands or small innominate grooves, particularly in the sigmoid colon, a spiculated appearance is
produced along the margins of the colon that simulates small
mucosal ulcers and sawtoothing (Fig. 14–21 *A, B*). The glands of

Lieberkühn are straight tubular glands with central crypts 0.5 to
0.7 mm. long. These are ordinarily perpendicular to the surface
and are regularly and profusely distributed over the mucosa of
the colon. The individual spicules may be scattered 3 to 5 mm.
apart, and they may be limited to a single segment or distributed
throughout the entire colon. Patients in whom this appearance
was seen have ranged in age from 2 ½ to 49 years. This should be
regarded as a transient, normal observation when the colon is
otherwise normal in length, caliber, and haustral pattern.

3. *The "Unused" Colon of a Neonate.* The gastrointestinal
tract in the healthy newborn infant has received considerable
study, but generally results are so variable that conclusions are
difficult (Henderson; Smith, 1959). The intestinal tract at birth is
longer in proportion to the length of the body than is the case in
adult life, and this disproportion is even more marked during the
second year of infancy. Apparently, all the glandular elements
found in the normal gastrointestinal mucosa of adults are present
at birth, although glandular structures are more shallow, especially at premature birth. In the newborn, the colon is redundant,
its haustrations are relatively shallow, and its musculature is
relatively active. Its capacity would appear to be between 6 and

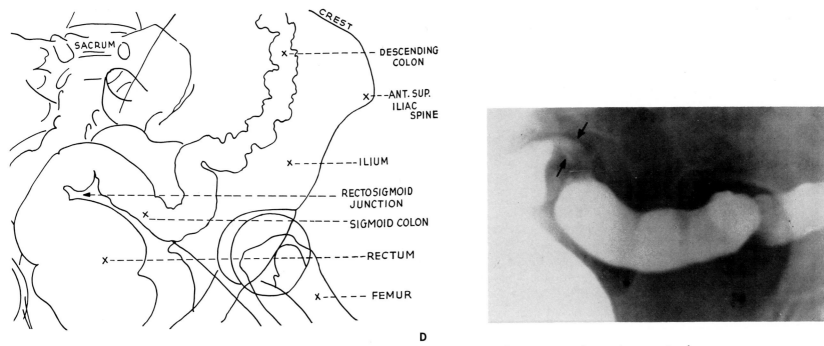

Figure 14-20 *Continued.* D. Oblique study of the rectosigmoid junction demonstrating a frequently encountered normal narrowness. A labeled tracing from another normal patient is shown for comparison.

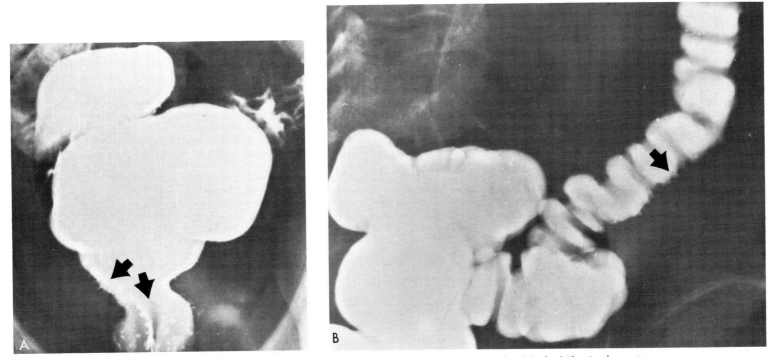

Figure 14-21. A. Radiograph demonstrating barium sulfate entering the glands of Lieberkühn in the rectum. When perpendicular to the surface, these present a dotlike pattern. B. Similar granular crypts demonstrated in profile in the region of the sigmoid simulating diverticulosis.

75 ml. of an opaque mixture. The neonatal intestine shows a relatively greater thickness of mucosa as compared to the muscle coats. Thus, the ratio of mucosa to muscle in the newborn subject is 23 to 26, whereas in the adult it is 27 to 41. The wall of the colon is relatively better developed than that of the small bowel.

There is no uniformity in the appearance of the colon; dogmatic descriptions are unwarranted and anatomic classification is highly variable. Generally, motility, especially of the stomach, is much more variable than it is in adults, and the stomach empties more slowly in the newborn period than at any other time of life. It is probable that the composition of the substance ingested is important since human milk leaves the stomach and reaches the large intestine more rapidly than does cow's milk in particular formulas. The jejunum in the newborn lacks sufficient muscle to throw the outline of its contents into the mucosal folds as is commonly observed in older subjects. Segmentation into isolated masses is therefore the most frequent observation, and "puddling" is the most frequent description of the ileum. Food eaten by a newborn infant requires from 3 to 6 hours at least before it begins to arrive at the cecum, and it appears in the stool in only a little more than 8 hours.

Meconium is first demonstrable in the bowel of the human fetus at 4 or 5 months gestation. The meconium tends to become increasingly firm, solid, and dark as gestational life progresses. At birth its amount is estimated to be from 60 to 200 grams, and it is described as "viscid, sticky, dark greenish-brown to black." In meconium ileus, the meconium is extremely viscid and it tends not to be propelled satisfactorily in the gastrointestinal tract. Hence, it is felt that pancreatic enzymes, which are lacking in meconium ileus, are responsible for the normally semifluid state of meconium. Usually, the normal infant passes some meconium within the first 10 hours of life, although failure to pass meconium in the presence of a normal alimentary tract may occur for over 24 hours after birth. Ninety per cent of normal infants will, however, pass meconium during the first 24 hours. The meconial characteristics disappear from the fecal mass by about the fourth day.

In a series of studies on the gastrointestinal tract from the small intestine to the colon in the newborn, it was noted that the caliber of the ileum and the colon after an opaque meal were so nearly the same that this measurement alone gave no clue to the location of the barium (Henderson). Often it was only when the barium was seen in the rectosigmoid colon that the examiner was certain that he had been observing barium-filled segments of the colon and not ileum. In antegrade studies in the newborn it is very difficult to outline the cecum, but by means of a barium enema the cecum begins to resemble its adult shape, although smaller.

The cecum at times appears to be separated from the ascending colon by a valvelike constriction at the ileocecal level. Although the appendix is not infrequently demonstrated by barium enema, it does not usually appear when the barium mixture has been orally administered.

When antegrade study of the colon is performed, the barium tends to be clumped as it is in the ileum, and it is not until 7 or 8 hours after a barium meal that one sees a continuously filled portion of colon; this usually appears in the descending and sigmoid area. Motility in the colon is generally more rapid in the infant than in the adult. In antegrade studies at the end of 24 hours, most of the barium meal has left the intestinal tract.

In studies utilizing a barium enema there is considerable variation in the total length and regional topography of an infant's colon compared with that seen in an adult. It is indeed difficult to fill the colon around to the cecum in the newborn infant. Colonic spasm occurs frequently. Marked variation in total length of the colon is seen; some are slightly redundant while in others there is a great deal of reduplication, sometimes to such an extent that it is difficult to follow the course of the bowel. The contour of the colon in the newborn is almost invariably smooth and its contents are "mushy." At times, meconium, adherent to the wall, imparts a ragged contour to the mucosa. Approximately four-fifths of infants studied will have some indication of a haustral pattern, although in most this pattern will be shallow. Haustrations are more evident after evacuation of the barium.

Although initially the "unused" or relatively unused colon may be of very small caliber and not redundant, it is apparent as additional barium flows into the colon that the sigmoid particularly is capable of much dilatation and apparent elongation; hence, the visible redundancy is dependent on the amount of mixture used. This is particularly true if the ileocecal valve is not relaxed.

A right-sided sigmoid is visible more often than one in the left abdomen, and in most cases the sigmoid is in the midline. The lumen size can be controlled by the amount of mixture used. The appearance of reduplication of the descending colon may be obtained in approximately a third of the cases, and the incidence of redundancy in the splenic flexure and in the transverse colon is about the same as it is in the descending portion (Henderson and Bryant).

The site of the ileocecal valve is much more clearly demarcated in the colon of the newborn infant than in the adult, and a definite separation is seen in the majority of infants. The fetal type of cecum can be anatomically described as conical, with the appendix arising from the apex of the cone and forming a continuation of the long axis of the colon. This is found quite frequently. It is probable that descent of the cecum is completed by the eighth month of fetal life (MacLean and Hertwig, quoted from Henderson and Bryant).

The accompanying illustrations (Fig. 14–19 *D, E, F*) show a barium enema in an "unused" colon in a neonate with a large peritoneal abscess, a photograph of a neonatal "unused" colon, and a barium enema in a neonate with jejunal atresia, but with meconium in the colon suggesting that complete obstruction by the jejunal atresia did not occur until at least some of the meconium content of the small bowel had passed into the colon. This conclusion, however, is not absolute, particularly since autopsy in stillborn infants reveals tenacious meconium adherent to the walls of the colon (Henderson and Bryant).

MOTILITY STUDY OF THE LARGE INTESTINE

The passage of a barium mixture in the adult as viewed fluoroscopically through the large intestine is usually slow and almost imperceptible. While the contents are still fluid, peristaltic activity and a constant head of pressure from the ileum force the barium column onward. When the barium mixture becomes semisolid or solid, it is a mass movement that forces the passage of the colonic contents. In a matter of seconds, the normal haustral pattern of the colon disappears, and an entire long segment of the large bowel appears to close down into a ribbonlike structure. This mass movement then gradually passes over the bowel distal to its site of origin and forces the bowel contents toward the rectum. It may reach the rectum in a matter of 15 or 20 seconds, and shortly thereafter, the original haustral markings once again make their appearance.

Normally, these mass movements do not occur many times during the day, but during a barium enema examination, especially in an irritable colon, they may be seen repeatedly, eventually forcing the evacuation of the colonic contents.

Some investigators, such as Wright, Cole and others, have described a haustral churning motion in which the haustra remain in evidence but change their size. This is a very slow movement, and can be detected ordinarily only in serial radiographic studies. This churning or mixing movement is the same as the segmentation movement previously described in the small intestine. About 2.5 cm. of the circular muscle contracts, sometimes constricting the lumen of the colon to almost complete occlusion. At the same time, the taeniae coli contract longitudinally. These latter haustral contractions reach a peak in about 30 seconds and then disappear during the next 60 seconds, and they may at times move slowly toward the anus during the period of contraction.

The rate of movement through the large intestine is very variable, but under ordinary circumstances the cecum is visualized in 1½ to 4 hours after the oral administration of barium. The head of the barium column will reach the hepatic flexure in 3 to 6 hours, and the splenic flexure in 6 to 12 hours. By 24 hours, usually about one-half of the barium has been evacuated and the remainder scattered in the colon. Ordinarily, the colon is virtually empty of barium in 48 hours, except for a few scattered foci. Variations from this sequence are very frequent, and caution must be exercised in the interpretation of abnormal motility of the large intestine.

Fluid is progressively absorbed from the colon until only

about 80 ml. of the 450 ml. daily load of chyme is lost in the feces (Guyton). The content of the colon tends to be fluid in the ascending colon normally, semifluid as it approaches the hepatic flexure, mushy in the transverse colon, and solid in the lower descending colon. Excess motility causes less absorption and diarrhea or loose feces.

Secretions of the Large Intestine. The surface epithelium of the large intestine contains a large number of goblet or mucus-secreting cells dispersed among the upper epithelial cells; the only significant secretion in the large intestine is mucus. When a segment of the large intestine becomes irritated, however, the mucosa then secretes large quantities of water and electrolytes in addition to the mucus, and this acts to dilute the irritating factors and causes rapid movement of the feces toward the anus. *The lost electrolytes, under these circumstances, contain an especially large amount of potassium (Guyton).*

TECHNIQUE OF RADIOLOGIC EXAMINATION OF THE SMALL INTESTINE (EXCEPT ANGIOGRAPHY)

Barium Meal. Many different types of barium meals have been tested and many different adjuvant agents have been employed. Generally, nonflocculating barium mixed with 50 per cent water is considered most satisfactory (Zimmer; Ardran et al.; Miller; Nelson et al., 1965b; Stacy and Loop).

Different volumes have been recommended—some have used 8 ounces, others, 19 ounces (Schlaeger); Marshak has recommended at least 16 ounces and at times 20 ounces (this has been corroborated by Caldwell and Flock).

Our own experience has favored the utilization of 8 ounces initially under fluoroscopic control. During this time the esophagus, stomach, and duodenum are examined, thereafter an additional 8 ounces are administered prior to the routine film studies. At predetermined intervals (30 to 60 minutes) each film is viewed before the next, and spot filming is done as necessary.

Acceleration of the Barium Meal. From time to time different drugs have been advocated to enhance motility and shorten the time of the small bowel examination. Marshak and Lindner recommend a subcutaneous or intramuscular injection of 0.5 mg. neostigmine. They do not, however, recommend the use of this drug in the elderly or in patients with heart disease, asthma, or mechanical intestinal or urinary tract obstruction. Atropine should be readily available in case a reaction should occur. Sovenyi and Varro have recommended the addition of 30 grams of sorbitol to a barium meal consisting of 400 cc. of water and 125 to 130 grams of nonflocculent barium for study of the small intestine. The small intestinal transit time is thereby shortened to approximately 40 to 60 minutes, and they claim that there is no apparent interference with accuracy of study.

Goldstein et al. compared various methods for acceleration of the small intestinal radiographic examination such as 0.5 mg. neostigmine methylsulfate, the right lateral decubitus position except during roentgenography, and the addition of Gastrografin to the barium mixture. They concluded that adding 10 ml. of Gastrografin to the barium mixture was the most effective method.

Other drugs have also been utilized but may tend to alter the size of the small intestine or its motility—hence, serious doubt is cast on the use of any medication to alter the procedure (Lumsden and Truelove; Holt et al.).

Cold isotonic saline has also been shown to hasten both motility of the small intestine and gastric evacuation (Weintraub and Williams). After the administration of barium sulfate in examination of the stomach and duodenum, the patient is given a glass of cold isotonic saline to drink. One half hour later he is given another glass of the saline. Under these circumstances the ileocecal region is reached in a half hour or an hour instead of the usual longer interval. In a variance of this basic technique, the second glass of isotonic saline is mixed with approximately 100 grams of barium which may enhance the contrast within the small intestine.

Conventional Small Intestinal Series. It is always desirable to have a film of the abdomen without contrast prior to the introduction of any contrast agent.

The patient is allowed no food or drink following the evening meal on the night before the examination.

A routine examination of the esophagus, stomach, and duodenum is carried out as previously described (Chapter 13). The barium column is watched as it passes into the jejunum. When it appears relatively stationary, it has been our practice to administer another 8 ounces of nonflocculent barium mixture as described above and then to obtain a film of the abdomen. Fifteen to thirty minutes later another film of the abdomen is obtained. This film is inspected, and time intervals are designated for the further examination of the passage of the barium in the small bowel. Usually these intervals are approximately 30 to 60 minutes. When the barium has reached the ileocecal region, the patient is examined fluoroscopically once again and spot-film compression studies of the ileocecal region are obtained.

If any abnormalities are seen in the course of the small intestinal series, the patient is restudied by fluoroscopy and the area in question is carefully compressed, palpated, and refilmed by spot-film compression techniques.

A representative routine series is shown in Figure 14–22.

If small bowel or large intestinal obstruction is suspected, a routine series of films for investigation of the abdomen without additional contrast is used prior to the small bowel series. These include chest film, supine anteroposterior view of the abdomen, and upright film of the abdomen or a lateral decubitus if the patient is unable to stand (see Chapter 15). If obstruction is suspected in the large intestine, we have preferred to administer a barium enema first to make certain of the site of the obstruction.

An obstruction in the small intestine is not considered a contraindication to examination with oral barium (Frimann-Dahl; Nelson et al., 1965b).

Small Intestinal Enema. Following the passage of a tube into the duodenum, 500 to 1000 cc. of thin barium solution may be given in a continuous stream by gravity. Thereafter, the entire small bowel is studied as this continuous stream of barium passes through it. Schatzki has indicated that barium reaches the cecum in about 15 minutes under these circumstances.

Modification of Technique with the Postoperative Partially Resected Stomach. The basic modification required for examination of a patient with a partially resected stomach is the study of the small intestine at more frequent intervals, particularly shortly after the administration of the oral barium. Motility through the proximal small intestine is more rapid than normal, but as the barium column reaches the ileum and beyond, motility occurs at normal time intervals.

Intubation Techniques for Study of Small Foci of Involvement. A Miller-Abbott or Cantor tube may be passed and allowed to move down the small intestine until it meets a point of delay or obstruction. The barium mixture is injected through the tube at this point, and the intestine at the site of obstruction is carefully studied without interference of adjoining loops. This technique is particularly useful for studying an area of obstruction, either partial or complete. A length of 6 to 8 feet of tubing is sufficient to extend from the pylorus to the cecum ordinarily. Approximately 3 hours are required for passage. The tube is withdrawn when it has reached the cecum if an obstruction is not present. The instillation of 4 to 8 cc. of liquid metallic mercury into the rubber balloon of the tube facilitates the passage of the tube through the pylorus and increases the rapidity with which the tube passes down the small intestine.

Radiologic Study of the Small Intestine with Water Soluble Iodinated Contrast Media. Various mixtures of water soluble iodide have been utilized for examination of the gastrointestinal tract both orally and rectally.

1. Forty per cent sodium diatrizoate solution (Hypaque) (Shehadi).

2. Forty per cent sodium diatrizoate with oxyphenisatin.

3. Twenty-five per cent diatrizoate solution plus an equal volume of barium sulfate suspension.

4. Forty per cent sodium diatrizoate or methylglucamine diatrizoate (Gastrografin).

5. Fifty grams of sodium diatrizoate dissolved in 75 cc. of sterile water to which 10 drops of a wetting agent such as Tween-80 have been added, to aid in the coating of the mucosa (Jacobson et al.). A flavoring agent must be added if this is used orally.

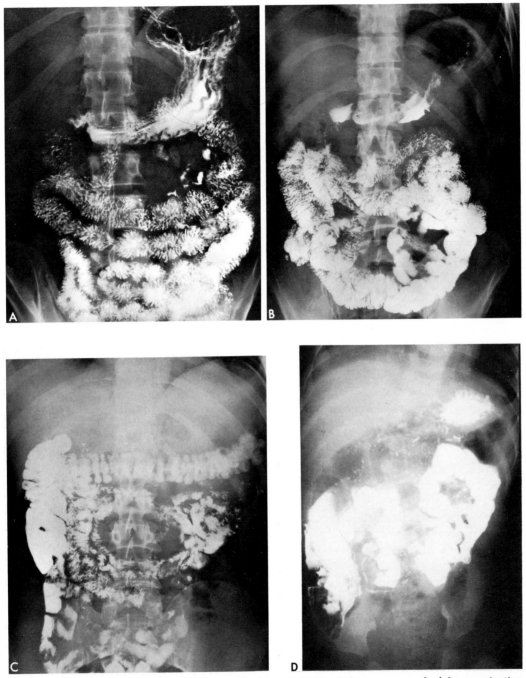

Figure 14–22. Illustrations to demonstrate frequent-interval film and fluoroscopy method for examination of small intestine: *A.* At 1 hour following administration of the barium; *B.* at 2 hours; *C.* at 3 hours. *D.* Representative small intestinal pattern of a normal infant on a predominantly milk diet. Note that the clumping and scattering are relatively normal for infants at this stage of development.

Because of the high tonicity of these water soluble agents, they have not been recommended, especially in children (Neuhauser; Nelson et al., 1965a). The high tonicity of these contrast agents has another result — they are diluted in the small intestine and become less radiopaque in the jejunum and ileum. However, in the colon water is reabsorbed and the contrast improves. The transit time is more rapid than with barium (30 to 90 minutes unless obstruction is encountered).

These water soluble contrast media may be particularly preferred in severely debilitated patients just prior to surgery, in the presence of suspected mesenteric occlusion, and in patients with known diverticulitis when there is a danger of impending perforation or the possibility of leakage of barium into the peritoneal space (Ostrum and Heinz). In general, however, it has been our preference to use the nonflocculent barium mixture described above.

Differences in Infants and Children. Small barium feedings of 1 to 3 ounces are utilized for infants and children. The transit time may be long in the very young (Lonnerblad). Fluoroscopy should be limited to the smallest possible field.

In the first weeks and months of life the normal feathery pattern of the small intestine does not appear. Distinct jejunal markings, however, are usually visible after the fifth month. Segmentation persists much longer (Fig. 14–22 D).

During the first year and until the infant assumes the erect posture, the small intestine lies almost entirely above the pelvis.

Large amounts of gas may be found in the jejunum and ileum during the first two or three years of life.

In general, clumping and segmentation of the barium column are so relatively common in the child (both healthy and sick) that this adult criterion of abnormality cannot be applied (Fig. 14–22 D). Also, the mucosal contours in the terminal segment of the ileum that are usually longitudinal and linear in the adult may normally have a cobblestone pattern in the child. They are probably caused by the greater abundance in the child of solitary and conglomerate lymph follicles, and are largest in the terminal ileum during preadolescence and adolescence.

Intestinal Biopsy Techniques (Wood et al.; Tomenius). In general, these instruments consist of flexible tubes at the lower end of which is a small metal cylinder provided with a circular lateral hole about 2 to 3 mm. in diameter. The capsule contains a circular knife blade. Suction applied with a vacuum pump or a large syringe aspirates a fragment of the mucosa through the opening of the capsule. The knife blade is released, cutting the mucosa fragment, which is then contained within the capsule. In the Crosby capsule the hole is somewhat enlarged, minimizing the occurrence of hemorrhagic artefacts. The capsule is removed as quickly as possible from the gastrointestinal tract, the terminal cylinder is unscrewed, and the mucosal fragments are collected and oriented on a small piece of wet lens paper with the cut surface downward. They are promptly immersed in 10 per cent formalin or a modified Bouin's solution and embedded in paraffin. They are thereafter stained with hematoxylin-eosin or by special staining techniques.

String Test for Bleeding in Upper Gastrointestinal Tract (Fig. 14–23). The original Einhorn string test of 1909 has been modified in two important ways: (1) the application of guaiac stains to the string, and (2) the administration of sodium fluorescein (20 ml., 5 per cent solution) intravenously and the withdrawal of the string 4 minutes thereafter. The string is then examined for fluorescence with a Wood's lamp. The string is a common type with a mercury bag tied to its end. There are small radiopaque gauze markers tied to the string at designated intervals. Approximately the first 40 cm. on the string lie in the esophageal area, 40 to 55 cm. in the gastric area, and beyond 55 to 60 cm. in the duodenal and jejunal areas. The total string length is approximately 150 cm. (Traphagen and Karlan; Smith; Haynes and Pittman).

According to Smith, the incidence of false negative tests is 1.2 per cent. False positive tests can be attributed to eating of meats, beets, tomatoes, gelatin, cherries (red), or chocolate, or to trauma in passing the string. The string must be withdrawn 4 minutes after the intravenous administration of the fluorescein, since fluorescein would be excreted by the major papilla (of Vater) if the procedure is prolonged.

ROENTGENOLOGIC VARIATIONS OF NORMAL

Variations With Age. During the first 3 or 4 months of life, while the infant is still on a milk diet, there is a tendency toward segmentation and lack of continuity of the barium column and delay of transit time. The stomach-to-colon time may be as long as 9 hours in the newborn (Fig. 14–22).

Gas in the small bowel is abnormal except in the very young and the very old (when not excessive). In the young it is due to air swallowing and in the old to a relative hypotonicity of the small intestine. Such changes begin to be particularly manifest beyond the age of 60 years.

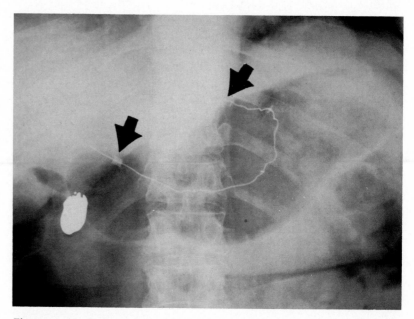

Figure 14–23. Radiograph demonstrating string test for gastrointestinal bleeding.

A persistent deficiency of gas in the small intestine of the newborn infant beyond the first day may be a cardinal sign of intestinal obstruction. However, there are other entities which may be responsible for this appearance, such as adrenal insufficiency, dehydration, diarrhea, and other interference with the normal transport mechanisms.

TECHNIQUE OF RADIOLOGIC EXAMINATION OF THE COLON (EXCEPT ANGIOGRAPHY)

The methods of examination are: (1) the plain radiograph of the abdomen; (2) the barium enema, under fluoroscopic visualization, and accompanied by spot-film compression radiography, in addition to certain routine film studies; (3) the barium meal, followed through until the colon is visualized, and thereafter at 6 hours, 24 hours, and further intervals if desired; and (4) the barium-air double contrast enema (see Fig. 14–24).

Preliminary Plain Radiograph of the Abdomen. If a film of the abdomen has not been obtained in the course of other studies prior to the barium enema, it is well to obtain a posteroanterior film of the abdomen prior to the introduction of any contrast agent. The routine base line film of the abdomen is not only useful from the standpoint of later evaluation after contrast is introduced, but in itself it may reveal significant abnormality (Rosenbaum et al.). Moreover, the appearance of dense inspissated fecal material may indicate the presence of a bowel obstruction. This appearance must also be differentiated at times from extraluminal gas which may produce a somewhat similar appearance.

The Routine Barium Enema

Preparation of the Patient. Thorough cleansing of the colon prior to the barium enema is essential, since any fecal material will obscure the normal anatomy and give rise to false filling defects and mucosal aberrations. This is best accomplished, in our experience, by the following routine:

1. Clear liquid diet for at least 24 hours prior to the examination forcing liquids.

2. One and one-half ounces of X-Prep liquid or its equivalent for catharsis, at 6 P.M. on the evening prior to the examination. As an alternative, a 10 ounce dose of liquid magnesium citrate (U.S.P.) may be administered at 8:00 P.M., followed by 4 Dulcolax tablets (5 mg. bisacodyl each) at 10:00 P.M. (Barnes). If magnesium citrate is used, the patient must drink about 6 glasses of water additionally before midnight.

3. Cleansing enemas prior to the barium enema examination until the returning fluid is clear, unless thorough cleansing of the colon has otherwise been accomplished following the catharsis. A Dulcolax suppository (10 mg.) in the rectum at 7:00 A.M. may be used.

Ordinarily the patient is examined without breakfast, as the breakfast meal will introduce gas in the stomach and occasionally in the colon.

Flocculent barium sulfate suspension is used (Barotrast or its equivalent) and is made by mixing the compounds in a 1 to 4 or up to 1 to 6 mixture, depending upon preference.

TANNIC ACID. Up until March, 1964 we had found it advantageous to introduce ½ to 1 tablespoon of tannic acid per quart of nonflocculating barium suspension in the mixture used for the barium enema. On March 17, 1964 the Commission of Food and Drugs indicated that the medical literature reported "a number of deaths associated with the addition of tannic acid to barium enemas." It indicated that tannic acid "is capable of causing diminished liver function and severe liver necrosis when absorbed in sufficient amounts." In view of these hazards, the Commission of Food and Drugs declared that "tannic acid for rectal use to enhance x-ray visualization is regarded as a new drug," and was not to be used in enemas until complete and further testing had established its safety (Federal Register, March 21, 1964; McAlister et al.). Various substitutes for tannic acid have been recommended, but none to our satisfaction has thus far been found (Reboul et al.). It is probable that adequate colon cleansing, a preparatory clear liquid diet, and the use of well-suspended barium preparations go far toward obtaining satisfactory studies.

At this time, the only tannic acid preparation that may be used as a colonic evacuant is Clysodrast (bisacodyl tannex).* This preparation must be used in accordance with directions. The dosage and administration according to the manufacturer's directions are as follows:

"It is important that the entire medical history and condition of the patient be considered in deciding the dosage regimen. Traumatizing procedures, such as repetition of enemas (with or without Clysodrast) should be kept at the minimum necessary to achieve the desired result.

"*Cleansing enema:* Prepare the cleansing enema by dissolving the contents of one packet (2.5 gm.) of Clysodrast in one liter of lukewarm water and administer.

"*Barium enema:* Prepare the barium enema by dissolving the contents of one or not more than two packets (2.5 gm. or 5.0 gm.) of Clysodrast in one liter of barium suspension. If more than one liter of barium suspension is prepared, it is important that the concentration of Clysodrast (bisacodyl tannex) never exceed 0.5 per cent (two packets per liter). The total dosage of Clysodrast for any one complete colonic examination, including the cleansing enema, should not exceed 7.5 gm. (three packets). No more than 10 gm. (four packets) of Clysodrast should be administered to any individual within a 72 hour period."

A cooperative efficacy study of Clysodrast suggests that in a 0.25 per cent concentration it probably plays an insignificant role

---

*Barnes-Hind Diagnostics, Inc.

in the cleansing of the colon when administered as a preparatory enema (Lasser et al.). It is likely that the completeness of filling of the colon outweighs any other consideration including the ingredients of the agent, in determining the adequacy of a preparatory enema. However, there is good evidence that the Clysodrast in the concentration utilized promoted a more complete contraction of the colon than did any placebo and that the evaluation of mucosal detail of the empty colon was enhanced by the Clysodrast. It has been our impression that this is indeed the main efficacy of the 0.25 per cent tannic acid–barium enema. It should, however, be utilized exactly as directed above. The chemistry of tannic acid, its analysis and toxicology have been reviewed by Krezanoski and the student is referred to this article for greater detail.

For *double contrast enemas* only barium sulfate specially processed for this purpose should be used. The Clysodrast may be added to this barium enema examination as described earlier, but (to repeat) *no more than four packets (10 gm.) of Clysodrast should be administered to any individual within a 72 hour period.* In this instance air without barium may be used following evacuation of the barium enema containing Clysodrast in order to obtain the double contrast.

The manufacturer further states that "Clysodrast is contraindicated in patients under the age of 10 and safe usage in pregnancy of Clysodrast has not been established with respect to the adverse effects upon fetal development. Therefore, it should not be used in women of child-bearing potential, particularly during early pregnancy, except where, in the judgment of the physician, the potential benefits outweigh the possible hazards."

In general, preparation of the patient begins with a residue-free diet the day before the examination. One to two ounces of castor oil (or its equivalent) is administered approximately 16 hours before the examination. On the day of the examination the Clysodrast cleansing enema is given and expelled as described above; it may be repeated if necessary. The patient is then given a barium enema and Clysodrast may be incorporated into the barium sulfate mixture as described above.

Order of the Barium Enema Examination. It has been our preference to perform the barium enema examination *prior* to the study of the upper gastrointestinal tract to avoid any possibility of barium lodging above an unsuspected obstruction in the colon.

We prefer also to examine the urinary tract and biliary system *prior* to the administration of barium orally or by rectum. Telepaque will, of course, introduce opaque material into the colon, and for the best results, the examination of the colon cannot be carried forward on the same day as oral cholecystograms (with Telepaque). In the *massively* bleeding patient, angiograms should be performed before the introduction of any opaque material in the abdomen.

Administration of the Enema. A plastic disposable enema tip and tube are strongly recommended, combined if possible with an enema reservoir. The enema reservoir may also be disposable, or a suitable cap provided between the enema tip and the reservoir to prevent contamination. The reservoir is elevated 3 feet above the table top in adults (or 18 inches in the newborn). For adults the enema reservoir usually contains 2 quarts of the mixture, which is usually adequate for most patients. Occasionally, additional barium must be used. In the newborn infant, 90 ml. of the barium mixture should be more than adequate since the average volume required is 70 mm. Volumes between these two extremes are utilized in the reservoir for different age groups.

The barium is introduced slowly and the examiner should allow the patient to accommodate small increments of the barium as it is introduced. Such slow introduction also allows the examiner to keep "ahead of the barium column" and thus to detect patterns of flow, blockage, filling defects, and mucosal pattern to best advantage. The routine of introduction of the barium and positioning of the patient as well as spot filming is shown in Figure 14–24.

Debilitated patients and those with a relaxed anal sphincter may require an enema tip with a retaining balloon. Great caution must be exercised in the insertion and inflation of such a balloon, since injury to the rectum may result. It is best for the examiner to perform a rectal examination prior to insertion of the balloon, to inflate the balloon very carefully, and to study its position and size fluoroscopically immediately following its insertion. In the presence of a low rectal carcinoma or ulcerative colitis, a balloon is definitely contraindicated. In any case, the use of the balloon should rarely be necessary, since most patients, when properly prepared, experience no difficulty in retaining the enema.

The Fluoroscopic-Radiographic Equipment. The radiographic equipment should be capable of high kilovoltage and high milliamperage with short exposure times. The kilovoltage should be at least 120 Kv. to permit overpenetration of the barium. Photo-timing for spot films is desirable. Image amplifier fluoroscopy is also preferred.

It is our preference to use one hand (left) for manipulation of the exposures and the fluoroscopic screen; the right hand, protected by a heavy lead glove, and kept over the heavy column of barium or outside the direct beam, is used to palpate the patient's abdomen.

Routine for Fluoroscopy. The routine for fluoroscopy is as follows:

1. The patient's abdomen and chest are initially surveyed.
2. Following this survey, the examination is carried out as detailed in Figure 14–24 *A*. The patient first lies on his left side, at an angle of about 60 degrees to the table. The barium mixture is allowed to flow slowly into the rectum to permit the patient to adjust to the liquid mixture being introduced. It should have been warmed to body temperature prior to introduction.

A spot film of the rectosigmoid junction is obtained when this

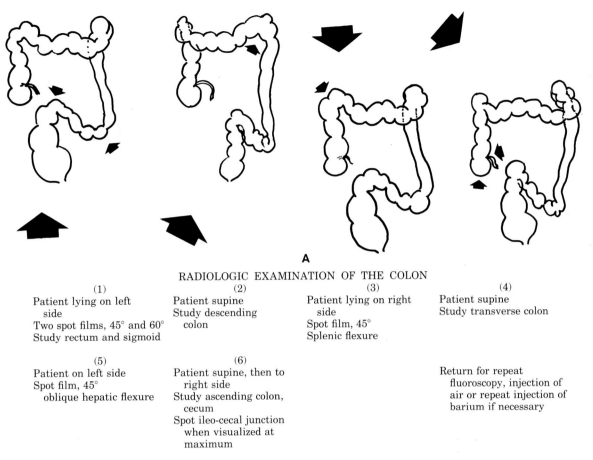

A

RADIOLOGIC EXAMINATION OF THE COLON

(1)
Patient lying on left
    side
Two spot films, 45° and 60°
Study rectum and sigmoid

(2)
Patient supine
Study descending
    colon

(3)
Patient lying on right
    side
Spot film, 45°
Splenic flexure

(4)
Patient supine
Study transverse colon

(5)
Patient on left side
Spot film, 45°
    oblique hepatic flexure

(6)
Patient supine, then to
    right side
Study ascending colon,
    cecum
Spot ileo-cecal junction
    when visualized at
    maximum

Return for repeat
    fluoroscopy, injection of
    air or repeat injection of
    barium if necessary

Figure 14–24.   A. Technique of fluoroscopic examination and spot filming of the colon.

Figure 14–24 continued on the following page.

junction is observed to fill and the barium flow momentarily stops (Fig. 14–24 *B*).

The patient is then lowered slightly to a 45 degree angle and a small amount of barium is introduced so that the entire sigmoid and lower descending colon are filled. Once again there is a cessation of the barium flow and a second spot film is obtained to demonstrate the entire sigmoid and junction with the descending colon (Fig. 14–24 *C*).

The patient then is turned on his back, fully supine, and the barium mixture is again allowed to flow until the descending colon to the level of the splenic flexure can be carefully examined.

The patient is then slowly turned to his right side as the barium mixture is allowed to flow around the splenic flexure, and again the flow ceases while a spot film is obtained of the splenic flexure (Fig. 14–24 *D*).

With the patient supine once more the barium is allowed to flow to fill the transverse colon and the beginning of the ascending colon around the hepatic flexure. The patient is then turned on his left side at an angle of approximately 45 degrees so that the

hepatic flexure is completely unwound, and another spot film is obtained (Fig. 14–24 *E*).

With the patient once again supine, the barium flow continues until the entire cecum is identified and reflux into the ileum through the ileocecal junction is obtained if possible. The patient is turned so that the ileocecal junction is seen to best advantage without interference from adjoining loops of bowel. A spot film is obtained (Fig. 14–24 *F*).

Usually the patient will experience moderate discomfort once the barium column has passed the hepatic flexure into the ascending colon, and the examination must be carried forward expeditiously at this point. Routine films are immediately obtained after the filling and reflux into the distal ileum.

Each of the films must be carefully inspected before the patient is allowed to leave. A repeat study may be undertaken if any questionable areas are seen during the film review. Air may also be injected at this time if necessary, although the ideal double contrast barium enema is a separate examination, as pointed out later.

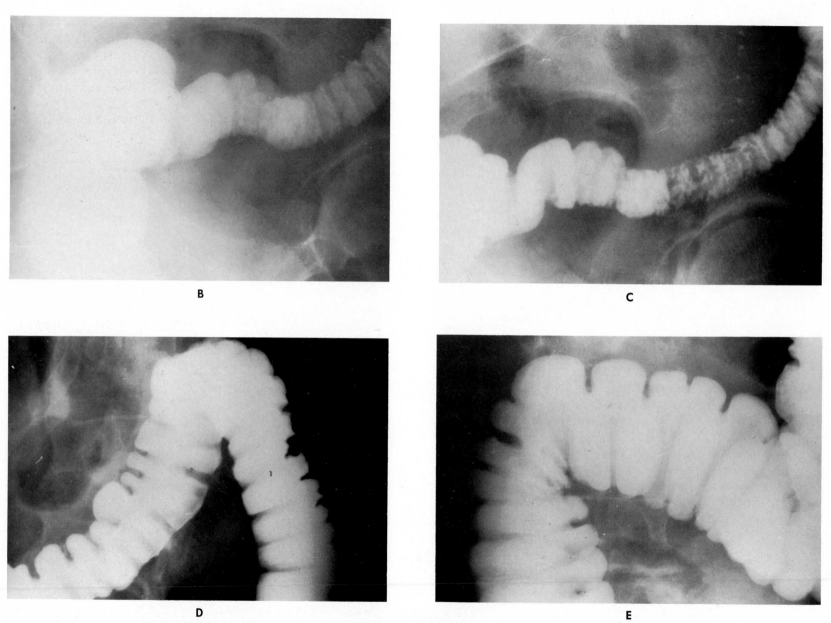

Figure 14–24 *Continued.*   *B* to *F.* Examples of spot films obtained during fluoroscopy of the rectosigmoid, sigmoid, splenic flexure, hepatic flexure, and ileocecal junction.

Figure 14–24 continued on the opposite page.

Routine films following fluoroscopy and spot filming are taken as follows: (1) a high kilovoltage posteroanterior view of the entire colon (Fig. 14–25), (2) a right or left lateral film of the colon centered at the rectosigmoid (Fig. 14–26 *A, B, C*). Oblique films are ordered as required. The spot films may be adequate for this purpose (Fig. 14–27).

Special studies of the rectosigmoid, such as the Chassard-Lapiné view of the rectum and sigmoid may be employed to "unravel" a tortuous and redundant sigmoid (Fig. 14–28). An alternate oblique study of the rectosigmoid and sigmoid colon may be obtained as shown in Figure 14–29 *A* and *B*. Here, the patient lies prone and the central x-ray beam, centered at the level of the anal canal, is directed approximately 35 degrees cephalad. A view very similar to the Chassard-Lapiné view is thereby obtained.

Following colonic evacuation, another posteroanterior prone film of the empty colon is obtained. If the evacuation has not been sufficient, the patient is asked to return after further evacuation for more film studies of the empty colon (Fig. 14–17).

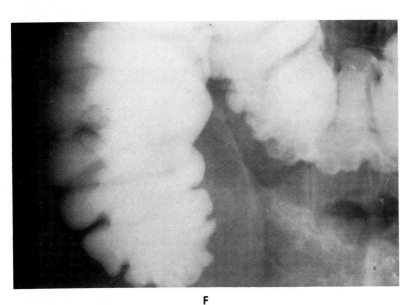

F

Figure 14–24 *Continued.   F. See opposite page for legend.*

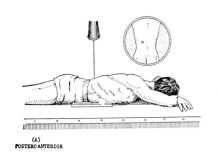

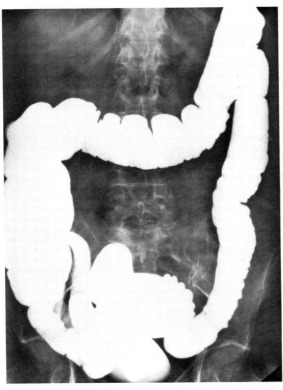

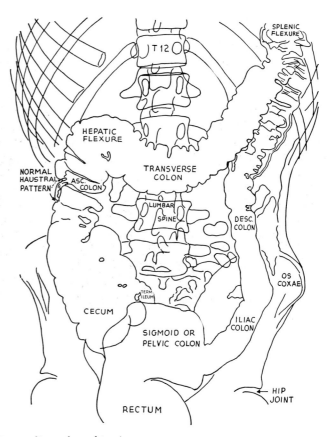

Figure 14–25.   Colon distended with barium: positioning of patient, radiograph, and tracing.

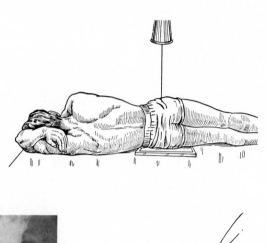

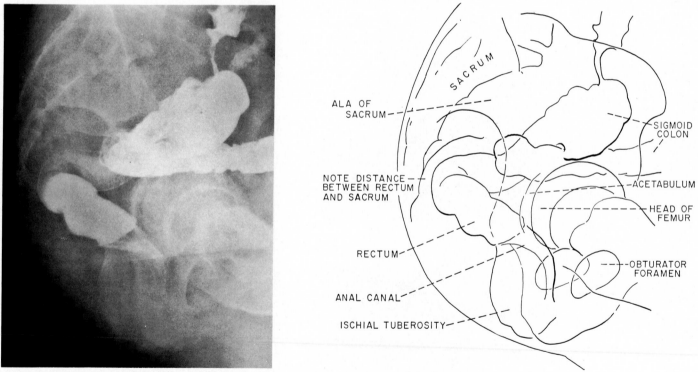

Figure 14–26. Lateral view of the rectosigmoid: positioning of patient, radiograph, and tracing.

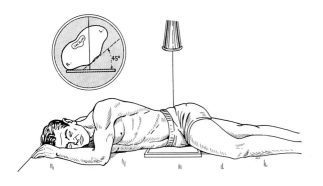

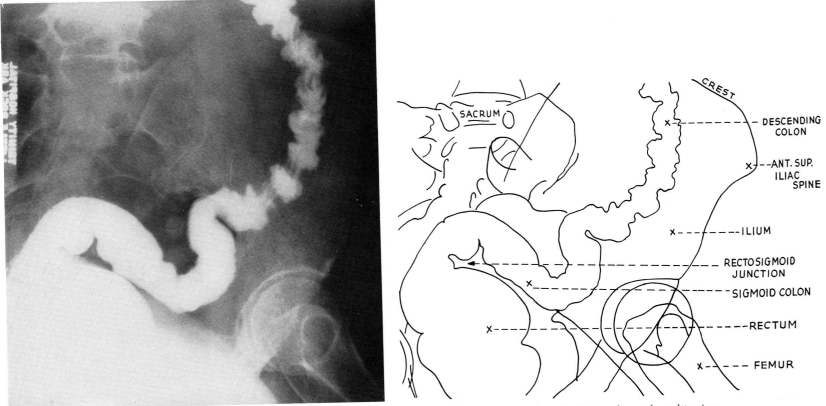

Figure 14-27.   Oblique study of pelvic and iliac colon showing position of patient, radiograph, and tracing.

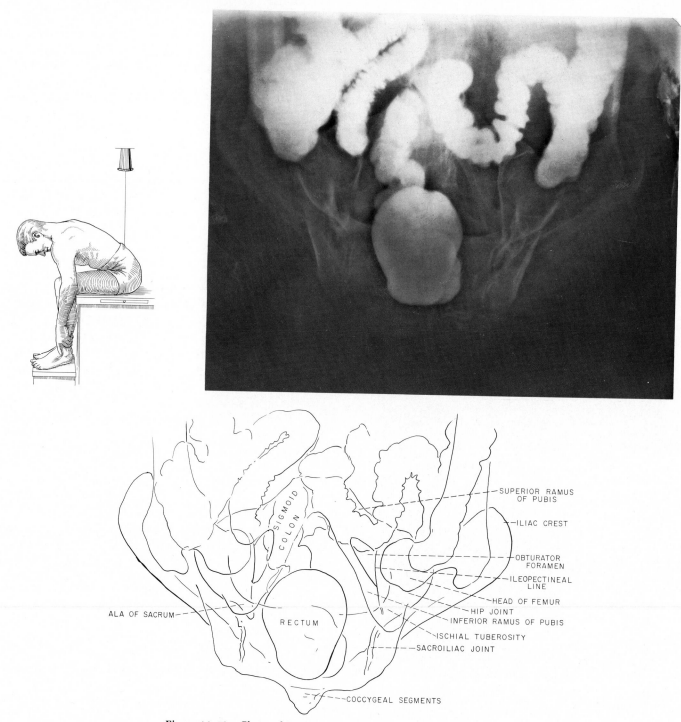

Figure 14–28. Chassard-Lapiné view of the rectum and sigmoid colon.

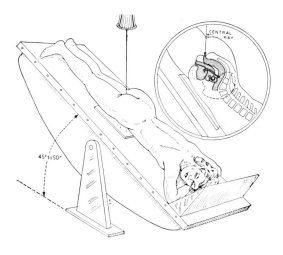

A

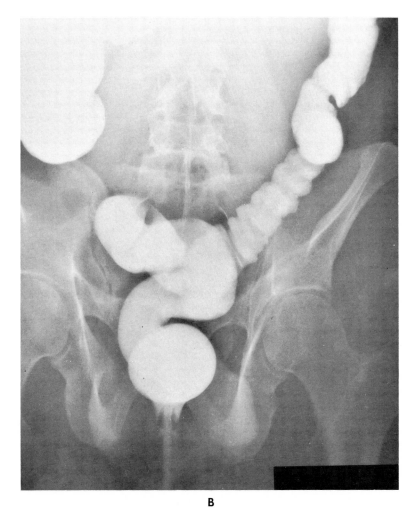

B

Figure 14–29.   Distorted view of sigmoid colon. *A.* Position of patient in relation to central x-ray beam. *B.* Radiograph so obtained.

If indicated, air may be introduced at this juncture for optimal visualization of questionable polypoid defects. *This adjunct is not necessarily a substitute for a properly performed barium-air double contrast enema which will be described later.*

Limitations of the Routine Barium Enema.   The barium enema examination should not be considered a substitute for the digital or sigmoidoscopic examination of the rectum. The rectum is often obscured by its voluminous barium content, or by a balloon, if such was employed, and in the postevacuation study the sigmoid and rectal loops may fold over one another in such a way as to mask a lesion.

Redundancy and overlapping of portions of the colon may obscure one of the anatomic parts—hence, a complete examination of all flexures in the fluoroscopic visualization is essential. Occasionally, such complete examination is virtually impossible and careful notation of this inadequacy should be made.

Haustral points of narrowness and the rectosigmoid junction may give the impression of abnormal areas of narrowness unless the examiner is thoroughly conversant with the wide variation in the normal appearance of the colon.

Unless the terminal ileum or appendix has been visualized, it is difficult to be completely certain that the cecum has been seen, and for that reason caution must be exercised in assuming that the colon has been completely filled when the terminal ileum and appendix have not been visualized. Unfortunately, it is sometimes impossible to fill the terminal ileum and appendix, so experience must dictate when the colon has been entirely distended with barium.

Fluoroscopy is not as accurate as film studies for revealing minute mucosal changes such as those seen in the earliest aberrations of mucosal structure. It is important to become familiar with the normal appearance of both the full and empty colon in this regard, so that minimal abnormalities may be recognized on the film.

When patients are unable to retain the enema and evacuation is forced before complete filling of the colon and cecum, it must not be assumed that an obstructive abnormality of an organic type necessarily exists in the colon. A repeat examination, especially with the aid of a carefully inserted rectal balloon, may be necessary.

The diagnosis of small polyps is fraught with difficulty. Moreton et al. have pointed out some of these difficulties. They found that in 267 colons studied by the double contrast method 63, or 23.5 per cent, showed fictitious polyps.

The importance of proctosigmoidoscopy is shown by the fact that this adjunctive study may permit observation of: thromboulcerative colitis; ulcerations occurring in amebic, bacillary, and tuberculous colitis; 90 per cent of the organic pathology occurring in the colon; 70 per cent of the nonmalignant tumors; 75 per cent of the malignant tumors originating in the colon; factitial prostatitis and lymphogranuloma venereum; foreign bodies; rectovesical and rectourethral fistulas; and perforation of the rectum or sigmoid by foreign bodies.

Complications of a Barium Enema

Perforation or rupture of the colon, which may be either *intra- or extraperitoneal.*

Perforation of the colon into the venous system (Rosenberg and Fine; Zatzkin and Irwin).

Water intoxication, especially in children (Steinbach et al.).

Colonic intramural barium (Seaman and Bragg). This complication results from mucosal rupture, which permits the barium to dissect into the colonic wall. The outstanding roentgen feature is a transverse striated pattern that is probably produced by the inner layer of circular muscle fibers.

Examination of the Colon Through a Colostomy. In preparation of the patient, a low residue diet for 24 to 48 hours and thorough cleansing of the colon through the colostomy is ordinarily sufficient.

If a Foley catheter is employed as the enema tip in order to prevent spillage of the barium out of the colostomy, the inflation of the Foley bag must be carried out with great caution and under careful fluoroscopic control. Perforation of the bowel may result (Seaman and Wells). Some have urged that a Foley catheter with a long tubular section ahead of the balloon be employed, the balloon being applied with pressure on the outside of the colostomy to prevent spillage (Margulis). Various other techniques for preventing spillage have been advocated.

The introduction of the barium and the rolling of the patient from one side to the other is very much the same as previously described for the routine barium enema. Spot films are taken as necessary. Likewise, the routine filming following the enema through the colostomy is very similar, care being exercised once again to obtain the films as quickly as possible after the filling to prevent spillage.

Barium-Air Double Contrast Enema. There are two types of double contrast barium-air enemas. After a conventional barium enema with a nonflocculating Barotrast-type mixture and after evacuation of the conventional barium enema, air may be insufflated. Results from this type of enema are not usually as good as those from a double contrast enema performed as a separate examination as follows.

The preparation of the patient must be especially carefully done under these circumstances. We have preferred placing the patient on a low residue diet for a period of 2 days, and on 2 successive nights prior to the morning of the examination we have recommended the administration of 1½ ounces of X-Prep liquid. *If 2 ounces of castor oil are used, they should be given on only one occasion, the evening before the examination as in the routine barium enema examination.*

Breakfast is omitted on the morning of the examination and *further cleansing enemas may be given if it is thought necessary.* It has been our usual experience that after 2 such consecutive days of preparation (sometimes 3), the colon is thoroughly cleansed and no further cleansing enemas are necessary.

The colloidal barium mixture (Barotrast may be utilized) is introduced to the mid-descending colon or lower descending colon, and this is followed immediately by forceful insufflation of air, with rotation of the patient first to the left prone position and then to the right prone to accomplish proper dispersion of the heavy barium mixture.

Another variant of this technique requires that the colloidal barium mixture be introduced into the splenic flexure or the middle of the transverse colon and aspirated into a special bag, after which air is injected.

There are various colloidal barium sulfate preparations available, each with specific directions for mixing. Some of these are Baroloid, which is easy to mix, Barotrast, Baridol, and Stabarium. Since the colloidal barium mixture is viscous, pressure is required to force it through the enema tubing. This may be done by elevation of the barium reservoir, by "milking" the tube, by piston-type syringes, or by pumping devices.

When suction and control drainage are required, various devices are available—the three-way valve box (designed by Templeton and Addington) which is attached to a sink and works on a Venturi siphon principle, or simple Y-tube and clamp devices which permit drainage through one branch of the Y and injections through the other.

The films we have obtained routinely are both oblique views, prone and supine films, and both horizontal, lateral, and decubitus films (Fig. 14–30). Chassard-Lapiné views and other special views of the rectosigmoid may be obtained as necessary.

It is our preference to utilize this special method of double contrast visualization of the colon only if the routine examination of the colon does not yield all information necessary.

It is unfortunate that both the routine barium enema examination and this special double contrast type cannot be done on the same day to best advantage. They are best done 1 or 2 days apart as indicated by the clinical history.

The Importance of the Lateral View of the Rectum and Sigmoid Colon. The direct lateral view of the rectosigmoid (Fig. 14–26 *A*) is important for the study of the soft tissue space between the rectum and sacrum; and in the infant, to determine the lowest point of obstruction, particularly in patients with Hirschsprung's disease. The retrorectal soft tissue space ordinarily measures between 0.2 and 1.6 cm. (mean, 0.7 cm.) and ordinarily does not exceed 2 cm. It may on occasion, however, even in a normal patient, exceed this measurement and still be of no pathologic significance.

Apart from detection of infiltration of the retrorectal space in patients with ulcerative colitis, this view is especially useful for visualization of retrorectal masses and sacral tumors.

Examination of the Colon After a Barium Meal. The barium

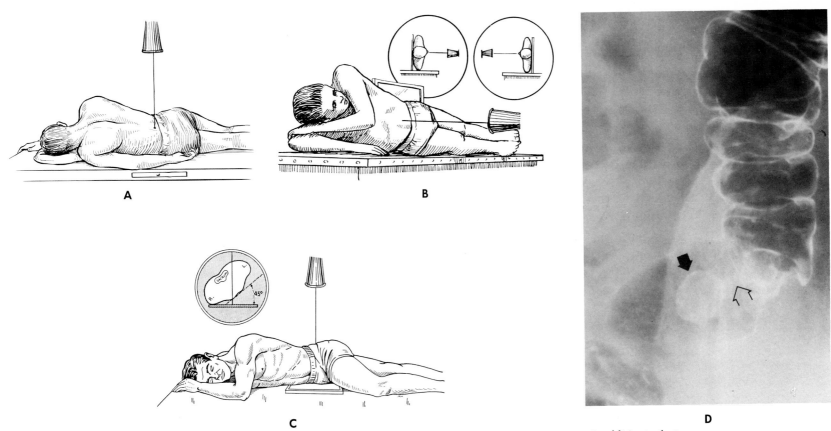

Figure 14–30. *A, B, C.* Positioning of patient for film studies with a double-contrast enema. In addition to the two oblique and the two horizontal beam views shown, straight posteroanterior and left lateral views are also obtained. *D.* Polyp in the colon as seen by double contrast. The closed arrow demonstrates the polyp; the open arrow shows the stalk.

meal method for examination of the colon is employed only if a barium enema is not feasible. It should never be employed unless it is certain that no colonic obstruction exists. When the barium reaches the distal portions of the colon, it is usually dehydrated and caked, giving rise to inaccurate analysis of the colonic structures.

It is possible that a more accurate concept regarding the irritable or spastic colon is obtained by this method.

When oral barium is used, films of the abdomen are taken at 2 and 6 hours, and at 12 and 24 hours if full visualization of the colon has not been obtained by the 6 hour interval. Usually a 24 hour study is necessary.

Silicone Foam in the Diagnosis of Lesions of the Rectum and Sigmoid. Cook and Margulis have employed a radiopaque silicone elastomer introduced into the rectum and sigmoid under fluoroscopic control for study of the rectum and sigmoid. The mixture utilized is spongy and capable of expanding into small crevices. Approximately 50 cm. of the distal colon is filled; 5 minutes later the foam sets and radiographs of the lower colon are obtained. Neostigmine (0.5 ml.) is then given subcutaneously (unless clinically contraindicated), and the patient expels the mold within a few minutes. Generally a balloon is used to fill the rectal ampulla, permitting a painless spontaneous expulsion of the foam mold. The addition of uniformly distributed barium sulfate or Hypaque powder to the silicone mixture before it is introduced into the colon results in radiopacity and allows fluoroscopic control of the filling of the rectum and sigmoid. The method should not be utilized in the presence of a tight or fibrotic anal sphincter, or if there is suspected perforation of the colon. Likewise, patients who have suffered from chronic constipation should not be so examined.

The Water Enema Examination for Lipoma. The water enema examination for identification of lipomas (Margulis and Jovanovich) is based upon the concept of a difference of absorption coefficients of water and fat in roentgenograms obtained in a lower kilovoltage range. This examination is performed only after a routine study has revealed a lesion suspected of being a lipoma.

ANGIOGRAPHY OF THE SMALL AND LARGE INTESTINES

Basic Arterial Anatomy

The *superior mesenteric artery* is the second unpaired branch of the abdominal aorta (Fig. 14–31). It arises from the front of the abdominal aorta from 1 to 23 mm. below the celiac trunk (preponderantly 1 to 6 mm.), usually opposite the lower third or middle of the first lumbar vertebra. It may arise anywhere from the lower border of the twelfth thoracic to the disk between the second and third lumbar vertebrae. It may arise as a common trunk with the celiac artery; indeed, it may give rise to the splenic or to both the splenic and hepatic arteries, or to the right gastroepiploic. For example, the right hepatic artery is a branch of the superior mesenteric in about 14 per cent of cases.

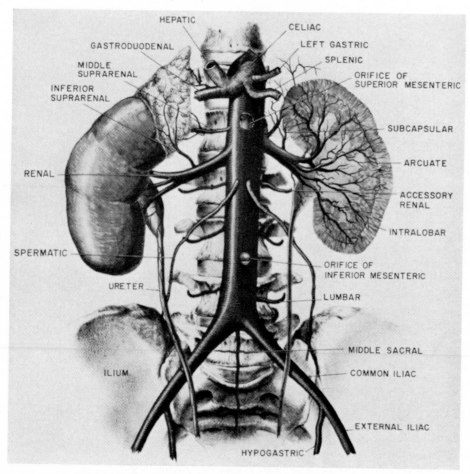

Figure 14–31. Abdominal aorta and its branches. (From Bierman, H. C.: Selective Arterial Catheterization. 1969. Courtesy of Charles C Thomas, Springfield, Illinois.)

The superior mesenteric artery crosses the duodenum and enters the mesentery following the route of the mesentery, and crossing the aorta, inferior vena cava, right ureter, and psoas major muscle. Its branches are: the *inferior pancreaticoduodenal*, feeding the duodenum and head of the pancreas; *intestinal; middle colic; right colic;* and *ileocolic*. It has a number of inconstant important branches to the pancreas (such as the *dorsal* or *transverse pancreatic artery*) in perhaps 14 to 20 per cent of cases, and a *right hepatic branch* in about 14 per cent of cases (Fig. 14–32). Other variations may occur.

The inferior pancreaticoduodenal arteries help form an arcade along the head of the pancreas and third part of the duodenum (see Chapter 13).

The *intestinal arteries*—branches of the superior mesenteric—arise from the left convex side of the superior mesenteric artery and number anywhere from 12 to 20, radiating into the mesentery. There are three to seven purely jejunal branches and eight to seven below the origin of the ileocolic artery that supply the jejunum, ileum, and proximal half of the colon. They form arcades by uniting and anastomosing in and around these organs. The arcades for the jejunum tend to be less tiered and multiplex when compared with those for the ileum. The *straight terminal arteries* alternate to one side or the other of the small intestine; their number increases as one proceeds distally along the intestine (Fig. 14–32 *A*).

The first intestinal artery anastomoses with the inferior pancreaticoduodenal artery (Fig. 14–32 *B*) may originate this artery. The terminal branches of the first intestinal artery also anastomose with the ileal branch of the ileocolic.

The *middle colic artery* arises somewhat variably from the superior mesenteric distal to the origin of the inferior pancreaticoduodenal artery and below the pancreas, but proximal to the jejunal or ileocolic branches (Fig. 14–32). It divides into right and left branches coursing along the margin of the colon. The *right branch* forms an anastomosis with the ascending branch of the right colic, and the *left branch* an anastomosis with the ascending branch of the left colic artery. The left colic is a branch of the inferior mesenteric.

Considerable variation exists in respect to the middle colic artery. It may be single; it may arise from a common stem with the right colic; or accessory middle colics may arise from any part of the superior mesenteric branching system (Netter).

The *right colic artery* crosses the ureter and gonadal vessels and divides into ascending and descending branches near the ascending colon. The *ascending branch* forms an anastomosis with the right branch of the middle colic; the *descending branch* forms an anastomosis with either the ascending or the colic branch of the ileocolic artery. Again, considerable variation exists in its relationship to the superior mesenteric or adjoining branches. The right colic artery is absent in 13 per cent of individuals.

The *ileocolic artery* arises in the root of the mesentery on the

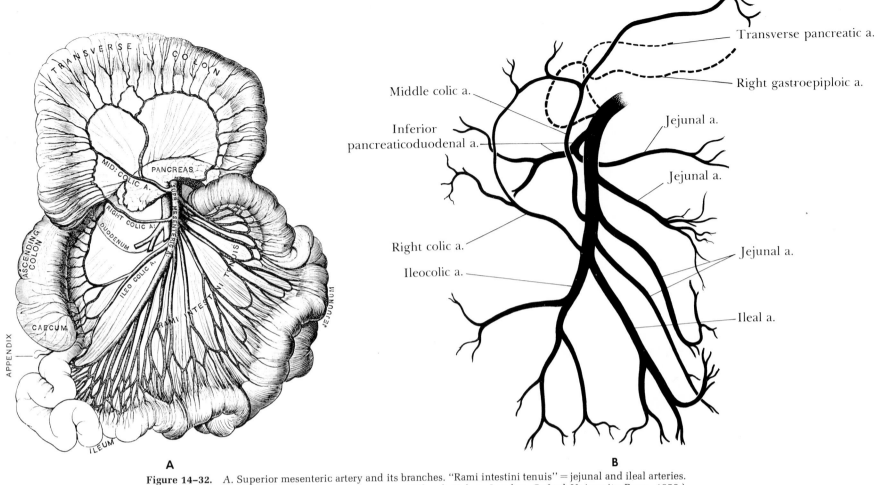

Figure 14–32. *A.* Superior mesenteric artery and its branches. "Rami intestini tenuis" = jejunal and ileal arteries. (From Cunningham's Manual of Practical Anatomy, 12th ed. Vol. 2. London, Oxford University Press, 1958.) *B.* Superior mesenteric artery and its branches. Constant branches are shown in solid lines, inconstant branches in interrupted lines. (From Ruzicka, F. F., and Rossi, P.: Radiol. Clin. N. Amer., 8:3–29, 1970.)

concave side of the superior mesenteric and its course crosses the psoas major muscle, gonadal vessels, and ureter. It may even cross the third part of the duodenum if it arises sufficiently high. It may arise independently from the superior mesenteric. When it reaches the cecum, the artery divides into approximately five branches supplying their corresponding regions: the *ileal, ascending colic, anterior cecal, posterior cecal,* and an *appendicular artery* (Fig. 14–33).

Figure 14–33. Blood supply of caecum and vermiform appendix (modified from Jonnesco, 1895.) The illustration on the left is from the front, the right from behind. In the latter the appendicular artery and the three taeniae coli springing from the root of the appendix should be specially noted. (From Cunningham's Textbook of Anatomy, 10th ed. London, Oxford University Press, 1964.)

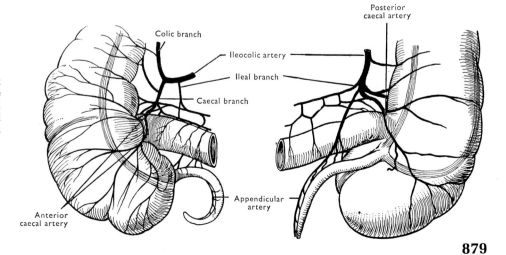

The *inferior mesenteric artery* is the third unpaired branch in the abdominal aorta, arising opposite the lower third of L3 vertebra (Fig. 14–31). This is usually about 4 cm. above the aortic bifurcation. It runs obliquely downward to the left behind the peritoneum and crosses the lower part of the abdominal aorta, the left psoas muscle, and the left common iliac artery. It descends into the pelvis in the sigmoid mesacolon and terminates on the rectum as the *superior rectal artery* (Figs. 14–34 *A, B;* 14–35).

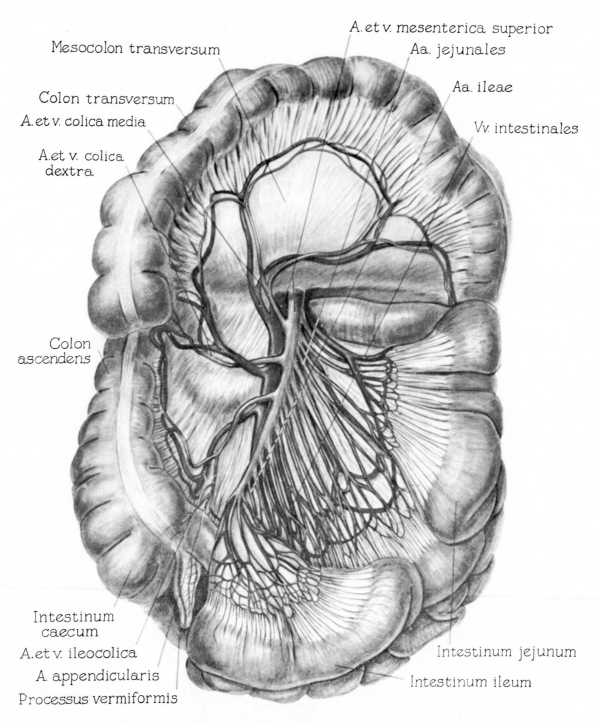

Mesocolon transversum

Colon transversum

A. et v. colica media

A. et v. colica dextra

Colon ascendens

A. et v. mesenterica superior

Aa. jejunales

Aa. ileae

Vv. intestinales

Intestinum caecum

A. et v. ileocolica

A. appendicularis

Processus vermiformis

Intestinum jejunum

Intestinum ileum

A

Figure 14–34.   A. Blood supply of the intestines. The transverse colon is lifted to show the patterns of distribution of the intestinal and colic branches of the superior mesenteric artery, and the accompanying venous tributaries to the portal vein. (From Warren, Handbook of Anatomy, Harvard University Press.)

Figure 14–34 continued on the opposite page.

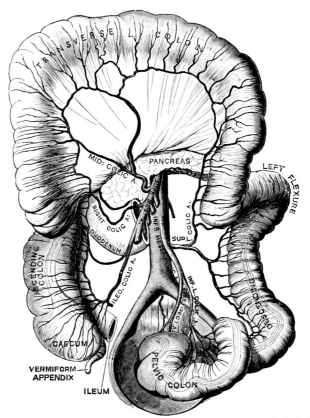

Left branch of middle colic a.

Accessory middle colic a.

Arc of Riolan

Superior mesenteric a.

Ascending branch
of left colic a.

Marginal artery
of Drummond

Inferior mesenteric a.

Left colic a.

Superior rectal
(hemorrhoidal) a.

Sigmoid a.

Middle colic a.

Right colic a.

Ileocolic a.

B

Figure 14–34 *Continued. B.* Superior and inferior mesenteric arterial systems, showing the arc of Riolan and the marginal artery of Drummond. The arc of Riolan is made up of the accessory middle colic artery, the ascending branch of the left colic artery, and an anastomotic branch between the two. The marginal artery of Drummond is shown here as a continuous vessel from sigmoid to cecum. In actuality, it is often interrupted, especially in the right colon. (From Ruzicka, F. F., and Rossi, P.: Radiol. Clin. N. Amer., 8:3–29, 1970.)

The branches of the inferior mesenteric artery are: the *left colic,* which ascends to anastomose with a branch of the accessory middle colic artery and forms another tier which in turn anastomoses with a branch of the middle colic artery itself, the *sigmoid,* and the *superior rectal.* These are indicated in diagram in Figure 14–34 *B.* They supply the corresponding portions of the rectum and colon. In about 27 per cent of persons the ascending branch of the left colic artery extends to the descending colon. In the remainder the ascending branch is directed toward the splenic flexure. There are numerous anastomoses between the left colic and sigmoid arteries in various arcades.

The *superior rectal artery* is actually the continued trunk of the inferior mesenteric artery (Fig. 14–35), and as it bifurcates it forms an arcade around the rectum continuous with similar arcades around the sigmoid.

Along their course, the branches of the superior rectal artery anastomose with branches of the middle and inferior rectal and middle sacral arteries which participate in supply of the two lowest segments of the intestinal tract, the rectum and anus, and thereby communicate with branches of the abdominal aorta more inferiorly.

The *middle rectal arteries* have a varied origin but most commonly arise from the anterior division of the hypogastric or internal iliac arteries.

The *middle sacral artery* is a single vessel originating from the posterior surface of the aorta, a little more than 1 cm. above the aortic bifurcation, and extending to the tip of the coccyx.

Figure 14–35. Superior and inferior mesenteric arteries and their branches. Usually, there is more than one inferior left colic (sigmoid) artery. (From Cunningham's Manual of Practical Anatomy, 12th ed. Vol. 2. London, Oxford University Press, 1958.)

881

Marginal Artery of Drummond. One of the significant arcades is formed by a continuous channel, the *marginal artery of Drummond* (Fig. 14–34 *B*), which links the blood stream of all the vessels sustaining the various portions of the colon, including the rectum. It acts as a terminal arcade from which smaller vessels permeate the colon perpendicularly. It begins with the terminal portion of the colic branch of the ileocolic artery and ends in the region of the upper sigmoid. Unfortunately, the *arteriae rectae* (perpendicular branches from the marginal artery) constitute an element of danger in so far as gangrene is concerned because these arteries are widely spaced and gangrene may result when two or more of them are severed.

Venous Drainage of the Small and Large Intestines

Generally, the veins involved in the drainage of the small and large intestines follow a design similar to that of the arteries. The exception to this rule is the right gastroepiploic vein, which drains directly into the superior mesenteric just before the latter enters the portal vein. However, the other tributaries of the superior mesenteric vein such as the *inferior pancreaticoduodenal, dorsal pancreatic, transverse pancreatic, jejunal, ileal, ileocolic,* and the *right and middle colic veins* follow a course almost identical with that of the arteries.

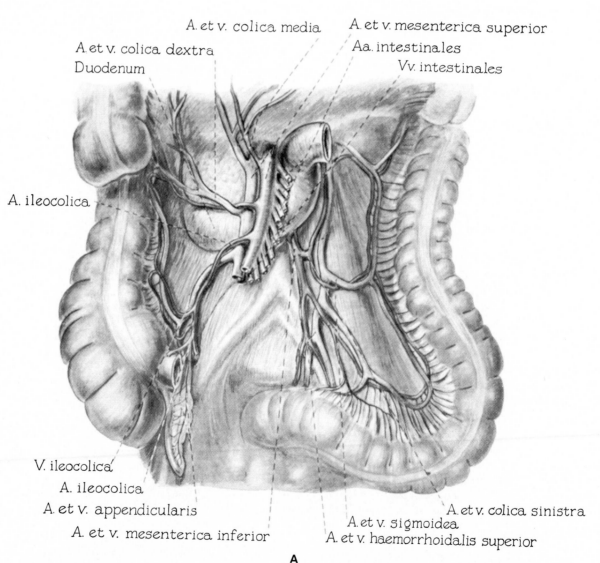

A

Figure 14–36. A. Blood supply to the large intestine. The jejunal and ileal divisions of the small intestine have been removed in order to expose the arterial branches of the inferior mesenteric and the corresponding veins of colic drainage. (From Warren: Handbook of Anatomy, Harvard University Press.)

Figure 14–36 continued on the opposite page.

The *pancreaticoduodenal arcades* are similar in respect to arteries and veins (see Chapter 13). Starting in the terminal ileum and taking in the root of the mesentery, the *superior mesenteric vein* lies to the right and somewhat in front of the corresponding artery. Both vessels are convex toward the left, and both cross in front of the third portion of the duodenum. The *inferior mesenteric vein* is similarly arranged, with the tributaries following closely corresponding arteries mostly to their left. *However, when the left colic and the upper sigmoid arteries take their origin from the inferior mesenteric artery, the corresponding vein follows a separate course.* The vein moves directly upward, ascending behind the peritoneum over the psoas muscles and to the left of the fourth part of the duodenum. It drains into the splenic vein behind the body of the pancreas. The course of the inferior mesenteric vein varies considerably, however, and it occasionally enters the superior mesenteric, in some individuals joining both the superior mesenteric and splenic veins (Fig. 14–36 *A, B*).

The *splenic vein* is formed by large veins from the hilus of the spleen, and it traverses the superior border of the pancreas ventral to the aorta, caudal to the celiac trunk, joining the superior mesenteric vein behind the head of the pancreas—the portal vein proper. It receives such tributaries as the *short gastric, left gas-*

troepiploic, and *pancreatic veins.* In about 60 per cent of cases the inferior mesenteric vein may join the splenic vein.

The *portal vein* is a thick trunk, 7 or 8 cm. long, originating just dorsal to the pancreas and opposite the right aspect of L2 vertebra. It passes between the layers of a hepatoduodenal ligament and dorsal to the hepatic artery and common bile duct proper. It enters the porta hepatis and divides into right and left branches.

The portal vein receives a *prepyloric vein, right and left gastric veins,* and the *posterior superior pancreaticoduodenal vein.* There may be other tributaries. In the liver, it corresponds in course and distribution to the hepatic artery and biliary duct. There are usually three portal branches to the caudal lobe.

The three structures—hepatic artery, portal vein, and biliary duct—are enclosed within the liver in a connective tissue sheath called the *perivascular fibrous capsule.*

The *hepatic veins* are quite large in diameter but have a short intra-abdominal length. Three hepatic veins begin within the liver and converge toward the inferior vena cava. Although they are relatively constant, *they do not parallel the intrahepatic course of the portal vein, hepatic artery, and bile duct,* but rather lie in intersegmental planes draining adjacent segments. *In the event of obstruction of the intrahepatic portal system, there are im-*

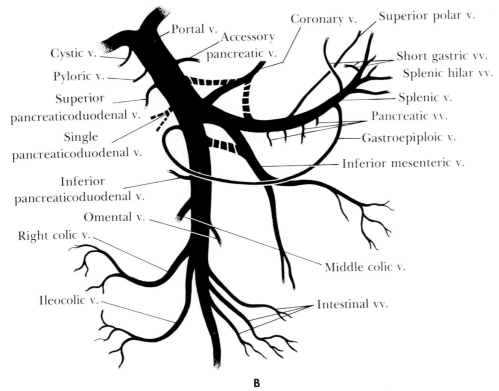

B

Figure 14–36 *Continued.* B. Portal venous system. Solid line drawing represents the most frequent pattern. Interrupted lines show variations of coronary, inferior mesenteric, and pancreaticoduodenal veins. When the pancreaticoduodenal vein is single, it empties into the right wall of the portal vein just above the confluence of the splenic and superior mesenteric veins. (From Ruzicka, F. F., Jr., and Rossi, P.: Radiol. Clin. N. Amer., 8:3–29, 1970. Modified from Douglass, B. E., Baggenstoss, A. H., and Hollinshead, W. H.: Surg., Gynec., Obstet., 91:562–576, 1950, by permission of Surgery, Gynecology, and Obstetrics.)

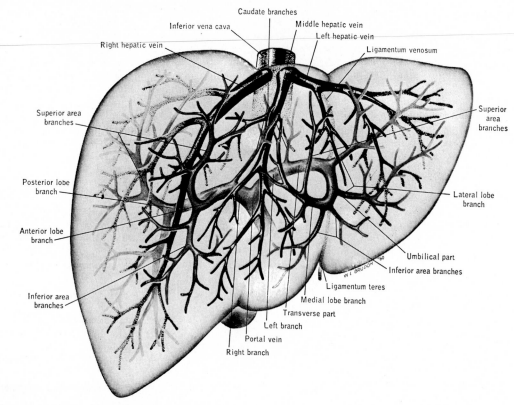

Figure 14–37. Intrahepatic distribution of the hepatic and portal veins. (From Anson, B. J. (ed.): Morris' Human Anatomy, 12th ed. Copyright © 1966 by McGraw-Hill, Inc. Used by permission of McGraw-Hill Book Company.)

portant bypass tributaries such as: (1) those between esophageal veins that are tributaries to the azygos and to the left gastric vein; (2) those between superior rectal veins that are tributary to the inferior mesenteric, and between middle and inferior rectal veins that are tributary to the internal iliac veins; (3) those between retroperitoneal, posterior, abdominal wall veins (such as those around the kidney, the inferior phrenic, and the azygos system) and the veins of the pancreas, duodenum, and liver; and (4) those between the epigastric anastomosis around the umbilicus, and the left branch of the portal vein by means of its periumbilical tributary.

When these collateral channels are used because of portal obstruction, varicosities and tortuous enlargements are produced which on occasion may bleed.

Illustrative angiograms of the celiac trunk, superior mesenteric artery, inferior mesenteric artery, and portal venous system are provided in Figures 14–38 to 14–41.

Some Variations of Arterial Patterns

The Celiac, Superior, and Inferior Mesenteric Trunks. Extensive studies have been made after dissection of the hepatic,

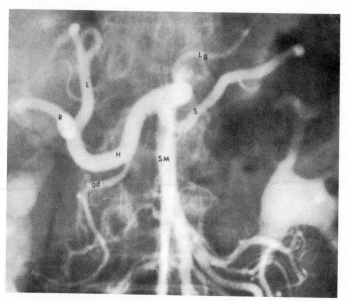

Figure 14–38. Simultaneous selective celiac and superior mesenteric artery injections show type I pattern (see Figs. 14–42 and 14–43 and text). Anteroposterior view. (S) Splenic artery, (SM) superior mesenteric, (gd) gastroduodenal, (H) proper hepatic, (R) right hepatic, (L) left hepatic, (Lg) left gastric. (From Ruzicka, F. F., Jr., and Rossi, P.: Radiol. Clin. N. Amer., 8:3–29, 1970.)

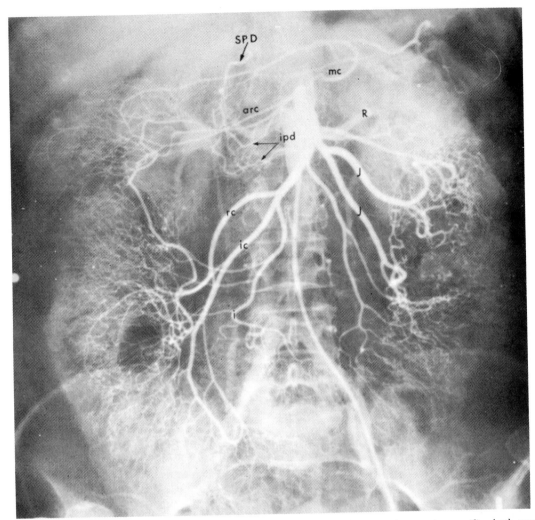

Figure 14-39. Superior mesenteric arteriogram. Some reflux of contrast agent into aorta opacifies both renal arteries. Note filling of pancreaticoduodenal arcades and superior pancreaticoduodenal artery from inferior pancreaticoduodenal arteries. *(R)* Renal, *(J)* jejunal artery, *(i)* ileal artery, *(ic)* ileocolic artery, *(rc)* right colic, *(mc)* middle colic, *(arc)* accessory right colic, *(ipd)* inferior pancreaticoduodenal, *(SPD)* superior pancreaticoduodenal artery. (From Ruzicka, F. F., Jr., and Rossi, P.: Radiol. Clin. N. Amer., 8:3-29, 1970.)

celiac, superior mesenteric, and inferior mesenteric arteries, and these variations do have practical significance in the interpretation of angiograms (Odnoralov).

As pointed out by Ruzicka and Rossi, if the main celiac trunk and the superior mesenteric artery are considered together, *six different basic types* can be proposed that include most of the variations encountered (Fig. 14-42). The classical pattern, illustrated here, occurs in approximately 93 per cent of cases. In a few instances, as shown, there is a separate origin for (1) the left gastric artery, (2) the splenic artery, and (3) the common hepatic artery. In another pattern, the left gastric and the splenic arise from the celiac artery, and the common hepatic arises from the superior mesenteric. In this instance there is a single common trunk for both the celiac and superior mesenteric branches. There are minor variations of each of these patterns.

Hepatic Artery. A number of hepatic artery variations occur also. For example, the most common type is Type 1, illustrated in Figure 14-42. In this instance the common hepatic artery arises from the celiac artery and the gastroduodenal artery in turn arises from it.

One variation of the hepatic artery is Type 5, shown in Figure 14-42, where the entire arterial blood supply of the liver arises from the superior mesenteric artery. As a further variation, the left hepatic may arise from the common hepatic, which

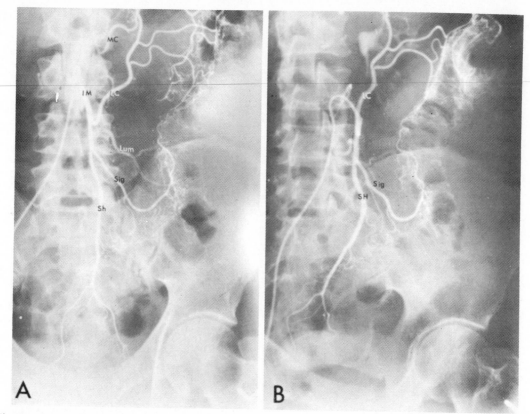

Figure 14–40. Selective inferior mesenteric arteriogram. *A.* Anteroposterior view. Middle colic artery fills via communications (not shown) with left colic branches. A small amount of reflux defines adjacent aorta, and lumbar artery is also opacified because of this reflux. *(MC)* Middle colic, *(LC)* left colic, *(Lum)* lumbar artery, *(Sig)* sigmoid, *(Sh)* superior hemorrhoidal, *(IM)* inferior mesenteric artery. *B.* Left posterior oblique view. (From Ruzicka, F. F., Jr., and Rossi, P.: Radiol. Clin. N. Amer., 8:3–29, 1970.)

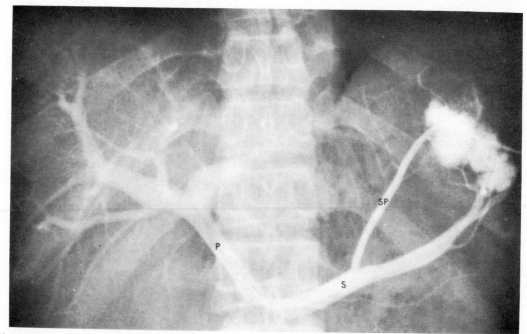

Figure 14–41. Normal splenoportogram. Injection into the splenic pulp results in visualization of splenoportal axis. Superior polar vein *(SP)* is part of splenoportal axis. Tributaries are not visualized normally by this technique. However, capsular veins of spleen and adjacent small vessels may fill during splenic injection in the normal patient. *(S)* Splenic vein, *(P)* portal vein. (From Ruzicka, F. F., Jr., and Rossi, P.: Radiol. Clin. N. Amer., 8:3–29, 1970.)

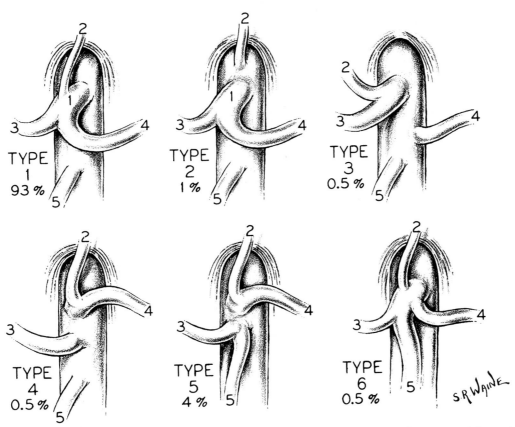

Figure 14–42. *(1)* Celiac trunk, *(2)* left gastric artery, *(3)* common hepatic artery, *(4)* splenic artery, *(5)* superior mesenteric artery, *(6)* right hepatic artery, *(7)* left hepatic artery, *(8)* gastroduodenal artery, *(9)* proper hepatic artery. (From Ruzicka, F. F., and Rossi, P.: N.Y. State J. Med., 23:3032–3033, 1968, reproduced with permission.)

in turn arises from the celiac artery. Probably the fourth most frequent variation is one in which the right hepatic arises from the common hepatic but the left hepatic arises from a left gastric. Four of the most frequent variations in patterns of arterial blood supply to the liver are shown in Figure 14–43.

Splenic Artery.   There are also numerous variations of the splenic artery and its branches (Michels). Apart from the splenic artery's pancreatic branches, which will be separately considered, the terminal branches of this artery need further comment. The superior polar artery, one of the terminal branches, may be short or long – 12 cm. or more. It may arise separately from the celiac axis and appear as a second splenic artery. There are also many short gastric arteries that may arise from either the splenic or any of its branches, and these help supply the posterior and anterior aspects of the cardia and fundus of the stomach.

PANCREATIC ARTERIAL DISTRIBUTION

The classical pattern of pancreatic arterial distribution has been described in Chapter 13. It will be recalled that the main ar-

terial blood supply for the pancreas is derived from: (1) the splenic artery, (2) the retroduodenal branch of the gastroduodenal artery, (3) the superior pancreaticoduodenal from the gastroduodenal artery, and (4) the inferior pancreaticoduodenal artery – a branch of the superior mesenteric.

The *dorsal pancreatic artery,* a branch of the splenic, is probably the principal nutrient vessel of the pancreas. The *transverse pancreatic artery,* at the inferior margin of the pancreas, is usually a branch of the dorsal. Branches of the great pancreatic artery (from the splenic artery) and the caudal artery anastomose with the transverse (Fig. 14–44). The *pancreatica magna* or large artery of the pancreas is indeed often smaller than the dorsal pancreatic artery, but it does constitute the principal blood supply to the tail of the pancreas. The dorsal pancreatic artery may, in turn, act as a collateral route between celiac and superior mesenteric arteries (Fig. 14–44 *C*).

Although the transverse pancreatic artery is in 90 per cent of the cases a branch of the dorsal pancreatic, it may take origin from the gastroduodenal, the right gastroepiploic, or the superior

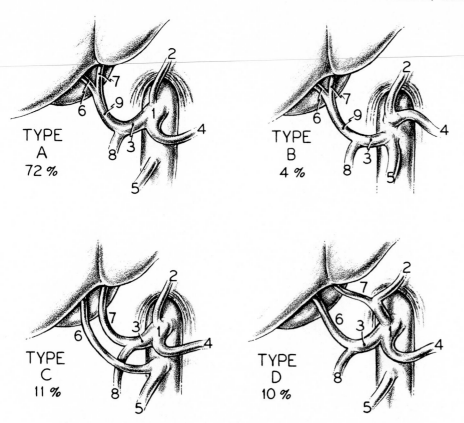

Figure 14–43. (1) Celiac trunk, (2) left gastric artery, (3) common hepatic artery, (4) splenic artery, (5) superior mesenteric artery, (6) right hepatic artery, (7) left hepatic artery, (8) gastroduodenal artery, (9) proper hepatic artery. (From Ruzicka, F. F., and Rossi, P.: N.Y. State J. Med., 23:3032–3033, 1968, reproduced with permission.)

pancreaticoduodenal (Michels). Indeed, at times there may be two transverse pancreatic arteries.

One of the most important variant branches of the superior mesenteric artery is an aberrant hepatic artery (Type C, Fig. 14–43). Other normal variations already mentioned are the dorsal pancreatic and transverse pancreatic arteries originating from the superior mesenteric instead of the splenic.

Occasionally, the right gastroepiploic arises from the superior mesenteric artery directly or from one of the branches.

Other variations of normal are seen around the origin of the middle colic and acessory middle colic arteries. The reader is referred to an excellent succinct review of the major anastomotic patterns of these vessels of the abdominal viscera by Ruzicka and Rossi; see also Michels.

Neonatal Umbilical Catheterization and Angiography

Basic Anatomy. The *umbilical vein* ascends to reach the liver by way of the falciform ligament, entering the *left portal vein* opposite the ductus venosus. If the latter is patent, a catheter may pass directly to the inferior vena cava, right atrium, and ultimately through the septum into the left atrium.

The paired umbilical arteries in the fetus are the main channels from the aorta to the placenta by way of the umbilical cord. The proximal parts of this main channel are the common iliac and internal iliac arteries. Atrophy of the umbilical artery leading to the internal iliac artery is incomplete, and a superior vesical artery arises as a result. A schematic drawing of the umbilical vein and umbilical arteries is shown in Figure 14–45. A catheter in the umbilical vein rises directly beneath the anterior abdominal wall toward the liver, joining the portal vein in the ductus venosus (Fig. 14–46 A). A catheter in the umbilical artery, however, descends to the pelvis minor and enters the aorta via either the common iliac or internal iliac artery (Fig. 14–46 B).

Injections of contrast media may be made into the catheter in the umbilical vein for visualization of the liver (transumbilical portography).

Selective catheterization of the abdominal branches of the newborn is possible through the umbilical artery. This method is often used to study vascular masses in the liver or kidney of the newborn. Failure to visualize renal arteries by this route is often confirmatory evidence of renal agenesis — another application of this kind of angiography.

Prolonged neonatal therapeutic canalization of umbilical vessels may lead to an acquired arteriovenous connection, which must be avoided. Short-term catheterization of these vessels presents no serious problems. Unfortunately, however, catheterization of the umbilicus is attended by thrombosis and intravascular clotting. Introduction of a catheter into the portal vein may lead to portal thrombosis with later portal hypertension and esophageal varices. Hence, this technique is reserved for cases in which special information or important therapeutic canalization is required (Kessler et al.; Salerna et al.; Emmanoulides et al.).

THE BILIARY TRACT

The radiographic examination of the gallbladder is at the same time a means of visualization of the anatomic structures of the gallbladder and cystic duct, and a test of hepatobiliary function. One can hardly be considered without the other, and a detailed knowledge of both is essential if we are to carry out the examination with accuracy.

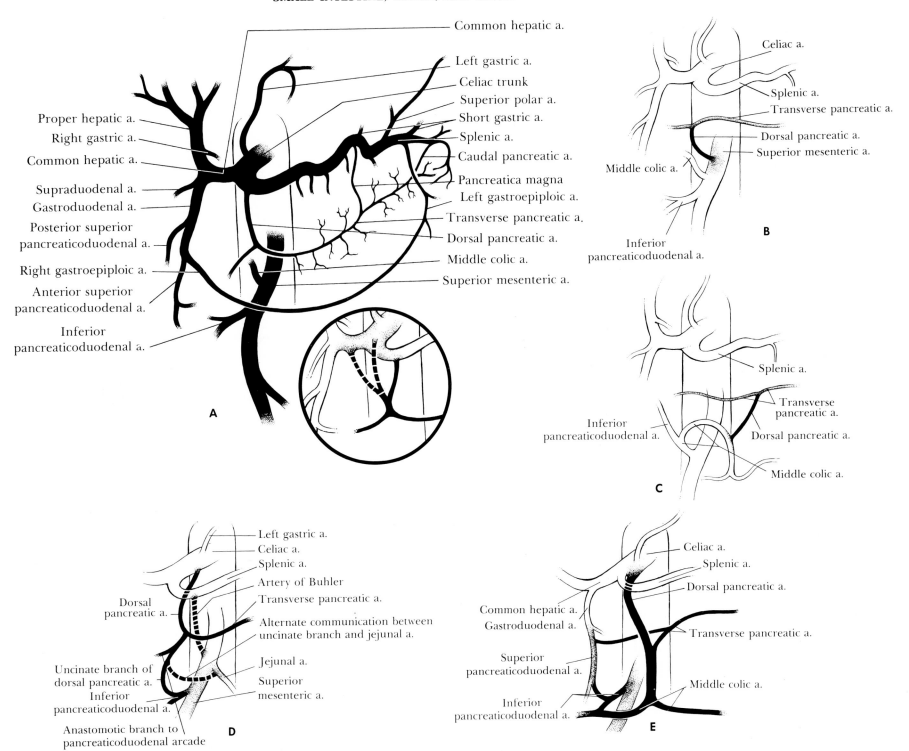

Figure 14–44. Pancreatic artery variations. The classical pattern of pancreatic arteries, as well as the major branches of the celiac system, are shown in *A.* Inset demonstrates the more usual variations of the dorsal pancreatic artery. Vessels portrayed by interrupted lines are alternate routes. Unusual sites of origin of the dorsal pancreatic artery are shown in *B* and *C. D* and *E.* The dorsal pancreatic artery as a major anastomotic channel. Two variations of this role are shown. The artery of Buhler, which is distinct from the dorsal pancreatic artery, similarly joins the celiac and superior mesenteric systems. (From Ruzicka, F. F., Jr., and Rossi, P.: Radiol. Clin. N. Amer., 8:3–29, 1970.)

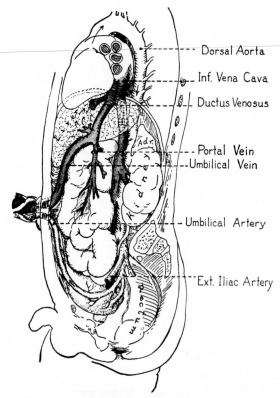

Figure 14–45 labels: Dorsal Aorta, Inf. Vena Cava, Ductus Venosus, Portal Vein, Umbilical Vein, Umbilical Artery, Ext. Iliac Artery

Figure 14–45. Semischematic drawings to show the vestiges in the adult of the umbilical vessels of the fetus. (From Cullen, The Umbilicus and Its Diseases, *in* Anson, B. J. (ed.): Morris' Human Anatomy, 12th ed. Copyright © 1966 by Mc-Graw-Hill, Inc. Used by permission of McGraw-Hill Book Company.)

The Microscopic and Gross Anatomy of the Biliary Tract (Figs. 14–47, 14–48). The liver is composed of many hundreds of units called lobules, and each lobule is composed of radial columns of parenchymal cells. Between these columns of cells lie the bile capillaries, the walls of which are the liver cells themselves. On the opposite side of these cells are the stellate cells of the lymph channels and reticulodenothelial system, and the endothelium of the venules leading into the central vein. The bile capillaries empty into interlobular bile ducts, which enter in their turn into larger bile ducts, until finally two chief branches are obtained: a large branch from the right, and a small branch from the left lobe of the liver, called the right and left hepatic ducts respectively (Fig. 14–48). These ultimately unite to form the common hepatic duct.

The common hepatic duct passes downward, and just beyond the porta hepatis, it is joined by the cystic duct from the gallbladder (a pear-shaped enlargement lying distal to the cystic duct) to form the common bile duct. The common hepatic duct is about 25 to 30 mm. in length, and about 6 mm. in diameter.

The cystic duct is about half the diameter of the hepatic duct but somewhat longer—about 30 to 37 mm. in length. It pursues a course backward and medially to join the hepatic duct.

The spiral constriction at the neck of the gallbladder (to be described below) is continued into the proximal portion, called the valvular portion of the cystic duct, in contrast to the nonvalvular portion, or pars glabra.

The common bile duct is about 7.5 cm. in length and about the same diameter as the hepatic duct. It passes downward between the two layers of the hepatoduodenal ligament, with the portal vein behind and the hepatic artery to its left. It then passes behind the superior part of the duodenum and runs in a groove between the duodenum and head of the pancreas. Joining the pancreatic duct (still maintaining a separate lumen), it pierces the descending part of the duodenum in its midportion, to open

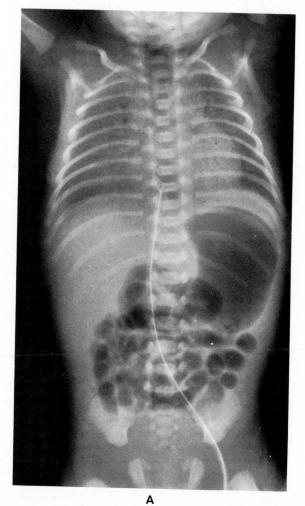

A

Figure 14–46. *A.* Anteroposterior view of newborn whose umbilical vein has been catheterized.

Figure 14–46 continued on the opposite page.

obliquely into the lumen at the duodenal papilla. Two common variations at the juncture with the duodenum are indicated in Figure 14–50.

The gallbladder is arbitrarily divided into four parts (Fig. 14–49): the distal end or *fundus* usually reaches the anterior border of the liver; the *body* runs backward, upward, and to the left; the *infundibulum* is situated between the body and neck, and consists of that portion tapering toward the neck; the *neck* is curved medially toward the porta hepatis and contains spiral crescentic folds around the interior of its lumen, forming the spiral valve of Heister. The neck of the gallbladder usually curves sharply like the letter "S." This continues into the valvular portion of the cystic duct as previously described. Smooth muscle fibers are found in the fundus and infundibulum but are almost completely absent in the body; conversely, there is much elastic

tissue in the body and very little in the fundus and infundibulum. The muscle fibers are longitudinal and oblique in the fundus but circular in the infundibulum, and this circular conformation is continued into the spiral valves.

The gallbladder, when measured angiographically, is 2 to 3 mm. thick, less than 35 sq. cm. in area, and 5 cm. or less in width (Rösch et al.; Deutsch; Redman and Reuter). The gallbladder may often appear larger than this in oral cholecystograms when distended and magnified, but a gallbladder that is somewhat enlarged and concentrates well is difficult to interpret.

Usually the gallbladder is not covered with peritoneum on its hepatic side, but occasionally it is suspended from the liver by a short peritoneal ligament. The gallbladder usually rests on the transverse colon in front, and its neck is usually in close proximity with the duodenum.

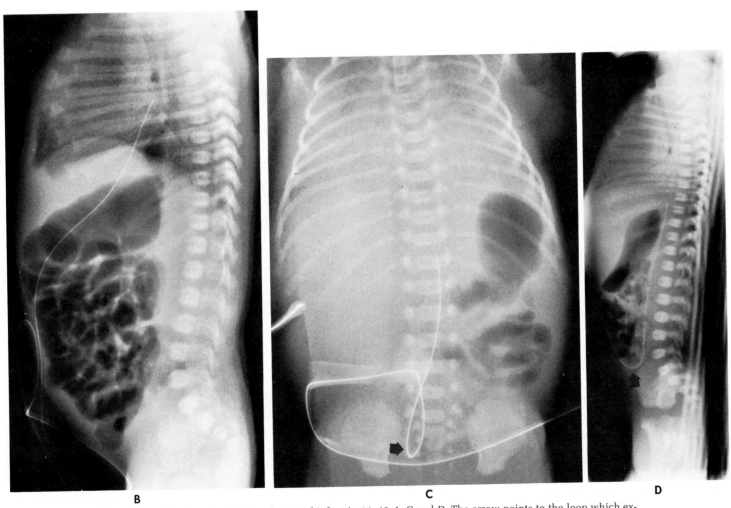

B   C   D

Figure 14–46 *Continued.* B. Lateral view of infant in 14–46 A. C and D. The arrow points to the loop which extends down to the hypogastric artery, which in frontal perspective establishes the arterial position of the catheter.

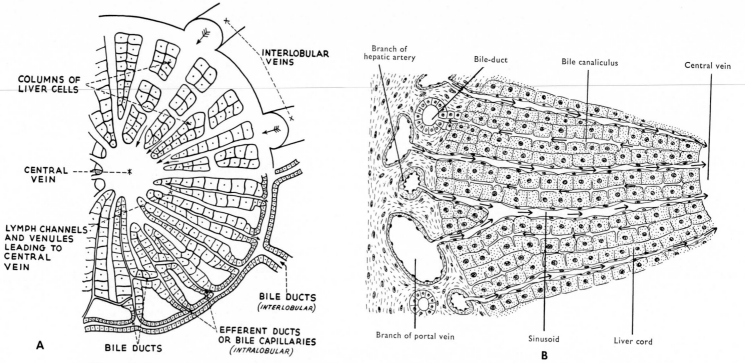

Figure 14–47. *A.* Diagram illustrating the structure of a liver lobule. (Modified from Cunningham's Textbook of Anatomy, 10th ed. London, Oxford University Press, 1964.) *B.* The structure of the liver lobule (human). (From Cunningham's Textbook of Anatomy, 10th ed. London, Oxford University Press, 1964.)

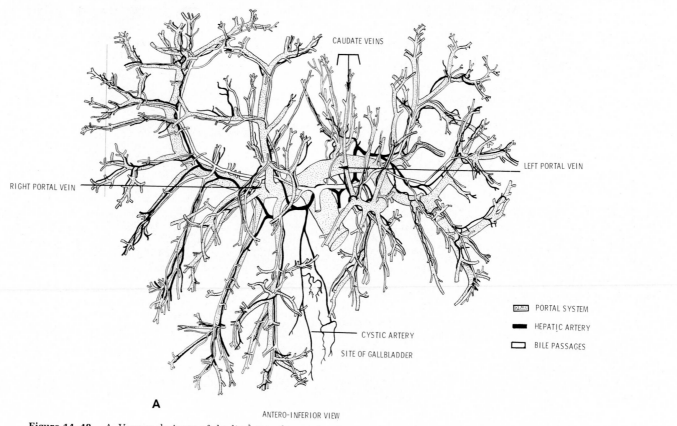

Figure 14–48. *A.* Venous drainage of the liver into the caval system as compared with the portal venous system.

Figure 14–48 continued on the opposite page.

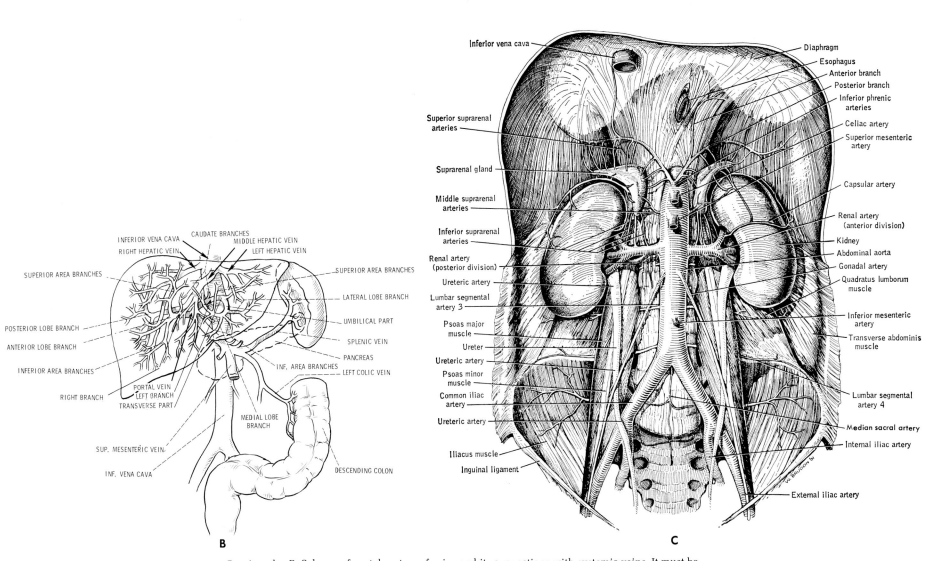

Figure 14-48 *Continued.* B. Schema of portal system of veins and its connections with systemic veins. It must be remembered that the systemic blood carried by the hepatic artery also enters the capillaries of the liver, and the hepatic veins contain therefore both portal and systemic blood. (Modified from Cunningham's Manual of Practical Anatomy, 11th ed. Vol. 2. London, Oxford University Press, 1949.) C. Abdominal aorta and its branches. (From Anson, B. J. (ed.): Morris' Human Anatomy, 12th ed. Copyright © 1966 by McGraw-Hill, Inc. Used by permission of McGraw-Hill Book Company.)

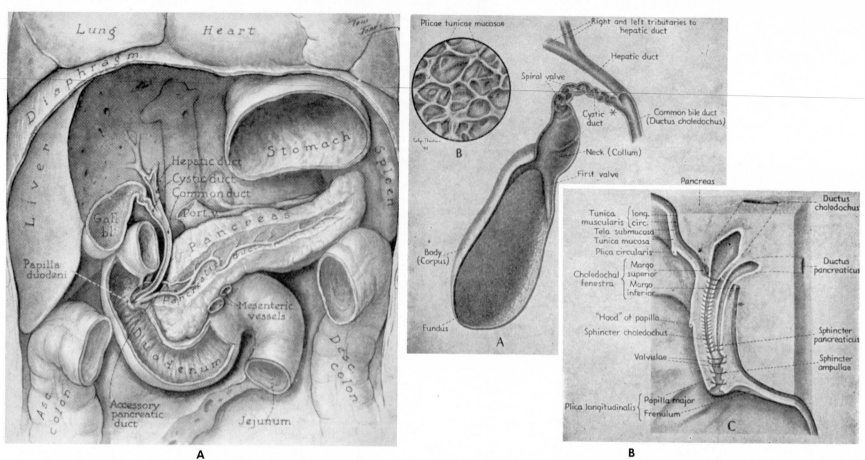

A

B

C

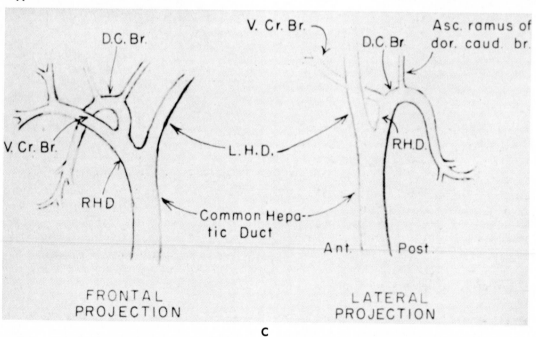

C

Figure 14–49. *A.* The gross anatomy of the biliary system. (From Jones, T.: Anatomical Studies. Jackson, Michigan, S. H. Camp and Co., 1943.) *B.* Gross anatomy of biliary tract. *(A)*, Interior of the gallbladder and cystic duct; *(B)*, surface of the mucosa of the gallbladder showing plicae; *(C)*, diagram of frontal section through duodenum at the inferior duodenal flexure showing the structure and relations of the papilla major (duodenal papilla). (After Boyden in Surgery. From Jackson, C. M., and Blount, R. F., in Jackson (ed.): Morris' Human Anatomy. New York, The Blakiston Co.) *C.* Schematic composite of the roentgen anatomy of the hepatic ductal system in its most common configuration. (D.C.Br.) Dorsocaudal branch, (V. Cr. Br.) ventrocranial branch. (From Schein, C. J., Stern, W. Z., and Jacobson, H. G.: Surgery, *51*:718–723, 1962.)

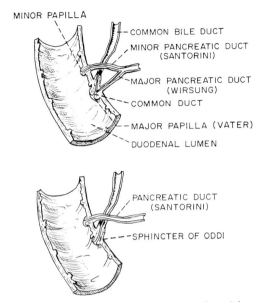

Figure 14–50. Anatomic sketch depicting the relationship of the major and minor papillae, the common bile duct, and the pancreatic duct. (After Daves.)

Variations of the Gallbladder (Fig. 14–51). The major variations of the gallbladder may be classified as follows:

1. *Variations in Shape.* The gallbladder may be ovoid, spherical or elongated.

2. *Variations in Position.* The gallbladder may be deeply embedded in the liver, or it may have a mesentery and lie in the iliac fossa. Its position also varies in relation to the spine. No definite pathologic function has been associated with these unusual locations.

3. *Construction by Mucosal or Serosal Folds.* These folds may produce a sacculation of the gallbladder and the so-called Phrygian cap. This does not have pathologic significance. Also, the gallbladder may be divided longitudinally into separate gallbladders and possess separate cystic ducts.

4. *Absence of the Gallbladder.* Rarely, the gallbladder is absent, and in such instances the hepatic ducts have usually been found to be dilated.

5. *Variations in Length of Ducts.* Variations in the length of the hepatic ducts, cystic duct and common bile duct may occur.

6. *Separate Openings.* The common bile duct and pancreatic duct may open separately into the duodenum.

Function of the Gallbladder. The functions of the gallbladder may be summarized as follows:

The Reservoir Function. A part of the bile secreted by the liver is stored in the gallbladder.

The Concentration Function. Water and salts are absorbed in the gallbladder, whereas the bile pigments are not, and as a result, bilirubin is concentrated about 20 times; cholesterol,

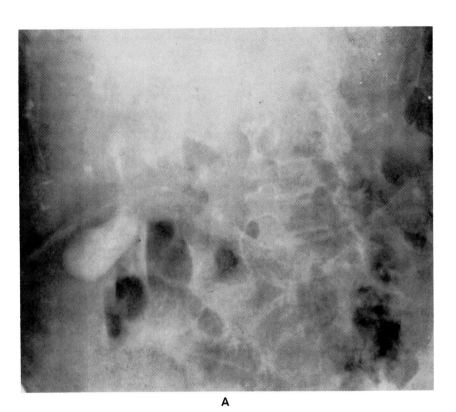

A

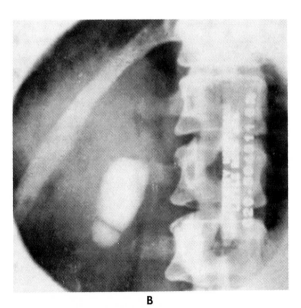

B

Figure 14–51. Variations in gallbladder of radiographic significance. A. Ptotic gallbladder lying in the iliac fossa. B. Mucosal or serosal fold of gallbladder, known as a Phrygian cap.

bile salts and calcium about 5 to 10 times (Rous and McMaster). In disease of the gallbladder, this concentration function is readily impaired. A contrast agent introduced in an inflamed gallbladder is reabsorbed in sufficient volume to prevent adequate concentration for visualization (Berk and Lasser). When a second dose of contrast agent is administered visualization may be possible. It has been postulated that many of the serum and tissue protein-binding sites are occupied in this second dose, thus leading to a more sustained elevation of the available opaque material in the blood and to an inhibition of reabsorption of the contrast material through the marginally inflamed gallbladder wall. As a result, more of the contrast agent is excreted in the bile and more remains in the gallbladder so that visualization may become possible (Rous and McMaster; Boyden).

The Emptying Mechanism. The exact mechanism involved is not completely understood. It is claimed by some that there is a reciprocal innervation of the gallbladder and sphincter of Oddi, so that vagal stimulation causes contraction of the gallbladder and relaxation of the sphincter. There is also a hormonal influence—when practically any acid or food substance, particularly fats and fatty acid, comes into contact with the duodenal mucosa, cholecystokinin is formed, which is absorbed into the blood stream and causes the gallbladder to contract (Boyden) (Fig. 14–52).

The Secretory Function. The gallbladder apparently secretes constituents of the bile, such as cholesterol and mucin.

Functions of Bile. The main functions of bile can be summarized as follows: (1) it is an important accessory agent in digestion because it accelerates the action of pancreatic enzymes; (2) it aids materially in the digestion of fats by decreasing surface tension, activating lipase, increasing the solubility of soaps and fatty acids, and materially aiding fatty absorption; (3) it forms a means of eliminating nitrogenous and toxic waste substances; (4) it helps to regulate acid-base and calcium balance in the blood stream.

(5) When fats are not absorbed adequately, the fat-soluble vitamins are not absorbed satisfactorily either. Therefore, in the absence of bile salts, vitamins A, E, D, and K are poorly absorbed. Vitamin K is usually not stored in the body and a deficiency of vitamin K results. This in turn leads to deficient formation by the liver of factor VII and prothrombin, which results in serious impairment of blood coagulation.

(6) Approximately 94 per cent of bile salts are reabsorbed from the intestine—on the average these salts make the circuit from intestine to liver and back to intestine some 18 times before being carried out in the feces (this is the enterohepatic circulation). The quantity of bile secreted by the liver is dependent on bile salts to a great extent, and hence, if there is a loss of bile salts

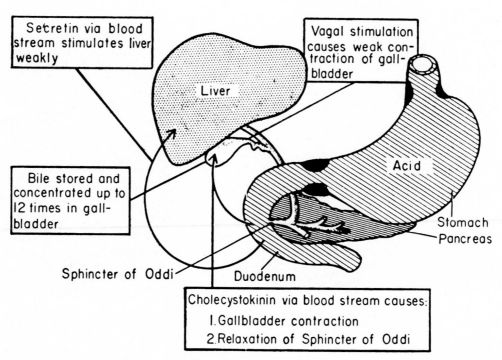

Figure 14–52. Mechanisms of liver secretion and gallbladder emptying. (From Guyton, A. C.: Textbook of Medical Physiology. 4th ed. Philadelphia, W. B. Saunders Co., 1971.)

TABLE 14–1 SELECTION OF PATIENTS FOR ORAL CHOLANGIOGRAPHY AND CHOLECYSTOGRAPHY

Test	Values	Probability of Success
Serum bilirubin		
(Mandel)	< 5 mg.%	{ Worth trying
	>10 mg.%	{ Failure
(Shehadi)	< 1 mg.%	Excellent
	< 2 mg.%	Satisfactory
	3 mg.% or	Poor or unlikely
	> 4 mg.%	Not possible
Bromsulphalein (BSP) retention		
(Etess and Strauss)	5–20%	Should not interfere
	>20–23%	Failure
(Blornstrom and Sandstrom)	>40%	Failure

through a fistula, for example, the volume of liver secretion is also depressed. (With a bile fistula, however, the liver increases its production of bile salts as much as ten-fold in an effort to increase bile secretion to normal.)

Jaundice. Jaundice causes a yellowish tint to the body tissues that results from large quantities of bilirubin in the extracellular fluids. The skin begins to appear jaundiced when the concentration rises to about three times normal, normal being 0.5 mg. per 100 ml. Borderline jaundice occurs at 1.5 mg. per 100 ml.

The common causes of jaundice are: (1) excessive destruction of red cells with release of bilirubin into the blood, or (2) obstruction of the bile ducts or damage to the liver cells so that bilirubin cannot be excreted by the liver.

Type 1 jaundice is *hemolytic* jaundice; Type 2 is *obstructive* jaundice. An understanding of these and other liver functions is inherent in the selection of patients for radiological gallbladder studies; Table 14–1 is presented as an aid in these judgments. Table 14–2 presents a battery of liver function studies helpful in the differential diagnosis of jaundice (Shehadi). It will be noted that generally gallbladder study by cholecystography is probably of no value when the serum bilirubin exceeds 10 mg. per cent; to insure reasonable success requires a serum bilirubin of less than 2 mg. per cent.

Gallstone Formation (Fig. 14–53). Bile salts are formed by

TABLE 14–2 LIVER FUNCTION STUDIES IN DIFFERENTIAL DIAGNOSIS OF JAUNDICE*

	Normal Values	Hemolytic Jaundice (Prehepatic)	Hepatocellular Jaundice (Hepatic) Medical	Obstructive Jaundice (Posthepatic) Surgical
Significant pathologic process	– –	Red blood cell destruction	Liver cell impairment	Bile flow interference
Cephalin cholesterol flocculation	0 to 1	Normal	Elevated	Normal or slightly elevated
Thymol turbidity	0 to 4	Normal	Elevated	Normal or slightly elevated
Zinc sulfate turbidity	0 to 4	Normal	Elevated	Normal or slightly elevated
Serum alkaline phosphatase	1 to 4 Bodansky units 5 to 13 King-Armstrong units	Normal	Normal or elevated	Markedly elevated
Brumsulfalein retention	5 per cent or less at 45 min.	Normal	Increased retention	Increased retention
Serum bilirubin	Up to 1.0 mg. per 100 ml.	Slight increase	Increase in proportion to degree of liver damage	Elevated
Icteric index	8 to 10	Elevated	Elevated	Elevated
Visualization of the gallbladder and bile ducts by means of cholecystography, oral and intravenous		Adequate Density may be slightly decreased	Possible but not satisfactory until B.S.P. retention is 5 per cent or below	None Sometimes possible in intermittent type, as jaundice is clearing, or between phases of obstruction

Icteric index 10 or below
Possible but faint up
  to 15
Bilirubin below 2 mg.,
  preferably 1 mg.
Poor or unlikely above
  3 mg.
Not possible above 4 mg.

*From Shehadi, W. H.: Clinical Radiology of the Biliary Tract. New York, McGraw-Hill Book Company, 1963.

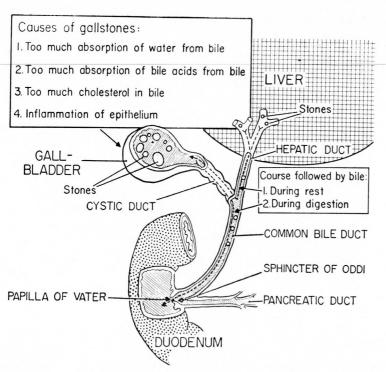

Causes of gallstones:

1. Too much absorption of water from bile
2. Too much absorption of bile acids from bile
3. Too much cholesterol in bile
4. Inflammation of epithelium

LIVER

Stones

GALL-
BLADDER

HEPATIC DUCT

Stones

Course followed by bile:
1. During rest
2. During digestion

CYSTIC DUCT

COMMON BILE DUCT

SPHINCTER OF ODDI

PAPILLA OF VATER

PANCREATIC DUCT

DUODENUM

Figure 14–53. Formation of gallstones. (From Guyton, A. C.: Textbook of Medical Physiology. 4th ed. Philadelphia, W. B. Saunders Co., 1971.)

ROENTGENOLOGIC EXAMINATION OF THE BILIARY TRACT

Introduction. Prior to the gallbladder examination, it is well to remove as much gas and fecal material from the gastrointestinal tract as possible. Cascara sagrada or enemas given at least 24 hours before the examination may be of considerable assistance. Pitressin may be employed intravenously (0.5 to 1 cc.) in those patients in whom it is not contraindicated on the basis of hypertension or arteriosclerosis.

It is also well to obtain a plain film of the entire right side of the abdomen in the posteroanterior projection prior to the administration of any dye. The gallbladder itself is not usually delineated with accuracy on such films, but if it should contain calcareous structure, this would immediately be evident from this preliminary study.

A visualization of the gallbladder requires that some form of contrast substance be introduced into it. Tetrachlorphenolphthalein had long been known as a bile secretion and had been used as a test for liver function. Graham and Cole (in 1924) introduced first the bromine radical and thereafter the heavier iodine radical

liver cells from cholesterol, and a small amount of cholesterol escapes with the bile salts in the bile. The bile salts, fatty acids, and lecithin in bile are responsible for the solubility of cholesterol in the bile. Abnormally, however, the cholesterol will precipitate and form gallstones (Fig. 14–53). As shown in this illustration, the causes of such precipitation are: (1) too much absorption of water from the bile, (2) too much absorption of bile acids from bile, (3) excessive cholesterol in bile, and (4) inflammation of the epithelium of the gallbladder. Inflammation permits excessive absorption of water, bile salts, and other substances through the epithelium of the gallbladder, and as a result cholesterol is no longer kept in solution.

Most cholesterol gallstones themselves are radiolucent (80 to 85 per cent) unless there are crevices in the gallstones, most likely containing excessive fat. These appear as "crow's feet" (Fig. 14–54). Calcium sometimes precipitates with some of the substances involved in the formation of cholesterol gallstones in the form of calcium carbonate—hence, these gallstones are radiopaque (Fig. 14–55). Since most stones in the gallbladder are radiolucent, however, special radiographic studies using iodinated contrast agents that may be concentrated in the gallbladder are necessary. These will be discussed shortly.

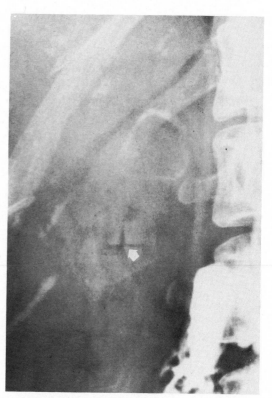

Figure 14–54. "Crowfoot" sign showing crevices which appear radiolucent in a gallstone, giving the appearance of a crow's foot.

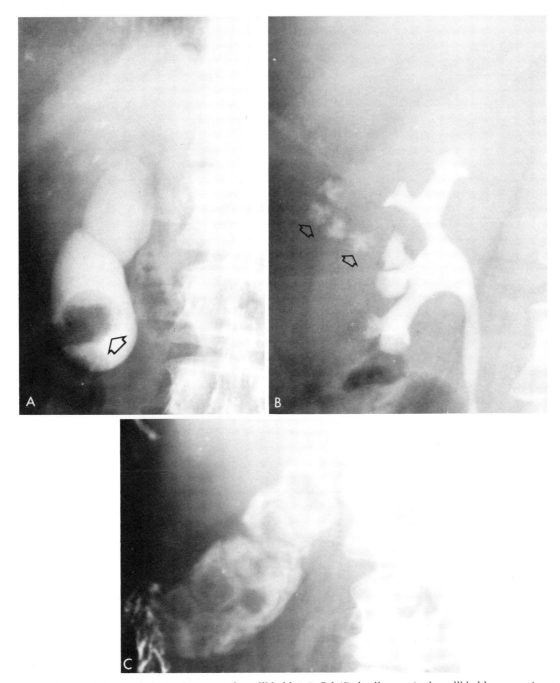

Figure 14–55. *A.* Large cholesterol stone in the gallbladder. *B.* Calcified gallstones in the gallbladder, assuming a "mulberry" appearance. *C.* Partially calcified stones in a partially calcified gallbladder.

instead of the chlorine in this compound, and thus obtained a substance which was secreted by the liver in the bile, and concentrated with the bile in the gallbladder. This made it possible to render the bile radiopaque.

In recent years new compounds such as Priodax, Telepaque,

Teridax, Monophen, and Cholografin (see Table 14–3) have been introduced which accomplish the same thing without many of the undesirable side effects attributed to the earlier contrast medium. Each of the newer compounds has certain contraindications and some adverse effects which are listed in Table 14–3.

TABLE 14–3 COMPARISON OF SOME OF THE MAJOR COMPOUNDS EMPLOYED FOR GALLBLADDER VISUALIZATION

Year of Introduction	Compound	Pharmacology	Contraindications	Accuracy and Adverse Effects
1940	Priodax	Phenylpropionic acid derivative Insoluble in water but soluble in alkali 51.38% iodine Excreted mostly by kidneys	Acute nephritis Uremia	35% less opacity than Telepaque 60% { nausea, diarrhea, dysuria } vs. 21.4% with Telepaque More patients require second dose (40%); fails to visualize 12% of gallbladders visualized with Telepaque
1949	Telepaque	Ethyl propanoic acid derivative Insoluble in water; soluble in alkali and 95% alcohol 66.68% iodine Excreted mostly via gastrointestinal tract	Acute nephritis Uremia Gastrointestinal diseases with disturbed absorption	Fails only in 3% of normal gallbladders or less with one dose Side reactions less than with Priodax Great opacity may obscure some gallstones
1953	Teridax	Triiodoethionic acid (ethyl propionic acid derivative) Insoluble in water; soluble in alkali 66.5% iodine Excreted mostly by kidneys	Acute nephritis Uremia	Failure after one examination not always indicative of disease; but after second dose approaches 100% accuracy Not as well worked out as to side reactions as Priodax or Telepaque Said to produce density intermediate between Priodax and Telepaque
	Monophen	Carboxylic acid derivative Insoluble in water 52.2% iodine Excreted mostly by kidneys	Acute nephritis Uremia	60% no adverse signs or symptoms 12% nausea 1% vomiting 9% diarrhea 9% cramps 3% dysuria Accuracy stated to be better (?) than Priodax
1953–1955	Cholografin	Iodipamide (triiodobenzoic acid derivative) For intravenous use (photosensitive) 64% iodine With normal liver 90% excreated in feces, 10% in urine With poor liver function: mostly excreted by kidneys (hence pyelograms)	Primary indication: Postcholecystectomy syndrome Contraindications: Iodine sensitivity Combined urinary and hepatic disease	Sensitivity high Side effects minimal with slow injection 77–85% successful biliary tree visualizations Visualization faint; usually gallbladder visualization too faint for significant accuracy Serious reactions: 2.5% Lesser reactions: 38.8%
	Orabilex (disapproved by Food and Drug Administration in U.S.A.)	Bunamiodyl (sodium acrylate derivative) 57% iodine Excreted in bile, but mainly by kidneys (70%): 30% by intestine	Renal disease Gastrointestinal diseases which would hamper absorption Double dose never to be used —may lead to acute renal failure	No advantage gained by second dose 12.5% nausea 8.9% vomiting 5.9% diarrhea 6.5% dysuria Approaches 100% accuracy
1959	Ipodate (Oragrafin) (Biloptin) (Solu-Biloptin)	Triiodohydrocinnamic acid derivatives (sodium or calcium salt) 61% iodine 42–48% excreted in bile in 24 hrs., equally in urine	Iodine sensitivity Combined renal-hepatic disease Severe kidney disorders Gastrointestinal disorders or liver disorders	Mild and transient nausea: vomiting; diarrhea

Methods of Study. There are several possible roentgenologic techniques that can be used to study the biliary system. These are:

1. Plain film of the abdomen.
2. Oral cholecystograms (including opacification of bile duct calculi).
   a. Rectal cholecystography.
3. Intravenous cholangiography.
4. Percutaneous transhepatic cholangiography.
5. Operative and postoperative cholangiography.
6. Biliary angiography.
   a. Liver.
   b. Gallbladder.

Plain Film of the Abdomen. The plain film of the abdomen should always precede contrast studies involving any organs contained in the abdomen.

In the case of the biliary tract, this should consist of: (1) KUB (kidney, ureter, bladder) film as described in Chapter 15, and (2) a 10 × 12 inch film of the right upper quadrant of the patient, with the patient in either the right posterior oblique or left anterior oblique projection (the same projection that is utilized subsequently in oral cholecystography). This film should extend from the iliac crest as close as possible to the right hemidiaphragm. The entire right lobe of the liver is usually included.

Oral Cholecystograms

Major Compounds Employed. Graham and Cole devised percutaneous, intravenous, and oral cholecystograms first, utilizing *tetrabromphenolphthalein* and later *sodium phenoltetraiodophthalein.* The compounds used later and some of the pharmacologic data are given in Table 14–3.

The pharmacodynamics of biliary contrast media have undergone considerable investigation (Shehadi, 1966a; Lasser et al.). By virtue of their chemical constitution, these agents are primarily "bile directed" rather than "urine directed."

The compound most frequently employed for oral study is *Telepaque,* a moderately lipid-soluble substance that is poorly soluble in an aqueous system. (*Cholografin,* the compound used in intravenous application, is freely soluble in an aqueous solution but is not appreciably absorbed from the gastrointestinal tract. This contrast agent will be discussed under intravenous cholangiography.)

After administration of Telepaque, there is a circulating level of 1 to 16 mg. per cent within 2 hours. Some patients, particularly those with less than 4 mg. per cent at 2 hours, show a rise at the 14 hour period. Shehadi has indicated that there are two distinct peaks in the absorption curve, one at 4 hours and a second, higher peak at 10 hours, and it is for this reason that the 10 hour interval is assumed to be the optimum time for film study for most patients.

Berk and Lasser have demonstrated the following cycle: the Telepaque is absorbed in the gastrointestinal tract, whereupon it is delivered to the liver. It is thereafter excreted in the bile, and if the extrahepatic biliary passages are open, it finds its way to the gallbladder. In the gallbladder the contrast agent and bile are concentrated above the level of the original bile. If, however, the gallbladder is inflamed or its mucosa is otherwise pathological, the contrast medium is absorbed from the gallbladder, and concentration of the agent does not occur sufficiently for roentgenologic visualization. When Cholografin is used, it accumulates in the gallbladder in the same form in which it is administered in sufficient concentration usually for visualization, although it is not as opaque as Telepaque. (For an understanding of the chemistry and conjugations involved, reference should be made to the original articles.)

Although many investigators may prefer one or another of these agents, preference in recent times has generally remained with Telepaque. There are some advantages and disadvantages of Telepaque versus *Oragrafin* (White and Fischer). The degree of opacification of the gallbladder and visualization of the biliary ducts is similar with both these oral cholecystographic agents. Calculi are more often demonstrated with Telepaque, but on the other hand, stones are not as often concealed by the lesser density of Oragrafin. The incidence of diarrhea is much higher and that of nausea and cramps slightly higher with Telepaque. There is also a lesser side effect with a double dose technique of Oragrafin as compared with Telepaque.

Technical Aspects of Oral Cholecystography

PREPARATION OF THE PATIENT. Prior to examination, it should be determined that: (1) the patient is not sensitive to iodine-containing contrast agents, and (2) the patient has been on a diet which might reasonably have produced previous evacuation of the gallbladder by fatty stimulation.

If possible, there should be at least one fat-containing meal the day prior to the cholecystographic examination in order to empty a distended gallbladder.

On the evening prior to the examination, the meal should be fat-free and may consist of fruit or fruit juice, fresh vegetables cooked without butter, a small portion of lean meat, toast or bread with jelly, coffee or tea but no milk, cream, butter, eggs, or any foods containing fat. Nothing should be eaten after the evening meal, although water may be taken in moderate amounts.

At about 10 P.M. six Telepaque tablets (3 grams) should be swallowed, each with one or two mouthfuls of water, a total of at least one full glass of water. To avoid nausea or vomiting, an interval of 5 minutes after each tablet may elapse. If roentgen examination is scheduled for 9 A.M., the best time for administration of Telepaque is between 9 and 11 P.M. on the night preceding the examination.

On the following morning, breakfast should be omitted.

The patient may be given an enema if it is discovered that

the contrast agent in the gastrointestinal tract interferes with adequate visualization of the gallbladder.

DOSE CONSIDERATIONS.   It is probable that 3 grams of Telepaque are sufficient for all adults irrespective of weight (Whitehouse and Martin). With some patients we have used doses as high as 6 grams (12 tablets) within a period of 24 hours. Different studies on the renal toxicity of contrast medium in patients with hepatorenal damage have called attention to the danger of larger doses of oral cholecystographic media (Seaman, Cosgriff and Wells). It has therefore been recommended that a dose of 6 grams not be exceeded within a period of 24 hours, and if such a dose has been employed, that it not be repeated for a period of at least 1 week.

Pediatric patients may be given proportionately smaller doses (Harris and Caffey).

Salzman et al. have found that biliary stones can, at times, be visualized by administering 1 gram of Telepaque three times a day for 4 days, and this opacity may persist for as long as 2 to 14 days. It is thought that this gallstone opacification phenomenon is due to a reaction between biliverdin on the surface of the stones and the contrast medium in the bile.

Caution must be exercised not to use this technique in patients who have impaired hepatorenal function.

FILM AND FLUOROSCOPIC TECHNIQUES.   On the morning after the patient has taken the contrast medium, films are repeated in the left anterior oblique projection (patient prone) with various degrees of obliquity. Each film should be studied until satisfactory visualization of the gallbladder is obtained. The gallbladder should be completely clear of interfering gas or other opaque shadows. Sufficient kilovoltage should be employed so that the contrast agent will not in itself obscure filling defects within the gallbladder (Fig. 14–56).

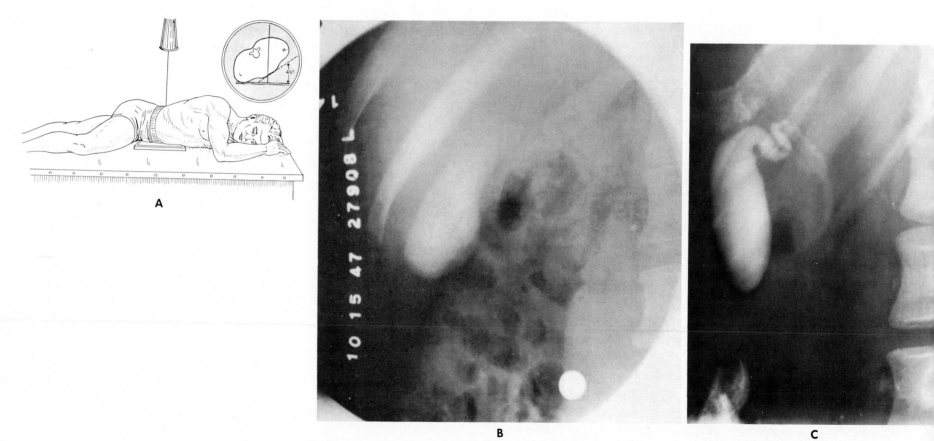

Figure 14–56.   Radiograph of gallbladder before fatty stimulation. *A.* Position of patient. *B.* Radiograph. *C.* Representative scout film of the gallbladder region extending from the iliac fossa to the diaphragm and from the left portion of the spine to the outer flank region.

Upright or lateral decubitus films are also obtained routinely to determine possible stratification or mobility of filling defects within the gallbladder (Fig. 14–58). Fluoroscopy with compression spot-film studies may be employed for this purpose.

Following this first part of the examination, the patient is given a meal consisting of foods with a high fat content such as eggs, butter, toast or cream; or a synthetic cholagogue such as Bilevac may be employed.

After the fatty meal or fat stimulation is administered, the films of the right upper quadrant are repeated in identical positions (Fig. 14–57). Body section radiography may be employed at any time in the procedure to obtain better visualization of the gallbladder proper or of the ductal system.

When the customary dose of six tablets is used, visualization of the extrahepatic ducts can be obtained in most patients in 5 to 20 minutes after the fat meal. However, if visualization of the extrahepatic ducts is especially indicated a somewhat higher dose of Telepaque (6 grams) may be required.

Variations of this general procedure may be undertaken as follows: (1) The Telepaque may be taken earlier in the evening and castor oil may be administered five hours after the Telepaque tablets (Mauthe). However, if the gallbladder is not visualized the morning following administration of the Telepaque, the examination is repeated in a day or so without the castor oil. Repetition of the examination under these circumstances is important. (2) In order to overcome biliary stasis (one of the common causes of nonvisualization or delayed visualization of the gallbladder) the use of bile acid for 5 to 30 days before repeating the cholecystographic examination has been recommended (Berg and Hamilton).

SIDE EFFECTS. Whitehouse and Martin have reported the following side effects from 3 gram doses of Telepaque in 400 patients; diarrhea, 25.3 per cent (of which 2.5 per cent were severe); dysuria, 13.7 per cent; mild nausea, 5.8 per cent; and mild vomiting 1.5 per cent. There were other side effects in 2.8 per cent of the cases and no side effects were noted in 62.5 per cent of the cases.

Patients with hepatorenal dysfunction constitute a group subject to potential hazards from oral cholecystography. Doses of Telepaque larger than those recommended earlier should be employed with caution. There are advantages and disadvantages to each of the various compounds, and a careful choice must be

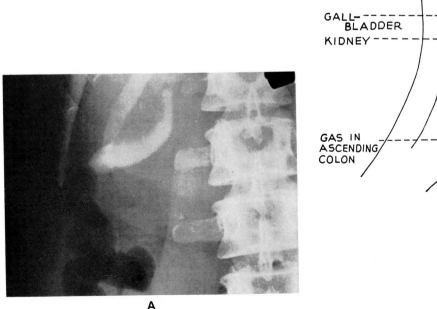

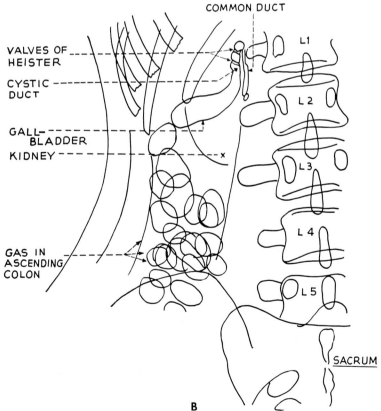

Figure 14–57. Gallbladder after fatty stimulation. *A.* Radiograph. *B.* Labeled tracing of *A.*

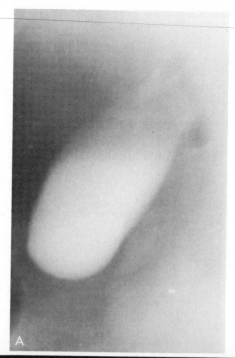

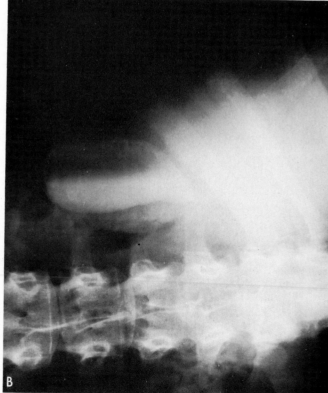

Figure 14–58. Layering of Telepaque that may occur normally in the gallbladder. *A.* Erect. *B.* Lateral decubitus with patient lying on left side.

made with full knowledge of all aspects of the contrast agent employed as well as the importance of the clinical evaluation in the case at hand.

VISUALIZATION OR NONVISUALIZATION. It is well documented also that repeat examinations of the gallbladder following initial failures of visualization, or inadequate visualization, without evidence of gallstones will be interpreted as normal. In Rosenbaum's series of 450 consecutive patients examined by cholecystography, there were 66 visualizations in which evidence of gallstones was initially absent or inadequate. After the second dose of Telepaque and repeat roentgen study, findings were interpreted as normal in 10 per cent of those with initial nonvisualization and in 64 per cent of those with initially inadequate visualization.

A gallbladder that is consistently small or large but has good concentration and no other abnormalities is difficult to interpret. It is assumed, however, that a gallbladder that is visualized well and contains no stones is normal (Fig. 14–56). Distended gallbladders should be studied further.

VARIATION IN NUMBER. A double gallbladder and duplication of the cystic duct may occur (Fig. 14–59). Triplication of the gallbladder is a rare anomaly which has also been described (Ross and Sachs). The congenital folded fundus of the gallbladder or variation of a Phrygian cap gallbladder, which represents a mucosal or serosal fold of the gallbladder, must be carefully differentiated by a number of oblique views (Fig. 14–51 *B*).

THE SIGNIFICANCE OF NONVISUALIZATION OF THE GALLBLADDER IN PATIENTS WITH INTACT GALLBLADDER. ABNORMALITY OF FUNCTION. There are certain basic assumptions that must be verified as far as possible in order to interpret oral cholecystograms:

1. That the patient actually has taken the contrast agent.

2. That adequate absorption of the agent has occurred (no esophageal, gastric, or intestinal obstruction) (Fig. 14–60).

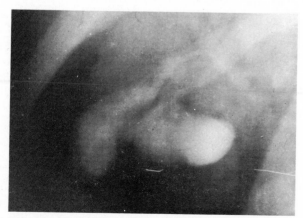

Figure 14–59. Cholecystogram demonstrating a double gallbladder. Note that even the cystic duct in this instance is duplicated.

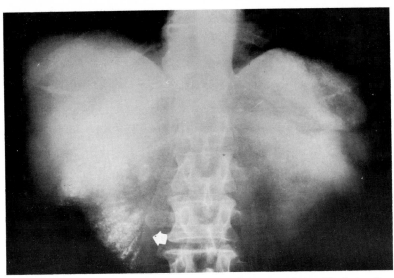

Figure 14–60. Nonvisualization of the gallbladder in a patient with obstruction of the duodenum. Note all of the contrast agent retained above the level of obstruction; this indicates inadequate absorption.

3. That the liver function is adequate for secretion of the test compound.

4. That the ductal system above the level of the gallbladder is not obstructed.

5. That the common bile duct is not obstructed (in which case there may be some associated gallbladder disease).

The oral cholecystogram is fundamentally a function test. It must not, however, be assumed that nonvisualization necessarily indicates abnormal function in certain rare instances. Complete absence of the gallbladder is a rare anomaly but can occur.

A surprisingly high proportion of men with cholelithiasis are asymptomatic (70 per cent of men with stones and 86 per cent of a control group have no symptoms) (Wilbur and Bolt). Of 30 per cent of patients with gallstones, two-thirds had only the unreliable signs and symptoms of dyspepsia and epigastric pain, symptoms which are found in 10 per cent of normal controls. Also, typical biliary colic can be a misleading description, since it is found in about 3.6 per cent of those with no stones and in 0.9 per cent of normal men.

Evaluation of Oral Cholecystography. Many investigators have compared the accuracy of the diagnosis following Telepaque cholecystography with the diagnosis established at surgery in patients undergoing surgery of the biliary tract.

In their series of 1207 cholecystographic examinations, in which all diagnoses were subjected to surgical and pathologic verification. Baker and Hodgson found only 1.9 per cent of all diagnoses to be in error. Of cases designated as normal preopera-

tively, 98.3 per cent were so found at surgery. Gallbladders designated as "poorly functioning" were found to be diseased. Of cases diagnosed as cholelithiasis, 98 per cent were confirmed. Gallbladders showing nonvisualization were found to be abnormal in 97.8 per cent of the cases. Alderson reported a 99 per cent accuracy in 315 patients.

Extrahepatic duct visualization was obtained in a high percentage of cases (85 per cent) when a synthetic cholagogue such as Bilevac was used (Norman and Saghapoleslami).

Dann et al. have reported that in 200 patients whose gallbladders were not visualized by oral cholecystography, the common bile duct was visualized in 30 per cent. Of this group, 28 patients were operated upon and all exhibited definite pathologic conditions in the gallbladder.

Rosenbaum, in a series of 400 consecutive patients examined by cholecystography, found that visualization was initially absent or inadequate without evidence of gallstones in 66. After a repeat dose and roentgen study, findings were normal in 10 per cent of those with initial nonvisualization and in 64 per cent of those with initially inadequate visualization.

Repeat dose, consecutive dose, or second dose cholecystography was also investigated by Berk. He studied 396 patients whose gallbladders were visualized poorly or not at all on initial cholecystograms employing Telepaque. Fifty per cent of these showed no improvement in concentration on the second study, 20 per cent showed moderate improvement, and 30 per cent showed marked improvement. Of these original 396 patients, 160 showed poor visualization on the initial study. Of these, a second or consecutive dose led to no improvement in 20 per cent, moderate improvement in 30 per cent, and marked improvement in 50 per cent. Of the 236 patients whose gallbladders were not visualized on the initial examination, 75 per cent showed no increase in opacification, 10 per cent showed moderate increase, and 15 per cent showed a marked increase. Hence, the "consecutive dose phenomenon" is more frequent in patients with initially faint visualization than in those with initial nonvisualization.

It is interesting to note that 38 of the 119 patients who demonstrated this phenomenon were restudied by follow-up cholecystograms 1 to 4 years later, and a majority of these failed to reproduce the same effect. Actually, in 33 of the 38 patients, the opacification of the gallbladder was normal with a single dose of Telepaque on the follow-up study.

It is thought by others, however, that if additional doses of Telepaque are justified, it may be best to follow the oral examination by an intravenous one to avoid some of the complications in relation to Telepaque (Whitehouse).

Morbidity Following Oral Cholecystography. Serious and even fatal reactions to gallbladder contrast media have been described by a number of authors. Increasing reports of renal complications have caused the withdrawal of Orabilex from active clinical use. Reports of renal insufficiency following the use of such a medium, especially in double dosage, have been made by a number of authors (Rene and Mellinkoff). The occurrence of thrombocytopenia following the administration of Telepaque was described by Bishopric in 1964. There would appear to be no way to predict the occurrence of thrombocytopenia despite the possibility of a previous similar reaction to another drug. Sensitivity to iodine may be a causative factor. Once again it should be emphasized that, as with all oral iodinated contrast media, these should not be administered in the presence of combined renal and hepatic disease or severe kidney impairment.

Modified Cholecystography. Various techniques have been devised for potentiating cholecystography.

1. The injection of cholecystokinin (75 Ivy dog units) intravenously has been advocated to enhance diagnostic accuracy in patients who apparently have gallbladder disease and yet are pronounced "normal" in routine cholecystography (Nathan et al.).

2. A rapid oral method for roentgenographic visualization has been investigated by Fischer et al., utilizing Oragrafin.

The student is referred to the original articles for further evaluation of these experimental techniques.

3. Certain pharmacologic agents are thought to enhance the diagnosis of biliary tract disease. For example, the combination of atropine and amyl nitrite may be utilized to differentiate a spasm of the sphincter of Oddi from an organic stenosis at this site. This is accomplished by the subcutaneous injection of 0.5 mg. of atropine sulfate about 1½ hours after the intravenous injection of contrast medium, with simultaneous inhalation of amyl nitrite. The two together may be used for relaxation of spasm of the sphincter of Oddi.

4. The intravenous or intramuscular injection of 0.01 gram of morphine may cause a contraction of the sphincter of Oddi and this, too, may prolong the persistence of the contrast agent in the bile duct. However, the routine use of morphine results in paralysis of the gallbladder and inhibits its contraction following administration of a cholagogue.

5. Prostigmine (0.5 mg. intravenously) has a less spastic effect on the sphincter of Oddi and does not affect the gallbladder.

6. Cholecystokinin may also be used. This agent causes contraction of the gallbladder and permits assessment of the dynamics of the biliary tract. Films are obtained approximately 5 to 35 minutes after the intravenous injection of this agent (75 Ivy units or 0.04 mg. of the dessicated material per kilogram of body weight). This time-span permits evaluation of gallbladder motility and sphincteric action.

7. Cholecystokinin may be combined with morphine also (Garbsch).

Rectal Cholecystography. This technique may be used when oral or intravenous methods are not practical or are contraindicated.

Orgrafin in a dose of 6 grams in a special rectal kit is utilized. The rectum must be thoroughly cleansed in advance. The contrast agent is dissolved in sterile distilled water immediately before use, and is slowly instilled in the rectum at bedtime over a period of 20 minutes. The examination of the gallbladder is carried forward as in the case of the oral cholecystogram 10 to 12 hours later. Calcium Oragrafin may be better for this purpose than the sodium preparation.

To be effective, the contrast agent must be retained by the patient. If expelled, the examination will be unsatisfactory.

The limiting factors for use of this technique are the relative unpredictability of rectal absorption and some rectal irritation.

Intravenous Cholangiography. *Contrast Medium.* The contrast agent, sodium iodipamide (Biligrafin in Germany), was replaced in 1955 by iodipamide methylglucamine and introduced in the United States under the trade name of Cholografin methylglucamine. The standard dose for the adult is 20 ml. of the latter compound. This dose contains approximately 5 grams of iodine. Approximately 90 per cent of the compound is excreted by the liver and 10 per cent by the kidneys. In patients with liver damage, a greater percentage will be excreted by the kidney. Wise has reported that in 12 years of experience with over 5000 injections, there have been no fatal reactions in the Lahey Clinic. Normal reactions such as nausea, vomiting, hypotension, or urticaria have, on occasion, occurred. (A dose greater than 20 ml. is contraindicated and may be toxic.)

Criteria and Indications for Intravenous Cholangiography. *When serum bilirubin levels are 1 mg. per 100 ml. or less, opaci-*

SITUATIONS JUSTIFYING USE OF INTRAVENOUS CHOLANGIOGRAPHY

1. Nonvisualization of gallbladder by oral route.
2. Need to distinguish gallbladder disease and obstructive disease of the distal common duct.
3. Evaluation of the postcholecystectomy syndrome.
4. Preoperative examination to demonstrate calculi in the common bile duct before cholecystectomy.
5. History of biliary abnormality in infants and children.
6. Emergencies in which speed is a factor.
7. Suspicion of a tumor near the porta hepatis.
8. Recent or subsiding jaundice in which bilirubin and BSP levels are appropriate to help differentiate infective hepatitis and common duct stones.
9. Functional biliary disorders in which a study of the duct system may help differentiate organic disease.

Figure 14–61.

fication of the ducts may be expected in 92.5 per cent of cases. If serum bilirubin values are above 4 mg. per 100 ml., opacification may be expected in only 9.3 per cent.

When BSP (bromsulphalein) retention level is below 10 per cent after 45 minutes, opacification may be expected in 96 per cent of injections, but if retention level is above 40 per cent, opacification may be expected in 26.2 per cent (Wise).

With these basic criteria in mind, *intravenous cholangiography is indicated in the following situations* (Fig. 14–61):

1. Nonvisualization by the oral route. According to Wise, 12 per cent of these patients were found to have gallbladders which appeared normal and in which no calculi were visualized. Of 201 patients with intact gallbladders not visualized by the oral route, visualization was accomplished in 70 by the intravenous method, and 24 of these were considered normal. All of those whose gallbladders were not visualized by the intravenous method were found later to be diseased.

2. Differentiation of gallbladder disease and obstructive disease of the distal common duct. (a) If the common duct is less than 7.0 mm. in diameter, nonvisualization of the gallbladder is due to cystic duct obstruction or primary gallbladder disease. (b) If the common duct is dilated, the cause of nonopacification may be common duct obstruction alone or a combination of cystic duct obstruction and common duct obstruction.

Further indications are listed in Figure 14–61.

Technique of Intravenous Examination. 1. Good catharsis on the night prior to the examination.

2. A plain film of the right upper quadrant in the right posterior oblique (and in some instances, left anterior oblique).

3. A preliminary subcutaneous injection of 5 mg. of para-bromdylamine is given. The patient is examined in the hydrated and nonfasting state.

4. A test dose of 1 cc. of Cholografin is administered intravenously, and a 3 minute interval is allowed to elapse until the remaining 19 cc. are injected over a minimum period of 10 minutes ("minor" reactions occur in 4.3 per cent). Drip infusion may be employed.

5. The first film is obtained following the completion of the injection in the supine position with the left side elevated approximately 15 degrees. Low kilovoltage is used.

6. Repeat films are obtained at 10 to 20 minute intervals thereafter for 40 to 60 minutes.

7. If no visualization is obtained at 60 to 90 minutes in a patient in whom the gallbladder has not been removed, a film of the right upper quadrant is made at 4 hours and if possible at 24 hours for visualization of the gallbladder.

8. Once a film giving the best possible visualization is obtained, films are made at 20 minute intervals in order to evaluate radiodensity, particularly if it appears that the duct is dilated and partially obstructed. (If the density and retention of the contrast medium in the bile ducts is greater at 120 minutes than at 60

minutes, partial obstruction of the common bile duct or main biliary tract is present.) If the duct is normal in size without evidence of obstruction and good drainage is seen, the study may be terminated in 60 to 90 minutes.

9. *Body section radiography should be performed as an additional adjunct when ductal visualization is optimum* (Fig. 14–62 B).

10. In children with suspected anomalies of the extrahepatic biliary system, between 0.6 and 1.6 cc. of 20 per cent sodium iodipamide (Cholografin) per kilogram of body weight was injected slowly by Hays and Averbrook and exposures made at intervals over a 4 hour period. This intravenous injection was preceded by a test dose for sensitivity of 0.5 cc. (Methylglucamine iodipamide should require half this dosage.)

Some Radiographic Signs of Abnormality in Intravenous Cholangiography

ABNORMALITIES OF THE GALLBLADDER. When the gallbladder is visualized, the abnormalities previously described in respect to oral cholecystograms also apply here.

When, however, the biliary tree is not visualized, a specific interpretation is not possible. Wise has reported a visualization of bile ducts in approximately 90 per cent of cases after cholecystectomy in which patients' serum bilirubin levels have been below 1 mg. per 100 ml. and BSP retention has been 10 per cent or less after 35 minutes.

In patients with an intact gallbladder and nonvisualization by oral cholecystography, Wise visualized 35 per cent of 201 gallbladders. In 12 per cent the gallbladder was considered normal by this technique.

When the bile ducts were visualized but the gallbladder was not, approximately 70 per cent of the patients were shown to have primary gallbladder disease. Approximately 10 per cent were shown to have primary common duct or pancreatic disease, and 20 per cent had combined gallbladder and common duct or pancreatic disease.

ABNORMALITIES IN SIZE OF THE COMMON BILE DUCT. In a postmortem study of the common bile duct Nazareno et al. reported that, with the usual cholangiographic technique and with the inherent magnification in most radiographic procedures, the upper limit of the diameter of the magnified common bile duct was 10 mm. in 97.5 per cent of normal people. The actual anatomic measurement was approximately two-thirds of that obtained roentgenographically. Others have indicated slightly different measurements (Wise; Shehadi, 1963b; McClenahan et al.). In a postcholecystectomy state, a "normal" bile duct is less than 19 mm. in diameter (Wise). The size, therefore, is such a variable criterion that the physician, in caring for his patient, must first decide whether or not obstruction exists, and then make a judgment, on this basis, whether abnormality is indicated.

ABNORMALITY OF CONTOUR OF THE COMMON BILE DUCT. Or-

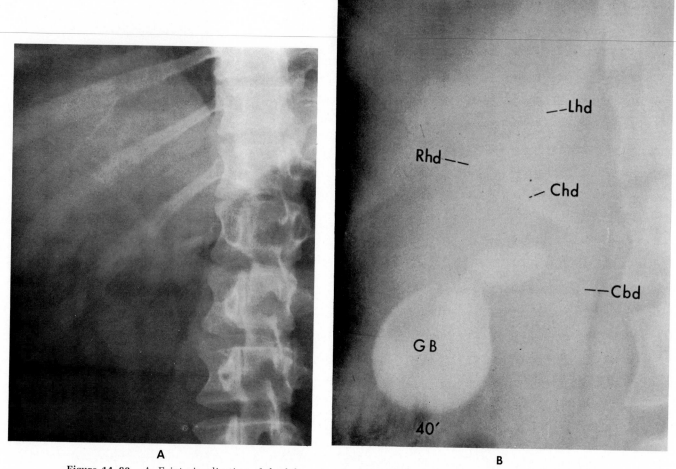

A   B

Figure 14–62. *A.* Faint visualization of the biliary tree by intravenous cholangiography with the aid of intra-venous Cholografin. Ordinarily a visualization of this order of density is obtained. Enhancement of detail is obtained by tomography. *B.* Normal intravenous cholangiogram–tomogram.

Figure 14–62 continued on the opposite page.

dinarily the two hepatic ducts and common hepatic duct are approximately equal in size and do not taper significantly. However, the common bile duct begins to taper near its origin at the level of the cystic duct to the ampulla. Absence of tapering must be regarded with suspicion as indicative of possible abnormality.

Normally, the common bile duct is gently convex toward the left (Fig. 14–62). A reversal of this convexity suggests an abnormal contour and displacement.

In response to obstruction, the hepatic radicals may also change their normal contour and size and become progressively dilated and increasingly opacified (Fig. 14–63).

ABNORMALITIES OF FUNCTION. Wise and O'Brien have proposed the time-density retention concept as applied to intravenous cholangiography and have shown a composite curve illustrating the relative density of contrast substance and drainage rates of unobstructed versus obstructed ducts (Fig. 14–64). In this curve maximum density in unobstructed cases is achieved at 45

minutes. Thereafter the density tends to diminish in unobstructed cases up to 2 hours after the beginning of the study. In obstructed cases, the density remains relatively constant at a maximum level during the 45 to 120 minute interval.

Evaluation of Intravenous Cholangiography in Patients with Intact Gallbladders. Wise reports an overall accuracy of specific diagnoses based on intravenous cholangiography in 79.4 per cent of cases. False positive predictions were made in 8.6 per cent of cases.

Wise also analyzed 694 injections of patients with intact gallbladders and found that the duct was visualized in 621; the presence of common duct calculi was proved in 39 of these cases. In only one of these 39 cases was the common duct stone found to be associated with a normal gallbladder in an otherwise normal common duct.

The usefulness of the intravenous cholangiogram in patients with intact gallbladders was also investigated by Eckelberg et al.

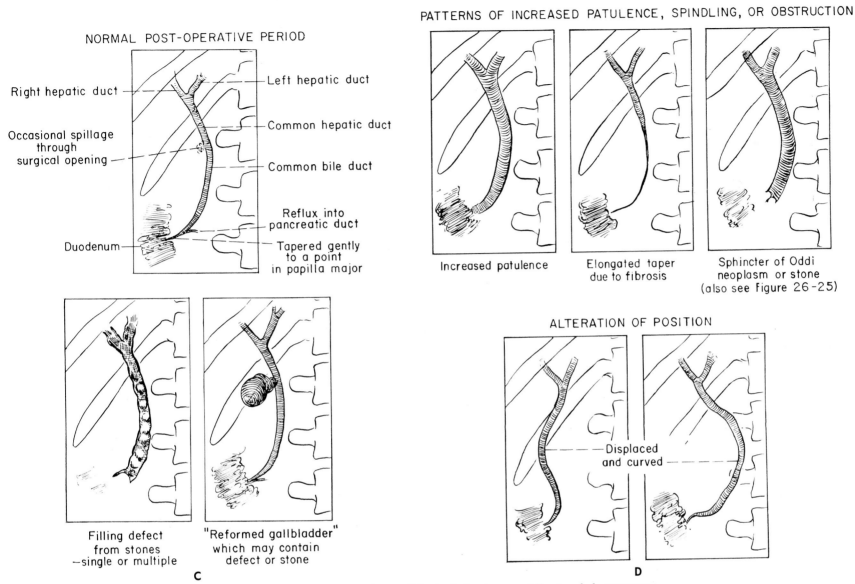

NORMAL POST-OPERATIVE PERIOD

Right hepatic duct

Left hepatic duct

Common hepatic duct

Occasional spillage
through
surgical opening

Common bile duct

Reflux into
pancreatic duct

Duodenum

Tapered gently
to a point
in papilla major

PATTERNS OF INCREASED PATULENCE, SPINDLING, OR OBSTRUCTION

Increased patulence

Elongated taper
due to fibrosis

Sphincter of Oddi
neoplasm or stone
(also see Figure 26-25)

Filling defect
from stones
—single or multiple

"Reformed gallbladder"
which may contain
defect or stone

ALTERATION OF POSITION

Displaced
and curved

C   **D**

Figure 14–62 *Continued.*   *C* and *D.* Abnormalities in cholangiograms, following cholecystectomy.

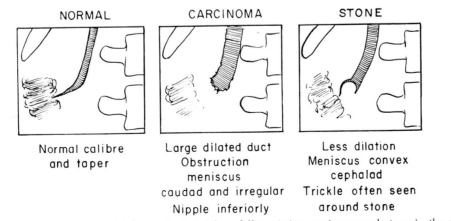

NORMAL

CARCINOMA

STONE

Normal calibre
and taper

Large dilated duct
Obstruction
meniscus
caudad and irregular
Nipple inferiorly

Less dilation
Meniscus convex
cephalad
Trickle often seen
around stone

Figure 14–63.   Roentgen signs which may be helpful in differentiating carcinoma and stone in the common duct in cholangiography.

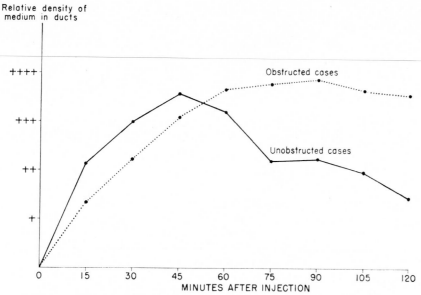

Figure 14–64. Composite curve illustrating the relative density of contrast substance, and drainage rates of an obstructed vs. a nonobstructed common bile duct. (From Wise, R. E., and O'Brien, R. G.: J.A.M.A., *160*:822, 1956. Copyright 1956, American Medical Association.)

They studied 133 patients and found that with intravenous cholangiography the gallbladder was visualized in 66 per cent. The longest interval before visualization was 135 minutes, and the average time for initial visualization was 33 minutes (but since 44 of the 133 examinations were terminated at 25 minutes, it is difficult to interpret this finding). The biliary ducts were visualized in 91 per cent, with the initial visualization occurring at 25 minutes in almost all patients. The longest interval for initial visualization of the ducts, however, was 50 minutes. The presence or absence of the contrast agent in the kidney-collecting system had no bearing upon the quality of visualization of the biliary tract.

Opacification of the bile duct accompanying nonvisualization of the gallbladder was found to be caused by complete mechanical obstruction of the cystic duct by stone or edema in about a third of the 57 patients for whom surgical exploration was done. Of the remaining patients most were found to have free gallstones at operation, but in about an eighth of the cases there was no discoverable anatomic reason to explain why the gallbladder had not filled with contrast media. Moreover, delay in opacification of the gallbladder beyond 25 minutes did not seem to be influenced by the presence or absence of stones in the gallbladder. In some cases, gallstones not demonstrated by oral cholecystography were disclosed by the intravenous examination.

Evaluation of Intravenous Cholangiograms in Postcholecystectomy Patients. Beargie et al. in 1962 presented their experience with intravenous cholangiography in the evaluation of 1956 patients with symptoms referable to the upper portion of the ab-

domen after cholecystectomy. They found, as did Wise, that a satisfactory visualization of the biliary tree correlated most closely with the results of serum bilirubin and bromsulphalein (BSP) retention studies. It was also reliably related to the values of alkaline phosphatase. They also concluded from a comparison of the radiologic cholangiographic findings with subsequent surgical findings that intravenous cholangiography provided an accuracy of diagnosis in 90 to 95 per cent of the patients. The diagnostic value of a delayed passage of contrast medium through the sphincter was a good sign of partial obstruction of the common bile duct.

Wise reported 1340 postcholecystectomy injections. Visualization of 1194 ducts was reported and common duct calculi were proved at surgery in 77 of these. In 51 of these there was no associated pathologic change. In 11 of those with calculi there were associated strictures; in 14, fibrosis of the sphincter of Oddi; and in 1, chronic pancreatitis. Of the 77 cases with proved common duct calculi 42 were visualized directly; in 29 the diagnosis was suspected by the indirect demonstration of abnormality in the common duct; and 6 were not diagnosed radiologically.

HAZARDS OF INTRAVENOUS CHOLANGIOGRAPHY. Accidents during gallbladder studies with Cholografin were studied by Frommhold and Braband. They collected data on 22 deaths attributed directly or indirectly to its administration. This death rate, even including doubtful and delayed deaths, represented a figure of 0.00035 per cent. This compares favorably with the death rate due to intravenous urography reported by Pendergrass — 0.0009 per cent in a review of 12,200,000 excretory urograms performed over a 27 year period. The sensitivity tests were negative in 5 of the 22 recorded fatalities with intravenous cholangiography.

Percutaneous Cholangiography. Under normal circumstances, puncture of the liver with an exploratory needle will fail to produce bile. Bile is obtained if extrahepatic obstruction is present. Percutaneous cholangiography may be employed in the differential diagnosis of jaundice in certain selected cases, provided normal clotting factors are present and broad spectrum antibiotics are given for one day prior to the examination in case operation is necessary (Flemma et al; Mujahed and Evans). It is contraindicated in hemorrhagic diathesis and vitamin K-resistant hypoprothrombinemia or in patients with febrile cholangitis.

Information elicited by percutaneous cholangiography is of value mainly in the following situations (Mujahed and Evans):

1. Differentiation between obstructive and nonobstructive jaundice.

2. Demonstration of the presence and site of carcinoma of the biliary system.

3. Demonstration of the number of calculi in the biliary system and their location.

4. Study of the biliary tree in congenital biliary atresia.

5. Decompression of the biliary tree prior to surgery.

Procedure. The percutaneous puncture is performed under local anesthesia and proper asepsis, with a 7 inch, 20 or 21 gauge needle with a stylet. The patient lies supine on a fluoroscopy table.

Mujahed and Evans restrict the procedure to patients scheduled for surgery and it is performed an hour or two beforehand.

The stylet is removed when the liver has been entered and a 20 cc. syringe is applied to the needle. Gentle aspiration is applied as the needle is advanced until bile is withdrawn freely. As much bile is withdrawn as is necessary to decompress the liver and for bacterial culture. As much as 60 cc. of 50 per cent methylglucamine diatrizoate (Renografin) may be necessary to fill the obstructed biliary tree.

The aspiration syringe is then replaced by a syringe containing 20 cc. of Renografin-60 or 75 per cent Hypaque. A polyethylene catheter may be threaded over the needle in advance to minimize trauma to the liver. The injection is carried out under television monitor control and satisfactory spot filming is obtained.

Usually the needle reaches a bile duct about 4 to 5 inches below the skin. If bile appears in the syringe at a skin distance of 2 to 2.5 inches, the needle is probably in the gallbladder.

If no bile ducts are entered after four punctures over the liver, extrahepatic obstruction is probably excluded. Occasionally, emergency operative intervention is necessary in patients with extrahepatic jaundice when there is bile leakage or internal bleeding as a result of the procedure.

If the injection of test substance puddles, usually it is in the liver. Occasionally the test injection disappears very quickly, in which case the injection was made into a vein; when slow movement of the contrast agent is noted, the injection was probably made into nondilated, branching, and tubular ducts.

Roentgen Signs of Abnormality in Percutaneous Cholangiography. These can be divided into the following categories: (1) filling defects caused by calculi; (2) obstructed duct (convexity upward) is usually due to a calculus; (3) smooth narrowness of a short segment indicates stricture; (4) duct rigid and irregular indicates carcinoma; (5) dilatation of the duct with an uneven and ragged obstruction pattern indicates carcinoma of ampulla or pancreas (dilatation usually greater with pancreatic pathology; (6) smooth, flat, shallow obstruction with dilatation of the duct indicates ampullary carcinoma; (7) tortuous and marked dilatation of ducts indicates pancreatic carcinoma. Obstructed end may be rounded, bulbous, tapered, or notched.

Evaluation of Percutaneous Cholangiography (Mujahed and Evans). In this study of 140 patients, procedures were successful with 74 per cent. Carcinoma of the pancreas was detected correctly by cholangiography in 34 of 41 cases, or 87 per cent, whereas, in a gastrointestinal series, it was suspected in 15 of 41 cases, or 37 per cent. Carcinoma of the ampulla of Vater was diagnosed from cholangiograms in 7 of 7 cases (100 per cent), but in the gastrointestinal series the rate of success was 55 per cent (4 of 7 cases). Complications from the study can be summarized as follows: (1) one death occurred out of the 140 patients; the authors noted that, in 800 procedures performed by others, four deaths had occurred; (2) subphrenic abscess occurred in 2 patients; and (3) bile and blood (500 to 1000 cc.) in the peritoneum was noted in 7 patients.

Pain following transcutaneous cholangiography may persist in the right upper quadrant for 6 to 8 hours. Surgery is performed 1 to 5 days after the procedure when indicated.

In a report by Flemma et al. complications in a total group of 27 cases consisted of three cases of bile peritonitis and three of gram negative septicemia. The peritonitis patients underwent immediate surgery, and the infected ones responded well to antibiotic therapy.

Direct Cholangiography. There are two types of direct cholangiography: (1) operative cholangiography (at the time of operation); and (2) postoperative or T-tube cholangiography (during the postoperative period) (Fig. 14–65).

Cholangiography at the time of surgery, in the opinion of Edmunds et al., should be performed in all cholecystectomy patients without selection except in those with serious debility. Clinical indications for common duct exploration as presently accepted are not sufficiently accurate to reduce the number of negative explorations. There are, indeed, many reports of common duct stones revealed by operative cholangiograms when no clinical indications for exploration were present (Hight et al.). Fully 95 per cent of all secondary operations on the biliary tract are for intraductal stones that may have been overlooked.

Also, the performance of cholangiography at the time of operation gives the surgeon an opportunity to make certain that all calculi have been removed from, or are no longer present in, the biliary tree.

Cholangiography at the time of operation provides a means of recognizing noncalculus obstruction of the common duct also (Partington and Sachs).

The T-tube cholangiogram allows a study of the common bile duct in the postoperative period prior to removal of the T-tube. In this way, a determination of patency of the common bile duct is determined.

Technique. Twenty-five to 50 per cent methylglucamine diatrizoate or sodium diatrizoate (Renografin or Hypaque) is directly injected into the biliary tree (in approximately 5 ml. fractions) either at the time of operation by means of a polyethylene tube inserted into the common duct or through a T-tube that has been previously introduced into the common hepatic duct at surgery. The contrast agent is warmed to body temperature before use.

For the *operative cholangiogram,* the contrast agent may be injected in three or four fractions of approximately 5 cc. each, and films obtained in sequence during the injection of each fraction.

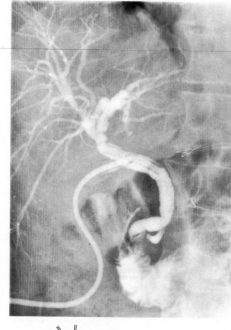

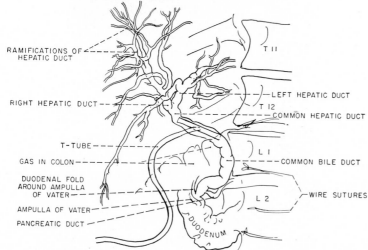

RAMIFICATIONS OF
HEPATIC DUCT

T II

RIGHT HEPATIC DUCT

LEFT HEPATIC DUCT

T 12

COMMON HEPATIC DUCT

T-TUBE

GAS IN COLON

L I

COMMON BILE DUCT

DUODENAL FOLD
AROUND AMPULLA
OF VATER

AMPULLA OF VATER

L 2

WIRE SUTURES

PANCREATIC DUCT

DUODENUM

Figure 14–65. Thirty-five per cent Renografin T-tube cholangiogram and its tracing. This contrast medium gives a more complete visualization of all hepatic radicles. This is extremely important since stones may be concealed in the hepatic radicles only to descend later and cause a recurrence of symptoms.

The films are numbered so that the sequence can be identified at the time of viewing. Care is exercised to remove all air bubbles from the syringe and connecting tube prior to injection. A cassette tunnel placed beneath the patient prior to surgery to allow proper positioning of the cassette under sterile conditions is important. A grid-cassette (or Bucky grid) beneath the table is also necessary to enhance detail. Diaphragmatic movement is suspended by the

anesthetist just prior to exposure and the exposures are made as rapidly as possible.

The films must be viewed immediately, so that additional studies may be taken as necessary.

The *postoperative cholangiogram* through the T-tube is performed as follows: a needle on the end of a long transparent catheter is carefully inserted into the end of the rubber T-tube and held vertically so that air that may not have been entirely expelled will rise to the surface. Every care must be exercised to avoid the injection of air into the biliary tree, since interpretation in respect to filling defects may thereby be complicated.

Approximately 5 cc. of the contrast agent is injected under fluroscopic control and a spot film is obtained in the anteroposterior projection. The patient is then rotated into the left posterior oblique position and the procedure repeated with an additional 5 cc. injection. A further injection is made when the patient is placed in the right posterior oblique, and finally, a fourth exposure is made with the patient supine once again in the straight anteroposterior. Ordinarily, a total of 20 to 25 cc. of the contrast agent is sufficient to obtain these several views. During this procedure the introduction of the fluid must be done gently and the rate slowed when necessary if resistance is met or if the patient complains of right upper quadrant discomfort. After the final injection, a right lateral film may be obtained if desired.

Also, if desired, another roentgenogram may be taken 15 minutes after the injection to visualize the emptying of the biliary tract. Depending upon the degree of delay, additional films may be taken at 15 minute or half-hour intervals until the patency of the biliary tract is determined (Hicken et al., 1959).

If an obstruction is encountered, it is recommended that withdrawal of as much of the contrast agent as possible be attempted prior to the removal of the injection apparatus.

An effort is made to visualize both the right and left hepatic ducts as well as the common bile duct in its entirety. At times, biliary calculi make their way into one or the other of the hepatic ducts after or during surgery and these would go unrecognized were it not for this procedure.

Complications. Edmunds et al. have reported that in 535 operative cholangiograms, there were four instances of complications which could possibly have been caused by these procedures. There were two cases of cholangitis, one case of acute hemorrhagic pancreatitis, and one case in which perforation of the common duct was thought to have occurred. All the patients survived their complications.

Value of Direct Cholangiography. Hampson and Petrie reported residual gallstones after cholecystectomy and common bile duct exploration in 7 per cent of primary operations and in 23 per cent of secondary operations for previously retained stones.

Hicken et al. (1950) reported the use of direct cholangiography with Hypaque in 350 patients. There were no local or constitutional reactions or complications which could be attributed to the contrast medium. Friesen has emphasized that the procedure is important in avoiding injury to the common duct at surgery. Operative cholangiography markedly decreases the risk of overlooking stones in seemingly normal common ducts at cholecystectomy. This possibility is estimated to occur in 10 to 18 per cent of cases (Vadheim and Rigos).

According to Chapman et al., normal operative cholangiographic findings are reliable evidence that the common bile duct does not contain stones or obstruction and therefore need not be explored.

Sachs has emphasized that unnecessary common duct exploration is reduced from 45 or 50 per cent to 4 or 5 per cent, and that overlooked stones are reduced from 16 or 25 per cent to 4 per cent.

Hess (1967) indicated an incidence of overlooked stones of 0.9 per cent in 650 cholangiograms.

Biliary Angiography (Deutsch; Farrell; Rösch et al.; Redman and Reuter). Selective celiac and mesenteric artery angiography for visualization of the gallbladder has been utilized for the diagnosis of gallbladder diseases which cannot be made by routine roentgenologic means.

Technique. The technique is similar to the Seldinger technique previously described for percutaneous transfemoral or brachial artery catheterization (see Chapter 10). Forty to 50 cc. of a contrast medium is injected directly into the celiac artery, or about half this quantity into the mesenteric artery. If selective catheterization of the cystic artery or hepatic artery can be accomplished, this route is desirable. Methylglucamine diatrizoate (Renografin) or sodium diatrizoate (Hypaque) is utilized. A pressure injector is employed so that the chosen volume is injected within 2 seconds, and exposures are made in rapid sequence—two per second for 4 seconds and one per second for 4 seconds thereafter. Thereafter ten exposures at 3 second intervals may be utilized. *Transjugular cholangiography* is a modification of the Seldinger technique, in which a catheter introduced via the jugular vein is directed into a hepatic vein (Weiner and Hanafee, for review). This technique avoids percutaneous liver entry and yet accomplishes a good visualization of an obstructed hepatic venous system (Fig. 14–66).

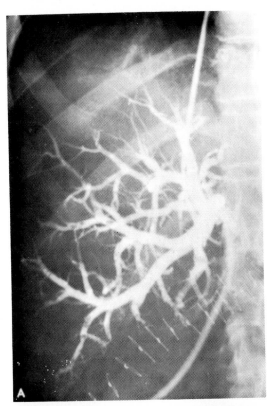

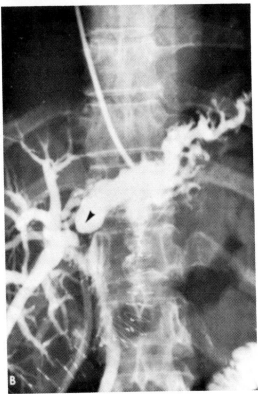

Figure 14–66. Operative exploration for obstructive jaundice in a 45 year old woman showed a mass obstructing the common hepatic duct near the bifurcation. A drainage catheter was placed from the common bile duct into the right ductile system, but the left system was completely obstructed and could not be entered. Biopsies were negative for neoplasm. Two weeks later she developed chills and fever.

One month postoperatively, transjugular cholangiogram was performed across a right hepatic vein, and showed visualization of the right ducts but no filling of the left system (*A*). The needle was then repositioned in a left hepatic vein; the left bile ducts were visualized and complete obstruction of the left system was demonstrated (*B*).

Subsequent biopsy at the time of surgery for reconstruction of the extrahepatic biliary tree revealed bile duct carcinoma. (From Weiner, M., and Hanafee, W. N.: Radiol. Clin. N. Amer., 8:61, 1970.)

Basic Anatomy. The basic anatomy of the cystic artery has already been described. It usually arises from the right hepatic artery near the origin from the common hepatic. Shortly after its origin it divides into an anterior branch, which is right-sided and peritoneal, and a posterior branch, which is left-sided and non-peritoneal. A rich capillary plexus communicates between these two main branches.

There are numerous variations of normal, well illustrated in the basic anatomy texts (Netter; Grant's *Atlas of Anatomy; Morris' Human Anatomy*). The most frequent of these are illustrated by Ruzicka and Rossi as shown in Figure 14–67. In about 25 per cent of the cases the two main branches of the cystic artery originate separately from the right hepatic artery. The cystic artery or one of its branches may also originate from the common

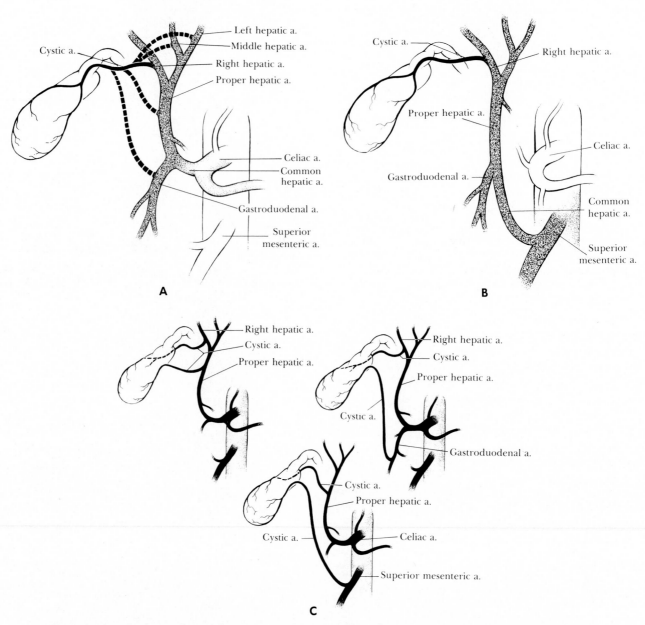

Figure 14–67. Cystic artery variations. In *A*, the solid vessel line indicates the most frequent site of origin of the cystic artery. The interrupted vessel lines show the more common variations. In *B*, the cystic artery arises from the right hepatic, which is a branch of the superior mesenteric artery. In *C*, three of the more common variations of double cystic arteries are shown. (From Ruzicka, F. F., Jr., and Rossi, P.: Radiol. Clin. N. Amer., 8:3–29, 1970.)

NORMAL GALLBLADDER MEASUREMENTS

The normal measurements of the gallbladder were derived angiographical-ly by Redman and Reuter from 25 normal gallbladders as follows:

	Mean Measurement	Range	Standard Deviation
Area	21.1 sq. cm.	11.4—33 cm.	5 cm.
Width	3.6 cm.	1.9— 5 cm.	0.77 cm.

Conclusions: Gallbladders measuring more than 35 sq. cm. or having a width of more than 5 cm. may be considered distended.

Figure 14–68.

hepatic artery, the left hepatic, the gastroduodenal, the celiac trunk itself, or the superior mesenteric.

Venous blood from the gallbladder is drained directly into the liver through a venous capillary plexus or into the portal venous system. Anastomoses with the choledochal and superior mesenteric veins occur.

Normal Gallbladder Measurements. The normal gallbladder has a wall thickness of 2 to 3 mm., 6 to 8 seconds after visualization of the cystic artery. Its measurements otherwise are shown in Figure 14–68. Generally, gallbladders measuring more than 35 sq. cm. or more than 5 cm. wide may be considered distended. An example of visualization of the gallbladder by cholecysto-angiography is shown in Figure 14–69.

Hepatic Angiogram. The basic anatomic variations of the hepatic artery have been previously described. These were shown to be closely related to variations of the celiac and superior mesenteric trunks (Fig. 14–67). The common hepatic artery is usually 3 to 6 cm. in length approximately, and is directed toward the right and superiorly toward the porta hepatis, where it divides into right and left hepatic arteries. These latter branches, in turn, divide into large interlobar arteries which follow along the connective tissue septa, subdividing repeatedly in the liver substance into smaller and smaller interlobular branches which run in the connective tissue between the lobules. Generally, the smaller vessels are straight and well defined, and approach the periphery of the liver in fairly predictable fashion. It will be recalled that the hepatic artery usually gives origin to the gastroduodenal, supraduodenal, and right gastric arteries. The hepatic artery then continues as the common hepatic artery before its division into right and left main branches. A middle hepatic artery sometimes arises from the left hepatic. The right hepatic passes behind the common hepatic duct to enter the "triangle of Calot" formed by the cystic duct, hepatic duct, and liver on its cephalad boundary.

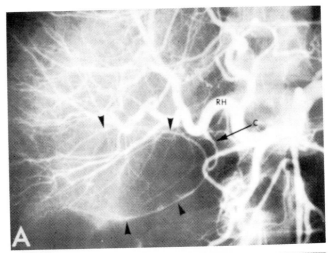
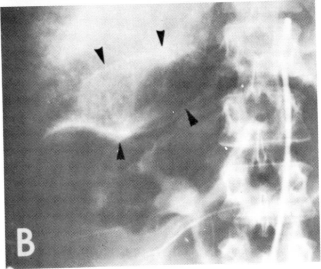

Figure 14–69. Celiac arteriogram. *A. (RH)* Right hepatic artery, *(C)* cystic artery. Arrowheads point out branches of cystic artery. *B.* Venous phase showing cystic veins. (From Ruzicka, F. F., Jr., and Rossi, P.: Radiol. Clin. N. Amer., 8:3–29, 1970.)

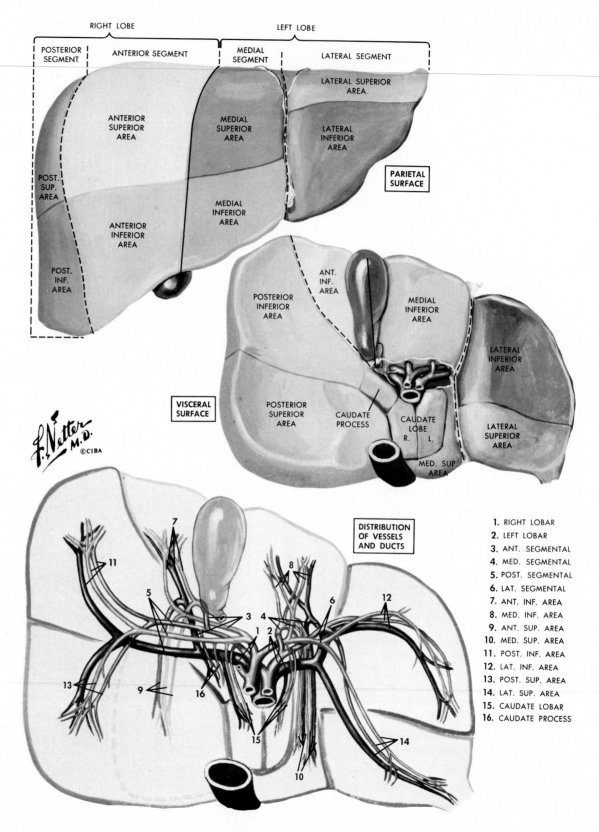

Figure 14-70. *See opposite page for legend.*

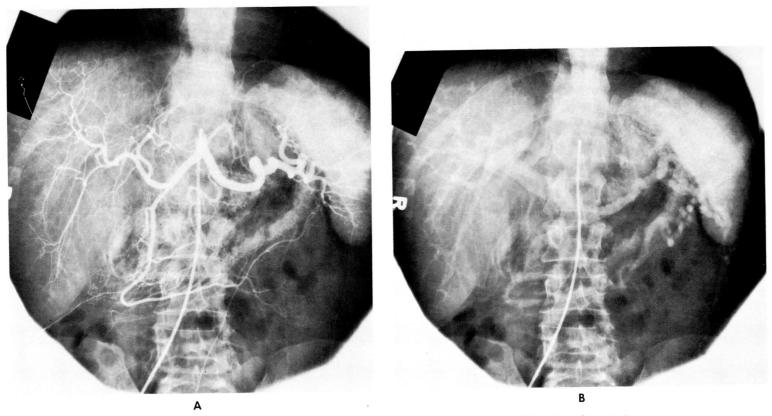

Figure 14–71. A. Normal hepatic arteriogram. B. Portal or splenoportal venogram following celiac arteriogram.

There is a distinct lobar and lobular composition of the liver, as illustrated in Figure 14–70, with the hepatic arteries, portal vein branches, and biliary ducts following parallel courses. The student is referred to Netter for a detailed description of the segmental division and lobar biliary ductal drainage of the liver.

An example of a normal hepatic arteriogram is shown in Figure 14–71. Hepatic arteriography is of significant value in the diagnosis and localization of a number of pathologic processes in the liver. These include malignancies, lymphomas, cirrhosis, cysts, hemangiomas, and vascular occlusions or aneurysm.

Visualization of the hepatic artery has also proven to be of considerable value in demonstrating the arterial blood supply as part of the management of continuous arterial infusion chemotherapy in the treatment of malignancies of the liver. The position of the infusion catheter is of great importance in that it must allow for selective chemotherapeutic treatment of the involved area. Also, hepatic arteriography provides a useful guide in determining the response of a lesion to this treatment.

Metastatic lesions or neoplasms may be better visualized by using epinephrine conjointly with the angiogram to obtain constriction of normal vessels, because abnormal vessels without vasomotor control do not respond to the adrenalin.

Portal Phlebography. The basic anatomy has been described previously (Fig. 14–48 A). The splenic and superior mesenteric veins comprise the main tributaries of the portal vein, with the inferior mesenteric usually draining into the splenic and the coronary vein terminating at the junction of the splenic and portal veins.

Techniques for Study. Percutaneous injection of the spleen results in opacification of the splenoportal trunk (Fig. 14–72).

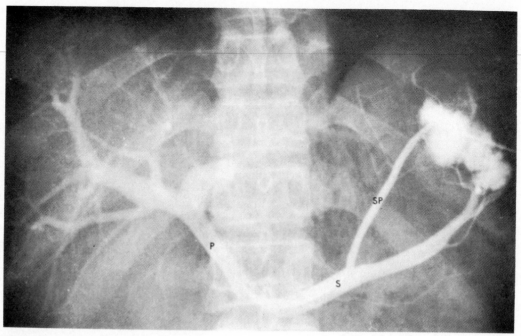

Figure 14–72. Normal splenoportogram. Injection into the splenic pulp results in visualization of splenoportal axis. Superior polar vein (SP) is part of splenoportal axis. Tributaries are not visualized normally by this technique. However, capsular veins of spleen and adjacent small vessels may fill during splenic injection in the normal patient. (S) Splenic vein, (P) portal vein. (From Ruzicka, F. F., Jr., and Rossi, P.: Radiol. Clin. N. Amer., 8:3–29, 1970.)

This procedure is performed by injection directly into the splenic pulp. Ordinarily 50 cc. of 70 per cent methylglucamine or sodium diatrizoate or its equivalent is employed. This volume is forcefully injected in 5 or 6 seconds, and exposures of one film per second for 12 to 15 seconds are usually adequate. The patient should be maintained in apnea during the injection and exposure. The following blood vessels are seen in rapid sequence: (1) the splenoportal trunk, (2) the intrahepatic portal branches, and (3) the sinusoidal system of the liver. The sinuosoidal phase reaches a maximum within 16 to 24 seconds and then fades, although it may persist for as long as 60 seconds.

The injection may be made directly into a cannulated branch of the portal system at surgery, and under these circumstances, the opacification is limited mostly to the vein injected along with the portal vein.

The splenic, superior mesenteric, and portal veins usually have approximately the same diameter and are confluent in the upper lumbar or lowermost thoracic region, which is usually projected over the spine. At the porta hepatis, the portal vein bifurcates into its two main branches. The coronary vein and the inferior mesenteric vein are also visualized, especially in the presence of increased resistance to flow within the liver (Fig. 14–73). Other tributaries of the portal system may also be shown, such as the gastroepiploic veins, the pancreatic veins, or even the

short gastric veins. The right main branch is usually readily detected along with its main ramifications, but there is a considerable superimposition of branches, making intimate detail difficult to obtain; the left main branch may be only partially visualized. It is thought that the better visualization of the right branch is due to its posterior position, and the effect of gravity of the contrast agent within the blood. The portal branches divide 5 to 7 times and almost any angle up to 90 degrees may be encountered, but branching occurs in a symmetrical manner and tapering of vessels is gradual. Although the more proximal vessels are straight, branches of the fourth to seventh order may be somewhat curved.

In the sinusoidal phase, the density of the contrast agent is fairly uniform. A spotted appearance is usually abnormal. There may, however, be some variation in density due to varying thicknesses of different parts of the liver. Since the left lobe is usually poorly opacified in this phase it cannot be evaluated accurately.

The other basic method of visualization of the extrahepatic portal venous system is by injection into the celiac artery and obtaining sequential studies during the venous phase. The splenoportal axis is usually fairly well defined (Fig. 14–74). Some of the veins that may be identified in this type of study are the gastric veins, coronary veins, gastroepiploic veins, and even the pancrea-

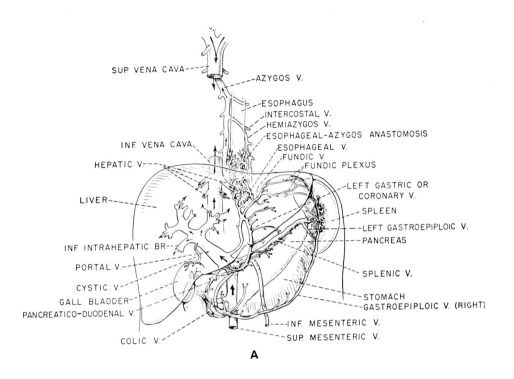

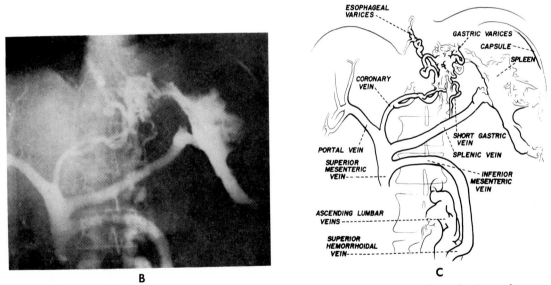

Figure 14–73. *A.* Anatomic diagram of the portal circulation and relationship to esophageal veins and azygos venous systems. *B.* Roentgenogram at 12 seconds demonstrates coronary vein, gastric and esophageal varices. The anastomosis between the inferior mesenteric vein and superior hemorrhoid plexus is demonstrated. The latter is also seen to drain into the vertebral venous plexus. *C.* Tracing of *B.* (From Evans, J. A., and O'Sullivan, W. D.: Amer. J. Roentgenol., *77*, 1957.)

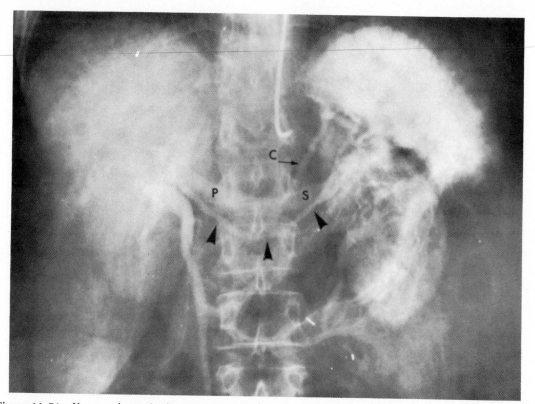

Figure 14–74. Venous phase of celiac artery injection. A double splenoportal axis is shown. The usual axis is made up of the splenic vein (S) and portal vein (P). Coronary vein (C) enters splenic vein. The anomalous axis (arrowheads) arises from a confluence of short gastric veins and splenic hilar radicles and passes parallel to the main S-P axis to enter the liver separately just below the portal vein. (From Ruzicka, F. F., Jr., and Rossi, P.: Radiol. Clin. N. Amer., 8:3–29, 1970.)

ticoduodenal veins. The rapidity of celiac injection and the volume of contrast agent employed will frequently determine the intensity of visualization. Usually the inferior mesenteric vein will not be seen unless the inferior mesenteric artery is selectively injected (Ruzicka and Rossi).

Diagrams illustrating the main routes of blood flow through regularly appearing tributaries of the portal system are shown in Figure 14–75. Thus, short gastric, pancreatic, inferior mesenteric, superior mesenteric, coronary, gastric, and esophageal dilated vessels become visible. This technique is particularly useful for demonstration of esophageal varices.

Summary of Circulation Through the Portal Venous System. Venous blood, carrying materials absorbed from the alimentary tract, passes into the liver through the portal vein and branches out progressively to reach the sinusoid in the individual liver lobules. The blood then reaches the central vein of the lobule. Arterial blood enters through the hepatic artery with oxygenated blood and it too enters the sinusoids to reach the central vein. The central veins are the actual beginnings of the hepatic venous system. The central veins from several lobules unite to enter sublobular veins, and these in turn merge to form increasingly larger trunks, finally converging to form three hepatic veins, which then enter the vena cava.

In the event of obstruction of the portal vein (Fig. 14–75 C) the most important collateral portal circulation is found in: (1) gastric veins of the portal and esophageal veins of the azygos system, (2) the inferior mesenteric of the portal and rectal veins of the internal iliac system, (3) branches along the falciform ligament which are tributaries of the portal vein and the superior and inferior epigastric veins, (4) intestinal veins of the portal system with retroperitoneal tributaries of the inferior vena cava. In the course of this collateral circulation, the region of anastomoses may become engorged and create esophageal varicosities, hemorrhoids, and a "caput medusae" owing to varicosities on the abdominal wall around the umbilicus.

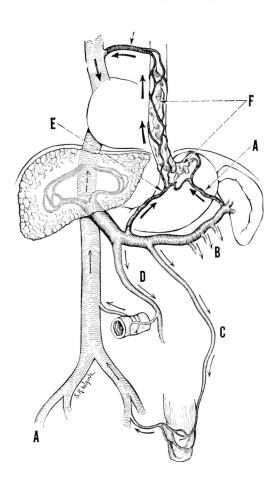

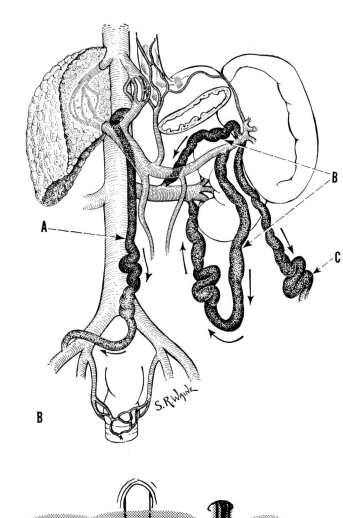

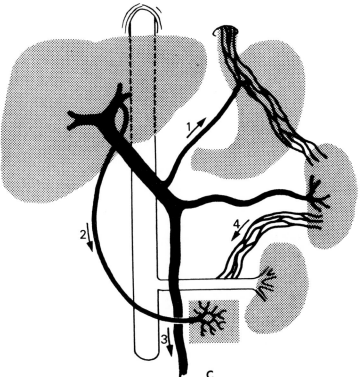

Figure 14–75. A. Diagram of main routes of hepato-fugal blood flow through regularly appearing tributaries of portal system. (A) Short gastric, (B) pancreatic, (C) inferior mesenteric, (D) superior mesenteric, (E) coronary, (F) gastric and esophageal varices.

B. Diagram showing hepatofugal flow through newly utilized, persisting embryonic channels between portal and systemic systems. (A) Transhepatic (parumbilical) collateral, (B) splenorenal collaterals, (C) collateral arising from spleen and communicating with systemic veins of the abdominal wall and/or retroperitoneum. Only one of several possible sites of termination of parumbilical collateral shown. (Modified from Rousselot, L. M., et al.: Studies on portal hypertension. IV. The clinical and physiopathologic significance of self-established (non-surgical) portal systemic venous shunts. Ann. Surg., *150*:3, 1959.) (From Schobinger, R. A., and Ruzicka, F. F., Jr.: Vascular Roentgenology. New York, The Macmillan Company, 1964.)

C. The most important venous collaterals in portal vein occlusion: (1) the coronary vein, (2) the umbilical vein, (3) links between mesenteric and systemic systems, and (4) splenorenal and splenogastric anastomoses. (From Wenz, W.: Abdominal Angiography. New York, Springer-Verlag, 1974.)

921

REFERENCES

Alderson, D. A.: The reliability of Telepaque cholecystography. Brit. J. Surg., *47*:655–658, 1960.

Anson, B. J. (ed.): Morris' Human Anatomy. 12th edition. New York, McGraw Hill, 1966.

Ardran, C. M., French, J. M., and Mucklow, E. H. B.: Relationship of the nature of the opaque medium to the small intestine radiographic pattern. Brit. J. Radiol., *23*:697–702, 1950.

Baker, H. L., and Hodgson, J. R.: Further studies on the accuracy of cholecystography. Radiology, *74*:239–245, 1960.

Beargie, R. J., Hodgson, J. R., Huizenga, K. A., and Priestley, J. T.: Relation of cholangiographic findings after cholecystectomy to clinical and surgical findings. Surg. Gynec. Obst., *115*:143–152, 1962.

Berg, A. M., and Hamilton, J. E.: A method to improve roentgen diagnosis of biliary disease with bile acids. Surgery, *32*:948–952, 1952.

Berk, J. E.: Persistence of symptoms following gallbladder surgery. Amer. J. Digest. Dis., *9*:295–305, 1964.

Berk, R. N.: The consecutive dose phenomenon in oral cholecystography. Amer. J. Roentgenol., *110*:230–234, 1970.

Berk, R. N., and Lasser, E. C.: Altered concepts of the mechanism of nonvisualization of the gallbladder. Radiology, *82*:296–302, 1964.

Bierman, H. C.: Selective Arterial Catheterization. Springfield, Illinois, Charles C Thomas, 1969.

Bishopric, G. A.: Athrombocytosis following oral cholecystography. J.A.M.A., *189*:771–772, 1964.

Boyden, E. A.: Effects of natural foods on the distention of the gallbladder. Anat. Rec., *30*:333, 1925.

Caldwell, W. L., and Flock, M. H.: Evaluation of small bowel barium motor meal with emphasis on effect of volume of barium suspension ingested. Radiology, *80*:383–391, 1963.

Chapman, M., Curry, R. C., and LeQuesne, L. P.: Operative cholangiography. Brit. J. Surg., *51*:600–601, 1964.

Chrispin, A. R., and Fry, I. K.: The presacral space shown by barium enema. Brit. J. Radiol., *36*:319–322, 1966.

Clark, R. H., Schmidt, F. E., and Hendren, T.: Retroperitoneal extravasation of barium enema. J. Louisiana Med. Soc., *113*:90–92, 1961.

Cohen, W. N.: Roentgenographic evaluation of the rectal valves of Houston in the normal and in ulcerative colitis. Amer. J. Roentgenol., *104*:580–583, 1968.

Cook, G. B., and Margulis, A. R.: The use of silicone foam for examining the human sigmoid colon. Amer. J. Roentgenol., *87*:633–643, 1962.

Cunningham, D. J.: Textbook of Anatomy. Tenth edition. London, Oxford University Press, 1964.

Dann, D. S., Rubins, S., and Bauernfeind, A.: Significance of visualization of the common duct in the non-visualized gallbladder. Amer. J. Roentgenol., *82*:1016–1019, 1959.

Dassel, P. M.: Innocuous filling of the intestinal glands in the colon during barium enema (spiculation) simulating organic disease. Radiology, *78*:799–801, 1962.

Deutsch, V.: Cholecysto-angiography. Visualization of the gallbladder by selective celiac and mesenteric angiography. Amer. J. Roentgenol., *101*:608–616, 1967.

Eckelberg, M. E., Carlson, H. C., and McIlrath, D. C.: Intravenous cholangiography with intact gallbladder. Amer. J. Roentgenol., *110*:235–239, 1970.

Edling, N. P. G., and Eklöf, O.: A roentgenologic study of the course of ulcerative colitis. Acta Radiol., *54*:397–409, 1960.

Edmunds, M. C., Emmett, J. M., and Clark, W. D.: Ten year experience with operative cholangiography. Amer. Surg., *26*:613–621, 1960.

Eklöf, O., and Gierup, J.: The retrorectal soft tissue space in children: normal variations and appearances in granulomatous colitis. Amer. J. Roentgenol., *108*:624–627, 1970.

Emmanoulides, G. C., and Hoy, R. C.: Transumbilical aortography and selective arteriography in newborn infants. Pediatrics, *39*:337, 1967.

Farrell, W. J.: Angiography of the liver: practical applications and demonstration of color subtraction technique. Radiol. Clin. of N. Amer., *4*:571–582, 1966.

Fischer, H. W., Galbraith, W. B., and Schroeder, A. F.: Rapid cholecystography with pharmacological assistance. Amer. J. Roentgenol., *84*:484–490, 1965.

Flemma, R. J., Capp, P., and Shagleton, W. W.: Percutaneous transhepatic colangiography. Arch. Surg., *90*:5, 1965.

Frimann-Dahl, J.: The administration of barium orally in acute obstruction: advantages and risks. Acta Radiol., *42*:285–295, 1954.

Frommhold, W.: A new contrast agent for intravenous cholecystography. (German text). Fortschr. Geb. Röntgenstrahlen, *70*:283–291, 1963.

Frommhold, W., and Braband, H.: Accidents during gallbladder studies with Biligrafin and their treatment. Fortschr. Geb. Röntgenstrahlen, *92*:47–59, 1960.

Garbsch, H.: The intravenous roentgenologic function study of the extrahepatic biliary tree. Radiologia Austriaca, *14*:131–158, 1963.

Goldstein, H. M., Poole, G. J., Rosenquist, C. J., Friedland, G. W., and Zboralske, F. F.: Comparison of methods for acceleration of small intestinal radiographic examination. Radiology, *98*:519–523, 1971.

Graham, E. A., and Cole, W. H.: Roentgenologic examination of the gallbladder: Preliminary report of a new method utilizing intravenous injection of tetrabromphthalein. J.A.M.A., *82*:613–614, 1924.

Guyton, A. C.: Textbook of Medical Physiology. Fourth edition. Philadelphia, W. B. Saunders Co., 1971.

Hampson, L. G., and Petrie, E. A.: The problem of stones in the common bile duct with particular reference to retained stones. Canad. J. Surg., 7:361–367, 1964.

Harris, R. C., and Caffey, J.: Cholecystography in infants. J.A.M.A., *153*:1333, 1953.

Haynes, W. F., Jr., and Pittman, F. E.: Application of fluorescein string test in 32 cases of upper gastrointestinal hemorrhage. Gastroenterology, *38*:690–697, 1960.

Hays, D. M., and Averbook, B. B.: Experience with intravenous cholecystography in infants and children. Surgery, *42*:638–641, 1957.

Henderson, S. G.: The gastrointestinal tract in the healthy newborn infant. Amer. J. Roentgenol., *48*:302–335, 1942.

Henderson, S. G., and Briant, W. W., Jr.: The colon in the healthy newborn infant. Amer. J. Roentgenol., *39*:261–272, 1942.

Hess, W.: Operative cholangiography. *In* Schinz, H. R., et al. (eds.): Roentgen Diagnosis. Vol. 1. New York, Grune and Stratton, 1967.

Hess, W.: Surgery of the Biliary Passages and Pancreas. Princeton, Van Nostrand, 1965.

Hicken, N. F., McAllister, A. J., Franz, B., and Crowder, E.: Technic, indications and value of postoperative cholangiography. Arch. Surg., *60*:1102–1113, 1950.

Hicken, N. F., McAllister, A. J., and Walker, G.: The problem of retained common duct stones. Amer. J. Surg., *97*:173–181, 1959.

Hicken, N. F., Stevenson, V. L., Franz, B. J., and Crowder, E.: The technic of operative cholangiography. Amer. J. Surg., *78*:347–355, 1949.

Hight, D., Lingley, J. R., and Hurtubise, F.: An evaluation of operative cholangiograms as a guide to common duct exploration. Ann. Surg., *150*:1086–1091, 1959.

Holt, J. F., Lyons, R. H., Neligh, R. B., Moe, G. K., and Hodges, R. J.: X-ray signs of altered alimentary function following autonomic blockade with tetraethylammonium. Radiology, *49*:603–610, 1947.

Jacobson, G., Berne, C. J., Meyers, H. I., and Rosoff, L.: The examination of patients with suspected perforated ulcer using a water soluble contrast medium. Amer. J. Roentgenol., *86*:37–49, 1961.

Kessler, R. E., and Zimmon, D. S.: Umbilical vein angiography. Radiology, *87*:841–844, 1966.

Kleinsasser, L. J., and Warshaw, H.: Perforation of the sigmoid colon during barium enema. Ann. Surg., *135*:560–565, 1952.

Krezanoski, J. Z.: Tannic acid: chemistry, analysis, and toxicology: an episode in the pharmaceutics of radiology. Radiology, *87*:655–657, 1966.

Lasser, E. C., and Gerende, L. J. (and others in cooperative study): An efficacy study of Clysodrast. Radiology, *87*:649–654, 1966.

Lonnerblad, L.: Transit time through the small intestine: Roentgenologic study of normal variability. Acta Radiol. (Suppl.), *88*:1–85, 1951.

Lumsden, K., and Truelove, S. C.: Intravenous Pro-banthine in diagnostic radiology of the gastrointestinal tract with special reference to colonic disease. Brit. J. Radiol., *32*:517–526, 1959.

Mandl, F.: Transcutaneous cholangiography in ichteric patients. Chirurg., *27*:341–343, 1956.

Margulis, A. R.: Examination of the colon. *In* Margulis, A. R., and Burhenne, H. J. (eds.): Alimentary Tract Roentgenology. St. Louis, C. V. Mosby Co., 1967.

Margulis, A. R., and Jovanovich, A.: Roentgen diagnosis of submucous lipomas of the colon. Amer. J. Roentgenol., *84*:1114–1120, 1960.

Marshak, R. H.: Regional enteritis: roentgenologic findings. *In* Bockus, H. L.: Gastroenterology. Vol. 2. Second edition. Philadelphia, W. B. Saunders Co., 1964.

Marshak, R. H., and Lindner, A. E.: Radiology of the Small Intestine. Philadelphia, W. B. Saunders Co., 1970.

Mauthe, H.: The accuracy of x-ray examination of the gallbladder. Wisconsin Med. J., *53*:473–476, 1962.

McAlister, W. H., Anderson, M. S., Bloomberg, F. R., and Margulis, A. R.: Lethal effects of tannic acid in the barium enema. Radiology, *80*:765–773, 1963.

McClenahan, J. L., Evans, J. A., and Braunstein, P. W.: Intravenous cholangiography in the postcholecystectomy syndrome. J.A.M.A., *159*:1353–1357, 1955.

Meyers, M. A.: Roentgen significance of the phrenicocolic ligament. Radiology, *95*:539–545, 1970.

Michels, A.: Blood Supply and Anatomy of the Upper Abdominal Organs. Philadelphia, J. B. Lippincott Co., 1955.

Miller, R. E.: Barium sulfate suspensions. Radiology, *84*:241–251, 1965.

Moreton, R. D., Stevenson, C. R., and Yates, C. W.: Fictitious polyps as seen in double contrast studies of the colon. Radiology, *53*:386–393, 1949.

Mujahed, Z., and Evans, J. A.: Percutaneous transhepatic cholangiography. Radiol. Clin. N. Amer., 4:535–545, 1966.

Nathan, M. H., Newman, A., Murray, D. J., and Camponovo, R.: Cholecystokinin cholecystography. Amer. J. Roentgenol., 110:240–251, 1970.

Nazareno, J. P., Studenski, E. V., and Pickren, J. W.: The cholangiogram: postmortem study. Radiology, 76:54–59, 1961 (14 ref).

Nelson, S. W., Christoforidis, A. J., and Roenigk, W. J.: Dangers and fallibilities of iodinated radiopaque media in obstruction of the small bowel. Amer. J. Surg., 109:546–559, 1965a.

Nelson, S. W., Christoforidis, A. J., and Roenigk, W. J.: A diagnostic physiologic sign of mechanical obstruction of the small intestine. Radiology, 84:881–885, 1965b.

Netter, F.: CIBA Collection of Medical Illustration. Vol. 3, Part 2. 1962.

Neuhauser, E. D. B., quoted in Sidaway, M. E.: The use of water soluble contrast medium in pediatric radiology. Clin. Radiol., 15:132–138, 1964.

Norman, A., and Saghapoleslami, M.: Oral extrahepatic cholangiography: a simple reliable technique. Radiology, 76:801–804, 1962.

Odnoralov, N. I.: Hepatic arteriography. In Schobinger, R. A., and Ruzicka, F. F., Jr. (eds.): Vascular Roentgenology. New York, The MacMillan Co., 1964. pp. 368–372.

Ostrum, B. J., and Heinz, E. R.: Small bowel obstruction versus adynamic ileus: A study using a water soluble oral contrast material (Hypaque sodium powder). Amer. J. Roentgenol., 89:734–739, 1963 (12 ref.).

Pansky, B., and House, E. L.: Review of Gross Anatomy. New York, The MacMillan Co., 1964.

Partington, P. F., and Sachs, M. D.: Routine use of operative cholangiography. Surg. Gynec. Obst., 87:299–307, 1948.

Pendergrass, E. P.: Symposium on contrast media reactions: introduction. Radiology, 91:61–62, 1968.

Reboul, J., Delorme, G., Marque, J., and Tavernin, J.: Results of the exploration of the colon by the double contrast method with Contalax lactose powder. Ann. Radiol., 6:283–296, 1963.

Redman, H. C., and Reuter, S. F.: The angiographic evaluation of gallbladder dilatation. Radiology, 97:367–370, 1970.

Rene, R. M., and Mellinkoff, S. M.: Renal insufficiency after oral administration of double dose of cholecystographic medium. New Eng. J. Med., 261:589–591, 1959.

Rösch, J., Grollman, J. H., Jr., and Steckel, R. J.: Arteriography in the diagnosis of gallbladder disease. Radiology, 92:1485–1491, 1969.

Rosenbaum, H. D.: The value of re-examination in patients with inadequate visualization of the gallbladder following a single dose of Telepaque. Amer. J. Roentgenol., 82:1111–1115, 1959.

Rosenbaum, H. D., Lieber, A., Hanson, D. J., and Pelligrino, E. D.: Routine survey roentgenogram of the abdomen on 500 consecutive patients over 40 years of age. Amer. J. Roentgenol., 91:903–909, 1964.

Rosenberg, L. S., and Fine, A. V.: Fatal venous intravasation of barium during a barium enema. Radiology, 73:771–773, 1959.

Ross, R. J., and Sachs, M. D.: Triplication of the gallbladder. Amer. J. Roentgenol., 104:656–661, 1968.

Rous, P., and McMaster, P. D.: The concentrating activity of the gallbladder. J. Exper. Med., 34:47, 1921.

Rubin, S., Dann, D. S., Ezekial, C., and Vincent, J.: Retrograde prolapse of the ileocecal valve. Amer. J. Roentgenol., 87:706–708, 1962.

Rudhe, U.: Roentgenologic examination of rectum in ulcerative colitis. Acta Paediat., 49:859–867, 1960.

Ruzicka, F. F., and Rossi, P.: Normal vascular anatomy of the abdominal viscera. Radiol. Clin. N. Amer., 8:3–29, 1970.

Sachs, M. D.: Routine cholangiography, operative and postoperative. Radiol. Clin. N. Amer., 4:547–569, 1966.

Salerno, F. G., Collins, O. D., Redmond, D., et al.: Transumbilical abdominal aortography in the newborn. J. Pediat. Surg., 5:40, 1970.

Salzman, E.: Opacification of bile duct calculi. Radiol. Clin. N. Amer., 4:525–533, 1966.

Salzman, G. F.: Solu-Biloptin (SH550) as a contrast medium for peroral cholegraphy. Acta Radiol., 52:417–425, 1960.

Sasson, L.: Entrance of barium into intestinal glands during barium enema. J.A.M.A., 173:343–345, 1960.

Schatzki, R.: Small intestinal enema. Amer. J. Roentgenol., 50:743–751, 1943.

Schlaeger, R.: Examination of the small intestine. In Margulis, A. R., and Burhenne, H. J. (eds.): Alimentary Tract Roentgenology. St. Louis, C. V. Mosby Co., 1967.

Schobinger, R. A., and Ruzicka, F. F., Jr.: Vascular Roentgenology. New York, The MacMillan Co., 1964.

Seaman, W. B., and Bragg, D. G.: Colonic intramural barium: complication of barium enema examination. Radiology, 89:250–255, 1967.

Seaman, W. B., Cosgriff, S., and Wells, J.: Renal insufficiency following cholecystography. Amer. J. Roentgenol., 90:859, 1963.

Seaman, W. B., and Wells, J.: Complications of the barium enema. Gastroenterology, 48:728–737, 1965.

Shehadi, W. H.: Clinical problems and toxicity of contrast agents. Amer. J. Roentgenol., 97:762–771, 1966a.

Shehadi, W. H.: Clinical Radiology of the Biliary Tract. New York, McGraw-Hill, 1963b.

Shehadi, W. H.: Oral cholangiography with Telepaque. Amer. J. Roentgenol., 92:436–451, 1954.

Shehadi, W. H.: Intravenous cholecystocholangiography. J.A.M.A., 159:1350–1353, 1955.

Shehadi, W. H.: Radiologic examination of the biliary tract: plain films of the abdomen; oral cholecystography. Radiol. Clin. N. Amer., 4:463–482, 1966b.

Shehadi, W. H.: Simultaneous intravenous cholangiography and urography. Surg. Gynec. Obst., 105:401–406, 1957.

Shehadi, W. H.: Studies of the colon and small intestines with water soluble iodinated contrast media. Amer. J. Roentgenol., 89:740–751, 1963a.

Smith, C. A.: The Physiology of the Newborn Infant. Third edition. Springfield, Illinois, Charles C Thomas, 1959.

Smith, V. M.: String impregnation test for lesions of the upper digestive tract. Ann. Intern. Med., 54:16–29, 1961.

Sovenyi, E., and Varro, V.: New method for x-ray studies of small bowel. Fortschr. Geb. Röntgenstrahlen, 91:269–270, 1959.

Stacy, G. S., and Loop, J. W.: Unusual small bowel diseases: methods and observation. Amer. J. Roentgenol., 92:1072–1079, 1964.

Steinbach, H. L., and Burhenne, H. J.: Performing the barium enema: equipment, preparation and contrast medium. Amer. J. Roentgenol., 87:644–654, 1962.

Stern, W. Z., Schein, C. J., and Jacobson, H. G.: The significance of the lateral view in T-tube cholangiography. Amer. J. Roentgenol., 87:764–771, 1962.

Templeton, A. W.: Colon sphincters simulating organic disease. Radiology, 75:237–241, 1960.

Tomenius, J.: A new instrument for gastric biopsies under visual control. Gastroenterology, 21:544–546, 1952.

Traphagen, D. W., and Karlan, M.: Fluorescein string test for localization of upper gastrointestinal hemorrhage. Surgery, 44:644–645, 1958.

Treves, V. F.: Anatomy of intestinal canal and peritoneum in man. Brit. Med. J., 1:580–583, 1965.

Vadheim, J. L., and Rigos, F. J.: Cholangiography as an aid to biliary surgery. Northwest Med., 51:400–402, 1952.

Weiner, M., and Hanafee, W. N.: Review of transjugular cholangiography. Radiol. Clin. of N. Amer., 8:53–68, 1970.

Weintraub, S., and Williams, R. G.: A rapid method of roentgenologic examination of the small intestine. Amer. J. Roentgenol., 61:45–55, 1949.

Weng, W.: Abdominal Angiography. Springer-Verlag, New York, 1974.

Whalen, J. P., and Riemenschneider, P. A.: An analysis of the normal anatomic relationships of the colon as applied to roentgenographic observations. Amer. J. Roentgenol., 99:55–61, 1967.

White, W. W., and Fischer, H. S.: Double blind study of Oragrafin and Telepaque. Amer. J. Roentgenol., 87:745–748, 1962.

Whitehouse, W. M., and Hodges, F. J.: Recent additions to radiographic techniques in biliary tract disease. Gastroenterology, 38:701–705, 1956.

Whitehouse, W. M., and Martin, O.: Clinical and roentgenologic evaluation of routine 2-gram Telepaque dosage in cholecystography. Radiology, 65:422–424, 1955.

Wilbur, R. S., and Bolt, R. J.: Incidence of gallbladder disease in "normal" men. Gastroenterology, 36:251–255, 1959.

Williams, I.: Diverticular disease of the colon without diverticula. Radiology, 89:401–412, 1967.

Wise, R. E.: Intravenous Cholangiography. Springfield, Illinois, Charles C Thomas, 1962.

Wise, R. E., and O'Brien, R. G.: Interpretation of the intravenous cholangiogram. J.A.M.A., 160:819–827, 1956.

Wood, I. J., Doig, R. K., Motteram, R., and Hughes, A.: Gastric biopsy: report on 55 biopsies using the new flexible gastric biopsy tube. Lancet, 1:18–21, 1949.

Zatzkin, H. R., and Irwin, G. H. L.: Nonfatal intravasation of barium. Amer. J. Roentgenol., 92:1169–1172, 1964.

Zimmer, E. A.: Radiology of the small intestine. I. Studies on contrast media for the x-ray examination of the gastrointestinal tract. Brit. J. Radiol., 24:245–251, 1951.

15

The Abdomen and Peritoneal Space

GROSS ANATOMY OF THE ABDOMINAL CAVITY

Boundaries and Subdivisions of the Peritoneal Cavity. The abdominopelvic cavity is that segment of the serous cavity of the trunk that lies below the diaphragm. The anterior wall is composed of the transversalis, internal oblique, and external oblique muscles, together with the rectus and pyramidal muscles, the skin and superficial fascia overlying these structures. The posterior wall is composed of the vertebral column, the posterior segment of the pelvis, the inferior portions of the diaphragm, and the quadratus lumborum and psoas muscles. The side walls of the abdomen are formed by the oblique and transverse muscles, and below by the iliacus muscles and the iliac bones.

The abdominal cavity is divisible into the abdominal cavity proper and the true pelvis or pelvis minor. The ribs cover approximately the same area of the abdomen as they do the thorax.

The true pelvis is bounded in front and at the sides by as much of the hip bones as lie below the level of the linea terminalis. These are partly clothed by the internal obturator muscle and pelvic fascia. The posterior wall is formed by the anterior aspect of the sacrum and coccyx, covered on each side by the pyriform muscle. The pyriform muscles pass out of the pelvis through the greater sciatic notch, thus closing these potential holes in the cavity. The floor of the pelvis is composed of the levator ani muscles, coccygeal muscles, and the endopelvic fascia.

There are certain openings in the abdominal walls that form potentially weak areas through which protrusions (herniations) may occur. These openings occur in the diaphragm to allow passage for the aorta, esophagus, and inferior vena cava; in the pelvic floor to allow passage for the urethra, rectum, and vagina; in the lower portion of the abdominal wall at the site of the inguinal canals through which the round ligaments and spermatic cords pass, and in the area of weakness formed by the femoral sheath, which contains the femoral arteries, veins, lymphatics, and femoral canal.

Ligaments and Mesenteric Folds of Peritoneum. The peritoneal cavity is, therefore, a potential space between the layers of the peritoneum. When all the viscera are cut away, there are certain lines of reflection of the peritoneum that demonstrate that the peritoneum is a continuous covering on the dorsal and ventral walls of the abdomen as well as on the diaphragm.

On the dorsal abdominal wall, proceeding caudad, the following ligamentous structures are encountered. The *falciform ligament* is continuous with the ventral layer of the *coronary* and *triangular ligaments* of the liver (Fig. 15–1). The anterior layer of the coronary ligament of the liver is continuous with the right side of the falciform ligament, at the place where the peritoneum is reflected from the diaphragm to the right lobe of the liver. The posterior layer of the coronary ligament of the liver extends from the back of the right lobe to the right suprarenal gland and kidney. The left and right triangular ligaments of the liver are situated where the anterior and posterior coronary ligaments meet (Fig. 15–2). The *anterior layer* of the triangular ligament is continuous with the left side of the falciform ligament anteriorly; also, the peritoneum is here reflected from the diaphragm to the left lobe of the liver. The *posterior layer* of the triangular ligament is dorsal to the anterior layer and is situated where the peritoneum is reflected from the left lobe of the liver to the diaphragm. The two layers of the triangular ligament join in a sharp fold at the left (Fig. 15–2).

The *dorsal layer* of the coronary and triangular ligaments is continuous with the lesser omentum at the abdominal end of the esophagus. The *lesser omentum* splits around the esophagus and stomach and then reunites and becomes continuous with the dorsal mesentery as the *lienorenal (splenorenal) ligament.* The *dorsal mesentery* is actually the *greater omentum* and it is fused to the transverse mesocolon. The *hepatogastric* and *hepatoduodenal ligaments* are mesenteric folds of peritoneum that form the lesser omentum and extend from the porta hepatis to the stomach and duodenum respectively.

The greater omentum passes around the pylorus and unites with the free edge of the lesser omentum. The *transverse mesocolon* posteriorly is continuous with the peritoneum covering the ascending and descending colon. The peritoneum of the descending colon caudally merges with the *sigmoid mesocolon* (Fig. 15–2). There is a *bare area of liver* which is not covered by peritoneum lying between the layers of the coronary ligament (Fig. 15–2).

926

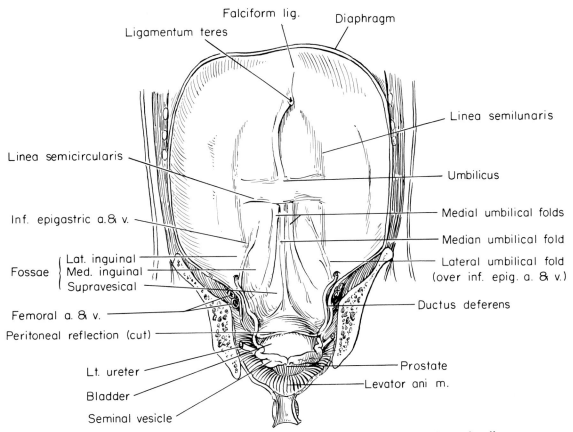

Figure 15–1. Peritoneal folds and relationships of the anterior (dorsal) abdominal wall.

The *greater omentum* is a double layer of peritoneum hanging from the greater curvature of the stomach, crossing over the transverse colon and descending in front of the abdominal viscera. There are three extensions from the greater omentum: (1) the *gastrocolic ligament,* which is the omentum between the stomach and transverse colon; (2) the *lienorenal ligament,* which is the mesentery from the left kidney to the spleen; and (3) the *gastrolienal ligament,* which is the dorsal mesentery joining the spleen to the stomach.

The *transverse mesocolon* is the dorsal mesentery of the transverse colon (see sagittal section, Figure 15–5). The *phrenicocolic ligament* is that fold of peritoneum extending between the left colic flexure to the diaphragm and helping to support the spleen (*sustentaculum* of the spleen). The *mesentery proper* is a broad fanlike fold of peritoneum extending from the posterior wall of the abdomen and suspending the entire jejunum and ileum from the dorsal body wall (Fig. 15–3).

The *omental bursa* or *lesser sac* is situated behind the stomach and communicates with the main cavity of the peritoneal space through the *epiploic foramen* (Figs. 15–4 and 15–5). As shown in the diagrams, the lesser sac is bounded

ventrally by the caudal lobe of the liver, the stomach, the greater omentum, and the lesser omentum; dorsally it is bounded by the greater omentum, transverse colon, and mesocolon as well as the left suprarenal and left kidney. To the right it opens into the greater sac. To the left are the phrenicocolic ligament, the hilum of the spleen, and the gastrolienal ligament (Fig. 15–4).

On the anterior abdominal wall moving cephalad above the umbilicus there is the *falciform ligament* containing the *ligamentum teres* (Fig. 15–1). On the ventral abdominal wall moving caudad to the umbilicus there is a fold extending from the umbilicus to the apex of the urinary bladder called the *median umbilical fold* which contains the obliterated urachus (Fig. 15–6). On either side of this middle umbilical plica or fold are *lateral folds* or *plicae* which cover ligamentous structures beginning at the umbilicus and extending to join the superior vesical branch of the internal iliac artery. These folds are remnants of the fetal umbilical arteries. More laterally and convexly toward the lateral abdominal margin are the *epigastric folds* or *plicae,* which are folds of peritoneum covering the inferior epigastric vessels (Fig. 15–1).

The *pelvic peritoneum* extends downward from the abdominal

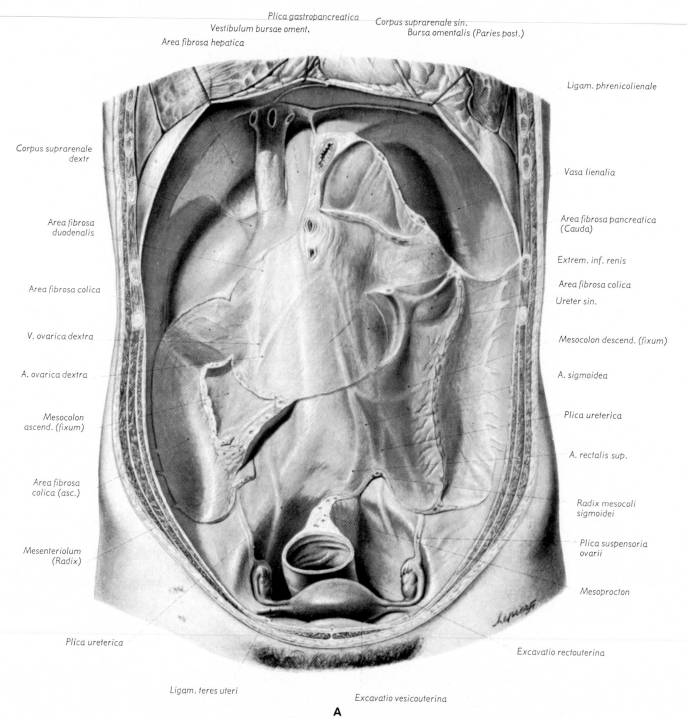

Figure 15–2.   A. Peritoneal relationships on the posterior abdominal wall.

Figure 15–2 continued on the opposite page.

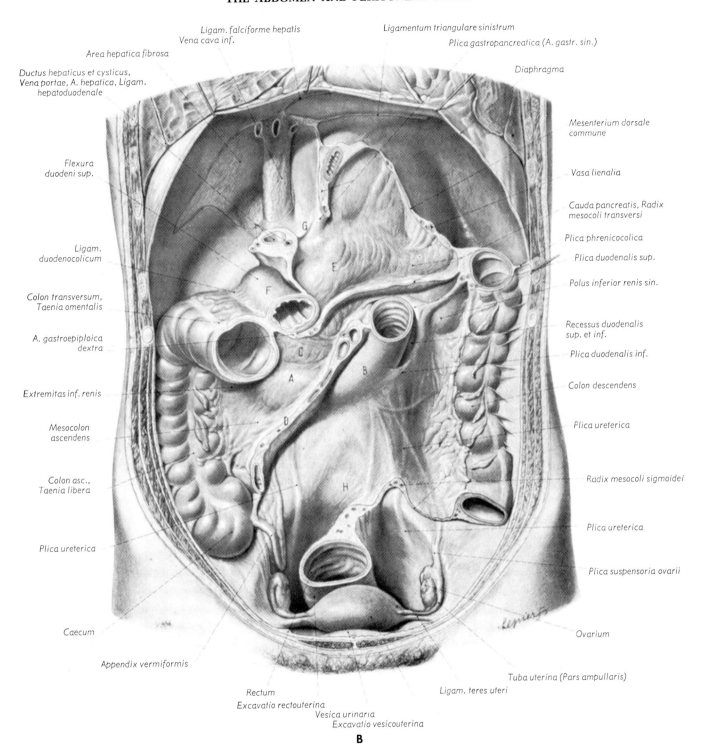

Ligam. falciforme hepatis
Vena cava inf.
Ligamentum triangulare sinistrum
Plica gastropancreatica (A. gastr. sin.)
Area hepatica fibrosa
Diaphragma
Ductus hepaticus et cysticus,
Vena portae, A. hepatica, Ligam.
hepatoduodenale
Mesenterium dorsale
commune
Flexura
duodeni sup.
Vasa lienalia
Cauda pancreatis, Radix
mesocoli transversi
Ligam.
duodenocolicum
Plica phrenicocolica
Plica duodenalis sup.
Colon transversum,
Taenia omentalis
Polus inferior renis sin.
A. gastroepiploica
dextra
Recessus duodenalis
sup. et inf.
Plica duodenalis inf.
Extremitas inf. renis
Colon descendens
Mesocolon
ascendens
Plica ureterica
Colon asc.,
Taenia libera
Radix mesocoli sigmoidei
Plica ureterica
Plica suspensoria ovarii
Plica ureterica
Ovarium
Caecum
Appendix vermiformis
Tuba uterina (Pars ampullaris)
Rectum
Ligam. teres uteri
Excavatio rectouterina
Vesica urinaria
Excavatio vesicouterina

B

Figure 15–2 *Continued.* B. Peritoneum on the posterior abdominal wall with the roots of the mesenteries and the posterior wall of bursa omentalis. Peritoneum covering duodenum, pancreas, and colon ascendens and descendens with mesocolon asc. and desc.

A, Pars tecta duodeni   E, Corpus pancreatis
B, Pars ascendens duod.   F, Pars horizontalis superior duod.
C, Caput pancreatis   G, Vestibulum bursae omentalis
D, Radix mesenterii   H, Promontorium

(From Pernkopf, E.: Atlas of Topographical and Applied Human Anatomy. Vol. 2. Philadelphia, W. B. Saunders Co., 1964.)

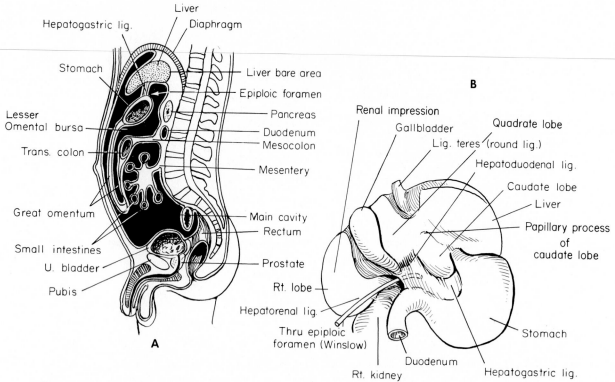

Figure 15–3. *A.* Sagittal section of abdominal cavity showing greater and lesser omental sacs with adjoining mesenteric attachments. *B.* View of hepatogastric ligament and epiploic foramen into lesser omental bursa, with adjoining structures.

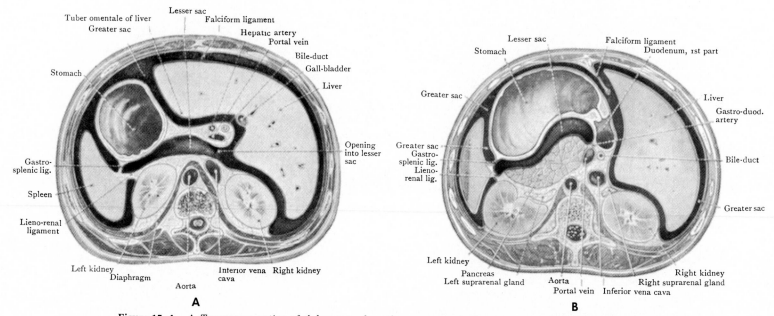

Figure 15–4. *A.* Transverse section of abdomen to show the arrangement of peritoneum at the level of the opening into lesser sac. *B.* Transverse section of abdomen to show the arrangement of the peritoneum immediately below the opening into the lesser sac.

Figure 15–4 continued on the opposite page.

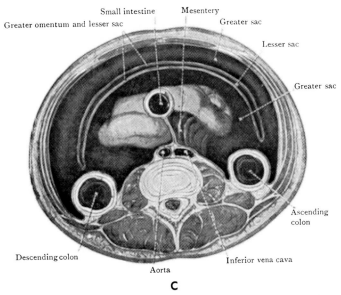

Figure 15–4 *Continued.* C. Transverse section of abdomen through the fourth lumbar vertebra, to show the arrangement of the peritoneum. (From Cunningham's Manual of Practical Anatomy, 12th ed. London, Oxford University Press, 1958.)

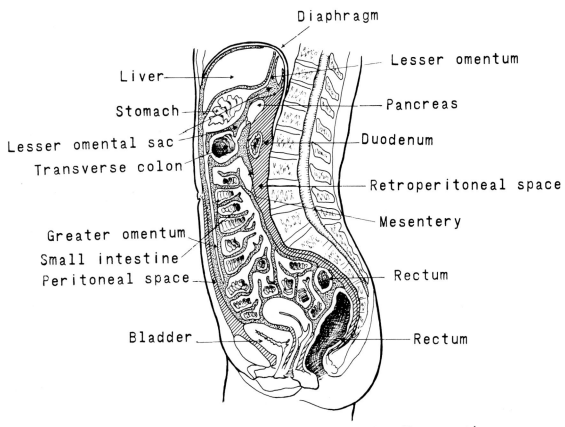

Figure 15–5. Sagittal diagram of abdomen showing relationships of lesser omental sac.

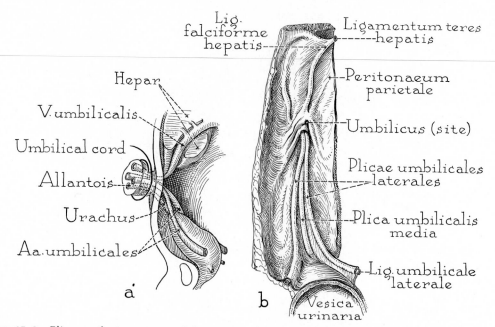

Figure 15–6. Plicae on the inner aspect of the anterior wall occasionally visualized in the posteroanterior view. Umbilical blood vessels and remnant of the urachus, and the serous folds caused by their presence on the internal aspect of the anterior abdominal wall. The obliterated umbilical vein occupies a fold of peritoneum, the falciform ligament of the liver, which, arising from the upper part of the anterior abdominal wall, runs to the umbilical incisura of the liver. Below the level of the umbilicus the urachus, persisting as a ligamentous strand, lifts the peritoneum in the median plane to produce a middle umbilical fold. Over the umbilical arteries the peritoneum projects, to each side of the midline, as a lateral umbilical fold. These *plicae*, together with lesser serous elevations over the functional inferior epigastric vessels, form boundaries of *foveae* on the internal aspect of the wall. (From Anson, B. J.: An Atlas of Human Anatomy. Philadelphia, W. B. Saunders Co., 1963.)

walls, covering the pelvic viscera and the anatomic structures contained therein. There is a vesicouterine pouch in the female between the urinary bladder and the uterus and a rectouterine pouch (pouch of Douglas) between the uterus and the rectum posteriorly. The relationship of these pouches to the vagina is evident in Figure 15–7. In the male the pelvic peritoneum extends on the posterior aspect of the urinary bladder into the rectum, creating a rectovesical pouch (Fig. 15–8).

Contents of the Abdomen. The following structures are found within the abdominopelvic cavity: (1) the peritoneum, mesenteries, omenta, and ligaments, (2) the liver, (3) the spleen, (4) the pancreas, (5) the adrenal glands, (6) the urinary tract, (7) the reproductive organs, (8) the gastrointestinal tract and (9) the blood vessels, lymphatics, and nerves.

The gastrointestinal tract, genitourinary tract, and cardiovascular system are considered separately.

RADIOLOGIC ANATOMY OF THE PERITONEAL SPACE

Lesser Peritoneal Sac. Anatomic drawings illustrating the anterior wall of the lesser sac and the posterior wall with the stomach partially removed are shown in Figures 15–9 and 15–10. The *anterior wall* is composed of the lesser omentum, the posterior surface of the stomach and duodenal bulb, and the gastrocolic ligament (Fig. 15–9). The *posterior wall* is bounded by peritoneum covering the pancreas, left adrenal gland, a part of the upper anterior surface of the left kidney, and portions of the posterior diaphragm (Fig. 15–10). Note the large fold of peritoneum raised from the posterior abdominal wall by the left gastric and left hepatic arteries. This fold divides the lesser sac into two compartments. The upper recess on the right is limited by the diaphragm and is caudad to the liver (also see Fig. 15–5). On the left aspect of

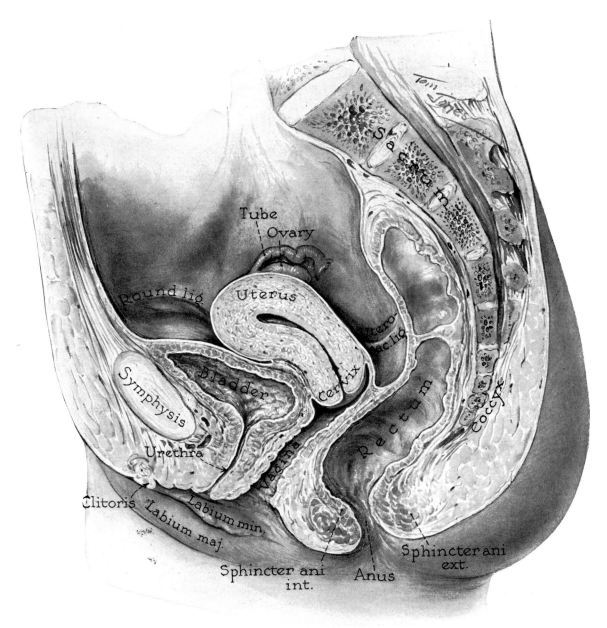

Figure 15–7. Female pelvis, sagittal section, showing the relations of the organs and the course of the peritoneum. The peritoneum ascends over the bladder to cover the vesical surface of the body of the uterus, from which it is continued lateralward as the anterior layer of the broad ligament; the shallow trough-like recess thus formed is the vesicouterine excavation (uterovesical pouch). The peritoneal layer next covers the fundus of the uterus, investing all of the posterior uterus and a small upper segment of the vaginal wall; from the uterus it is again draped lateralward to form the posterior layer of the broad ligament of the uterus. From the uterus and the ligament the peritoneum passes to the front of the rectum, forming a deeper sac, the rectouterine excavation. The peritoneum reaches the rectum approximately at the junction of its lower and middle thirds; in the middle third it covers only the front of the tube, while in the upper third it clothes the sides as well; the layers of the two sides then meet above to form a mesenteric support for the sigmoid colon. In partially investing the rectum the peritoneum forms paired pouches, the pararectal fossae, bounded on each side by a crescentic fold of peritoneum, the rectouterine fold (fold of Douglas). (From Anson, B. J.: An Atlas of Human Anatomy. Philadelphia, W. B. Saunders Co., 1963.)

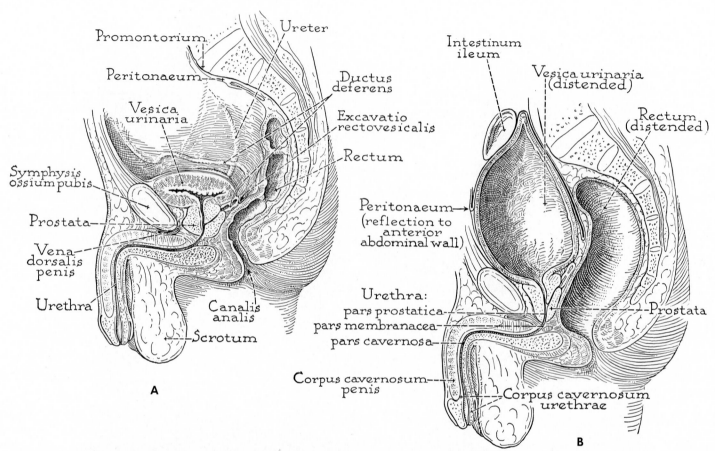

Figure 15–8. Sagittal section through the lower abdomen and pelvis, demonstrating the urinary bladder and rectum. *A.* Showing the organs in the empty condition. In sagittal section the bladder is three-sided. The superior surface faces upward; the posterior surface is directed both backward and downward; inferiorly, the bladder rests upon the pelvic floor, the levitor ani muscles, and the pubic symphysis. *B.* The bladder and rectum distended. The distended bladder rises above the space just described, projecting into the true abdominal cavity. It assumes a bulbous form and loses its triangular configuration. (From Anson, B. J.: An Atlas of Human Anatomy. Philadelphia, W. B. Saunders Co., 1963.)

this recess, the peritoneum of the posterior wall of the lesser sac is reflected from the diaphragm onto the posterior surface of the fundus of the stomach. This reflection is called the *gastrophrenic ligament* and is continuous laterally with the gastrosplenic and lienorenal ligaments. Inferiorly the lesser peritoneal space is limited by the transverse mesocolon, the root of which crosses the head of the pancreas and extends along its inferior margin (Fig. 15–10). The *right margin* of the lesser sac is formed by the peritoneal reflection over the inferior vena cava. The *foramen of Winslow* described previously in Chapter 13 is only large enough to admit one finger but this size may vary.

In the living, the lesser sac is very distensible but it can expand only to the left inferiorly and anteriorly, since the liver, diaphragm, and posterior abdominal wall prevent expansion in the other directions (Walker and Weens). Pneumoperitoneum of the lesser sac, herniations, and abscesses may be responsible for such distention and may be recognized by the anatomic boundaries given.

Differentiation of Peritoneal Organs from Retroperitoneal Organs. An organ only partly covered by peritoneum is referred to as a "retroperitoneal" organ. An organ that is completely covered by peritoneum except for entrance of vessels is called a "peritoneal" organ. The various ligaments or folds of mesentery previously described connect the completely peritonealized organs to the abdominal wall. The opening from the general peritoneal cavity into the lesser peritoneal cavity through the foramen of Winslow has been described earlier. In addition, in the female there are two minute apertures in the peritoneal cavity at the openings of the uterine tubes. As will be shown in Chapter 17, injections into the uterine cavity and uterine tubes communicate with the pelvic peritoneal space.

Some of these relationships of peritoneal and retroperitoneal organs are best seen in cross-sectional diagrams of the abdomen. For example, at about the *level of the fourth lumbar vertebra* or the umbilicus (Fig. 15–4 C): the descending and ascending colon are only partially peritonealized and therefore are partially retroperitoneal. There is a mesenteric band extending approximately from the midline to the small intestine which contains the major mesenteric vessels and nerves; hence the small intestine is completely peritonealized. The aorta and inferior vena cava are retroperitoneal and are posterior to the mesentery containing the major blood vessels to the small intestine.

At the level of the *first and second lumbar vertebrae* (Fig. 15–4 B), the reflections of the peritoneum are somewhat more complex. Here the epiploic foramen of Winslow connecting the general peritoneal cavity and omental bursa can be identified. The omental bursa is just dorsal to the stomach; its vestibule is that portion of this space that lies just dorsal to the hepatoduodenal ligament. The omental bursa is limited ventrally by the liver, the lesser omentum, the stomach, and the greater omentum; dorsally by the abdominal wall, the left suprarenal glands, the pancreas,

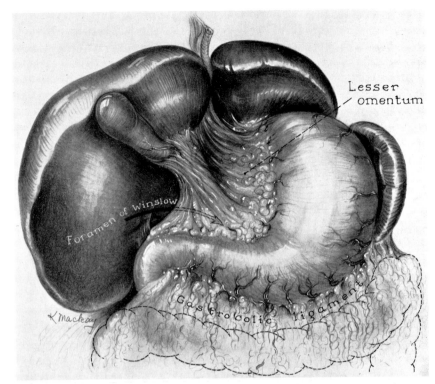

Figure 15–9. Anatomic drawing illustrating anterior wall of lesser sac; composed of lesser omentum, posterior surface of stomach and duodenal bulb, and gastrocolic ligament. (From Walker, L. A., and Weens, H. S.: Radiology, 80:727, 1963.)

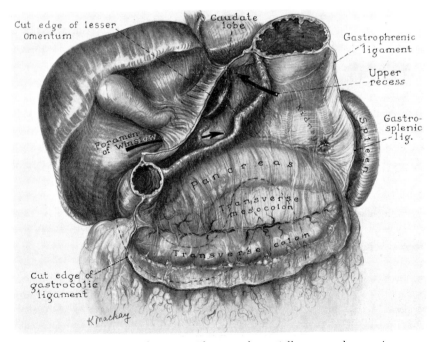

Figure 15–10. Anatomic drawing with stomach partially removed, exposing posterior wall of lesser sac. Note fold of peritoneum raised by left gastric and hepatic arteries. (From Walker, L. A., and Weens, H. S.: Radiology, 80:727, 1963.)

the transverse mesocolon, and at times the dorsal portion of the greater omentum. At this level, the spleen is largely peritoneal, although there is a small segment dorsally adjoining the kidney which is not completely invested by peritoneum. The spleen is connected with the stomach by a ligamentous mesenteric structure called the gastrosplenic ligament (gastrolienal). The pancreas, both kidneys, the aorta, and superior vena cava are all retroperitoneal structures. On the ventral aspect of the pancreas at this level is the lesser omental bursa.

Along the *right aspect of the lesser omental bursa* are the root structures of the liver or portal triad which are invested partly by peritoneum from the greater peritoneal cavity and partly by the lesser omental bursa. These structures are mainly the *portal vein, hepatic artery,* and *common bile duct*—the structures of the portal triad. The foramen of Winslow in cross section is situated on the dorsal aspect of the kidney adjoining the liver, which at this level is completely invested by peritoneum and lies in the peritoneal space. The falciform ligament appears to suspend the liver from the anterior abdominal wall.

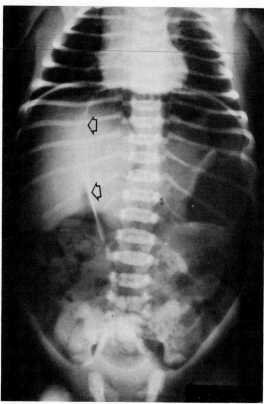

Figure 15–12. "Air dome" or "football sign" indicating a large amount of free air in the abdomen. Arrows point to falciform ligament—the "lacing" on the "football."

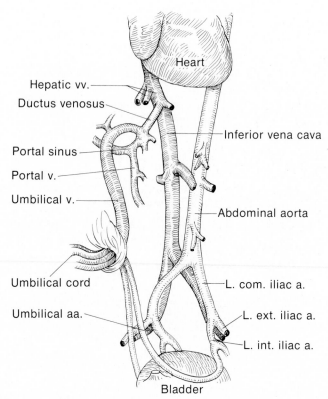

Heart

Hepatic vv.
Ductus venosus
Portal sinus
Portal v.
Umbilical v.
Inferior vena cava
Abdominal aorta
Umbilical cord
Umbilical aa.
L. com. iliac a.
L. ext. iliac a.
L. int. iliac a.
Bladder

Figure 15–11. Neonatal umbilical circulation. (From Sapin, S. O., Linde, L. N., and Emmanouilides, G. C.: Pediatrics, *31*:946–951, 1963.)

In sagittal section, Figure 15–5, other special relationships can be noted. The liver is almost completely invested by peritoneum except for a small area on its superior and posterior aspects. The omental bursa in part lies posterior to the liver, whereas the general peritoneal cavity is otherwise anterior to the liver and the hepatogastric ligament. The stomach is partially invested by the peritoneum of the omental bursa dorsally, and by the peritoneum of the general peritoneal cavity ventrally. The bands of mesentery extending to the colon and small intestine from the posterior abdominal wall are also shown in diagram. The greater omentum is a sac-like structure which extends down from the greater curvature of the stomach and then folds back upon itself to continue with the posterior wall of the lesser omental bursa and the anterior aspect of the transverse colon.

The *general peritoneal cavity* continues downward to the upper aspect of the urinary bladder and the uterus in the female, and it dips down once again between the uterus and the rectum, investing the anterior aspect of the rectum. Since the sigmoid colon is completely surrounded by peritoneum it is connected by a mesentery with the posterior wall of the abdomen, and is called the "mesosigmoid" or "mesocolon." We have previously noted the vesicouterine pouch and the rectouterine pouch between the uterus and anterior abdominal wall, and the uterus and colon respectively (Figs. 15–7 and 15–8).

The falciform ligament previously described contains the remains of the left umbilical vein of the fetus, and, as pointed out in Chapter 14, it is an important route for venous catheterization in the newborn (Fig. 15–11). The falciform ligament is readily identified in pneumoperitoneum of the infant (Fig. 15–12).

When air is introduced into the peritoneal space the abdominal organs separate from the abdominal wall and the cavity becomes visible.

The Folds of Peritoneum and Fossae of the Pelvis in the Female. The folds and fossae of the pelvis, especially that of the female, are of considerable significance in radiologic anatomy. The *transverse vesicle fold* extends from the urinary bladder lat-

erally to the pelvic wall (Fig. 15–13; this is the same in the male and female). Likewise, there is a *ureteral fold* overlying the ureter in both sexes. In the female, however, there is a *broad ligament* which incompletely divides the pelvic cavity into anterior and posterior compartments by folds of peritoneum draped over the uterine tubes and ovaries (Fig. 15–13). This will be described further in Chapter 17. A third fold in the female is the *rectouterine fold,* which extends from the rectum to the uterus. There is also a strong ligamentous structure extending between the uterus and the sacrum called the *uterosacral ligament* (see Chapter 17).

Potential Peritoneal Spaces. The various reflections in the peritoneal cavity described above create certain potential spaces which can be considerably significant, particularly with inflammatory processes. Thus, the supraomental region contains four recesses: (1) a *right subphrenic recess,* which lies between the right lobe of the liver and the diaphragm and is bounded by the

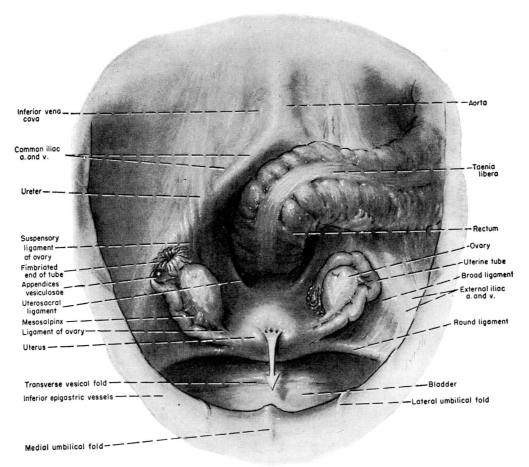

Figure 15–13. Female pelvic organs, anterior view. The uterus is retracted slightly ventrad in the direction of the arrow. (From Anson, B. J. (ed.): Morris' Human Anatomy, 12th ed. Copyright © 1966 by McGraw-Hill Inc. Used by permission of McGraw-Hill Book Company.)

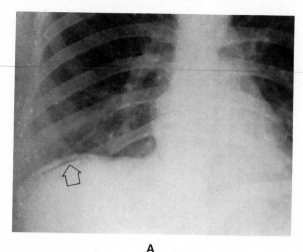

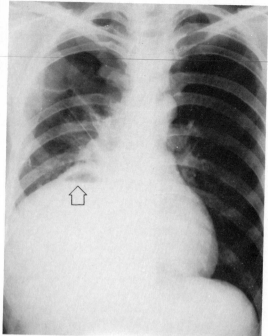

A

B

Figure 15–14. *A.* Free air beneath the right hemidiaphragm producing a crescentic shadow. *B.* Greater elevation beneath the right hemidiaphragm due to a subphrenic abscess, likewise with free air.

falciform ligament and the coronary ligament. A subphrenic abscess or free air from a ruptured hollow viscus may accumulate here (Fig. 15–14 *A* and *B*); (2) a *subhepatic recess*, which lies between the liver and the other abdominal viscera. Abscess accumulation is prone to occur here also (Fig. 15–15); (3) a *left subphrenic recess*, which is anterior and perigastric and lies between the dome of the diaphragm, the left lobe of the liver, the stomach, the spleen, and the greater omentum. It is also bounded

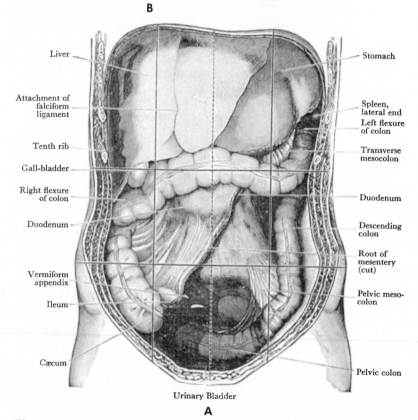

Figure 15–16. Abdominal viscera after removal of the jejunum and ileum, demonstrating the three infraomental patential spaces: two created by the root of the mesentery (cut), and the third being the pelvic cavity proper. (From Cunningham's Manual of Practical Anatomy, 12th ed. Vol. 2. London, Oxford University Press, 1958.)

Figure 15–16 continued on the opposite page.

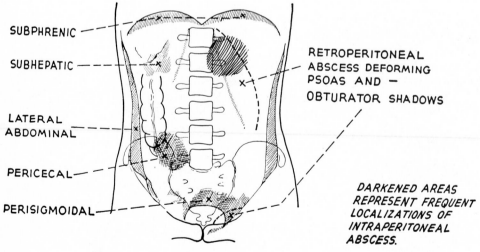

SUBPHRENIC

SUBHEPATIC

RETROPERITONEAL
ABSCESS DEFORMING
PSOAS AND —
OBTURATOR SHADOWS

LATERAL
ABDOMINAL

PERICECAL

PERISIGMOIDAL

DARKENED AREAS
REPRESENT FREQUENT
LOCALIZATIONS OF
INTRAPERITONEAL
ABSCESS.

Figure 15–15. Diagram illustrating the various localizations of intraperitoneal and retroperitoneal abscesses.

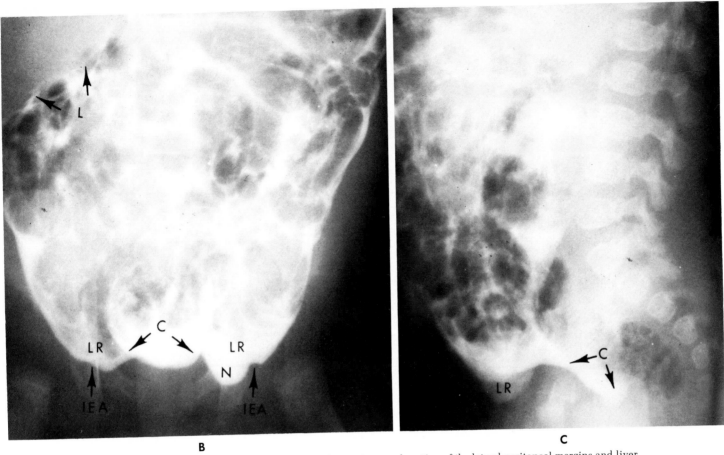

Figure 15–16 *Continued.* *B* and *C.* Normal study. *B.* Note good coating of the lateral peritoneal margins and liver edge (*L*). The contrast material has pooled in the normal lateral recesses (*LR*) and cul-de-sac (*C*). Note the notch due to the inferior epigastric artery (*IEA*) and the normal extension of the peritoneal sac medial to it (*N*).

C. Lateral view (not a necessary part of the examination) showing location of the lateral recesses (*LR*) and cul-de-sac (*C*). (From Swischuk, L. E., and Stacy, T. M.: Radiology, *101*:139–146, 1971.)

by the falciform ligament; (4) the *omental bursa,* which some anatomists regard as a diverticulum from the subhepatic fossae, communicating with the general peritoneal cavity through the epiploic foramen.

The infraomental region contains three potential spaces; two of these spaces are created by the division of the posterior abdominal cavity along the root of the mesentery extending from the duodenojejunal flexure to the right iliac fossa (Fig. 15–16). The infraomental compartment communicates with the supraomental compartments in the neighborhood of the hepatic or splenic flexures of the colon on the right and left sides respectively. The third infraomental potential space is the pelvic cavity proper.

Position of Abdominal Viscera. The usual position of the abdominal viscera as visualized roentgenographically is illustrated in Figures 15–16, 15–17 and 15–18. There is a wide normal range in both form and position of abdominal viscera in the liv-

ing. These may be altered by gravity, physiologic changes, or constitutional variations. Even with retroperitoneal structures considerable variation may be noted during life. The urinary and genital tracts will be described in greater detail in Chapters 16 and 17, and the alimentary tract has already been described in Chapters 13 and 14. These organs may all be visualized in part in plain film surveys of the abdomen without additional contrast media by virtue of the fatty envelope or tela subserosa, which surrounds these various organs, or by gas which may be found normally or abnormally in the hollow viscera. Abnormally, calcification in some form may further intensify the image of one or another of these several organs.

The Properitoneal Fat Layer or Tela Subserosa. Between the transverse fascia, which covers the inner surfaces of the abdominal muscles, and the peritoneum lies a considerable quantity of extraperitoneal areolar tissue, which contains a variable amount of fat (Fig. 15–19). This is called the *tela subserosa* and

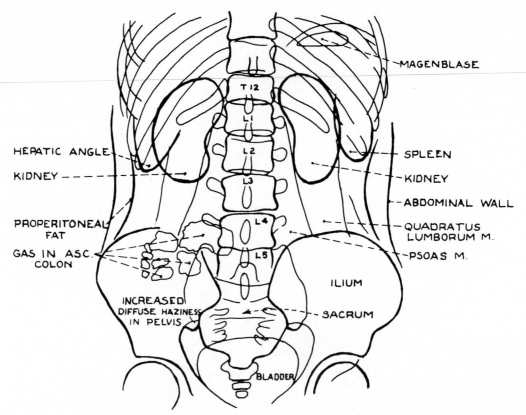

Figure 15–17. Routine for examination of the recumbent film of the abdomen.

its parietal component is called the *properitoneal fat layer*. At times an intraperitoneal fat component is visualized as well. These layers are of considerable importance radiologically, since their identification may reflect intra- or extrainflammatory or neoplastic processes of the abdomen. Moreover, the tela subserosa continues posteriorly, and is particularly abundant around the kidneys, giving rise to a considerable perirenal fat layer. It is this continuation of the tela subserosa around the kidneys ("Gerota's" capsule) that permits a fairly accurate visualization of these organs without the necessity for contrast media (Figs. 15–17, 15–19, and 15–20).

The introduction of a gas such as air in the tela subserosa often separates the fatty layer from the corresponding organ and allows a clear depiction of this organ (Fig. 15–21). Thus, the kidneys and the suprarenal glands can be accurately identified. Somewhat similar depiction, although not as clearly defined, may be obtained by retroperitoneal tomography (Fig. 15–22).

Further Correlative Studies of the Properitoneal Fat Layer (extraperitoneal perivisceral fat pad [EPFP]) (Whalen et al., 1969). Whalen et al. have demonstrated schematically, by comparative cross sections with cadavers, the relationships of the extraperitoneal perivisceral fat pad ("properitoneal fat layer" in other terminology). In Figure 15–23 the extraperitoneal perivis-

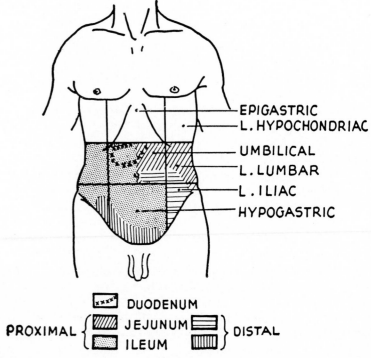

Figure 15–18. Approximate distribution of the small intestine within the abdomen.

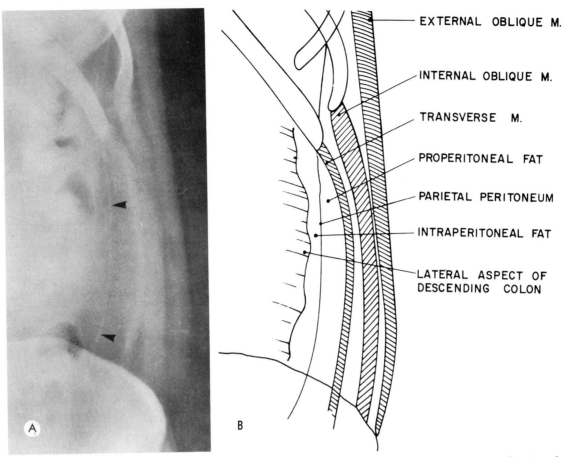

EXTERNAL OBLIQUE M.

INTERNAL OBLIQUE M.

TRANSVERSE M.

PROPERITONEAL FAT

PARIETAL PERITONEUM

INTRAPERITONEAL FAT

LATERAL ASPECT OF
DESCENDING COLON

A

B

Figure 15–19. A. Normal roentgenographic anatomy in the flank. There is unusually extensive visualization of parietal peritoneum (arrows). B. Diagram of roentgenogram. (From Budin, E., and Jacobson, G.: Amer. J. Roentgenol. 99:62, 1967.)

ceral fat pad is shaded, showing an intimate contact of the posterior portions of the liver and spleen with the perivisceral fat. The structures in Figure 15–23 A and B which are not in contact with this fatty layer are rarely visualized on plain films of the abdomen, whereas those below the indicated horizontal line are consistently identifiable on plain films in older children and adults. The associated schematic frontal view of the liver is also shown.

Schematic frontal and lateral views of the liver (Fig. 15–24) show the fatty layer behind the liver and between it and the right kidney. Whalen and his associates believe that the anterior portions of the right lobe and the entire left lobe are not related to the extraperitoneal perivisceral fat pad, but do relate closely to the colon and stomach respectively. Similarly, in Figure 15–25, a schematic frontal view of the spleen demonstrates the relationship of anterior and posterior margins of the spleen to the fatty layer as well as the splenic angle. The reason for poor correlation between radiological and clinical evaluation of liver and spleen size is explained by the fact that the fatty layer delineates the posterior margin but not the anterior margin of these organs.

The Hepatic Angle and Splenic Angle. The tela subserosa and properitoneal fat not only delineate the flank regions as shown in Figure 15–19 but normally surround the liver and spleen, creating the so-called hepatic angle and splenic angle as shown diagrammatically in Figure 15–23. As shown in diagrams in previous discussions of the anatomy of the liver and spleen, these organs are almost completely enclosed by peritoneum and may therefore be clearly identified by the properitoneal fatty envelope of tela subserosa.

The flank not only has a specific structural pattern but is generally concave between thorax and iliac crest; asymmetry in this shape is clinically significant, since mass or inflammatory lesions may cause a bulging of the flank on one side or the other. Indeed, accurate measurements of the spleen and liver may be made for demonstration of possible abnormalities contained in these organs (see later discussions of the spleen and liver).

A representative abnormality of the right flank and hepatic angle is illustrated in Figure 15–27. In this instance irregularity of the properitoneal fat line and fracture of the right lower ribs in-

(Text continued on page 945.)

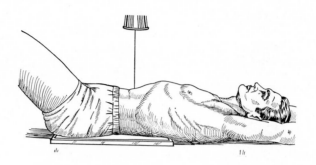

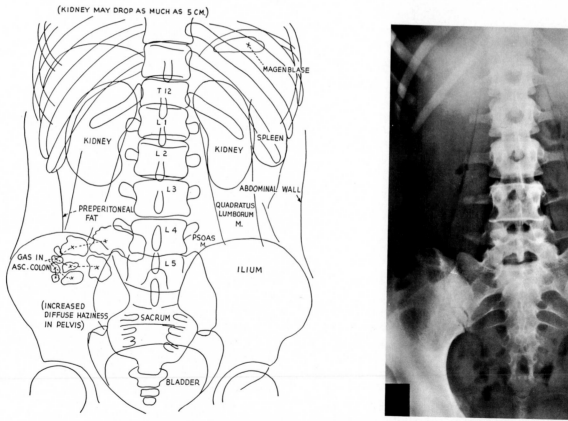

Figure 15–20. Anteroposterior view of abdomen (KUB film).

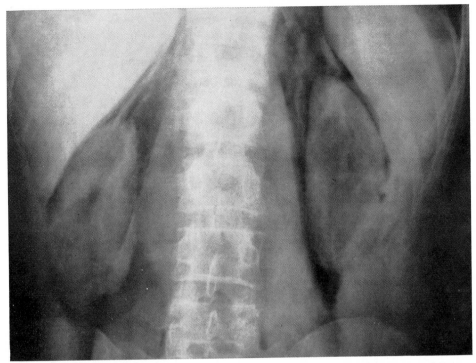

Figure 15–21. Normal retroperitoneal pneumogram. (From McLelland, R., Landes, R. R., and Ransom, C. L.: Radiol. Clin. N. Amer., 3:115, 1965.)

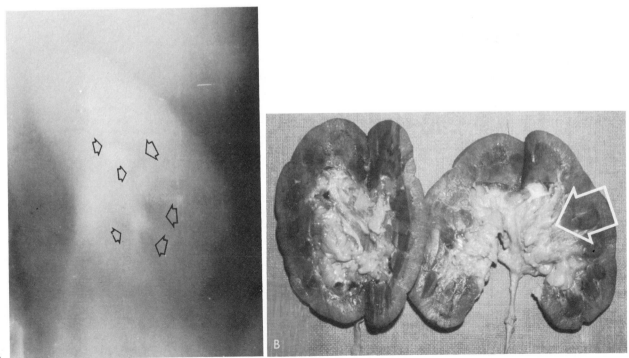

A

Figure 15–22. Renal fibrolipomatosis. *A.* Excretory urogram (tomogram) showing excessive fat around renal pelvis and calyces. *B.* Specimen.

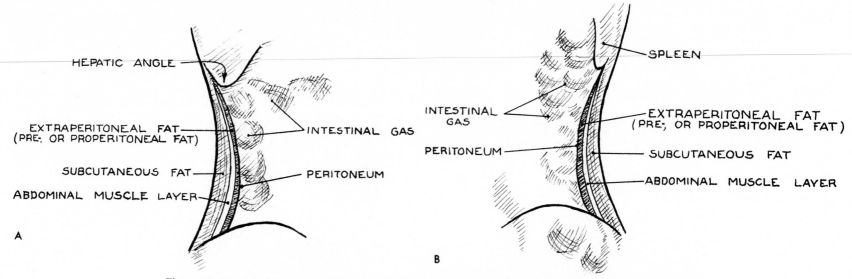

Figure 15–23.　*A* and *B*. Diagrams demonstrating flank anatomy, showing the relationship of the properitoneal fat layer to the rest of the abdominal wall.

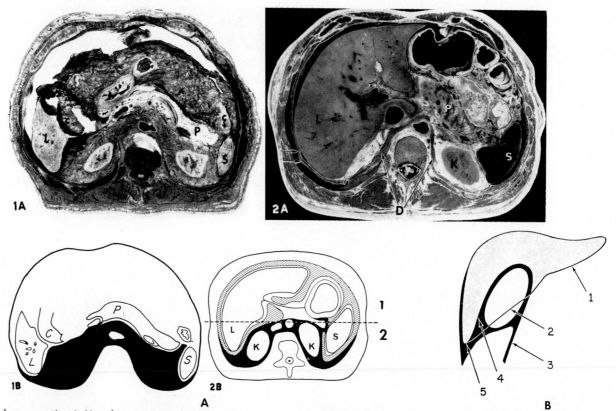

Figure 15–24.　*A*. Horizontal cross section (1A) and tracing (1B) of cadaver at the level of the lower border of liver. The "extraperitoneal perivisceral fat pad" is shaded. Note the deep indentation and intimate contact of the posterior portions of liver and spleen with the perivisceral fat. Code: (L) Liver, (S) spleen, (P) pancreas, (C) colon, (D) diaphragmatic crura, (K) kidney.

Horizontal cross section (2A) and schematic drawing (2B) of another cadaver at the level of the upper portion of liver. The structures above the horizontal line (1) which are not in contact with e.p.f.p. are rarely visualized on plain films. The structures below this line (2) and intimate with e.p.f.p. are consistently identifiable on plain films.

Note the diaphragmatic crura buried in the e.p.f.p. (A) and the large fat pad adjacent to the posterior liver and spleen, which is well shown in this specimen.

Observe paucity of e.p.f.p. where diaphragm (⌒) contacts the liver. The properitoneal fat lines terminate here.

B. Schematic frontal view of liver. E.p.f.p. shown in black. (1) Left lobe of liver, (2) anterior portion of right lobe of liver, (3) e.p.f.p. outlining psoas muscle, (4) posterior portion of liver, (5) hepatic angle.

Figure 15–24 continued on the opposite page.

year have at least some fat present (Fig. 15–28). Likewise, the splenic outline was not noted in neonates but it was seen in 50 per cent of children over 1 year of age. The psoas muscle margin (to be discussed below) was seen in only one of 23 neonates, but in 56 per cent of the 1 to 5 year age group and in 100 per cent of the 11 to 15 year age group.

The Roentgenology of the Paracolic Gutter. The ascending and descending colon are partially retroperitoneal as shown in Figure 15–4 C. When the patient is in the supine position a "paracolic gutter" is created. Normally, the peritoneal gutter either is empty or may contain intestine or omentum; the lines of contrast in the anteroposterior projection are shown in Figure 15–29 A. The opposing visceral and parietal peritoneal surfaces may be visualized radiographically as a hair line separating the serosal and retroperitoneal structures. Figure 15–29 B shows what happens in the anteroposterior projection when a small amount of fluid is free within the gutter. When increasing amounts of fluid in the gutter (c) spill over into the main peritoneal cavity these roentgen appearances are further modified. Figure 15–29 C and D illustrates the result of turning the patient first on one side and then on the other, allowing gravity to move the fluid that is free within the peritoneal space out of the gutter; the fluid that is fixed in the retroperitoneal tissues remains immobile (Fig. 15–30). Somewhat similar demonstrations are shown in Figure 15–30 B and C. "Dog ears" in the pelvis refers to mass densities superior and lateral to the urinary bladder that are sec-

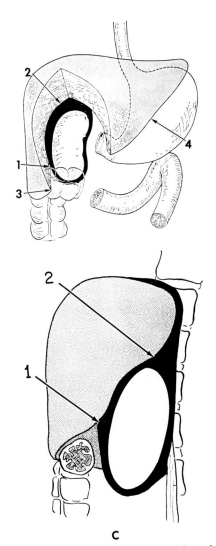

C

Figure 15–24 Continued. C. Schematic frontal and lateral views of the liver. Upper, a section of the liver is absent to show the e.p.f.p. behind the liver and between it and right kidney.

Any surface of the liver between points 1 and 2 may cast a recognizable shadow, depending upon the path of the central ray and the shape of the renal fossa of the liver.

The anterior portions of the right lobe (3) and the entire left lobe (4) are *not* related to the e.p.f.p. and do relate to colon and stomach respectively. (A, B, and C from Whalen, J. P., Berne, A. S., and Riemenschneider, P. A.: Radiology, 92:466–472, 1969.)

dicate an impact over the liver with blood presenting itself in the flank between the fat line and the ascending colon.

Hepatic Angle and Splenic Angle as a Function of Age. Franken has demonstrated that our ability to visualize these angles in children varies depending upon their age. The visualization is related directly to the extent of development of extraperitoneal fat. Only 47 per cent of neonates have a demonstrable properitoneal flank stripe, whereas all children above the age of 1

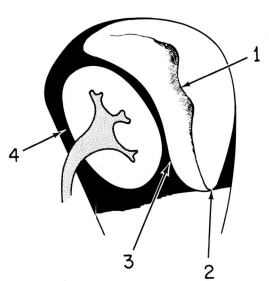

Figure 15–25. Schematic frontal view of spleen. E.p.f.p. shown in black. (1) Anterior portion of spleen, (2) splenic angle, (3) posterior portion of spleen, (4) e.p.f.p. outlining psoas muscle. (From Whalen, J. P., Berne, A. S., and Riemenschneider, P. A.: Radiology, 92:466–472, 1969.)

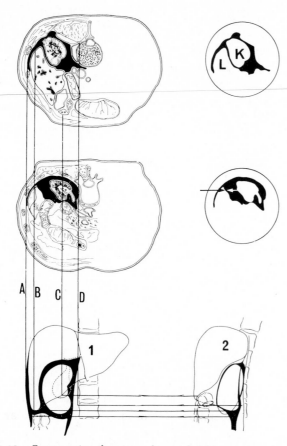

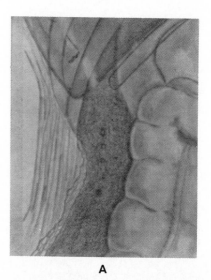

Figure 15–26. Cross-section drawings of normal right upper quadrant, showing that the contour of the pliable e.p.f.p. (black) conforms to the shape and size of the organs indenting it. The roentgen shadows which represent the e.p.f.p. in conventional anteroposterior and lateral views are diagrammed below (1 and 2).

(→ ←) demonstrates the significant anterior-posterior fat-soft-tissue interface which occurs normally. (K) Kidney, (L) liver, (A) properitoneal fat line, (B) posterior portion of liver, (C) anterior portion of liver, (D) spine. (From Whalen, J. P., and Berne, A. S.: Radiology, 92:473–480, 1969.)

ondary to intra-abdominal fluid in the peritoneal recesses lateral to the rectum (Fig. 15–30 *D*).

Importance of Peritoneal Reflections and Mesenteric Attachments. As discussed earlier, the transverse mesocolon is a major barrier dividing the abdominal cavity into supra- and inframesocolic compartments. The root of the small bowel mesentery further divides the lower compartment into two unequal infracolic spaces.

The external paracolic gutters represent potential channels of spread between the upper and lower abdominal compartments. The left infracolic space is more anatomically continuous with the pelvic cavity. The right paracolic gutter is continuous with the right subhepatic space. This is called "Morrison's pouch," in its posterosuperior extension. The right paracolic gutter may also be continuous with the right subphrenic space, in which case Mor-

rison's pouch is more dependent when the body is in a supine position. The most dependent recess in Morrison's pouch is formed by a peritoneal groove between the lateral aspect of the descending duodenum and the underlying right kidney just above the transverse mesocolon.

The falciform ligament separates the right and left subphrenic spaces. The left subphrenic and subhepatic spaces communicate with one another freely around the smaller left lobe of the liver (Meyers, 1970). This space is also continuous with the perisplenic space.

Variations in the position of the appendix, as pointed out in

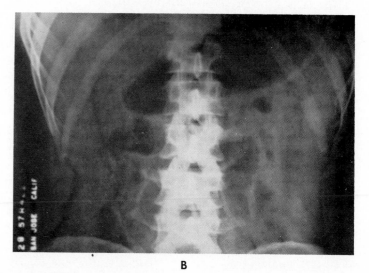

Figure 15–27. *A* and *B*. Irregularity of the properitoneal fat line and fracture of the right lower ribs indicating impact over the liver. Blood is present in the flank between the fat line and the ascending colon. A mild adynamic ileus is present. At operation there were three lacerations of the liver and a large amount of free blood in the peritoneal cavity. (From McCort, J. J.: Radiology, 78:49, 1962.)

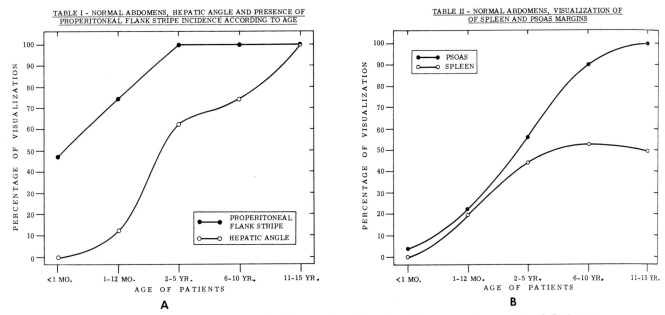

Figure 15-28. *A.* Table showing normal abdomens, hepatic angle and presence of properitoneal flank stripe incidence according to age. *B.* Normal abdomens, visualization of spleen and psoas margins. (From Franken, E. A.: Radiology, *102*:393–398, 1972.)

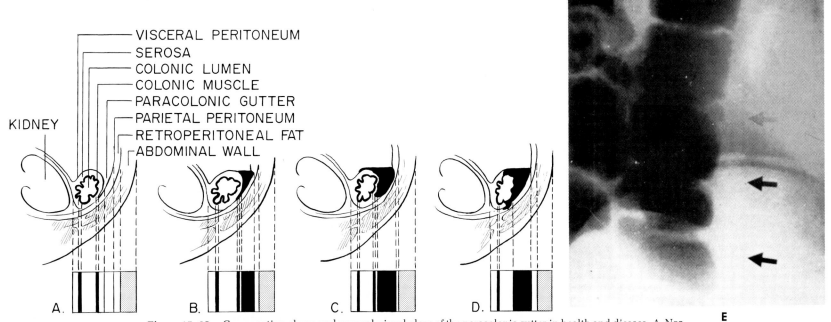

Figure 15-29. Cross section above and coronal view below of the paracolonic gutter in health and disease. *A.* Normal. The peritoneal gutter either is empty or may contain intestine or omentum. The opposing visceral and parietal peritoneal surfaces may be visualized radiographically as a hair line separating the serosal and retroperitoneal masses, both of which may vary greatly in thickness. *B.* Small amount of fluid free within the gutter. *C.* More fluid within the gutter spilling over into the main peritoneal cavity (as with rupture of the spleen or liver). *D.* The fluid (or blood) arising from the retroperitoneal tissues infiltrating the serosa gives a radiographic picture similar to *C,* but should be differentiated from free fluid by various gravity techniques. *E.* Thickened "wall" of colon between gas medially suggested free peritoneal fluid from injured spleen. Surgery demonstrated that the thickened "wall" originated in serosal infiltration from a massive retroperitoneal hematoma. Scoliosis of spine, present in this patient, is not characteristic of ruptured spleen and points more to a retroperitoneal irritation. (*A–E* from Cimmino, C. V.: Radiology, *90*:761, 1968.)

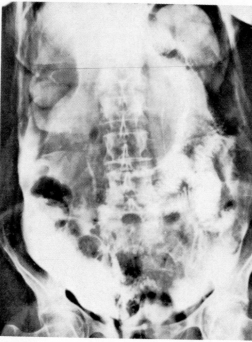
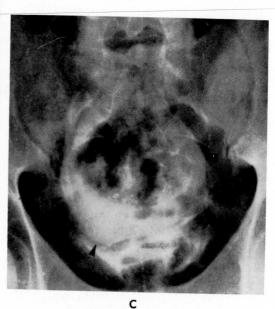

A

B

C

Figure 15-30. *A.* Roentgenogram of the pelvis in a patient with ascites demonstrates the "dog ears" sign. Fluid in peritoneal recesses on either side of the rectum produces "ears" superior and lateral to the bladder shadow. *B.* Extensive leakage of Hypaque during examination of perforated duodenal ulcer demonstrates extent of peritoneal cavity in abdomen; lateral borders represent margins of paracolonic fossae. *C.* Spill of Hypaque during study of ruptured bladder demonstrating pelvic fossa (arrows) just above bladder. (From Budin, E., and Jacobson, G.: Amer. J. Roentgenol., 99:62, 1967.)

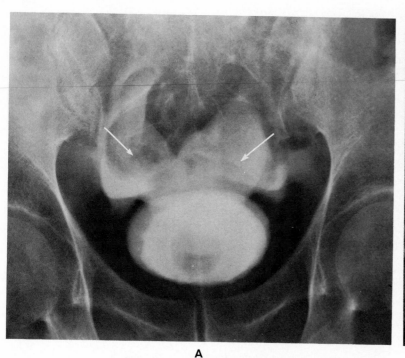

A

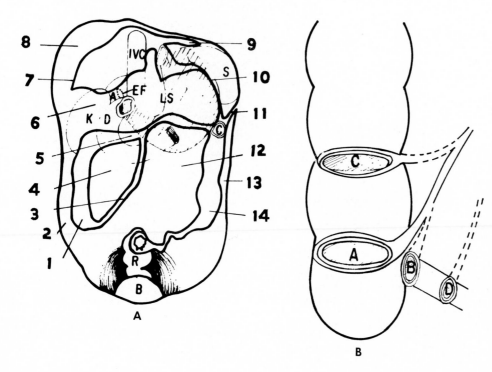

B

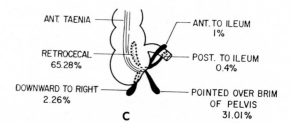

C

Figure 15-31. *A.* Diagram of posterior peritoneal reflections and recesses. (S) Spleen, (LS) lesser sac, (IVC) inferior vena cava, (EF) epiploic foramen, (K) right kidney, (D) duodenum, (A) adrenal gland, (C) splenic flexure of colon, (R) rectum, (B) urinary bladder, (1) attachment of peritoneal reflections of ascending colon, (2) right paracolic gutter, (3) root of mesentery, (4) right infracolic space, (5) root of transverse mesocolon, (6) area of Morrison's pouch, (7) right triangular ligament, (8) right subphrenic space, (9) left triangular ligament, (10) gastrolienal ligament, (11) phrenicocolic ligament, (12) left infracolic space, (13) left paracolic gutter, (14) attachment of peritoneal reflections of descending colon.

B. Diagram showing variations in the insertion of the lower end of the small-bowel mesentery. The commonest insertion is at the cecocolic junction (A), but possible variations include the ileocecal valve (B), the ascending colon (C) or the terminal ileum (D). (After Testut and Latarjet).

C. Diagram showing the incidence of variations in position of the appendix, as determined by Wakeley. The majority of the retrocecal appendices are also intraperitoneal. (A, B, and C from Meyers, M. A.: Radiology, 95:547–554, 1970.)

Chapter 14, are also important from the standpoint of determining potential inflammatory foci in the peritoneal space. These relationships are documented by Meyers in Figure 15–31 *A* and *B*. Thus, a knowledge of these basic anatomic attachments becomes of considerable significance in plotting the diagram of pathways of flow of intraperitoneal fluid or exudates.

Displacement of Abdominal Organs by Mass Lesions. A knowledge of the cross-sectional anatomy of the abdomen is particularly important in evaluation of displacement phenomena (Whalen et al., 1971, 1972). Displacement of abdominal organs by

mass lesions is an important indicator in differential diagnosis. Analysis of mass displacements that can occur in the left upper quadrant reveals the following distinguishing characteristics (Fig. 15–32):

1. *Enlargements of the spleen* displace the stomach medially when the enlargement involves the anterior aspect of the spleen, but when the posterior aspect is enlarged, the kidney is depressed.

2. *Suprarenal enlargements* ordinarily increase the size of the triangular space above the kidney, depress the kidney, and

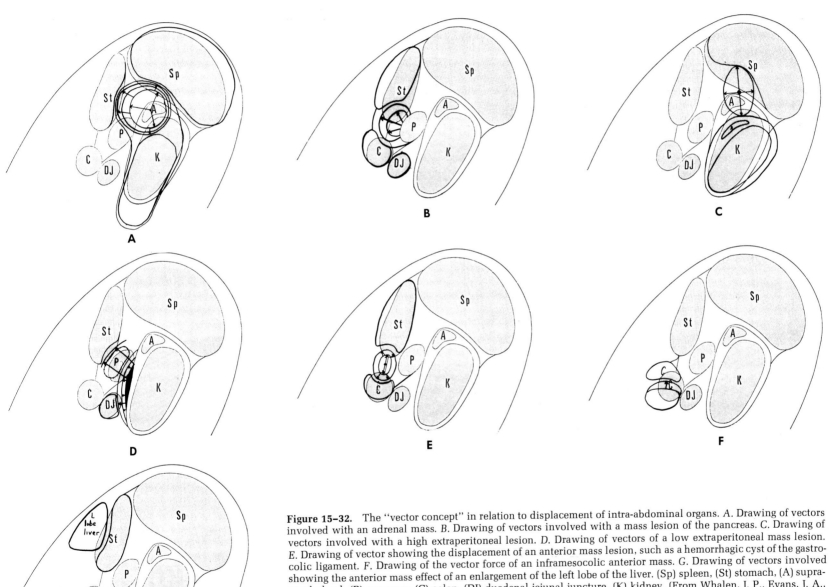

Figure 15–32. The "vector concept" in relation to displacement of intra-abdominal organs. *A*. Drawing of vectors involved with an adrenal mass. *B*. Drawing of vectors involved with a mass lesion of the pancreas. *C*. Drawing of vectors involved with a high extraperitoneal lesion. *D*. Drawing of vectors of a low extraperitoneal mass lesion. *E*. Drawing of vector showing the displacement of an anterior mass lesion, such as a hemorrhagic cyst of the gastrocolic ligament. *F*. Drawing of the vector force of an inframesocolic anterior mass. *G*. Drawing of vectors involved showing the anterior mass effect of an enlargement of the left lobe of the liver. (Sp) spleen, (St) stomach, (A) suprarenal gland, (P) pancreas, (C) colon, (DJ) duodenal-jejunal juncture, (K) kidney. (From Whalen, J. P., Evans, J. A., and Shanser, J.: Amer. J. Roentgenol., 113:104, 1971.)

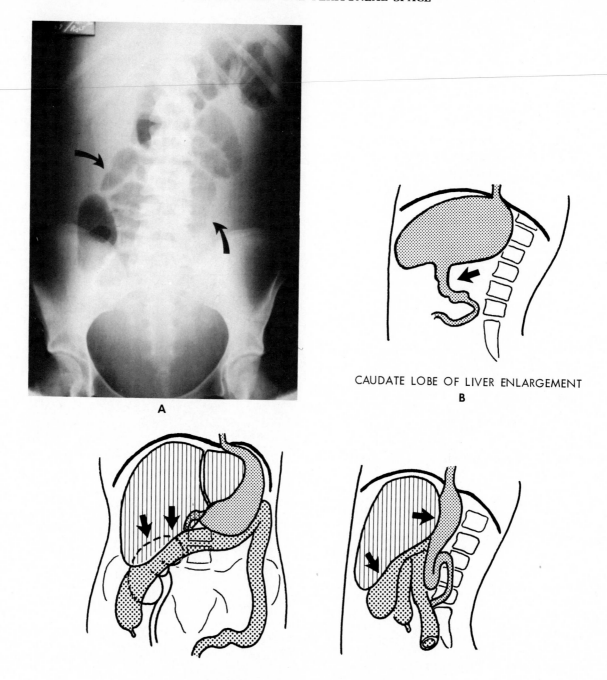

A

CAUDATE LOBE OF LIVER ENLARGEMENT
B

RIGHT LOBE OF LIVER ENLARGEMENT

DISPLACEMENT OF STOMACH TO LEFT AND POSTERIORLY
DOWNWARD DISPLACEMENT OF RIGHT KIDNEY
NO DISPLACEMENT OF SECOND PART OF DUODENUM
DOWNWARD DISPLACEMENT OF TRANSVERSE COLON
DOWNWARD AND POSTERIOR DISPLACEMENT OF HEPATIC FLEXURE
NO DISPLACEMENT OF DUODENOJEJUNAL FLEXURE

B

Figure 15–33.   A. Anteroposterior view of the abdomen: hepatoma with ascites and floating loops of bowel. B. Diagrams showing changes with enlargement of the right lobe and caudate lobe of the liver.

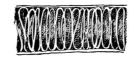 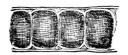 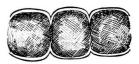

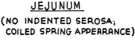

Figure 15–34. Schematic illustration of distended bowel, showing differences between jejunum, ileum, and colon.

possibly impress or elevate the spleen. The splenic artery may be elevated on arteriography but the renal artery may or may not be depressed.

3. *Pancreatic masses* are more anterior than renal or adrenal masses, and they do not usually separate the kidney and spleen unless there is an unusually large pseudocyst or cyst of the pancreas. The duodenojejunal junction is depressed and the stomach is elevated. The splenic artery is not elevated but flattened.

4. *Renal enlargements* produce a variable appearance depending upon the portion of the kidney from which enlargement arises.

5. *Extraperitoneal mass lesions* that are high in the left abdomen simulate adrenal tumors but not as predictably. The kidney is often displaced laterally or downward, and the spleen and kidney may be separated by an inordinate distance.

6. *Low extraperitoneal masses* may simulate superficially pancreatic masses. The stomach is pushed forward and the duodenum is displaced forward, but the duodenojejunal junction may not be depressed.

7. *Mass lesions arising in the gastrocolic ligament* displace the stomach upward and the colon downward without displacement of any posterior structures such as the kidney.

8. *Masses arising in the intraperitoneal cavity* that are *inframesocolic* and tend to elevate the colon, are often near the midline and displace only anterior structures.

9. The *left lobe of the liver* is the most anterior structure in the abdomen. It displaces the stomach posteriorly or downward when enlarged; occasionally the colon will also be displaced downward and posteriorly as well.

10. *Generally, the properitoneal fat or extraperitoneal fat layer defines posterior structures better than the anterior structures;* thus, the suprarenal portion of the spleen, the adrenal, renal, and some extraperitoneal mass lesions are better defined than those that are anteriorly situated.

11. Similarly, Figure 15–33 demonstrates what might occur *when the right lobe of the liver enlarges.* Usually the stomach is displaced to the left and posteriorly, and the hepatic flexure is displaced downward. With caudate lobe of liver enlargement, the pyloric antrum and adjoining duodenal bulb are displaced anteriorly.

There are many other indicators that are outside the scope of this text. These few, however, emphasize the importance of a careful knowledge of the anatomy of the abdomen for radiologic interpretation.

Gas Patterns of the Abdomen. Normally, except in the very young and the very old, gas is not contained in the small intestines. However, it can readily be visualized in the region of the stomach and colon. Often intermixed with the gas shadows in the colon are shadows representing fecal material. In the newborn, gas is ordinarily visualized throughout the gastrointestinal tract by at least 24 hours after birth, but early in the newborn period

such is not the case. The schematic illustrations applying to barium-containing loops of bowel (Chapters 13 and 14) also apply to loops containing only gas. Thus, the valvulae conniventes impart a spiral appearance to the gas shadows of the jejunum, and the spiral loops tend to be close to one another high in the small intestine. In the ileum, however, the valvulae are more widely separated, but can be differentiated from the haustrations of the colon because of the lack of indented serosa at these sites (Fig. 15–34). The gas pattern of the stomach follows closely that pattern that might be expected from our previous descriptions of the barium-filled stomach (Fig. 15–35). Mass lesions impressing themselves on the gas-filled stomach may produce outright roentgen evidence of abnormality resembling the barium-filled stomach (Fig. 15–36).

Abnormal gas patterns in the abdomen are an important indicator of disease, either when they are found outside the usual distribution in the gastrointestinal tract (Fig. 15–37, for example), or when they are so bizarre that they suggest some other pathologic process (Fig. 15–38).

CHANGES IN APPEARANCE OF GAS-CONTAINING STOMACH

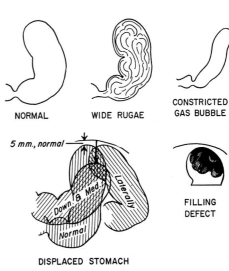

Figure 15–35.

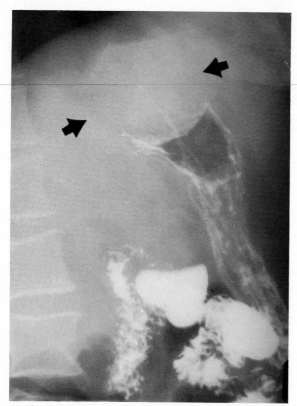

Figure 15–36. Carcinoma of the liver displacing the fundus of the stomach downward from the left hemidiaphragm. This carcinomatous involvement of the liver was thought to be secondary to a carcinoma of the pancreas.

Abnormal gas patterns in the abdomen are of course outside the scope of the present text but are shown here as examples of this important appearance.

Erect or Lateral Decubitus Films for Study of Gas Patterns (horizontal x-ray beam study).   As will be shown in our description of films obtained in study of the abdomen, a horizontal x-ray beam is employed with the patient either erect or lying on one side or the other (lateral decubitus) to allow gas to rise to the uppermost level and fluid to gravitate to a lower level, thus frequently giving better definition of (1) free air in the abdominal cavity, or (2) gas-to-fluid interfaces. Moreover, unusual mobility is an indication at times of abnormality, and fixation may likewise indicate the presence of an inflammatory or neoplastic process.

For example, gas bubbles contained in an abscess will move very little when the patient moves, and thus can be differentiated from gas intermixed with feces which will tend to gravitate dependently. When air has escaped into the peritoneal space, it will rise to the highest possible level, and unless there are adhesions preventing such a rise, this gas will accumulate under the diaphragm in relation to its point of origin as described in previous sections (Fig. 15–39). In the upright film, the soft tissue

structures of the pelvis minor are less clearly defined, and, in general, structural detail is less distinct than in the recumbent film.

However, in the recumbent film, a large fluid-containing mass with only a very small amount of gas may not be indicated at all because its water density blends with adjoining structures. In the erect position, the fluid level is an important indicator of this mass lesion. A comparison of these appearances is shown in Figure 15–40.

At times gas can be demonstrated in the cecum and ascending colon in an abnormal position in the abdominal cavity, providing an important clue to an abnormality in rotation of the gastrointestinal tract. When the midgut is first withdrawn into the abdominal cavity from the umbilical cord, it occupies a position in the left half of the abdomen with the cecum and ascending colon in the left lower quadrant. Normally, the cecum and ascending colon gradually ascend toward the right to their final position (Fig. 15–41). In a child abnormality of gastrointestinal rotation is a particularly important finding since it may be associated with intermittent or markedly debilitating episodes of intestinal obstruction. Even in the adult it may be an important indicator of such pathology. (The barium-filled gastrointestinal tract is shown in Figure 15–41.)

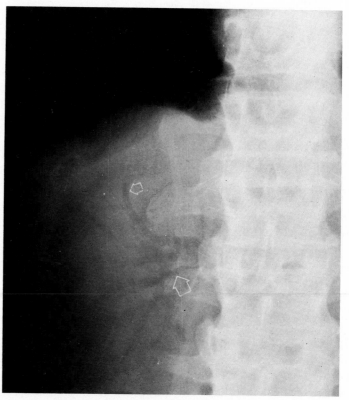

Figure 15–37. Free air in the biliary tract resulting from a surgical communication produced between the gallbladder and the duodenum.

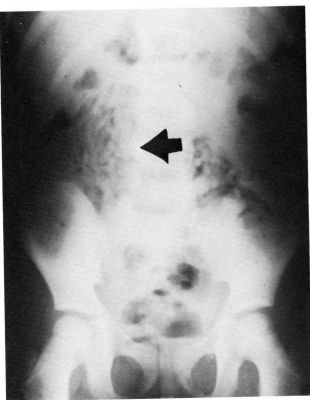

Figure 15–38. Anteroposterior view of the abdomen demonstrating the coiled gas appearance of worm infestation in the gastrointestinal tract.

Prone Position in Study of Gas Patterns. The prone position, particularly in a child, may at times be more advantageous for diagnostic purposes than the supine (Berdon et al.). Marked gaseous distention of the small intestine is frequent in infants due to air swallowing. The prone position may result in markedly improved visualization of the small intestine and the retroperitoneal structures such as the kidneys. In the supine position, sometimes a fluid-filled fundus of the stomach has the appearance of a left suprarenal mass. Likewise, in an infant, the duodenal bulb, when full of fluid, may simulate a mass. When the infant is prone, on the other hand, gastric air fills the fundus (Fig. 15–42) and other posterior loops of alimentary tract, and the central abdomen appears relatively free of gas. The kidneys and adrenal areas may be better seen.

The Psoas Shadows. The fatty tissue contained in the capsule of the iliac and psoas muscles as well as in the region of the obturator fascia permits an accurate delineation of these retroperitoneal structures in most instances (Fig. 15–43). The quadratus lumborum muscle is usually also visible. The aortic shadow, in an adjoining retroperitoneal location, is ordinarily not seen unless it is aneurysmal or contains abnormal calcium deposits from atherosclerosis. Identification of these fascial planes is particularly significant in determination of certain types of retroperitoneal mass lesions such as hemorrhage, inflammation, neoplasm, and aneurysm.

Obliteration of the psoas shadow is likewise important. When the fascial envelope of the psoas muscle is infiltrated by an

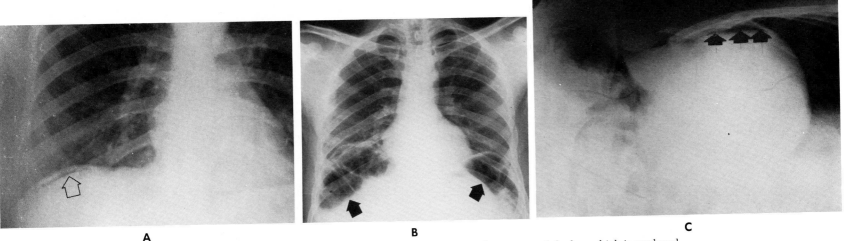

A   B   C

Figure 15–39. A. PA film of the chest indicating the rather typical semilunate type of shadow which is produced under the right hemidiaphragm by free air under the diaphragm. B. PA film of the chest demonstrating the appearance of interposition of colon under the right hemidiaphragm. This appearance must not be confused with free air under the diaphragm and can usually be distinguished by the appearance of haustrations within the gas pattern. C. Free air on the lateral decubitus film study. The free air is above the liver and beneath the right hemidiaphragm.

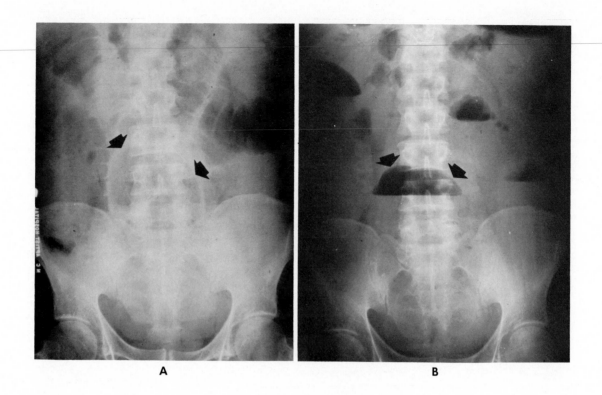

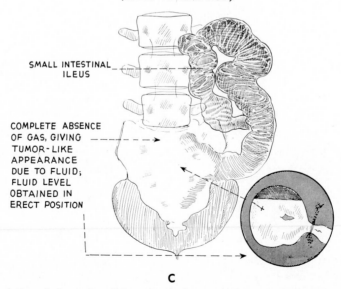

STRANGULATION
(SUPINE APPEARANCE)

SMALL INTESTINAL
ILEUS

COMPLETE ABSENCE
OF GAS, GIVING
TUMOR-LIKE
APPEARANCE
DUE TO FLUID;
FLUID LEVEL
OBTAINED IN
ERECT POSITION

C

Figure 15–40. Strangulation of a loop of small intestine producing mechanical obstruction. The strangulation was due to internal herniation. *A*. Supine study. *B*. Erect study. *C*. Line tracing. Note the complete absence of gas in the pelvis minor (pseudotumor appearance). The gas in the strangulated bowel is best seen in the erect position.

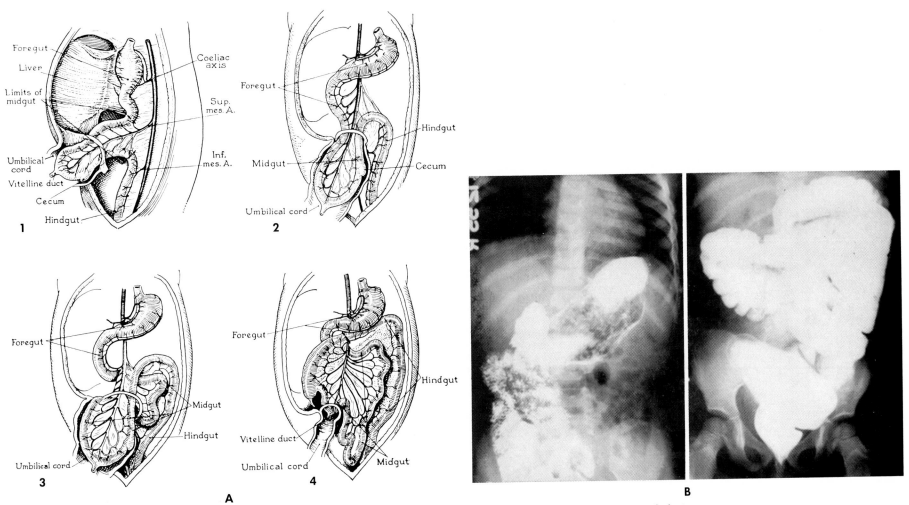

Figure 15–41   *A. 1 to 4.* Normal fetal rotation of the gastrointestinal tract. (Modified from Golden: Radiologic Examination of the Small Intestine; *in* Caffey, J.: Pediatric X-ray Diagnosis, 4th ed. Chicago, Year Book Medical Publishers, 1961.) *B.* Barium-filled gastrointestinal tract demonstrating nonrotation of the small intestine and colon.

inflammatory or neoplastic process, the normal psoas stripe may be obscured. This sign, of course, must be interpreted with caution since overlying gas or intestinal content may give the false impression of such obliteration. A diagram and radiograph illustrating the normal and abnormal obturator fascial planes are shown in Figure 15–43.

Hernia.   Hernia may be defined as "the protrusion of any organ or part of an organ from its normal enclosure." Abdominal hernias are quite frequent, and although they are in the realm of the pathological, a brief word about their roentgen anatomy is in order here.

Abdominal hernias may involve any of the abdominal viscera and any of the actual or potential foramina surrounding the general peritoneal cavity. Internal hernias are formed by protrusion

of the gut, usually into certain peritoneal fossae within the abdominal cavities. Usually this is related to a faulty fixation of the mesentery. Thus, there may be a hernia of intestine through the epiploic foramen into the omental bursa. Retroperitoneal hernia may occur at the site of the inferior duodenal recess, and intersigmoid hernia may protrude through the sigmoid mesocolon. Likewise, hernia may occur between unfused components of the transverse mesocolon as well as in the retrocecal or retrocolic region. The incidence of internal herniation as given by Hansmann and Morton is: paraduodenal fossae, 53 per cent; pericecal, 13 per cent; transverse mesocolon, 8 per cent; epiploic foramen into omental bursa, 8 per cent.

The most usual presentation of internal hernias is that of partial or complete obstruction of the small intestine, although

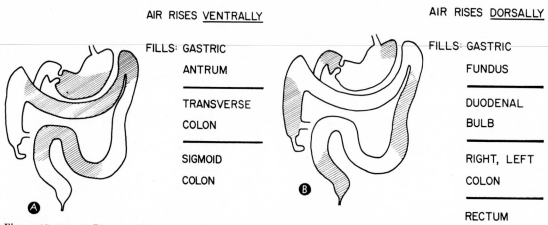

SUPINE

PRONE

AIR RISES <u>VENTRALLY</u>

AIR RISES <u>DORSALLY</u>

FILLS: GASTRIC
ANTRUM

TRANSVERSE
COLON

SIGMOID
COLON

FILLS: GASTRIC
FUNDUS

DUODENAL
BULB

RIGHT, LEFT
COLON

RECTUM

Figure 15–42. *A.* Diagram of supine abdomen showing localization of air. Note obscuration of renal areas leading to confusion of the transverse and sigmoid colon with the small bowel. *B.* Diagram of prone abdomen showing shift of air with resultant clearing of the renal areas, and improved separation of the colon gas from the small bowel gas. (From Bendon, W. B., Baker, D. H., and Leonidas, J.: Amer. J. Roentgenol., *103*:444, 1968.)

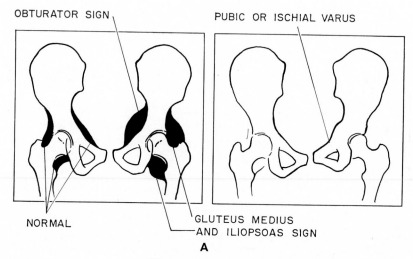

OBTURATOR SIGN

PUBIC OR ISCHIAL VARUS

NORMAL

GLUTEUS MEDIUS
AND ILIOPSOAS SIGN

A

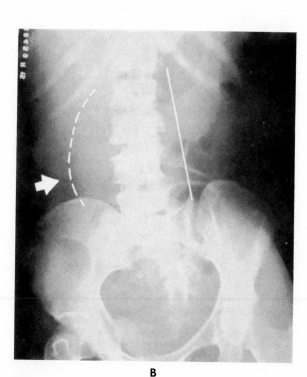

B

Figure 15–43. *A.* Diagram illustrating the normal and abnormal obturator and iliopsoas fascial planes of the pelvis and hips. *B.* Radiograph demonstrating the appearance of the widened psoas shadow resulting from a large retroperitoneal abscess. Note the loss of detail in the flank shadow region. (Lines added to show psoas margins.)

the patient may be asymptomatic and diagnosed incidentally during the evaluation of other abdominal symptoms. With a right paraduodenal hernia, almost all of the small intestine is imprisoned in a peritoneal sac behind the ascending and transverse colon, occupying the right half of the abdomen and opening just to the left and near the duodenojejunal junction at the ligament of Treitz. A left paraduodenal hernia occurs on the left side of the abdomen in the mesentery of the transverse descending and sigmoid colon, with the mouth of the sac opening to the right. The left paraduodenal hernia occurs much more frequently than the right in the ratio of approximately 3 to 1. Paraduodenal hernias, in most series, account for more than half of internal hernias.

External hernias are protrusions through gaps or weaknesses in the muscular wall, usually covered by parietal peritoneum. Thus, hernia may occur externally through the diaphragm into the chest, through the lumbar triangle, the greater sciatic foramen, the perineum in the pelvic diaphragm, the obturator foramen, the umbilicus, the inguinal canal, the femoral canal, and ventrally, through surgical defects or through the linea alba above the umbilicus. Of these, the inguinal, femoral, diaphragmatic, and umbilical hernias are the most frequent types.

The Kidneys, Ureters, or Urinary Bladder Without Adequate Contrast. On the plain film, the kidneys are studied from the standpoint of size, position, radiodensity, contour, architecture of the renal fascia, and the presence or absence of calcific shadows. The normal features of these aspects of the kidney as well as the special identification of collecting structures following the introduction of contrast media are postponed for a full description to Chapter 16 (Fig. 15–44).

BLOOD SUPPLY OF THE ABDOMEN

The Abdominal Aorta. The abdominal aorta has been shown in cross section at various levels in Figure 15–4. Its main branches have been described in Chapters 13 and 14. The longi-

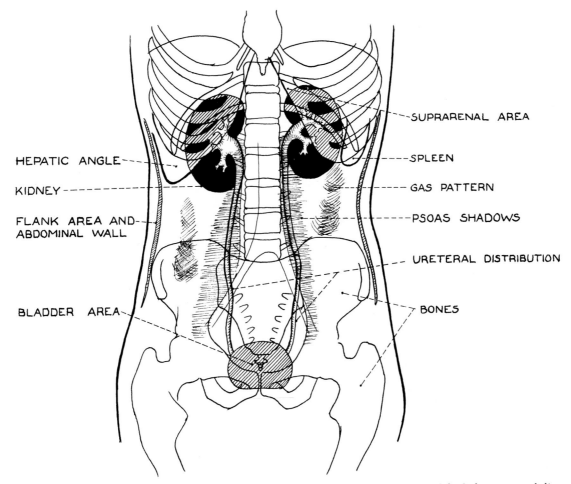

Figure 15–44. Areas where roentgen abnormalities may be visualized on plain films of the kidney, ureteral distribution, and bladder region, apart from calcification (shown later).

tudinal appearance of the abdominal aorta and its primary proximal branches are shown in Figure 15–45. Since the branches have already been described in considerable detail, Table 15–1 is included here as a summary of the arterial supply of the abdomen. The abdominal aorta begins at the aortic hiatus of the diaphragm, usually at the lower level of the twelfth thoracic vertebra, and extends caudad just to the left of the midline. It ends opposite the L4 vertebra by dividing into right and left common iliac arteries. At its origin the aorta is approximately 20 mm. in diameter; just below the renal arteries it is 16.5 mm. in diameter; and at its termination opposite the L4 vertebral body it reduces slightly to 15.9 mm. On its right aspect lies the inferior vena cava, which is ventral to it at the level of L1 and dorsal to it at L4. The aorta is retroperitoneal throughout.

Throughout its length it lies on the anterior longitudinal liga-

ment of the lumbar spine, L1 to L4. The lumbar segmental arteries and the middle sacral artery are all dorsal to the aorta. There are numerous para-aortic lymph nodes along its entire length (the lymphatics will be described more fully later).

The branches of the aorta are shown in Table 15–1 and usually occur in the following descending order: right and left inferior phrenic, celiac, right and left middle suprarenal, right and left first lumbar, superior mesenteric, right and left renal, right and left testicular or ovarian, right and left second lumbar, inferior mesenteric, right and left third lumbar, right and left fourth lumbar, median sacral, and right and left common iliac.

Measurements of the abdominal aorta in the living obtained during the course of intravenous aortography in adults are shown in Table 15–2. In this table, the degree of magnification is not clearly described, and it is suggested that body surface area deter-

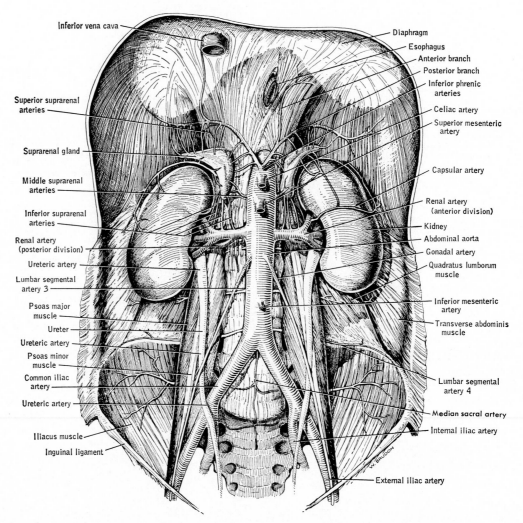

Figure 15–45. Abdominal aorta and its branches. (From Anson, B. J. (ed.): Morris' Human Anatomy, 12th ed. Copyright © 1966 by McGraw-Hill, Inc. Used by permission of McGraw-Hill Book Company.)

TABLE 15–1   ARTERIAL SUPPLY OF THE ABDOMEN*

Distribution	Artery	Origin	Distribution	Artery	Origin
Phrenic Artery, Right and Left			Spleen, pancreas, stomach, greater omentum	Splenic	Celiac
Right crus of diaphragm, central tendon of diaphragm	Inferior phrenic (right and left)	Abdominal	Left portion, greater curvature of stomach	Short gastric	Splenic
Anastomoses with left phrenic, internal mammary and pericardiophrenic arteries	Anterior branch (right and left)	Phrenic	*Superior Mesenteric Artery*		
Anastomoses with intercostals	Posterior branch (right and left)	Phrenic	Pancreas, duodenum	Inferior pancreaticoduodenal	Superior mesenteric
Suprarenal gland, branches to vena cava, liver and pericardium	Superior suprarenal (right and left)	Phrenic	Ileum, jejunum	Intestinal	Superior mesenteric
			Transverse colon	Middle colic	Superior mesenteric
			Ascending colon	Right colic	Superior mesenteric
Suprarenal Arteries, Right and Left			Cecum, appendix, ascending colon	Ileocolic	Superior mesenteric
Suprarenal gland (right and left)	Middle suprarenal (right and left)	Aorta	Mesentery of vermiform appendix	Appendicular	Ileocolic
Lumbar Arteries, I, II, III, IV			*Renal Arteries, Right and Left*		
Bodies of vertebrae and ligaments	Vertebral	Lumbar	Kidney	Renal	Abdominal aorta
Psoas, quadratus lumborum, oblique muscles of abdomen	Muscular	Lumbar	Suprarenal gland	Inferior suprarenal	Renal
			Kidney capsule and perirenal fat	Capsular	Renal
Longissimus dorsi and multifidus spinae	Dorsal	Lumbar	Upper end of ureter	Ureteral	Renal
			Kidney	Terminal branches	Renal
Multifidus	Lateral branch	Dorsal			
Sacrospinalis	Medial branch	Dorsal	*Internal Spermatic and Ovarian Arteries*		
Vertebral canal	Spinal	Dorsal	Testis	Internal spermatic	Abdominal aorta
			Ureter, adjacent retroperitoneal tissue	Ureteral	Internal spermatic
Celiac Axis			Cremaster muscle	Cremasteric	Internal spermatic
Esophagus, lesser curvature of stomach	Left gastric	Celiac	Epididymis	Epididymal	Internal spermatic
Anastomoses with branches from thoracic aorta	Esophageal branches	Left gastric	Terminal branches to testis	Testicular	Internal spermatic
Stomach, greater omentum	Left gastroepiploic	Splenic	Ovary, ureter, uterus, tubes	Ovarian	Abdominal aorta
Pancreas	Pancreatic	Splenic	*Inferior Mesenteric Artery*		
Stomach, pancreas, liver, duodenum	Common hepatic	Celiac	Lower half of descending colon, sigmoid, rectum	Inferior mesenteric	Abdominal aorta
Lesser curvature of stomach	Right gastric	Hepatic	Descending colon	Left colic	Inferior mesenteric
Right lobe of liver	Right hepatic	Hepatic proper	Sigmoid flexure of colon	Sigmoid	Inferior mesenteric
Left lobe of liver	Left hepatic	Hepatic proper	Upper part of rectum	Superior hemorrhoidal	Inferior mesenteric
Gallbladder, undersurface of liver	Cystic	Hepatic proper			
Stomach, duodenum, pancreas	Right gastroepiploic	Gastroduodenal			

*From Bierman, H. C.: Selective Arterial Catheterization. Springfield, Ill., Charles C Thomas, 1969. Table 11.1.

TABLE 15–2   AVERAGE AGE AND DIAMETER IN MM. OF ABDOMINAL AORTA AT SITES MEASURED*

Sex	No. of Cases	Age	At 11th Rib	Above Renal Arteries	Below Renal Arteries	At Bifurcation of Aorta	Difference between 11th Rib and Bifurcation of Aorta
Male	29	53.9 ± 13.7	26.9 ± 3.96	23.9 ± 3.92	21.4 ± 3.65	18.7 ± 3.34	8.14 ± 2.14
Female	44	56.9 ± 14.3	24.4 ± 3.45	21.6 ± 3.16	18.7 ± 3.96	17.5 ± 2.52	6.80 ± 4.54

*From Steinberg, C. R., Archer, M., and Steinberg, I.: Measurement of the abdominal aorta after intravenous aortography in health and arteriosclerotic peripheral vascular disease. Amer. J. Roentgenol., *95*:703, 1965.

Element of magnification not indicated. Target-film distance is 48 inches.

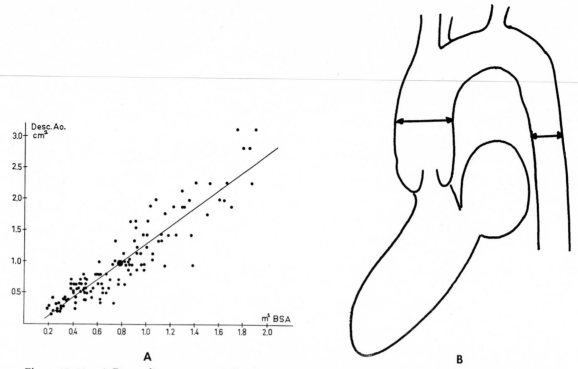

Figure 15–46. *A.* Descending aorta in cm² plotted against body surface area in m². All diagnostic groups are plotted together since no statistical difference between the groups was found in the co-variance analysis. *B.* Schematic drawing of lateral angiocardiogram. The points of measurements for the ascending and descending aorta are marked by horizontal lines. All measurements were performed on films exposed in systole. (From Arvidsson, H.: Acta Radiol. (Diag.), 1:981–994, 1963.)

minations are not significant. The average of the abdominal aorta was larger for men than for women in this study (Steinberg et al.). For comparison, the measurements of the descending thoracic aorta recorded by Arvidsson are shown in Figure 15–46. Here, the measurements in square centimeters are plotted against body surface area in square meters, resulting in virtually a straight line regression. Thus, a measurement of the descending thoracic aorta of approximately 2.25 sq. cm. is indicated for an average body surface area of 1.7 sq. meters. (It should be noted that this measurement is in square centimeters, in contrast to the measurements by Steinberg et al. which are in linear millimeters.)

Collateral Circulation of the Abdominal Aorta. There are two general anatomic systems of collateral circulation which develop in response to the gradual occlusion of the abdominal aorta (Bron). These have been designated as collaterals extending between the viscera and systemic circulation as well as from one systemic vessel to another. Schematic illustrations of the more common anastomotic channels are presented in Figure 15–47. The main anastomotic pathway from the viscera to the systemic circulation is a single vessel continuing from the superior mesenteric artery to the internal iliac arteries, via the middle colic artery through the left colic branch of the inferior mesenteric arte-

ry. This vessel passes into the pelvis as the superior hemorrhoidal artery and communicates ultimately with the internal iliac artery.

The anastomotic channels allowing for communication from one systemic branch to another around the aorta are also shown in this figure. This is a rich plexus of vessels involving the flanks, back, and abdominal wall, and consisting of intercostal, lumbar, internal mammary, deep circumflex iliac, and inferior epigastric arteries—all providing blood to the internal and external iliac arteries. In contrast with these vessels are the arterial collaterals (Fig. 15–48 *A, B*) which develop during high and low obstruction of the thoracic aorta (Grupp et al.).

The Inferior Vena Cava. The inferior vena cava has been shown in cross section in Figure 15–4 *A, B,* and *C.* It is formed by the union of the right and left common iliac veins opposite the L5 vertebral body, passing cranially ventral to the lumbar vertebrae to the right of the abdominal aorta through the caval opening in the diaphragm, and ending in the inferior part of the right atrium of the heart usually opposite the T8 vertebra. In the lower abdomen it is slightly dorsal to the aorta but in the upper abdomen it is on a plane ventral to the aorta, separated from it by the right crus of the diaphragm and the caudate lobe of the liver.

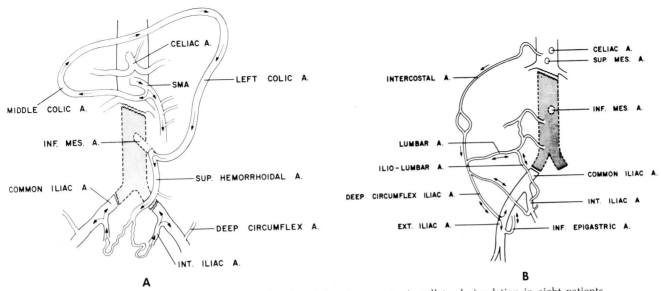

Figure 15–47. A. Composite schematic drawing of the viscerosystemic collateral circulation in eight patients with aortic occlusion at the renal level. The shaded area represents the occluded portion of the aorta. B. Composite schematic drawing of the systemic–systemic collateral pathways in abdominal aortic occlusion. The shaded area represents the occluded portion of the aorta. (From Bron, K. M.: Amer. J. Roentgenol., 96:887–895, 1966.)

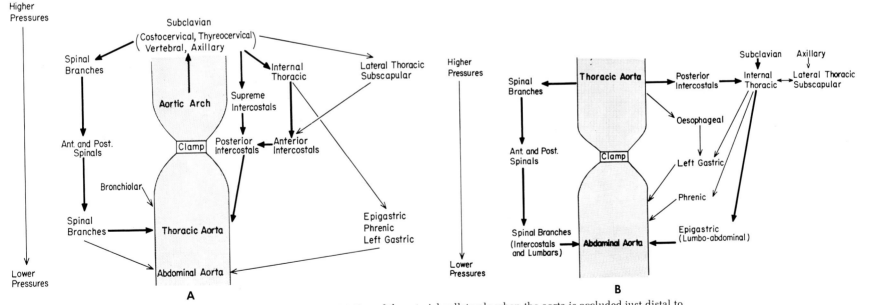

Figure 15–48. A. Diagrammatic representation of the arterial collaterals when the aorta is occluded just distal to the left subclavian artery (high occlusion). Heavy lines indicate the direction of preferred flow. B. Diagrammatic representation of the arterial collaterals when the aorta is occluded between the origin of the 8th and 9th posterior intercostal arteries (low occlusion). Heavy lines indicate the direction of preferred flow. (From Grupp, G., Grupp, I. L., and Spitz, H. B.: Amer. J. Roentgenol., 94:159–171, 1965.)

Lymphatic channels draining the pelvis and abdomen are in close apposition to the inferior vena cava throughout its course in the retroperitoneal space.

Tributaries to the inferior vena cava generally correspond with branches of the abdominal aorta except for those contributing to the portal vein. The following are the main tributaries:

right testicular or ovarian, renal, right suprarenal, inferior phrenic, and hepatic (which indirectly receives blood from the portal vein). It also receives other smaller tributaries.

A schematic representation of the relationships of the inferior vena cava with surrounding anatomic structures in frontal and lateral views is shown in Figure 15–49 *A* and *B*.

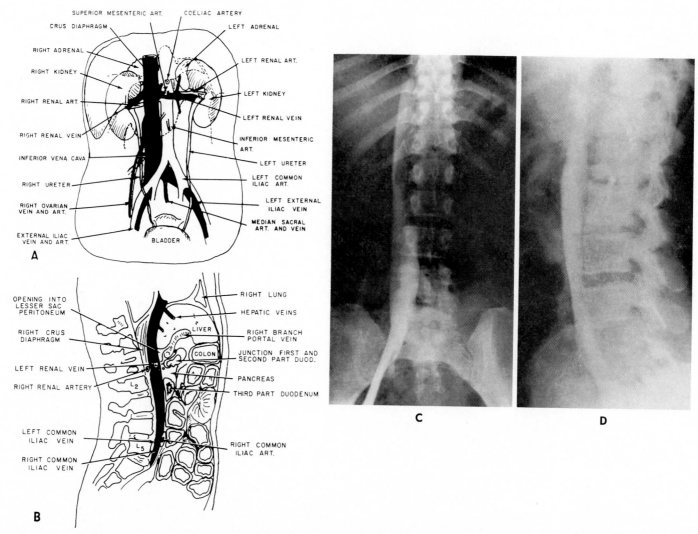

Figure 15–49. Schematic representation of the relationships of the inferior vena cava (shown in black) with the surrounding anatomic structures. *A.* In the anteroposterior view notice the relationships of the vena cava to the course of the external iliac vein and artery, the right ureter, and the relation of the right renal artery, as it crosses from the aorta behind the vena cava, to the right kidney. *B.* In the lateral view the compression of the vena cava by the right renal artery is demonstrated at the level of the interspace between L-1 and L-2. A slight anterior indentation at the lower end of the vena cava caused by anterior compression from the right common iliac artery is also shown. The pancreas and third portion of the duodenum lie just anterior to the vena cava. *C* and *D.* Anteroposterior and lateral inferior vena cavograms in a normal subject. *C.* Note that the course of the right external iliac vessel is smooth and straight and the lateral border of the inferior vena cava in the anteroposterior projection is smoothly outlined. The column of Hypaque shows some dilution from the renal vessels on the left. *D.* In the lateral projection there is a small indentation at the level of the L/1–2 interspace, where the right renal artery indents the vena cava as it crosses from the aorta to enter the right kidney. A slight anterior compression of the upper end of the vena cava is caused by the liver mass. (From Hillman, D. C., Tristan, T. A., and Bronk, A. M.: Radiology, *81:*416, 1963.)

In view of the low pressure and thin wall of the inferior vena cava it is rather readily displaced, distorted, or obstructed by external pressure from adjoining masses. Hence, investigation of the inferior vena cava has a significant place in the diagnostic armamentarium.

The inferior vena cava can be readily examined by means of an injection of approximately 30 cc. of 50 per cent methylglucamine diatrizoate or sodium diatrizoate (Hypaque), manually injected during a 3 second period into a femoral vein, a blood pressure cuff having occluded the opposite femoral vein. The femoral vein may be catheterized, if desired, percutaneously. Alternatively, both femoral veins may be catheterized percutaneously by the Seldinger method and 30 cc. of the contrast agent injected simultaneously through each catheter. The bilateral injection probably gives better results than unilateral injection.

Anteroposterior and lateral views may be obtained simultaneously or in sequence. Six exposures are made, one every three-fourths of a second with a film changer, during which time the patient is directed to suspend breathing and expiration and not to perform a Valsalva maneuver.

The column of contrast medium may appear slightly diluted, particularly opposite the renal region, because blood containing no contrast enters the inferior vena cava at these levels.

These studies are particularly helpful in detecting abnormal mass lesions involving lymph nodes or contiguous organs.

The Inferior Vena Cava After Ligation (Ferris et al.; Grupp et al.). Surgical procedures to obstruct or filter the blood returning to the heart via the inferior vena cava have been utilized to prevent thrombi from moving through the inferior vena cava into the heart in the course of recurrent embolization. The anatomic routes of venous return after occlusion of the inferior vena cava are numerous, and Ferris et al. have divided these into the following groups:

1. CENTRAL CHANNELS (Fig. 15–50 *A*). The central channels consist of the ascending lumbar, internal and external vertebral venous plexuses, hemiazygos-azygos system, and the inferior vena cava above the level of occlusion.

2. INTERMEDIATE CHANNELS. These consist of the ovarian-testicular veins, the ureteric veins, and the left renal–azygos system (Fig. 15–50 *B*). The ureteric veins under these circumstances may attain such a large size that they produce a notching of the ureters radiographically.

3. THE PORTAL SYSTEM (Fig. 15–50 *C*). The portal system fills via the superior hemorrhoidal anastomoses with the middle and inferior hemorrhoidal plexus. Also, abdominal wall veins may communicate with a patent umbilical vein, thus forming another means of filling the portal veins.

4. SUPERFICIAL ROUTES. These are very extensive (Fig. 15–50 *C*) and involve many veins, such as the inferior epigastric draining into the internal mammary; the superficial epigastric and circumflex iliac veins draining into the thoraco-abdominal veins; and the lateral thoracic draining into the axillary veins.

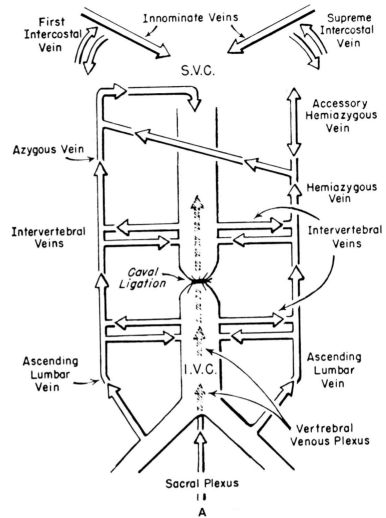

Figure 15–50. A. Central channels. The semidiagrammatic sketch shows the central routes of venous return after caval occlusion. The ascending lumbar veins and the vertebral venous plexus are connected at multiple levels by intervertebral veins. These latter permit flow in either direction. (From Ferris, E. J. et al.: Radiology, 89:1–10, 1967.)

Figure 15–50 continued on the following page.

Another diagrammatic representation of the collaterals between the inferior and superior vena cava is shown in Figure 15–50 *E*.

ABDOMINAL LYMPHATICS

The abdominal lymphatics may be discussed under two main categories: (1) the parietal lymph nodes, and (2) the lymphatic drainage of viscera.

Parietal Lymph Nodes. The parietal lymph nodes are largely divided into two main groups: (1) the *epigastric parietal* lymph nodes, which are situated along the inferior epigastric vessels, and (2) the *lumbar parietal* lymph nodes, which are situated

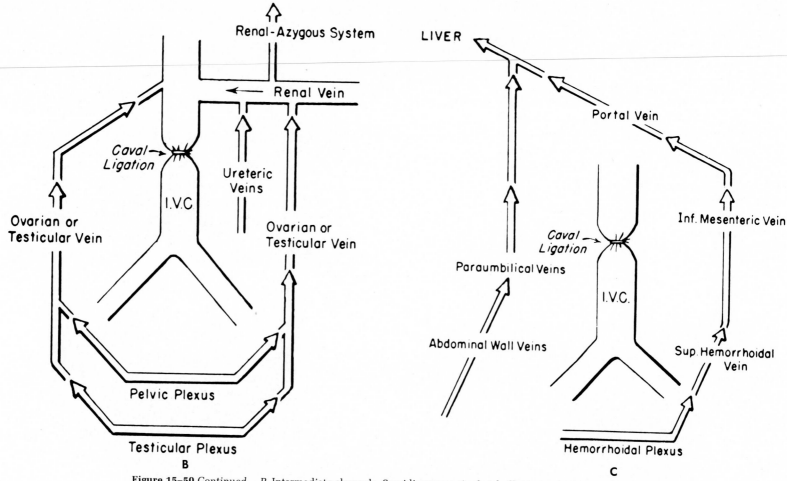

Figure 15–50 *Continued.* B. Intermediate channels. Semidiagrammatic sketch illustrates the intermediate bypass routes of the occluded inferior vena cava. The ovarian or testicular veins usually drain into the renal vein on the left and into the cava on the right. Ureteric veins are included in the intermediate group.

C. Portal route. Semidiagrammatic sketch of the routes of the portal vein filling in obstruction of the inferior vena cava. (From Ferris, E. J. et al.: Radiology, 89:1–10, 1967.)

Figure 15–50 continued on the opposite page.

to the right or left of the aorta, in front of it (preaortic), or behind it (retroaortic). Those to the right of the aorta are generally ventral to the inferior vena cava or dorsal to it, with afferent channels coming from common iliac nodes, gonads, kidneys, and suprarenal and abdominal muscles. Those situated to the left of the aorta are similar to these except that their origins are in the region of the left psoas muscle and left crus of the diaphragm. Those lymph nodes in front of the aorta are mainly clustered around the three major arterial branches: celiac, superior mesenteric, and inferior mesenteric. Those behind the aorta are found largely on the bodies of the third and fourth lumbar vertebrae.

Other groups of lymph nodes of the ilio-pelvic-aortic region are divided as follows: (1) an *external iliac group* situated around the external iliac vessels, (2) a *hypogastric group* near the origin of the different branches of the hypogastric artery in the angles formed by their separation, (3) a *common iliac group* around the common iliac artery, and (4) the *abdominoaortic group* located around the abdominal aorta as described earlier. All of these form the four chains to the right and left, in front of, and behind the aorta (Fig. 15–51).

Lymphatic Drainage of the Pelvic Organs. Figure 15–51 illustrates not only the usual basic anatomy of lymphatics and lymph nodes but also the primary lymphatic drainage of the urinary bladder and testicle. In most instances, the drainage will find its way to the juxta-aortic group. A somewhat similar general pattern of lymphatic drainage exists for the ovary and body of the uterus. The important primary echelon for the pelvic organ is the external iliac, common iliac, and juxta-aortic lymph nodes.

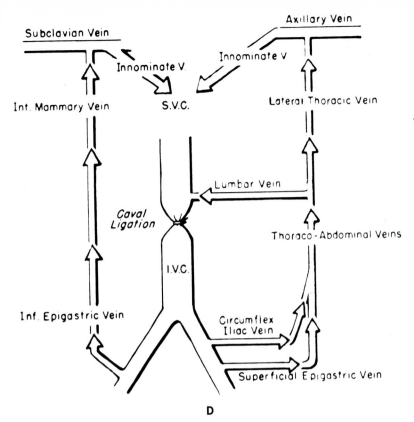

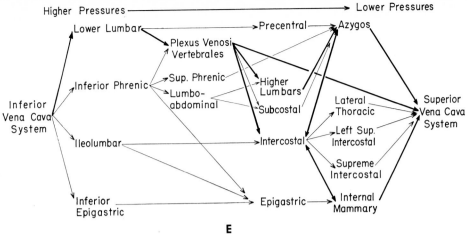

Figure 15–50 *Continued.* *D.* Superficial routes. Semidiagrammatic sketch depicts some of the superficial routes of venous return of the occluded inferior vena cava. (From Ferris, E. J. et al.: Radiology, 89:1–10, 1967.) *E.* Diagrammatic representation of the venous collaterals when the inferior vena cava is occluded just above the diaphragm. Heavy lines indicate the direction of preferred flow. (From Grupp, G., Grupp, I. L., and Spitz, H. B.: Amer. J. Roentgenol., 94:159–171, 1965.)

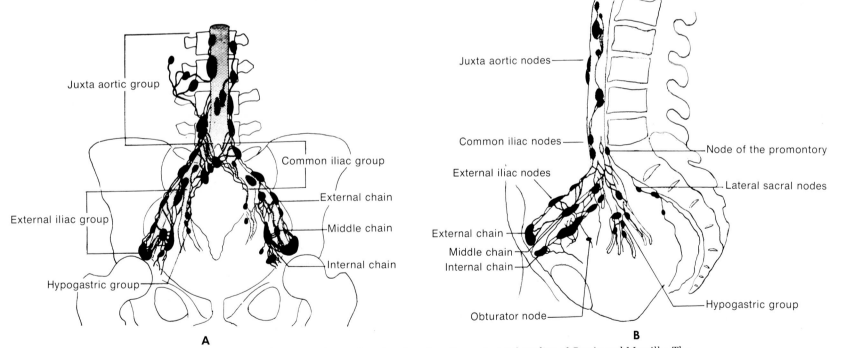

Figure 15–51. *A.* Semidiagrammatic anterior view based on the anatomical studies of Cunéo and Marcille. The three-chain arrangement of the iliac groups is well shown, and the major node groupings are outlined. *B.* Semidiagrammatic lateral view of the right iliopelvic lymphatic system, again showing the three-chain arrangement of the external and common iliac groups. A small satellite node, which is the true anatomical "obturator" node, is designated. (From Herman, P. G., Benninghoff, D. L., Nelson J. H., Jr., and Mellins, H. Z.: Radiology, 80:82–193, 1963.)

Figure 15–51 continued on the following page.

965

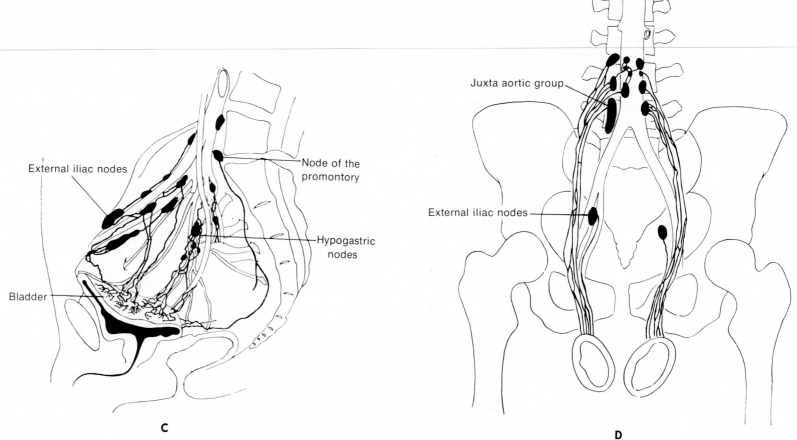

C

D

Figure 15–51 *Continued.*   *C.* Lymphatic drainage of the urinary bladder based on the anatomical studies of Cunéo and Marcille. Note the three lymphatic pedicles leading to the primary echelon of lymphatic drainage of the bladder. The major pedicle leads to the external iliac, while accessory pedicles lead to the common iliac and the hypogastric groups. The same pattern of lymphatic drainage applies to the prostate, rectum, cervix, and the vagina above the hymen. *D.* Lymphatic drainage of the testicle based on the anatomical studies of Rouvière. Note two lymphatic pedicles: a major pedicle leading to the juxta-aortic group and a minor pedicle leading to an external iliac node. (From Herman, P. G., Benninghoff, D. L., Nelson, J. H., Jr., and Mellins, H. Z.: Radiology, *80:*82–193, 1963.)

Figure 15–51 continued on the opposite page.

Generally, the hypogastric nodes are less important in this respect.

The *uterine cervix* has additional clinical significance because the lymphatic drainage is achieved by three main pathways leading to: (1) the *external iliac lymph nodes,* (2) the *hypogastric lymph nodes,* and (3) the *common iliac lymph nodes.* A middle node of the internal chain of the external iliac group has been named by some the *principal node,* and by others the *obturator node* because of its location between the iliac vein and the obturator nerve in the "obturator fossa." This usually adjoins the acetabulum on its inner aspect, or is close to it (Herman et al.).

It is interesting to note that the radiologic demonstration of

lymph nodes corresponds very closely to the classical anatomic descriptions.

Lymphatic Drainage of Viscera (Fig. 15–52). As previously pointed out in the description of the *stomach* (Chapter 14), there are three major zones and flow of the lymphatics in this region: (1) to the superficial gastric lymph nodes, (2) along the inferior gastric, and (3) to the splenic nodes. These in turn drain to the preaortic celiac nodes.

The main drainage of the *liver* is to retrosternal and anterior thoracic nodes, to hepatic nodes, and to preaortic nodes as well as to nodes along the inferior vena cava.

The *pancreas* drains to pancreaticosplenic nodes and from

(Text continued on page 973)

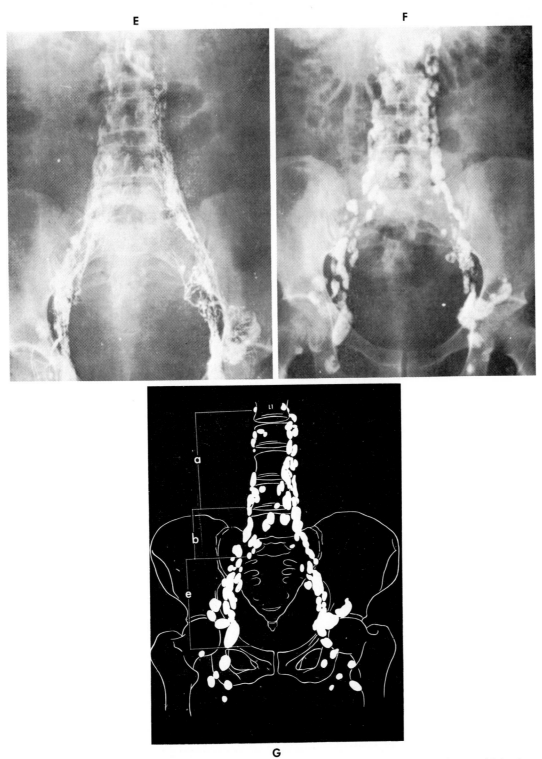

Figure 15–51 *Continued.* E. Anteroposterior roentgenogram made immediately after completion of injection of contrast medium. Lymphatic channels are primarily filled, while the lymph nodes are incompletely opacified.

F. Anteroposterior roentgenogram showing the lymph nodes, taken 24 hours after E. The striking similarity to Fig. 15–51 A is apparent.

G. Tracing of E, illustrating the major node groups. (a) Juxta-aortic, (b) common iliac, (e) external iliac. (From Herman, P. G., Benninghoff, D. L., Nelson, J. H., Jr., and Mellins, H. Z.: Radiology, *80*:82–193, 1963.)

Figure 15–51 continued on the following page.

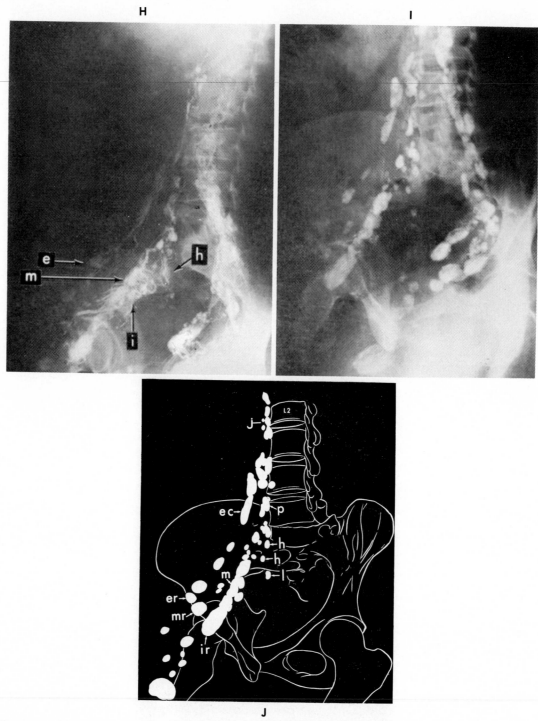

Figure 15–51 *Continued.* *H.* Right posterior oblique roentgenogram made immediately after completion of injection. Lymphatic channels are filled, while the lymph nodes are incompletely opacified. (e) External chain of the external and common iliac groups, (m) middle chain of the external and common iliac groups, (i) internal chain of the external and common iliac groups, (h) channels connecting hypogastric with external and common iliac groups.

I. Right posterior oblique roentgenogram showing lymph nodes as they appeared 24 hours after *H.*

J. Tracing of *I.* (er) External retrocrural node, (mr) middle retrocrural node, (ir) internal retrocrural node, (m) middle node of the internal chain, (l) lateral sacral node of the hypogastric group, (h) hypogastric nodes, (j) juxta-aortic nodes, (p) node of the promontory, (ec) common iliac node. (From Herman, P. G., Benninghoff, D. L., Nelson, J. H., Jr., and Mellins, H. Z.: Radiology, *80*:82–193, 1963.)

Figure 15–51 continued on the opposite page.

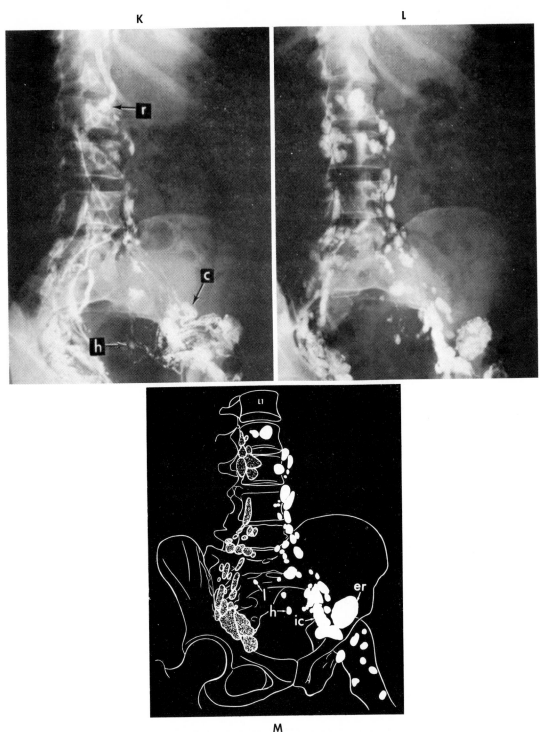

Figure 15–51 *Continued.* K. Left posterior oblique roentgenogram made immediately after completion of injection. Lymphatic channels again dominate the picture, while the nodes are incompletely filled. (h) Hypogastric tributaries connecting with the external and common iliac chains, (c) communications between external and middle chains of the external iliac group, (r) receptaculum chyli.

L. Left posterior oblique roentgenogram showing lymph nodes as they appear 24 hours after K.

M. Tracing of L. (er) External retrocrural node, markedly enlarged. (ic) internal chain, represented by a closely packed group of nodes, (h) hypogastric nodes, (l) lateral sacral nodes of hypogastric group. (From Herman, P. G., Benninghoff, D. L., Nelson, J. H., Jr., and Mellins, H. Z.: Radiology, 80:182–193, 1963.)

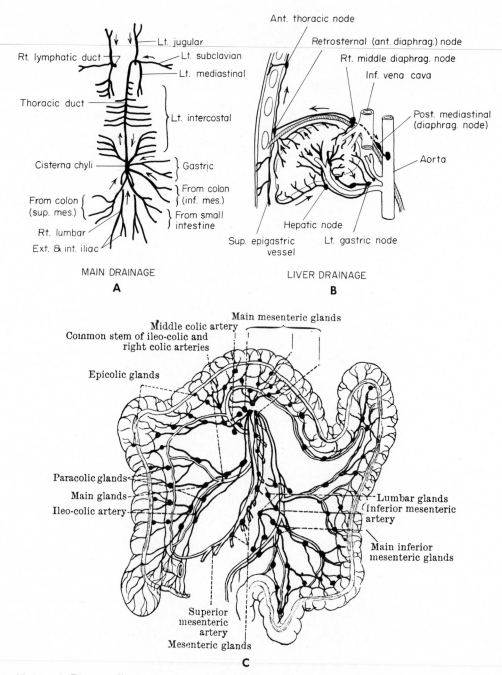

Figure 15–52. *A.* Diagram illustrating the main lymphatic drainage from the lumbar region to the jugular. *B.* Lymphatic drainage of the liver. *C.* Diagram of the lymph glands and lymph vessels of the large intestine. (After Jamieson and Dobson.) (From Cunningham's Textbook of Anatomy, 6th ed. London, Oxford University Press, 1931.)

Figure 15–52 continued on the opposite page.

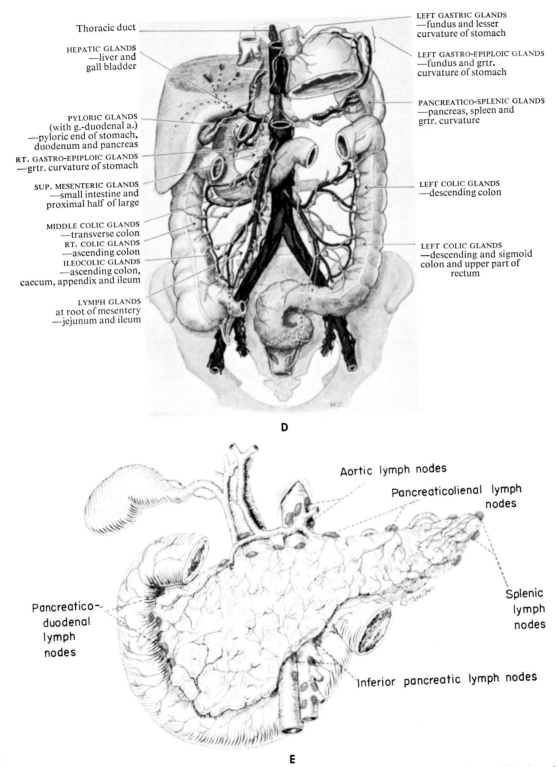

Thoracic duct

HEPATIC GLANDS
—liver and
gall bladder

PYLORIC GLANDS
(with g.-duodenal a.)
—pyloric end of stomach,
duodenum and pancreas

RT. GASTRO-EPIPLOIC GLANDS
—grtr. curvature of stomach

SUP. MESENTERIC GLANDS
—small intestine and
proximal half of large

MIDDLE COLIC GLANDS
—transverse colon
RT. COLIC GLANDS
—ascending colon
ILEOCOLIC GLANDS
—ascending colon,
caecum, appendix and ileum

LYMPH GLANDS
at root of mesentery
—jejunum and ileum

LEFT GASTRIC GLANDS
—fundus and lesser
curvature of stomach

LEFT GASTRO-EPIPLOIC GLANDS
—fundus and grtr.
curvature of stomach

PANCREATICO-SPLENIC GLANDS
—pancreas, spleen and
grtr. curvature

LEFT COLIC GLANDS
—descending colon

LEFT COLIC GLANDS
—descending and sigmoid
colon and upper part of
rectum

D

Aortic lymph nodes

Pancreaticolienal lymph
nodes

Pancreatico-
duodenal
lymph
nodes

Splenic
lymph
nodes

Inferior pancreatic lymph nodes

E

Figure 15–52 *Continued.* D. Abdominal lymph nodes with their main drainage areas. Lumbar and iliac lymph vessels, and nodes, black; portion of aorta removed to show cisterna chyli. (Reprinted by permission of Faber and Faber Ltd. from *Anatomy of the Human Body*, by Lockhart, Hamilton, and Fyfe: Faber & Faber, London, J. B. Lippincott Company, Philadelphia.) E. Lymphatics of pancreas and duodenum. (From Anson, B. J. (ed.): *Morris' Human Anatomy*, 12th ed. Copyright © 1966 by McGraw-Hill, Inc. Used by permission of McGraw-Hill Book Company.)

Figure 15–52 continued on the following page.

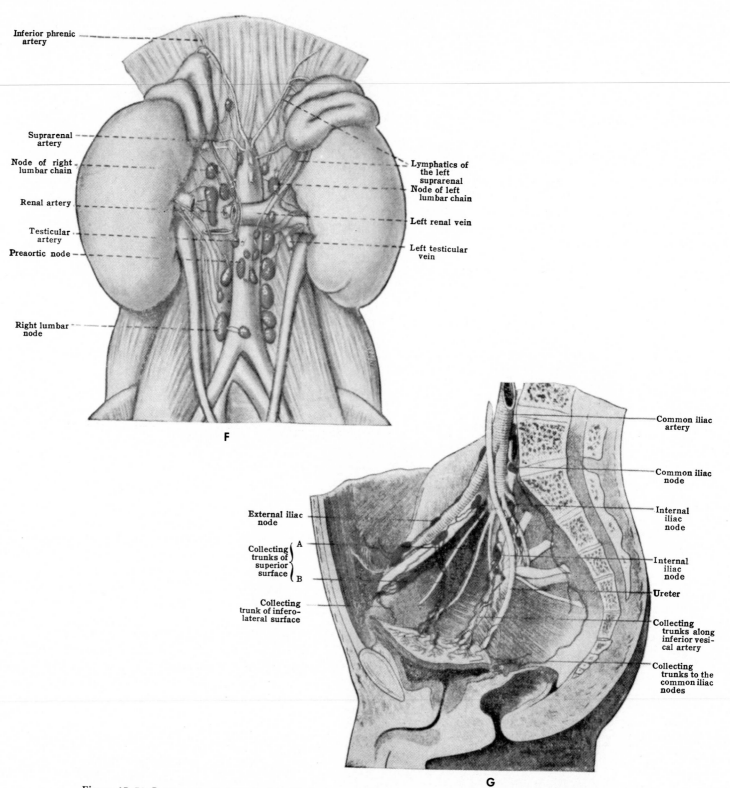

Inferior phrenic
artery

Suprarenal
artery

Node of right
lumbar chain

Renal artery

Testicular
artery

Preaortic node

Right lumbar
node

Lymphatics of
the left
suprarenal
Node of left
lumbar chain

Left renal vein

Left testicular
vein

F

Common iliac
artery

Common iliac
node

Internal
iliac
node

Internal
iliac
node

Ureter

Collecting
trunks along
inferior vesi-
cal artery

Collecting
trunks to the
common iliac
nodes

External iliac
node

Collecting
trunks of
superior
surface

Collecting
trunk of infero-
lateral surface

A

B

G

Figure 15–52 *Continued. F.* Lymphatics of kidneys and suprarenal glands. (After Poirier and Cunéo.) *G.* Lymphatics of bladder. (After Cunéo and Marcille.) (From Anson, B. J. (ed.): Morris' Human Anatomy, 12th ed. Copyright © 1966 by McGraw-Hill, Inc. Used by permission of McGraw-Hill Book Company.)

Figure 15–52 continued on the opposite page.

there to celiac nodes of the preaortic group, to pancreaticoduodenal nodes, and to superior mesenteric nodes in the preaortic group.

The lymphatics of the *small intestine* are the lacteal to mesenteric nodes in the mesentery; from these lymph flows on to the superior mesenteric group of preaortic nodes.

The *colon* has a lymphatic drainage corresponding closely to its blood supply, with the ascending and transverse colon draining to the superior mesenteric group of preaortic lymph nodes, and the descending and sigmoid colon draining ultimately to the inferior mesenteric group of preaortic lymph nodes.

The *cisterna chyli* is located in front of the second lumbar vertebra behind and to the right of the aorta, just beside the right crus of the diaphragm. It is formed by the right and left lumbar trunks and intestinal trunk. At its termination it narrows down and passes through the aortic hiatus of the diaphragm to become the *thoracic duct* (see Chapter 12).

Diagnostic Criteria for Normal Lymph Nodes

Architecture of Nodes. Lymph nodes generally have a very fine reticular internal architecture. They should normally have no significant filling defects. In the presence of some of the lymphomas (malignant lymphosarcomas), a lymph node often will take on a marked foaminess in its architecture—this must be regarded as abnormal. Moreover, the replacement of more than one-third of a lymph node by a filling defect is an indicator of abnormality.

Lymphatic Channels. The persistence of multiple channels on the 24 hour film is an indicator of lymphatic obstruction. Moreover, excessive filling of channels is sometimes an indicator of partial obstruction.

Measurements. Abrams has advocated three measurements to aid diagnosis of normal lymph nodes (Fig. 15–53). The right lateral spine-to-node distance (measurement B) is the measurement from the right lateral border of a lumbar vertebral body at its midpoint to the most lateral border of the right juxtacaval node group. Measurement C is the left lateral spine-to-node distance similarly obtained. Measurement A is obtained from the lateral view and represents the distance to the most anterior margin of the lymph node chain from the twelfth to the second lumbar vertebrae.

Single lymph nodes were also measured for size, care being taken not to measure clusters but rather isolated nodes. These measurements, as recommended by Abrams, are shown in Table 15–3. The 95 per cent confidence limit for the maximum size of a lymph node is shown to be 2.7 cm.; for measurement A it is 3.2 cm.; for measurement B it is 1.8 cm.; and for measurement C it is 2 cm. Abrams has proposed a maximum normal measurement for lymph node size of 2.6 cm.; a maximum for A of 3 cm.; for B of 2 cm.; and for C of 2 cm. These measurements are based upon 60 normal and 60 abnormal cases.

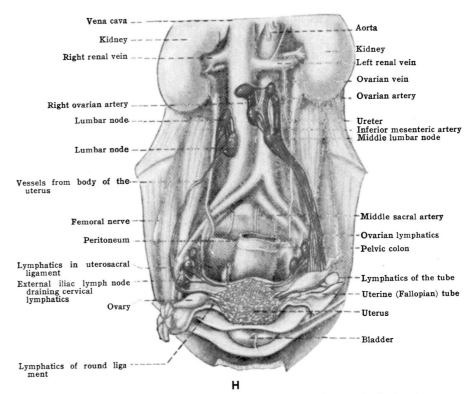

Figure 15–52 *Continued.* H. Lymphatics of internal genital organs in the female. (After Poirier.) (From Anson, B. J. (ed.): Morris' Human Anatomy, 12th ed. Copyright © 1966 by McGraw-Hill, Inc. Used by permission of McGraw-Hill Book Company.)

Lymphographic Technique. This technique has been previously described in Chapter 5. A superficial lymphatic vessel on the medial aspect of the dorsum of the foot is cannulated and the contrast material, usually Ethiodol, is slowly injected over a period of approximately 2 hours. (Ethiodol is the ethyl ester of poppyseed oil and contains approximately 37 per cent iodine.) Usually 5 cc. (but as much as 10 cc. can be used on occasion) is injected on each side by a special pumping device.

Generally, 6 to 24 hours after the injection, the Ethiodol concentrates in the lymph nodes, and disappears from the lymphatic channels proper. The lymph nodes retain the contrast material for several months.

Roentgenograms are taken immediately after the injection and then 24 and 48 hours later. The roentgenograms obtained are the anteroposterior, oblique, and lateral projections as well as a posteroanterior view of the chest. At times, at the 24 or 48 hour period it may be desirable to combine this study with intravenous pyelograms. Pelvic arteriograms or venograms may be obtained following the lymphograms for better topographic evaluation.

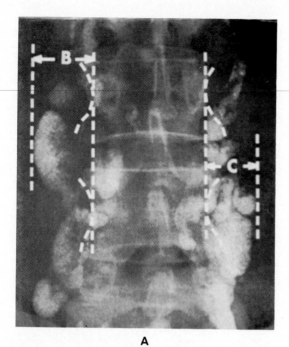

A

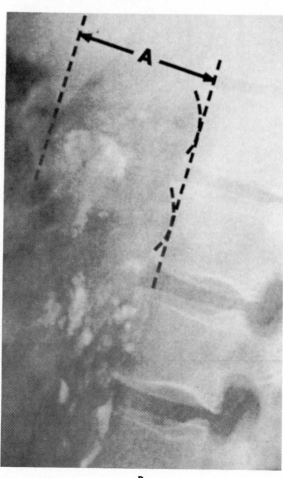

B

TABLE 15–3   SIZE AND POSITION OF LYMPH NODES
IN LYMPHOMA*

(a comparison of 60 normal and 60 abnormal cases)

	Mean	± 1 S. D.	± 2 S. D.	Proposed Maximum Normal
Size of Node				
Normal	1.9	0.42	2.7	2.6
Abnormal	3.1	0.96		
Measurement A				
Normal	2.0	0.61	3.2	3.2
Abnormal	3.3	1.32		
Measurement B				
Normal	0.9	0.47	1.8	2.0
Abnormal	1.8	1.24		
Measurement C				
Normal	1.0	0.52	2.0	2.0
Abnormal	2.2	1.17		

*From Abrams, H. L.: Angiography, Vol. 2. 2d ed. Boston, Little, Brown & Co., 1971. Table 80–4.

Radiographic Study of the Peritoneal Space and Abdominal Wall

1. **Anteroposterior Film of the Abdomen, Recumbent.**   This is also commonly referred to as a "KUB" film, since it is usually employed in examinations of the urinary tract, and the letters symbolize "kidney, ureter, and bladder." The structures delineated in this examination are shown in Figures 15–54 and 15–56. It will be seen that several layers can be identified in the lateral abdominal wall above the iliac crests: the skin and subcutaneous tissues, the muscular layer, the properitoneal fat layer, and finally the abdominal viscera. The tela subserosa is continued around the kidney, permitting the outline of that organ to be seen; the psoas muscle shadow and quadratus lumborum muscle shadows are likewise differentiated on both sides. The posterior inferior margin of the liver casts a rather well-defined shadow beneath both lower poles of the kidneys and under the peritoneum above the iliac crests. The obturator fascial planes can be clearly delineated on the inner aspect of the pelvic inlet, and often the dome of the urinary bladder, when distended with urine, can be clearly demonstrated by its tela subserosa.

Figure 15–53. *A* and *B*. Three of the four basic measurements that are obtained to show lymphatic size. The fourth measurement is the maximum size of individual lymph nodes. (From Abrams, H.: Angiography, Vol. 2. 2d ed. Boston, Little, Brown & Co., 1971.)

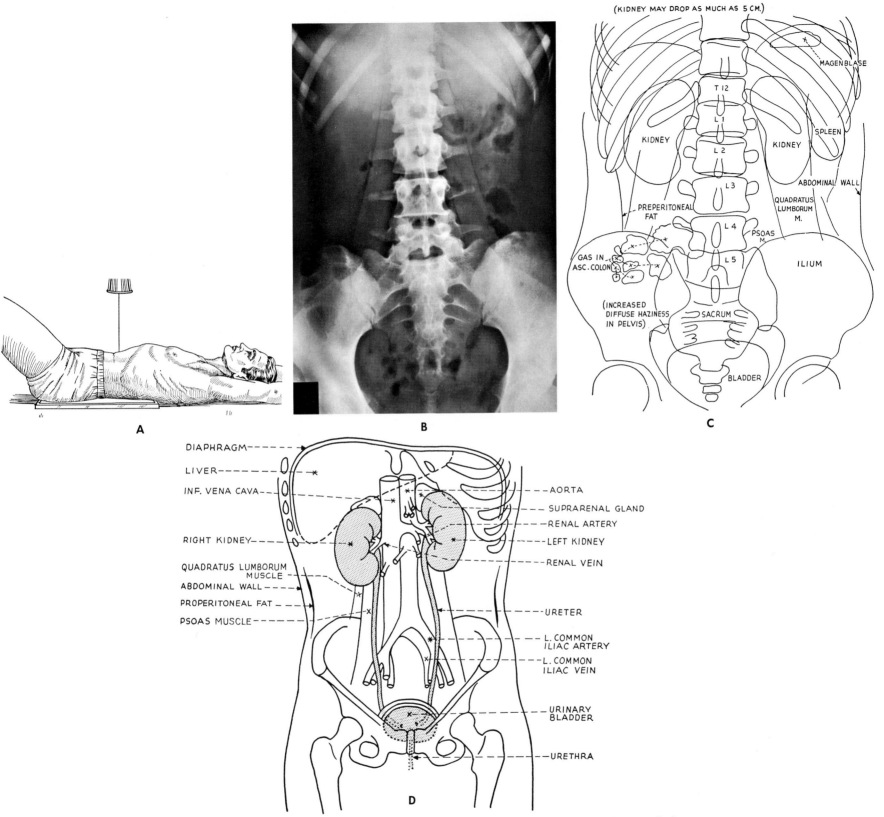

Figure 15–54. Anteroposterior view of abdomen (KUB film). *A.* Position of patient. *B.* Radiograph (intensified). *C.* Labeled tracing of *B. D.* Diagram intensifying the urinary tract and indicating other anatomic relationships.

There are variable gas shadows and fecal shadows in the colon and stomach in the adult, and in the small intestine as well in the infant. These tend to obscure soft tissue detail considerably, as well as the detail of the bony structure of the lumbar spine and pelvis. For that reason, if it is desired that such interference be eliminated, and if the patient can be prepared for this examination, it is well to give the patient a good cathartic such as 2 tablespoonfuls of castor oil the night before the examination. If the examination is an emergency, such preparation is of course impossible.

2. **Anteroposterior Film of the Abdomen, Erect.** In this study, most of the abdominal viscera tend to descend owing to the action of gravity. Unusual mobility is an indication of abnormality, but the limits of normal in this respect are fairly great. If there is fluid in the gastrointestinal tract as well as gas, fluid levels are obtained. In the small intestine, such fluid levels are frequently an indication of mechanical obstruction. Abnormally, also, air which has escaped into the peritoneal space may be present, in which case it will rise to the highest possible level. Unless there are adhesions which prevent such rise, this gas will usually accumulate under the diaphragm. In obtaining this film, it is important that the diaphragm be absolutely motionless—otherwise a thin stripe of free air will be obscured and may escape detection. *A rapid exposure technique should always be employed if free air under the diaphragm is suspected, and in our laboratory we employ a separate chest exposure, or lateral decubitus film of the abdomen* (patient lies on his side and a horizontal x-ray beam is employed to obtain a frontal view of the abdomen), as well as the upright film of the abdomen. The chest film allows for simultaneous examination of that portion of the trunk and helps to exclude referred disease—a very important consideration whenever one is confronted with abdominal complaints.

In the upright film, the soft tissue structures in the anatomic pelvis are less clearly defined, and in general, structural detail is less distinct than in the recumbent film.

3. **Patient Supine; Horizontal X-ray Beam.** In this film study, the patient lies supine, and a horizontal x-ray beam is directed at the abdomen from the patient's side. The main purpose of this examination is to demonstrate free air under the xiphisternum, and also to see any fluid levels which may be present in the small or large intestine. All other detail is generally obscured.

4. **Patient on Side; Horizontal X-ray Beam.** In this examination, the patient lies on one side, and a horizontal x-ray beam is directed at the abdomen from the anterior aspect. Ordinarily, a Potter-Bucky diaphragm is employed, if possible, to obtain better detail. The viscera tend to drop by gravity, but if there are fluid levels present, once again they can be readily demonstrated, and any free air in the peritoneal space rises to the uppermost part of the abdomen where it can be seen. This examination is also helpful when it is desired to eliminate gaseous shadows from one side

of the abdomen, since the gas-containing loops of bowel will tend to drop away from the side which is uppermost. Kirklin has shown that this can be used efficaciously in gallbladder studies.

Recommended Routine for Study of the Acute Abdomen (Fig. 15–55). The pathologic abdomen is out of the realm of this text, but in this connection it may be pointed out that in the study of a patient for acute abdominal disease, it is well to obtain both a recumbent and an erect film of the abdomen, a chest film, and frequently an additional study with the patient on his side, employing a horizontal x-ray beam.

It is also important to note the degree of separation of the gas-containing loops of bowel, since peritoneal disease will often widen the space between adjoining loops of bowel, which is normally about 2 mm. Indeed, this phase of the study is just as important, if not more so, as the examination for the relative clarity of the properitoneal fat line.

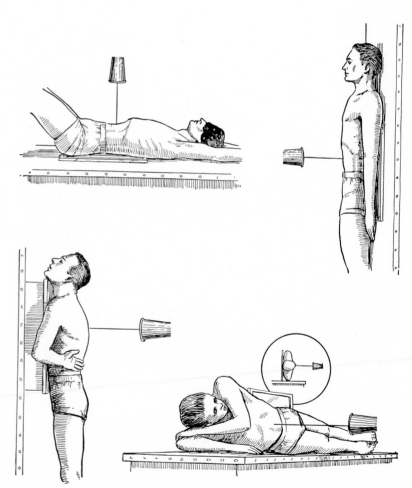

Figure 15–55. Routine film studies obtained for plain film survey of abdominal disease. Note that a PA chest film is part of this routine. (Decubitus left lateral may be preferable.)

A useful routine to follow in examining a KUB film is summarized in Figure 15–56. The following sequence may be used: (1) the kidneys are studied for size, position, contour, density and architecture; (2) the ureteral distribution is postulated and outlined, and any opacities are particularly noted; (3) the urinary bladder area is identified and also the adjoining obturator fascia; (4) the psoas shadows and shadows of the quadratus lumborum muscles are clearly identified; (5) the flank area and abdominal

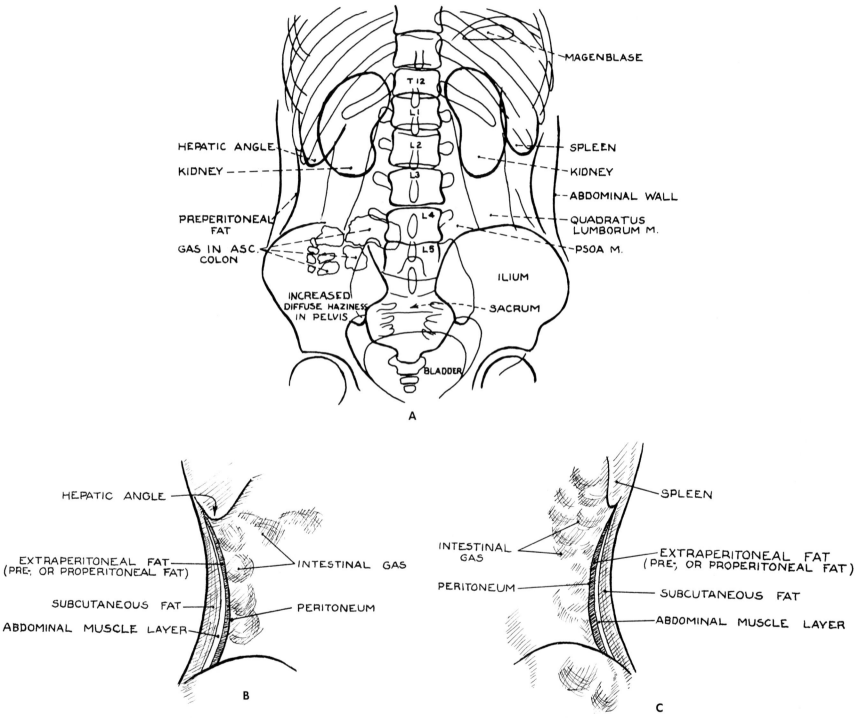

Figure 15–56. Routine for examination of the recumbent film of the abdomen. *B* and *C*. Diagrams demonstrating flank anatomy, showing the relationship of the properitoneal fat layer to the rest of the abdominal wall.

wall are carefully studied (see Fig. 15–56 *B* and *C*); (6) the bony structures are carefully examined for intricate detail and configuration as well as density; (7) the gas pattern is carefully defined; (8) the hepatic and splenic angles are clearly defined if possible; (9) any abnormal masses are described, with particular attention to their size, position, contour, density, and architecture; (10) any opaque shadows in the abdomen are noted and identified etiologically, if possible.

THE LIVER

The basic and radiologic anatomy of the liver and pancreas have been described in Chapter 14 because of the close relationship of these structures to the alimentary tract. Only those aspects pertinent to this section on the abdomen without added contrast will be included here.

Surface Topography; Gross Anatomy. A line connecting the lower border of the fifth rib on the left with the upper border of this rib on the right usually forms the upper border of the superior surface of the liver. This border is ordinarily slightly concave under the xiphisternum. As seen from the front, the lower margin of the liver is found under the costal margin on the right and passes obliquely upward to the eighth or ninth costal cartilage on the left (Fig. 15–54 *D*).

The liver maintains this relationship in the recumbent position, but when erect it drops a variable distance of several centimeters. The position of the liver also varies with the body habitus and the position of the patient.

The falciform ligament on the anterior and superior surface of the liver divides the liver into a large right lobe and a small left lobe. The quadrate and caudate lobes on the inferior surface of the liver are subdivisions of the right lobe, and are important in that they impart an irregularity to the inferior margin of the liver as it is seen on the plain radiograph of the abdomen.

The left lobe of the liver is contained under the cupola of the left diaphragm and overlies the stomach and the spleen.

Although the liver can be moderately well outlined on the plain radiograph, nevertheless it is rather difficult to detect with certainty even with moderate degrees of enlargement.

Areas of calcification as well as bronchovascular markings from the lung may be projected into the liver area from the posterior costophrenic angle of the chest. These must not be misinterpreted as liver abnormalities.

Pneumoperitoneum (Fig. 15–57). The introduction of air into the peritoneal space provides a means of delineating the viscera separately from the abdominal wall. The location, size, mobility, outline, and attachments of the various abdominal organs can be detected in this manner.

Normally, there is a fairly wide range of mobility of the liver,

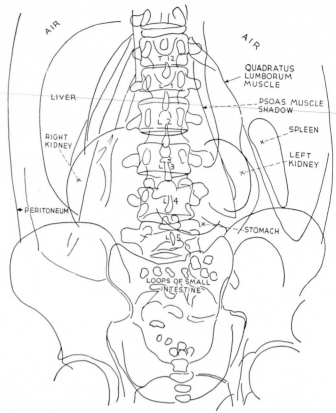

Figure 15–57.   Tracing of a radiograph demonstrating pneumoperitoneum in the erect anteroposterior view of the abdomen.

spleen, and other intra-abdominal organs, and any restriction in motion can be readily detected. Examination of the patient while on his left side allows the air to rise over the right lobe of the liver, and the liver drops into the left abdomen, allowing a clear visualization of the right kidney. When the patient lies on his right side, the left kidney, spleen, splenic flexure, and descending colon are visible. When the patient lies prone, with the abdomen suspended between two supports under the thigh and chest, the air rises to the prevertebral space, outlining the structures here.

In the erect position, the liver drops away from the diaphragm and any subphrenic space-occupying lesion becomes readily demonstrable.

Pelvic pneumoperitoneum will be described separately (Chapter 17).

Pneumoperitoneum is somewhat painful and even somewhat dangerous if there is a communication through the diaphragm into the chest. A pneumothorax may result when a marked shift of the mediastinum produces considerable respiratory and cardiovascular embarrassment. Immediate relief of such a pressure pneumothorax is a necessity. There is some question as to whether the information gained is worth the inconvenience of the examination.

Peritoneography. Peritoneography is the double contrast examination of the peritoneal cavity and its contents using a water-soluble positive contrast medium and gas. The technique proceeds as follows (Meyers, 1973a): The patient is given a laxative on the night prior to the examination to cleanse the gastrointestinal tract; cleansing enemas and emptying of the bladder are performed just prior to positioning the patient for examination. The patient should be supine at the time the local anesthetic is administered and during the transabdominal puncture, which is performed in the left supraumbilical area, lateral to the border of the left rectus abdominis muscle. A Rochester needle with a stylet is employed. After the needle has been appropriately inserted and it is certain that a blood vessel or bowel has not been punctured, the inner metallic needle is withdrawn and the flexible plastic outer cannula is allowed to remain in place. Under fluoroscopic control, a small amount of air or meglumine diatrizoate is injected to document the position of the needle in the peritoneal cavity. Approximately 1200 to 1500 ml. of nitrous oxide, recommended as the gas of choice, is introduced during a period of several minutes into the peritoneal cavity. Thereafter, 150 to 200 ml. of 60 per cent meglumine diatrizoate diluted with 50 to 75 ml. of normal saline is instilled into the abdominal cavity. A test dose is first introduced and the patient is observed for any adverse reactions. An open intravenous drip is maintained throughout the procedure and vital signs are monitored. An obturator is then inserted into the cannula, which is taped to the skin to prevent dislodgement.

Roentgenograms of the abdomen are obtained in various positions, supplemented by image amplifier fluoroscopic observation. Increments of 50 to 75 ml. of meglumine diatrizoate can be utilized thereafter to enhance visualization.

Following radiography, as much gas as possible is withdrawn from the abdomen; thereafter the patient remains recumbent for about 30 minutes to 1 hour to allow further absorption of the gas and to minimize abdominal distress.

This examination may be combined with simultaneous upper gastrointestinal study with barium sulfate or intravenous cholangiography. It may also be combined with tomography for more accurate visualization of a given anatomic area.

The structures routinely visualized include the peritoneal reflections and ligaments, such as the parietal peritoneum, greater omentum, lesser omentum, and transverse mesocolon, and the ligaments of the upper abdomen and those surrounding the liver, such as the coronary, falciform, splenorenal, gastrosplenic, phrenicocolic, and umbilical ligaments. No contrast medium apparently gains entrance to the lesser peritoneal sac. The thickness of the wall of portions of the alimentary tract can be described in detail.

Some illustrative radiographs are shown here: (1) In the prone position, peritoneography shows the right lobe of the liver, the gallbladder, greater omentum, the walls of bowel loops, falciform ligament, and spleen (Fig. 15–58 A).

The double contrast examination provides clear visualization of the perisplenic compartment and structures since the spleen is suspended in the left upper quadrant posteriorly by its ligamentous reflections (see Chapter 14 and Figure 15–58 B, C, D). The anterior notched border of the spleen is well outlined (Fig. 15–58 E). The tail of the pancreas may also thereby be seen.

The contrast medium may also gravitate to the pelvic cavity where visualization of the urinary bladder and female reproductive organs may be obtained.

The films recommended by Meyers are: frontal and both oblique projections in the prone Trendelenburg position (20 to 30 degrees), posteroanterior, anteroposterior, right and left lateral with the table horizontal, and frontal and both oblique views in the supine Trendelenburg position. Since the contrast medium gravitates to the pelvic recesses, the earlier phases of the examination are carried out in the prone Trendelenburg position.

About 80 per cent of the nitrous oxide is absorbed within 2 hours. Experimentally, the ascites induced by this intraperitoneal injection of the hypertonic water-soluble contrast agent is completely resorbed in 2 to 24 hours.

Related study of the pelvic structures will be described in Chapter 17.

Herniagram in an Infant (White et al.; Swischuk and Stacy, 1971). Hernias have already been described; they are of primary interest in this text from the standpoint of their anatomic and roentgen presentations. Demonstration of an inguinal hernia in an infant is often difficult. The technique of the herniagram is carried out as follows: With the patient in the supine position, 10 to 15 ml. of 60 per cent meglumine diatrizoate is injected transperitoneally. The injection is usually made in the midline about 1 to 2 cm. below the umbilicus, after a trial aspiration for possible penetration of the bowel or urinary bladder is made. The contrast medium is thereafter instilled and the child is held erect until a single upright anteroposterior roentgenogram of the lower abdomen, penis, and upper thighs is obtained about 5 to 10 minutes later (Fig. 15–59).

There are several advantages to this procedure: (1) It accomplishes the demonstration of occult bilateral hernias. (2) It provides a full delineation of the anatomy of the peritoneal sac before it is distorted by operative manipulation. (3) In addition to the inguinal herniagram, an excretory urogram can be obtained because the contrast agent is so readily absorbed from the peritoneal space. The excretory urogram can be obtained approximately 45 minutes following the instillation of the contrast material into the peritoneal cavity. (4) It requires only a single pelvic roentgenogram with its consequent radiation. (5) It demonstrates at an early age a cryptorchid testis (abdominal testis) associated with the hernia.

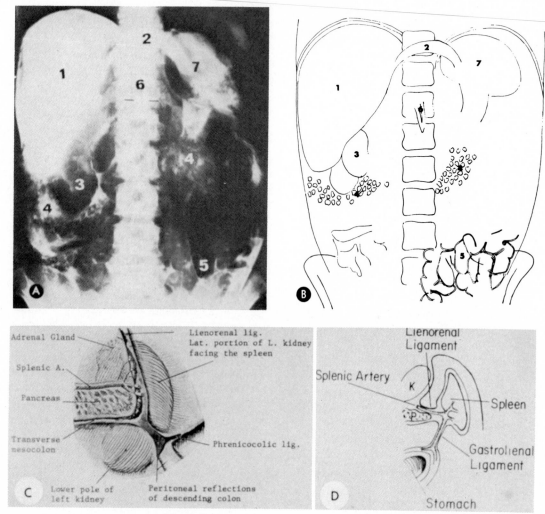

Figure 15–58.   *A* and *B.* Prone peritoneography. (1) Positive contrast medium coats the ventral surface of the right lobe of the liver. (2) The arcuate collection resides within the median subphrenic space, anterior to the stomach beneath the central tendinous portion of the diaphragm. (3) The gallbladder displaces the positive contrast medium and is outlined as a "filling defect." (4) The greater omentum presents a characteristic honey-combed appearance. (5) The walls of bowel loops are outlined by contrast medium in the peritoneal cavity and intraluminal gas. (6) The falciform ligament. (7) The spleen. *C.* Posterior peritoneal attachments of the left upper quadrant (after Corning). The spleen has been removed. *D.* Diagrammatic transverse section with emphasis on the peritoneal attachments. The tail of the pancreas (P), anterior to the left kidney (K), resides within the lienorenal ligament. The perisplenic space is bounded by this and the gastrolienal ligament. (From Meyers, M. A.: Amer. J. Roentgenol., *117:353–363,* 1973.)

Figure 15–58 continued on the opposite page.

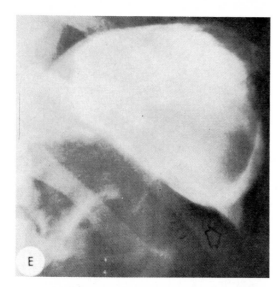

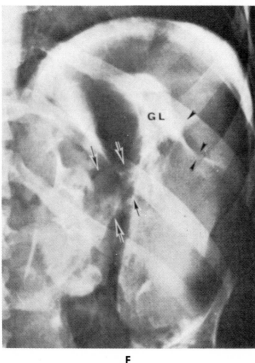

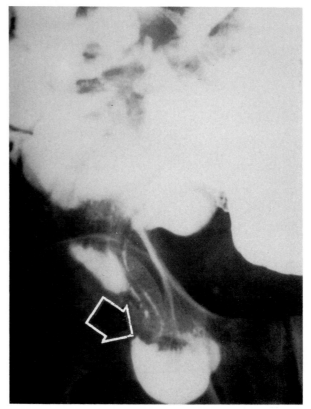

Figure 15–59. Inguinal hernia filled with barium.

Figure 15–58 *Continued.* E. Supine peritoneography. Selective opacification outlines the margins of the spleen to the level inferiorly of the phrenicocolic ligament (arrow). (From Meyers, M. A.: Radiology, 95:539–545, 1970.) F. Prone peritoneography. The tail of the pancreas, ensheathed within the leaves of the lienorenal ligament, is outlined (arrows). It is directed toward the splenic hilus, between the anterior notched border of the spleen (arrowheads) indicated by contrast medium apposing the gastrolienal ligament (GL) and the more medial posterior margin in relationship to the left kidney. Compare to diagram in C. (From Meyers, M. A.: Amer. J. Roentgenol., 117:353–363, 1973.)

In most cases, absorption of the meglumine diatrizoate from the peritoneal cavity occurs within 4 to 8 hours.

It is probably prudent to test for sensitivity to the contrast agent as if it were being injected intravenously.

A normal study is shown for comparison (Fig. 15–60). There is usually a good coating of the lateral peritoneal margin and even the liver edge. The contrast material collects in a pool in normal lateral recesses and cul-de-sacs. A notch caused by the inferior epigastric artery and the normal extension of the peritoneal sac medial to it may be noted.

SPECIAL RADIOGRAPHIC STUDY OF THE LIVER

Hepatolienography with Thorotrast. This is now a historic method since the Food and Drug Administration no longer permits the use of Thorotrast, owing to its inherent alpha radiation and toxicity (Rösch). However, because some patients may have Thorotrast in the liver and spleen even at the present time, it is of clinical interest and utility to recognize its appearance in the abdomen.

Thorotrast is a stable suspension of 25 per cent thorium dioxide which, when introduced intravenously, is stored in the re-

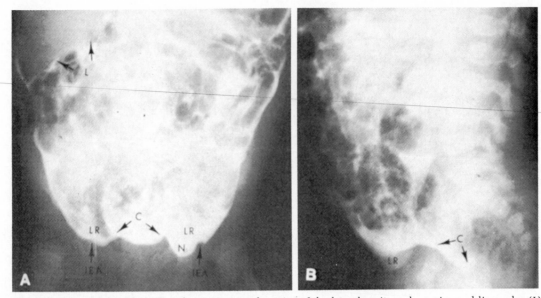

Figure 15–60. *A* and *B*. Normal study. *A*. Note good coating of the lateral peritoneal margins and liver edge (*L*). The contrast material has pooled in the normal lateral recesses (*LR*) and cul-de-sac (*C*). Note the notch due to the inferior epigastric artery (*IEA*) and the normal extension of the peritoneal sac medial to it (*N*).

B. Lateral view (not a necessary part of the examination) showing location of the lateral recesses (*LR*) and cul-de-sac (*C*). (From Swischuk, L. E., and Stacy, T. M.: Radiology, *101*:139–146, 1971.)

ticuloendothelial system. *Because of its long-lived radioactivity, it had the potential to induce late degenerative, fibrotic, and even malignant changes in the liver and spleen.* It was supplied in 25 cc. ampules, and was freely miscible with water or saline. A total dose of 50 to 75 cc. was necessary over a period of several days, given intravenously. The initial dose did not exceed 10 or 15 cc., but in the absence of symptoms, this was increased to 25 cc. intravenously in 1 day. The radiographic examination was made 1 or 2 days after the last dose.

Because the thorium salts were fixed by the reticuloendothelial cells of the liver and spleen, these organs were clearly outlined on the radiograph (Fig. 15–61). Lymph nodes near the porta hepatis may also be seen. Any space-occupying lesions within the liver or spleen were clearly demarcated since they did not become impregnated.

The injection of short-lived radioactive material such as technetium-99m-labeled sulfur colloids has replaced long-acting radioactive material for visualization of the spleen and liver following the advent of various imaging devices in nuclear medicine. The student is referred to textbooks in Nuclear Medicine for further detail.

Hepatic Angiogram.   See Chapter 14.

THE SPLEEN

The spleen lies in the left upper quadrant posterior to the stomach and immediately under the diaphragm. It varies in size considerably, but ordinarily does not project significantly below the horizontal plane at the level of the left costal margin. The diaphragm separates it from the ninth, tenth, and eleventh ribs on the left. The medial surface of the spleen is in contact with the tail of the pancreas (Fig. 15–4), and the lower pole of the spleen is in contact with the splenic flexure of the colon. The anteromedial portion of the spleen is in contact with the greater curvature of the stomach (Fig. 15–4 *A* and *B*).

The spleen is supported by *three main ligamentous attachments:* (1) the *phrenicosplenic* ligament, which is a reflection of the peritoneum running from the diaphragm and ventral aspect of the left kidney to the hilum of the spleen, and which contains splenic vessels; (2) the *gastrosplenic* (or gastrolienal), which is actually a dorsal mesentery between the spleen and the stomach, and contains the short gastric and left gastroepiploic artery; and (3) the *phrenicocolic* ligament, which lies beneath the caudal end of the spleen.

The *primary functions* of the spleen are: (1) the *storage of red*

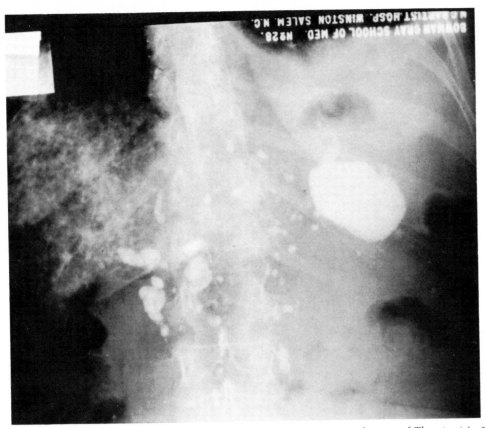

Figure 15–61. Thorotrast hepatolienography following intravenous injection of 60 cc. of Thorotrast in 3 days. This film was obtained 1 week following the last injection. Note deposition in upper abdominal lymph node caudad to the liver. (The use of Thorotrast is no longer permitted for these purposes by the FDA.)

blood cells that may be forced back into the circulation in a respiratory crisis by contraction of the smooth muscle in the capsule and trabeculae; (2) *destruction of worn-out red blood cells;* (3) *removal of foreign material* from the blood stream; (4) *production of mononuclear leukocytes;* and (5) it is an important part of the reticuloendothelial defense mechanism and system.

Normal Blood Supply (Fig. 15–62). The normal vascular supply of the spleen is extremely varied, to the extent that, in one study of 100 dissections, no two vascularization patterns were exactly alike (Michels, 1942). Measurements of the splenic artery have revealed an average length of 13 cm., with a range of 8 to 32 cm., and an average width of 7.5 mm., with a range of 5 to 12 mm. Tortuosity is frequent. There are four main segments of the *splenic artery:* (1) the *suprapancreatic*—the first 1 to 3 cm.; (2) the *pancreatic,* which is usually found in the dorsal surface of the pancreas and supplies small pancreatic branches; (3) *prepancreatic,* which runs obliquely along the anterior surface of the tail of the pancreas and usually branches into a superior and an inferior ter-

minal artery, but occasionally into a medial terminal artery as well; (4) *prehilar,* which is found between the tail of the pancreas and the spleen.

The *dorsal pancreatic artery* originates from the splenic artery in about 40 per cent of dissections. It may arise from the celiac, hepatic, or superior mesenteric artery, and it supplies the dorsal and ventral surfaces of the pancreas in the region of the neck. It has two branches, one which anastomoses with the superior pancreaticoduodenal artery and one which supplies the uncinate process.

A left branch of the splenic artery, the *transverse pancreatic,* runs along the inferior surface of the pancreas until it anastomoses with the arteria pancreatic magna and the caudal pancreatic vessels.

An additional branch may arise from the dorsal pancreatic which communicates with the superior mesenteric artery and provides a collateral pathway between celiac and superior mesenteric channels.

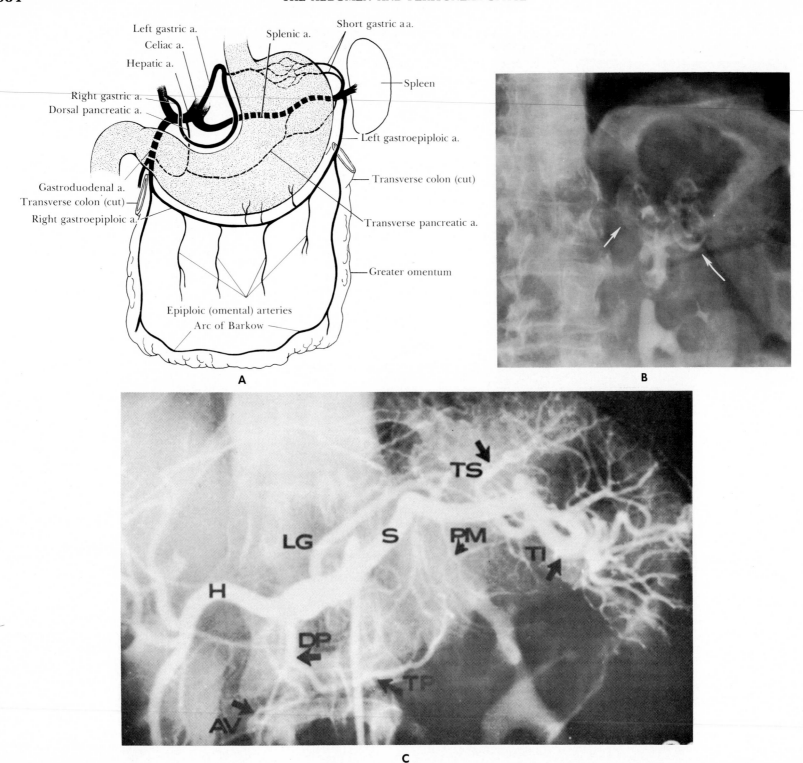

Figure 15–62. *A.* Line drawing representing celiac arterial axis as related to stomach and greater omentum. (Modified from Ruzicka, F. F., Jr., and Rossi, P.: Radiol. Clin. N. Amer., 8:3–29, 1970.) *B.* Dilated and tortuous calcified splenic artery. *C.* Normal splenic arterial anatomy. This 40-year-old female patient was investigated for abdominal pain. Hepatic artery (*H*); left gastric artery (*LG*); splenic trunk (*S*). Superior terminal (*TS*) and inferior terminal (*TI*) vessels supply numer-ous branches to the splenic parenchyma. The dorsal pancreatic branch (*DP*) is well visualized originating from the proximal splenic and divides into the transverse pancreatic (*TP*) and anastomotic vessels (*AV*) which supply the head of the pancreas and anastomose with the pancreaticoduodenals. The pancreatica magna (*PM*) originates from the second segment of the splenic trunk. (*C* from Abrams, H. L.: Angiography, 2d ed. Vol. 2. Boston, Little, Brown & Co., 1971.)

The *arteria pancreatic magna* is the largest arterial branch of the pancreas, measuring about 2 to 4 mm. in width and arising from the distal third of the splenic artery. It supplies the tail of the pancreas and anastomoses with the transverse pancreatic and with the caudal pancreatic vessels.

The *caudal pancreatic artery* originates from the distal splenic trunk or from the left gastroepiploic artery. It supplies the tail of the pancreas or a small accessory spleen when present. It anastomoses with the transverse pancreatic and arteria pancreatic magna.

There is considerable variation in the terminal splenic branches. They average about 4 cm. in length but may vary from 1 to 12 cm.

The *left gastroepiploic* arises from the splenic artery in about 72 per cent of dissections, 1 to 4 cm. proximal to the primary terminal division. It descends along the right aspect of the greater curvature of the stomach, anastomosing with the right gastroepiploic. There are various branches to the spleen from this vessel. An important branch is the *left epiploic* which originates from the left gastroepiploic near the spleen and descends in a posterior layer of the greater omentum below the transverse colon.

A *superior polar artery* is found in about 65 per cent of dissections, most commonly arising from the splenic trunk proximal to its primary division. It may vary in length from 2 to 12 cm. and in width from 1 to 5 mm. Occasionally, it arises directly from the celiac artery, forming a double splenic artery.

An *inferior polar branch* is found in 82 per cent of dissections, most frequently originating from the left gastroepiploic artery. It varies in length from 3 to 8 cm.

For a detailed discussion of angiographic analysis of normal vessels, their origin and incidence of visualized branches, the student is referred to Abrams' comprehensive review of this subject. The vessel diameters recorded by Abrams were as follows:

Tortuosity and increased length of the pancreatic artery increases somewhat with age but is not necessarily associated with atherosclerosis (Michels, 1955).

TABLE 15-4 DIAMETER OF THE SPLENIC ARTERY
IN ITS VARIOUS PORTIONS

Vessel	Average Diameter in mm.	Maximum Diameter in mm.	Minimum Diameter in mm.
Celiac origin	10.9	21	8
Splenic origin	8.2	14	6
Splenic midportion	7.3	11	5
Splenic hilum	6.5	10	3

TABLE 15-5 THE LENGTH OF THE SPLENIC ARTERY
AND ITS SEGMENTS

Splenic Artery	Average Length in cm.	Maximum Length in cm.	Minimum Length in cm.
Total	17.3	33	8.5
Suprapancreatic segment	2.5	7	1
Pancreatic segment	10.4	22.5	5
Prepancreatic segment	2.5	6	0.4
Prehilar segment	1.5	4.5	0.3

The *splenic vein* emerges from the hilum of the spleen, runs in a groove on the dorsum of the pancreas below the splenic artery, and usually joins the superior mesenteric vein behind the neck of the pancreas to form the portal vein (see Chapter 14).

The *lymphatics of the spleen* drain into the pancreaticosplenic lymph nodes.

The splenic artery and vein run in the phrenicolienal ligament to the hilus and, as noted previously, the artery's course is often tortuous.

To summarize, the significant branches from the splenic artery and vein are: (1) a *left gastroepiploic,* which may or may not anastomose with the right gastroepiploic; (2) *pancreatic branches;* and (3) *short branches to the stomach;* and all of these may provide collateral circulation for the spleen. Because of the end-organ relationship of the arteries, the spleen is subject to infarction.

Ordinarily, the spleen creates a slight impression upon the splenic flexure of the colon and the greater curvature of the stomach.

Calcification (Fig. 15–63) is frequent in the region of the spleen, and this may be due to phleboliths, tubercles, calcified infarcts, splenic artery aneurysms, and certain cysts (hydatid), but this subject is outside the scope of this text. Subcapsular calcification may also occur, but this is also most likely a pathologic degenerative change.

Apart from lobulation, accessory spleens are not infrequently found. These are usually in the neighborhood of the main organ but sometimes they may be distributed elsewhere in the abdominal cavity.

A congenital absence of the spleen may also occur, particularly in relation to some types of congenital heart disease.

Techniques of Examination. The usual techniques of visualization of the spleen are: (1) *plain film studies,* especially anteroposterior or posteroanterior views of the left upper quadrant; (2) *contrast visualization* of the *stomach, kidneys,* or *splenic flex-*

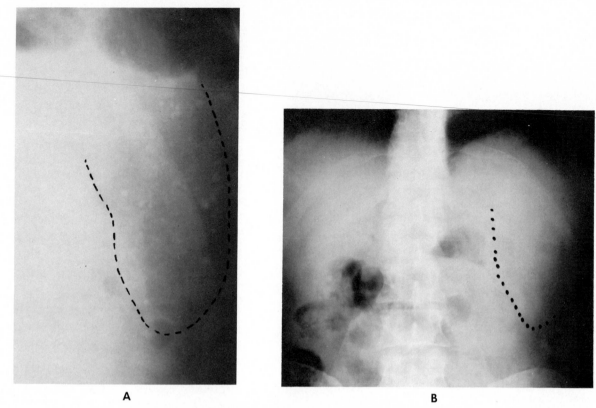

A   B

Figure 15–63.   A. Numerous calcified tubercles or phleboliths in the spleen.

ure of the colon, together with a visualization of the *diaphragm;* (3) *pneumoperitoneum;* (4) *angiography* (arteriography and venography) through an aortic route; (5) *splenoportography;* (6) *radioisotopic scanning techniques,* using labeled compounds that are taken up selectively by the reticuloendothelial system, such as technetium-99m sulphur colloid (which is also taken up by the liver), crenated red cells labeled with chromium-51, or colloidal gold.

Retroperitoneal air studies with laminagraphy in the anteroposterior projection may be helpful. The spleen is seen best at a distance of 4 to 11 cm. from the back.

The Spleen in the Anteroposterior Film of the Abdomen. The splenic shadow can usually be identified along the left upper lateral aspect of the stomach as a tonguelike structure, the tip of the tongue normally extending to the left costal margin (Fig. 15–17). Only the inferior one-half or one-third of the spleen is visible radiographically on a plain film of the abdomen. Small 3 to 5 mm. calcific tubercles or phleboliths may frequently be recognized within the spleen. Rarely, the splenic capsule itself is calcified (Fig. 15–63). In older age groups, the splenic artery is often seen

as a tortuous calcific aneurysmal structure arising from the celiac trunk medial to the spleen and projected over the stomach.

Measurement of Splenic Size.   The caudal tip of the splenic shadow forms a good basis for measurement, as shown in Figure 15–63 *B*. Measurement of the spleen 2 cm. above its tip should not exceed 3.5 cm. (Wyman).

Whitley et al. have demonstrated by means of a computer approach to the prediction of splenic weight from routine films, that the parameters L and W, as indicated on a routine film, provide the most accurate basis for predicting the weight of the spleen (Fig. 15–64 *B*). L is estimated by a vertical line from the tip of the spleen to the intercept with the diaphragm, and W is the width of the spleen at the midpoint of L or as close to this point as this measurement can be made. In their study, the measurement of the spleen 2.5 cm. above the tip was the least accurate and has the lowest correlation coefficient. The product of L and W alone offered a fairly accurate first approximation of splenic weight. Actually, the measurement of L alone is in itself quite accurate and was the single best indicator found by these investigators: "On a routine abdominal film in an average sized adult, an L of more than 11.3 cm. can give a 70 per cent probability, and an L above 15 cm., a 98 per cent probability of the spleen being enlarged. . . .

"If the product of L and W is obtained, correcting for magnification: if this product is 50 or more, the probability is 75 per cent that the spleen's weight is more than 200 grams; and if this product is 75 or more, the probability is 98 per cent that the spleen's weight is more than 200 grams."

THE PANCREAS

Gross Anatomy (Figs. 15–65, 15–66). The pancreas has already been described in relation to the stomach and duodenum (see Chapter 13). It lies transversely and obliquely on the posterior abdominal wall, its right end in the concavity of the duodenum and its left end touching the spleen. The greater part of the pancreas lies behind the stomach.

Anatomically, it is subdivided into a head, body, and tail having the following relationships. The head, which is largely retroperitoneal, is in contact superiorly with the pylorus and proximal portion of the duodenum; on the right with the descending duodenum and terminal portion of the common bile duct; caudally with the horizontal portion of the duodenum; and on the left with the terminal ascending portion of the duodenum. The inferior vena cava and abdominal aorta lie behind it. The body crosses to the left where it tends to pass upward slightly and posteriorly as it traverses the spine, left kidney, and adrenal gland.

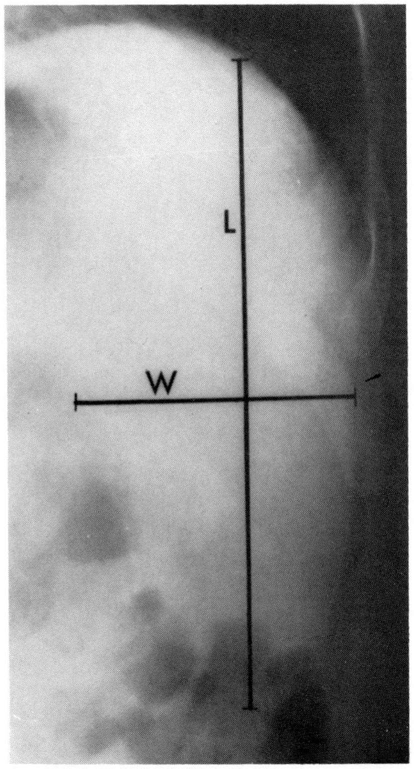

Figure 15–64. Anteroposterior radiograph of the left upper abdomen illustrating the parameters L and W superimposed on the image of the spleen. (From Whitley, J. E., Maynard, C. D., and Rhyne, A. L.: Radiology, 86:73–76, 1966.)

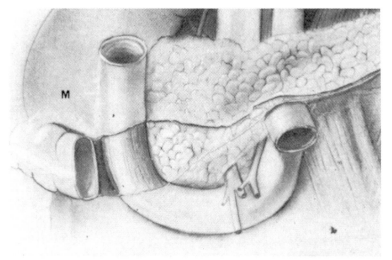

Figure 15–65. Drawing showing the root of the transverse mesocolon, extending across the infra-ampullary portion of the duodenum and the lower border of the pancreas. Note the relationships of the anterior hepatic flexure of the colon and of the duodenojejunal junction. M marks the location of Morison's pouch, the intraperitoneal posterior extension of the right subhepatic space. (From Meyers, M. A., and Whalen, J. P.: Amer. J. Roentgenol., 117:263–274, 1973.)

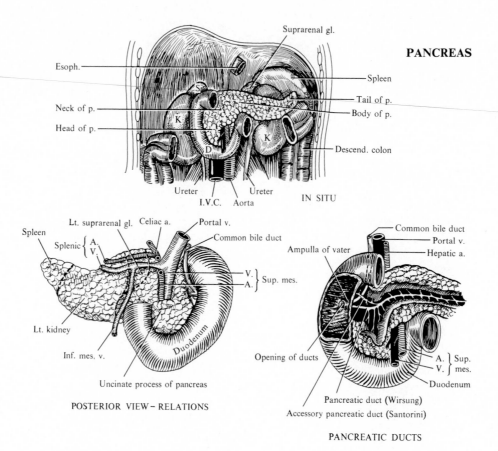

PANCREAS

IN SITU

POSTERIOR VIEW – RELATIONS

PANCREATIC DUCTS

TRANSVERSE SECTION – RELATIONS

MAIN BLOOD VESSELS

Figure 15–66. Summary of anatomic details of the pancreas: *in situ*, from posterior view, pancreatic ducts, transversely, and main arterial supply and venous drainage. (K) kidney, (D) duodenum, (I.V.C.) inferior vena cava, (a.) artery, (v.) vein, (aa) arcades. (From Pansky, B., and House, E. L.: Review of Gross Anatomy. New York, Macmillan Company, 1964.)

It forms the posterior wall of the lesser omental bursa. The tail of the pancreas projects into the splenorenal ligament and is in contact laterally with the medial aspect of the spleen, and caudally with the splenic flexure of the colon.

As noted previously, the pancreaticoduodenal arteries are situated on the ventral aspect of the head of the pancreas along with pancreaticoduodenal veins and superior mesenteric vessels. The splenic artery runs along the superior margin or border of the body of the pancreas. The root of the transverse mesocolon extends across the middle of the head of the pancreas and lower border of the body. The splenic vessels cross ventral or dorsal to the tail of the pancreas on their way to join the spleen (Fig. 15–66).

These relationships of the pancreas are important radiographically since it is only by displacement of contiguous structures that abnormalities of this organ can be recognized.

The relationships of the pancreatic duct and accessory pancreatic duct have been previously described in conjunction with the biliary system (Chapter 13).

Accessory or supernumerary nodules of pancreatic tissue are not rare, and they may occur anywhere in the foregut. They are most common in the duodenum and are usually situated in the postbulbar region on the right aspect of the second part of the duodenum.

At times a ring of glandular tissue from the head of the pancreas surrounds the descending duodenum, forming an annular pancreas. The aberrant pancreas can usually be recognized by the smoothness of the filling defect produced and by the dimple centrally related to a supernumerary pancreatic duct draining into the adjoining gastrointestinal tract.

METHODS OF EXAMINATION OF PANCREAS

Plain Posteroanterior Film of the Abdomen. This is useful only if the pancreas contains abnormal calcific deposits, or if there is obvious displacement of the stomach as seen by the gas contained within it.

Barium Meal. The stomach and duodenum are outlined with barium, and displacement of these organs as seen in the posteroanterior and lateral projections is of significance in detecting abnormality in the pancreas.

Passage of Radiopaque Tube into the Stomach and Duodenum. This method basically involves the same principle as the barium meal in that displacements of the tube are interpreted in the light of enlargement of the pancreas or lesser omental bursa. This method has the advantage of not requiring the introduction of an opaque medium; thus, interference with the presence of calcium in the pancreas is avoided. The stomach and duodenum are not outlined as accurately as they are with barium, however.

Introduction of Air into the Stomach. Air may also be used to outline the stomach, but it does not provide as clear visualization as does barium. Posteroanterior and lateral views of the abdomen are taken as before, and displacements of the stomach detected by this means.

Other Methods

Laminagraphy with retroperitoneal air, combined with gaseous distention of the stomach and duodenum. This technique has not received wide acceptance.

Hypotonic duodenography (see Chapter 13).

Angiography (see Chapter 13).

Radioisotopic techniques are generally considered of only moderate usefulness and are outside the scope of this text.

Peroral pancreaticobiliary ductography (see Chapter 13).

Transduodenal pancreatic ductography (see Chapter 13).

THE ADRENAL GLANDS (SUPRARENALS)

Gross Anatomy. The adrenal glands are two small glands that lie upon the superior poles of each kidney, and are 3 to 5 cm. in height, 3 cm. in width, and 1 to 2 cm. in anteroposterior thickness. Each is composed of a thick cortex, a medulla of chromaffin tissue, and each lies within Gerota's capsule, which also surrounds the kidney.

The right adrenal is rather pyramidal in shape, having its anterior surface laterally in contact with the liver and with the inferior vena cava, its posterior surface with the diaphragm, and its base with the kidney below. Both of its sides are concave and its general appearance is that of a "cocked hat."

The left gland is more semilunar in shape. Anteriorly it is in contact with the stomach above, the pancreas below, and the diaphragm posteriorly; its base touches the left kidney below it. The left adrenal lies as much medial to the left kidney as above it, in contrast to the right adrenal, which caps the kidney. The amount of peritoneum covering the gland is variable. The right gland is more medial and lower in relation to the spine than the left.

The dimensions, weight, and area of the suprarenal gland as gathered from the literature are summarized in Table 15–6. It is

TABLE 15–6 DIMENSIONS, WEIGHT, AND AREA OF THE SUPRARENAL GLAND

Reference	Length	Width	Thickness	Weight	Area Right	Area Left
Herbut	3–5 cm.	2–4 cm.	0.4–0.6 cm.	3.5–5 Gm.		
Soffer	4–6 cm.	2–3 cm.	0.2–0.8 cm.	3–5 Gm.		
Steinbach and Smith					2.0–7.8 (aver. 4.2) sq. cm.	2.0–8.7 (aver. 4.3) sq. cm.

apparent from these tabular notations that although the normal suprarenal gland may vary considerably in size, its shape is fairly well preserved and its margins are practically always concave (Meyers, 1963). Occasionally, the normal medial border of the left suprarenal gland may be minimally convex.

The adrenals, unlike the kidneys, are firmly fixed at their apices and hence, in the erect position there is a tendency for the renal structures to separate from the suprarenal.

In the infant, the adrenal gland is relatively large—the fetal cortex in particular is larger in proportion to the rest of the gland during the prenatal months, beginning with approximately the seventh month. The cortex gradually diminishes proportionately to age 2, when its relationship to the medulla is stabilized and remains relatively constant thereafter. The decrease in weight of the gland is rapid during the first months of extrauterine life but it slows down after this period. After the first postnatal year the glands enlarge slowly and continue to grow progressively until puberty, with final weights of approximately 5 gm. (Warwick

and Williams). The female suprarenal gland usually is slightly larger than that of the male. The left gland is usually slightly larger than the right (Anson).

Blood Supply (Fig. 15–67).   The suprarenal glands receive an abundant blood supply, and this has become increasingly important clinically. There are three arteries or groups of arteries supplying the glands: (1) single or multiple branches *from the phrenic artery,* (2) single or multiple branches directly *from the aorta* (the middle suprarenal), and (3) single or multiple renal branches directly *from the renal arteries* on each side.

Most of the branches are short. The middle suprarenal arising from the aorta may be absent and there may be variable branches from the gonadal arteries or arteries from the renal pelves or cortex as well.

One large vein arises from a central part of the medulla of each gland and drains most of the blood from each suprarenal gland. Blood from the left gland empties into the left renal vein, whereas blood from the right gland empties directly into the infe-

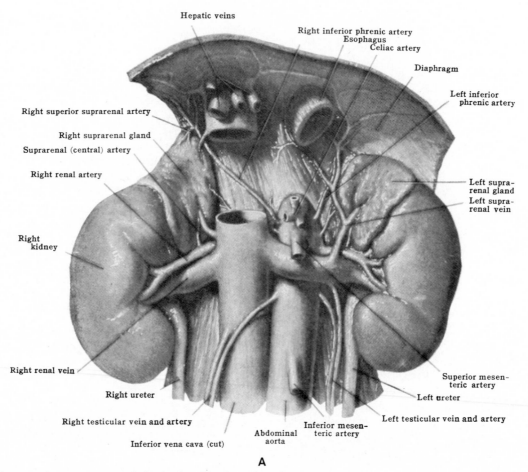

A

Figure 15–67.   A. Suprarenal glands, their blood supply and relationships to adjacent retroperitoneal structures. (From Anson, B. J. (ed.): Morris' Human Anatomy, 12th ed. Copyright © 1966 by McGraw-Hill, Inc. Used by permission of McGraw-Hill Book Company.)

Figure 15–67 continued on the opposite page.

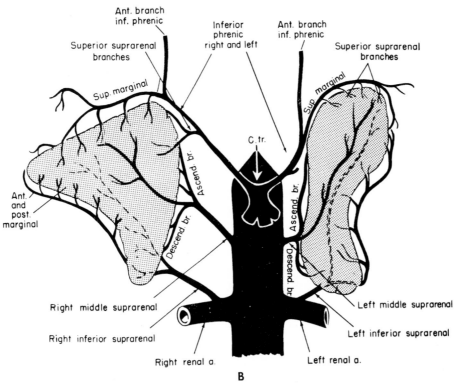

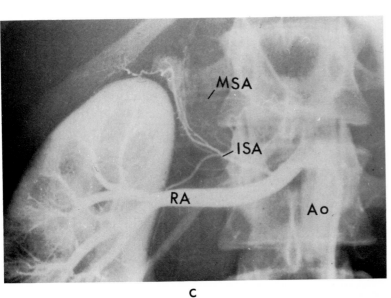

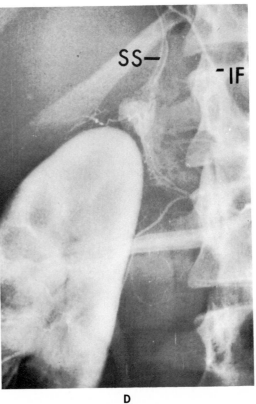

Figure 15–67 *Continued.* B. Schematic diagram of adrenal circulation. After Gérard. Some of the variations are discussed in the text. (From Kahn, P. C., and Nickrosz, L. V.: Amer. J. Roentgenol., *101:*739–749, 1967.) C to E. Close-up views of adrenal arterial supply and capillary phase.

Figure 15–67 continued on the *following* page.

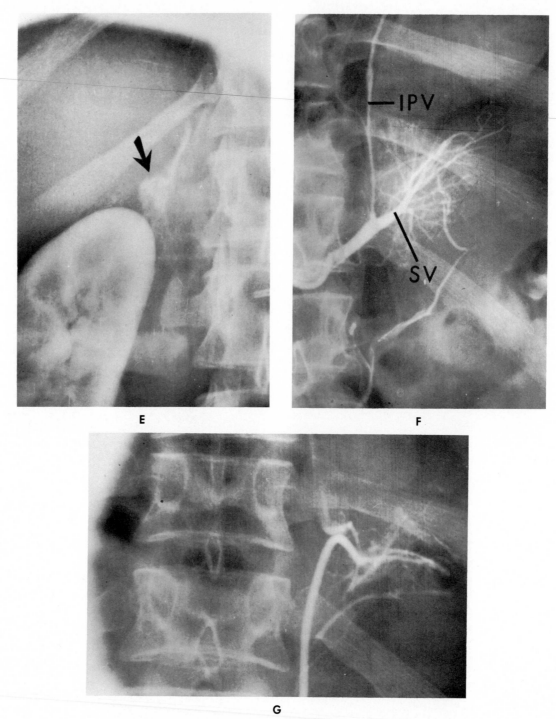

Figure 15–67 *Continued.*　*F* and *G*. Close-up views of adrenal vein.

rior vena cava. Because of the greater constancy and relative simplicity of the topography of the suprarenal veins, they are considered by some investigators to be more significant for investigation than the arteries. Displacement of these vessels or alterations in the branching pattern or types of vessels provide clues to the abnormal morphology of the suprarenal gland.

Method of Study by Perirenal Air Insufflation (Fig. 15–68). This method involves the introduction of air, oxygen, or carbon dioxide directly into the perirenal areolar tissue by needle puncture through the lumbar triangle. Several hundred cubic centimeters are usually necessary, and 12 to 24 hours must elapse to allow for proper distribution of air around the kidney and adrenal gland. Stereoscopic anteroposterior and lateral films are obtained at 24 hour intervals for approximately 3 days. Occasionally, the gas diffuses over to the opposite side, and a bilateral visualization is obtained.

When oxygen is used, the examination must be carried out more quickly, since most of this gaseous medium will be absorbed in about 6 hours. Carbon dioxide has been proposed as the safest gaseous medium to employ, since large volumes of this gas can be introduced directly into the blood stream without untoward results. However, the absorption of carbon dioxide is so rapid that diagnostic radiographic detail is impaired. With proper technique, carbon dioxide may well be the best medium to employ for this purpose.

The presacral route has achieved greater popularity for insufflation of gases around the renal and suprarenal areas (Fig. 15–68). In this technique, the needle is inserted through the skin outside the anus into the tela subserosa between the rectum and the sacrum. A finger is placed in the rectum during the needle insertion to help guide its positioning. Approximately 1000 cc. of gas are introduced. During the next 2 hours, the patient is rotated frequently.

When air is used, an initial film of the suprarenal area is obtained at the 2 hour interval and hourly thereafter until maximal visualization is obtained. At this time, it is well to perform intravenous pyelograms, and once again appropriate films of the suprarenal area are obtained. Oblique and stereoscopic films as well as body section radiographs (5 to 10 cm. from posterior) are now used to aid in the diagnosis.

The adrenal gland on the right is thereafter seen as a pyramidal structure capping the right kidney, and the left adrenal as a semilunar-shaped structure partially capping and medial to the left kidney.

Gas embolism has been described as one of the unfortunate complications of this procedure and, for that reason, it cannot be used indiscriminately as it is never completely without hazard.

In the survey reported by McLelland et al., in a total of 11,422 procedures there were 122 cases of severe gas embolism, of which 58 ended fatally (Ransom et al.).

With *retroperitoneal pneumography* the films recommended by Meyers are: (1) both supine posterior obliques, (2) anteroposterior erect, (3) body section radiographic cuts at 1 cm. intervals between 6 and 12 cm. from the posterior, and (4) a 24 hour film if oxygen is used. If air or oxygen is used, a scout film centered over the suprarenals is obtained 2 hours after the injection and hourly thereafter until maximum visualization is obtained. Excretory urograms and nephrotomograms may be combined with this procedure at this time.

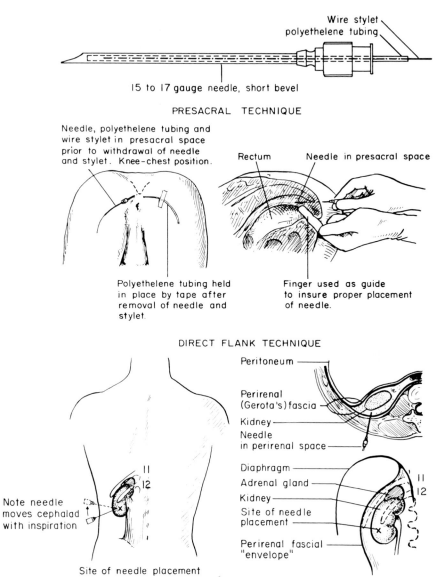

Figure 15–68. Diagrams illustrating the direct flank and presacral techniques for retroperitoneal pneumography. (From McLelland, R., Landes, R. R., and Ransom, C. L.: Radiol. Clin. N. Amer., 3:116, 1965.)

Normal retroperitoneal pneumograms are illustrated in Figure 15–69.

Adrenal Arteriography. Although generally the three adrenal arteries already described represent the main blood supply of the adrenal gland, more than one adrenal branch arises directly from the aorta in approximately 30 per cent of cases. There are a number of other variations (Gagnon). The *middle* adrenal artery traverses laterally to the posterior surface of the adrenal gland where it breaks up into a number of twigs (4 or 5) just barely visible on the radiograph. The *superior* adrenal arteries supply the

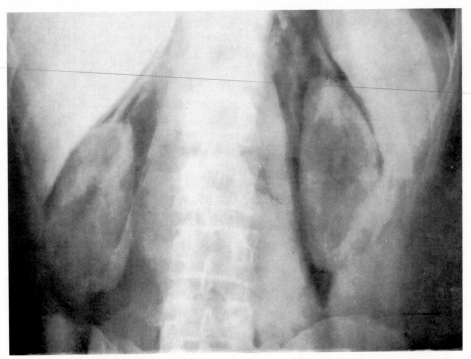

Figure 15–69. Normal retroperitoneal pneumogram. (From McLelland, R., Landes, R. R., and Ransom, C. L.: Radiol. Clin. N. Amer., 3:115, 1965.)

upper pole of the adrenal gland and arise principally from the inferior phrenic arteries. These branch off the aorta just above the celiac axis usually. At times, however, the inferior phrenic arises below the celiac or even from the renal artery itself. The adrenal arteries are actually a number of twigs arising from the inferior phrenic and its posterior division. The inferior adrenal arteries arise from the renal arteries either directly or with the superior renal capsular branch. Other adrenal branches may arise from the gonadal arteries.

Technique. Midline abdominal aortograms may be sufficient for opacification of the adrenal arteries and glands. The Valsalva maneuver improves this visualization by slowing down the aortic blood flow, and by separating to some extent the kidneys and adrenals. Intra-arterial epinephrine or norepinephrine may also improve visualization. This is particularly helpful because it reduces the vascularization of surrounding organs that might interfere. Unfortunately, epinephrine may produce undesirable effects by constriction of the spinal arteries.

Selective catheterization of the three main blood vessels of supply is feasible.

A series of 6 to 8 films spaced over 8 to 12 seconds is usually sufficient for the purpose and the frontal projection may be supplemented by a right posterior oblique for the right adrenal gland, and left posterior oblique for the left.

The Normal Adrenal Arteriogram. The cortex of the adrenal gland can usually be identified as a dense blush about 2 mm. wide. The medulla is relatively less opaque, and the adrenal vein appears later in the film sequence. Examples are shown in Figure 15–67. Multiple injections are usually required to opacify the entire adrenal gland. Unfortunately, confusing shadows caused by opacification of surrounding organs may occur.

Adrenal Venography. Since each adrenal gland drains by only one vein (Figs. 15–67 and 16–70) injection of the adrenal veins is a valuable study, particularly for demonstration of filling defects within these glands.

There are no valves in adrenal veins. On the right side there are three main tributaries to the renal vein—inferolateral, ventromedial, and posterior. The junction of these three veins occurs near the top or the middle of the gland, thus forming the adrenal vein, usually about 3 mm. in diameter and rarely exceeding 10 mm. in length. The right adrenal vein usually drains into the inferior vena cava about 3 to 4 cm. above the right renal vein and near the T12 vertebra. This occurs in very close proximity to or in conjunction with the hepatic vein. On the left side there are four main venous trunks: inferolateral, ventral, medial, and posterior. The left adrenal vein is usually 20 to 40 mm. long, and it is joined by the left inferior phrenic vein about 15 to 20 mm. below the left adrenal gland. A renal capsular vein often joins the adrenal, and communications occur to other veins such as the gonadal, lumbar, and hemiazygos. The left adrenal vein therefore empties into the left renal vein on its upper surface to the left of the aorta near the point at which the renal vein crosses the lateral border of the vertebral body.

Technique. Superselective adrenal vein catheterization is different on each side and special configuration of the catheter has to be devised. For percutaneous femoral catheterization, two catheters each different in design must usually be employed (Kahn). For specifics of technique the student is referred to Kahn.

The contrast agent should be injected gently to avoid rupture of the gland, even though this causes some inevitable discomfort to the patient. The volume varies from 0.5 to 5 ml., depending on the location of the catheter tip. Single films or short serial sequential films are utilized. Frontal and oblique projections are recommended. On the right side in the right oblique view, the inferior vena cava is superimposed over the gland and in the left oblique, the spine is superimposed, unfortunately. Adrenal vein ruptures may occur in 5 to 10 per cent of cases, even in experienced hands.

Normal Adrenal Venograms. The adrenal veins are very thin and sinuous. The adrenal glands can be measured by means of venography—normally the area should be less than 17 sq. cm. (Reuter et al.). Usually some veins outside the adrenal are also seen. Unfortunately, also, a hepatic vein may be injected by mistake and great care must be exercised so that a false interpretation does not result.

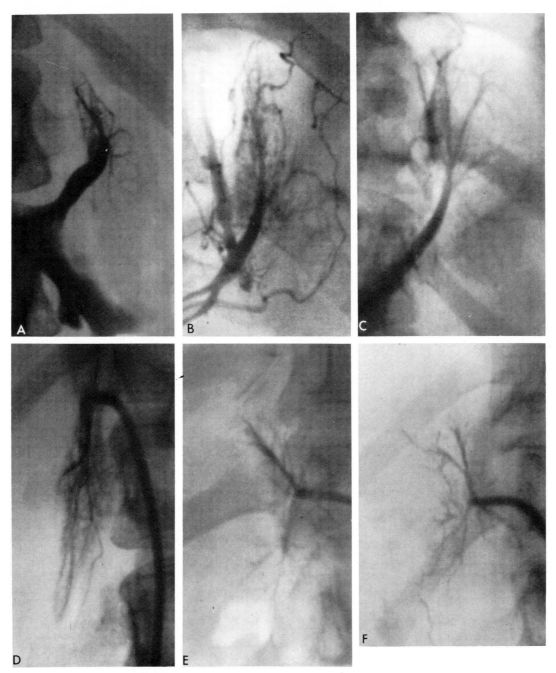

Figure 15–70.   Adrenal venography in the anteroposterior projection. Appearance of normal left adrenal glands. *A.* Small normal gland (4 cm.²) in a 90 lb. woman without biochemical evidence of adrenal abnormality. *B.* Larger normal gland with single central vein (9.4 cm.²) in a 165 lb. man. The gland was removed because of primary aldosteronism. A nodule 2 mm. in diameter was found. The gland weighed 9.3 g. The large vein medial to the adrenal gland is the inferior phrenic vein. *C.* Large normal gland with two central veins (16.7 cm.²) in a 209 lb. woman without biochemical evidence of adrenal abnormality.

Adrenal venography in the anteroposterior projection. Appearance of normal right adrenal glands. *D.* The main adrenal vein drains the length of the gland and exits at the top. *E.* A main adrenal vein exiting at the mid-portion of the gland receives two primary branches. *F.* A main adrenal vein exiting at the mid-portion of the gland receives three primary branches. (From Reuter, S. R., Blair, A. J., Schteingart, D. E., and Bookstein, J. J.: Radiology, *89:805–814*, 1967.)

REFERENCES

Abrams, H. L. (ed.): Angiography, Vol. 2. Second edition. Boston, Little, Brown & Co., 1971.

Anson, B. (ed.): Morris' Human Anatomy, 12th edition. New York, McGraw-Hill, 1966.

Arvidsson, H.: Angiocardiographic measurements in congenital heart disease. Acta Radiol. (Diag.), *1*:981–994, 1963.

Berdon, W. E., Baker, D. H., and Leonidas, J.: Advantages of prone positioning in gastrointestinal and genitourinary roentgenologic studies in infants and children. Amer. J. Roentgenol., *103*:444–455, 1968.

Bierman, H. C.: Selective Arterial Catheterization. Springfield, Ill., Charles C Thomas, 1969.

Bron, K. M.: Thrombotic occlusion of the abdominal aorta. Amer. J. Roentgenol., *96*:887–895, 1966.

Budin, E., and Jacobson, G.: Roentgenographic diagnosis of small amounts of intraperitoneal fluid. Amer. J. Roentgenol., *99*:62–70, 1967.

Campbell, R. E.: Roentgenologic features of umbilical vascular catheterization in the newborn. Amer. J. Roentgenol., *112*:68–76, 1971.

Cimmino, C. V.: Further experiences with the roentgenology of the paracolonic gutter. Radiology, *90*:761–764, 1968.

Coopwood, T. B., and Bricker, D. L.: Paraduodenal hernias. South. Med. J., *65*:1138–1141, 1972.

Cunningham, D. J.: Manual of Practical Anatomy, Vol. 2. 12th edition. London, Oxford University Press, 1959.

Ferris, E. J., Vittimberga, F. J., Byrne, J. J., Nabseth, D. C., and Shapiro, J. H.: The inferior vena cava after ligation and plication. Radiology, *89*:1–10, 1967.

Franken, E. A.: Ascites in infants and children. Radiology, *102*:393–398, 1972.

Gagnon, R.: The arterial supply of the human adrenal gland. Rev. Canad. Biol., *16*:421, 1957.

Gagnon, R.: Middle suprarenal arteries in man: a statistical study of 200 human adrenal glands. Rev. Canad. Biol., *23*:461, 1964.

Grupp, G., Grupp, I. L., and Spitz, H. B.: Collateral vascular pathways during experimental obstruction of aorta and inferior vena cava. Amer. J. Roentgenol., *94*:159–171, 1965.

Hansmann, G. H., and Morton, S. A.: Intra-abdominal hernia, report of a case and review of the literature. Arch. Surg., *39*:973–986, 1939.

Herbut, P. A.: Urologic Pathology, Vol. 2. Philadelphia, Lea and Febiger, 1952.

Herman, P. G., Benninghoff, D. L., Nelson, J. H., Jr., and Mellins, H. Z.: Roentgen anatomy of the ilio-pelvic-aortic lymphatic system. Radiology, *80*:182–193, 1963.

Hillman, D. C., and Tristan, T. A.: Inferior cavography in the detection of abdominal extension of pelvic cancer. Radiology, *81*:416–427, 1963.

Kahn, P. C.: Adrenal venography. *In* Abrams, H. L. (ed.): Angiography, Vol. 2. Second edition. Boston, Little, Brown & Co., 1971. Pp. 941–950.

Kahn, P. C., and Nickrosz, L. V.: Angiography of the adrenal glands. Amer. J. Roentgenol., *101*:739–749, 1967.

McLelland, R., Landes, R. R., and Ransom, C. I.: Retroperitoneal pneumography: A safe method using carbon dioxide. Radiol. Clin. N. Amer., *3*:113–128, 1965.

Meyers, M. A.: Diseases of the Adrenal Gland: Radiological Diagnosis. Springfield, Ill., Charles C Thomas, 1963.

Meyers, M. A.: Peritoneography. Amer. J. Roentgenol., *117*:353–363, 1973.

Meyers, M. A.: The spread and localization of acute intraperitoneal effusions. Radiology, *95*:547–554, 1970.

Meyers, M. A., and Whalen, J. P.: Roentgen significance of the duodenal colic relationships: an anatomic approach. Amer. J. Roentgenol., *117*:263–274, 1973.

Michels, N. A.: The variational anatomy of the spleen and splenic arteries. Amer. J. Anat., *70*:21, 1942.

Michels, N. A.: Blood Supply and Anatomy of the Upper Abdominal Organs. Philadelphia, J. B. Lippincott Co., 1955.

Pansky, B., and House, E. L.: Review of Gross Anatomy. New York, Macmillan, 1964.

Ransom, C. L., Landes, R. R., and McLelland, R.: Air embolism following retroperitoneal pneumography: a nationwide survey. J. Urol., *76*:664, 1956.

Reuter, S. R., Blair, A. J., Schteingart, D. E., and Bookstein, J. J.: Adrenal venography. Radiology, *89*:805–814, 1967.

Rösch, J.: Roentgenologic possibilities in spleen diagnosis. Amer. J. Roentgenol., *94*:453–461, 1965 (27 references).

Soffer, L. S.: Diseases of the Endocrine Glands. Philadelphia, Lea and Febiger, 1951.

Steinbach, H. L., and Smith, K. L.: Extraperitoneal pneumography in diagnosis of retroperitoneal tumors. Arch. Surg., *70*:161–172, 1955.

Steinberg, C. R., Archer, M., and Steinberg, I.: Measurement of the abdominal aorta after intravenous aortography in health and arteriosclerotic peripheral vascular disease. Amer. J. Roentgenol., *95*:703–708, 1965.

Swischuk, L. E., and Stacy, T. M.: Herniography: radiologic investigation of inguinal hernia. Radiology, *101*:139–146, 1971.

Walker, L. A., and Weens, H. S.: Radiological observations on the lesser peritoneal sac. Radiology, *90*:727–737, 1963.

Warwick, R., and Williams, P. L.: Gray's Anatomy. 35th British edition. London, Faber and Faber, 1973.

Whalen, J. P., Berne, A. S., and Riemenschneider, P. A.: The extraperitoneal perivisceral fat pad. 1. Its role in the roentgenologic evaluation of abdominal organs. Radiology, *92*:466–472, 1969.

Whalen, J. P., Berne, A. S., and Riemenschneider, P. A.: The extraperitoneal perivisceral fat pad. 2. Roentgen interpretations of pathologic alterations. Radiology, *92*:473–480, 1969.

Whalen, J. P., Evans, J. A., and Shanser, J.: Vector principle in the differential diagnosis of abdominal masses. 1. The left upper quadrant. Amer. J. Roentgenol., *113*:104–124, 1971.

Whalen, J. P., Evans, J. A., and Meyers, M. A.: Vector principle in the differential diagnosis of abdominal masses. 2. Right upper quadrant. Amer. J. Roentgenol., *115*:318–333, 1972.

White, J. J., Parks, L. C., and Haller, J. A.: The inguinal herniagram: a radiologic aid for accurate diagnosis of inguinal hernia in infants. Surgery, *63*:991–997, 1968.

Wyman, A. C.: Traumatic rupture of the spleen. Amer. J. Roentgenol., *72*:51–63, 1954.

16

The Urinary Tract

The urinary tract consists of the following major structures: (1) the kidneys—one on each side, (2) the ureters, (3) the urinary bladder, and (4) the urethra.

CORRELATED GROSS AND MICROSCOPIC ANATOMY OF THE URINARY TRACT

The Kidneys

The kidneys are paired, retroperitoneal, bean-shaped organs lying on each side of the vertebral column. The exact relationships of the kidney to the vertebral column are indicated in Figure 16–1. Thus, the distance in centimeters cranially and caudally of the poles of normal adult kidneys from the middle of L2 vertebra in plain roentgenograms is shown for both male and female (plus or minus two standard deviations). Usually the left kidney is slightly higher than the right and the upper pole is approximately 4 cm. closer to the midline than the lower pole. The angle between the longitudinal axis of the kidneys and the midline within two standard deviations is shown in Figure 16–1 C for both male and female. On the right side in the male this approximates 19.4 degrees; on the left side, 18.9 degrees. For the female, on the right side, the angle of the longitudinal axis of the kidneys to the midline approximates 17.1 degrees, and on the left side, 15.8 degrees.

Normal Kidney Size. The right kidney is usually slightly smaller than the left. A number of different methods of measurement of the kidneys are available.

Table 16–1 shows the normal adult renal size in absolute measurements, plus or minus two standard deviations.

Simon has reported the ratio of renal adult cephalocaudad lengths to height of the second lumbar vertebral body (plus disk) to be 3.7 ± 0.37, with a statistical range of normal values between 3.0 and 4.4 cm. (Meschan, Martin).

Normal measurements in adults and children in relation to body height and age are indicated in Table 16–2. Kidney length increases with age until approximately age 20 in both men and women, and begins to diminish somewhat in the cephalocaudad

dimension from about age 50. In children, kidney length increases progressively with body height; and in adults, similarly, kidney length is related to body height but with a lesser angle of inclination.

These data summarize renal size as studied by Hodson in normal children. The mean kidney length in children varies from 6 cm. with a body height of 24 inches to 12 cm. with a body height of 72 inches. The size of the kidney depends largely on the size of the child. Body height is probably the most reliable guide, since it is less liable to rapid fluctuation than is body weight. Between 4 and 15 years, there is a steady mean increase per year of 0.35 cm. and 5 cm. in kidney length and body height, respectively.

Friedenberg et al. utilized a *renal index* for measurement of kidney size, as shown in Figure 16–2. The renal index in this instance is defined as the product of the length and width of the kidney divided by the body surface area of the patient in square meters.

The left and right renal indices for children are shown in Figure 16–3 A and B. The left-minus-right renal index for children is shown in Figure 16–3 C. Similarly, the left and right renal indices and the left-minus-right index for adult males are shown in Figure 16–4. Figure 16–5 contains similar information for adult females.

Currarino related the length in centimeters of four lumbar vertebral bodies to kidney length for various age groups in children and found (Fig. 16–6) that the length of each kidney corresponded closely to the length of this segment of the lumbar spine plus or minus 1 cm. throughout childhood, with the exception of the first 1 to 1½ years of life in which the length of a normal kidney was greater.

It is important to compare the kidney size on each side of the patient. Discrepancies between the two kidneys of greater than 1 cm. are of considerable significance. Generally, a difference in length of the two kidneys up to 1 cm. may occur normally, especially in children (Currarino). Elkin, in comparing the kidneys of the two sides, found that the average left kidney measurement is greater than the right—the difference between the two sides varying from 1 to 9 per cent. This calculation is based upon the product of the horizontal and vertical measurements of the

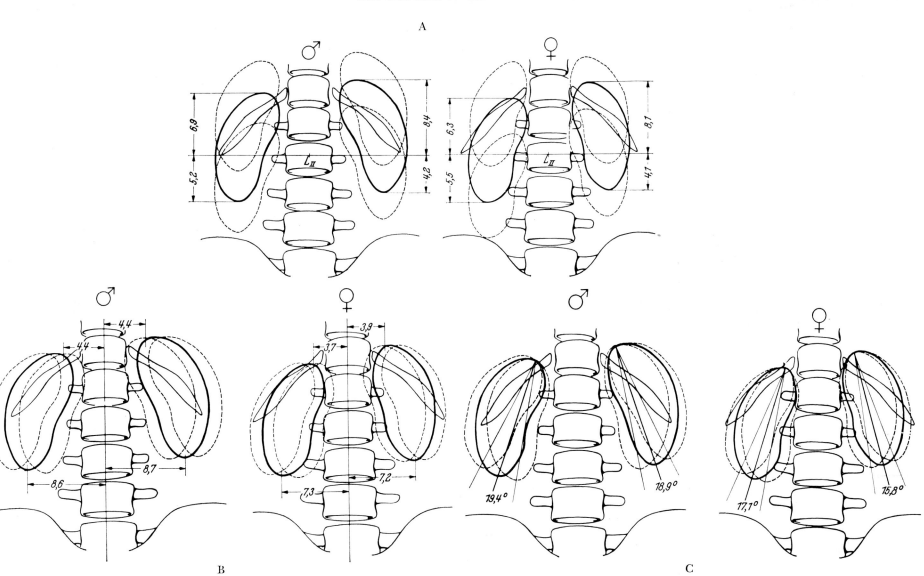

Figure 16–1. A. Distances in centimeters cranially and caudally from the middle of vertebra L-II, of the poles of normal adult kidneys in plain roentgenograms. Dotted lines indicate ± 2s. B. Distances in centimeters of the cranial and caudal poles of normal adult kidneys from the midline in plain roentgenograms. Dotted lines indicate ± 2s. C. The angle between the longitudinal axis of the kidneys and the midline. Dotted lines indicate ± 2s. (After Moell, H.: Acta Radiologica, 46:640–645, 1956.)

TABLE 16–1 NORMAL ADULT RENAL SIZE
(THE MEAN PLUS OR MINUS TWO STANDARD DEVIATIONS)[a]
(Modified after Moell)

Male:	Right kidney	Vertical: 11.3–14.5 cm.
		Width: 5.4– 7.2 cm.
	Left	Vertical: 11.6–14.8 cm.
		Width: 5.3– 7.1 cm.
Female:	Right kidney	Vertical: 10.7–13.9 cm.
		Width: 4.8– 6.6 cm.
	Left	Vertical: 11.1–14.3 cm.
		Width: 5.1– 6.9 cm.

[a]Standard deviation = 0.8 cm. for vertical dimension.

two kidneys in centimeters. Because this measurement was developed particularly to note kidney size in acute ureteral obstruction, it was arbitrarily determined that differences of greater than 11 per cent were significant. However, if the right kidney were larger than the left by a smaller percentage, this could also present a criterion for enlargement.

Kidney Mobility. There is considerable mobility of the kidneys during respiration. Normally, the range of movement is about 3 cm. less on the right side than on the left and is somewhat larger for women than for men. However, on deeper inspiration excursion up to 10 cm. may be recorded.

TABLE 16–2*

RADIOGRAPHIC SIZE OF THE KIDNEY

Department of X-ray Diagnosis
University College Hospital
London, England

NORMAL MEASUREMENTS IN ADULTS AND CHILDREN

This chart is published in response to considerable demand by radiologists and clinicians for graphic data on the size of normal kidneys as determined from radiographs. The size of a normal kidney varies widely from person to person, depending on the number and distribution of calyces and the actual shape of the organ, making accurate estimation of the size of an individual kidney difficult. However, knowledge that a kidney is larger or smaller than average has considerable significance.

Good radiographic definition of the renal outline of a majority of patients is a simple matter, provided the patient is prepared properly.
Good definition of the renal outline of infants and bedridden patients is more difficult to obtain, however, and usually tomography or localized abdominal compression must be used.

The graphs have been found useful in the interpretation of radiographs, especially those of children. Statistically, the graphs are valid.
In particular, the one relating to children shows an unusually close relation between the length of the kidney and the height of the body throughout the period of growth. The simple relation of length of kidney to height of body or to age and sex was chosen because statistically this measurement is as satisfactory as others more complicated.[1,2]

TECHNICAL POINTS

A. The data were derived using a target-film distance of 36 inches (91.5 cm). Radiographs made at a target-film distance of 40 inches (101.8 cm) would show a 2 percent reduction in the size of the kidney.

B. For the normal kidney, 68 percent of the readings lie within the range of mean plus or minus 1 standard deviation; 99.5 percent lie within the range of mean plus or minus 2½ times the standard deviation.

REFERENCES

1. Karn, M. N.: Radiographic Measurements of Kidney Section Area. **Ann. Hum. Genet., 25**:379-385, May, 1962.

2. Hodson, C. J.; Drewe, J. A.; Karn, M. N., and King, A.: Renal Size in Normal Children. A Radiographic Study During Life. **Arch. Dis. Child., 37**:616-622, December, 1962.

BIBLIOGRAPHY

Hodson, C. J.: Radiology of the Kidney. In Black, D. A. K. (editor): **Renal Disease.** Published by F. A. Davis Company, Philadelphia, Pennsylvania, and Blackwell Scientific Publications, Oxford, England, 1962, pp. 388-417.

Möell, H.: Kidney Size and Its Deviation from Normal in Acute Renal Failure. A Roentgenographic Study. **Acta Radiol.**, Supp. 206, 1961, pp. 5-74.

Panichi, S., and Bonechi, I.: Il volume del rene in condizioni normali. **Boll. Soc. Medicochir. Pisa, 26**:611-614, November-December, 1958.

Vuorinen, P.; Anttila, P.; Wegelius, U.; Kauppila, A., and Koivisto, E.: Renal Cortical Index and Other Roentgenographic Renal Measurements. **Acta Radiol.**, Supp. 211, 1962, pp. 5-54.

EASTMAN KODAK COMPANY
Radiography Markets Division
Rochester, N.Y. 14650

Kidney Length/Body Height—Adults
Men—Standard Deviation = 1.098 cm   Women—Standard Deviation = 0.993 cm

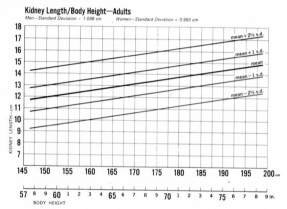

Kidney Length/Age—Men
Standard Deviation = 1.02 cm

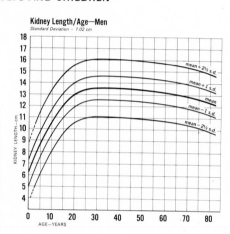

Kidney Length/Body Height—Children
Standard Deviation = 1.529 cm

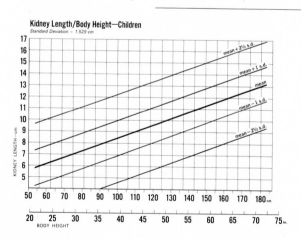

Kidney Length/Age—Women
Standard Deviation = 1.02 cm

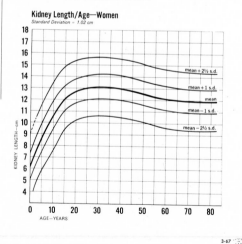

M4-8A   3-67

*Courtesy Radiography Markets Division, Eastman Kodak Company.

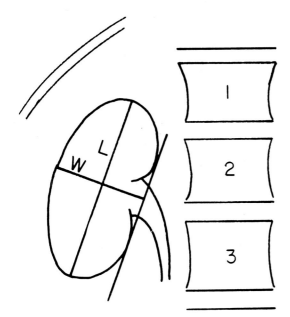

Figure 16-2. Line drawing of the right kidney region to demonstrate the method of measuring renal size (see text). Length of kidney in centimeters is indicated by *L* and width in centimeters by *W*. Renal index is calculated as follows: $RI = L \times W/BSA$, where *BSA* is the body surface area of the patient in square meters. (From Friedenberg, M. J. et al.: Radiology, 84:1022–1029, 1965.)

A maximum excursion of 5 cm. (or 1½ vertebral bodies) occurs in the change from the recumbent to the erect position.

Gondos has recommended that measurements of the kidneys be made from a film taken with the patient prone, suggesting that in this position renal rotation is reduced or eliminated.

Renal Shape. Normally, the kidney is bean-shaped. Fetal lobulation (Fig. 16-7), however, is frequently encountered in children and tends to occur in three basic patterns, as illustrated in Figure 16-12 *A* (Cooperman and Lowman): (1) there may be a local bulge of the lateral border of the left kidney; (2) the left kidney may be triangular, and somewhat enlarged; (3) there may be a diffuse multilobulated form that is either unilateral or bilateral.

Additionally, lobulation may indicate partial or complete duplication of one kidney that may be without special pathologic significance. To make absolutely certain of this, usually complete study, sometimes including nephrotomography and arteriography, is necessary.

The medial border of the kidney is concave and contains a slitlike aperture, the hilus. This is the orifice of a cavity called the *renal sinus*, which is about 2.5 cm. in depth and contains the following structures: (1) the renal *pelvis* and *calyces;* (2) the branches of the *renal artery* before their entrance into the actual substance of the kidney, and the tributaries of the *renal vein* after their exit; (3) the *lymph vessels* and *nerves* of the kidney; and (4) small amounts of *fat* around and among the other structures (Fig. 16-8).

There are usually 8 to 10 *renal papillae* which protrude into the renal sinus, but there may be as few as 4 or as many as 18 (Anson).

The "Edge Pattern" of the Kidney. The surface of the kidney is invested by a thin but strong fibrous capsule. External to it is a considerable quantity of fat tissue known as the *adipose capsule* (Gerota's capsule). It is this fatty tissue envelope that permits identification of the kidney on plain radiographs, since it is considerably more radiolucent than the surrounding muscular structures. On the other hand, perirenal inflammations or neo-

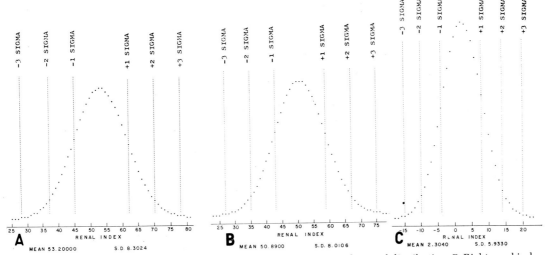

Figure 16-3. *A.* Left renal index—children. Frequency plot of theoretical normal distribution. *B.* Right renal index—children. Frequency plot of theoretical normal distribution. *C.* Left minus right renal index—children. Frequency plot of theoretical normal distribution. (From Friedenberg, M. J. et al.: Radiology, 84:1022–1029, 1965.)

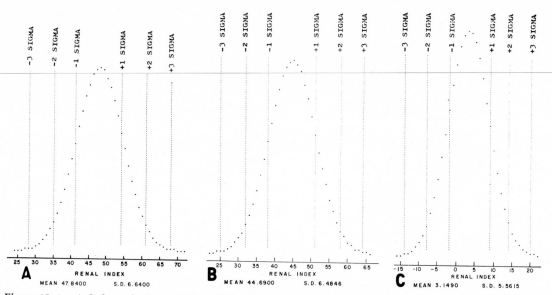

Figure 16–4. *A.* Left renal index—adult males. Frequency plot of theoretical normal distribution. *B.* Right renal index—adult males. Frequency plot of theoretical normal distribution. *C.* Left minus right renal index—adult males. Frequency plot of theoretical normal distribution. (From Friedenberg, M. J. et al.: Radiology, *84:*1022–1029, 1965.)

plasms may invade this fatty envelope and impair good detail, and this is a roentgen sign of abnormality. It is this adipose capsule which is continuous with the tela subserosa and which is insufflated with air or oxygen in the performance of perirenal air insufflation studies.

Relationship of the Kidney to Other Retroperitoneal Structures. Each kidney is retroperitoneal alongside the last thoracic and upper three lumbar vertebrae, the left usually being higher than the right.

Posteriorly, the kidneys lie on a muscle bed composed of the

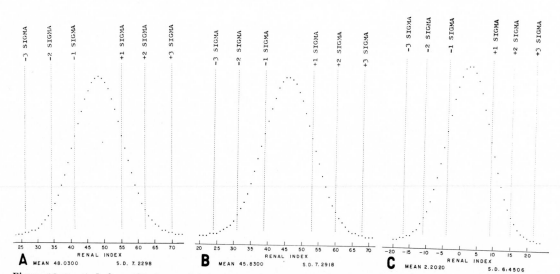

Figure 16–5. *A.* Left renal index—adult females. Frequency plot of theoretical normal distribution. *B.* Right renal index—adult females. Frequency plot of theoretical normal distribution. *C.* Left minus right renal index—adult females. Frequency plot of theoretical normal distribution. (From Friedenberg, M. J. et al.: Radiology, *84:*1022–1029, 1965.)

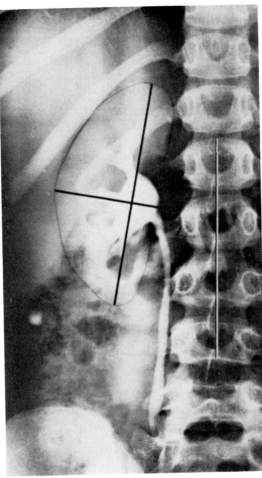

A

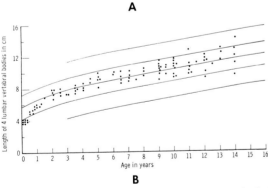

B

Figure 16–6. *A.* Comparative measurement of the length of the kidney and the length of a segment of the lumbar spine, comprising the four upper lumbar vertebral bodies and the three intervertebral spaces between them. *B.* Graph of the length of the comparative lumbar spine segment, as measured by the method shown in *A,* superimposed on the graph for kidney length of Hodson et al. (*A* and *B* from Currarino, G.: Amer. J. Roentgenol., *93*:464, 1965.)

diaphragm, the psoas major, quadratus lumborum, and transversus abdominis muscles. The structures intervening between the quadratus lumborum and the kidney are the subcostal vessels and nerves such as the ilio-hypogastric and ilio-inguinal. The dia-

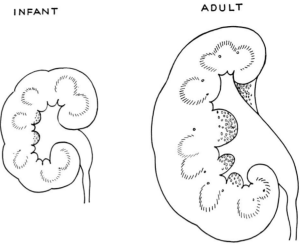

Figure 16–7. Infantile renal lobulation and its comparison with the adult renal contour. (After Caffey.)

phragm separates the upper part of the kidney from the pleura and the twelfth rib.

Anteriorly, the right kidney has the following relationships: the suprarenal gland overlaps its upper end, especially medially, and the duodenum overlaps it along its hilus. The hepatic flexure

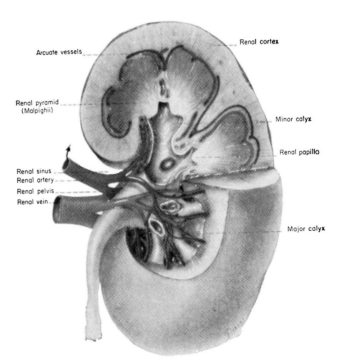

Figure 16–8. Dissection of anterior half of right kidney, showing structures in the renal sinus. (From Anson, B. J. (ed.): Morris' Human Anatomy, 12th ed. Copyright © 1966 by McGraw-Hill, Inc. Used by permission of McGraw-Hill Book Company.)

of the colon covers a considerable part of the lower end of the kidney. Between the colon and the lower part of the duodenum, a small part of the lower end of the kidney is contiguous to the jejunum (Fig. 16–9). The right lobe of the liver tends to overlie the right kidney as well as the other structures named.

The *left kidney anteriorly* has the following relationships (Fig. 16–9 C): the suprarenal gland caps its upper and medial portion, and the spleen borders upon its upper lateral aspects. The body of the pancreas with the splenic vessels lies across the kidney at or near its midsection. The left half of the transverse colon crosses the kidney below the pancreas, and the descending colon overlaps its lower part laterally. A small portion of the lower pole of the left kidney is in contact with the colon but the rest of its anterior surface is covered by the peritoneum. The stomach, the transverse colon, and the jejunum are all separated from the kidney by the peritoneum, and although the spleen is also separated by peritoneum it is attached at one point by the lienorenal ligament.

Longitudinal Section Through the Kidney (Coronal Section) (Fig. 16–10). The substance of the kidney as revealed by

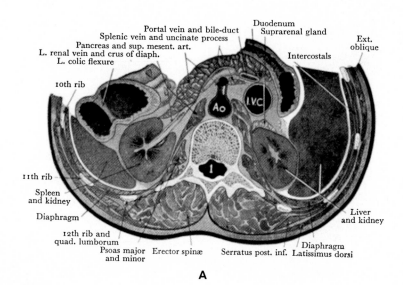

Figure 16–9. *A.* Transverse section through abdomen at the level of the first lumbar vertebra. *B.* Right kidney and duodenum. The relation of the duodenum and the right flexure to the kidney is not so extensive as usual. *C.* Relations of left kidney and pancreas. (From Cunningham's Manual of Practical Anatomy, 12th ed., Vol. 2. London, Oxford University Press, 1958.)

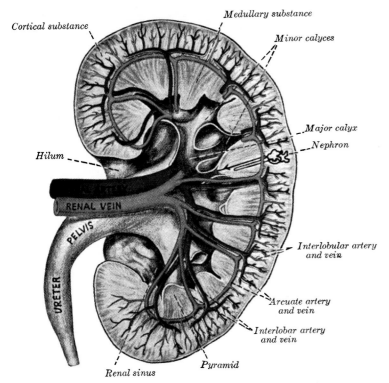

Cortical substance

Medullary substance

Minor calyces

Major calyx

Nephron

Hilum

RENAL VEIN

PELVIS

URETER

Interlobular artery and vein

Arcuate artery and vein

Interlobar artery and vein

Renal sinus

Pyramid

Figure 16–10. Longitudinal section through a normal kidney. (From Gray's Anatomy of the Human Body, 29th ed. Goss, C. M. (ed.) Philadelphia, Lea & Febiger, 1973.)

together are spoken of as a *renal (malpighian) corpuscle*. The renal corpuscles are found only in the cortex and renal columns of the kidney. Extending inward from the glomerular capsule is a *proximal convoluted tubule* which twists considerably before it passes into the *descending limb of Henle's loop* (Fig. 16–11 *B*). Henle's loop extends into the medullary pyramid, but thereafter it reverses its direction, increases in size, and becomes the *ascending limb of Henle's loop*. It then leaves the pyramid to re-enter the cortex and once again twists about as the *distal convoluted tubule*. The tubule becomes narrower and opens with other similar tubules into a *straight* or *collecting tubule*, which descends into the medullary pyramid and unites with other collecting tubules, and then finally it opens as a *papillary duct* into a *renal calyx* at the summit of a papilla.

The *renal pelvis* is a reservoir contained within the renal sinus. Usually it contains two main subdivisions or *major calyces*. The major calyces divide into *minor calyces*, each of which terminates in relation to one, two, or sometimes three renal papillae. The protrusion of papillae into the calyces impart a characteristic cup-shaped appearance to the calyces. Considerable variation occurs in the number of major and minor calyces and shape of the renal pelvis (Fig. 16–12); the pelvis may be *intrarenal* where it lies entirely within the renal sinus, or *extrarenal* where it lies like a dilated sac largely outside the kidney proper (Fig. 16–12 *B*).

Blood Vessels of the Kidney

Arteries. The renal arteries arising from the aorta usually divide into *two main branches* directed anteriorly and posteriorly to the kidney (Fig. 16–13). The *posterior* or *dorsal* branch usually arises first and is somewhat smaller in caliber than the *anterior* or *ventral* branch. Secondary branches from the dorsal and ventral branches supply the *five main renal arterial segments* of the kidney as shown in Figure 16–14. The *apical segment* is usually supplied largely by the posterior or dorsal branch of the renal artery, whereas the *lower segment* is supplied mostly by the anterior or ventral branch. Furthermore, *upper and middle branches* of the anterior segment can usually be identified. This segmental distribution within the kidney takes on practical significance if a surgeon contemplates removal of a small part of the kidney. The renal arteries thereafter branch into *interlobar arteries* between the pyramids (Fig. 16–10). At the bases of the pyramids, the interlobar arteries unite to form the *arcuate* arteries. The arcuate arteries, in turn, send branches into the cortex as the *interlobular arteries,* and these give rise to *afferent glomerular arteries* and some *nutrient* and *perforating capsular arteries*. Arising out of the glomerulus are the *efferent glomerular arteries* which form a capillary network around the nephrons but also give rise to a few *arteriolae rectae*, which enter the medulla and run directly toward the pelvis.

Measurements of the Renal and Splenic Arteries. The renal and splenic arteries may be measured at the place where they in-

this section has three main parts—an external cortex, an internal medulla, and the renal tubules. The *external cortex* is approximately 12 mm. thick and contains numerous renal corpuscles, convoluted tubules, and minute vessels. The cortex is actually composed of two portions: (1) a *peripheral layer*, the cortex proper; and (2) processes called *"renal columns"* which dip inward between renal pyramids to reach the bottom of the sinus of the kidney (Fig. 16–8).

The *internal medulla* contains approximately eight structures called *renal pyramids*. The apices of these pyramids project into the bottom or side of the renal sinus, and into minor calyces of the renal pelvis (Fig. 16–8). The bases of the pyramids form a margin with the cortical substance. Each pyramid contains strandlike structures which converge upon the apex, called the *papilla*, which in turn protrudes into a calyx. The papilla contains a variable number of minute apertures which represent the terminations of *papillary ducts*. The urine passes from these ducts into the renal calyces and thereafter, into the renal pelvis.

The *renal tubules* with their associated glomeruli of blood vessels constitute the essential units of the kidney (Fig. 16–11). Each tubule is composed of a *glomerular capsule* invaginated by a *glomerulus* of blood vessels; the glomerulus and its capsule

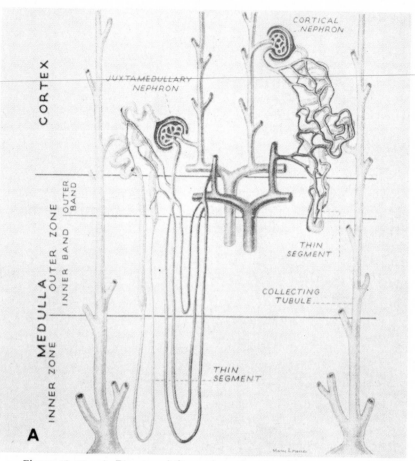

Figure 16–11. A. Diagram of the nephron showing those portions which are situated in the cortex as against those situated in the medulla. The cortical nephron and juxtamedullary nephron are separately shown. (From Smith, H. W.: Principles of Renal Physiology. New York, Oxford University Press, 1956.)

Figure 16–11 continued on the opposite page.

tersect a line 2 cm. from, and parallel to, the lateral border of the aorta, as shown in Figure 16–13 B. When the renal artery bifurcates at a point closer than 2 cm. from the aorta it is measured just proximal to this bifurcation. When a kidney receives more than one artery from the aorta, the equivalent diameter (D) is obtained from the equation:

$$D = 4 \times \sqrt{D1^4 + D2^4 + \ldots Dn^4}$$

in which D1 and D2 are the diameters of two such arteries, and Dn the diameter of the nth such artery.

The *ratio of the internal diameter of the renal artery* to the splenic artery is indicated in the accompanying table. The normal ratio of the renal artery to the splenic artery should be greater than 1. The tabular values are shown within one standard deviation (Maluf).

A narrow renal artery is always indicative of reduced renal function but not renal ischemia; an artery of normal caliber does not necessarily imply normal renal function.

Veins. The renal veins (Fig. 16–13 C) begin in the plexuses around the tubules and correspond closely to the arteriolae rectae and the interlobular, arcuate, and interlobar arteries. There are, however, some veins contained in the fibrous capsule of the kidney known as the *stellate venules* that open into the interlobular veins, and communicate with the veins of the fatty capsule around the kidney.

Anastomoses between the renal and systemic vessels occur in the fat around the kidney where the perforating capsular arteries join branches from suprarenal, gonadal, superior, and inferior mesenteric arteries. The renal veins terminate in the inferior vena cava. The *left* renal is longer than the right, crossing the ventral side of the aorta just below the superior mesenteric artery and opening into the inferior vena cava above the right renal vein. It receives as tributaries the *left inferior phrenic,* the *left internal spermatic,* and the *left suprarenal.* It usually lies above the level of the right renal vein, and dorsal to the renal vein, the body of the pancreas, and splenic vein; the inferior mesenteric vein crosses it ventrally.

The *right* renal vein is short and lies in front of the renal artery with no extrarenal tributaries ordinarily.

Blood Vessels of the Adrenal Glands

As indicated previously, the *arteries of the adrenal glands* are derived from three sources: a *superior* artery *from the phrenic;* a *middle* artery *from the aorta;* and an *inferior* artery *from the renal* itself on each side (see Chapter 15).

The veins generally follow the arteries with *one main vein* from each suprarenal gland derived from its medullary portion.

Lymphatic Channels of the Kidney (Rawson; Lilienfeld et al.). The distribution of the lymphatic channels of the human kidney is shown diagrammatically in Figure 16–13 C. The lymphatic vessels generally follow closely the arterial and venous channels, with the exception of the afferent and efferent arterioles

Figure 16–11 *Continued.* B. Scheme of tubules and vessels of the kidney. (From Anson, B. J. (ed.): Morris' Human Anatomy, 12th ed. Copyright © 1966 by McGraw-Hill, Inc. Used by permission of McGraw-Hill Book Company.)

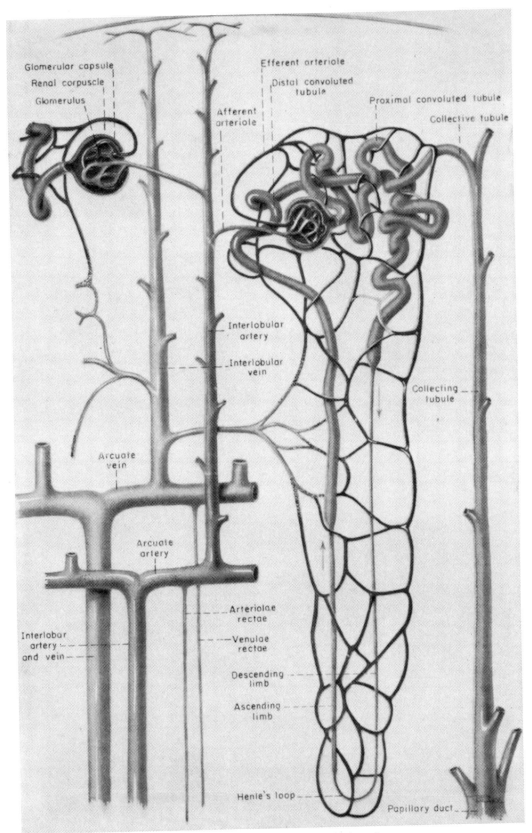

Glomerular capsule
Renal corpuscle
Glomerulus
Efferent arteriole
Distal convoluted tubule
Proximal convoluted tubule
Collective tubule
Afferent arteriole
Interlobular artery
Interlobular vein
Collecting tubule
Arcuate vein
Arcuate artery
Interlobar artery and vein
Arteriolae rectae
Venulae rectae
Descending limb
Ascending limb
Henle's loop
Papillary duct

B   **Figure 16–11.**   *See opposite page for legend.*

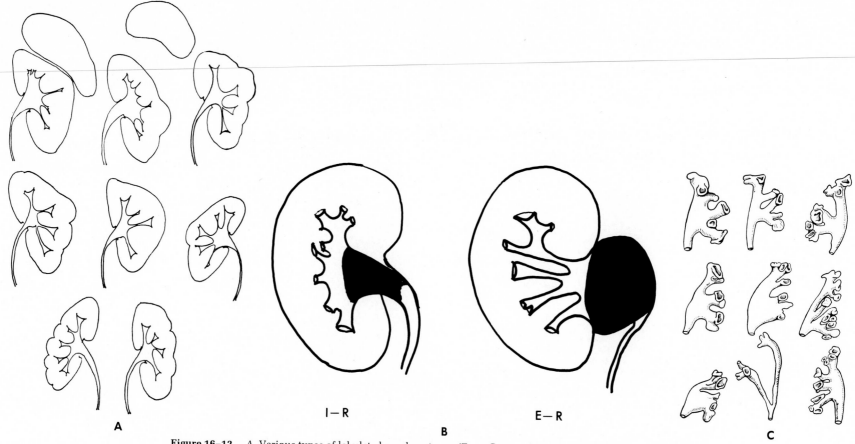

A

I—R   B   E—R

C

Figure 16–12. A. Various types of lobulated renal contours. (From Cooperman, L. R., and Lowman, R. M.: Amer. J. Roentgenol., *92*:273, 1964.) B. Intrarenal (I-R) and extrarenal (E-R) pelvis of kidney (pelvis in solid black). The demarcation of the junction of the intrarenal pelvis and the ureter is not distinct. C. Variations in configuration of normal renal pelves and calyces.

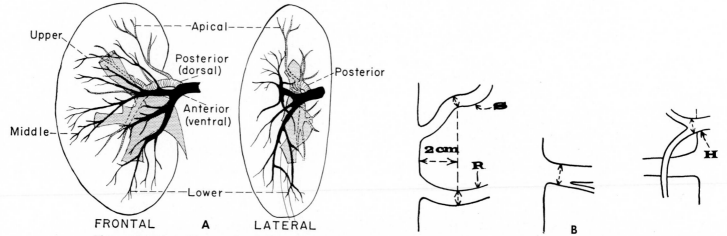

FRONTAL   A   LATERAL   B

Figure 16–13. A. Diagram illustrating the renal artery and its segmental branches in frontal and lateral perspectives, showing the relationship to the pelvocalyceal system. (After Boijsen, E.: Acta Radiol. (Suppl.), *183*:51, 1959.) B. Drawings illustrating method of measuring internal diameter of renal, splenic, and hepatic arteries. *Left,* The renal (R) and splenic (S) arteries are measured where they intersect a line 2 centimeters from and parallel to the lateral border of the aorta. The measurements are made at right angles to the longitudinal axis of the vessel at the 2 centimeter intersection. *Center,* When the renal artery bifurcates at a point closer than 2 centimeters from the aorta it is measured proximal to this bifurcation. *Right,* The hepatic artery (H) is measured proximal to its bifurcation into the hepatic artery, proper, and into the pancreaticoduodenal artery. Target-to-film distance 32 inches. Measurements are reduced by 10% for distortion. (From Atlas of Roentgenographic Measurement, 3rd ed., by Lusted, L. B., and Keats, T. E. Copyright © 1972 by Year Book Medical Publishers, Inc., Chicago. Used by permission. [Redrawn from Maluf, N. S. R.: Surg., Gynec., & Obstet. *107*:415, 1958.])

Figure 16–13 continued on the opposite page.

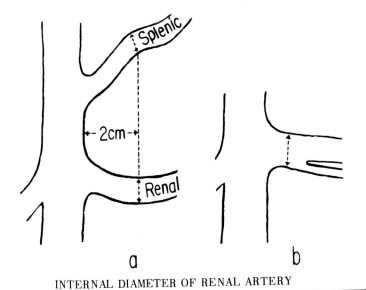

INTERNAL DIAMETER OF RENAL ARTERY

		S.D.
Two normal kidneys	6.5 — 6.7 mm.	0.75 — 0.88
One healthy hyper-trophied kidney	8.4 — 8.6 mm.	0.71 — 0.83

$$\text{Normal ratio:} \quad \frac{\text{Diameter of renal artery}}{\text{Splenic artery}} = \; > 1$$

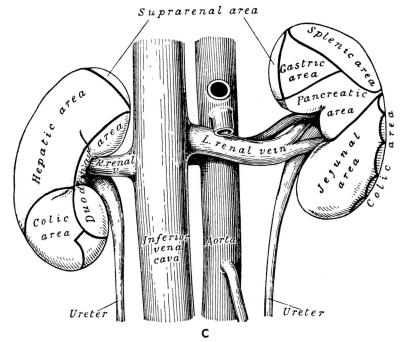

C

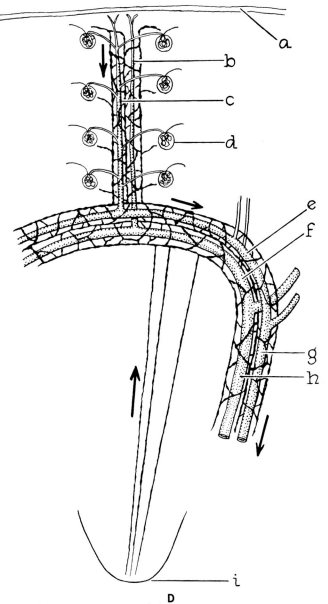

D

Figure 16–13 *Continued.* C. Gross relationships of renal veins to inferior vena cava and anterior surface relationships of the kidneys. (From Warwick, R., and Williams, P. L.: Gray's Anatomy. 35th British edition. London, Longman [for Churchill-Livingstone], 1973.) D. Lymphatic channels of the human kidney (diagrammatic). Two separate systems are demonstrable. One begins in the cortex and accompanies the interlobular vessels toward the corticomedullary junction; the other starts at the papilla and ascends to join the cortical system at the corticomedullary junction. From there large trunks follow the arcuate and interlobar vessels to leave the kidney at the hilus. Arrows show the probable direction of the lymph flow. The structures shown are: (a) tunica fibrosa, (b) interlobular vein, (c) interlobular artery, (d) glomerulus, (e) arcuate artery, (f) arcuate vein, (g) interlobar artery, (h) interlobar vein, and (i) papilla. (From Rawson, A. J.: Arch. Path., 47:283–292, 1949. Copyright 1949, American Medical Association.)

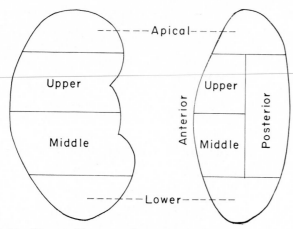

Figure 16–14. Diagram illustrating the segmental distribution of the renal artery. The apical segment is usually supplied largely by the posterior or dorsal branch of the renal artery, whereas the lower segment of the kidney is supplied by the anterior or ventral branch of the renal artery for the most part. (After Boijsen, E.: Acta Radiol. (Suppl.), *183*:10, 1959.)

of the glomeruli, which apparently are not accompanied by lymphatic vessels. The lymphatic channels are more plentiful in the cortex than in the medulla. *Two separate systems* of channels are present: one system begins as tiny blind-ending vessels lying in close contact with Bowman's capsule. These channels gradually enlarge, forming a network around the arterial and venous vessels of the cortex beginning near the terminal branching of both arteries and veins. Lymphatic channels wind loosely around the arteries and veins, frequently coming in chance contact with a convoluted tubule. Those channels that lie in close proximity to large thin-walled venous vessels are prominent, particularly in the outer half of the cortex. The lymphatic channels accompany the interlobular vessels and progress toward the hilus, winding around the arcuate vessels and interlobar arteries and veins. They finally leave the kidney at the hilus, terminating in lymph nodes on either side of the aorta.

Another system of lymphatic channels begins blindly as a network beneath the mucosa of the papilla. These channels ascend in a rather straight line, gradually increasing in size and running parallel to the small blood vessels of the medulla. They empty into the larger lymphatic channels that surround the arcuate arteries and veins.

Generally, increased renal blood flow augments urinary output and increases lymph flowing from the kidneys.

In some respects this double renal lymphatic system corresponds closely to the two hemic circulations demonstrated in the kidney by Trueta et al. These two hemic systems, a greater and a lesser, originate close to the arcuate arteries. The *greater circulation for blood* consists of: interlobular arteries, afferent arterioles, glomerular capillaries, efferent arterioles, capillaries of the medullary rays, capillaries around the convoluted tubules, collecting veins, and interlobular veins.

The *lesser circulation for blood* consists of afferent arterioles of the juxtamedullary glomeruli, these glomeruli themselves, their efferent arterioles, and the vasa recta, arterial and venous, of the medulla.

Variations of the Normal Kidney. The kidneys of different individuals vary considerably as to *size* as noted previously, but generally they are proportional to the size of the body (with numerous exceptions, however).

Variations in *shape* of the kidney are numerous also: they may be elongated or lobulated; they may appear double or may actually be completely duplicated on one side, each with a separate renal pelvis and ureter. In the infant or fetus lobulations are frequent—being found much less frequently in the adult.

Variations in *position* of the kidney have already been described (see Figure 16–1).

There may be *multiple renal arteries* in approximately 25 per cent of normal individuals.

Absence of one kidney is quite rare, occurring on an average of only once in 2400 persons (Anson). Likewise, an extra kidney may sometime be found caudal to the normal one and either attached to it or completely separate (Fig. 16–15). When there are two ureters arising from such a duplex kidney, they usually cross so that the ureter draining the upper renal portion implants itself in the urinary bladder at a lower level than the other.

VARIATIONS IN RENAL SIZE OR NUMBER

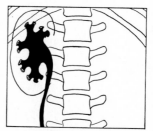

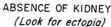 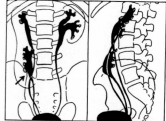

ABSENCE OF KIDNEY
(Look for ectopia)

SUPERNUMERARY KIDNEY

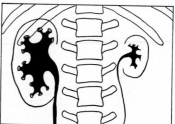 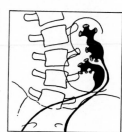

COMPENSATORY HYPERPLASIA
OF ONE KIDNEY WITH APLASIA
OF THE OTHER

UNILATERAL FUSED
KIDNEY

Figure 16–15.

Ureters

Introduction. The ureter is a tubular connection between the kidney and the urinary bladder, extending downward from the renal pelvis in extraperitoneal tissue. It is approximately 5 mm. in diameter and 25 cm. in length. It is fairly uniform in size except for three slight constrictions: (a) at the *ureteropelvic junction* (superior isthmus); (b) at the place where the *ureter crosses the pelvic brim* (inferior isthmus); and (c) at the extreme lower end of the ureter as it passes through the urinary bladder wall (called an *intramural constriction*) (Fig. 16–16). The ureter is slightly longer on the left side than on the right, and longer in the male than in the female. It has two portions—the *superior abdominal portion* and the *inferior pelvic portion.*

The *abdominal portions* of the ureters on both sides are embedded on the medial aspect of the psoas major muscles and pass ventral to the common or external iliac artery to enter the true pelvis. They lie ventral to the transverse processes of the third, fourth, and fifth lumbar vertebrae, and both are crossed by the spermatic or ovarian vessels. The right abdominal portion of ureter is covered by descending duodenum and is situated to the right of the inferior vena cava. It is crossed by right colic and ileocolic vessels, the mesentery, and terminal ileum. The left abdominal ureter is crossed by left colic vessels and sigmoid mesocolon. The left ureter is ordinarily separated from the aorta by a space which ranges from 2.5 cm. cranially to 1.5 cm. opposite the bifurcation of the aorta.

The *pelvic portion* of the ureters must be described separately for males and females. In the *male,* this portion of the ureter begins at the pelvic brim, courses caudad close to the internal iliac artery along the ventral border of the greater sciatic notch. It lies medial to the obturator, inferior vesicle, and middle rectal arteries. It turns medially to reach the lateral angle of the urinary bladder at the level of the lower part of the greater sciatic notch. Here, it lies ventral to the seminal vesicles. The vas deferens crosses over it as it approaches the urinary bladder.

In the *female,* the pelvic ureter forms the dorsal boundary of the ovarian fossa. It runs medially and ventrally on the lateral aspect of the cervix and upper part of the vagina to the fundus of the urinary bladder. As it runs ventrally it passes inferior to the uterine artery.

At the level of the urinary bladder the two ureters on each side are about 5 cm. apart in both male and female.

The *intramural* portion of the ureters runs obliquely through the urinary bladder for a distance of approximately 2 cm. and opens into the urinary bladder through two slitlike apertures, the *ureteral ostia,* which are about 2.5 cm. apart in the empty bladder but may be as much as 5 cm. distant from each other when the bladder fills. The ureteral ostia together with the urethral opening of the urinary bladder consitute the *bladder trigone.*

The ureters are not provided with a definite valve at their junction with the urinary bladder, but these slitlike openings ap-

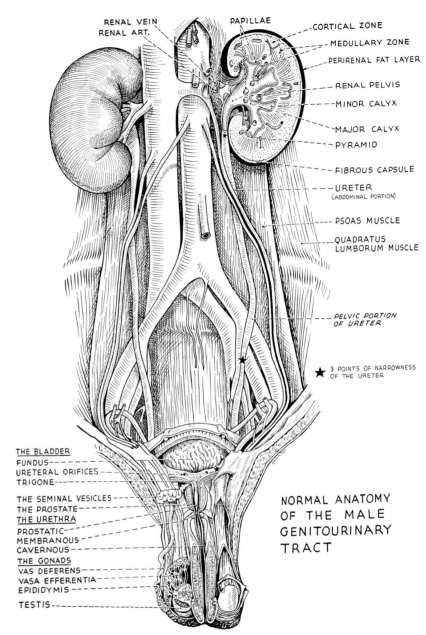

Figure 16–16. Gross anatomy of the urinary tract.

pear to have a valvelike action, so that ureteral reflux from the urinary bladder is considered abnormal. However, on occasion, reflux of urine from bladder to ureter probably takes place normally. Reflux is particularly important in the presence of recurrent infection, in which case pyelonephritis may ensue. The ureter is constantly undergoing peristalsis and hence its lumen is variable in size.

The course of the ureter varies somewhat and tends to be redundant in some individuals, particularly following pregnancy.

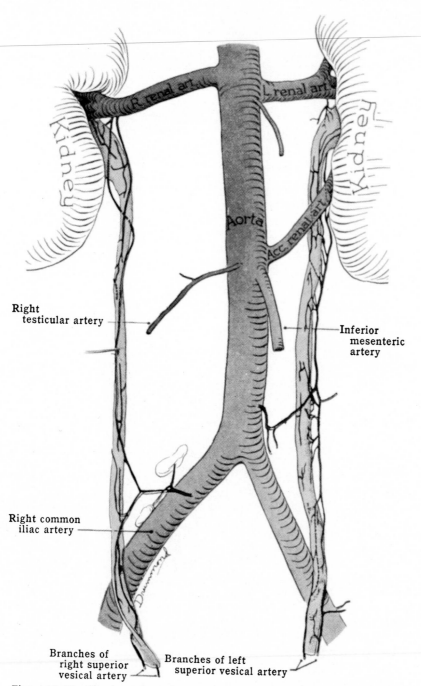

Right
testicular artery

Right common
iliac artery

Branches of
right superior
vesical artery

Branches of left
superior vesical artery

Inferior
mesenteric
artery

Figure 16–17. Blood supply to the ureter. The arterial system was injected with latex by way of the femoral artery. (Dissection by W. R. Mitchell.) (Reproduced by permission from J. C. B. Grant: An Atlas of Anatomy, 5th ed. Copyright © 1962, The Williams and Wilkins Company.)

Vessels of the Ureter

Arteries. The arteries of the ureter are branches of the renal, internal spermatic, superior, and inferior vesicle arteries.

The *veins* follow correspondingly named arteries and terminate in correspondingly named veins.

The *lymphatics* pass to the lumbar and internal iliac nodes (Fig. 16–17).

Variations of Normal. Apart from variations in length and diameter, the ureter varies with body height, sex, and variations in the positions of the kidneys and urinary bladder. Unilateral absence is usually accompanied by absence of the kidney on the same side. At times there are supernumerary or double ureters that may be complete or incomplete, unilateral or bilateral.

As noted previously, if a ureter is duplicated on one side, the ureter from the superior pelvis terminates inferior to that from the inferior pelvis. Duplication of the ureter occurs in approximately 3 per cent of all individuals (Anson). It occurs slightly more often in females than in males and is more frequently unilateral than bilateral. It is more often complete than incomplete.

Congenital kinking of the ureter is infrequent but may occur, particularly as an accompaniment to ectopia of a kidney. However, kinking of the ureter may also occur over an anomalous vessel.

Anomalies of implantation of the ureteral ostium also occur, most frequently in the female urethra. In the male this formation may occur in the ejaculatory ducts, seminal vesicles, ductus deferens, prostatic utricle, or vestibule. In the female, abnormalities of implantation may also occur in the vagina, uterus, or uterine tubes.

The Urinary Bladder

Introduction. The urinary bladder is a strong, muscular hollow viscus which receives the urine from the kidneys through the ureters, retains it for a period of time, and ultimately expels it through the urethra by micturition. It lies anteriorly, posterior and superior to the pubic symphysis, below the peritoneum and surrounded by extraperitoneal fatty tissue. In the adult, when empty, it lies in the pelvis, but when distended, it balloons upward.

In a *child,* even when empty, it is in contact with the abdominal wall, and is located almost entirely in the abdomen proper. By 6 years of age the greater part of the urinary bladder is ordinarily accommodated by the pelvis, but it is not wholly a pelvic organ until shortly after puberty.

In the male, the seminal vesicles and deferent ducts lie on the lower part of the *posterior surface* of the urinary bladder (Fig. 16–18 *A, B*). The bladder is separated from the rectum by the rectovesical septum, seminal vesicles, and vas deferens (bilaterally).

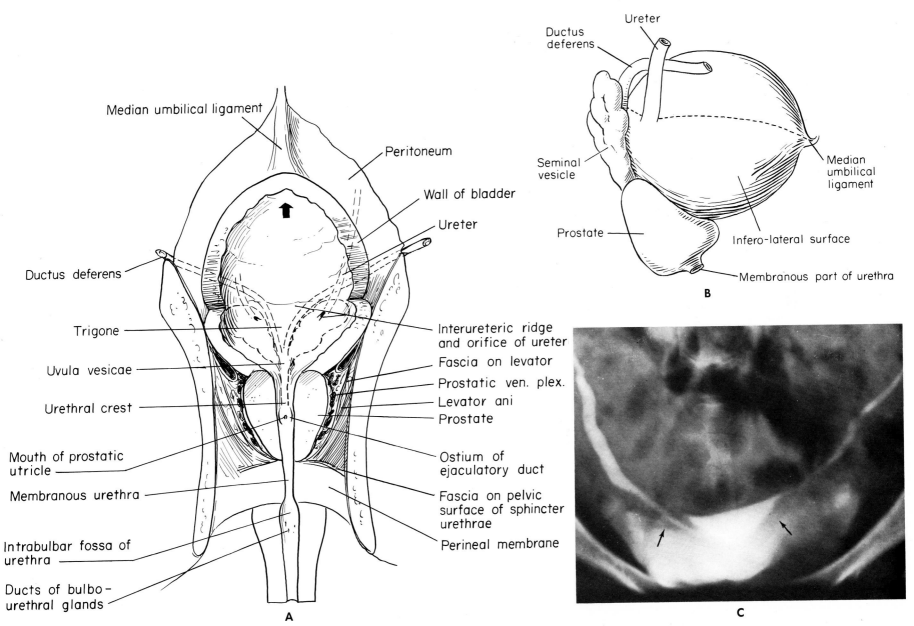

Figure 16–18. *A.* Urinary bladder in frontal perspective, showing relationship to ductus deferens, prostate, ureters, and male urethra. *B.* Urinary bladder hardened in situ showing relationship to ureters, ductus deferens, seminal vesicles, and prostate in lateral view. (From Cunningham's Manual of Practical Anatomy, 12th ed., Vol. 2. London, Oxford University Press, 1958.) *C.* Radiograph of urinary bladder cystogram showing interureteric ridge.

In the *female,* the posterior surface is separated from the uterus by the peritoneum.

In the male, the pelvic colon and coils of the distal ileum rest on the *upper surface* of the urinary bladder, whereas in the female, the upper surface is related closely to the overhanging uterus and a loop of ileum.

In the *infant,* a median umbilical ligament extends up the abdominal wall from the apex of the urinary bladder to the umbilicus. This represents the urachus.

The *neck* of the urinary bladder is about 2 to 3 cm. behind the pubic symphysis, a little above its lower border. Pubovesical ligaments are attached in front and at the sides. In the female it narrows abruptly to become continuous with the urethra. In the male it is continuous with the prostate which surrounds the first part of the urethra, and posteriorly it is in contact with the commencement of the ejaculatory ducts (Fig. 16–18 *A*).

The *inferolateral surface* of the bladder is separated from the pubis by a prevesical cleft and is spoken of as the *retropubic space of Retzius.*

In the female, the *fundus* of the urinary bladder is separated from the ventral surface of the uterus by a vesicouterine pouch below; behind, it is proximal to the cervix and the upper vaginal wall. The inferior surface of the bladder rests on pelvic and urogenital diaphragms.

Interior of Urinary Bladder. When the bladder is full its mucous coat is smooth. When empty, it is wrinkled except over the *trigone,* which is a smooth triangular area above the urethral orifice. The three points of reference for the trigone are the two *ureteric orifices* dorsolaterally and the *internal urethral orifice* ventrally. The base of the triangle is formed by the *interureteric ridge* between the orifices (Figs. 16–18 *A* and 16–19). The internal urethral orifice, placed at the apex of the trigone, presents a very slight elevation, the *uvula vesicae,* caused by the middle lobe of the prostate (Fig. 16–18 *A*).

Vessels and Nerves. The arteries supplying the bladder are the superior, middle, and inferior vesical, which are derived from the anterior trunk of the hypogastric artery (Fig. 16–19). The obturator and inferior gluteal arteries also supply small visceral branches to the bladder. In the female additional branches are derived from the uterine and vaginal arteries.

The *veins* consist largely of a plexus on the inferolateral surface, the plexus communicating with the prostatic plexus. Several veins drain this plexus and pass into the internal iliac vein.

The *lymphatics* drain toward the external, internal, sacral, and median common iliac lymph nodes.

The nerves on the bladder are supplied *via* the inferior hypogastric and vesical plexuses.

Variations of Normal. The urinary bladder varies in shape considerably in different individuals—it may be ellipsoid, triangular, conical, or spherical. At times, the urinary bladder is deformed by adjoining tissues or masses.

The Male Urethra

The male urethra extends from the internal urethral orifice of the urinary bladder to the external urethral orifice at the end of the penis. It is divided into three portions: *prostatic, membranous,* and *cavernous* (Fig. 16–20 *B*).

The *prostatic portion* is somewhat dilated, measuring about 3 cm. in length. In transverse section it is horseshoe shaped with a convexity directed forward. The *urethral crest* (verumontanum) is a longitudinal ridge on its posterior wall. It is about 3 mm. in height and 15 to 17 mm. long. A depressed fossa, the *prostatic sinus,* lies on either side of the crest. These fossae are perforated by numerous apertures which are the orifices of the prostatic ducts from the lateral lobes of the prostate. The ducts of the middle lobe open behind the crest.

At the distal end of the urethral crest is another elevation, the *colliculus seminalis,* which contains the orifices of the prostatic utricle and the slitlike openings of the ejaculatory ducts.

The *membranous portion* of the urethra is short and narrow with a very slight anterior concavity between the apex of the prostate and the bulb of the urethra. It represents that portion of the urethra which perforates the urogenital diaphragm about 2.5 cm. below and behind the pubic symphysis. The membranous portion of the urethra is surrounded by a sphincter.

The *cavernous portion* is approximately 15 cm. long and extends from the membranous portion to the external urethral orifice. It begins just below the urogenital diaphragm and bends downward and forward, measuring about 6 mm. in diameter. It is slightly dilated proximally within the bulb and again distally within the glans penis, where it forms the *fossa navicularis* of the urethra.

The *external urethral orifice* is a vertical slit about 6 mm. long bounded on either side by two small labia.

There are numerous mucous glands which open on the floor of the cavernous portion of the urethra called the *urethral glands of Littré.* There are small pitlike recesses or lacunae of different sizes between these glands. One of the lacunae is larger than the rest and situated in the fossa navicularis (Fig. 16–20).

The Female Urethra

The *female urethra* is about 4 cm. long and extends from the internal to the external urethral orifice. Located behind the pubic symphysis and embedded in the wall of the vagina, it is approximately 6 mm. in diameter and perforates the urogenital diaphragm. Its external orifice is situated in front of the vaginal opening about 2.5 cm. from the glans of the clitoris. A prominent feature is a slight elevation or fold which is called the *urethral crest.* Many small urethral glands open into the urethra, the largest of which are the *paraurethral glands of Skene* (Fig. 16–21).

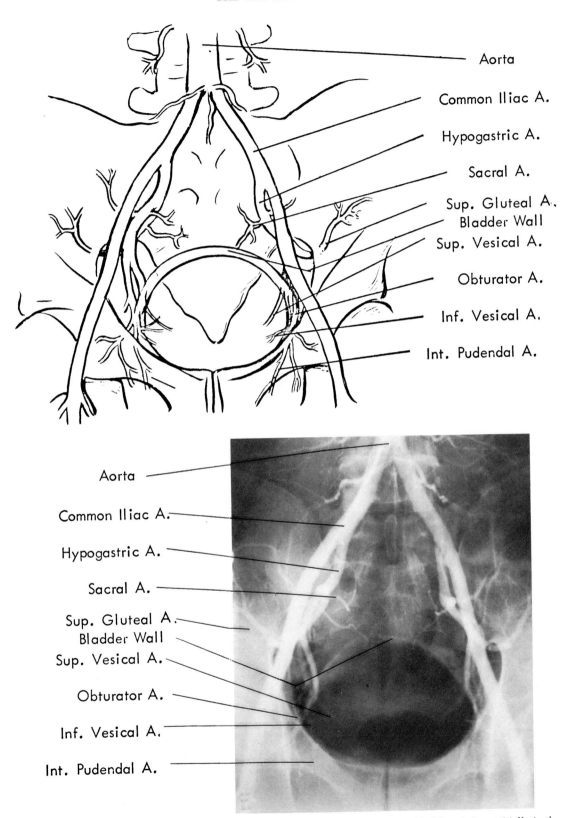

Aorta

Common Iliac A.

Hypogastric A.

Sacral A.

Sup. Gluteal A.
Bladder Wall
Sup. Vesical A.

Obturator A.

Inf. Vesical A.

Int. Pudendal A.

Aorta

Common Iliac A.

Hypogastric A.

Sacral A.

Sup. Gluteal A.
Bladder Wall
Sup. Vesical A.

Obturator A.

Inf. Vesical A.

Int. Pudendal A.

Figure 16–19. Triple contrast study of the urinary bladder, with air in the urinary bladder, air interstitially in the urinary bladder wall, and arterial angiograms for demonstration of the urinary bladder arterial blood supply.

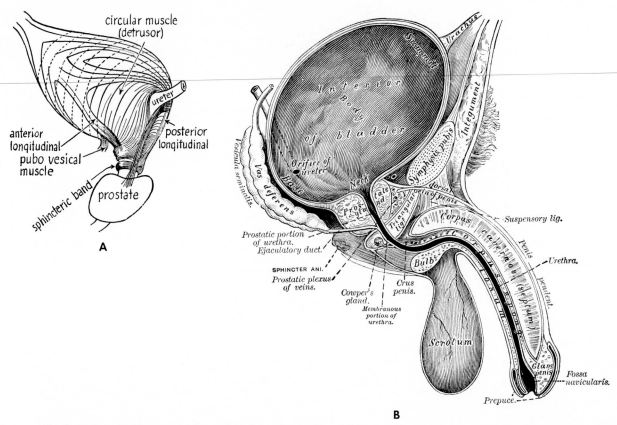

Figure 16–20. *A.* Diagram of the muscles of the bladder (after McCrea). *B.* Vertical section of bladder, penis, and urethra. (*A* from Gray's Anatomy of the Human Body, 29th ed. Goss, C. M. (ed.) Philadelphia, Lea & Febiger, 1973. *B* from 24th ed., 1942, edited by W. H. Lewis.)

GENERAL COMMENTS REGARDING URINARY BLADDER FUNCTION

The Trigonal Canal (Shopfner and Hutch). Radiologic study during the late stages of voiding of the bladder base and urethra in an oblique or lateral position has revealed two primary anatomical units of the bladder: the *vault* and the *base plate*. The *base plate* extends from a point 2 cm. anterior to the internal urethral orifice to another point about 2 cm. posterior to the interureteric ridge (Fig. 16–22 *A*). As indicated by Shopfner and Hutch, a slight constriction or contraction ring is present at the superior margin of the base plate in some patients (Fig. 16–22 *F*). This represents the division between the base plate below and the vault above. There is considerable variation in the contour of the base plate. The internal urethral orifice is slightly anterior to its center, and its anterior edge is the most dependent part of the urinary bladder. That portion of the base plate extending from its anterior edge to the urethrovesical junction is designated the *an-*

terior trigonal plate, whereas the part between the urethrovesical junction and the interureteric notch is the *posterior trigonal plate*. The base plate is flat regardless of the degree of bladder distention but increases slightly in length as bladder filling increases. The segment above the interureteric notch is the *nontrigonal portion* of the base plate and this corresponds to the fundus ring (Fig. 16–22). The nontrigonal portion may droop over the flat posterior trigonal plate if the bladder is not maximally filled or is not contracting vigorously (Figs. 16–23, 16–24).

Physiologically it would appear that the base plate functions independently of the vault of the urinary bladder. The base plate appears to dilate slightly in the early stages of voiding, apparently to receive the contents of the vault. It appears first to be shaped like a funnel, and then finally, a tube. After voiding, the trigonal canal gradually returns to its normal flat position to await refilling of the urinary bladder.

In *children under two years of age*, the base plate is convex inferiorly and funnel-shaped rather than flat as in the older child.

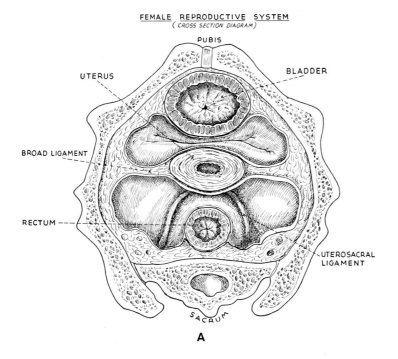

FEMALE REPRODUCTIVE SYSTEM
(CROSS SECTION DIAGRAM)

PUBIS

UTERUS

BLADDER

BROAD LIGAMENT

RECTUM

UTEROSACRAL
LIGAMENT

SACRUM

A

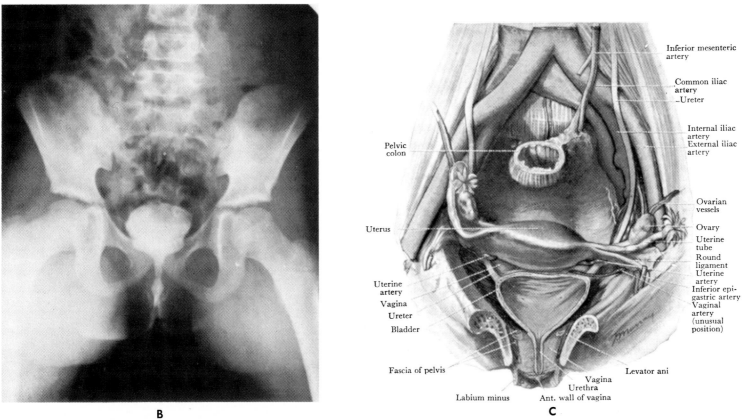

B

Inferior mesenteric
artery

Common iliac
artery

Ureter

Internal iliac
artery

External iliac
artery

Pelvic
colon

Ovarian
vessels

Ovary

Uterus

Uterine
tube

Round
ligament

Uterine
artery

Inferior epi-
gastric artery

Uterine
artery

Vaginal
artery
(unusual
position)

Vagina

Ureter

Bladder

Fascia of pelvis

Levator ani

Vagina

Urethra

Labium minus

Ant. wall of vagina

C

Figure 16–21. *A.* Gross anatomy of the female reproductive system. Superior cross-sectional diagram. *B.* Normal female urethrogram. *C.* Dissection of pelvis of a multiparous female, showing the relations of bladder to uterus and vagina, of vagina to urethra and broad ligaments, and of ureters to broad ligaments and vagina. (From Cunningham's Manual of Practical Anatomy, 12th ed., Vol. 2. London, Oxford University Press, 1958.)

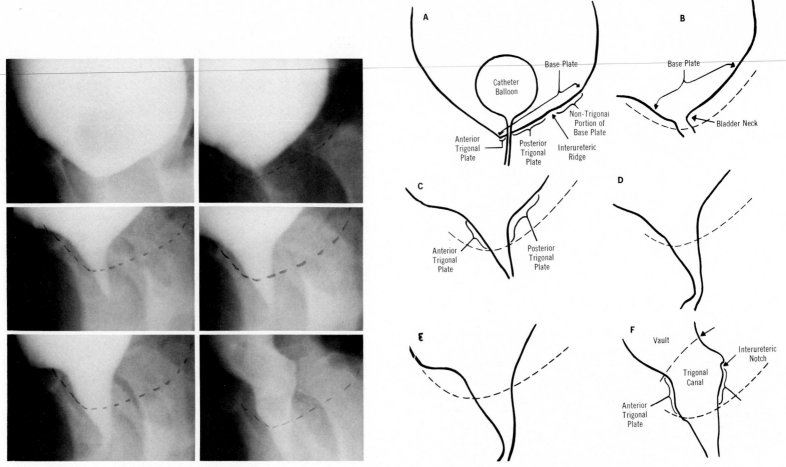

Figure 16–22. Voiding sequence in a 4 year old female. The landmarks of the base plate are shown in A. The contraction ring in F indicates the division between the base plate below and the vault above. Progressive cephalic movement of the anterior and posterior trigonal plates creates the trigonal canal which is continuous with the posterior urethra. The contraction ring is above the interureteric ridge, indicating that the trigonal canal is formed by the entire base plate and not by the trigonal plates alone. (From Shopfner, C. E., and Hutch, J. A.: Radiology, 88:209–221, 1967.)

The specific demonstration of the trigonal canal is feasible in perhaps only 55 per cent of patients (Shopfner and Hutch). However, it may be demonstrated in higher percentages in those with mature bladder bases.

Anatomic Changes in the Normal Urinary Tract in the Change from the Supine to the Prone Position (Riggs et al.). Although individual variations occur, the majority of patients show the following changes in the prone position as compared with the supine (Fig. 16–25). (1) There is a bilateral increase in renal length due to magnification and transverse axial rotation. (2) The right kidney tends to move cephalad and medially while the left kidney tends to move caudad. (3) Both kidneys tend to become more parallel to the spine in both frontal and lateral perspectives. (4) Both kidneys tend to rotate about their long axes with the renal pelves moving posteriorly. (5) Both kidneys tend to move anteriorly except in infants. (6) The contrast medium in the urinary bladder gravitates cephalad and anteriorly, creating a more convex, denser, and higher dome. (7) Although many adults

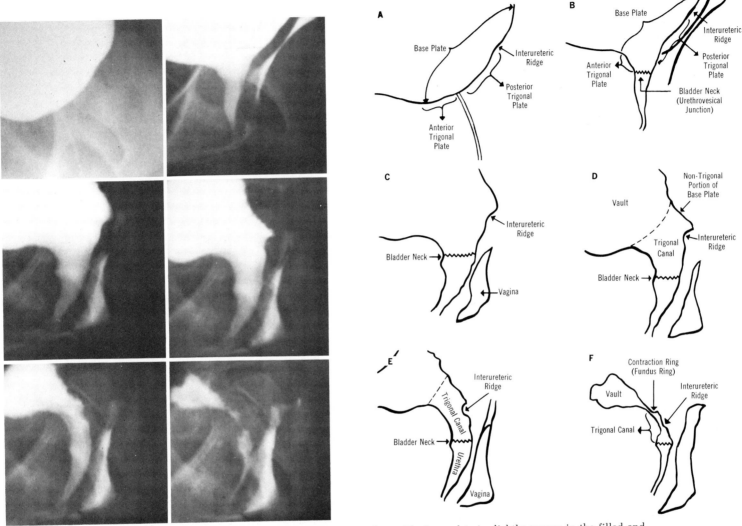

Figure 16–23. Voiding sequence in a 5 year old female. *A.* The base plate is slightly convex in the filled and resting bladder. *B.* During early voiding, the trigonal plates have moved to an oblique position but the base plate has changed little in size. *C* and *D.* Progressive decrease in the size of the vault and base plate is occurring. In *D,* the trigonal canal is beginning to develop and extends well above the interureteric notch. A distinct difference in caliber exists between the base and the vault. *E.* The trigonal plates are vertical and the trigonal canal is well-developed and continuous with the posterior urethra. *F.* Voiding has almost ceased and the canal has reduced in width during the urethral stripping process. A distinct constriction exists between the base plate and the vault, above the interureteric ridge. (From Shopfner, C. E., and Hutch, J. A.: Radiology, 88:209–221, 1967.)

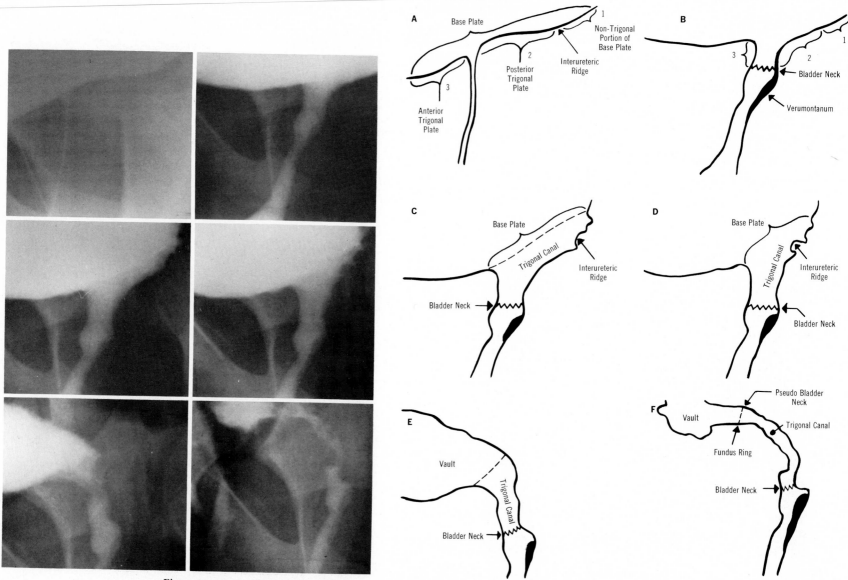

Figure 16–24. Voiding sequence in a 13 year old male. *A.* The trigonal plates are flat in the filled and resting bladder. The nontrigonal portion of the base plate droops over the posterior trigonal plate (bracket #1). *B.* Voiding has started and the trigonal plates have moved to an oblique position. *C* and *D.* The vault and base plate are becoming smaller as voiding progresses and the trigonal canal is already well-developed. *E.* During the late stages of voiding, the trigonal canal has become narrower and longer as the plates have moved to a vertical position. *F.* A contraction ring marks the division between the trigonal canal and the vault and acts as a pseudo-bladder neck. The canal has decreased in width but increased in length during urethral stripping. (From Shopfner, C. E., and Hutch, J. A.. Radiology, *88:*209–221, 1967.)

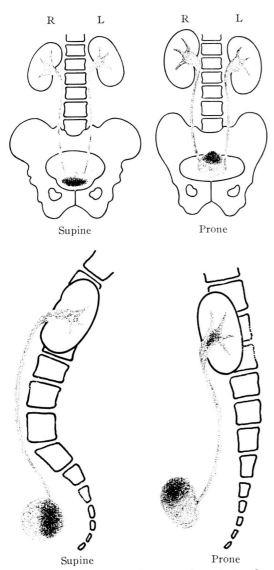

face of the upper pole. This is more common on the left side. It is thought to be caused by a knuckle of renal cortex of indefinite size which bulges down into the upper pole of the renal sinus (Fig. 16–26).

2. There may be a *"normal" large kidney* with unilateral localized renal enlargement and without contralateral diminution of renal size.

3. The liver and spleen may alter the "normal" renal shape by *pressure.* A renal bump in the midsegment has been described in approximately 10 per cent of patients that is caused by pressure from the spleen (Frimann-Dahl). This has been called the "dromedary kidney" by Harrow and Sloane and has also been described by Doppman and Shapiro.

4. *Double renal hilus.* The renal hilus is usually central but may on occasion be eccentric, lying closer to either the upper or lower pole. When there is a duplication of the collecting system, two hili can be visualized, especially by nephrotomography. There is apparently no relationship between the double hilus and multiple renal arteries.

5. There may be *venous impressions* on the calyceal system as shown in Figure 16–27. Generally, these are wide, smooth filling defects involving the proximal portion of the superior infun-

Figure 16–25. Summary of anatomic changes in the majority of cases. *Upper,* In the prone view both kidneys appear larger and are more parallel to the spine. The profile of the renal pelves is better, i.e., wider. Right kidney is higher and more medial, but the left kidney is slightly lower. Dome of the bladder is higher and more convex.

Lower, In the prone view the spine shows straightening of lumbar lordosis. Both kidneys are more parallel to the spine. There is a slight tendency to anterior movement. Pelves appear more true lateral. Bladder appears higher and more anterior. (From Riggs, W., Jr., Hagood, J. H., and Andrews, A. E.: Radiology, 94:107–113, 1970.)

show only minimal change, the findings are most pronounced and consistent in infants. (8) The upper portion of the left kidney in adults is often better seen on the prone film.

GENERAL URINARY TRACT VARIANTS

1. *Suprahilar bulge.* There may be a localized bulge of renal parenchyma just above the hilus continuous with the medial sur-

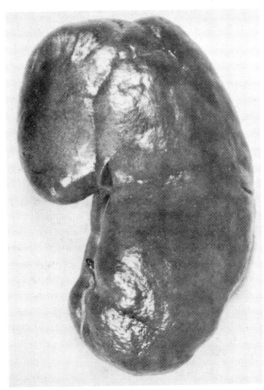

Figure 16–26. Photograph of a left kidney directly *en face* in the anteroposterior position showing a prominent suprahilar bulge (necropsy specimen). (From Doppman, J. L., and Shapiro, R.: Amer. J. Roentgenol.: 92:1380–1389, 1964.)

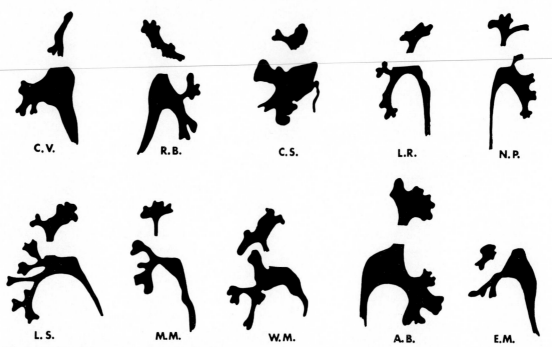

Figure 16–27. Intravenous urographic findings in the ten cases with apparent renal vein impression of the upper infundibulum. Angiographic studies in all revealed no arterial branching in the region of the wide, smooth defect. In three cases the renal veins were opacified and appeared responsible for the impressions. (From Meng, C-H., and Elkin, M.: Radiology, *87*:878–882, 1966.)

dibulum. They present a curved venous trunk on angiography, crossing the filling defect.

6. *Arteries* supplying the kidneys may also *cause pressure defects* of the calyces or infundibula because of the intimate relationship of these intrarenal structures. These defects appear as radiolucent bands roentgenologically, not exceeding 2 to 3 mm. in width ordinarily (Fig. 16–28) (Meng and Shapiro; Weisleder et al.).

7. *Arterial impressions on the ureters and renal pelvis* (Baum and Gillenwater; Chait et al.). Arterial impressions similar to those in the intrarenal collecting system may also be found in the renal pelvis and ureters. At times these are related to normal accessory renal arteries that arise low on the aorta, and sometimes they produce extrinsic pressure defects on the medial or lateral aspect of the ureter. Vessels crossing the ureteral pelvic junction may indeed be implicated with ureteropelvic partial obstruction.

8. *Compression by the iliac artery* may produce its impression on the ureters also at the level at which the ureters cross the iliac vessels.

9. *Renal artery stenosis* may, by backup of blood, cause dilatation of the ureteral artery and perfusion of the kidney by ure-

teral arterial twigs feeding into the renal artery distal to the stenosis (Fig. 16–29).

10. *Normal gonadal vein crossing defect on the ureter.* Both ureters may be crossed by normal gonadal veins (Fig. 16–30). Proximally this may occur a short distance below the ureteropelvic junction, and distally at about the level of the lumbosacral junction. Crossing defects may be seen at each of these locations. An aberrant dilated right ovarian vein has been said to be responsible for urinary tract infection in a previously gravid woman, this being called the *right ovarian vein syndrome.*

11. Other abnormalities *associated with venous distention* may be responsible for *indentation and impressions* on the ureters, such as: varicoceles and varices of the broad ligament; occlusions of the inferior vena cava; renal vein occlusions; occlusion of the azygos vein; occlusion of the superior vena cava; portal hypertension; and carcinoma of the pancreas. In each instance, venous dilatation and impression upon the ureter is postulated.

12. *Retroperitoneal tumors and enlarged lymph nodes may also displace or impress the ureters.* In each instance, careful roentgen diagnostic study is necessary to differentiate the various possibilities (Chait et al.).

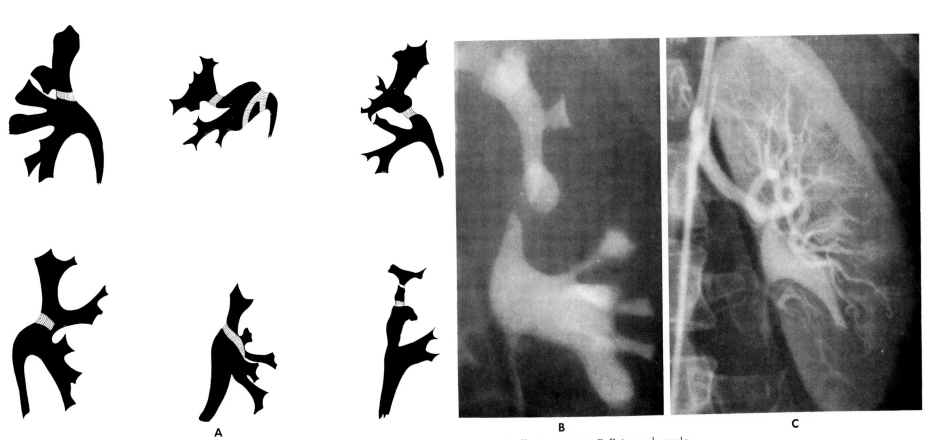

Figure 16–28. *A.* Schematic drawings of arterial impressions on the renal collecting system. *B.* Retrograde pyelogram showing arterial impression on the superior calyceal infundibulum. *C.* Tracing of the arteriogram. The renal and ventral branches are black; the dorsal branches striped; the collecting system gray. (From Weissleder, von H., Emmrich, J., and Schirmeister, J.: Fortschr. Geb. Roentgenstr. Nuklearmed., 97:703–710, 1962.)

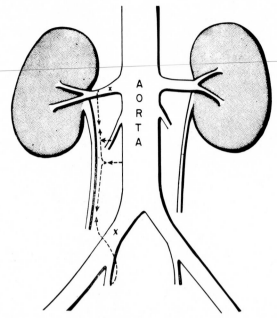

Figure 16–29. Sketch of the arterial supply of the ureter. The ureter normally receives its arterial supply from branches of the renal artery, gonadal artery, directly from the aorta, from lumbar arteries, directly from the internal iliac artery, or from branches of the internal iliac artery. As each of these twigs reaches the ureter, it branches into an ascending and descending limb and joins with its neighbors to form a continuous channel. Flow is normally *to* the ureter from all sources, but direction of flow is responsive to pressure changes. Renal artery stenosis (upper X) may cause dilatation of the ureteral artery and perfusion of the kidney by ureteral arterial twigs feeding into the renal artery distal to the stenosis. Similarly, aortic occlusion or occlusion of the common or internal iliac artery (lower X), with resultant lowered pressure in the pelvis, may result in ureteral artery dilatation; flow in this case, however, is *from* the renal artery *to* the pelvis. (From Chait, A., Matasar, K. W., Fabian, C. E., and Mellins, H. Z.: Amer. J. Roentgenol., *111*:729–749, 1971.)

Basic Physiology of the Kidneys

The Nephron. Figure 16–11 illustrates diagrammatically the nephron, which is the basic functioning unit of the kidney. It contains an afferent and an efferent arteriole leading into and out of the glomerulus; juxtaglomerular cells lie at the junction of the afferent and efferent arteriolar system with the glomerular capillary. It has been suggested that the juxtaglomerular cells (JGA) have an endocrine function, or that perhaps they act like the glomus cells elsewhere in the body. It is true that these cells become heavily granulated in pyelonephritis associated with hypertension, as well as in the early stages of experimental ischemia and hypertension. The degree of granulation parallels the width of the zona glomerulosa of the adrenal cortex and varies inversely with the levels of plasma sodium in animals and man. It

has also been suggested that JGA cells synthesize and store renin.

Blood Supply. The basic blood supply of the kidney has already been described. Approximately 70 per cent of all kidneys are supplied by a single renal artery originating from the aorta; two or more arteries supply the remainder.

Multiple renal arteries are significant since, in some cases, the supplemental artery may supply as much as half the blood supply to the kidney. The most common and important artery is

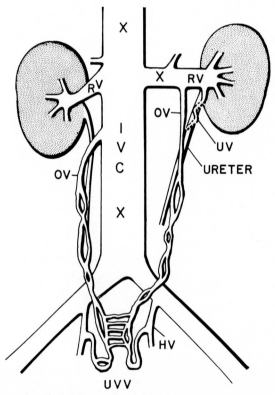

Figure 16–30. Sketch of abdominal, renal, and periureteric venous anatomy. The left gonadal vein (ovarian vein in the sketch) almost invariably empties into the left renal vein, while the right empties into the inferior vena cava below the right renal vein. The ureteral veins generally empty into the renal veins at a location peripheral to the site of gonadal emptying. Either of these two latter structures is capable of causing ureteral notching either of a serpentine nature or of a simple extrinsic pressure type. Free communication between them has been noted on multiple occasions. The ovarian veins are in free communication in the broad ligament with the uterine veins and therefore with the hypogastric and iliac veins, It will be seen therefore that occlusion or stenosis of the inferior vena cava above the renal veins, below the renal veins, or in the renal veins (sites marked X) is capable of altering flow in the gonadal or ureteric veins and thereby accounting for vascular notching. (RV) renal vein, (OV) ovarian (gonadal) vein, (UV) ureteral vein, (HV) hypogastric vein, (UVV) uterine veins, (X) sites of occlusion. (From Chait, A., Matasar, K. W., Fabian, C. E., and Mellins, H. Z.: Amer. J. Roentgenol., *111*:729–749, 1971.)

the supplemental vessel to the inferior portion of the kidney; it may supply as much as 20 to 50 per cent of the renal parenchyma.

In the arcuate veins, the pressure is about 25 mm. of mercury. Beyond these, the pressure suddenly drops to approximately 7 mm. of mercury because of "cushions" or sinusoids which serve as contractor mechanisms at the junction of the arcuate and interlobar veins.

Renal Function.   The function of the kidney may be outlined as follows (Fig. 16–31):

1. *Filtration* of the blood plasma and removal of some of its solutes such as potassium chloride sulfate, sodium, urea, glucose, amino acid and the like.
2. *Selective tubular reabsorption.*
3. *Tubular synthesis and excretion.*
4. *Acid-base regulation.*
5. *Volume regulation* of the fluid environment of the body.
6. *Osmolality regulation.*
7. *Maintenance of a normal blood pressure.*
8. *Erythropoiesis.*

As the result of an effective filtration pressure gradient in the glomerulus, the walls of the glomerular capillaries act as a sieve, allowing particles of certain sizes to filter through and retaining larger ones.

The renal tubules, on the other hand, are primarily concerned with: (1) *water reabsorption* from the glomerular filtrate; (2) *reabsorption* of certain *threshold substances* and ions necessary for the equilibrium of the organism; (3) *excretion* of some organic and inorganic compounds in substances; (4) *synthesis* of certain metabolites; and (5) *excretion of the final waste products* into the collecting system, after an appropriate regulation of acid-base balance and osmolality. It is probable that water is absorbed from both proximal and distal convoluted tubules.

In addition, approximately 14 per cent of water is reabsorbed in the collecting tubules under the control of an antidiuretic hormone derived from the pituitary gland (ADH). To some extent this reabsorption is accomplished by the hyperosmotic environment of the interstitial fluid in the medulla of the kidney involving and surrounding the loops of Henle. This is part of the so-called counter-current phenomenon.

Glomerular filtration and tubular secretion and excretion are the two renal functions especially identified by roentgenologic techniques. Contrast agents such as Hypaque, Miokon, and Renografin are in large measure excreted normally by glomerular filtration, much as is inulin. These compounds, therefore, offer the opportunity for physiologic tests of glomerular filtration. Paraamino hippurate and Hippuran are largely excreted (or secreted) via the tubules and are useful in measuring tubular secretion or excretion. Previously used compounds such as Diodrast more closely resemble the latter group of compounds although not exclusively so. Diodrast is also excreted by the liver as well as by glomerular filtration.

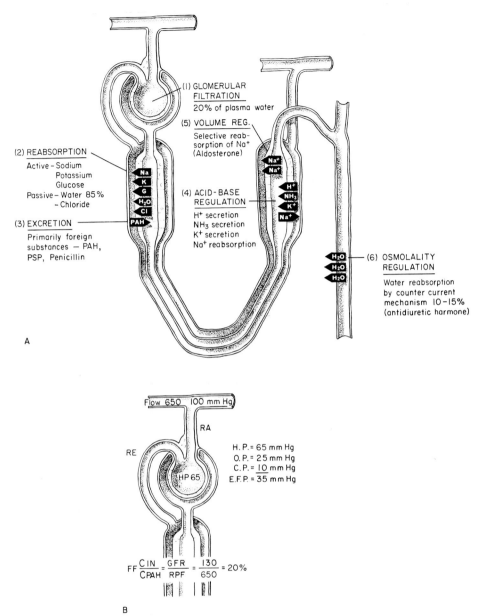

Figure 16–31. *A.* Physiology of the nephron. The various functions of the nephron in regulation of the internal environment of the body are diagrammatically illustrated. *B.* Diagrammatic illustration of glomerular hemodynamics in the maintenance of filtration pressure. (H.P.) Hydrostatic pressure, (O.P.) osmotic pressure, (C.P.) capillary pressure, (E.F.P.) effective filtration pressure, (RA) afferent arterioles, (RE) efferent arterioles, (FF) filtration fraction, (CIN) clearance of inulin, (CPAH) clearance of para-aminohippurate, (GFR) glomerular filtration rate, (RPF) renal plasma flow. (From Meschan, I.: Radiol. Clin. N. Amer., 3:18, 1965.)

Sodium diatrizoate (Hypaque) is excreted at the rate of approximately 65 per cent in 2 hours and 88 per cent in 6 hours. This is more rapid than the excretion of Diodrast and Urokon.

Kidney function is routinely studied in a dehydrated body

state. This, of course, is not a normal physiologic state and therefore cannot accurately be related to conventional clearance studies by inulin or para-amino hippuric acid techniques. If clearance of these compounds is to be studied, the body must be in a hydrated state, equilibrated, and at normal rest.

In a subsequent section, a "washout" test for renovascular hypertension will be described. The basis for this test is as follows: in patients with kidneys responsible for renovascular hypertension, dilution of the contrast agent does not occur during the washout phase. This so-called hyperconcentration results from excessive, obligated tubular water reabsorption and a low-flow phenomenon in the kidney nephron.

Normal Intrarenal Circulation Time. Circulation times of 6 to 8, 8 to 10, and 10 to 12 seconds have been published (Becker et al.). Generally, an intrarenal circulation time of less than 5 seconds is considered abnormal when a bolus of 8 ml. of contrast material is used, delivered in 1 second.

Gallbladder Visualization Following the Injection of Diatrizoate. Excretion of pyelographic agents via the bile and into the gallbladder with incidental opacification of the gallbladder may occur in unusual circumstances. As a general rule, when this phenomenon occurs with the diatrizoates, renal dysfunction with delayed excretion of contrast material occurs, and creatinine and blood urea nitrogen values are elevated (Segall).

TABLE 16–3 CONTRAST MEDIA USED IN UROGRAPHY AND ANGIOGRAPHY

Trade Name	Organic Compound	Per Cent Iodine W/V	Concentration of Drug in Commercially Available Solution	Manufacturer's Suggested Dosage			
				Adult Dose	Children's Dose	Subcutaneous Administration	Intramuscular Administration
Neo-Iopax[a]	Sodium iodomethamate	25.8 38.6	50% 75%	20 cc. of 50% 30 cc. of 50% 20 cc. of 75%	10 cc. of 50%	10% solution (dilute 14 cc. of 75% solution to 100 cc. with normal saline)[e]	Not recommended
Diodrast[b]	Iodopyracet, U.S.P.	17.5 (35% in 70% solution)	35% (70% also available)	20–30 cc. of 35%	0– 6 mo.: 5 cc. 7–12 mo.: 6– 7 cc. 1– 3 yr.: 7–10 cc. 4– 6 yr.: 10–16 cc. 7– 8 yr.: 16–20 cc.	7% solution (dilute 20 cc. of 35% solution to 100 cc. with normal saline)[e]	35% solution Children: 10–20 cc. Adults: 20–30 cc.
Hippuran[c]	Sodium iodohippurate	7 (in 20% solution)	Powder only available. Mix 12 gm. with 60 cc. of distilled water to make 20% solution	60 cc. of 20%	0–12 mo.: 6 gm.+ 9.55 cc. water 1– 4 yr.: 8 gm.+ 12.5 cc. water 4– 8 yr.: 10 gm.+ 21 cc. water	Not recommended	Not recommended
Urokon[c]	Sodium acetrizoate, U.S.P.	19.74 (46.06% in 70% solution)	30% 70% for difficult cases only or aortography or nephrotomography	25 cc. of 30% 25 cc. of 70%	<4 yr.: 0.7 cc. of 30% solution >4 yr.: 25 cc. of 30% solution	Not recommended	Not recommended
Miokon[c]	Sodium diprotrizoate, U.S.P.	28.7	50%	20 cc. of 70% 25 cc. of 50% 30 cc. of 50%	<3 mo.: 6 cc. 3– 6 mo.: 6– 8 cc. 6–12 mo.: 8–10 cc. 1– 2 yr.: 10–15 cc. 2– 6 yr.: 15–20 cc. >6 yr.: 20–25 cc.	Not recommended	Not recommended
Hypaque-50[b]	Sodium diatrizoate, U.S.P.	30	50% for excretory urography	30 cc. of 50%	0– 6 mo.: 5 cc. 6–12 mo.: 6– 8 cc. 1– 2 yr.: 8–10 cc. 2– 5 yr.: 10–12 cc. 5– 7 yr.: 12–15 cc. 7–11 yr.: 15–18 cc. 11–15 yr.: 18–20 cc.	Dilute with equal quantities of distilled water[e]	Inject undiluted or diluted with equal parts distilled water
Hypaque-75[b]	Sodium diatrizoate, U.S.P.	39.3	75% 90% for nephrotomography	50 cc. or more	Infants: 5–10 cc. Older children: 15–20 cc.	Not recommended	Not recommended
Hypaque-90[b]	Sodium diatrizoate, U.S.P.	46	75% 90% for nephrotomography	50 cc. or more	Infants: 5–10 cc. Older children: 15–20 cc.	See text	See text

[a]Schering
[b]Winthrop Laboratories
[c]Mallinckrodt Pharmaceuticals
[d]E. R. Squibb and Sons

[e]Subcutaneous injections are given in divided doses over each scapula. Intramuscular injections are given in divided doses into each gluteal region. To increase the rate of absorption, the addition of hyaluronidase to the solution is recommended (150–200 turbidity units on each side for children, 500 for adults).

Table 16–3 continued on opposite page.

Contrast Media Used in Urography and Angiography

The most commonly used contrast media in urography and angiography are indicated in Table 16–3, with the manufacturer's suggested dosage. In Figure 16–32, the structural formula of the more common of these agents is compared.

Various physiologic evaluations of the dose of contrast medium for intravenous urography have been carried out (Dure-Smith), as for example with Urografin, a mixture of sodium and methylglucamine diatrizoate in the ratio of 10 to 66 (Renografin,

U.S.P.). From this study, the following conclusions may be drawn: (1) There is a good correlation between the dose of contrast medium and plasma concentration. This is initially largely independent of renal function. (2) The minimum concentration of contrast agent in the glomerular filtrate necessary to produce an appreciable nephrogram is probably in the range of 70 mg. iodine per cent. This can apparently be attained with 20 cc. of Urografin 76 per cent in 1 to 2 seconds. If 140 cc. of Urografin-76 is infused slowly, levels well above this are maintained for well over 60 minutes.

The mean plasma concentration of Urografin occurs at iden-

TABLE 16–3 CONTRAST MEDIA USED IN UROGRAPHY AND ANGIOGRAPHY (*Continued*)

Trade Name	Organic Compound	Per Cent Iodine W/V	Concentration of Drug in Commercially Available Solution	Manufacturer's Suggested Dosage			
				Adult Dose	Children's Dose	Subcutaneous Administration	Intramuscular Administration
				Retrograde pyelograms:			
Renografin-30[d]	Diatrizoate methyl-glucamine, U.S.P.	15	30%	15 cc. (unilateral)	Proportionately smaller for children	Not used	Not used
Renografin-60[d]	Methylglucamine diatrizoate, U.S.P.	29	60%	25 cc. of 60% (over 15 yrs.)	Under 6 mo.: 5 cc. 6–12 mo.: 8 cc. 1– 2 yr.: 10 cc. 2– 5 yr.: 12 cc. 5– 7 yr.: 15 cc. 8–10 yr.: 18 cc. 11–15 yr.: 20 cc.	Not used	Not used
Renografin-76[d]	Diatrizoate methyl-glucamine	37	76%	20–40 cc. of 76% (over 15 yrs.)	Under 6 mo.: 4 cc. 6–12 mo.: 6 cc. 1– 2 yr.: 8 cc. 2– 5 yr.: 10 cc. 5– 7 yr.: 12 cc. 8–10 yr.: 14 cc. 11–15 yr.: 16 cc.	Not used	Not used
Renovist[d]	Sodium and methyl-glucamine diatrizoate	37	69%	25 cc. of 37% solution (over 15 yrs.)	Under 6 mo.: 5 cc. 6–12 mo.: 8 cc. 1– 2 yr.: 10 cc. 2– 5 yr.: 12 cc. 5– 7 yr.: 15 cc. 7–10 yr.: 18 cc. 10–15 yr.: 20 cc.	Not used	Not used
				Retrograde pyelography:			
Retrografin	Neomycin sulfate solution with methyl glucamine diatrizoate	15	25% neomycin 30% methylgluca-mine diatrizoate	15 cc. (unilateral)	Proportionately smaller for children	Not used	Not used
Ditriokon[c]	Sodium diprotrizoate and diatrizoate	40	68.1%	40–50 cc. (over 12 yrs.)	0.5–1 cc./kg. body weight	Not used	Not used
Conray-60[c]	Meglumine iothalamate	28.2	60%	25–30 cc. (14 yrs. and over)	Under 6 mo.: 5 cc. 6–12 mo.: 8 cc. 1– 2 yr.: 10 cc. 2– 5 yr.: 12 cc. 5– 8 yr.: 15 cc. 8–12 yr.: 18 cc. 12–14 yr.: 20–30 cc.	Not used	Not used
Conray–400[c]	Sodium iothalamate 66.8%	40	66.8%	40–50 cc. (over 14 yrs.)	0.5–1 cc./kg. under 14 yrs.	Not used	Not used

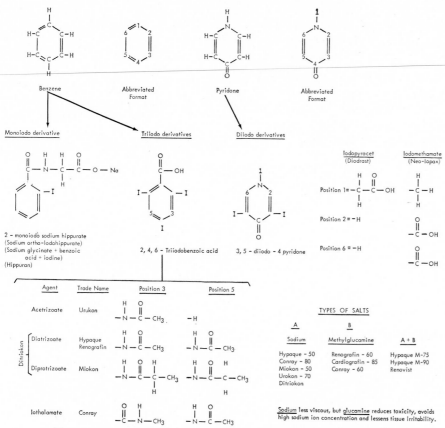

Figure 16–32. The organic structure of the iodinated derivatives of benzene and pyridone which are used in the radiographic visualization of the kidneys. (Modified from Potsaid.)

tical rates regardless of the rapid intravenous injection of 20 cc. or the slow infusion of 140 cc. of Urografin.

If a contrast medium is injected slowly over 8 to 10 minutes, the peak plasma concentration is not reached until 15 minutes, and this should indeed be the period of maximum density of the nephrogram and optimum period of nephrotomography.

The contrast medium itself acts as a simple osmotic diuretic. The concentration of contrast medium in the urine is accurately reflected by the diuresis.

In patients with normal renal function who have been deprived of fluid for some 12 hours, the concentration of contrast medium in the urine continues to increase with increasing doses up to 140 cc. of Urografin-76, despite the increasing diuresis.

The better the dehydration of the patient, the higher will be the "optimal" dose for this patient. Maximum dehydration, however, is not achieved within the usual period of 8 to 12 hours of fluid restriction before urography. The optimal dose of contrast medium, or one which will produce no further increase in concen-

tration of contrast medium in the urine, will depend on the state of hydration of the patient at the start of the procedure.

Even in high dose urography, dehydration will improve the concentration of contrast medium in the urine in patients with normal renal function. *Actually, however, drip infusion pyelography probably offers no advantage over high dose urography in which equivalent doses of the undiluted contrast medium are injected. A rapid injection usually causes a higher peak of the plasma concentration and a denser nephrogram than a slower injection.*

O'Connor and Neuhauser (1963) described a method of total body opacification with relatively large doses of intravenously injected radiopaque contrast media—2 to 4 cc. per kilogram of body weight in infancy. The mechanism of this is thought to be opacification of the entire blood vascular compartment in less than 60 seconds. The added density of the various tissues is proportional to the blood supply. An avascular or hypovascular lesion will be radiolucent in contrast to the adjacent structures with a greater blood supply. The method is limited in differentiating a chronic or poorly vascularized neoplasm from a cyst, but it is particularly useful in defining cystic, hemorrhagic, and chronic lesions.

Apparently, untoward reactions are not dose-related in the dose ranges employed, but *it is probable that the intravenous injection of any such contrast media should not be performed when hyperbilirubinemia is present in the newborn.*

An investigation of higher volumes of contrast material to improve intravenous urography has been carried out by Friedenberg and Carlin. These investigators arbitrarily chose certain volumes with respect to body surface area as shown in Table 16-4. There was a slight increase in the frequency of side effects, which were, however, mild and well tolerated by the patients. Generally, the use of higher volumes of the contrast material improved the quality of intravenous urograms significantly. It increased the diagnostic accuracy of the examination and reduced the need for retrograde pyelography with its attendant hazards.

TABLE 16–4 DOSAGE SCHEDULE TESTED FOR HIGH-VOLUME UROGRAPHY*

Body Surface Area (sq. meters)	Volume (ml.)
Less than 1.30	30
Less than 1.50	40
Less than 1.70	50
Less than 1.90	60
Less than 2.10	70
Less than 2.25	80
Less than 2.40	90
Greater than 2.40	100

*From Friedenberg, M. J., and Carlin, M. R.: Routine use of higher volumes of contrast material. Radiology, *83*:405–413, 1964.

No effort was made in this study to determine the relative merits of injecting the contrast material in single versus divided doses, but from other data in the literature it would appear that this probably would not be a significant factor.

RADIOLOGIC METHODS OF STUDY

Preparation of the Patient. The patient should have a small supper or no meal at all on the night prior to the examination, with nothing by mouth after this meal. Dehydration for at least 12 hours prior to the examination is highly desirable and enhances the concentration in the kidney with either single-dose or infusion techniques.

Catharsis with preparations such as 45 cc. of X-Prep liquid, 1 or 2 oz. of castor oil, or a full dose of magnesium citrate U.S.P. at approximately 6:00 P.M. on the evening prior to the examination is preferred. Some investigators have preferred cleansing enemas on the morning of the examination, but often this will introduce gas into the gastrointestinal tract that will interfere with the clarity of the examination. Suppositories to stimulate colonic evacuation on the morning of the examination may be employed. Aloin, cascara sagrada, or phenolphthalein may be utilized in lieu of the cathartics mentioned above.

Plain Film, Patient Supine (Fig. 16–33). *An anteroposterior film in suspended respiration with the patient supine must precede any contrast study of the urinary tract.* In the pediatric age groups, some physicians may prefer a prone film instead, either prior to the study or during the procedure (Baker) (see previous comparison of prone and supine films of the urinary tract). If the supine position is employed, the abdomen may be compressed with an inflated rubber bag, provided this does not cast an opaque shadow on the roentgenogram. These films should include the entire area from the diaphragm to the pubic symphysis.

Such film studies must be done immediately prior to the injection of contrast media, since any opacities in the urinary pathways may change position in short intervals of time. Moreover, the introduction of opaque material into the urinary tract will obscure calcific structures.

Since one film in the erect position may also be obtained in

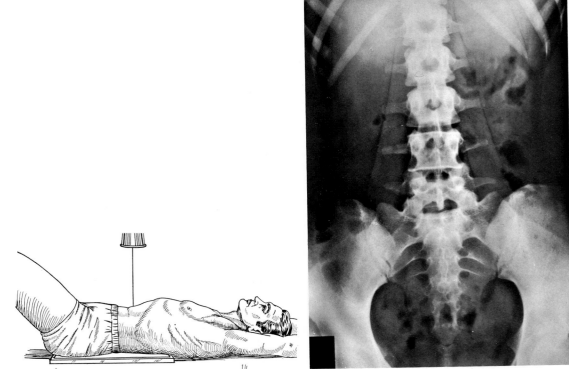
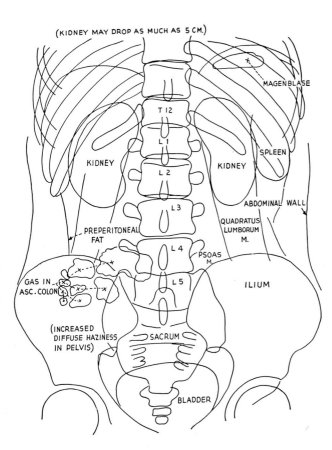

Figure 16–33. Anteroposterior view of abdomen (KUB film).

the course of the entire study, an anteroposterior view of the abdomen in this position prior to the injection of the contrast medium may also be desired.

Single Injection Excretory Urogram (IVP) (Fig. 16–34 *A* and *B*).

Immediately before injection of any contrast medium the patient is instructed to *void*.

Contrast media which have been and are being used are listed in Table 16–3. The most commonly used at this time are: 50 per cent sodium diatrizoate; 60 per cent meglumine diatrizoate; 60 per cent meglumine iothalamate; and occasionally, 66.8 per cent sodium iothalamate.

The *usual intervals* for taking of films after intravenous injection of the opaque medium are: 4 to 5 minutes; 8 to 15 minutes; 25 to 40 minutes; 60 minutes; 90 minutes; 2 hours; and delayed urography at hourly intervals if necessary up to 8 hours following the intravenous injection if so indicated. If only four films are utilized in the entire examination (three films in addition to the plain film), the recommended time intervals for use with the diatrizoates are 4 minutes, 8 minutes, and 15 to 30 minutes.

In some instances, *oblique films* will also be taken, and usually the best time for these is immediately following maximal visualization of the ureters (10 to 20 minutes).

If the lower ureters are not accurately visualized in the supine position the patient may then be turned in the *prone position* and a repeat study obtained at an optimum time interval.

Dose. Many radiologists employ doses larger than those suggested by the manufacturer as indicated in Table 16–3. For example, in infants 6 months or younger, 10 cc. of the diatrizoate are employed; in older children, a minimum dose of 2 to 3 cc. per pound is usually employed; in adults, the usual dose is often 1.5 cc. per pound or even greater, to a maximum of 150 cc. if necessary.

Delayed Films. If excretion and concentration are delayed, it is well to keep obtaining films until a good concentration of the medium is seen in the urinary bladder. At times even 8 to 24 hour films may be helpful.

Cystogram and Voiding Urethrogram. If, in addition, a cystogram is desired by this excretory method, oblique studies of the urinary bladder are obtained. Urethrograms require an oblique

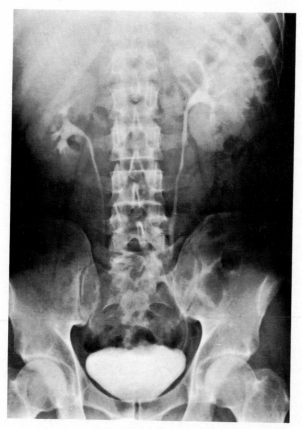
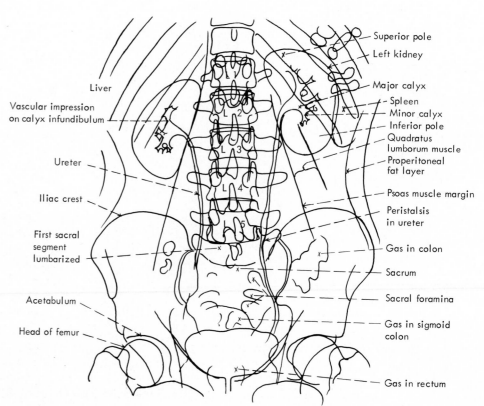

Figure 16–34. Representative excretory urogram (also called intravenous pyelogram) obtained 15 minutes after the intravenous injection of a suitable contrast agent (25 ml. 50 per cent Hypaque).

RADIOLOGIC METHODS OF STUDY OF THE URINARY TRACT

1. Preparation of patient.
2. Plain film, patient supine (KUB).
   a. Prone film in infants.
3. Single injection excretory urogram.
4. Infusion excretory urogram.
5. Hypertension study pyelogram—rapid sequence dehydrated urogram, combined with a hydrated pyelogram.
6. Nephrotomography.
7. Retrograde pyelography.
8. Cystography and cystourethrography.
   a. With voiding urethrogram.
   b. Retrograde urethrogram.
   c. Cystogram (with excretory or retrograde pyelogram).
   d. With double contrast (air).
   e. Triple contrast—angiography plus pneumocystogram plus interstitial air in wall of urinary bladder.
   f. "Chain" cystourethrogram—investigation of stress incontinence.
9. Renal arteriography and aortography.
10. Phlebography and inferior vena cavography.
11. Roentgen evaluation of the surgically exposed kidney.
12. Cineradiography of the upper urinary tract and cystourethrography.
13. Perirenal air insufflation.
14. Seminal vesiculography.
15. Reactions to contrast media.

Figure 16–35

study of the urethra while the patient is urinating into a suitable receptacle (voiding cystourethrogram). Usually it is more satisfactory to perform urethrograms following instillation of the medium directly into the bladder (Fig. 16–36).

In infants it has been customary to administer a carbonated cola drink to distend the stomach and thus portray the left kidney more clearly; some, however, advise against this procedure because the gas soon passes farther into the gastrointestinal tract and makes accurate visualization difficult (Baker).

If intravenous injection is unsuccessful, gluteal intramuscular injection may be used together with an injection of hyaluronidase to promote absorption (Fainsinger). Hypaque and Renografin (sodium diatrizoate and meglumine diatrizoate) may also be given intramuscularly (Emmett).

Infusion Excretory Urography. Infusion excretory urography is the technique of opacifying the urinary tract by means of a large amount of contrast medium introduced by continuous intravenous drip. The technique, described by Harris and Harris, involves the intravenous infusion of 140 cc. of 50 per cent sodium diatrizoate (Hypaque) mixed with an equal amount of physiologic salt solution and allowed to run freely through a 19 gauge hypodermic needle. After 225 cc. has been introduced the infusion is slowed in order to maintain an open needle for the duration of the study. The first roentgenogram is made 20 minutes following commencement of the infusion. Thereafter, any other radiographs may be obtained as necessary.

A rapid infusion of 100 ml. of Renografin-76 plus 1 ml. of isotonic dextrose solution per pound of body weight may be similarly employed.

The main advantage of this technique is the increased clarity with which the collecting system and ureters may be identified, sometimes avoiding the necessity for retrograde pyelography. Moreover, body section radiographs can be obtained when nephrotomography might be indicated, such as the differentiation of renal cysts and neoplasms (Fig. 16–37).

The Rapid Sequence Dehydrated Excretion Urogram Combined with a Hydrated Pyelogram. The Hypertension Pyelogram (Fig. 16–38). At the onset of an excretory urogram, the patient is decidedly dehydrated. Normally, hydration of a patient undergoing an excretory urogram will produce a marked dilution of the contrast agent within a normal kidney and some dilatation of the calyces, so that the visualization of the calyces may be indistinct. In patients with renovascular hypertension, such dilution of the contrast agent does not ordinarily occur, and hydration may actually enhance the visualization of an otherwise poorly seen collecting system.

To facilitate hydration, urea diuresis has been recommended as follows: a slow-drip intravenous infusion of 40 grams of urea in 500 ml. of 5 per cent dextrose (rather than isotonic saline as in the Amplatz method) is begun through an 18 gauge needle. This is momentarily clamped off and 50 cc. of 75 per cent Hypaque-M is introduced as rapidly as possible through this needle (within 30 seconds). Films are obtained immediately thereafter and then at 1 minute intervals for 6 minutes. The slow drip is continued only to keep the needle from being obstructed by a blood clot. An additional film is obtained at 8 minutes. Following exposure of the 8 minute pyelogram, at which time the renal collecting systems are usually at their peak of opacification, a more rapid infusion of the urea-dextrose mixture is begun so that the entire infusion occurs

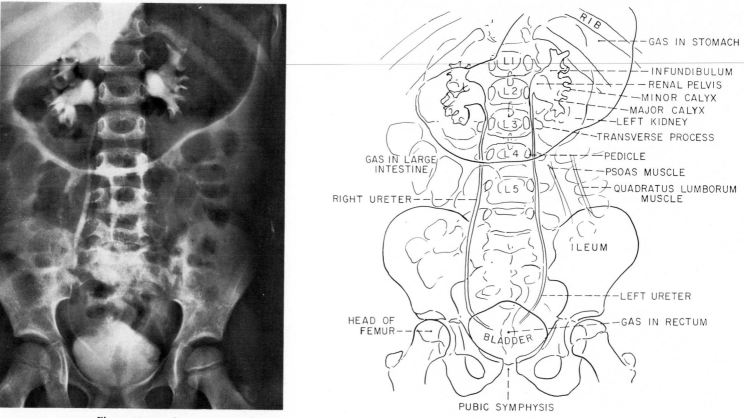

Figure 16–36. Intravenous pyelogram on a child. The upper urinary tract is demonstrated clearly through the gas-distended stomach.

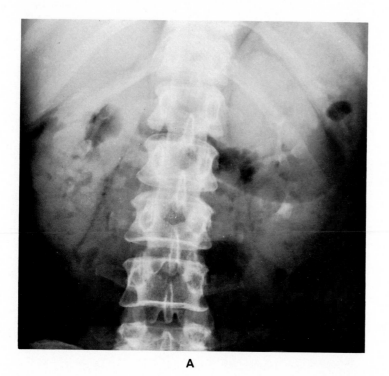

A

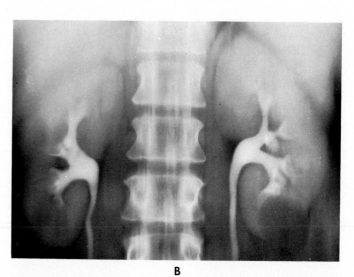

B

Figure 16–37. Value of drip-infusion urogram with tomogram. *A.* Excretory urogram, showing poor visualization of renal pelvis and calyces. *B.* Drip-infusion urogram with tomogram. Excellent visualization of renal parenchyma and collecting system. Previously unsuspected mass (simple cyst) is present in lower pole of left kidney. (From Emmett, J. L., and Witten, D. M.: Clinical Urography. 3rd ed., Vol. 1. Philadelphia, W. B. Saunders Co., 1971.)

in 10 to 15 minutes. Thereafter films are obtained at 5 minute intervals for a total of 20 minutes. The best washout phenomenon appears on the 15 and 20 minute films ordinarily.

A 5 per cent solution of Mannitol may be substituted for the urea-dextrose mixture to produce diuresis and is probably easier to manage than the urea.

The first phase of this study has been called the minute pyelogram or rapid sequence intravenous pyelogram. The latter phase has been called the "washout" study. The latter is a radiologic adaptation of the Howard and Stamey tests.

Nephrotomography (Fig. 16–39 *A* and *B*). Body section radiographs (see Chapter 1) allow the radiologist to focus on any plane of the body which is parallel to the table top on which the patient is lying. Nephrotomography may be readily applied during infusion pyelography during the so-called nephrographic phase. This is the period when opacification of the renal parenchyma is at its best.

Good nephrographic opacification is obtained by the rapid injection of large doses of the contrast agent (Weens et al.; Evans et al., 1954).

Various techniques have been described to obtain maximum concentration of the contrast agent in the nephrogram phase at the time the various "cuts" are obtained. The complete series of films should be exposed within 60 to 90 seconds following the rapid intravenous injection of the large bolus of contrast agent.

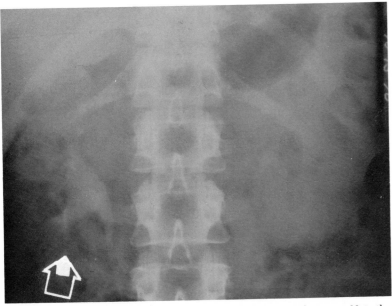

Figure 16–38. Renovascular hypertension with a positive washout test. Note the hyperconcentration of the right renal pelvis and calyces even after the left renal collecting system is completely washed out. The blood pressure in this patient was 190/120. The above film was obtained 15 minutes after the injection of a large volume diuretic (Mannitol).

Although simple cysts or tumors may be diagnosed by this method with 90 to 95 per cent accuracy (Evans), renal arteriography is usually employed subsequently for greater reliability.

Better quality nephrotomograms may be obtained following renal arteriography or midstream aortograms when the injection is made at the level of, or just below, the origin of the renal arteries.

Retrograde Pyelography (Fig. 16–40). Patient preparation for retrograde pyelography is much the same as for intravenous pyelography.

This method requires that catheters be introduced into the ureters by cystographic manipulation. Most urologists prefer opaque ureteral catheters. Ordinarily the tip of the catheter is introduced well into the renal pelvis, but care must be exercised not to penetrate the renal calyces because local infarction may result.

It is customary to obtain a plain film of the abdomen after the introduction of the ureteral catheters and prior to the injection of the opaque medium. Oblique studies are taken if necessary, especially if ureteral calculi are suspected.

Following the initial studies, an opaque medium is injected through the ureteral catheter. This may be an organic iodide preparation such as Hippuran (sodium orthoiodohippurate dihydrate), Skiodan, or a 12 per cent solution of sodium iodide or bromide. Skiodan is combined with the antibiotic Neomycin in Retropaque as an antibacterial medium. The organic iodide media are preferred and 20 to 30 per cent solutions of any of these are quite satisfactory. Too great an opacity is undesirable since calculi may be obscured.

When the injection is made, overdistention of the pelvis and calyces should be avoided. A good method of introduction is by means of gravity or carefully controlled pressure (46 cm. of water). Ordinarily 5 to 10 cc. of medium will make a satisfactory pyelogram. Films are developed immediately to assure good filling and good visualization of the various anatomic structures. Special films may be taken as necessary following these exploratory studies.

Following this initial injection and after satisfactory visualization of the renal calyces and pelvis, a film is obtained while withdrawing the catheter, all the while injecting the opaque medium. This permits a complete visualization of the ureter as well as the pelvis and kidney calyces.

When ureteral obstruction is expected, a delayed pyelogram is sometimes desired. This may be obtained in the erect position to visualize the point of obstruction to better advantage.

Cystography and Cystourethrography

Excretory Cystograms and Cystourethrograms (Fig. 16–41). Following the excretory urogram, an excretory cystogram may be obtained, although usually the urinary bladder is not completely distended at this time. One should hesitate to express a final

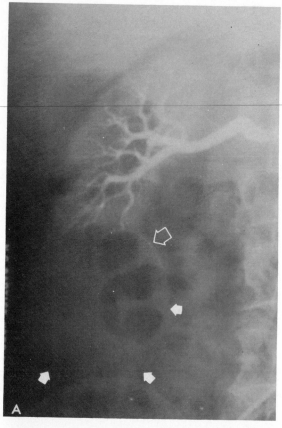

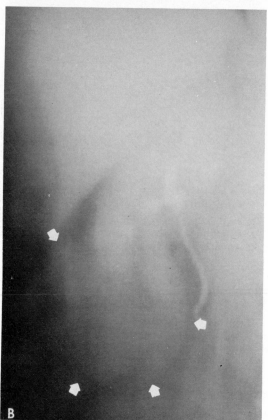

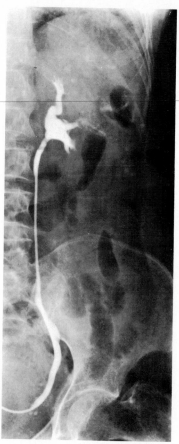

Figure 16–40. Representative retrograde pyelogram with ureteral catheter in situ.

opinion on such films. Excretory cystourethrograms can be made during the act of voiding as a final part of the excretory urographic study.

These tests are most important in a pediatric practice since often vesical, ureteral, or urethral dysfunction or morphologic abnormality may be discovered thereby. Vesicoureteral reflux that may be missed during conventional studies may be easily recognized with a voiding cystourethrogram.

The Simple Retrograde Cystogram (Fig. 16–42). The procedure is performed as follows: after the patient has completely voided, the urinary bladder is catheterized and the residual urine measured. Thereafter 150 to 200 ml. of a 10 to 30 per cent solution of any of the diiodinated or triiodinated compounds used for excretory urography are instilled in the urinary bladder through the catheter and the catheter is removed. The urinary bladder is

Figure 16–39. Renal cyst. *A.* Arteriogram. *B.* Nephrotomogram. Renal angiogram in a patient with renal cyst involving the inferior pole of the right kidney: solid arrows, wall of the cyst; open arrow, capsular artery of the cyst producing the thin-walled appearance of renal cyst. Nephrotomogram has solid arrows outlining the renal cyst and contrast agent in the collecting system and right ureter.

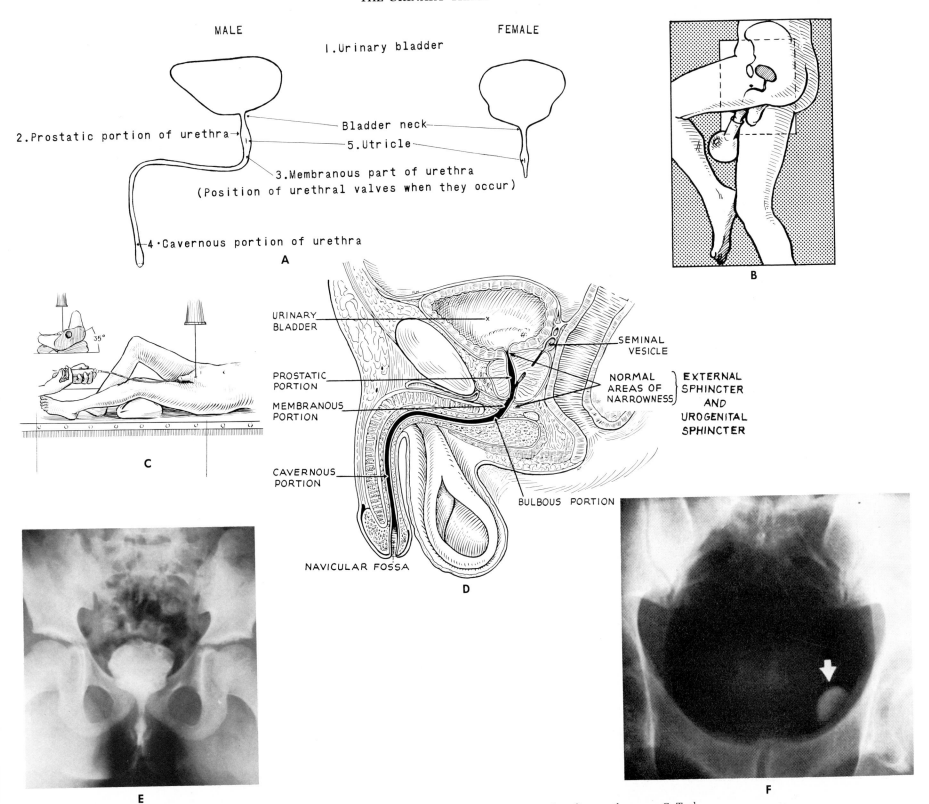

Figure 16–41. *A.* Male and female cystourethrogram anatomy. *B.* Technique of voiding urethrogram. *C.* Technique of retrograde urethrogram. *D.* Anatomy of male urethra. *E.* Female urethrogram. *F.* Air cystogram of the urinary bladder demonstrating a filling defect due to a small sessile bladder carcinoma.

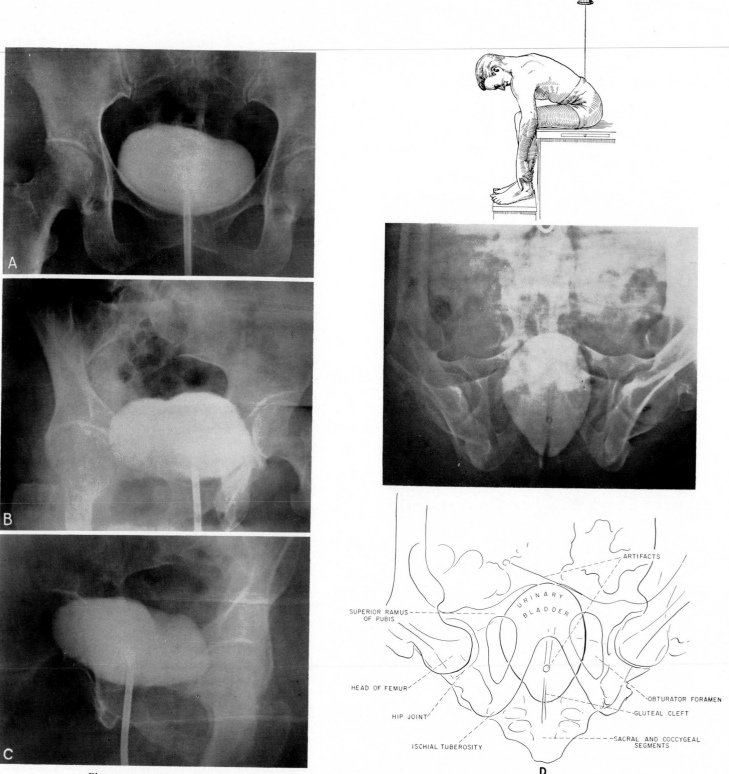

Figure 16–42. Representative normal cystograms. *A.* Anteroposterior view. *B.* Left posterior oblique view. *C.* Right posterior oblique view. A lateral view may also be employed. *D.* Chassard-Lapiné view of urinary bladder (also called sitting, squat, or jackknife view).

filled within the limits of comfort to the patient. The views obtained are shown in Figure 16–42. The oblique and profile studies are necessary to distinguish diverticula or filling defects which otherwise might be obscured. Finally, the patient is encouraged to void as completely as possible, but if unable to void the bladder is evacuated by catheter. The *postvoiding study* is of some value to demonstrate: (a) vesical diverticula, (b) filling defects caused by neoplasm, and (c) vesicoureteral reflux. The demonstration of the latter requires that a full 14 × 17 inch film be utilized to include both ureters and kidneys as well as the urinary bladder. Under normal conditions it is not unusual for 10 to 20 cc. to remain in the urinary bladder after the patient has apparently voided completely.

The Air Cystogram (Fig. 16–41 *F*). Approximately 100 to 200 cc. of air are introduced by catheter. Vesical tumors may produce a soft tissue density within the air cystogram. Air cystography may be enhanced by double contrast by using opaque media in addition to air. In the presence of a rupture of the urinary bladder air will enter the abdominal cavity or soft tissue space surrounding the urinary bladder. Fatal air embolism has been described as a complication of air cystography (Emmett and Witten).

The Polycystogram and Superimposition Cystography (Fig. 16–43 *A* and *B*). This procedure is utilized to help determine the degree of fixation of the urinary bladder against adjacent structures. The bladder is filled with approximately 200 ml. of the contrast agent and three serial exposures are made in the anteroposterior projection, each exposure being one-third of the normal exposure time without changing the cassette. After the first exposure, the contrast agent is removed in two steps: approximately 120 ml. the first time and 50 ml. the second time, and the vesical outline is compared in these three instances (Cobb and Anderson). If the entire vesical wall is not fixed, there is a tendency for the outlines of the urinary bladder to show fixation by convergence of the contrast agent on all three exposures.

The Triple-Voiding Cystogram (Lattimer, Dean, and Furey). Voiding in three installments often permits better emptying of a large atonic bladder. The films obtained after each voiding are called the triple-voiding cystogram. Usually the patient is allowed to walk around for approximately 2 minutes after each voiding episode. This technique provides a mechanism for measuring residual urine as well as for demonstrating vesicoureteral reflux.

Delayed Cystography for Children. This method is of par-

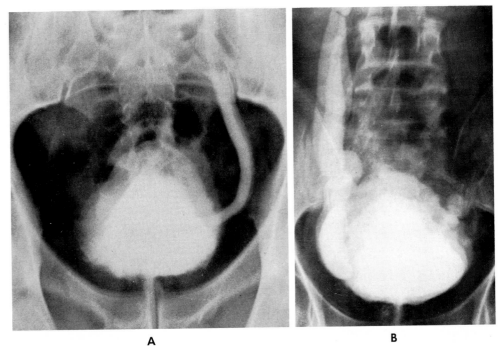

A	**B**

Figure 16–43. *A.* Polycystogram of man, with *transitional cell epithelioma of bladder wall* on the right side. Retrograde cystogram with three exposures on one film, each for one third of usual exposure time, with 200, 80, and 30 ml. of contrast medium, respectively, in bladder. Note concentricity of outlines as evidence of noninfiltrating tumor. Bilateral vesicoureteral reflux, particularly on the left side. *B.* Polycystogram of man, 75 years of age, with prostatic hypertrophy and vesical tumor. Tumor on right side of bladder wall is shown by concentric outlines. Bladder wall in area of tumor is not fixed. Note right vesicoureteral reflux and small vesical diverticulum on left. (Courtesy of Dr. H. W. ten Cate, *in* Emmet, J. L., and Witten, D. M.: Clinical Urography, 3rd ed. Philadelphia, W. B. Saunders Co., 1971.)

ticular value in children in order to check urinary retention, particularly since children are often unable to void on command. Vesicoureteral reflux that has not been visible by other methods may be demonstrated thereby. Indeed, excretory urography and cystoscopy may be misleading, and this diagnosis may be missed without evidence from a delayed cystogram.

Micturition Cystourethrogram (voiding cystourethrogram). Voiding cystourethrography usually distends the prostatic urethra sufficiently to demonstrate the external urethral sphincteric mechanism. The anterior urethra is also thereby visualized. In very young children, who cannot void on command, *expression cystourethrography* may be necessary under anesthesia.

The Retrograde Cystourethrogram (Fig. 16–41). The simple retrograde urethrogram is of less value than a voiding cystourethrogram for unimpeded visualization of the vesical neck and prostatic urethra. Voiding cystourethrography ordinarily permits a good visualization of the posterior as well as the anterior urethra. This procedure is of particular importance in children in whom valves of the urethra and vesicoureteral reflux are best demonstrated by voiding cystourethrography. Films in an oblique position with the patient standing are preferred if at all feasible.

Kjellberg et al. have recommended the utilization of a suspension of barium sulfate with sodium carboxymethylcellulose. They have warned, however, that this should not be used for retrograde urethrography, since fatal venous embolism has been described secondary to retrograde use of barium suspensions in the urethra; moreover, vesicoureteral reflux has, on occasion, resulted in barium impaction of the ureter. However, this is a very favorable medium in respect to its density and nonirritating attributes.

Kjellberg et al. have used simultaneous biplane sequential films with automatic filming at 3 to 5 second intervals, depending on the rate of micturition. Waterhouse, on the other hand, has reduced the technique by making only one x-ray exposure with the patient lying in the right oblique posterior position, thus diminishing x-ray exposure. Cineradiography has also been extensively employed (Dunbar).

"Chain" Cystourethrography (Fig. 16–44). Urethrocystograms have proved to be of value in some female patients under treatment for stress incontinence (Green; Calatroni et al.). This is carried out as follows. With the help of a probe, a chain of metallic beads is introduced into the urinary bladder through the urethra, the probe is withdrawn, and one end of the chain remains in the bladder, while the other is taped to the inner surface of the thigh. Thereafter, 50 cc. of 10 to 15 per cent solution of sodium iodide (or equivalent in organic iodine) is introduced into the urinary bladder by means of a No. 10 Nelaton catheter. Once the catheter is withdrawn, the patient is instructed to stand upright, whereupon frontal and lateral x-ray films centered over the lower pubis are taken. These radiographs are taken serially so that different

degrees of stress are registered. The posterior urethrovesical angle (PUV) is measured, as well as the angle of inclination to the perpendicular of the upper urethra. The normal PUV angle is 90 to 100 degrees, and the normal angle of inclination of the upper urethra to the perpendicular is 30 degrees with the patient in the erect position and straining. The normal and various examples of abnormal angles are illustrated in Fig. 16–44.

Renal Arteriography and Aortography (Fig. 16–45). Visualization of the renal arteries, their major ramifications, nephrograms, renal collecting systems, and to a limited extent, renal veins, may be accomplished by (1) translumbar aortography, (2) percutaneous aortography by catheter techniques, and (3) selective renal arteriography (Colapinto and Steed). Translumbar aortograms may be employed in patients with severe aortoiliac disease in whom retrograde catheterization may be impossible or hazardous. On the other hand, transbrachial or axillary artery catheterization may be attempted for selective catheterization in some of these cases. We have considered these techniques as special procedures outside the scope of this text and the student is referred to extensive monographs on these subjects (Schobinger and Ruzicka).

Percutaneous transfemoral renal arteriography is probably the procedure of choice. Not only can the individual single or multiple renal arteries be selectively visualized, but midstream injection into the aorta may help determine the multiplicity of renal arteries for greatest accuracy. The use of a mechanical injector and rapid film sequencing equipment permits a dynamic study of the arterial blood supply of the kidney and allows an accurate assay of the pathology and physiology as well as anatomy.

Patterns of Collateral Flow in Renal Ischemia (Abrams and Cornell; Paul et al.). The vessels supplying the renal collaterals are usually the lumbar, internal iliac, testicular or ovarian, inferior adrenal, renal capsular, and intercostal arteries as well as the aorta itself. *The third lumbar artery is the commonest source of anastomotic flow to the kidney.* Ordinarily these collaterals are not demonstrable in the absence of renal ischemia. Usually the collateral vessels are coiled and tortuous and lengthened by comparison with the normal. They may also be dilated. Abrams and Cornell have divided the renal collateral circulation into three categories: (1) a capsular system (Fig. 16–45), (2) a peripelvic system, and (3) a periureteric system. As noted in Figure 16–45, the capsular system consists of the first four lumbar arteries, branches of the internal iliac, and the intercostal arteries. Not shown in the diagram are the inferior adrenal and capsular branches of the kidney which themselves may make major contributions.

The peripelvic system consists largely of the aorta itself, the inferior adrenal, the first three lumbar, the gonadal, and the gonadal branches. Occasionally there are direct capsular branches from the renal artery proximal to the stenosis when such exists.

The periureteric system consists mainly of the internal iliac artery with other contributing arteries being the second, third and fourth lumbar, gonadal, and direct aortic branches.

Thus, although it is usually considered that after vessels perforate the renal sinus they are "end" arteries, nevertheless, a renal collateral circulation is able to maintain function and viability of involved renal parenchyma in many cases.

Within the kidney there are perforating capsular branches which arise from the interlobular arteries and terminate by communicating with the adipose-capsular arteries in the retroperitoneal arterial plexus of Turner. Arterial communications in the retroperitoneal plexus are numerous (Paul et al.). Additional basic references on this subject are those by Merklin and Michels, and Graves.

Phlebography and Inferior Vena Cavography (Fig. 16–46). Generally, the techniques employed for selective phlebography are similar to those for renal arteriography, except that the catheter must be preformed in accordance with the anatomy of the renal veins. The femoral vein is the site of insertion of the catheter except where a block in the inferior vena cava is encountered. Under these circumstances, the catheter may be introduced into an arm vein, passed through the superior vena cava, right atrium, and then into the inferior vena cava.

The inferior vena cava may be demonstrated in similar fashion.

Other variations of left renal phlebography have been described, such as left spermatic phlebography.

Visualization of the renal veins has become increasingly important in the diagnosis of invasive malignancies of the kidneys and their prognostic evaluation. Renal vein thrombosis may be differentiated in this manner. As indicated previously the anatomy of the renal venous system may be subdivided into: (a) extrarenal venous structures, and (b) intrarenal venous structures.

Extrarenal Venous Structures. The *right renal vein* may be

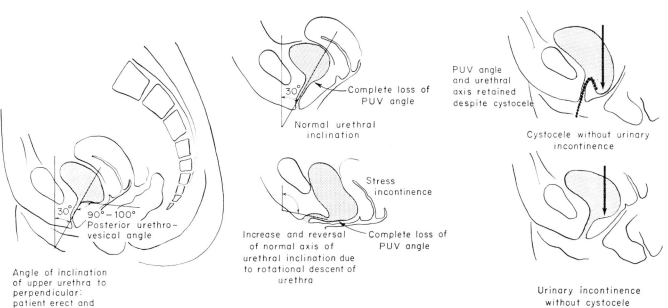
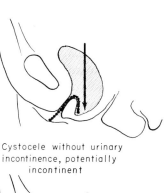
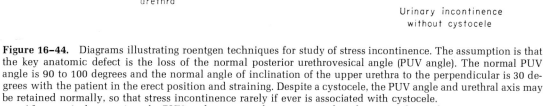

Figure 16–44. Diagrams illustrating roentgen techniques for study of stress incontinence. The assumption is that the key anatomic defect is the loss of the normal posterior urethrovesical angle (PUV angle). The normal PUV angle is 90 to 100 degrees and the normal angle of inclination of the upper urethra to the perpendicular is 30 degrees with the patient in the erect position and straining. Despite a cystocele, the PUV angle and urethral axis may be retained normally, so that stress incontinence rarely if ever is associated with cystocele.

After surgical correction, the PUV angle may vary between 55 and 95 degrees with an adequate segment of the bladder base posterior to the urethral junction participating in the formation of the new angle. The angle of inclination of the urethral axis is usually 5 to 15 degrees but may vary up to 25 degrees with respect to the vertical in the standing position. There must also be a correction of the tendency to funnel formation of the vesical neck area of the bladder base. Note that a chain of metallic beads is introduced into the bladder through the urethra. When the probe is withdrawn, one end of the chain remains in the bladder while the other is taped to the inner surface of the thigh. Sixty ml. of a 10 to 15 per cent solution of sodium iodide are introduced into the bladder and the catheter is withdrawn. The patient is instructed to stand upright, and frontal and lateral radiographs are taken of this area. (Modified from Calatroni, C. J., et al.: Amer. J. Obstet. Gynec., *83:*649–656, 1962; and Green, T. A.: Amer. J. Obstet. Gynec., *83:*632–648, 1960.)

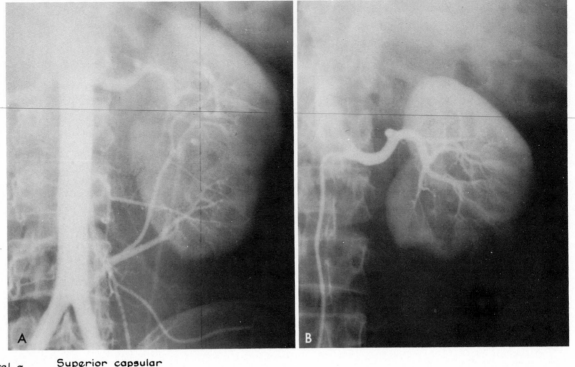

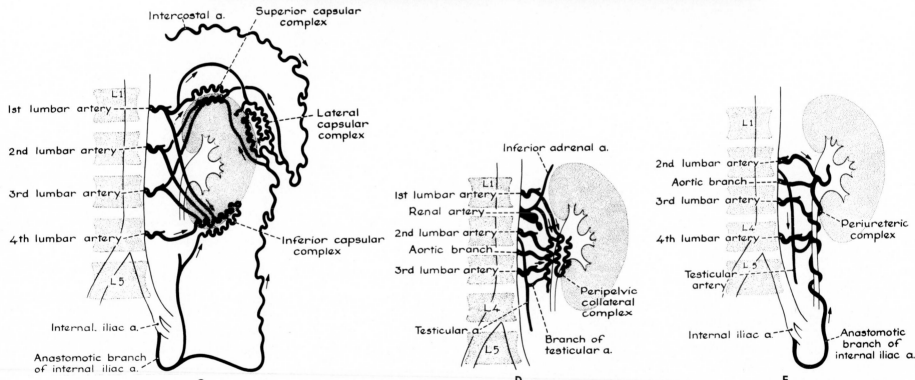

Figure 16–45. Selective arteriogram showing the appearance with a double renal artery supplying one kidney when both left renal arteries are filled (*A*), and when only the upper is filled (*B*). *C–E*. Renal Collateral Circulation. Diagrammatic representation. *C. The capsular system:* The first four lumbar arteries, branches of the internal iliac, and the intercostal arteries contributed significantly to the capsular complex. In addition, not pictured here, the inferior adrenal and capsular branches proximal to the stenosis also made major contributions. Note that a separate "lateral" capsular complex has been indicated; this represents a continuation of the superior capsular system, but has been designated "lateral" because of its location and mode of filling.

D. The peripelvic system: The aorta directly, the inferior adrenal, first three lumbar, and testicular (or ovarian) arteries all supplied branches to the peripelvic system. Additional important pathways were direct capsular branches from the renal artery proximal to the stenosis.

E. The periureteric system: The internal iliac artery was the single most common source of periureteric collaterals. The second, third, and fourth lumbar, testicular, and direct aortic branches were also large and important components of this collateral pathway. (From Abrams, H. L., and Cornell, S. H.: Radiology, 84:1001–1012, 1965.)

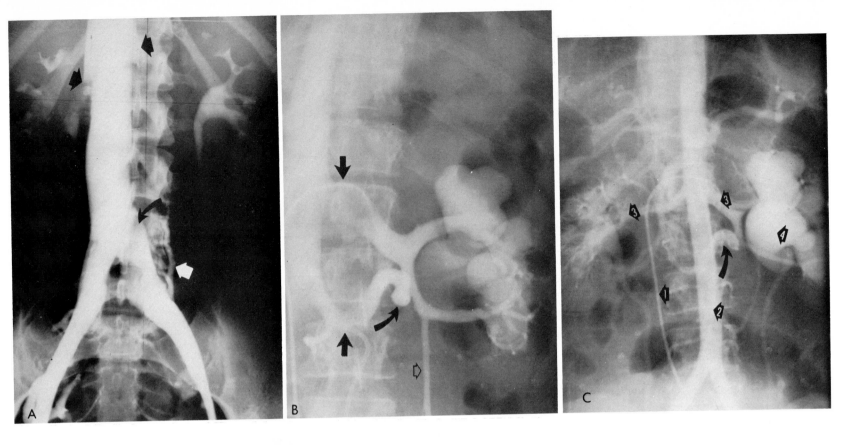

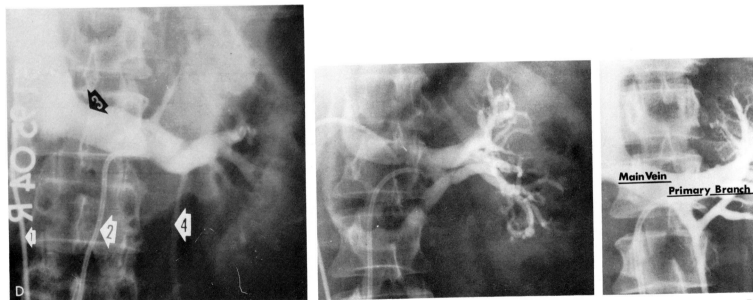

Figure 16–46. *A.* Renal venogram and inferior vena cavagram (black curved arrow). Black straight arrows point to origin of renal veins. White arrow shows paravertebral veins. *B.* Inferior vena cavagram with filling of the circumaortic renal vein, and associated hydronephrosis. Open arrow shows left spermatic vein. *C.* Aortogram in same patient as *B*: (1) Catheter in inferior vena cava, (2) catheter in abdominal aorta, (3) renal arteries, (4) hydronephrotic kidney. Curved black arrow shows circumaortic left renal vein retaining contrast agent. *D.* Left normal renal venograms. (1) Catheter in inferior vena cava, (2) catheter in aorta and left renal artery, (3) left renal vein, (4) left spermatic vein. (Courtesy University of Iowa, Department of Radiology.) *E.* Left renal phlebogram—bifid main left renal vein. *F.* Normal renal venous anatomy. (*E* and *F* by kind permission of the Honorary Editor of Clinical Radiology. Sorby, W. A.: Renal phlebography. Clin. Radiol. *20*:166–172, 1969. Published by E. & S. Livingstone, Ltd.)

bifid, trifid, or plexiform and quite short—1 to 2 cm. There are rarely any anastomotic veins adjoining it. It adjoins the inferior vena cava at an acute angle. The *left renal vein* is longer, 4 to 6 cm., and its junction with the inferior vena cava usually forms a right angle. A large *left ovarian* or *testicular vein* usually joins it. The inferior *left adrenal vein* and a number of anastomotic channels to the lumbar paraspinal plexus also join the left renal vein.

Apart from the utilization already mentioned, catheterization of the renal veins is useful in assessing the patency of splenorenal shunts and in estimation of renal blood flow, by measuring the rate of clearance of a contrast agent from the renal venous system.

Intrarenal Venous Structures. The normal intrarenal venous anatomy is shown in Figure 16–46 *F*. The main renal vein may have three to four primary tributary veins and these in turn have two to three interlobar veins coursing between the calyces and medullary pyramids. The interlobar veins are linked by arcuate veins running between the cortex and medulla. Fine, parallel cortical veins drain the outer surface, flowing into the arcuate veins. There are a few subcapsular stellate veins as well. The veins are not segmental end vessels, unlike the renal arteries. Communications between veins are free and numerous. Of interest is the distortion of the venous system by cysts in the kidney. The thickness of the renal cortex may also be measured accurately by virtue of the cortical veins (Sorby; Kahn).

Implacements upon, deformity, or displacements of the inferior vena cava also have assumed greater importance in diagnosis, particularly in relation to malignancies which involve the central axis of the body (lymphomas or metastasizing carcinomas).

Triple Contrast Study of the Urinary Bladder (Fig. 16–47). This study consists of (1) oxygen or air injected in the perivesical tissue space; (2) air injected into the urinary bladder via catheter; and (3) retrograde femoral arteriography for visualization of the blood supply of the urinary bladder.

The patient is placed supine on the x-ray table in the Trendelenburg head down position, an 18 gauge needle is inserted in the extraperitoneal space just outside the urinary bladder, and approximately 300 cc. of air is instilled. The urinary bladder wall may be seen when 300 to 500 cc. of air is injected into the urinary

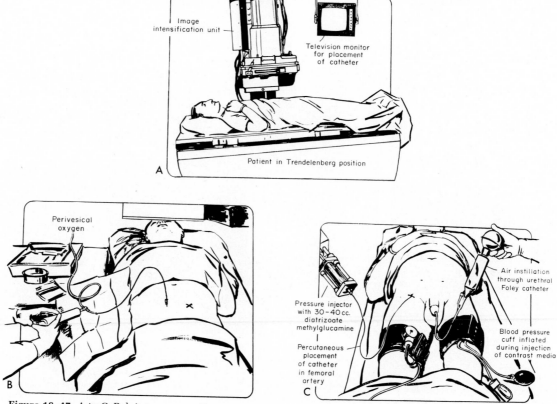

Figure 16–47. *A* to *C.* Pelvic pneumoperitoneum, air cystography, and arterial angiography of the urinary bladder (triple contrast). (Courtesy Drs. S. C. Lacy, C. E. Cox, W. H. Boyce, and J. E. Whitley, Departments of Urology and Radiology. The Bowman Gray School of Medicine.)

Figure 16–47 continued on the opposite page.

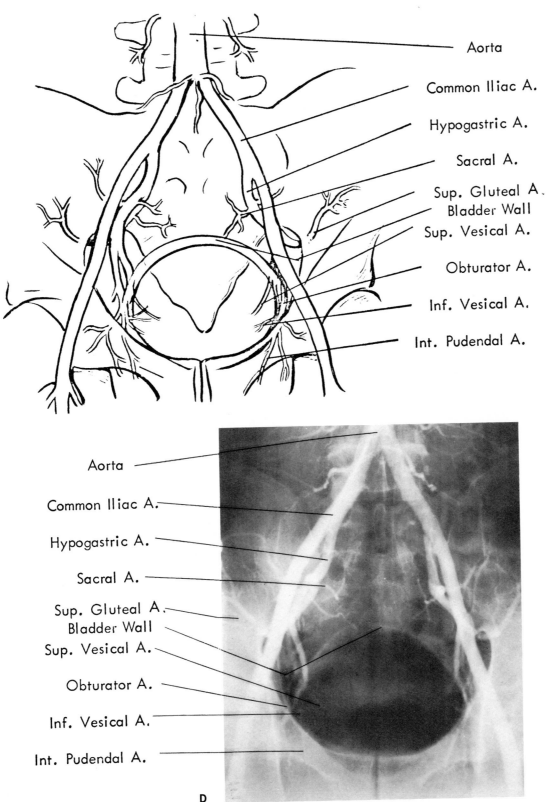

Aorta

Common Iliac A.

Hypogastric A.

Sacral A.

Sup. Gluteal A.
Bladder Wall
Sup. Vesical A.

Obturator A.

Inf. Vesical A.

Int. Pudendal A.

Aorta

Common Iliac A.

Hypogastric A.

Sacral A.

Sup. Gluteal A.
Bladder Wall
Sup. Vesical A.

Obturator A.

Inf. Vesical A.

Int. Pudendal A.

D

Figure 16–47 *Continued.* D. Radiograph obtained in normal triple contrast study of urinary bladder and labeled tracing of same.

bladder through a Foley catheter. The femoral artery is catheterized by the Seldinger technique as in aortography. Pressure injection and serial filming are accomplished so that the arterial distribution to the urinary bladder and to any tumor contained within its wall is shown. Any spreading to, or invasion of, contiguous structures in the pelvis may also be demonstrated. The triple contrast technique is particularly helpful for assessment of total spread and degree of involvement of the urinary bladder by malignancy. This, too, is a special procedure beyond the scope of this text.

Roentgen Examination of the Surgically Exposed Kidney (Fig. 16–48). Radiography of the surgically exposed kidney, particularly during removal of renal stones, may be accomplished by wrapping a suitably sized film in black paper and packing it in a

sheet of sterile rubber to be placed next to the kidney during its radiography at the time of surgery. Sterile packs are commercially available for this purpose. The films may be placed in a sterile rubber glove at the time of radiography also. A special cassette utilizing intensifying screens has also been devised for this technique (Olsson).

Cineradiography (Dux et al.). Cineradiography of the excretory urogram may be readily accomplished with image amplification and cinematography. Urine is transported toward the urinary bladder as a result of the active coordinated contraction of muscle groups in the renal pelvis, major and minor calyces, and ureter. Emptying of the renal pelvis depends on its shape and size, on flow from individual calyceal groups, and on filling pressure (the pressure changes in the ureter). Peristalsis or antiperi-

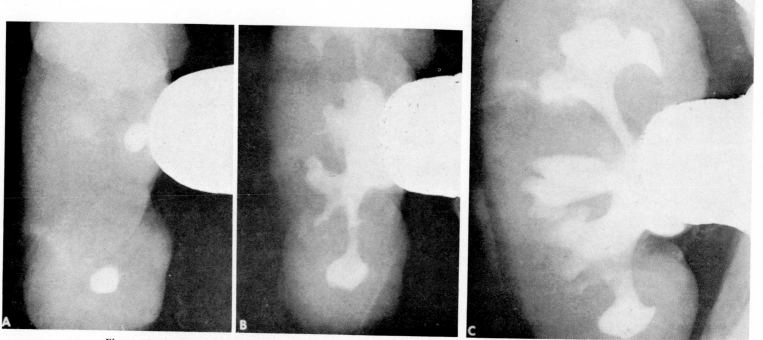

Figure 16–48. Renal organography during surgery. All exposures are 15 milliampere/second with average of 65 Kvp. *A.* Exposure with central ray passing from convex surface through the hilus of the kidney. Four calculi are visible, one in the pelvis and three in the inferior calyx. Only the two larger calculi were visualized on preoperative roentgenograms. Note clearly visible untreated cotton umbilical tapes which support the relatively small kidney at each pole. Large kidneys may require two films to cover the entire organ. The use of two properly placed films will remove the "blind spot" occasioned by the notch in the film which accommodates the renal pedicle. *B.* Same position as *A* after occluding the ureter with a rubber-shod spring clamp and filling the pelvis with contrast medium through a 23 gauge needle. *C.* Same as *B* with central ray traversing the short axis of the kidney. Such rotational exposures permit accurate localization of small calculi and assist in planning plastic revisions of a strictured calyx (calycotomy), calycectomy, excision of intrarenal diverticula or cysts, and partial nephrectomies.

Angiography by this technique is accomplished by temporary occlusion of the primary renal artery and filling with dilute contrast medium through a 23 or 25 gauge intracatheter needle inserted into the renal artery distal to the point of occlusion. (From Boyce, W. H.: Radiol. Clin. N. Amer., 3:101, 1965.)

stalsis cannot ordinarily be demonstrated in the normal renal pelvis. In the ureter, on the other hand, urine transport appears to depend upon pure peristaltic contraction.

Cineradiography may also be employed as an adjunct to urethrocystograms, but because of the greater radiation exposure of the gonads by this technique single or selected rapid film sequences on 70 to 105 mm spot films are usually preferred.

Pneumograms of the Urinary Bladder and Pneumopyelograms. Air may be injected through a ureteral catheter for the latter purpose. Unfortunately, small bubbles of air will simulate

calculi or small polypi, and hence the constancy of a finding must be interpreted with caution. Filling defects, however, are sometimes demonstrated to excellent advantage by this technique. The danger of air embolism must be considered.

Perirenal Air Insufflation (Fig. 16–49). Perirenal air insufflation, direct or by means of the introduction of presacral air, may be utilized (Cocchi). When introduced presacrally, the air rises in the tela subserosa and follows along the fascial planes, giving rise to a delineation not only of the kidney but also of the suprarenal structures. This method is particularly useful for the

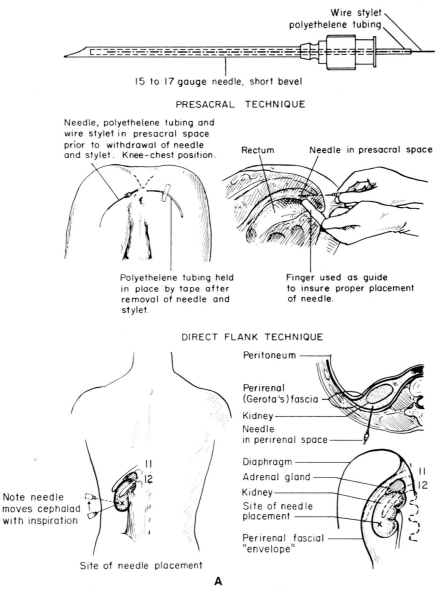

Figure 16–49. A. Diagrams illustrating the direct flank and presacral techniques for retroperitoneal pneumography.

Figure 16–49 continued on the following page.

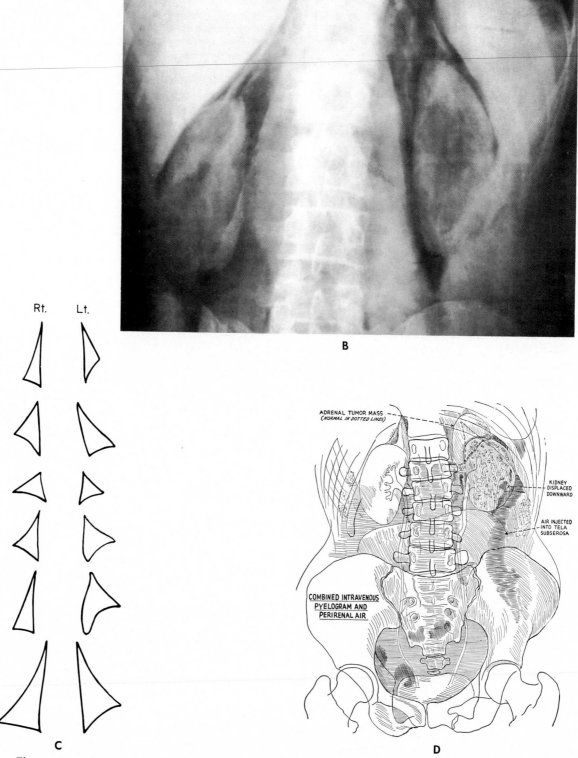

B

Rt.   Lt.

C

ADRENAL TUMOR MASS
(NORMAL IN DOTTED LINES)

KIDNEY
DISPLACED
DOWNWARD

AIR INJECTED
INTO TELA
SUBSEROSA

COMBINED INTRAVENOUS
PYELOGRAM AND
PERIRENAL AIR

D

Figure 16–49 *Continued.* B. Normal retroperitoneal pneumogram. C. Tracings of six normal retroperitoneal pneumograms. (A, B, and C from McLelland, R., Landes, R. R., and Ransom, C. L.: Radiol. Clin. N. Amer., 3:115, 1965.) D and E. Perirenal air insufflation around the left kidney and suprarenal area, demonstrating an adrenal tumor mass in this region. This proved to be adrenal cortical carcinoma. D. Labeled tracing of radiograph shown in E.

Figure 16–49 continued on the opposite page.

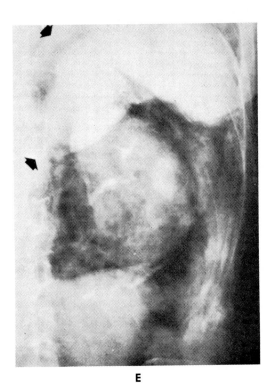

E

Figure 16–49 *Continued.* E. Radiograph coned down over renal and suprarenal areas.

delineation of suprarenal tumor masses. It is of special value when it is combined with intravenous or retrograde pyelograms and body section radiographs.

Seminal Vesiculography. Seminal vesiculography is a specialized procedure not frequently employed. It is utilized primarily to study the appearance of the seminal vesicles and the vas deferens, and occasionally in relation to prostatic carcinoma (Emmett et al.) (Fig. 16–50 *A* and *B*).

The Normal Kidney's Reaction to Intravenous Pyelography (Arkless). (1) Kidneys will ordinarily enlarge after the injection of contrast material, reaching a maximum increase of approximately 0.5 cm. at about 5 minutes following completion of the injection. When films are exposed and measured from the beginning of the injection, the maximum size is reached at about 2.5 to 3 minutes if 25 cc. is used, whereas if 50 cc. is employed it tends to be earlier. (2) The time required for calyceal visualization also varies somewhat according to the amount of contrast material injected. Calyceal visualization is usually accomplished at 2 minutes when 50 cc. is employed, but there may be a ½ to 1 minute further delay when only 25 cc. is utilized.

Comparison of Renal Tests. Wigh et al. have compared sodium diatrizoate (Hypaque) intravenous pyelograms with other renal tests, including blood urea nitrogen levels, phenolsulfonphthalein excretion rates and creatinine clearance values. The accompanying scattergrams (Fig. 16–51) are presented to com-

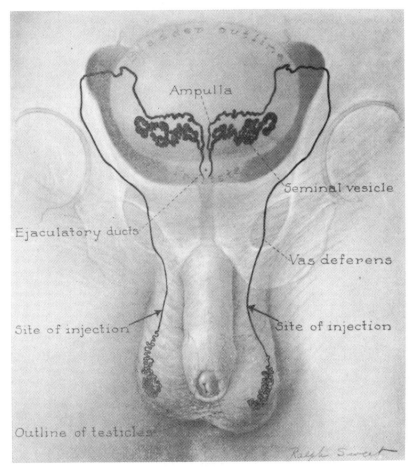

A

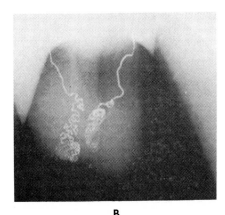

B

Figure 16–50. *A.* The male genital tract. The sites of exposure of the vasa deferentia are indicated, into which injections of the contrast media are made upward and frequently downward. *B.* Filling of the distal portions of the epididymides has been achieved. Greater filling has been obtained on the right than on the left. (From Tucker, A. S., Yanagihara, H., and Pryde, A. W.: Amer. J. Roentgenol., 71:490–500, 1954.)

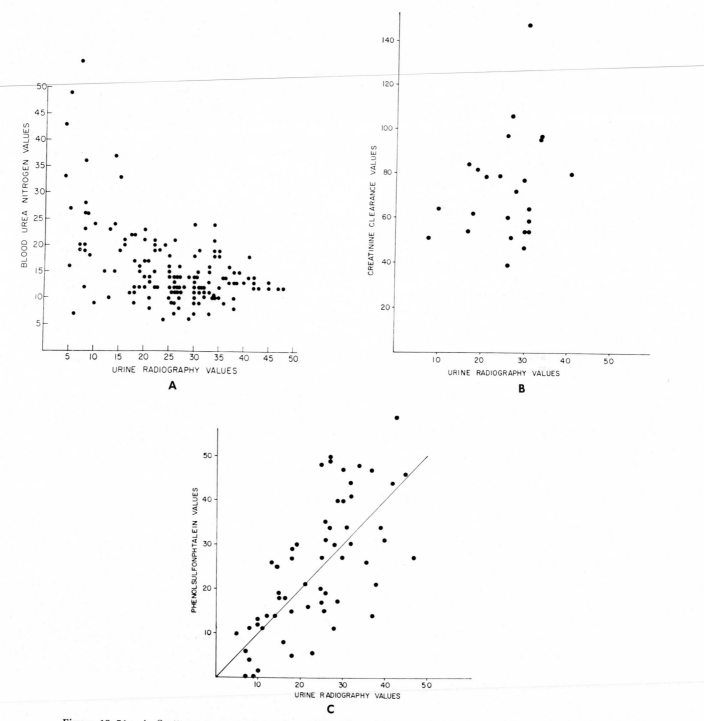

Figure 16–51. *A.* Scattergram comparing urine radiography values—per cent of excreted sodium diatrizoate (Hypaque 50%)—with blood urea nitrogen determinations in mg. per cent in 143 patients. *B.* Graph plotting urine radiography values against creatinine clearance expressed in ml./min. for 24 patients. *C.* Comparison of urine radiography determinations with phenolsulfonphthalein tests, expressed as per cent voided in fifteen minutes for 59 patients. (From Wigh, R., Anthony, H. F., Jr., and Grant, B. P.: Radiology, *78:*869–878, 1962.)

pare the urine radiography values with those of one of the other tests. In each case in which incomplete micturition occurred, the urine radiography percentage was connected to take into account residual bladder Hypaque. This estimate was derived from a post-voiding radiograph.

Blood Urea Nitrogen. A plot of the percentage of organic iodide excretion in 30 minutes against the blood urea nitrogen in milligrams per cent is shown in Figure 16–51 *A*. On the assumption that 24 mg. per cent might be the upper limit of normal for blood urea nitrogen excretion (BUN), the patients who excreted 20 per cent or more of the Hypaque were placed in this category. Generally, with higher BUN levels less than 20 per cent of the injected Hypaque was excreted in 30 minutes. There were, however, 29 patients (in this group of 143) who excreted less than 20 per cent of the contrast agent and who had blood urea nitrogen levels between 8 and 24 mg. per cent—values in the normal range. Generally, then, one may conclude that a fair urogram may be anticipated in patients with BUN levels up to 20 mg. per cent, although some exceptions will be found to this rule. Of course, many extrarenal factors play a part in BUN levels, and a good correlation, therefore, between BUN and excretory urography cannot be expected.

Creatinine Clearance. A scattergram indicating the relationship of creatinine clearance to urine radiography values is shown in Figure 16–51 *B*. The graph shows only in a very general way that the better the Hypaque clearance, the greater the clearance of creatinine.

Phenolsulfonphthalein Determinations. Figure 16–51 *C* shows a comparison of the phenolsulfonphthalein determinations with urine radiography. This demonstrates the closest correlation of any of the three tests presented. Average phenolsulfonphthalein values are 35 per cent in 15 minutes; 35 per cent Hypaque excretion, on the other hand, reflects a high value rather than an average one.

There is therefore no absolute index as to which of the tests is necessarily best. Since the patient is in a dehydrated state for the excretory urograms, the comparison itself rests on a physiologically abnormal condition.

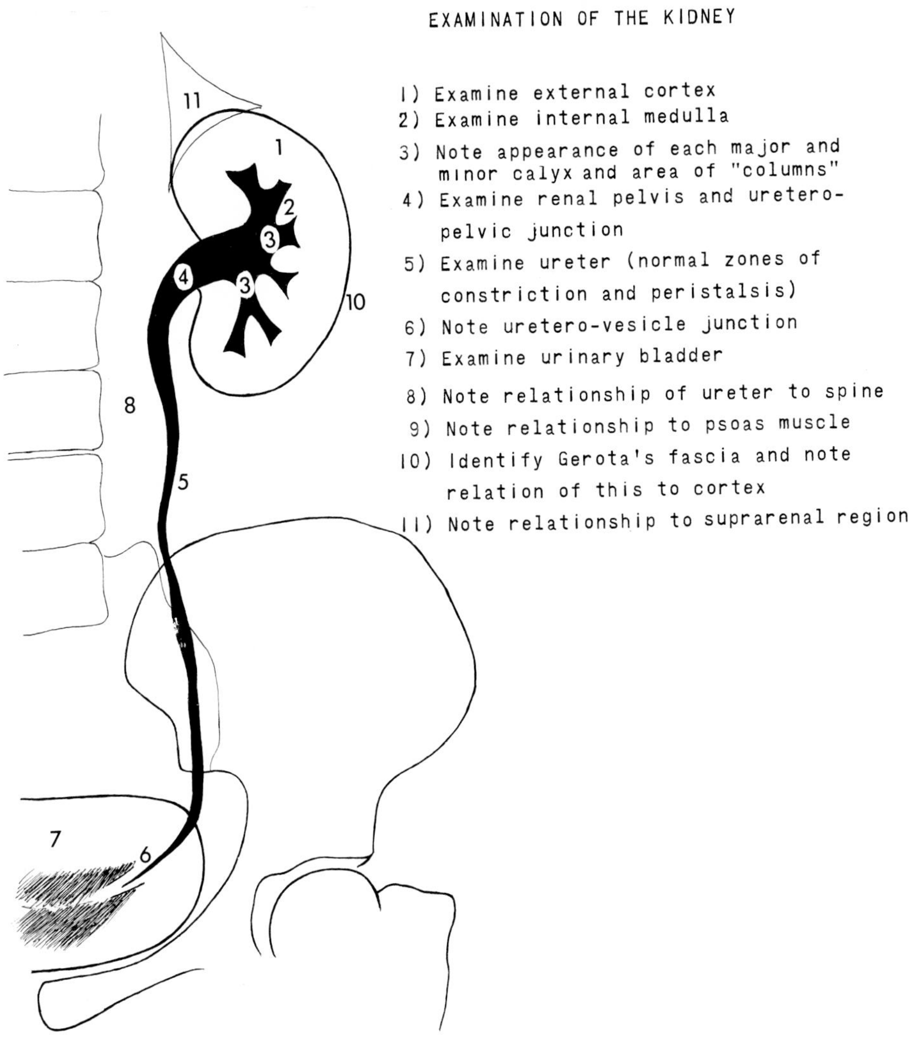

Reactions to Contrast Media

General Comments. Reactions to the intravenous injection of contrast media are common. Mild reactions include warmth and flushing, nausea, vomiting, tingling, numbness, cough, and local pain in the arm, especially if the injection is carried out slowly. Serious reactions may include conjunctivitis, rhinitis, urticaria, facial edema, glottic edema, and even shocklike reactions with dyspnea, convulsions, cyanosis, shock, and even

EXAMINATION OF THE KIDNEY

1) Examine external cortex
2) Examine internal medulla
3) Note appearance of each major and minor calyx and area of "columns"
4) Examine renal pelvis and ureteropelvic junction
5) Examine ureter (normal zones of constriction and peristalsis)
6) Note uretero-vesicle junction
7) Examine urinary bladder
8) Note relationship of ureter to spine
9) Note relationship to psoas muscle
10) Identify Gerota's fascia and note relation of this to cortex
11) Note relationship to suprarenal region

Figure 16–52. Kidney collecting system with excretory urography. Method of studying films.

occasional death. It has been estimated that there has been an incidence of 6.6 deaths per million examinations (Pendergrass et al., 1958). Approximately 90 per cent of fatal reactions occurred during or immediately after injection, and hence it is vital that medications to counteract reactions be immediately available to the physician who performs the injection.

Generally, a pre-injection dose of the contrast agent is performed, allowing several drops of the contrast agent to enter the blood stream with a delay of 30 to 60 seconds indicated thereafter. A longer delay of 4 to 5 minutes is advised if there is a strong history of allergy or sensitivity in the patient. If no untoward reaction then occurs, the entire dose is injected. The best protection against serious reactions is a careful history to elicit any record of severe allergies, drug reactions, asthma, hay fever, sensitivity to iodine, previous reactions to excretory urography and related conditions.

Although results are variable in relation to the prior administration of antihistamine drugs, it appears that the preliminary intravenous injection of antihistamines, 3 to 5 minutes prior to the injection of the contrast medium, may reduce the incidence or severity of a reaction. Fifty milligrams of Benadryl (diphenhydramine hydrochloride) or 20 milligrams of Chlor-Trimeton (chlorpropheniramine-maleate) are perhaps most widely used.

In treatment of reactions the following must be judiciously employed:

1. Immediate subcutaneous or intramuscular administration of 0.5 cc. of 1 in 1000 epinephrine; this may be repeated in 10 to 15 minutes. Blood pressure must be watched closely for hypotension and impending shock.

2. One hundred per cent oxygen may be administered immediately through a face mask. If there is inadequate airway, an anesthesiologist should be called to introduce an endotracheal tube. Artificial respiration then may be carried out as necessary.

3. If shock is profound, epinephrine may be administered slowly intravenously in a dose of 0.25 cc.

4. Benadryl (20 mg.) or hydrocortisone (100 mg.) or both, may be administered intravenously at once.

5. Asthma and pulmonary edema may be combatted with 0.5 grams of Aminophylline, given intravenously over a period of 5 to 20 minutes.

6. Hypotension may be treated with the intravenous administration of vasopressor drugs such as phenylephrine hydrochloride (Neo-Synephrine), 0.5 mg.; or methoxamine hydrochloride (Vasoxyl), 5 to 10 mg. If there is no response, levarterenol bitartrate (Levophed), 4 to 8 cc. in 500 cc. of 5 per cent glucose, should be given intravenously, the rate of administration being governed by the blood pressure.

7. Convulsions or laryngospasm or both may be controlled with the intravenous injection of 2 to 3 cc. of 2.5 per cent solution of thiopental sodium. Laryngeal edema, if not controlled by epinephrine, may require an emergency tracheotomy.

Risk of Excretory Urography in Multiple Myeloma. It has been postulated that urinary contrast media may be a precipitating or exciting factor which sets the stage for precipitation of hyaline casts in the kidney in patients with multiple myeloma. It is thought that this may be obviated by alkalinization of the urine and adequate hydration. A few reports of fatal anuria following excretory urography in patients with multiple myeloma have appeared.

Advantages and Disadvantages of Excretory Urography as Opposed to Retrograde Pyelography. These are summarized in Table 16–5. Intravenous and retrograde pyelography are complementary or supplementary procedures and one does not exclude the utilization of the other.

TABLE 16–5 ADVANTAGES AND DISADVANTAGES OF EXCRETORY UROGRAPHY AS OPPOSED TO RETROGRADE PYELOGRAPHY

Excretory Urograms	Retrograde Pyelograms
Greater comfort to patient; no risk of infection.	Great discomfort and risk of infection
Does not require ureteral catheterization.	Requires ureteral catheterization.
Yields some information regarding renal function and may allow selectivity in retrograde study.	No information regarding renal function.
Probably of no value when BUN is elevated above 50 mg. per cent but may be tolerated when small doses of contrast agent are employed (Davidson et al.).	May precipitate anuria in some medical diseases such as pyelonephritis, glomerulonephritis, and arteriolar nephrosclerosis.
Detail fair when infusion pyelograms are employed but usually not as good as in retrograde study.	Structural detail optimal, but artificial distention of the collecting structures of the kidney usually occurs.
Safe in the presence of obstructing ureteral calculus.	Inadvisable to inject contrast medium above a point of obstruction, since a severe reaction in the patient may ensue.
Dangerous in cases with strong history of allergy or iodine sensitivity.	May be utilized with caution.
Possibly dangerous in patients with multiple myeloma and related disorders.	May be utilized with caution.
Should not be utilized when in vivo studies of thyroid by radioactive iodine are contemplated.	May be utilized.

Summary: **Excretory and retrograde studies are complementary and supplementary. One does not exclude the utilization of the other.**

METHOD OF ANALYSIS OF FILMS OF URINARY TRACT

Each part of the roentgenologic examination of the urinary tract plays a special role, and the method of examination of the films is closely related to this factor.

KUB Film. A routine for analysis of the anteroposterior film of the abdomen without added contrast has been previously described (Chapter 15). This film becomes an integral part of the examination of the urinary tract. The radiographic description of the kidney must concern itself with the exact outline, size, position, mobility, general configuration and relationship to contiguous structures. The numerous variations within normal limits must be recognized. For example, infantile renal lobulation may sometimes be found in an adult renal contour, and it is important to exclude the possibility of renal pathology when this occurs.

Excretory Urogram. (Fig. 16–52). In infusion pyelography, a reasonably good *nephrographic phase* can be obtained and this may be further intensified by nephrotomography.

Following the nephrographic phase, the *collecting system* is visualized, which, as shown, includes the major and minor calyces and the renal pelvis. By means of nephrotomography one can determine the relationship of these collecting structures to other internal medullary structures, such as the area of the columns. There is a wide variation in the appearance of the kidney, pelves, and calyces. A normal kidney pelvis permits an equal drainage from all parts of the kidney and allows a free flow into the ureters and bladder. There is usually a common pelvis, two to three major calyces, and six to fourteen minor calyces. The superior calyces are usually in a direct line with the ureter, whereas the inferior calyces are horizontally placed. On occasion, however, the ureter divides almost immediately into the calyces, with no common renal pelvic basin. The average capacity of the renal pelvis is 7.5 cc. of fluid, but this may be as high as 20 cc. and still not be considered pathologic.

The major calyces are merely channels, whereas the minor calyces consist of a neck with an expanded cupped distal end. The cupping is formed by the projection of the minor papillae into the calyces. The edges of the cup must be clean-cut and sharply demarcated. It is important, however, not to mistake the rounded shadow of the calyx seen end-on for a clubbed calyx, since the latter appearance is definitely abnormal.

Serial studies may show that there are changes in the size and contour of the calyces, owing to contraction and relaxation of the renal pelvis and ureter. These changes must be considered physiologic. Impressions by arteries and veins have already been described.

Other confusing pyelographic appearances are shown in Figures 16–53 and 16–54. Thus, the ureteropelvic junction may appear somewhat abnormal depending upon anomalies of rotation of the kidney. The extrarenal pelvis as against the intrarenal, duplicity of the renal pelvis, and backflow phenomena all may contribute to some confusion.

Backflow Phenomena. (Figs. 16–53 and 16–54). Occasionally, the dye will enter the collecting tubules, renal veins, or lymphatics when introduced in retrograde pyelography. The causes of this phenomenon are not known. Part of the reason may be increased pressure resulting from introduction of the contrast agent, but this may not be the sole cause. There are five types of backflow: (1) pyelotubular, (2) pyelolymphatic, (3) pyelovenous, (4) pyelosinus, and (5) pyelointerstitial.

Pyelotubular backflow is manifest by the dye radiating in straight diverging lines from a minor calyx. Pyelolymphatic backflow appears as irregular lines arising from the region of the hilus and passing inward to the region of the renal lymph nodes. Pyelovenous backflow has the appearance of thick cobwebs or hazy streaking around the major calyx and adjoining neck of the minor calyx. The veins visualized are the venous plexuses into

CONFUSING PYELOGRAPHIC APPEARANCES

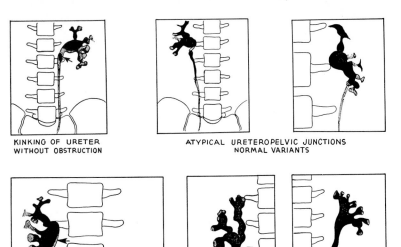

KINKING OF URETER WITHOUT OBSTRUCTION

ATYPICAL URETEROPELVIC JUNCTIONS NORMAL VARIANTS

EXTRARENAL PELVIS

NORMAL VARIANTS OF RENAL CALYCES

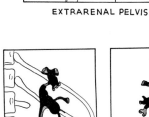
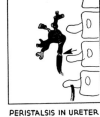
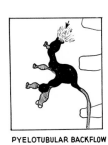
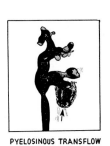

CALYCEAL NORMAL VARIANTS

PERISTALSIS IN URETER

PYELOTUBULAR BACKFLOW

PYELOSINOUS TRANSFLOW

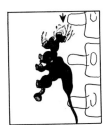
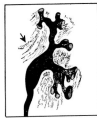
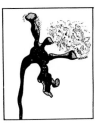
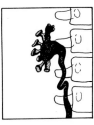

PYELOVENOUS BACKFLOW

PYELOLYMPHATIC BACKFLOW

PYELO-INTERSTITIAL BACKFLOW

URETERAL KINKING WITHOUT OBSTRUCTION

Figure 16–53.

which the interlobar veins of the kidney drain, since the tissue separating the calyces from the endothelium at these points is extremely thin and easily ruptured.

Often there is an accumulation of fat surrounding the renal

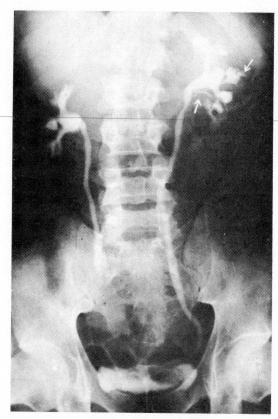

Figure 16–54. Intensified radiograph demonstrating backflow phenomena.

The Rapid Sequence and Washout Pyelogram (Fig. 16–49 *D*, *E*). This requires some additional features for study.

1. The time of appearance of the collecting system in the rapid sequence phase is normally no later than 3 minutes. Delayed appearance is significantly abnormal.

2. Careful comparison of the two kidneys must be made. Differences between them may be of pathologic importance.

3. Features such as shape and comparative size of the two kidneys become of increased importance. Differences of 1.5 cm. or greater in the cephalocaudal dimension of the two kidneys are of considerable significance.

4. By the 8 or 10 minute film in the rapid sequence study, every detail of the kidney collecting system should be visualized. In this concentrated phase of kidney function the kidney calyces are not distended.

5. In the *washout phase,* ordinarily by 10 minutes, the concentration of the contrast media becomes faint and kidney calyces may be slightly distended. If by any chance the concentration is enhanced by the 10 or 15 minute interval, an abnormal situation exists, pointing strongly toward hypertensive renopathy.

The Ureters. The ureter usually leaves the renal pelvis at its most dependent point and passes directly downward into the urinary bladder. Rotation of the kidney will cause some variation in this appearance, and this rotation can be recognized by the appearance of the calyces. The important factor to bear in mind is the presence or absence of interference to drainage from the kidney pelvis or any potential for such interference.

Constant peristalsis occurs over the length of the ureter, and portions of the ureter may not be visualized in excretory urography, depending upon this factor. If an area of constriction is abnormal, it is constant and is associated with a persistent dilatation of the ureter above this level. Normal areas of narrowness occur in three locations described above, namely the *ureteropelvic junction,* the *bifurcation of the iliac vessels,* and the point of *entrance of the ureter into the urinary bladder.*

Slight irregularities in the anatomic course of the ureter are of no significance if ureteral obstruction is manifest. A mild degree of tortuosity occurs with deep inspiration also. Displacement of the ureter, however, takes on considerable significance when contiguous masses are suspected.

The Urinary Bladder. In the anteroposterior recumbent projection the neck of the bladder lies just below the upper border of the pubic symphysis, and the fundus rises to a variable distance above the symphysis, depending upon the degree of distention. The distended bladder is ellipsoid in the adult, but in the child it tends to be elongated on its long axis, extending outside the pelvis minor. The outline of the bladder is usually smooth when distended, but may be irregular in the partially collapsed state, and this appearance should not be regarded as abnormal

pelvis and extending somewhat into the hilus of the kidney upward toward the renal columns. This fat is found normally but may exist in abnormal concentration, particularly in the presence of renal atrophy. This is best shown by nephrotomography (renal fibrolipomatosis).

Infusion Pyelogram. The infusion pyelogram ordinarily does not distend the collecting system, and the concentration of the contrast media is excellent so that in many instances detail is sufficiently adequate to obviate the necessity for retrograde pyelography. On the other hand, if minute detail is required in respect to the collecting system or the ureters or bladder, retrograde cystography, ureterography, or pyelography becomes essential.

In the excretory urogram the calyces are normally cupped with sharp pointed margins surrounding the renal papilla. In the retrograde pyelogram, a different standard of normal is used, since often the calyces are moderately distended under positive pressure.

unless the degree of distention is inadequate. Often the thickness of the urinary bladder can be differentiated, since the outer wall of the urinary bladder is delineated by perivesical fat.

In the male, a minimal rarefaction may be apparent at the neck of the bladder resulting from the impression of the medial lobe of the prostate. When this impression is more than slight, it is usually but not always an indication of abnormal enlargement of the prostate or seminal vesicles.

In the undistended bladder indentations of the dome are visible. They likewise may have no significance since they are usually caused by pressure from contiguous organs, such as the pelvic colon, rather than by pathologic entities.

The Urethra. The prostatic urethra is slightly spindle-shaped and is 2 to 4 cm. in length. It joins the base of the urinary bladder abruptly. The narrowness of the membranous portion extends for a distance of 1 to 1.5 cm. The outline of the cavernous part of the urethra is fairly uniform throughout. Occasionally, there is a slight reflux into the ejaculatory duct as it opens into the prostatic urethra.

The female urethra is approximately 5 cm. in length and resembles closely the proximal one-third of the male urethra. Normally its walls are small and smooth, with a minimum lumen of about 3 mm. and a maximum of 8 mm. Irregularity, dilatation, or outpouching is of pathologic significance.

REFERENCES

Abrams, H. L., and Cornell, S. H.: Patterns of collateral flow in renal ischemia. Radiology, *84*:1001–1012, 1965.

Anson, B. J. (ed.): Morris' Human Anatomy. 12th edition. New York, McGraw-Hill, 1966.

Arkless, R.: The normal kidney's reaction to intravenous pyelography. Amer. J. Roentgenol., *107*:746–749, 1969.

Baker, H. L., Jr., and Hodgson, J. R.: Further studies on accuracy of oral cholecystography. Radiology, *74*:239–245, 1960.

Baum, S., and Gillenwater, J. Y.: Renal artery impressions on the renal pelvis. J. Urol., *95*:139–145, 1966.

Becker, J. A., Canter, I. E., and Perl, S.: Rapid intrarenal circulation. Amer. J. Roentgenol., *109*:167–171, 1970.

Calatroni, C. J., Poliak, A., and Kohan, A.: A roentgenographic study of stress incontinence in women. Amer. J. Obst. Gyn., *83*:649–656, 1962.

Chait, A., Matasar, K. W., Fabian, C. E., and Mellins, H. Z.: Vascular impressions on the ureters. Amer. J. Roentgenol., *111*:729–749, 1971.

Cobb, O. E., and Anderson, E. E.: Superimposition cystography in the diagnosis of infiltrating tumors of the bladder. J. Urol., *94*:569–572, 1965.

Cocchi, U.: Retropneumoperitoneum and Pneumomediastinum. Stuttgart, Georg Thieme Verlag, 1957.

Colapinto, R. F., and Steed, B. L.: Arteriography of adrenal tumors. Radiology, *100*:343–350, 1971.

Cooperman, L. R., and Lowman, R. M.: Fetal lobulation of the kidneys. Amer. J. Roentgenol., *92*:273, 1964.

Cunningham, D. J.: Manual of Practical Anatomy, Vol. 2. 12th edition. London, Oxford University Press, 1958.

Currarino, G.: Roentgenographic estimation of kidney size in normal individuals with emphasis on children. Amer. J. Roentgenol., *93*:464–466, 1965.

Dickinson, R. L.: Human Sex Anatomy. Second edition. Baltimore, Williams and Wilkins Co., 1949.

Doppman, J. L., and Shapiro, R.: Some normal renal variants. Amer. J. Roentgenol., *92*:1380–1389, 1964.

Dunbar, J. S.: Personal communication.

Dure-Smith, P.: The dose of contrast medium in intravenous urography: a physiologic assessment. Amer. J. Roentgenol., *108*:691–697, 1970.

Dux, A., Thurn, P., and Kisseler, B.: The physiological emptying mechanism of the urinary tract in the roentgen cinematogram. Fortschr. Geb. Röntgenstrahlen, *97*:687–703, 1962.

Elkin, M.: Radiological observations in acute ureteral obstruction. Radiology, *81*:484–491, 1963.

Emmett, J. L.: Clinical Urography. Second edition. Philadelphia, W. B. Saunders Co., 1964.

Emmett, J. L., and Witten, D. M.: Clinical Urography: An Atlas and Textbook of Roentgenologic Diagnosis. Third edition. Philadelphia, W. B. Saunders Co., 1971.

Evans, J. A.: Nephrotomography in investigation of renal masses. Radiology, *69*:684–689, 1957.

Evans, J. A.: Specialized roentgen diagnostic techniques in the investigation of abdominal disease. Radiology, *82*:579–594, 1964.

Evans, J. A., Dubilier, W., Jr., and Monteith, M. C.: Nephrotomograph.: Amer. J. Roentgenol., *71*:213–223, 1954.

Fainsinger, M. H.: Excretory urography in the young subject: hyaluronidase and tomography as aids. South Afr. Med. J., *13*:418–420, 1950.

Friedenberg, M. J., and Carlin, M. R.: The routine use of higher volumes of contrast material to improve intravenous urography. Radiology, *83*:405–413, 1964.

Friedenberg, M. J., Walz, B. J., McAlister, W. H., Locksmith, J. P., and Gallagher, T. L.: Roentgen size of normal kidneys. Radiology, *84*:1022–1029, 1965.

Frimann-Dahl, J.: Normal variations of left kidney: anatomic and radiologic study. Acta Radiol., *55*:207–216, 1955.

Gondos, B.: Rotation of the kidney around its transverse axis. Radiology, *74*:19–25, 1960.

Gondos, B.: Rotation of the kidney around its longitudinal axis. Radiology, *76*:615–619, 1961.

Gondos, B.: Roentgenographic evaluation of the size and shape of the kidneys. M. Ann. Dist. Col., *31*:158–161, 1961.

Grant, J. C. B.: Atlas of Anatomy, Baltimore, Williams and Wilkins Co., 1962.

Graves, F. T.: The anatomy of the intrarenal arteries and its application to segmental resection of the kidney. Brit. J. Surg., *42*:132–139, 1954.

Gray, H.: Gray's Anatomy of the Human Body. 29th edition. Philadelphia, Lea and Febiger, 1973.

Green, T. A.: Development of a plan for the diagnosis and treatment of stress incontinence. Amer. J. Obst. Gyn., *83*:632–648, 1962.

Harris, J. H., and Harris, J. H., Jr.: Infusion pyelography. Amer. J. Roentgenol., *92*:1391–1396, 1964.

Harrow, B. R., and Sloane, J. A.: Dromedary or humped left kidney: lack of relationship to renal rotation. Amer. J. Roentgenol., *88*:144–152, 1962.

Hodson, C. J.: The radiological contribution toward the diagnosis of chronic pyelonephritis. Radiology, *88*:857–871, 1967.

Kahn, P. C.: Selective venography in renal parenchymal disease. Radiology, *92*:345–349, 1969.

Kjellberg, S. R., Ericsson, N. D., and Rudhe, U.: The Lower Urinary Tract in Childhood: Some Correlated Clinical and Roentgenologic Observations (Erica Odelberg, trans.). Chicago, Ill., Almqvist Yearbook Pub. Inc., 1957.

Kurlander, G. J., and Smith, E. E.: Total body opacification in the diagnosis of Wilms' tumor and neuroblastoma. A note of caution. Radiology, *89*:1075–1076, 1967.

Lattimer, J. K., Dean, A. L., Jr., and Furey, C. A.: The triple voiding technique in children with dilated urinary tracts. J. Urol., *76*:656–660, 1956.

Lilienfeld, R. M., Friedenberg, R. M., and Herman, J. R.: The effect of renal lymphatics on kidneys and blood pressure. Radiology, *88*:1105–1109, 1967.

Martin, J. F.: Newer basic concepts of renal anatomy of radiologic interest. Radiol. Clin. N. Amer., *3*:3–11, 1965.

Martin, J. F., Deyton, W. E., and Glenn, J. F.: The minute sequence pyelogram. Amer. J. Roentgenol., *90*:55–62, 1963.

McLelland, R., Landes, R. R., and Ransom, C. L.: Retroperitoneal pneumography: A safe method using carbon dioxide. Radiol. Clin. N. Amer., *3*:113–128, 1965.

Meng, C-H, and Elkin, M.: Venous impressions on the calyceal system. Radiology, *87*:878–882, 1966.

Merklin, R. J., and Michels, N. A.: The variant renal and suprarenal blood supply with data on the inferior phrenic, ureteral and gonadal arteries: a statistical analysis based on 185 dissections and review of the literature. J. Internat. Coll. Surg., *29*:41–76, 1958.

Meschan, I.: Background physiology of the urinary tract for the radiologist. Radiol. Clin. N. Amer., *3*:13–28, 1965.

Moell, H.: Kidney size and its deviation from normal in acute renal failure. A roentgen diagnostic study. Acta Radiol. (Suppl.), *206*:1–74, 1961.

Moell, H.: Size of normal kidneys. Acta Radiol., *46*:640–645, 1956.

O'Connor, J. F., and Neuhauser, E. B. D.: Total body opacification in conventional and high dose venous urography in infancy. Amer. J. Roentgenol., *90*:63–71, 1963.

Olsson, O.: Roentgen examination of the kidney and ureter. *In* Flocks et al. (eds.): Encyclopedia of Urology. Berlin, Springer-Verlag, 1962, pp. 1–365.

Paul, R. E., Jr., Ettinger, A., Fainsinger, M. H., Callow, A. D., Kahn, P. C., and Inker, L. H.: Angiographic visualization of renal collateral circulation as a means of detecting and delineating renal ischemia. Radiology, *84*:1013–1021, 1965.

Pendergrass, H. P., Tondreau, R. L., Pendergrass, E. P., Ritchie, D. J., Hildreth, E. A., and Askovitz, S. I.: Reactions associated with intravenous urography: Historical and statistical review. Radiology, *71*:1–12, 1958.

Rawson, A. J.: Distribution of the lymphatics of the human kidney as shown in a case of carcinomatous permeation. Arch. Pathol., *47*:283–292, 1949.

Riggs, W., Jr., Hagood, J. H., and Andrews, A. E.: Anatomic changes in the normal urinary tract on urograms. Radiology, *94*:107–113, 1970.

Schobinger, R. A., and Ruzicka, F. F., Jr.: Vascular Roentgenology. New York, The Macmillan Co., 1964.

Segall, H. D.: Gallbladder visualization following the injection of diatrizoate. Amer. J. Roentgenol., *107*:21–26, 1969.

Shopfner, C. E., and Hutch, J. A.: The trigonal canal. Radiology, *88*:209–221, 1967.

Simon, A. L.: Normal renal size: An absolute criterion. Amer. J. Roentgenol., *92*:270–272, 1964.

Sorby, W. A.: Renal phlebography. Clin. Radiol., *20*:166–172, 1969.

Trueta, J., Barclay, A. E., Daniel, P. M., Franklin, K. J., and Prichard, M. M. L.: Studies of the renal circulation. Springfield, Ill., Charles C Thomas, 1947.

Waterhouse, K.: Voiding cystourethrography: a simple technique. J. Urol., *85*:103–104, 1961.

Weens, H. S., Olnick, H. M., James, D. F., and Warren, J. V.: Intravenous nephrography: A method of roentgen visualization of the kidney. Amer. J. Roentgenol., *65*:411–414, 1951.

Weissleder, H., Emmrich, J., and Schirmeister, J.: Gefassebedingte Kontrastmittelaussparungen im urographischen Bild. Fortschr. Geb. Röntgenstrahlen, *97*:703–710, 1962.

Whalen, J. P., and Ziter, F. M. H.: Visualization of the renal fascia—a new sign in localization of abdominal masses. Radiology, *89*:861–863, 1967.

Wigh, R., Anthony, H. F., Jr., and Grant, B. P.: A comparison of intravenous urography, urine radiography and other renal tests. Radiology, *78*:869–878, 1962.

17

The Genital System

THE MALE GENITAL SYSTEM

Related Gross Anatomy. Each *testis* (Fig. 17–1) is formed by numerous lobules, each containing coiled tubules called seminiferous tubules. The spermatozoa are formed in these tubules. These lobules and tubules converge posteriorly toward the rete testis, which consists of a network of tubules which empty by coiled ducts into the head of the *epididymis*. Here the duct of the epididymis is formed and extends in very tortuous fashion to the tail of the epididymis where it becomes the *ductus deferens*. This latter is a cordlike structure which traverses the posterior aspect of the spermatic cord, and in the vicinity of the trigone of the urinary bladder undergoes slight bulbous dilatation to form the *ampulla of the ductus deferens*. Near the lower margin of this ampulla, there is a diverticulumlike structure which extends cepha-

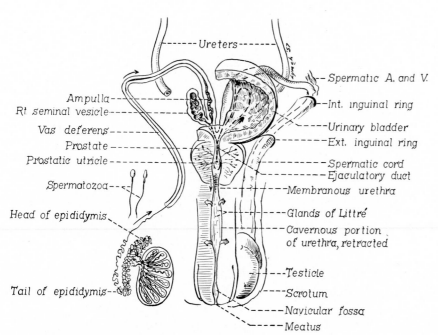

Figure 17–1. The male reproductive system. (Modified from Dickinson, Atlas of Human Sex Anatomy. Baltimore, The Williams & Wilkins Co.)

1056

lad, and appears racemose in configuration. This is the *seminal vesicle*. The continuation of the ampulla of the ductus deferens beyond the point of junction with the seminal vesicle is called the *ejaculatory duct,* and this empties into the lower posterior aspect of the prostatic urethra, one opening on either side of the *prostatic utricle*. In its course, the ejaculatory duct traverses about two-thirds of the length of the prostate. (Fig. 16–18 *A*)

The *prostate gland* is a conical structure, its base directed craniad and in contact with the caudal surface of the urinary bladder, and its apex pointing caudad, just superior to the superior fascia of the urogenital diaphragm. Anteriorly it is separated from the pubic symphysis by the pudendal plexus of veins and adipose tissue; posteriorly it is separated from the rectum by fascia which is continued over the seminal vesicles and over the pelvis laterally.

The posterior surface is separated from the rectum by the *rectovesical septum*. The *urethra* enters the prostate near its anterior surface and descends almost vertically within it so that the greater part of the prostate is posterior to the urethra. Its cross-sectional pattern and relationship to the bladder and urethra are shown in Figure 17–2. In cross section the prostate gland has four lobes, the *lobes anterior and posterior* to the urethra, the *lateral lobes* on either side of the urethra, and the *middle lobe* lying between the posterior aspect of the urethra near its junction with the urinary bladder and the ejaculatory duct. The *anterior lobe* is small and nonglandular and lies in front of the urethra. The *lateral lobes* extend not only laterally but also anterior to the urethra. The *middle lobe* contains the subtrigonal and cervical glands (Albarran's glands). As shown previously, the prostatic urethra contains a longitudinal ridge on its dorsal wall called the *urethral crest,* depressions on the sides of the crest into which the prostatic ducts open called the *prostatic sinuses*, and a *seminal colliculus* that is the summit of the urethral crest on which the ejaculatory ducts open. This colliculus also contains a median blind-ending sac, the *prostatic utricle*.

The *seminal vesicles* are bilateral lobulated sacs consisting of irregular pouches. They lie against the fundus of the bladder ventrally, and their dorsal surfaces are separated from the rectum by rectovesical fascia. Superiorly they are closely related to the *vas*

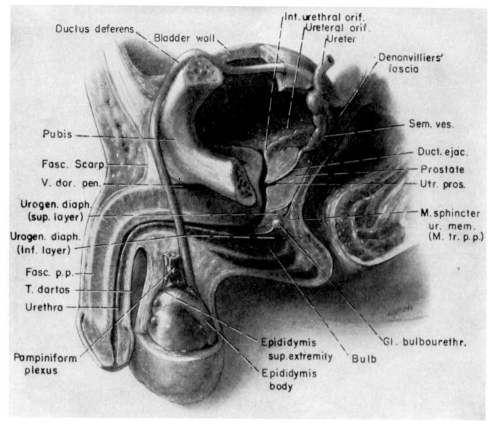

Figure 17–2. Midsagittal section of male pelvis. *Gl. bulbourethr.*, bulbourethral gland; *Fasc. p. p.*, deep perineal fascia; *T. dartos*, dartos tunic; *Duct. ejac.*, ejaculatory duct; *M. tr. p. p.*, m. sphincter urethrae membranaceae (m. transversus perinei profundus); *Fasc. Scarp.*, Scarpa's fascia; *Sem. ves.*, seminal vesicle; *Utr. pros.*, prostatic utricle; *V. dor. pen.*, v. dorsalis penis. (From Anson, B. J. (ed.): Morris' Human Anatomy, 12th ed. Copyright © 1966 by McGraw-Hill, Inc. Used by permission of McGraw-Hill Book Company.)

deferens and *ureters*. Inferiorly, the seminal vesicles join the vas deferens from either side on the posterior surface of the prostate (Figs. 17–2 and 17–3).

The course of the vas deferens and relationship to the pelvis and seminal vesicles is indicated in Figure 17–5.

The vessels and nerves of the vas deferens, seminal vesicles and prostate include: the middle rectal and inferior vesical arteries, the prostatic plexus of veins to the internal iliac veins, and lymphatics terminating in the internal iliac and sacral nodes predominantly.

The most important lobes of the prostate clinically are the median lobe, enlargement of which leads to urinary tract obstruction with encroachment on the urethra; and the lateral lobes, hypertrophy of which causes urinary obstruction. It is the posterior lobe which is encountered by rectal digital examination.

The relationships of the *male urethra* with cross sections of the penis at different levels are shown in Figure 17–6. The urethra and its examination have been previously discussed with the urinary tract in Chapter 16.

The *bulbourethral glands* or *Cowper's glands* are two small glands that lie on each side of the membranous portion of the urethra (Fig. 17–6), embedded between the two fascial layers of the urogenital diaphragm. The duct from this gland traverses the substance of the *corpus spongiosum of the penis* and opens on the floor of the bulbar portion of the urethra. This gland can be clinically significant in that occasionally a cyst may occur or accessory glands may be demonstrated distal or proximal to the main ductal openings.

Technique of Examination. There are only certain portions of the male genital system which can be examined radio-

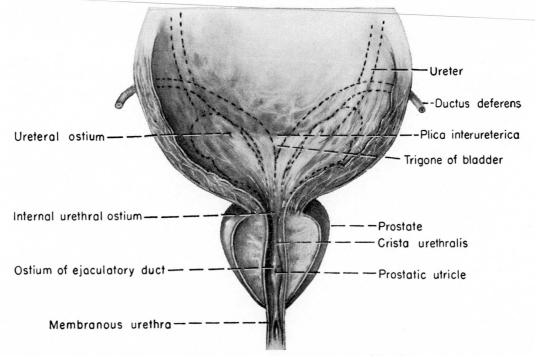

Ureter

Ductus deferens

Ureteral ostium

Plica interureterica

Trigone of bladder

Internal urethral ostium

Prostate

Crista urethralis

Ostium of ejaculatory duct

Prostatic utricle

Membranous urethra

Figure 17–3. Trigone of bladder and floor of prostatic urethra. (From Anson, B. J. (ed.): Morris' Human Anatomy, 12th ed. Copyright © 1966 by McGraw-Hill, Inc. Used by permission of McGraw-Hill Book Company.)

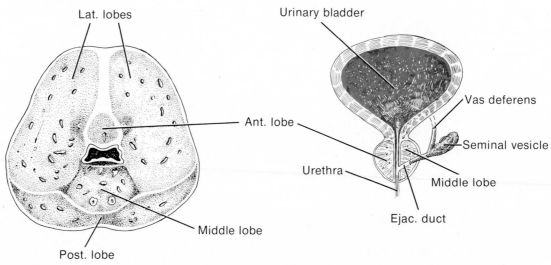

Lat. lobes

Urinary bladder

Ant. lobe

Vas deferens

Seminal vesicle

Urethra

Middle lobe

Ejac. duct

Middle lobe

Post. lobe

Figure 17–4. Cross section and sagittal section of prostate gland, showing relationship to urethra and urinary bladder.

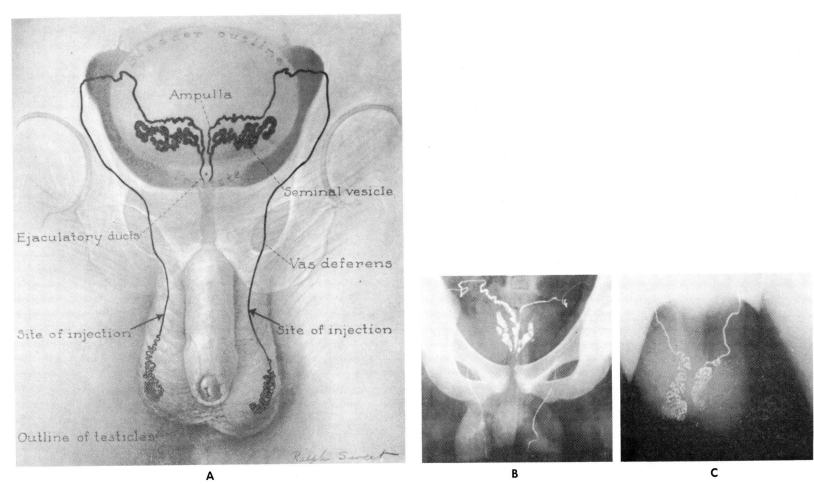

Figure 17-5. *A.* The male genital tract. The sites of exposure of the vas deferens are indicated, into which injections of the contrast media are made upward and frequently downward. *B.* Normal seminal vesiculogram (with Umbrathor). The distal segment of the right vas deferens is larger than that of the left. The right seminal vesicle is slightly better filled than the left. The injection of the left vas was made 24 hours before this film, and that of the right 4½ hours before this film. *C.* Same patient as above with filling of the distal portions of the epididymides achieved at the same time as *B.* Greater filling has been obtained on the right than on the left. (From Tucker, A. S., Yanagihara, H., and Pryde, A. W.: Amer. J. Roentgenol., 71:490–500, 1954.)

graphically by presently known methods. The examination is confined to a soft tissue study of the prostate, seminal vesicles, and scrotal contents, and the direct injection of opaque media into the lumen of the seminal vesicles, vas deferens, and ejaculatory duct via the vas deferens.

The usual method employed in the direct injection depends on the exposure of the vas through a small inguinal incision under local anesthesia. This injection is first directed upward to fill the vesicles and then downward to the epididymis to fill the tubules (Fig. 17-2). Either an iodized oil, such as Ethiodol, or diatrizoate (Renografin or Hypaque) may be used. Urethroscopic catheterization has also been employed by a few. The latter

method also does not permit visualization of the vas deferens, and serves only to outline the ejaculatory ducts and seminal vesicles.

Radiographic Appearances. On a plain radiograph the prostate may be visualized when enlarged as an impression directed upward at the base of the urinary bladder. Calculi may be seen within the prostate, but the outline of the gland cannot be delineated.

Using contrast material, the numerous racemose or diverticulumlike tubes of the seminal vesicles appear like an indefinite mass, and the ductus deferens may be seen as a tubular structure which conforms closely to the anatomic description just given (Fig. 17-5). The more distal tubules may be visualized,

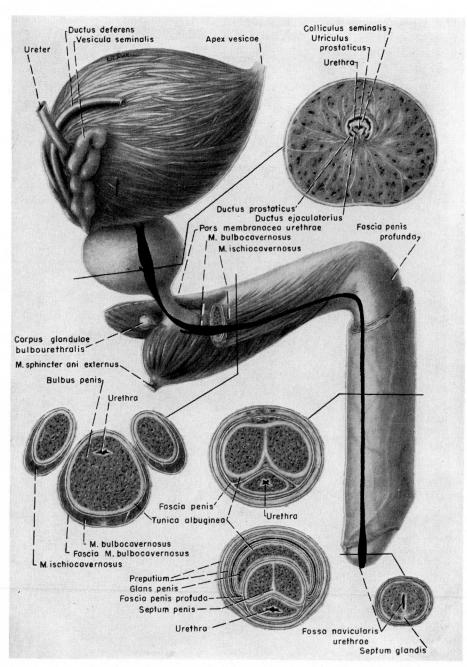

Figure 17–6. Relations of the male urethra with cross sections of the penis at different levels. Semidiagrammatic. (From Anson, B. J. (ed.): Morris' Human Anatomy, 12th ed. Copyright © 1966 by McGraw-Hill, Inc. Used by permission of McGraw-Hill Book Company.)

depending upon the efforts of the investigator, but they are examined infrequently.

In prostatic carcinoma, the ejaculatory duct may be invaded and occluded, but in the normal subject it may be seen extending beyond the junction of the ductus deferens and the seminal vesicles.

THE FEMALE REPRODUCTIVE SYSTEM

The soft tissue structures of this system will be described first and then a brief account will be given of the bony pelvis and its anatomic variations.

Soft Tissues.   The organs of the female genital system consist of two *ovaries,* two *oviducts,* the *uterus,* the *vagina* and the *external genitalia.* The suspensory and supplementary structures are the *broad ligaments* (and *mesosalpinx*) on either side, the *round ligament,* the *mesovarium* and *mesometrium* (Fig. 17–7).

The *broad ligament* is the transverse fold of peritoneum extending across the pelvis minor, dividing it into an anterior and a posterior compartment. This has frequently been compared with a "curtain draped over a clothesline." Projecting into the posterior compartment and attached a little below the upper margin of the broad ligament, is the *mesovarium,* with the ovary attached to its free edge. That portion of the broad ligament above this is called the *mesosalpinx,* and that below, the *mesometrium.* The relationship of the uterus and vagina in lateral perspective is shown in Figure 17–8.

The *ovaries* are two almond-shaped organs—one on either side of the pelvis. Their exact position in nulliparous women is somewhat variable but their long axis is usually vertical in the erect position. The right ovary is usually slightly larger than the left, and the length varies from 2.5 to 5 cm. The width is ordinarily one-half the length and the thickness one-half the width.

The *oviducts,* or *uterine tubes,* are two trumpet-shaped tubes which run in the superior border of the broad ligament between the uterine horns and the lateral pelvic walls. The dilated end lies over each ovary. Each oviduct is from 7 to 14 cm. in length. Ordinarily, the fimbriated end and mouth of the infundibulum rest upon the medial end of the ovary. The course of the oviducts is rather variable, and may be different on the two sides.

The *uterus* is a pear-shaped organ with a body or fundus and a downward extension, the cervix, which has supravaginal and vaginal sections. The cavity of the body is flattened transversely and has a triangular shape, being broad above where each cornua communicates with an oviduct and narrow below where it communicates with the canal in the cervix. The direction of the axis of the uterus is quite variable. Ordinarily a moderate degree of anteflexion is considered the normal position, making an angle of 80 to 120 degrees with the horizontal. There may also be a slight list to the right or to the left side.

The *vagina* extends from the uterus to the external genitalia where it opens to the exterior. Its course roughly parallels the anterior curvature of the sacrum and averages 5 to 7 cm. in length.

There is a deep depression between the rectum and uterus known as the *rectouterine pouch of Douglas.*

The ovarian vessels enter the broad ligament at its base and pass through the superior border of the suspensory ligament of the ovary.

The size of the uterus, which varies under normal conditions at various ages and in various physiologic states, is as follows: (1) adult virgin, 7 to 8 cm. in length, 4.5 to 5 cm. across its fundus; its anteroposterior thickness is 2 to 3 cm.; (2) in normal nonpregnant women, the depth of uterine and cervical cavities is 3 cm. approximately; (3) in the prepubertal period it is smaller; and (4) in women who have borne children it is larger.

Blood Supply of Female Genital System

Ovary. The *ovarian artery* supplies the ovary directly from the aorta, descending in the suspensory ligament of the ovary to the broad ligament and sending branches to the ovary and uterine tubes (Fig. 17–9). The *ovarian vein* travels with the ovarian artery, terminating on the right in the vena cava and on the left in the renal vein (Fig. 17–10).

Oviduct (Uterine Tube). The arterial supply to the oviduct is similar to that of the ovary. The venous drainage of the oviduct is likewise similar to that of the ovary, with some flow to the uterine plexus (Fig. 17–10).

Uterus. The uterus receives a number of arteries such as:

an *ovarian* branch and a *uterine* branch from the anterior division of the internal iliac artery which crosses the ureter to reach the side of the uterus through the broad ligament, where it ascends to the level of the uterine tube. This artery supplies the cervix, upper vagina, body of the uterus, uterine tube, and round ligament (Fig. 17–11).

The *veins* of the uterus are derived from a *uterine plexus,* which in turn communicates with a *vaginal plexus* that is drained chiefly by uterine veins ending in internal iliac veins (Fig. 17–10).

Vagina. The *vaginal artery* is derived from the internal iliac artery. It sends branches to the uterus and joins branches from the uterine artery to form the *azygos artery of the vagina.* The *veins* of the vagina drain from a plexus communicating with vesical, rectal, and uterine plexuses through a vaginal vein to empty into the internal iliac vein (Fig. 17–10).

The *lymphatic drainage* of these structures is shown in Figure 17–12. The *ovarian lymphatics* follow the ovarian artery, entering the lateral and preaortic lymph nodes. The *oviduct lymphatics* follow the ovarian and uterine drainage. In the uterus the cervical lymphatics drain to the external, internal, and common iliac nodes; those from the body and fundus follow an ovarian drainage to the lateral and preaortic nodes, some going to external iliac and some to superficial inguinal nodes.

The *vaginal lymphatics drain* to the external, internal, and common iliac nodes from the upper, middle, and lower portions respectively.

The *vulvar drainage* ends in superficial inguinal nodes for the most part.

Thus, the lymph nodes that are most concerned in draining

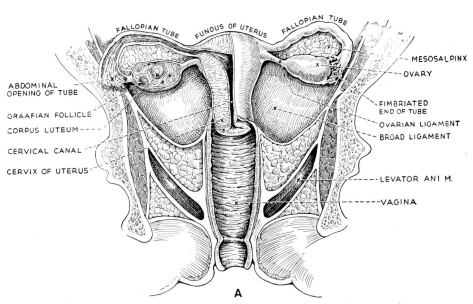

Figure 17–7. A. Gross anatomy of female reproductive system. A. Frontal view.

Figure 17–7 continued on the following page.

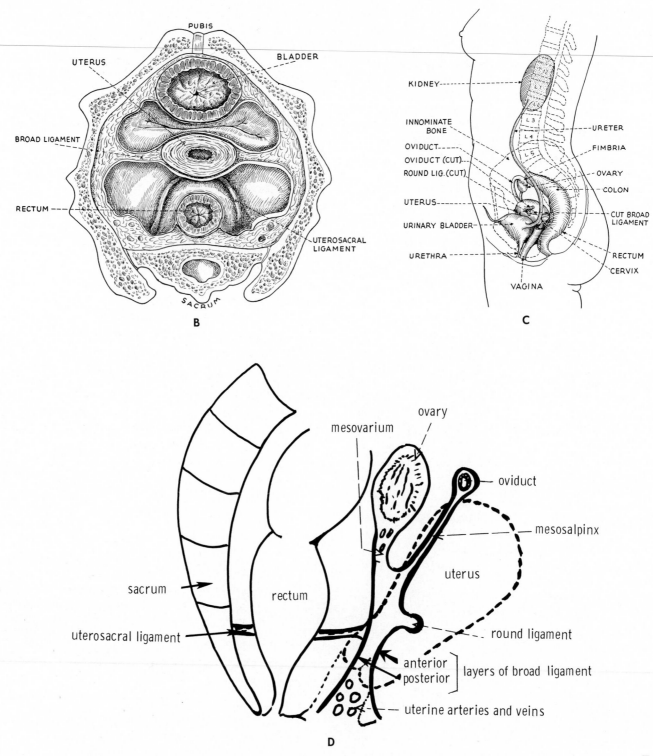

Figure 17-7 *Continued.* *B.* Superior cross-sectional diagram. *C.* Lateral relationships of genitourinary tract. *D.* Isometric view of broad ligament and its relationship to contiguous organs in the female pelvis.

Figure 17-7 continued on the opposite page.

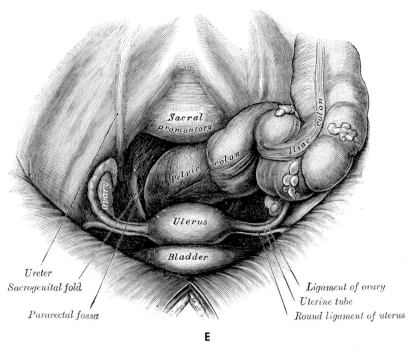

E

Figure 17–7 *Continued.*   E. Female pelvis and its contents, seen from above and in front. (From Gray's Anatomy of the Human Body, 29th ed. Goss, C. M. (ed.) Philadelphia, Lea & Febiger, 1973.)

the female genital system ultimately are the *common iliac*, the *external iliac*, and the *internal iliac* (Fig. 17–13).

Pelvic Architecture of the Female

Bony Pelvis.   In addition to the normal anatomic landmarks of the pelvis described in Chapter 5, certain areas should receive the attention of the radiologist as having an influence on the course of labor. Differences characteristic of male and female types should be borne in mind. These areas are as follows:

1. *The Subpubic Arch* (Fig. 17–14).   Note should be made of the bones of the pubic rami, whether they are delicate, average, or heavy; whether the pubic angle is wide or curved (female) or narrow and straight (male), and whether the side walls of the forepelvis are divergent, straight, or convergent. The configuration of the pelvic arch is a guide to the capacity of the true pelvis.

2. *The Ischial Spines.* These are classified as sharp, average, or anthropoid. Sharp spines are definitely a male characteristic and when present, direct the attention to the necessity for a more detailed examination of the pelvis, as they may be associated with converging side walls of the forepelvis. The anthropoid spines are blunt and shallow.

3. *The Sacrosciatic Notch and Sacrum.*   The capacity of the posterior pelvic inlet is related to the width of the sacrosciatic

notch and the configuration of its apex. The male pelvis shows a long narrow notch with a high rounded apex and the female a wide notch with a blunt apex.

The inclination of the sacrum directly affects the capacity of the birth canal since a forward tilt will offer a barrier to normal delivery. If the forepelvis is wide and divergent, compensation

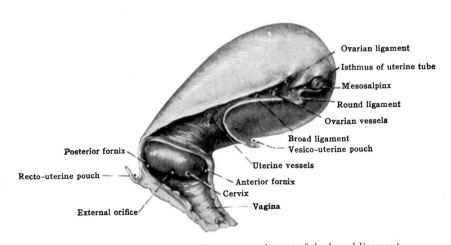

Figure 17–8.   Lateral view of uterus, showing attachment of the broad ligament. (From Anson, B. J. (ed.): Morris' Human Anatomy, 12th ed. Copyright © 1966 by McGraw-Hill, Inc. Used by permission of McGraw-Hill Book Company.)

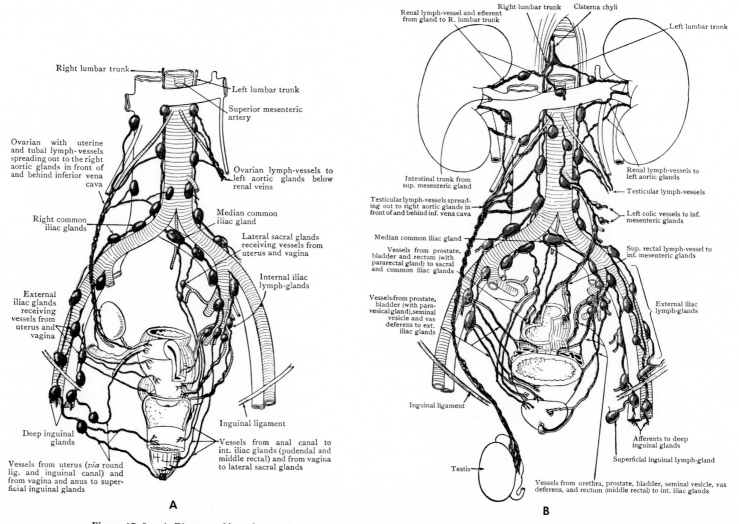

Right lumbar trunk
Left lumbar trunk
Superior mesenteric artery

Ovarian with uterine and tubal lymph-vessels spreading out to the right aortic glands in front of and behind inferior vena cava

Ovarian lymph-vessels to left aortic glands below renal veins

Right common iliac glands

Median common iliac gland

Lateral sacral glands receiving vessels from uterus and vagina

External iliac glands receiving vessels from uterus and vagina

Internal iliac lymph-glands

Deep inguinal glands

Inguinal ligament

Vessels from anal canal to int. iliac glands (pudendal and middle rectal) and from vagina to lateral sacral glands

Vessels from uterus (*via* round lig. and inguinal canal) and from vagina and anus to superficial inguinal glands

A

Right lumbar trunk   Cisterna chyli

Renal lymph-vessel and efferent from gland to R. lumbar trunk

Left lumbar trunk

Intestinal trunk from sup. mesenteric gland

Renal lymph-vessels to left aortic glands

Testicular lymph-vessels spreading out to right aortic glands in front of and behind inf. vena cava

Testicular lymph-vessels

Left colic vessels to inf. mesenteric glands

Median common iliac gland

Vessels from prostate, bladder and rectum (with pararectal gland) to sacral and common iliac glands

Sup. rectal lymph-vessel to inf. mesenteric glands

Vessels from prostate, bladder (with paravesical gland), seminal vesicle and vas deferens to ext. iliac glands

External iliac lymph-glands

Inguinal ligament

Afferents to deep inguinal glands

Superficial inguinal lymph-gland

Testis

Vessels from urethra, prostate, bladder, seminal vesicle, vas deferens, and rectum (middle rectal) to int. iliac glands

B

Figure 17–9. *A.* Diagram of lymph vessels and lymph glands of female pelvis and abdomen. *B.* Diagram of lymph vessels and lymph glands of male pelvis and abdomen. (From Cunningham's Manual of Practical Anatomy, 11th ed. London, Oxford University Press, 1949.)

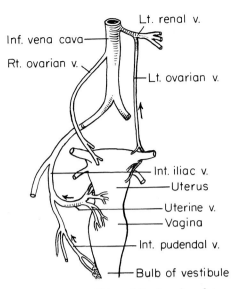

Figure 17-10. Veins of the female pelvis.

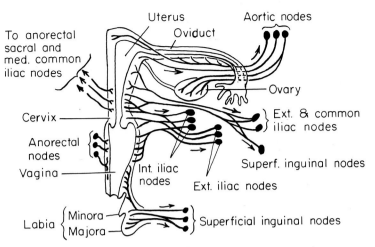

Figure 17-12. Lymph vessels of the female genitalia.

occurs but if convergent, a funnel pelvis will result. The female sacrum is wide and short compared with that of the male.

The curvature of the sacrum on the lateral projection is also important. Normally the sacrum is concave anteriorly. When this curvature is absent owing to any developmental aberration, the midpelvis is diminished and the progress of labor is impeded. The absence of this curvature will be readily apparent from measurements to be described later.

4. *The Pelvic Inlet.* The pelvic inlet with its variations can be classified into four major types (Fig. 17-15):

The inlet of the anthropoid pelvis is relatively long in anteroposterior measurements and narrow in transverse diameter.

The pelvic arch is usually wider than normal and the sacrosciatic notch is wide and shallow when seen in the lateral view. The anthropoid type is so called because it closely resembles the pelves found in the higher apes.

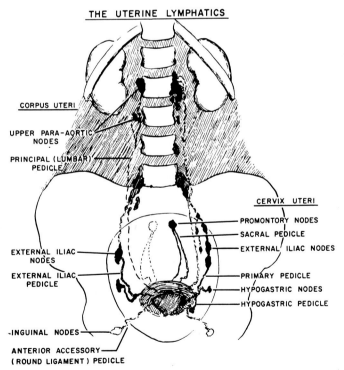

Figure 17-13. Diagrammatic sketch of the uterine lymphatic circulation. The solid lymph nodes and pedicles represent the visualized primary drainage areas, the shaded lymph nodes are secondary drainage areas, and the open lymph nodes are nonopacified lymph nodes in our case. (From Hipona, F. A., and Ditchek, T.: Amer. J. Roentgenol., 98:236–238, 1966.)

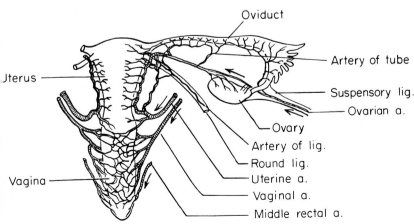

Figure 17-11. Arteries of the female genitalia.

A

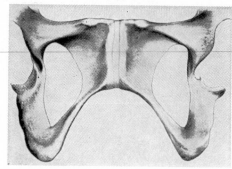

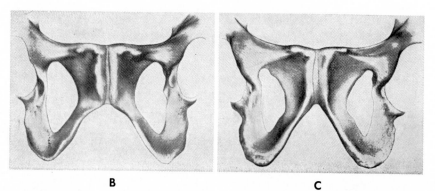

B   C

Figure 17–14. Variations in size and shape of the subpubic arch. *A.* Delicate bones, wide angle; well-curved female type of pubic rami. *B.* Average bones, moderate angle; average curvature of pubic rami. *C.* Heavy bones, narrow angle; straight masculine type of pubic rami. (From Golden, R.: Diagnostic Roentgenology, Vol. 2. Baltimore, Williams and Wilkins Co., 1963–1969.)

DIFFERENT PELVIC TYPES
(PELVIC INLET VIEW)

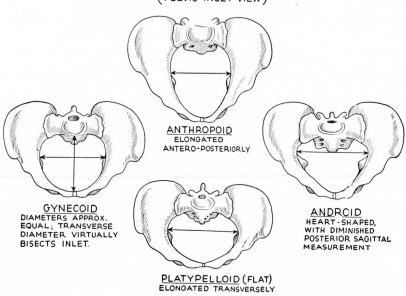

ANTHROPOID
ELONGATED
ANTERO-POSTERIORLY

GYNECOID
DIAMETERS APPROX.
EQUAL; TRANSVERSE
DIAMETER VIRTUALLY
BISECTS INLET.

ANDROID
HEART-SHAPED,
WITH DIMINISHED
POSTERIOR SAGITTAL
MEASUREMENT

PLATYPELLOID (FLAT)
ELONGATED TRANSVERSELY

Figure 17–15.

TYPICAL GYNECOID PELVIS

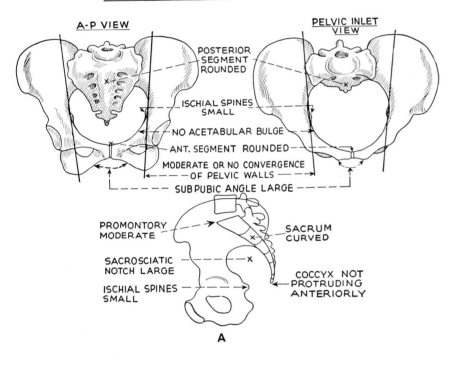

A-P VIEW

PELVIC INLET VIEW

POSTERIOR SEGMENT ROUNDED

ISCHIAL SPINES SMALL

NO ACETABULAR BULGE

ANT. SEGMENT ROUNDED

MODERATE OR NO CONVERGENCE OF PELVIC WALLS

SUBPUBIC ANGLE LARGE

PROMONTORY MODERATE

SACRUM CURVED

SACROSCIATIC NOTCH LARGE

ISCHIAL SPINES SMALL

COCCYX NOT PROTRUDING ANTERIORLY

A

FACTORS STUDIED IN PELVIC ARCHITECTURE

1. PELVIC INLET STUDY (*SEE DIAGRAMS OF DIFFERENT PELVIC TYPES*)

2. PROMINENCE OF ISCHIAL SPINES

3. CONVERGENCE OF LATERAL PELVIC WALLS

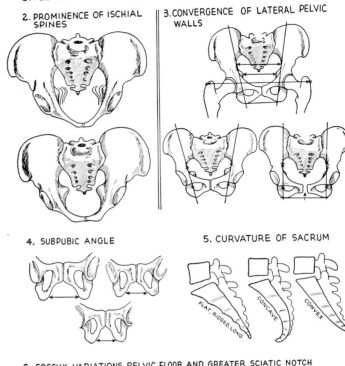

4. SUBPUBIC ANGLE

5. CURVATURE OF SACRUM

FLAT, RIDGED, LONG   CONCAVE   CONVEX

6. COCCYX VARIATIONS, PELVIC FLOOR AND GREATER SCIATIC NOTCH

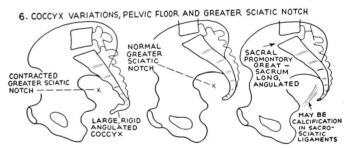

CONTRACTED GREATER SCIATIC NOTCH

NORMAL GREATER SCIATIC NOTCH

LARGE, RIGID ANGULATED COCCYX

SACRAL PROMONTORY GREAT — SACRUM LONG, ANGULATED

MAY BE CALCIFICATION IN SACRO-SCIATIC LIGAMENTS

7. UTERINE AXIS FACTOR IN RELATION TO SACRUM AND SACRAL PROMONTORY

A. AXIS OF UTERUS NEAR SPINE, GOOD FLEXION OF HEAD

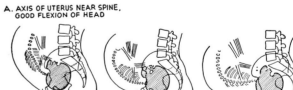

NORMAL - FLEXION OF HEAD SATISFACTORY

FLEXION FAIR

PENDULOUS UTERUS - FLEXION OF HEAD ABSENT

B

Figure 17–16.

The gynecoid pelvis is the average type as seen in the human female. The inlet is round or slightly oval, the pubic angle is wide, and the sacrosciatic notch is also wide. The cavity of the pelvis is ample in all directions (Fig. 17–16).

The android pelvis refers to a female pelvis which has marked masculine characteristics. These include what is described as a blunt heart-shaped or wedge-shaped inlet with narrow forepelvis, and the widest diameter is close to the sacral promontory. A narrow masculine type of sciatic notch is present and the sacrum is set forward in the pelvis. The pubic arch is usually narrow.

The platypelloid or flat pelvis is characterized by an inlet with a transversely oval shape. The anteroposterior diameter is short and the greatest transverse diameter is wide—this diameter occurring well in front of the sacrum. The angle of the forepelvis is wide also, but the sacrosciatic notch and subpubic angle vary in size.

It should be stated that gradations between all types are seen and individual variations should be described as they appear on the radiograph.

The reader is referred to the work of Caldwell and Moloy on this subject.

Methods of Study of the Female Genital System

In the entire description below of the applications and usefulness of radiographic techniques in investigation of obstetrical and gynecologic problems, the student must bear in mind those aspects of radiologic protection which pertain here (see Chapter 2). The information to be gained must justify the exposure of the patient (and the fetus, if one is present). In any case, radiation exposure of the patient and the fetus in the first trimester of pregnancy is to be avoided unless the problem at hand is a critical one.

Direct Radiography and Its Applications. Anteroposterior, lateral, and "inlet" views of the pelvis are obtained and a considerable amount of information is available from these views (Fig. 17–16).

The purposes of roentgen study of the female patient in obstetrics and gynecology may be outlined as follows:

1. **The study of the female pelvis and abdomen** (apart from pregnancy), including (a) the determination of an extrauterine fetus; (b) the study of pelvic soft tissues outside the uterus, particularly to determine if interference to parturition might result; (c) pelvic mensuration and description as a guide to determination of possible cephalopelvic disproportion; and (d) all those anatomic and pathologic possibilities in the abdomen and pelvis that exist regardless of the sex of the patient.

2. **Special gynecologic study of the nonpregnant female** for: (a) hysterosalpingography, or the detailed study of the uterine cavity and oviducts and determination of the patency of the latter; (b) pelvic pneumography—the study of the pelvic peritoneal space by introduction of gas into the space; (c) a combination of these; and (d) pelvic angiography.

3. **A study of the pregnant mother in respect to the fetus** for the purpose of: (a) determining the presence of a fetal skeleton *in utero* or intra-abdominally; (b) determining the presence of multiple fetuses; (c) determining fetal normalcy, age, and development; (d) determining fetal viability or death; or (e) describing the accurate presentation of the fetus.

4. **A study of the pregnant uterus apart from the fetus,** including: (a) the placenta—its size, position, and density; (b) the amniotic space (the amniotic space may be entered to withdraw fluid for special study, or may serve as a guide to fetal transfusion); or (c) general uterine density and normalcy of appearance.

5. **Genitography of the abnormal infant or child** (intersex problems).

STUDY OF THE FEMALE PELVIS AND ABDOMEN

Introductory Comments. The study of the pregnant mother for intra-abdominal abnormalities outside the uterus lies outside the scope of this text. The features of the extrauterine fetus, for example, tubal pregnancy, and the implantation of a placenta anywhere in the abdominal cavity are subjects which have been discussed in our companion text, *Analysis of Roentgen Signs*, and the student is referred for brief discussion to this reference. This applies to a consideration of the ruptured uterus also.

Study of Pelvic Soft Tissue Structures Outside the Uterus (especially to determine if interference to parturition may result). This, too, involves abnormalities in the retroperitoneal space such as tumors of the sacrum, inflammatory swellings, or urinary tract abnormalities. Similarly, abnormalities of the intestine may be considered here. These are outside the scope of this text and the student is referred to *Analysis of Roentgen Signs* for further discussion.

Cephalopelvic Disproportion and Pelvic Measurement. Many methods of measurement of the maternal pelvis and the fetal head have been proposed. These include such adjuncts as special rulers or grids which are projected over the pelvis in its midsection, special tables and graphs which provide for determination of the extent of magnification, special slide rules which facilitate determination of magnification, nomograms which help resolve the extent of magnification if the basic factors are known, and teleroentgenograms which minimize the extent of magnification to the point where the degree of accuracy possible is related largely to the degree of accuracy of the actual measurement.

In all these proposed methods the *basic concepts and objectives are to measure the important diameters of the pelvis and head,* eliminating as much as possible the elements of magnification and distortion; *to describe the pelvic architecture* as accurately as possible from the standpoint of parturition; and to *describe any other factors* in relation to the pelvis, fetus, or placenta such as have been previously indicated in this section.

It is important for the student to adopt that method of correction for magnification and distortion that is most feasible in his particular installation and to learn that method thoroughly rather than to be attracted to one proposal or another by various authors. If it is possible to obtain at least 72 inch target-to-film distance films (teleroentgenograms), one may assay the size of the pelvis and fetal head without difficulty, since a maximum magnification on the order of 10 per cent is thereby feasible. For those measurements such as the interischial spinous diameter, to be obtained in the middle of the pelvis, the magnification is on the order of only 5 per cent. Moreover, when nonengagement of the fetal head occurs in a pendulous abdomen, the distance between head and inlet is not as significant in the teleroentgenogram as in other proposed techniques. Fetal head and pelvic measurements are more easily obtained with breech presentations when teleroentgenograms are employed, since distortion is minimal.

Templeton has utilized high kilovoltage pelvimetry with a teleroentgenographic technique and a target-to-film distance of 10 feet; by using 150 Kv. and a 1 mm. focal spot, he was able to obtain anteroposterior and lateral roentgenograms with the patient standing against a grid cassette (100 lines per inch). He employed an angulation of 20 degrees toward the feet for the anteroposterior roentgenogram. Comparison of radiation exposure to the fetus and maternal pelvis was made using a pelvic phantom. Whereas the conventional kilovoltage technique averaged a total of 1020 milliroentgens to the midpelvis, this high kilovoltage technique averaged a total of 60 milliroentgens. Thus, radiation hazard was 17 times less with this high kilovoltage technique, and the teleroentgenograms made magnification correction unnecessary. All obstetric measurements were made readily on the two upright roentgenograms.

If methods other than the teleroentgenographic technique are employed, it is important to obtain both the lateral and anteroposterior views without moving the patient. This is important because the lateral view is employed to correct for magnification on the anteroposterior projection, and similarly the anteroposterior projection is employed to obtain certain measurements which are applied to the lateral view. If there is a difference in the position of the fetal head, for example, in these two views, the correction factors are much more complex and virtually nullified.

For this reason erect films are preferred by some. When the patient is standing, the position of the fetus with respect to the maternal pelvis is not apt to change when the patient moves from the anteroposterior to the lateral position. The erect standing film may also be preferred in order to obtain maximum gravitational effect of the fetus above the maternal pelvis.

Evaluation of Pelvicephalography in the Light of Radiation Hazard. Considerable confusion has resulted with respect to the indications and contraindications for the radiologic study of the female pelvis and fetal skull in pregnancy. While radiation is not the only genetic hazard in our environment which can result in increased mutations, every effort should be made to reduce this particular hazard as much as possible. Although it has not been absolutely proved in mammals, it is generally accepted that genetic aberrations from exposure to radiation can occur at virtually any dose level.

The reader is referred to Chapter 2 for a more detailed consideration of the many aspects of radiation protection. From these discussions, however, we may derive the following conclusions:

1. Roentgen pelvic encephalometry should not be considered a routine procedure. It must be employed only after thorough obstetrical examination and evaluation, and the information to be obtained must be of critical value. Nevertheless, this procedure must be undertaken with the full understanding that the radiologist cannot and should not by himself attempt to predict the outcome of delivery. The data obtained should permit a thorough study of the maternal pelvis in all its aspects and should provide some idea of the relative size, shape, and position of the fetal skull in relation to the maternal pelvis.

2. All precautions should be employed to minimize radiation exposure. These must include high kilovoltage techniques, fast films, fast screens, collimation, additional filtration, increased target-to-film distance, and superior darkroom processing so that repeated exposures are unnecessary.

3. The optimal time for roentgen pelvic encephalometry is during the last 2 weeks of pregnancy. Under these circumstances, with a cephalic presentation the fetal gonads may actually lie outside the primary beam of radiation if one concentrates on the maternal pelvis.

4. Although information regarding the fetus, including fetal maturity, age, and development, may be obtained, fetal weight predictions have proved inaccurate and unsatisfactory since no relationship has been established between fetal skull measurements and body weight (Ane et al.).

Pelvic and Fetal Measurements in Use. Regardless of the method employed for correction for magnification and distortion, the measurements that are most valuable are indicated in Figures 17–17 to 17–19. These are measurement of the pelvic inlet in both the anteroposterior and transverse diameters, measurement of the midpelvis in its anteroposterior diameter, the interischial spinous diameter, the posterior sagittal measurement of the midpelvis, the intertuberous diameter as a measurement of the pelvic outlet, and the two largest perpendic-

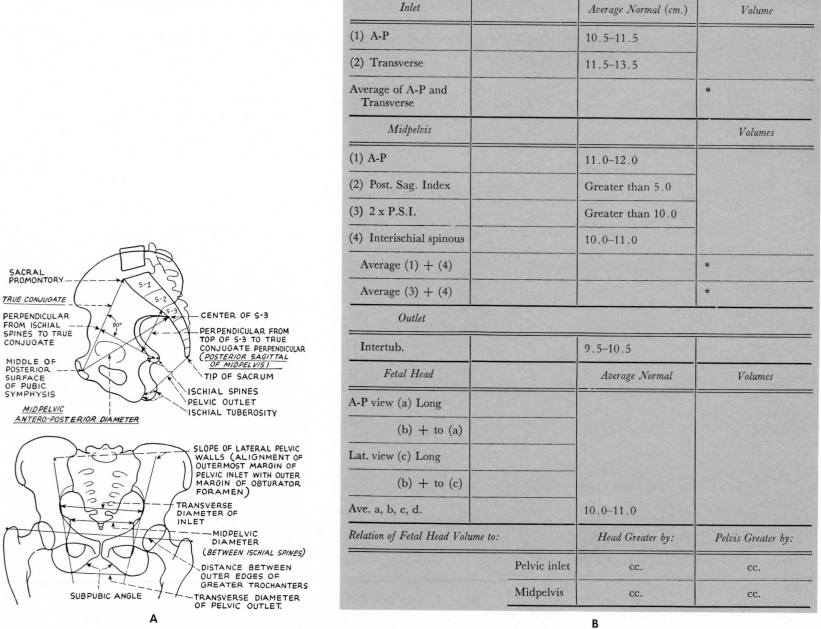

Format for Reporting Cephalopelvic Measurements			
Inlet		*Average Normal (cm.)*	*Volume*
(1) A-P		10.5–11.5	
(2) Transverse		11.5–13.5	
Average of A-P and Transverse			*
Midpelvis			*Volumes*
(1) A-P		11.0–12.0	
(2) Post. Sag. Index		Greater than 5.0	
(3) 2 x P.S.I.		Greater than 10.0	
(4) Interischial spinous		10.0–11.0	
Average (1) + (4)			*
Average (3) + (4)			*
Outlet			
Intertub.		9.5–10.5	
Fetal Head		*Average Normal*	*Volumes*
A-P view (a) Long			
(b) + to (a)			
Lat. view (c) Long			
(b) + to (c)			
Ave. a, b, c, d.		10.0–11.0	
Relation of Fetal Head Volume to:		*Head Greater by:*	*Pelvis Greater by:*
	Pelvic inlet	cc.	cc.
	Midpelvis	cc.	cc.

A

B

Figure 17–17. *A.* Diagrams illustrating the various measurements obtained from routine anteroposterior and lateral teleroentgenograms of the pelvis for pelvic measurement. *B.* Method of reporting pelvic measurements. (All measurements are recorded after correction for magnification.)

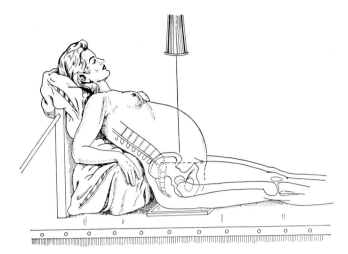

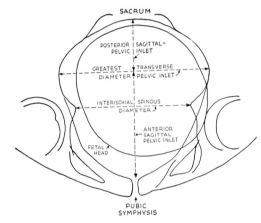

Figure 17–18. Tracing of radiograph routinely employed in pelvicephalometry. Special view of pelvic inlet, showing positioning of patient (note the pelvic inlet is parallel to the table top) and tracing of radiograph so obtained.

ular diameters of the fetal head in both the anteroposterior and lateral projections (it is well to add approximately 4 mm. to the average diameter in consideration of the scalp soft tissues) (Ball and Golden; Schwarz).

We have elected to describe in great detail one technique with which we have considerable experience, rather than to give a brief, cursory description of the many techniques which are available for the purpose of pelvicephalometry. This technique has been modified by the author for teleroentgenography, in which erect films are not as essential as they would be for shorter film-to-target distances.

Having obtained the various measurements the following procedure is utilized (modification of Ball method; Schwarz's classification):

All four diameters of the fetal head are averaged together,

and an average fetal head diameter is obtained (Fig. 17–19). From this average fetal head diameter, the tables are employed to obtain an average fetal head volume (computed from the formula $4/3\ \pi\ r^3$, where r is the average radius of the fetal head). The bottom scale on Fig. 17–20 can be used for this purpose.

The greatest transverse and anteroposterior diameters of the pelvic inlet are averaged together; utilizing this as a diameter, the volume of a sphere is obtained.

The anteroposterior diameter of the midpelvis and the interischial sp.nous diameter are averaged together and again the volume of a sphere is obtained, using this average diameter. Another method of finding midpelvis sphere volume is to double the posterior sagittal midpelvic index and to average this with the interischial spinous diameter. This becomes the average diameter of the midpelvis, and the volume of the associated sphere is thereby determined.

Thus, the volume of the fetal head, the volume of a sphere with an average diameter equivalent to the average diameter of the pelvic inlet, and the volume of a sphere having as its diameter the average diameter of the midpelvis have been computed. These three spheres are thereafter compared in volume. If the midpelvic and inlet volumes each exceed the volume of the fetal head, no further computation is necessary. This group would be considered as "no disproportion demonstrated," and the incidence of cesarean section, regardless of reason, would be about 4 per cent. Incidence for cephalopelvic disproportion in this group would prove to be about 1 per cent, based upon 350 patients (Schwarz).

A "borderline disproportion" group may be differentiated, in which the fetal head volume exceeds the volume capacity of the inlet by 70 cc. or less, or the volume capacity of the bispinous diameter by 50 to 220 cc. (In the latter instance, anything less than 50 cc. would fall into the "no disproportion" category.) Incidence of cesarean section in this group would prove to be about 33 per cent.

The "high disproportion" group consists of those patients with fetal head volumes exceeding the volume capacity of the inlet by more than 70 cc., or the bispinous diameter volume capacity by more than 220 cc. The incidence of cesarean section in this group would prove to be about 80 per cent for any reason, and the incidence of "difficult delivery" 87 per cent. Difficult delivery is defined as applying to deliveries requiring cesarean section, high or midforceps, or to infant death resulting from proved brain injury (Schwarz).

In all of these computations it is important to remember this basic principle: *Under no circumstances do any of these measurements indicate that spontaneous delivery will or will not occur.* These measurements are for purposes of comparison only. It is impossible by these measurements to predict the intensity of labor contractions, uterine atonia, and a host of other factors in the individual case which have not been reduced to mathematical terms.

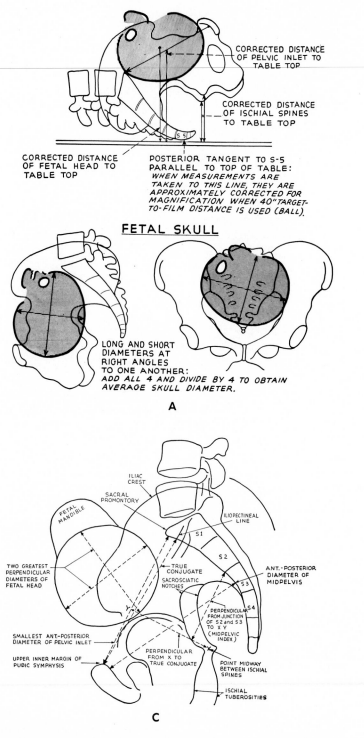

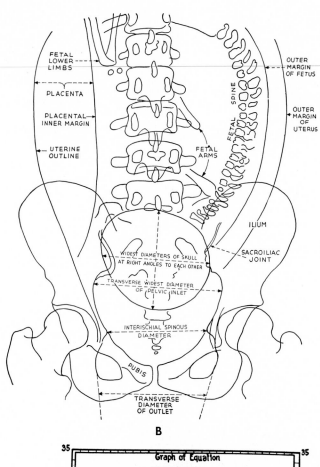

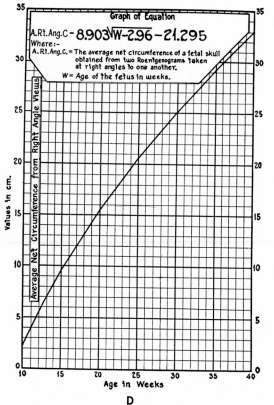

Figure 17–19. *A.* Diagrams illustrating the various measurements of the fetal head which are obtained and compared with the pelvic measurements. *B* and *C.* Tracings of radiographs routinely employed in pelvicephalometry. *B.* Anteroposterior (position same as KUB film). *C.* Lateral (position same as lateral abdomen or lumbar spine). *D.* Graph for computation of fetal age in weeks from average corrected circumference of skull obtained from two radiographs taken at right angles to one another. (From Hodges, P. C.: Amer. J. Roentgenol., 37:644–662, 1937.)

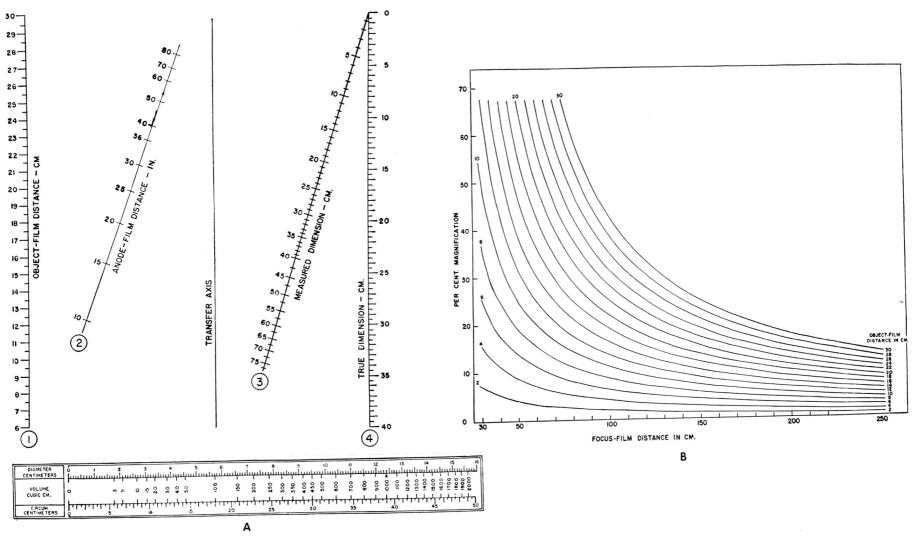

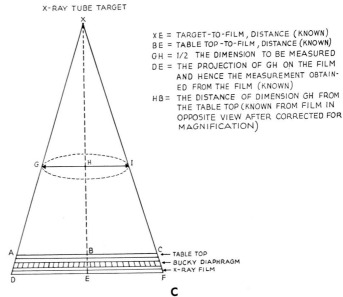

Figure 17-20. *A.* Nomograms for correction of magnification and for conversion of diameters to volumes. With a straight edge, a line is drawn from the object-film distance (1) of a certain dimension through the anode-film distance (2) used when the film was taken to the transfer axis. From this point on the transfer axis, a line is drawn through the dimension as measured on the film (3) which intersects (4) at the true, corrected dimension. With the table at the bottom of the nomogram a circumference or a diameter measurement in centimeters can be transposed directly to volume of a similar sphere in terms of cubic centimeters. (After Halmquest, from Golden, R.: Diagnostic Roentgenology. Baltimore, The Williams & Wilkins Co., 1963-1969.) *B.* Graph demonstrating the per cent magnification readily obtained when one knows the focus-film distance in centimeters and the object-film distance in centimeters. (Courtesy T. H. Oddie, D.Sc.) *C.* Triangulation method of determining radiographic magnification (see text).

Study of Pelvic Architecture

Pelvic Inlet. In addition to the anteroposterior and lateral views of the abdomen and pelvis, it may be routine in this radiographic study to obtain a special view of the pelvic inlet as illustrated in Fig. 17–18. With this special view, the pelvic inlet can be described as falling into one or another of at least four major pelvic types. There are, of course, many subtypes in these groups but at least these four major types must be understood (Figs. 17–14 and 17–15). Delivery of the fetus is most readily accomplished with the gynecoid pelvis (Fig. 17–16 *A*); difficulty is encountered with increasing frequency in the android, platypelloid, and anthropoid types.

If the posterior sagittal portion of the pelvic inlet is diminished, an occiput posterior presentation is favored.

The Sacrum. Following analysis of the pelvic inlet, the prominence of the sacral promontory and the curvature of the sacrum are studied for architecture (Fig. 17–16 *B*). The capacity of the posterior pelvic inlet is related to the width of the sacrosciatic notch and the configuration of its apex. Also the inclination of the sacrum directly affects the capacity of the birth canal, since a forward tilt offers a barrier to normal delivery. The female sacrum is wide and short compared with that of the male. Normally, also, the sacrum is concave anteriorly; when this curvature is absent because of any developmental aberration, the midpelvis is diminished and the progress of labor is impeded.

Size of the Sacrosciatic Notch. The capacity of the posterior pelvic inlet is related to the width of the sacrosciatic notch and configuration of its apex. The male pelvis shows a long narrow notch with a high rounded apex and the female a wide notch with a blunt apex.

Prominence of the Coccyx. A prominent coccyx interferes with the passage of the fetus through the birth canal.

Prominence of the Ischial Spines. Ischial spines are classified as sharp, average, or anthropoid. Sharp spines are definitely a male characteristic and may be associated with convergent side walls of the pelvis. Gynecoid spines are blunt and shallow.

Slope of Pelvic Walls. The slope of the pelvic wall is readily obtained by drawing a tangent along the outer aspect of the obturator foramen connecting with the outermost margin of the transverse diameter of the pelvic inlet. For maximum facility of delivery, the lines so drawn should be parallel. Convergent lines indicate a diminution in either midpelvis or pelvic outlet which may cause some difficulty in delivery.

Subpubic Angle. The pubic rami may be delicate, average, or heavy, and the pubic angle may be wide or curved as in the female or narrow and straight as in the male. The capacity of the pelvic outlet to a great extent is regulated by the subpubic angle and the pubic rami.

Diastasis of the Pubic Symphysis. In experimental animals there is a considerable diastasis of the pubic symphysis and resorption of bone along both sides of the pubic symphysis near term. This is an endocrine phenomenon. In the human such resorption of bone or actual diastasis does not ordinarily occur, but a relaxation of the ligaments across the pubic symphysis does occur, and occasionally diastasis persists following parturition. Such diastasis may facilitate delivery.

Extent of Acetabular Bulge. Occasionally in association with nutritional deficiencies or hereditary disorders of the bony pelvis, there is a bulging inward of the acetabulum, producing the so-called Otto pelvis or arthrokatadysis. Such abnormality may impede the passage of the fetus through the midpelvis.

Method of Reporting. In reporting, one section is devoted entirely to the various measurements; these are given in table form (Fig. 17–17 *B*). The theoretical fetal skull diameter, perimeter, and volume are also indicated relative to the dimensions of the pelvic inlet and midpelvis.

The second portion of the report should refer to pelvic architecture and details concerning fetus, placenta, and amniotic sac.

Method for Correction of Magnification. The degree of magnification will vary in accordance with the distance between the x-ray tube target and the film, and the distance between the diameter (or distance) to be measured and the film. If the dimension in question is parallel with the film surface, distortion is eliminated. If the target-to-film distance is known and also the object-to-film distance, it is possible to calculate accurately the true measurement of the part. This may be accomplished by graphs or nomograms (Fig. 17–20) (Ball, Snow), stereoscopic films (Caldwell and Moloy), metal notched rules placed next to the part being radiographed (Colcher-Sussman), or perforated metal plates superimposed on the radiograph (Thoms).

In those methods that employ calculation, graphs, or nomograms to determine the degree of magnification, the basic procedure is as follows:

1. The desired dimension is measured on the one radiograph, whether it be the anteroposterior or lateral view.

2. The distance that this dimension is placed from the film is determined from the other radiograph. Thus, to determine this object-to-film distance for dimensions measured on the anteroposterior view, the lateral radiograph is employed and vice versa.

3. There will, however, be an error of magnification on this second radiograph also, which must be corrected before it can be applied as the object-to-table-top distance.

4. In order to obtain object-to-film distance, the object-to-table-top distance is first calculated, and to this figure is added the known table-top-to-film distance (usually 5 cm.).

5. Only those dimensions in the central ray can be measured, unless the teleroentgenographic method is employed where beam divergence is negligible.

6. The following triangulation laws are applied (Fig. 17–20 *C*):

$$\frac{GH \text{ (unknown)}}{DE \text{ (known)}} = \frac{XH}{XE} = \frac{XE - (HB + BE) \text{ (known)}}{XE \qquad \text{(known)}}$$

From this equation, it is obvious that all factors are known except GH and hence, simple algebraic solution is possible. Snow's special calculator or Ball's nomograms allow this algebraic solution to be obtained directly.

STUDY OF THE NONPREGNANT FEMALE— GYNECOLOGIC RADIOLOGY

X-ray Appearance of Intrauterine Contraceptive Devices (Lehfeldt). Most intrauterine contraceptive devices are made of radiopaque materials. Three commonly employed devices are illustrated in Fig. 17-21. In rare cases pregnancy has occurred with the device *in situ*. No obstetric difficulties caused by the intrauterine devices have been reported.

X-ray evidence of the intrauterine contraceptive device in the pelvic area is no definite proof that it is within the uterine cavity. In the nonpregnant woman, the definite answer may be supplied by a hysterogram. In pregnancy, the presence or absence of the device should not be determined until the early part of the third trimester to avoid fetal exposure to radiation.

Perforation of the uterus occurs rarely. According to Shimkin et al., uterine perforation may occur in about 1 out of 2500 insertions of a coil or loop and in 1 out of 150 insertions of a bow. Perforation occurs especially at the time of insertion or occasionally at attempted blind removal. It may be partial or complete. Perforation at insertion is often asymptomatic and unrecognized.

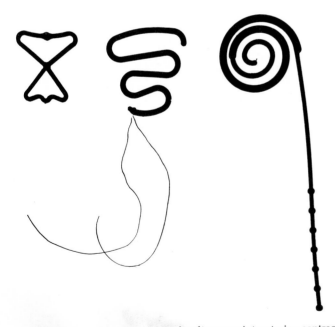

Figure 17-21. Most commonly employed radiopaque intrauterine contraceptive devices (left to right): Birnberg bow; Lippes loop with attached nylon string (nonopaque); Margulies coil with radiopaque cervicovaginal extension. (From Lehfeldt, H.: Fertility and Sterility, 16:502-507, 1965.)

Intestinal obstruction may occur by herniation of small bowel through an aperture of the device or by volvulus about a point of fixation due to adhesions around the device.

Hysterosalpingography. The main uses of this procedure are: (1) study of sterility problems; (2) investigation of uterine bleeding; (3) re-establishment of tubal patency; (4) visualization of abnormalities of the uterine cavity or oviducts; and (5) visualization of sinus tracts communicating with the female genital tract.

Technique of Examination. As with all contrast procedures, it is always advisable to obtain a preliminary scout film prior to the introduction of the contrast medium (Fig. 17-22 A). Areas of calcification and soft tissue masses can thereby be delineated prior to the introduction of the special medium. The lithotomy position over an x-ray Bucky table, preferably equipped with image amplification and closed circuit television fluoroscopy, is employed.

A cannula, preferably radiolucent, is inserted into the uterine cervical canal after visualization of the cervix through an appropriate speculum. It is best that the cannula be filled with contrast material so that all air bubbles are extracted prior to the insertion into the uterine cervical canal. The introduction of air bubbles may cause confusion in interpretation.

Under fluoroscopic control, while viewing the injection on a television monitor, a fractional injection of an appropriate contrast medium is begun (for example, Sinugrafin). A spot film may be obtained after each 2 cc. injection if so desired and a total of 6 to 10 cc. is employed (Fig. 17-22 B). The entire study may be done with video tape recording. The examination can cease after the investigator is satisfied that the entire genital tract has been visualized maximally. After the last injection, stereoscopic anteroposterior and lateral films are obtained.

If Sinugrafin or Salpix is employed, serial films may be obtained at 20 minutes, 60 minutes, 2 hours, and 3 hours (Fig. 17-22 D). Ordinarily, by 3 hours, the soluble absorbable medium has been resorbed and may be found in the urinary bladder. It is important at this time to note whether or not there is any residual dye in loculated areas within the pelvis such as may occur with hydrosalpinx.

Hysterosalpingography with Opaque Oily Substances (Fullenlove). Hysterosalpingography with opaque oily substances is preferred by some because of the denser image produced and because this method permits a 24 hour follow-up study which water soluble substances cannot provide (Fig. 17-23).

The technique is fundamentally the same; care must be exercised, however, to remove the speculum prior to injection so as not to obscure the cervical canal and internal os. The injection is made under image amplifier fluoroscopic control so that venous intravasation may be seen immediately.

Although practically all patients are examined for sterility or habitual abortion, many abnormalities may be visualized.

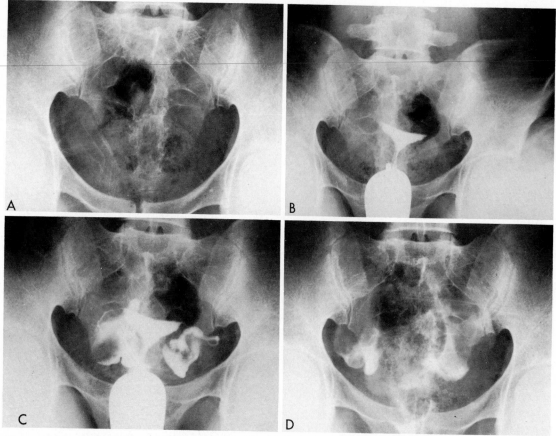

Figure 17–22.   Radiographs demonstrating routine films obtained by hysterosalpingography with soluble, absorbable medium. *A.* Preliminary scout film prior to the injection of the first medium. *B.* Film obtained after the insertion of the first 2 cc. fraction. *C.* Radiograph obtained after the fourth insertion of the 2 cc. fraction. This radiograph demonstrates spillage into the pelvic peritoneal space. *D.* Film obtained 20 minutes after the injection, showing the opaque medium to be still present in the pelvic peritoneal space, but already some of the medium has been absorbed and is appearing in the urinary bladder. Dotted areas indicate the impression of the ovaries upon the contrast medium.

These are summarized and illustrated in *Analysis of Roentgen Signs*.

The complications which can occur are hemorrhage, flare-up of an infection, and venous or lymphatic intravasation. The latter can be recognized immediately during fluoroscopy and the examination is stopped. The oil tends to disappear in from 1 to 3 days but may be recognized in lungs. Lymphatic intravasation occurs with about the same frequency as venous intravasation. There usually is no adverse reaction and it follows the same course as lymphangiography, disappearing over a period of 3 to 6 months.

Uterine Isthmus Insufficiency.   Brünner and Ulrich have employed the technique of hysterography with a balloon catheter for the visualization of the uterine isthmus. They indicate that the advantage of using this catheter for hysterography is the possibility of diagnosing incompetence of the uterine isthmus while the patient is not pregnant and thereby establishing the probable cause of habitual abortion.

Contraindications to Procedure.   Uterine bleeding at the time of injection, such as may occur with menstruation or with some abnormality, may predispose to emboli to the lung and elsewhere, and thus may be considered a contraindication. Actually, no fatalities have been reported, even when iodized oil has been demonstrated radiographically in the chest. Nevertheless, it is a complication to be avoided if possible.

During any active inflammatory phase in the pelvis, the procedure is to be avoided in order to obviate any further spread.

Pregnancy is probably a contraindication to the procedure. Abortions have been reported.

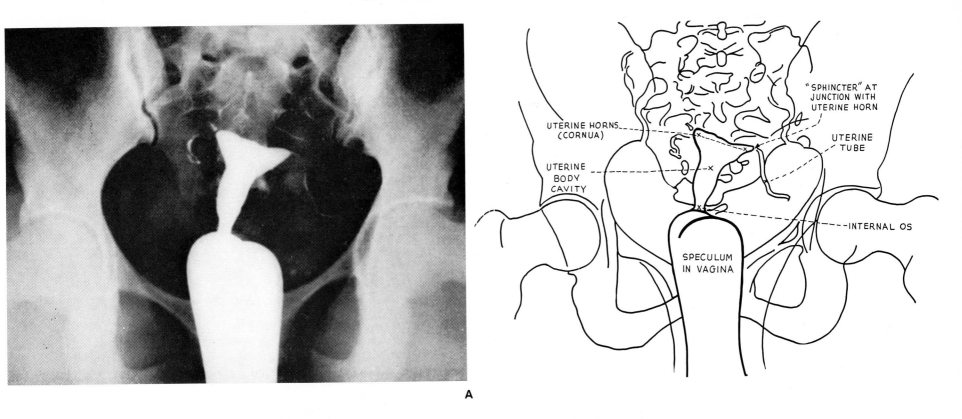

UTERINE HORNS
(CORNUA)

"SPHINCTER" AT
JUNCTION WITH
UTERINE HORN

UTERINE
TUBE

UTERINE
BODY
CAVITY

INTERNAL OS

SPECULUM
IN VAGINA

A

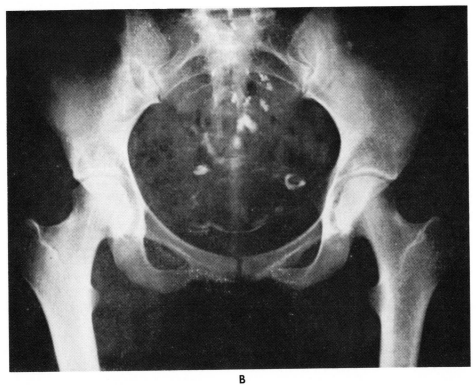

B

Figure 17–23. Hysterosalpingography with Lipiodol. *A.* Initial full film and tracing of same. *B.* Twenty-four hour film.

Normal Roentgen Findings (Fig. 17–24).   In the anteroposterior projection, the uterine cavity is ordinarily visualized as a triangular structure with the apex pointed downward toward the cannula. Occasionally a dimpling is noted at the top of the uterus, indicating the point of fusion of the two halves from which it is originally formed. Thin threadlike structures extend from both uterine horns, indicating filling of the oviducts and finally a spillage at the fimbriated ends of the oviducts into the anatomic pelvis (Fig. 17–25). The uterine horn is a narrow segment which may on occasion undergo spasm. The isthmus beyond the uter-

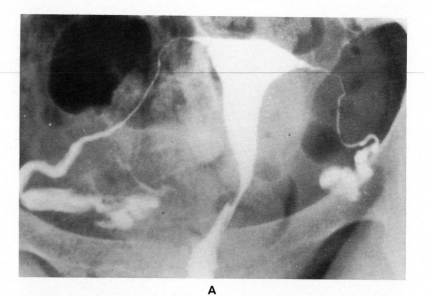

A

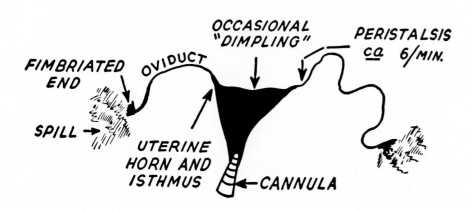

a. ANTEROPOSTERIOR

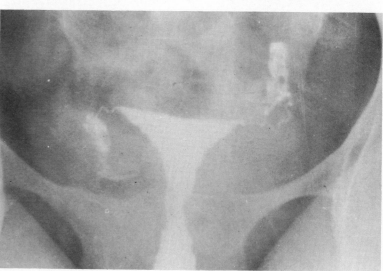

B

Figure 17–25.   A. Normal hysterosalpingogram using water soluble media. B. Hysterosalpingogram with slight endometrial hyperplasia.

Figure 17–25 continued on the opposite page.

b. LATERAL VIEW

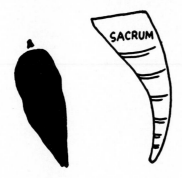

Figure 17–24.   Diagrams illustrating the normal roentgen findings in hysterosalpingography.

ine horn may likewise on occasion be slightly narrowed. On serial films peristalsis in the oviducts may be noted at a rate of approximately 6 per minute. In the lateral view the uterine cavity is carrot-shaped and in slight anteversion.

Abnormal Uterine Findings (Käser et al.). Abnormal roentgen anatomy is outside the scope of this text and the student is referred for a summary description of these abnormalities to *Analysis of Roentgen Signs.* Example illustrations, however, of some of the abnormalities encountered are shown in Figure 17–26.

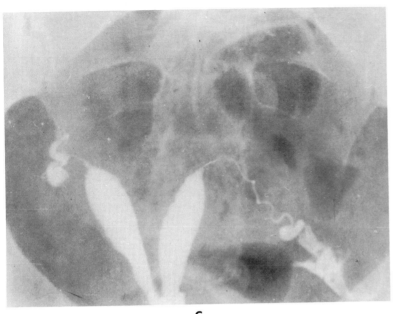

C

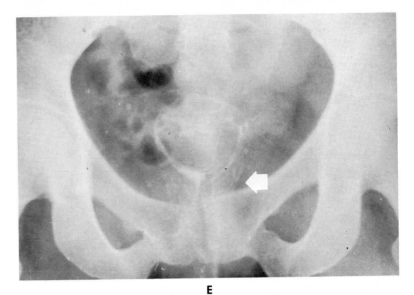

E

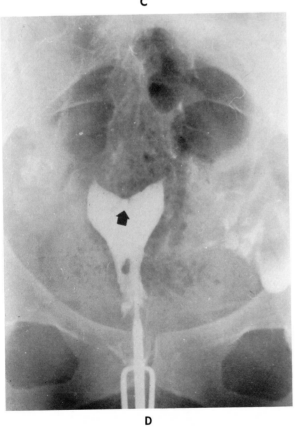

D

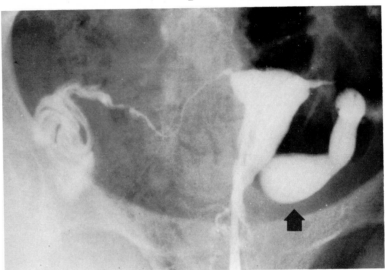

F

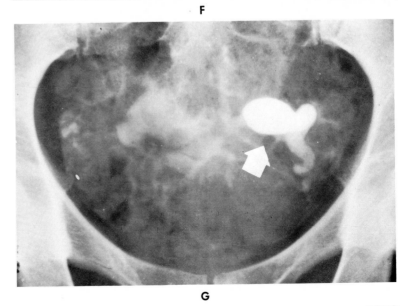

G

Figure 17–25 *Continued.* *C* and *D.* Bicornuate uterus surgically repaired with persistent scar formation. *E.* Vagina coated with contrast material (Sinugrafin) after hysterosalpingography. *F.* Appearance of hydrosalpinx on the left at time of initial injection. *G.* Appearance of hydrosalpinx on the 30-minute retention film taken afterward.

<u>UTERUS</u>

1. <u>SMALL SIZE</u>

    a. INFANTILE

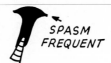 SPASM FREQUENT

2. <u>ABNORMALITIES OF POSITION</u>

    a. NORMAL RETRO- AND ANTE-FLEXION

    b. NORMAL SLIGHT DEFLECTION TO RIGHT OR LEFT FROM INSTRUMENTATION

    c. DISPLACEMENT BY ADJOINING PELVIC MASSES

3. <u>PROTRUSIONS OR SINUSES FROM UTERINE CAVITY</u>

    a. ADENOMYOSIS OR ENDOMETRIOSIS

4. <u>IRREGULARITY OF OUTER SMOOTH MARGIN</u>

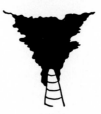

    a. BENIGN HYPER-PLASIAS OF MENOPAUSE

    b. ENDOMETRITIS

    c. RETAINED PLACENTA

    d. CARCINOMA

5. <u>FILLING DEFECTS</u>

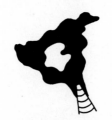

    a. FIBROMYOMA BEGINNING PREGNANCY POLYP INTRAUTERINE SYNECHIAE

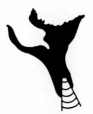

    b. CORPUS CARCINOMA RETAINED PLACENTA.

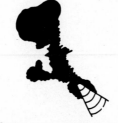

    c. CERVIX CARCINOMA

6. <u>DUPLICATION</u>

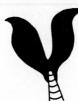

Figure 17–26. Diagrammatic tracings illustrating some abnormal roentgen findings within the uterus proper in hysterosalpingograms.

Gynecography (Pneumoperitoneum of the Pelvis) (Fig. 17–27). This technique allows visualization of the uterine fundus, ovaries, oviducts, and broad ligaments (Granjon).

Technique. 1000 to 2000 cc. of a gaseous medium (air, carbon dioxide, nitrous oxide) are slowly introduced under pressure not exceeding 12 cm. of water. Films are taken in the position shown in Figure 17–27.

Anteroposterior and lateral projections are employed. A normal appearance is shown.

Normal Anatomy. The pelvic pneumogram demonstrates the normal uterus and normal ovaries as smooth organs free of adhesions. The normal ovaries (Weigen and Stevens) vary in size from 3.7 to 14.6 square centimeters, with a mean of 9 square centimeters. The uterine fundus, broad ligaments, anterior surface of rectum, and dome of the urinary bladder may all be demonstrated clearly (Fig. 17–27).

Contraindications include peritoneal infection, massive hemorrhage, and large lesions.

Types of pathologic processes identified include malformed uterus, uterine hypoplasia, extrauterine pregnancy, abnormalities of site, formation, and volume of the ovaries (Stein-Leventhal syndrome), and ovarian tumor masses and cysts (Fig. 17–28) (see *Analysis of Roentgen Signs*).

In a series of 110 patients using nitrous oxide as the gaseous media, Buice and Gould reported no unusual complications.

The procedure was especially valuable in patients who could not be accurately evaluated by manual examination. These included young children, patients with congenital anomalies of the ovaries, tubes, or uterus, obese patients, and uncooperative patients.

Little et al. have used the term "gynecography" to indicate combined hysterosalpingography and pelvic pneumoroentgenography. Others have also employed this combined technique (Semin et al.). The gas may be introduced by transuterine inflation, cul-de-sac, or transabdominal puncture. The combination of the two procedures on a single film demonstrated the status of the uterine cavity, the tubal lumina, and the contours and relative sizes of the pelvic structures. They describe the primary contraindications to gynecography as being pregnancy, uterine bleeding, purulent cervical or uterine discharge, acute or subacute pelvic inflammatory disease, shock, localized or diffuse peritonitis, large tumor masses filling the pelvis, and elderly patients or those who are poor risks from the cardiac viewpoint. They indicate that the complications of pneumoperitoneum in pelvic pneumoroentgenography are relatively mild and transitory, but that the complications of hysterosalpingography are somewhat more serious when they occur. There may be allergic reactions to the contrast agent, venous extravasation of the dye, occasional pulmonary embolism, rupture of the uterus or tubes, and transportation of infection or tumor cells into the peritoneal cavity. Fortunately, these complications are rare.

Barium Vaginography (Rubin et al.). A standard rectal enema tip is thrust through the center of a sponge inserted into the introitus of the vagina with the patient supine on the fluoro-

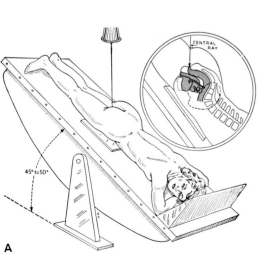

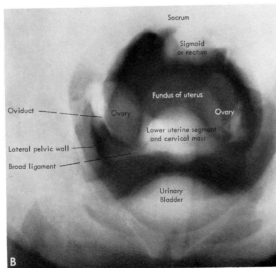

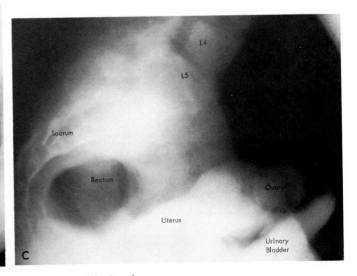

Figure 17–27. A. Position of patient (after instillation of gas) for radiography. Pneumoperitoneum of the female pelvis in posteroanterior (B) and lateral (C) projections. This patient was a 29 year old female with a Stein-Leventhal syndrome proved by surgery, but her ovaries are considered normal in size for a young woman. (Courtesy of Dr. Wilma C. Diner, Department of Radiology, University of Arkansas Medical Center, Little Rock, Arkansas.)

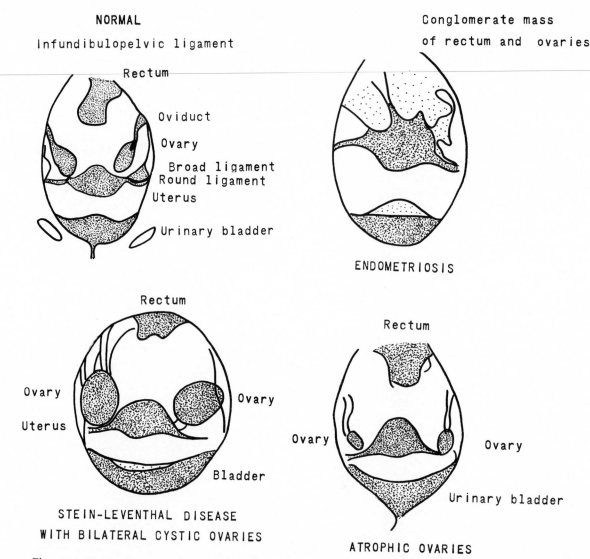

Figure 17–28. Stein-Leventhal syndrome, endometriosis, and atrophic ovaries, demonstrated by gynecography with normal for comparison. (Modified from Stevens, G. M.: Seminars in Roentgenology, 44:252–269, 1969. Used by permission.)

scopic table. The patient keeps her legs together and the enema tip is advanced into the vagina while the sponge approximates the labia. A thin solution of barium is instilled into the vagina and photofluorograms or spot films are exposed in the antero-posterior, oblique, and lateral projections.

The patient is then permitted to evacuate the barium and a double contrast study may be carried out thereafter if desired. Finally the patient is given a cleansing douche at the termination of the examination.

Utility of Method. The following pathologic states may be determined: (1) vaginal extension from cancer of the cervix; (2) vaginal extension from adjoining carcinomas or malignancies of the bladder, rectum, or other adjacent organs; (3) demonstration of fistulas (through the colon or through the urinary bladder); (4) enterovaginal fistulas following irradiation.

Generally this procedure may help, especially in tumor staging and treatment planning.

Angiography of the Pelvis. Percutaneous, transfemoral aortography by the Seldinger technique has permitted catheterization of major branches of the iliac arteries. The injections may be made in the aorta above the bifurcation of the iliac arteries or in selective branches.

This technique may be utilized for accurate placental visualization, or for visualization of neoplastic masses or other abnormalities in the pelvis. For example, this procedure has been found very useful in a study of the extension of carcinoma of the cervix, uterine tumors, adnexal tumors, problems of pregnancy and placentography. The placental circulation is usually identified as early as the second month in unruptured extrauterine pregnancy. It appears as a scattered, fine, mottled or cotton-fluff opacification. There is ordinarily a lingering density in the placenta due to slowing of the circulation in this area (Meng and Elkin).

The techniques of pelvic angiography and pneumoperitoneum have also been combined (Rådberg and Wickbom). Lymphangiography has also been used as an adjunct to gynecologic roentgenology (Howett). This has been discussed and illustrated in prior chapters.

Technique.   Reference is made to prior chapters for more detailed technical description. Using mild sedation, sterile technique, and local anesthesia a Seldinger needle is inserted into the femoral artery approximately 2 inches below the inguinal ligament. The needle is usually inserted through both walls of the artery. After the stylet in the needle is withdrawn, the cannula is carefully withdrawn through the posterior wall into the lumen of the femoral artery, when pulsating bleeding is encountered. The stylet is immediately inserted partially and the cannula threaded up the femoral artery a short distance. A long, specially coiled spring guide is then introduced through the cannula and advanced within the arterial lumen under fluoroscopic control. The spring guide must be introduced far enough so that when the cannula is withdrawn over it, it will remain in place. The cannula is then removed entirely and a length of appropriate catheter tubing is pushed over and along the guide into the femoral artery. Fluoroscopy is always employed during manipulation of the guide and tubing. The tip of the catheter is usually localized in the upper abdominal aorta for abdominal aortography and renal arteriography, or at the aortic bifurcation for pelvic arteriography.

The guide is then withdrawn and a few milliliters of heparin-saline solution (10 units of heparin per milliliter of normal saline solution) is injected through the tubing to prevent clotting.

During the injection for pelvic arteriography, blood pressure cuffs may be employed as tourniquets about both thighs to prevent the radiopaque agent, such as the diatrizoates, from running off into the leg arteries. The usual dose of contrast agent of 60 per cent methylglucamine or 89 per cent methalamate is 20 to 25 cc., depending upon the location of the catheter and the size of the vessel being injected. This material is injected rapidly and a series of films is obtained, usually two or three per second for the first 3 seconds, and 1 per second thereafter for 7 or 8 seconds.

A mechanical pressure injector is desirable to allow the rapid injection of large volumes of the agent. It is desirable usually to complete the injection within 1 second.

In the presence of pregnancy, for placental visualization for example, fluoroscopy should be minimal.

The catheter is removed following the procedure and hemostasis is obtained by constant pressure, followed thereafter by a pressure dressing to be removed in 2 to 4 hours. The patient should be kept under observation for a sufficiently long period to allow detection of recurrence of bleeding at the cannulation site.

Side Effects Noted by Patients.   Usually the injection of the contrast agent produces a sensation of heat in the area of distribution, and occasionally a sudden brief sharp or burning pain in the lower back may be encountered. Usually such pain persists for 10 to 15 seconds only. Care must be exercised that dissection of the artery has not occurred subintimally. Varying degrees of nausea may occur immediately after the injection in occasional patients, but vomiting rarely occurs and the nausea disappears spontaneously. During the week following the procedure, tenderness and ecchymosis are observed at the needle puncture site in the groin, but this may be minimized by prevention of hematoma formation during the procedure and an appropriate pressure dressing thereafter.

Repeated injections may be carried out with adequate time for excretion of the contrast agent in those patients who have normal renal function. Ordinarily, 120 ml. of the contrast agent can be tolerated in the course of 1 hour of such study in such patients. In the presence of disturbed or abnormal renal function, lesser volumes of contrast agent are usually utilized.

The Normal Pelvic Arteriogram.   In the straight anteroposterior projection centered over the midpelvis, the lower level of the abdominal aorta, its bifurcation, and the internal and external iliac arteries and their branches to the gluteus, pelvic organs, and legs present a symmetrical appearance except for a reactive constriction of the catheterized femoral and external iliac arteries in many cases.

Usually, the entire *uterine artery* can be studied from its point of origin on the internal iliac artery to its course in the parametrium and along the lateral margin of the uterus. It usually courses close to the easily identified outward-sweeping *superior gluteal arteries.* These are the only branches of the internal iliac arteries which in frontal projection cross the external iliac artery to give off their major branches. The uterine artery courses medially and caudad to the cervix and thereafter ascends upward along the lateral margin of the uterus as far as the fundus. Its course is tortuous lateral to the uterine body and numerous ramifications extend into the uterine wall with many fine branches terminating in the endometrium. Occasional branches of the uterine artery extend laterally to supply the adnexa on the same side. Considerable variation unfortunately exists as to size and appearance and even asymmetry in given pa-

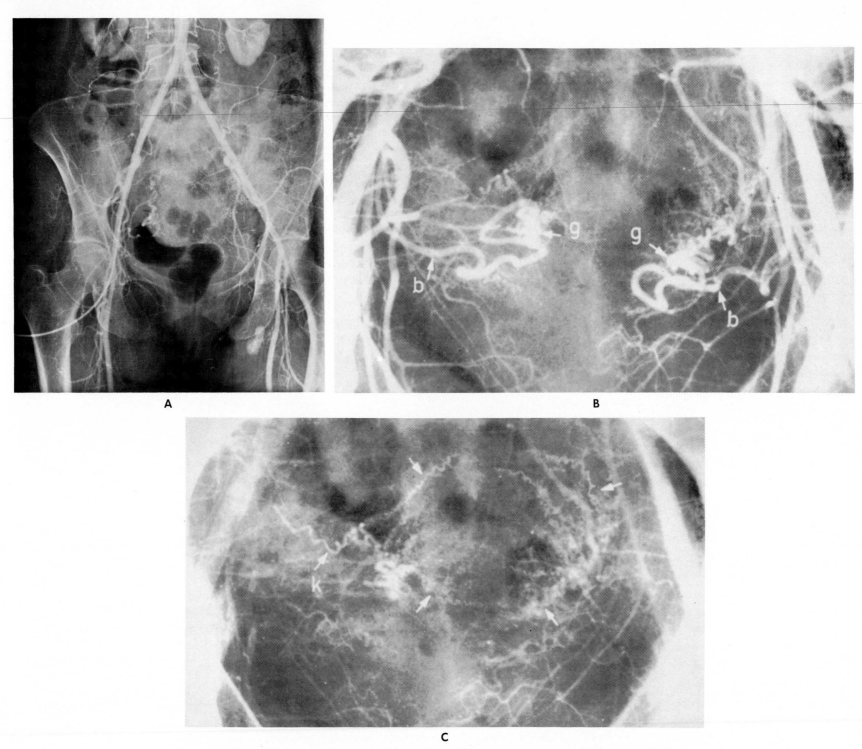

Figure 17–29. A. Originally, the Seldinger catheter is inserted above the bifurcation of the aorta and then withdrawn to the hypogastric arterial level, as shown in B and C (pelvic arteriograms). B and C. Normal arteriograms. Anteroposterior projection of the uterus. B. Film taken immediately after the injection of opaque medium. The uterine artery in the parametrium (b) and the uterine artery running along the lateral margin of the uterus (g) are visible. Small tortuous intramural arteries are beginning to opacify. C. Film taken two seconds after film B. The main trunk of the uterine artery is now faintly outlined. Numerous small, tortuous intramural arteries are visible within the uterus (arrows). The right adnexal branch (k) follows a tortuous course. (From Abrams, H. L.: Angiography, 2nd ed. Vol. 2. Boston, Little, Brown & Co., 1971.)

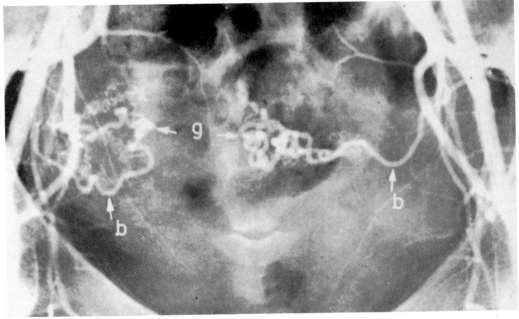

A

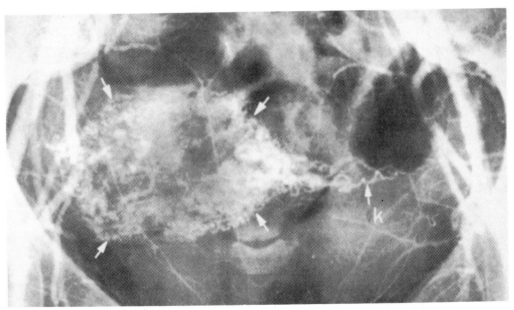

B

Figure 17–30. Normal arteriogram. Axial projection of the uterus. A. Film taken immediately after the injection of opaque medium. The uterine arteries in the parametrium (b) and along the lateral margin of the uterus (g) are seen. A few tortuous intramural arteries within the right half of the uterus begin to opacify. B. Film taken two seconds after film A. The main trunk of the uterine artery is now faintly outlined. Numerous small, tortuous intramural arteries are visible within the uterus (arrows). The left adnexal branch (k) follows a tortuous course. (From Abrams, H. L.: Angiography, 2nd ed., Vol. 2. Boston, Little, Brown & Co., 1971.)

tients. Occasionally, also, the entire adnexa and even the upper part or the entire uterus may be supplied by the *ovarian artery*.

Although placentography has been employed in the past for detection of placenta praevia, ectopic tumors, and placental tumors, the advent of ultrasound has diminished the need for arteriography in these conditions.

An angiogram in a normal intrauterine pregnancy of nine weeks duration is shown in Figure 17–32.

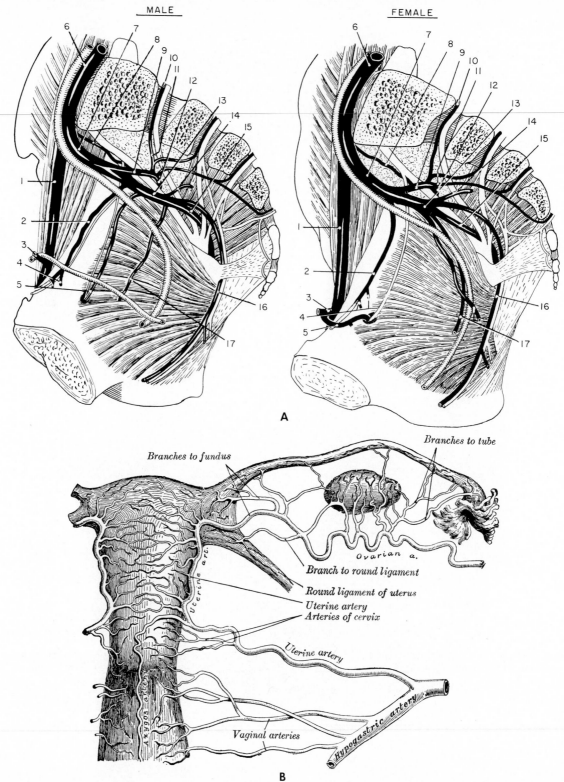

MALE

FEMALE

A

Branches to fundus

Branches to tube

Ovarian a.

Branch to round ligament

Round ligament of uterus

Uterine artery
Arteries of cervix

Uterine art.

Uterine artery

Vaginal arteries

Hypogastric artery

B

Figure 17–31. A. The arteries of the pelvic cavity in the male and female: (1) external iliac; (2) umbilical which terminates as the medial umbilical ligament; (3) inferior epigastric; (4) superior vesical; (5) obturator — in one arising from the anterior division of the internal iliac and in the other from the inferior epigastric branch of the external iliac; (6) common iliac; (7) internal iliac; (8) iliolumbar; (9) posterior division; (10) branch of lateral sacral entering sacrum; (11) lateral sacrals; (12) superior gluteal; (13) anterior division; (14) middle rectal; (15) inferior gluteal; (16) internal pudendal; and (17) inferior vesical in the male, and uterine and vaginal in the female. (From Roger C. Crafts, A Textbook of Human Anatomy. © 1966. The Ronald Press Company, New York. Modified and redrawn after Jamieson.) B. The arteries of the internal organs of generation of the female, seen from behind (after Hyrt). (From Gray's Anatomy of the Human Body, 29th ed. Goss, C. M. (ed.) Philadelphia, Lea & Febiger, 1973.)

1086

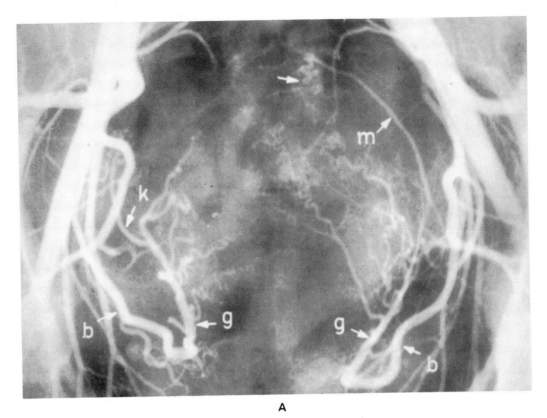

A

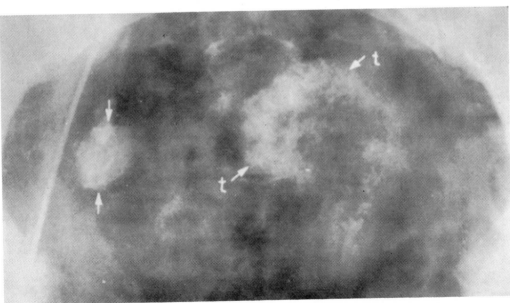

B

Figure 17–32. Normal intrauterine pregnancy of nine weeks' duration. *A*. Film taken immediately after the injection of opaque medium. The uterine arteries in parametrium (*b*) and along the lateral margin of corpus uteri (*g*) are visible. The fundal insertion of the placenta is beginning to opacify (*unmarked arrows*) Some intramural arteries (*m*) running toward the placenta show a partial loss of tortuosity. (*k*) Right adnexal branch. *B*. Two seconds after *A*. The intervillous space is opacified (*t*). *Unmarked arrows* point to the corpus luteum of pregnancy, supplied by the right adnexal branch (see *A*). (From Abrams, H. L.: Angiography, 2d ed. Vol. 2. Boston, Little, Brown & Co., 1971.)

As pregnancy progresses the uterine artery becomes more dilated and convoluted and in the last trimester, the uterine vessels begin to lengthen. At term they are quite straight. It has been demonstrated that the uterine artery is more prominent on one side than the other during gestation (Solish et al.), usually the side on which the placenta is implanted.

In placentography, the placental sinuses containing contrast agent have a scattered, fine, mottled or "cotton-fluff" appearance. Some density may be retained for a considerable period of time in the placental sinuses, allowing for easier identification of these structures (Benson et al.).

Visualization of the Ovarian Arteries. The ovarian arteries are usually so narrow that information of diagnostic value is rarely obtained from the radiologic appearance. Demonstration of these arteries does, however, occur in at least half of the angiograms.

Visceral Pelvic Venography in the Female. Generally, pelvic venography has not consistently produced good results for visualization of the female pelvic structures such as the uterus, vagina, and ovaries. Opacification by the usual methods occurs in no more than 15 to 20 per cent of cases with bilateral common iliac injection or selective internal iliac injections (Doppman and Chretien). Improvement has been achieved by some using catheterization of an ovarian vein, utilizing large volumes of contrast material, urinary bladder distention, and a 35 degree cranial angulation of the radiographic tube. Bilateral femoral vein catheterization was utilized by Doppman and Chretien for catheterization of the ovarian veins. These must be catheterized at least to the level of the iliac crest for success and it is also desirable that both ovarian veins be injected simultaneously (Fig. 17–33). Usually a large volume of contrast agent such as 80 ml. of meglumine iothalamate (Conray-60) is injected through a Y con-

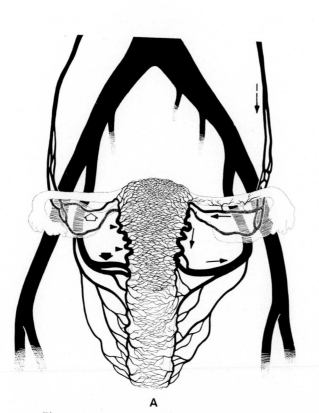

A

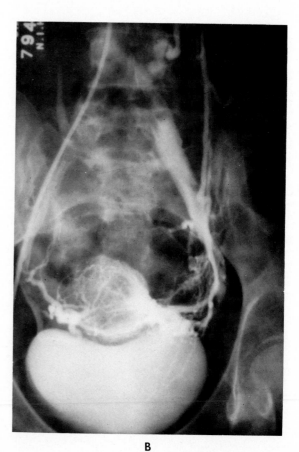

B

Figure 17–33. *A.* Diagrammatic sketch of the major visceral veins of the pelvis. The right ovarian pedicle (clear arrow), right uterine plexus (arrowheads), and right uterine pedicle or vein (solid arrow) are shown on the left. The direction of flow during retrograde ovarian venography, shown on the right, is down the ovarian vein, medially via the ovarian pedicle to the uterine plexus, down the uterine plexus, and laterally in the uterine pedicle to the internal iliac vein (arrows). This route is invariably demonstrated with satisfactory retrograde injection; filling of the uterine myometrial plexus is less constant.

B. Retrograde left ovarian venogram obtained without bladder distension or angulation of the radiographic tube. The uterus is projected axially above the bladder. (From Doppman, J. L., and Chretien, P.: Radiology, 98:406, 1971.)

nector at a rate of 10 to 15 ml. per second. "The Valsalva maneuver, balloon compression of the lower inferior vena cava, and the upright position seem to have no influence on pelvic vein filling; the most essential factor is the placement of the catheter tip deep in the ovarian vein, preferably below the level of the pelvic brim" (Doppman and Chretien).

It is recommended that the x-ray tube be angled 35 degrees cranially with distention of the urinary bladder so as to prevent superimposition of the ovarian pedicle, uterine plexus, and uterine pedicle. Distention of the urinary bladder with gas is to be preferred. One film every second for 15 seconds is adequate.

Combined Pelvic Angiography and Pneumoperitoneum in Gynecologic Diagnosis. These two methods are often complementary. The vascular structure of the pelvis combined with the morphological delineation of detail by pneumoperitoneum makes a valuable contribution to the diagnostic armamentarium (Rådberg and Wickbom).

STUDY OF THE PREGNANT MOTHER IN RESPECT TO THE FETUS

Introduction. Protection from radiation and potential radiation hazards take on greater significance in this field, since there are at least two or more lives involved (mother and fetuses) and not just that of the patient. The hazards of radiation must be carefully weighed against the benefits to be achieved.

Determination of a Fetal Skeleton in Utero. The viable fetus should not be exposed to irradiation during the first trimester of pregnancy. Hormonal tests are far more sensitive in any case for the detection of early pregnancy, since ossification of the fetal skeleton does not occur prior to the third month of gestation, and radiographically detectable fetal skeletal parts are difficult to find prior to the 13th or 14th week.

The indications for seeking fetal skeletal parts are (1) an enlarging uterus without other evidence of pregnancy; (2) an enlarging tumor mass of the pelvis that could conceivably be teratomatous or represent an extra-uterine pregnancy; (3) a previously suspected gravid uterus when the clinical situation has changed and pregnancy tests have ceased to be positive; and (4) an abnormal fetus that is strongly suggested by clinical appearances (hydrocephalus; anencephaly).

The fetal parts that lend themselves most readily to early detection are the segmental structures such as those of the spine and ribs; occasionally the extremities and head may be seen in faint outline.

The oblique views of the pelvis are often more helpful than straight anteroposterior views, since the fetal ossified parts may be projected over the sacrum and lost to view.

Determination of Multiple Fetuses. Study for multiple fetuses is not undertaken prior to the later stages of pregnancy, preferably late in the last trimester when radiation hazard to the fetus is minimal. Multiple fetuses can be ascertained, however, after approximately the fourteenth week when fetal ossification may be manifest radiographically. A differentiation of multiple fetuses is particularly useful in patients who have enlarged uteri because of pendulous abdomens, marked lordosis of the lumbar spine, or a tendency to polyhydramnios. The physician may not assume that the 14 week size uterus will necessarily reveal the skeletons of developing twins. The fetal skeletons may not be determinable at this early period, especially with twins.

Fetal Normalcy. Fetal normalcy is best studied late in the last trimester. In evaluating the fetal skeleton in utero, it is important to bear in mind the problems related to magnification and distortion. Before diagnosing an abnormal fetus, one must be certain of the finding by means of examinations in various projections and serial studies.

A thin black line surrounding the fetus on the radiograph is called the normal "fetal fat line." This is best developed after the eighth month when the deposition of subcutaneous fat occurs most rapidly. When the fetal fat line is thicker than normal, postmaturity of the fetus may be suspected.

Evidence of trauma to the fetus may also be detected on occasion in utero.

Fetal Age and Development. Fetal age determination should rarely be required prior to the third trimester of pregnancy. There are many different bases upon which fetal age can be estimated, but probably the most reliable are estimation of actual fetal length and determination of average fetal head diameter.

The determination of fetal length can be made by measuring the total length of the fetus, attempting correction for magnification and distortion. These are optimal on teleroentgenograms (6 foot film-to-target distance), but at best, distortion may be troublesome and lead to inaccuracy. After correction for magnification, if distortion is known to be negligible (Fig. 17–20), a simple rule in determination of fetal age according to fetal length is set up as follows; prior to the fifth month, the fetal age in months is indicated by the square root of the length in centimeters. After the fifth month, the length in centimeters is divided by five in order to obtain the fetal age in months.

Determination of average fetal head diameter can be accurate. There are several tables and graphs available for computing fetal age from roentgen measurements of the fetal skull, based on the anthropometric studies of Scammon and Calkins, Hodges, and others. These graphs indicate the fetal age in accordance with occipital-frontal diameter in centimeters, biparietal skull diameter, and average net circumference of the fetal skull obtained from two roentgenograms taken at right angles to one another (Fig. 17–19 D). The average diameter of the fetal skull is obtained by averaging the long and short perpendicular diameters (corrected for magnification) from anteroposterior and lateral teleroentgenograms of the fetal skull (average of two diameters for each view).

A graph is also available based upon the length of the femoral shaft; we consider this less valuable roentgenographically since distortion makes it very difficult to be certain that the true length has been obtained.

Prediction of Fetal Maturity. The following criteria are perhaps most important.

1. An ossification center is present in the distal end of the femur in 90 per cent of term fetuses.

2. Proximal tibial epiphyseal ossification is noted at term in 70 to 80 per cent of the newborn.

3. Less practical standards for ossification are (a) ossification of the hyoid bone should be complete; (b) ossification of the central parts of the vertebrae should appear; and (c) the first segments of the coccyx, the metacarpals, and the phalanges may be visualized.

With regard to reliability of some of these criteria, Schreiber et al. (1962) came to the following conclusions:

1. Visualization of the fetal distal femoral ossification centers indicated a mature fetus by several criteria in 92 to 98 per cent of cases, with an average of 96 per cent for all criteria.

2. Approximately one fetus in twenty with visualized distal femoral ossification centers was not mature.

3. Visualization of both the distal femoral and proximal tibial epiphyseal centers on antepartum abdominal films was a highly reliable indicator of fetal maturity. When these centers were present the fetus was mature in 95 to 100 per cent of cases with an average of 98 per cent for all criteria.

4. Presence of ossification centers for the distal femoral epiphyses on postpartum knee films was associated with a mature fetus in 93 per cent of cases. However, 58 per cent of the newborn with absent femoral epiphyseal centers were mature by the same criteria and 61 per cent were mature by clinical estimation.

Therefore, failure to visualize these centers on postpartum knee films was not ipso facto evidence of prematurity in their series. Failure to visualize the distal femoral epiphyseal ossification centers on the antepartum films was also a poor indicator of prematurity because of superimposition of structures and fetal movement during the radiographic exposure.

In a second study (1963) distal femoral epiphyseal ossification centers were demonstrated on abdominal films in 80 per cent of the cases in which they were visualized subsequently on postpartum films of the knees of the newborn. False positive demonstration of distal femoral epiphyses was obtained in 1.7 per cent of cases.

The determination of fetal maturity by whatever means is often an important decision, since very often it in turn will decide whether or not elective induction of labor or repeat cesarean section may be indicated.

In the unpublished data from the Vanderbilt Fetal Age Study, antepartum radiographic visualization of the fetal ossification centers about the knees was a better indicator of fetal maturity than estimated gestational age, uterine size, and other physical findings.

Fetal maturity may in part be estimated from measurements of the fetal skull and determination of fetal age (Figs. 17–19 *D* and 17–20 *B*).

Russell, in a study of 3606 maternity cases, found that radiologic assessment of fetal maturity predicted the delivery date more accurately than did the menstrual history. Parity, maternal age, sex of the child, socioeconomic status, fetal weight, and season of the year were without significant influence on the rate of radiologic development of the fetus. A twin pregnancy developed more slowly radiologically than did a single pregnancy. A single fetus was more likely to die perinatally if it was premature radiologically and if the radiologic age was appreciably less than the chronologic age. A postmature fetus was not at increased risk if the radiologic appearance did not indicate postmaturity.

Brosens et al. reported a cytologic test for fetal maturity in combination with a new radiologic method for estimation. They used a lipid contrast medium for intrauterine fetal visualization, which is accomplished by amniocentesis after ultrasonic localization of the placenta. A few milliliters of the amniotic fluid are aspirated and 6 ml. of Ethiodan are injected. An x-ray film is taken 8 to 24 hours later. After 6 to 8 hours Ethiodan outlines the fetal skin clearly through absorption on the vernix. The cytologic method involves counting lipid positive cells in amniotic fluid, using 0.1 per cent aqueous Nile-blue sulfate stain. At birth, maturity was estimated by the pediatrician using neurological parameters. No complications resulted from the injections. The histologic study of the lungs in live born infants who died soon after delivery showed no abnormalities attributable to Ethiodan inhalation.

Margolis and Voss obtained the fetal length indirectly after 34 weeks gestation (in women less than 180 pounds in weight) by measurement of the fetal lumbar vertebral length in utero. Films of the near-term pregnant woman were obtained with the patient prone and a target-to-film distance of 100 cm. The top of the first lumbar vertebra and the bottom of the fifth were marked on the film of the pregnant uterus so obtained. The distance through the middle of the vertebrae was measured to the nearest millimeter with a flexible ruler. The measured lumbar vertebral length could be related to the total newborn length ± 5 cm. Reference to an intrauterine growth chart yielded an approximation of fetal maturation.

Thus, a fetal lumbar vertebral length of 52 mm. or more indicated that 95 per cent of the group weighed over 2500 grams, with an actual total length of 49 cm. or more.

The lumbar vertebral length did not show significant correlation with the weight-length ratio, or with the duration of gestation as calculated by the date of the last menstrual period.

TABLE 17–1   PRESENCE OF SIX OSSIFICATION CENTERS IN ROENTGENOGRAMS OF NEWBORNS*

Ossification Center	Birth Weight, Gm.					
	Under 2000	2000–2499	2500–2999	3000–3499	3500–3999	4000 or More
Calcaneus						
White boys	100%					
girls	100					
Negro boys	100					
girls	100					
Astragalus						
White boys	72.7	100%				
girls	83.3	100				
Negro boys	90.9	100				
girls	100	100				
Dist. femoral epiphysis						
White boys	9.1	75.0	85.3%	100%	100%	
girls	50.0	91.7	98.0	100	100	
Negro boys	18.2	88.5	90.7	94.0	100	
girls	50.2	93.8	99.0	100	100	
Prox. femoral epiphysis						
White boys	0.0	18.8	52.9	78.8	84.1	97.1%
girls	0.0	54.2	75.5	85.7	90.7	90.5
Negro boys	0.0	38.5	62.7	76.0	80.0	92.9
girls	14.3	40.6	76.7	88.1	86.4	100
Cuboid						
White boys	0.0	6.2	14.7	39.8	44.3	60.0
girls	0.0	37.5	57.1	65.2	70.4	76.2
Negro boys	0.0	23.1	43.8	58.0	68.2	100
girls	21.4	37.5	68.0	78.2	81.8	75.0
Head of humerus						
White boys	0.0	7.7	13.8	41.9	49.0	59.1
girls	0.0	5.6	25.8	41.9	69.4	86.7
Negro boys	0.0	0.0	15.2	27.6	48.4	63.6
girls	0.0	10.7	22.7	52.6	38.9	100

*From Growth and Development of Children, 6th ed., by Lowrey, G. H. Copyright © 1973 by Year Book Medical Publishers, Inc., Chicago. Used by permission.

The relationship of six ossification centers in roentgenograms of the newborn to birth weight is indicated in Table 17–1 for white and Negro boys and girls. From this data, it can be seen that birth weight, sex, and race are highly significant factors.

Determination of Fetal Viability, Death, or Other Fetal Abnormalities.   This is considered outside the scope of this text and the student is referred to *Analysis of Roentgen Signs.*

Presentation of Fetus.   The position of the fetal head, small parts, and back is readily determined by consideration of the anteroposterior and lateral radiographs.

A "military" position of the head precludes engagement unless the head is very small and the pelvis is very large. This hyperextended position is more common with cephalopelvic disproportion or other factors that interfere with engagement, such as a distended bladder, pelvic mass, placenta previa, polyhydramnios, or a pendulous uterus. Atypical fetal presentations that can be recognized radiographically are face and brow presentation, transverse, shoulder or arm, breech, footling, or knee.

Roentgenographic pelvic measurements and fetal head mensuration play an important part in management decisions.

When the head is not engaged in a prima gravida, some possibilities to be considered are: obstructing masses in the pelvis such as ovarian cysts or fibroids; placenta previa centralis; a short umbilical cord, or more often a cord twisted around the fetus; fetal malformation such as hydrocephalus and cystic hygroma of the neck; or a pendulous uterus impairing the direction of uterine force.

STUDY OF THE PREGNANT MOTHER FOR UTERINE DETAIL OUTSIDE THE FETUS

Placenta (Fig. 17–35).   Various methods for study of the placenta radiologically are: (1) routine anteroposterior and lateral views of the abdomen, inclusive of the entire uterus; (2) a special lateral film employing a wedge filter when the placenta is anteriorly situated in the uterine fundus. (A "wedge filter" is an x-ray filter and medium interposed between the x-ray tube and the patient which will diminish the radiation over the patient's thinner parts so that this area on the radiograph will have equal clarity with the x-ray image of the thicker anatomic portions. This is particularly useful on the lateral view.) The placenta is situated on either the anterior or posterior surface of the uterine fundus in most instances and can usually be differentiated as a

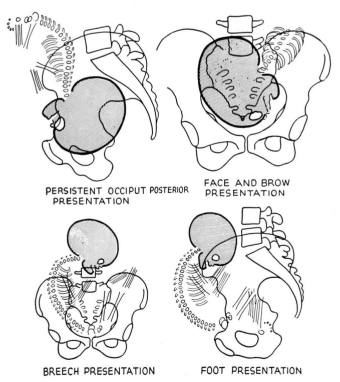

PERSISTENT OCCIPUT POSTERIOR PRESENTATION FACE AND BROW PRESENTATION

BREECH PRESENTATION FOOT PRESENTATION

Figure 17–34.   Diagrams illustrating various types of atypical presentation as they may be seen radiographically.

ROENTGEN STUDY OF THE PLACENTA

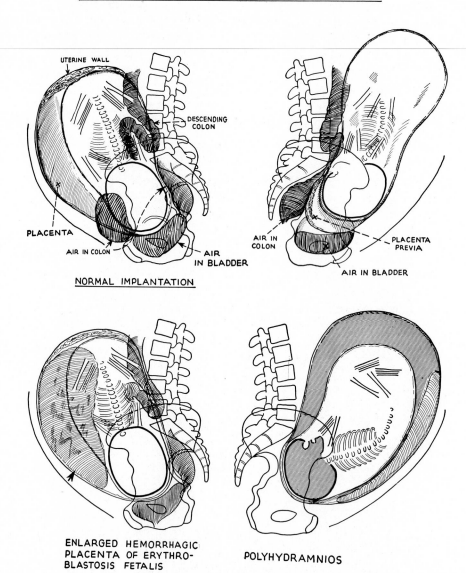

Figure 17–35. Radiographic appearance of normal placental implantation compared with appearances of abnormal implantations. The placenta previa is shown in good contrast by means of air distention of both the bladder and the rectum.

thick, crescentic, platelike structure with a central thickness of 6 to 8 cm. tapering to each side, and a diameter of approximately 25 cm. Contraction and blood loss after delivery diminish the size of the placenta postnatally. The fetus faces the placenta in about three-quarters of the cases. Occasionally, calcification can be identified within the placenta.

3. Radioisotopic techniques or ultrasound compound B scans

(outside the scope of this text) may be utilized for scanning the placenta.

4. Angiographic methods are seldom used in view of the radiation exposure required, but in rare instances they may also be employed.

Amniography

Technique. The maternal urinary bladder is emptied and the placenta localized, either radiographically or by image amplifier fluoroscopy. The maternal abdominal wall is punctured at a distance from the placenta so that entrance is made into the amniotic sac. Generally the dosage is 1.5 cc. of Renografin-60 per week of gestation, up to a total of 50 cc. (Blumberg et al.).

Anteroposterior and lateral films of the abdomen are obtained as early as 30 minutes following injection, or as late as 2 to 3 hours afterward.

Hazards, apart from x-ray radiation, may be (1) premature labor may be induced; and (2) in a series of 50 consecutive patients studied in this way for painless vaginal bleeding, the morbidity noted included needle marks in three infants, one of them infected, and postpartum maternal morbidity involving six patients (Blumberg et al.).

Purposes of Procedure

1. It provides a positive contrast outline of all structures within or impinging upon the amniotic sac. Thus the method may be used to detect placenta previa.

2. Fetal death can be distinguished with reasonable certainty. In films taken after 2 hours, some of the contrast agent should be detected in the fetal stomach or intestine. In a dead fetus, no swallowing will have occurred.

3. It can be a guide to fetography and intrauterine fetal transfusion.

4. It assists in diagnosis of uterine or fetal abnormalities.

5. Premature membrane rupture may be diagnosed by leakage of the contrast medium into the vagina.

6. Extrauterine pregnancy can be demonstrated.

7. Removal of the amniotic fluid under fluoroscopic guidance prior to delivery has also been very helpful in determining the onset of deterioration from erythroblastosis fetalis in the fetus.

After 29 weeks of gestation, the prognosis of impending fetal death on the basis of the rise of optical density of the amniotic fluid seems to be quite accurate. Prior to this time the significance of a given rise of optical density of the amniotic fluid is less certain. This has afforded an effective means of selection of fetuses for preterm delivery and postdelivery exchange transfusions (Queenan et al.; Liggans).

Amniography as a Guide to Fetography and Intrauterine Fetal Transfusions. During amniography, the fetus swallows the radiopaque medium when it is present in amniotic fluid, and this results in delineation of the fetal gastrointestinal tract.

In 1963 Liley demonstrated that he could pass a needle through the maternal abdominal wall, the uterine wall, and the abdominal wall of the fetus to instill Rh negative blood into the peritoneal cavity of the fetus. Blood so instilled was absorbed in the fetal peripheral circulation. Others who have repeated this technique have also reported success with it (Queenan et al.; Bowman and Friesen; Duggin and Taylor).

Image intensifier fluoroscopy is of course essential for such a procedure. It is apparently not unusual to make three or four attempts to enter the peritoneal cavity of a fetus 25 to 26 weeks of age before a successful intraperitoneal approach is achieved.

Technique for the Transuterine Infusion of Red Cells into the Fetus in Erythroblastosis Fetalis (Ferris et al.). An 8 inch No. 16 Touhy needle is introduced into the amniotic sac at a point approximating the anterior abdominal wall of the fetus (Fig. 17–36). The needle is thereafter inserted into the peritoneal cavity of the fetus. Five cc. of methylglucamine diatrizoate are injected to check the needle position. If the end of the needle is free, the opaque medium will outline the diaphragm of the fetus in a crescent shape that can usually be recognized fluoroscopically. Also, contrasted bowel loops of the fetus may be seen. Once the needle is definitely free, 50 to 100 cc. of packed red cells are injected into the peritoneal cavity of the fetus. In their phantom studies Ferris et al. showed that the radiation to the fetus was 228 milliroentgens.

Use of Carbon Dioxide as a Contrast Agent for Localization (Hanafee and Bashore). An injection of 2 to 5 cc. of carbon dioxide is made under fluoroscopic control. If the needle-catheter system is correctly placed, all the signs of free intraperitoneal air in the newborn are evident. If the needle is outside the fetus, gas will be spread over a wide arc.

A catheter replaces the needle after the correct position is ascertained, and the blood is allowed to drip in during the next 30 to 60 minutes.

Excessive quantities of carbon dioxide should not be employed since gas may stimulate the fetus to excessive position change.

A grid to aid in film localization of the needle in intrauterine transfusion has been recommended by Wade.

Prenatal Sex Determination. Fort and Riggs were able to outline the fetal labia in a fetus at 22 weeks of gestation during intrauterine fetal transfusion. Likewise, they were able to visualize a fetal testis in a male fetus. Thus, prenatal sex determination was possible.

GENITOGRAPHY IN INTERSEXUAL STATES (Shopfner)

The components of sexual differentiation consist of chromosomal, gonadal, internal genital anatomy, external genital anato-

my, hormonal aspects, environmental rearing, and sexual orientation or gender. The last two elements are largely governed by internal and external genital anatomy; in the case of the male, hormonal activity is required as well.

The clinical studies which are of assistance in the determina-

A

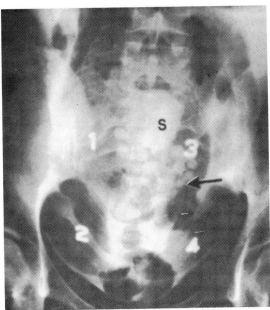

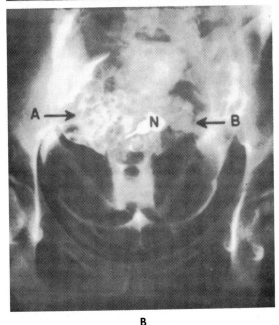

B

Figure 17–36. A. Complete breech presentation. Radiopaque material may be seen in the fetal stomach (S) and small intestine (arrow). Localizing lead markers surround fetal peritoneal cavity. B. Touhy needle (N) in fetal peritoneal cavity. intestine (B). (From Queenan, J. T.: J.A.M.A., *191*:944, 1965. Copyright 1965, American Medical Association.)

tion of these sexual components are sex chromatin pattern, a study of the external genital anatomy, a knowledge of the internal genital anatomy, urinary hormonal excretion, and the nature of the gonads as determined by biopsy.

Genitography is the simplest and best procedure for providing information regarding the internal genital anatomy, particularly prior to the time when knowledge of the nature of the gonads is not essential. Apparently genitography can provide anatomic information not afforded by other means.

The technique of genitography requires the filling of all genital cavities with opaque media. Two methods may be employed: a flushing technique, or a multiple catheter technique. The examination should be performed under fluoroscopy for proper control. The multiple catheter technique is employed when the flushing technique fails, since in placing a catheter into one cavity, one may miss other passages. The relationship of the urinary bladder may be simultaneously determined by excretory urography. It is suggested that the opaque medium employed be aqueous at first try; if success is not obtained, an oily medium may thereafter be employed.

A simple classification of intersex states is the following: true hermaphroditism, in which both ovaries and testes are present in the same individual; female pseudohermaphroditism, in which ovaries and a masculinized lower genital tract in external genitalia are present; and male pseudohermaphroditism, in which the testes are present but female external genitalia are noted. This classification does not include those instances with hypoplastic structures which do not communicate with the exterior of the body.

The basic principle in handling intersex problems is that it is easier to transform a sexually ambiguous person into a female than a male.

There are actually very few circumstances in which the intersex problem can be resolved by masculinization of the external genitalia. Hypospadias is one of these. Shopfner has recommended that genitography be employed, particularly in patients with hypospadias, in order to detect unsuspected müllerian remnants which would tend to counteract the benefits derived from correction of the hypospadias. Genitography also affirms the presence or absence of the vagina and shows the relationship of the urethra to it. Such information becomes important in assigning a practical sex to an intersexual patient.

For further detail in regard to this important subject, the reader is referred to Shopfner's comprehensive monograph.

REFERENCES

Anson, B. J. (ed.): Morris' Human Anatomy. 12th edition. New York, McGraw Hill, 1966.

Ball, R. P., and Golden, R: Roentgenographic obstetrical pelvicephalometry in the erect posture. Amer. J. Roentgenol., *49*:731–741, 1943.

Benson, R. C., Dotter, C. T., and Straube, K. R.: Percutaneous transfemoral aortography in gynecology and obstetrics. Amer. J. Obst. Gyn., *8*:772–789, 1963.

Blumberg, M. L., Wohl, G. T., Wiltchik, S., Schwarz, R., and Emich, J. P.: Placental localization by amniography. Amer. J. Roentgenol., *100*:688–697, 1967.

Borrell, U., and Fernstrom, I.: Uterine arteriography. *In* Abrams, H. N.: Angiography, Vol. 2. Second edition. Boston, Little, Brown & Co., 1971.

Bowman, J. M., and Friesen, R. F.: Multiple intraperitoneal transfusions of the fetus for erythroblastosis fetalis. New Eng. J. Med., *271*:703–707, 1964.

Brosens, I., Gordon, H., and Baert, A.: Prediction of fetal maturity with combined cytologic and radiologic method. J. Obst. Gyn. Brit. Comm., *76*:20–26, 1969.

Buice, J. W., and Gould, D. M.: Abdominal and pelvic pneumography. Radiology, *69*:704–710, 1957.

Bunner, F., and Ulrich, J.: Roentgenologic changes in uterine isthmus insufficiency. Amer. J. Roentgenol., *98*:239–243, 1966.

Caldwell, W. E., and Moloy, H. C.: Anatomical variations in the female pelvis and their effect in labor with a suggested classification. Amer. J. Obst. Gyn., *26*:479–503, 1933.

Crafts, R. C.: Textbook of Human Anatomy. New York, Ronald Press Co., 1966.

Doppman, J. L., and Chretien, P.: Visceral pelvic venography in carcinoma of the cervix. Radiology, *98*:406, 1971.

Duggin, E. R., and Taylor, W. W.: Fetal transfusion in utero. Report of case. Obst. Gyn., *24*:12–14, 1964.

Ferris, E. J., Shapiro, J. H., and Spira, J.: Roentgenologic aspects of intrauterine transfusions. J.A.M.A., *196*:635–644, 1966.

Fort, A. T., and Riggs, W. W.: Urographic prenatal sex determination during intrauterine fetal transfusion. J. Urol., *100*:699–700, 1968.

Fullenlove, T. M.: Experience with over 2000 uterosalpingographies. Amer. J. Roentgenol., *106*:463–471, 1969.

Granjon, A.: La gynécographie. Presse Méd., *61*:1765–1766, 1953.

Gray, H.: Gray's Anatomy of the Human Body. 29th edition. Philadelphia, Lea and Febiger, 1973.

Hanafee, W., and Bashore, R.: Carbon dioxide in horizontal fluoroscopy in intrauterine fetal transfusion. Radiology, *85*:481–484, 1965.

Hipona, F. A., and Ditchek, T.: Uterine lymphogram following hysterosalpingography. Amer. J. Roentgenol., *98*:236–238, 1966.

Hodges, P. C.: Roentgen pelvimetery and fetometry. Amer. J. Roentgenol., *37*:644–662, 1937.

Howett, M.: Lymphangiography as an adjunct to gynecologic roentgenology. Sem. in Roentgenol., *4*:289–296, 1969.

Käser, O., and Deuel, H.: Experience with hysterosalpingography (exclusive of determination of tubal potency in sterility). Radiol. Clin., *18*:349–360, 1949 (in German).

Lehfeldt, H.: X-ray appearance of intrauterine contraceptive devices. Fertility and Sterility, *16*:502–507, 1965.

Liggins, G. C.: Fetal transfusion by the impaling technique. Obst. Gyn., *27*:617–621, 1966.

Liley, A. W.: Intrauterine transfusion of foetus in haemolytic disease. Brit. Med. J., *2*:1107–1109, 1963.

Little, H. M., Jr., Hutchinson, J. F., Richey, L. E., and Schreiber, M.: The use of gynecography in pelvic diagnosis. South. Med. J., *54*:715–720, 1951 (15 ref.).

Margolis, A. J., and Voss, R. G.: Method for radiologic detection of fetal maturity. Amer. J. Obst. Gyn., *101*:383–389, 1968.

Meng, C. H., and Elkin, M.: Gynecologic angiography. Sem. in Roentgenol., *4*:267–279, 1969.

Meschan, I.: Analysis of Roentgen Signs. Philadelphia, W. B. Saunders Co., 1973.

Pansky, B., and House, E. L.: Review of Gross Anatomy. New York, The Macmillan Co., 1964.

Queenan, J. J., Anderson, G. G., and Mead, P. B.: Intrauterine transfusion by the multiple needle technique. J.A.M.A., *196*:664–665, 1966.

Rådberg, C., and Wickbom, I.: Pelvic angiography and pneumoperitoneum. Acta Radiol. (Diag.), *6*:133–144, 1967.

Rubin, S., Lambie, R. W., Davidson, K. C., and Herman, E. M.: Barium vaginography. Sem. in Roentgenol., *4*:212–217, 1969.

Russell, J. G. B.: Radiologic assessment of fetal maturity. J. Obst. Gyn. Brit. Comm., *76*:208–219, 1969.

Scammon, R. E., and Calkins, L. A.: The Development and Growth of the Human Body in the Fetal Period. Minneapolis, University of Minnesota Press, 1929.

Schreiber, M. H., Menachof, L., Gunn, W. G., and Beihusen, F. L.: Reliability of visualization of distal femoral epiphyses as a measure of maturity. Amer. J. Obst. Gyn., *83*:1249–1250, 1962.

Schreiber, M. H., Nichols, M. M., and McGanity, W. J.: Epiphyseal ossification center visualization: Its value in prediction of fetal maturity. J.A.M.A., *184*:504–507, 1963.

Schulz, E., and Rosen, S. W.: Gynecography, technique and interpretation. Amer. J. Roentgenol., *86*:866–878, 1961 (20 ref.).

Schwarz, G. S.: A simplified method of correcting roentgenographic measurements of the maternal pelvis and fetal skull. Amer. J. Roentgenol., *71*:115–120, 1954.

Schwarz, G. S.: Editorial. Radiology, *64*:874–876, 1955.

Schwarz, G. S.: Roentgenometric classification of cephalopelvic disproportion. Radiology, *64*:742, 1955.

Semin, R. N., Becker, M. H., Rachad, M. A., Fathy, A. M., and Kandil, O. F.: Combined pneumopelvigraphy and hysterosalpingography in benign gynecological conditions. Radiology, *86*:677–681, 1966.

Shimkin, P. M., Siegel, H. A., and Seaman, W. B.: Radiologic aspects of perforated intrauterine contraceptive devices. Radiology, *92*:353–358, 1969.

Shopfner, C. E.: Gynecologic roentgenology in children. Sem. in Roentgenol., *4*:218–234, 1969.

Shopfner, C. E.: Genitography in intersexual states. Radiology, *82*:664–674, 1964.

Snow, W.: Roentgenology in Obstetrics and Gynecology. Second edition. Springfield, Ill., Charles C Thomas, 1951.

Solish, G. I., Masterson, J. G., and Hellman, L. M.: Pelvic arteriography in obstetrics. Amer. J. Obst. Gyn., *81*:57, 1961.

Stevens, G. M.: Pelvic pneumography. Sem. in Roentgenol., *4*:252–266, 1969.

Templeton, A. W.: High kilovoltage pelvimetry. Amer. J. Roentgenol., *93*:943–947, 1965.

Watson, E. H., and Lowrey, G. A.: Growth and Development of Children. Fifth edition. Chicago, Year Book Medical Publishers, 1967.

Weigen, J. F., and Stevens, G. M.: Pelvic pneumography in the diagnosis of polycystic disease of the ovary, including Stein-Leventhall syndrome. Amer. J. Roentgenol., *100*:680–687, 1967.

AUTHOR INDEX

Note: this index includes first authors and single authors only.

INDEX

SUBJECT INDEX

For the most part, items in this index are listed only under the nouns and not under the descriptive adjective. For example, the term maxillary sinus will be found under *Sinus, maxillary,* rather than under *Maxillary sinus.*

Page numbers printed in **bold face** indicate major discussions; numbers in *italic* indicate illustrations.

For names of structures see under the proper headings, as Arteries, Nerves, Ligaments, Veins.

For names of structures see under the proper headings, as Arteries, Nerves, Ligaments, Veins.

For names of structures see under the proper headings, as Arteries, Nerves, Ligaments, Veins.

For names of structures see under the proper headings, as Arteries, Nerves, Ligaments, Veins.

For names of structures see under the proper headings, as Arteries, Nerves, Ligaments, Veins.

For names of structures see under the proper headings, as Arteries, Nerves, Ligaments, Veins.

For names of structures see under the proper headings, as Arteries, Nerves, Ligaments, Veins.

For names of structures see under the proper headings, as Arteries, Nerves, Ligaments, Veins.

For names of structures see under the proper headings, as Arteries, Nerves, Ligaments, Veins.

For names of structures see under the proper headings, as Arteries, Nerves, Ligaments, Veins.

For names of structures see under the proper headings, as Arteries, Nerves, Ligaments, Veins.

INDEX

For names of structures see under the proper headings, as Arteries, Nerves, Ligaments, Veins.

For names of structures see under the proper headings, as Arteries, Nerves, Ligaments, Veins.

For names of structures see under the proper headings, as Arteries, Nerves, Ligaments, Veins.

For names of structures see under the proper headings, as Arteries, Nerves, Ligaments, Veins.

For names of structures see under the proper headings, as Arteries, Nerves, Ligaments, Veins.

For names of structures see under the proper headings, as Arteries, Nerves, Ligaments, Veins.

For names of structures see under the proper headings, as Arteries, Nerves, Ligaments, Veins.

For names of structures see under the proper headings, as Arteries, Nerves, Ligaments, Veins.

For names of structures see under the proper headings, as Arteries, Nerves, Ligaments, Veins.

INDEX

For names of structures see under the proper headings, as Arteries, Nerves, Ligaments, Veins.

For names of structures see under the proper headings, as Arteries, Nerves, Ligaments, Veins.

For names of structures see under the proper headings, as Arteries, Nerves, Ligaments, Veins.

For names of structures see under the proper headings, as Arteries, Nerves, Ligaments, Veins.

For names of structures see under the proper headings, as Arteries, Nerves, Ligaments, Veins.

For names of structures see under the proper headings, as Arteries, Nerves, Ligaments, Veins.

For names of structures see under the proper headings, as Arteries, Nerves, Ligaments, Veins.

APPENDIX A

COMPUTED TOMOGRAPHY
OF THE
BRAIN AND ORBIT

APPENDIX B

COMPUTED
WHOLE BODY
TOMOGRAPHY

Computed Tomography of the Brain and Orbit

In 1972, Godfrey Hounsfield, electronic engineer and physicist, and Dr. James Ambrose, neuroradiologist (both of England), reported the first computed transverse axial x-ray scanning technique of the head. In essence, the machine they developed consisted of an x-ray device that produces a slitlike beam or thin sheet of x-rays, which passes through the head. The x-ray tube produces this beam at 1-degree intervals, eventually moving through 180 degrees. By careful collimation, this "sheet of x-rays" can delimit a slice of tissue from 0.4 to 1.3 cm. in width. At each degree pause, the "remnant radiation" emitted is detected by phosphorescent crystals, and the number of photons so recorded is transmitted to a computer. The volume of tissue traversed in the 180-degree arc is theoretically divided into thousands of small units (*volume elements*, or *"voxels"*). The absorption of x-ray photons in each of these voxels is related to the average tissue structure, or its average absorption coefficient. Tissues are now classified in relation to this absorption in so-called Hounsfield units, in an effort to relate the absorption coefficients of the voxels to water. The ultimate reconstruction of the image is made from the total photons absorbed by each voxel in the computer to a gray scale read-out device (*direct display console, or DDC*), by an appropriate algorithm and use of the computer language. Tissues with only minimally differing absorption coefficients may thereby be differentiated.

The diagrammatic representation of the scanning sequence is illustrated in Figure A–2, and a photograph of a patient in position for scanning is shown in Figure A–1. In early models, the patient's head was placed snugly in a water bag (Fig. A–3), contained within the so-called gantry in the photograph.

Water absorption is used as the basis for comparison with all other absorption values.

The scanning process may be started from any angle, moving 1 degree at a time, but it is usually begun with the x-ray tube in its lowermost position, with the patient "brow-up." The water in the bag must be pure and free from bubbles or air to avoid artefacts; and the patient must be motionless, with anesthesia required where the patient cannot cooperate to this extent.

With more recent water bag models, two slices are recorded simultaneously (omitting the slice between them). The slice omitted at each degree is thereafter included alternately, thereby speeding up the scan time.

The tomographic photographs reproduced here were obtained with a scan time of approximately 4½ minutes, for each two slices; that is, 10 slices are obtained in approximately 22½ minutes. If 'contrast enhancement" is required to demonstrate blood vessels and selective absorption across the "blood-brain barrier," 150 to 300 ml. of 25 per cent meglumine diatrizoate is injected by drip or rapidly, and the entire scanning sequence is repeated.

There should be full cognizance that some patients may have undesirable reactions to the contrast agent and may require immediate treatment, as described in the section on the urinary tract, since the agents used are identical.

A "window width" on the control panel adjusts the degree of contrast in the image. The "window level" control sets the center of the window width to any desired point on the scale of x-ray absorption coefficients.

In the usual settings, cerebrospinal fluid appears black; bone appears white; and the brain appears various shades of gray. With appropriate use of the controls, it is possible to measure the absorption coefficient of any given portion of the image to assist in interpretation.

For greater detail, the student is referred to the text on this subject by New and Scott[*] and to information provided by the manufacturer of the unit being utilized.

Currently, numerous improvements are being incorporated, such as replacement of the water bag, increase in the number of detector crystals, increase in computer capability, and improvement of the photographic image of the DDC.

The brief "atlas of anatomy" included in this Appendix is for introductory purposes only. A list of references on CT scanning is included at the end of Appendix B.

---

[*]New, P. F. J., and Scott, W. R.: Computerized Tomography of the Brain and Orbit (EMI Scanning). Baltimore, Williams & Wilkins Co., 1975.

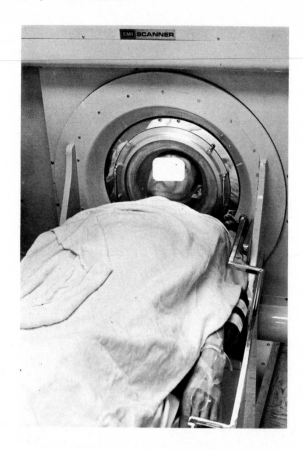

FIGURE A-1 Patient in position in the Emitronics Head Computed Tomographic (C/T) Unit. The water bag shown around the patient's head is being replaced in forthcoming models so that there will be greater accuracy in positioning of the patient and greater ease in study of the orbit and posterior fossa, as well as coronal scanning capabilities.

FIGURE A-2 Diagrammatic representation of scanning sequence, which comprises a series of 180 parallel traverses of the accurately aligned x-ray beam and two photon detectors, with 1 degree rotation of the gantry after each linear sweep. Each block of tissue in each of the two simultaneously scanned sections (slices) will have been scanned 180 times at the completion of a scan sequence, and the photon transmission measurements obtained are averaged for each small tissue block. The readings are digitized and fed to the computer, which solves 28,800 simultaneous equations for each slice to derive absorption (attenuation) values in each block. (From New, P. F. J., and Scott, W. R.: Computerized Tomography of the Brain and Orbit (EMI Scanning). Baltimore, Md., The Williams & Wilkins Co., 1975.)

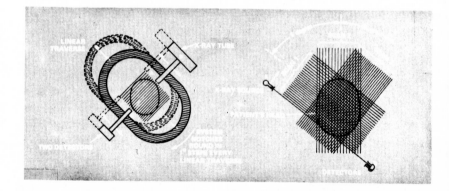

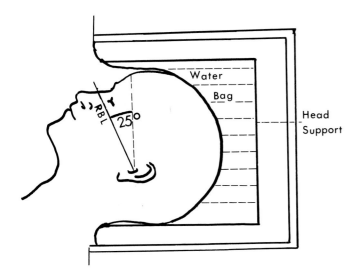

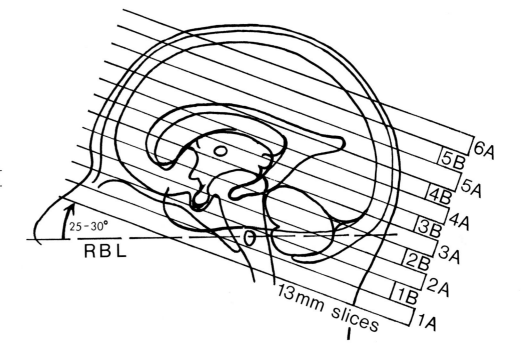

FIGURE A-3 Diagram illustrating patient in usual position in the water bag contained within the head gantry (replaced in newer models). Reid's base line (RBL) is 90 degrees to the horizontal when examination of the orbit or posterior fossa is required.

FIGURE A-4 Orientation for usual tomographic slices obtained and those illustrated in this chapter (25–30 degrees to RBL).

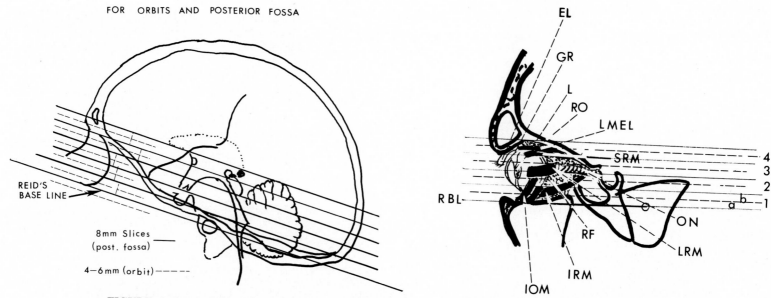

FIGURE A–5 *A.* Orientation for orbital and posterior fossa tomographic slices. Occasionally posterior fossa slices are taken at narrower intervals as well, but since a lesser number of photons is collected in each of the "voxels," the images so obtained are coarser. The window width and level usually require different settings for the orbit, as compared with posterior fossa brain settings (see manufacturer's manual for details).

B. Close-up diagram of the orbit and its contents, showing the anatomic structures in their usual relationship to the "tomographic cuts" obtained. (EL) eyelid, (GR) global rim, (L) lens of eye, (RO) roof of orbit, (LMEL) levator muscle of upper eyelid, (SRM) superior rectus muscle, (ON) optic nerve, (LRM) lateral rectus muscle, (RF) retrobulbar fat, (IRM) inferior rectus muscle, (IOM) inferior oblique muscle, (RBL) infraorbital meatal line (Reid's base line).

1, 2, 3, 4 represent the cuts shown; and "a" and "b" are subdivisions within these cuts. A total of eight cuts, approximately 5 mm. apart, is obtained usually.

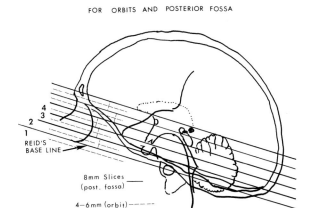

FOR ORBITS AND POSTERIOR FOSSA

REID'S
BASE LINE

8mm Slices
(post. fossa)

4—6mm (orbit)

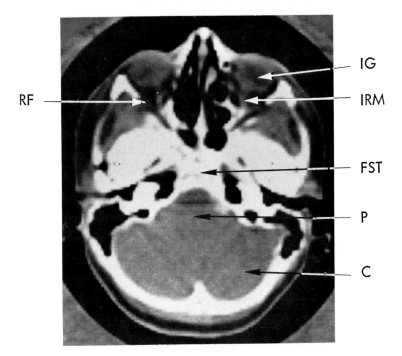

RF — FST

IG

IRM

P

C

RF   =   RETRO-ORBITAL FAT
IG   =   INF. GLOBE
IRM =   INF. RECTUS MUSCLE
FST =   FLOOR, SELLA TURCICA
P   =   PONS
C   =   CEREBELLUM

FIGURE A–7   Orbital section 21B (EMI settings: 5/200).

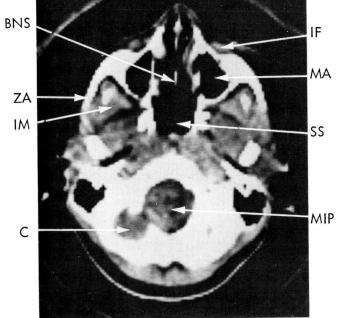

BNS

ZA

IM

C

IF

MA

SS

MIP

FIGURE A–6 Orbital section 21A (EMI settings: 18/75).

BNS =   BONE NASAL SEPTUM
ZA   =   ZYGOMATIC ARCH
IM   =   INFRATEMPORAL MUSCLES
C   =   CEREBELLUM
IF   =   INFRAORBITAL FAT
MA   =   MAXILLARY ANTRUM
SS   =   SPHENOID SINUS
MIP =   MEDULLA AND/OR INFERIOR PONS

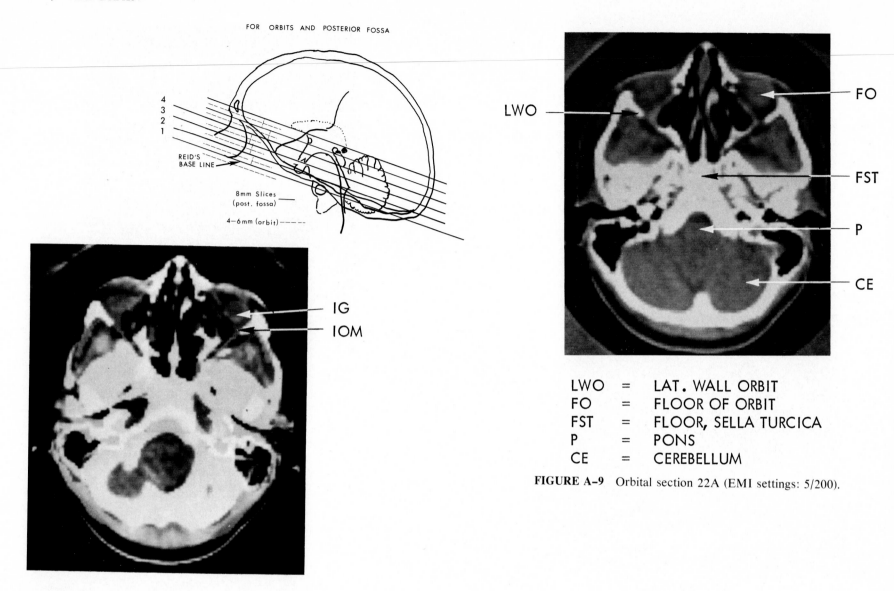

FOR ORBITS AND POSTERIOR FOSSA

REID'S BASE LINE

8mm Slices (post. fossa)

4–6mm (orbit)

IG
IOM

LWO

FO

FST

P

CE

LWO = LAT. WALL ORBIT
FO = FLOOR OF ORBIT
FST = FLOOR, SELLA TURCICA
P   = PONS
CE = CEREBELLUM

FIGURE A–9 Orbital section 22A (EMI settings: 5/200).

IG = INF. GLOBE
IOM = INF. OBLIQUE MUSCLE

FIGURE A–8 Repeat orbital section 21B on another patient for special visualization of inferior oblique muscle (EMI settings: 5/200). (Second cut.)

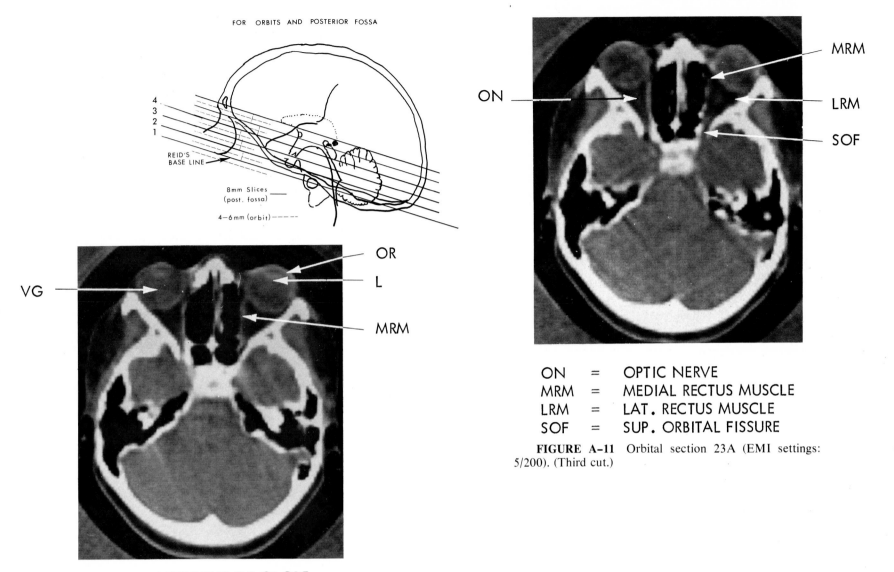

FOR ORBITS AND POSTERIOR FOSSA

REID'S BASE LINE

8mm Slices (post. fossa)

4–6mm (orbit)

FIGURE A–11 Orbital section 23A (EMI settings: 5/200). (Third cut.)

ON = OPTIC NERVE
MRM = MEDIAL RECTUS MUSCLE
LRM = LAT. RECTUS MUSCLE
SOF = SUP. ORBITAL FISSURE

VG = VITREOUS OF GLOBE
OR = OCULAR RIM
L = LENS
MRM = MEDIAL RECTUS MUSCLE

FIGURE A–10 Orbital section 22B (EMI settings: 5/200).

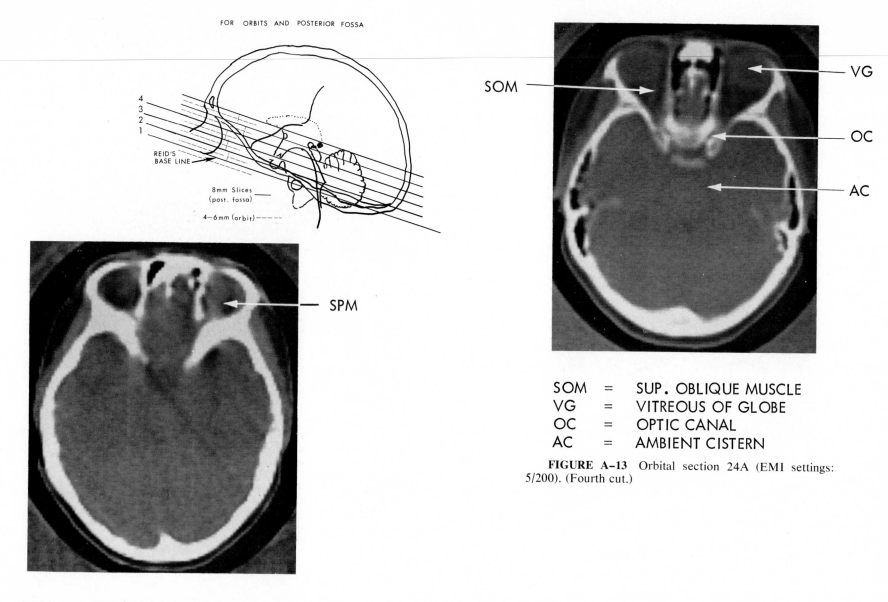

FOR ORBITS AND POSTERIOR FOSSA

4
3
2
1

REID'S
BASE LINE

8mm Slices
(post. fossa)

4–6mm (orbit)

SOM

VG

OC

AC

SPM

SOM = SUP. OBLIQUE MUSCLE
VG = VITREOUS OF GLOBE
OC = OPTIC CANAL
AC = AMBIENT CISTERN

FIGURE A–13 Orbital section 24A (EMI settings: 5/200). (Fourth cut.)

SPM = SUPERIOR PALPEBRAL MUSCLE

FIGURE A–12 Orbital section 23B (EMI settings: 5/200).

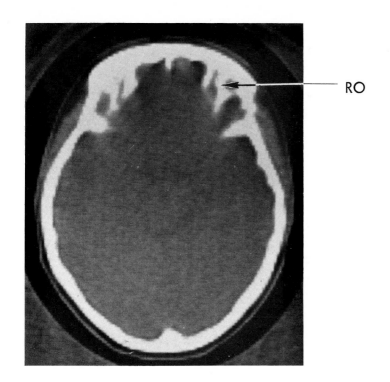

RO = ROOF OF ORBIT

FIGURE A–14 Orbital section 24B (EMI settings: 5/200).

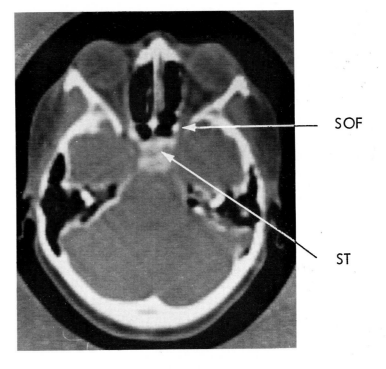

SOF = SUP. ORBITAL FISSURE
ST = SELLA TURCICA

FIGURE A–15 Orbital section 23A for superior orbital fissure (EMI settings: 0/400).

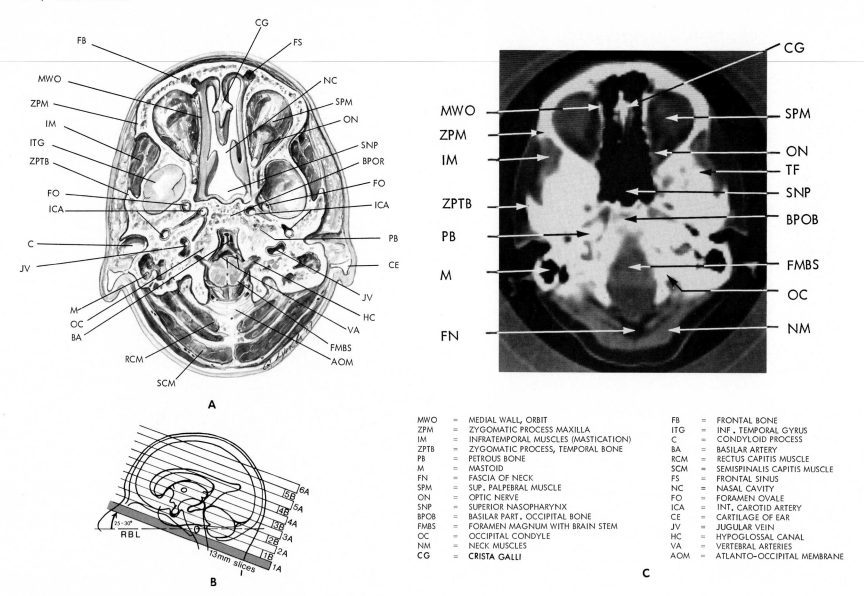

FIGURE A–16 *A*. Anatomic sketch equivalent to section 1A of brain scan. *B*. Miniature of Figure 7–67 for orientation. *C*. Labeled scan at this level.

MWO	=	MEDIAL WALL, ORBIT
ZPM	=	ZYGOMATIC PROCESS MAXILLA
IM	=	INFRATEMPORAL MUSCLES (MASTICATION)
ZPTB	=	ZYGOMATIC PROCESS, TEMPORAL BONE
PB	=	PETROUS BONE
M	=	MASTOID
FN	=	FASCIA OF NECK
SPM	=	SUP. PALPEBRAL MUSCLE
ON	=	OPTIC NERVE
SNP	=	SUPERIOR NASOPHARYNX
BPOB	=	BASILAR PART. OCCIPITAL BONE
FMBS	=	FORAMEN MAGNUM WITH BRAIN STEM
OC	=	OCCIPITAL CONDYLE
NM	=	NECK MUSCLES
CG	=	**CRISTA GALLI**

FB	=	FRONTAL BONE
ITG	=	INF . TEMPORAL GYRUS
C	=	CONDYLOID PROCESS
BA	=	BASILAR ARTERY
RCM	=	RECTUS CAPITIS MUSCLE
SCM	=	SEMISPINALIS CAPITIS MUSCLE
FS	=	FRONTAL SINUS
NC	=	NASAL CAVITY
FO	=	FORAMEN OVALE
ICA	=	INT. CAROTID ARTERY
CE	=	CARTILAGE OF EAR
JV	=	JUGULAR VEIN
HC	=	HYPOGLOSSAL CANAL
VA	=	VERTEBRAL ARTERIES
AOM	=	ATLANTO-OCCIPITAL MEMBRANE

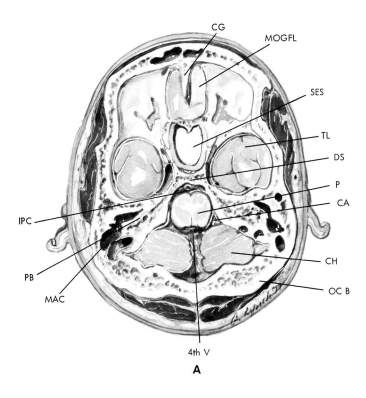

A

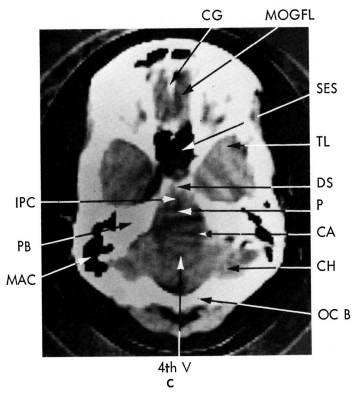

CG   MOGFL

SES

TL

DS

P

CA

CH

OC B

IPC

PB

MAC

4th V

C

IPC	=	INTERPEDUNCULAR CISTERN
PB	=	PETROUS BONE
MAC	=	MASTOID AIR CELLS
CG	=	CRISTA GALLI
MOGFL	=	MED. ORBITAL GYRUS-FRONTAL LOBE
SES	=	SPHENOID AND ETHMOID SINUSES
TL	=	TEMPORAL LOBE
DS	=	DORSUM SELLAE
P	=	PONS
CA	=	CISTERNA AMBIENS
CH	=	CEREBELLAR HEMISPHERE
OC B	=	OCCIPITAL BONE
4th V	=	4th VENTRICLE

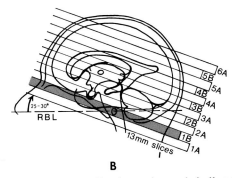

B

FIGURE A–17 *A*, Diagram of brain section and skull at 1B level. *B*, Miniature of Figure A–4 for orientation. *C*, Labeled computed tomograph at this level.

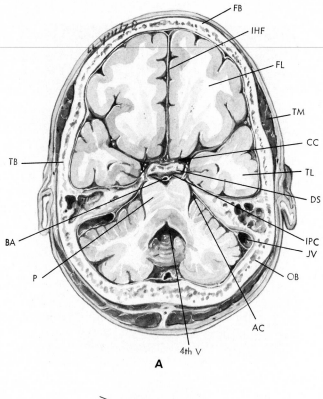

A

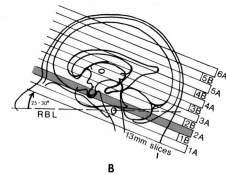

B

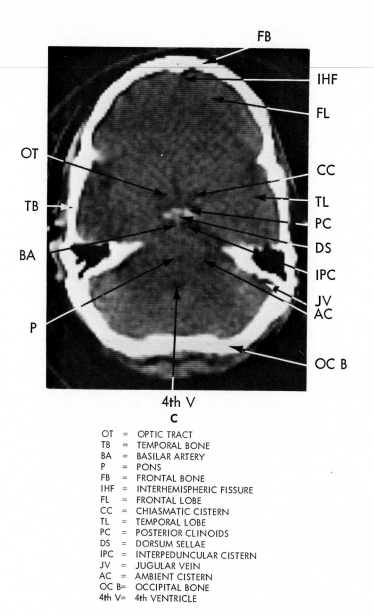

C

OT = OPTIC TRACT
TB = TEMPORAL BONE
BA = BASILAR ARTERY
P = PONS
FB = FRONTAL BONE
IHF = INTERHEMISPHERIC FISSURE
FL = FRONTAL LOBE
CC = CHIASMATIC CISTERN
TL = TEMPORAL LOBE
PC = POSTERIOR CLINOIDS
DS = DORSUM SELLAE
IPC = INTERPEDUNCULAR CISTERN
JV = JUGULAR VEIN
AC = AMBIENT CISTERN
OC B = OCCIPITAL BONE
4th V = 4th VENTRICLE

FIGURE A–18 *A.* Diagram of the brain at the 2A level. *B.* Miniature of Figure A–4 for orientation. *C.* Tomographic scan at the 2A level.

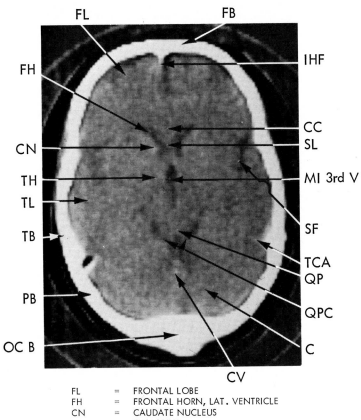

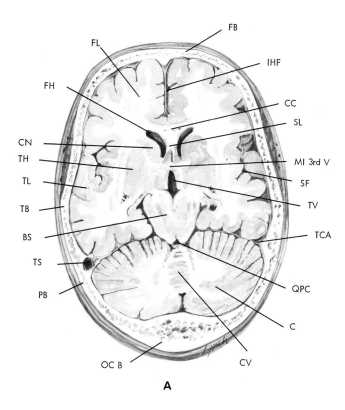

A

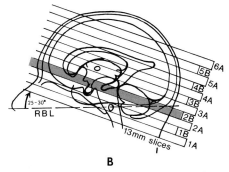

B

FIGURE A-19 *A*. Diagram of section through brain at 2B level. *B*. Miniature of Figure A-4 for orientation. *C*. Tomographic scan at the 2B level.

FL	=	FRONTAL LOBE
FH	=	FRONTAL HORN, LAT. VENTRICLE
CN	=	CAUDATE NUCLEUS
TH	=	THALAMUS
TL	=	TEMPORAL LOBE
TB	=	TEMPORAL BONE
BS	=	BRAIN STEM
TS	=	TRANSVERSE SINUS
PB	=	PARIETAL BONE
OC B	=	OCCIPITAL BONE
FB	=	FRONTAL BONE
IHF	=	INTERHEMISPHERIC FISSURE
CC	=	CORPUS CALLOSUM
SL	=	SEPTUM LUCIDI
MI 3rd V	=	MASSA INTERMEDIA IN 3rd VENTRICLE
SF	=	SYLVIAN FISSURE
TV	=	THIRD VENTRICLE
TCA	=	TENTORIUM CEREBELLI ATTACHMENT
QP	=	QUADRIGEMINAL PLATE
QPC	=	QUADRIGEMINAL PLATE CISTERN
C	=	CEREBELLUM
CV	=	CEREBELLAR VERMIS

C

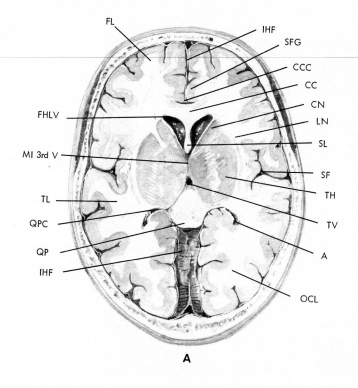

A

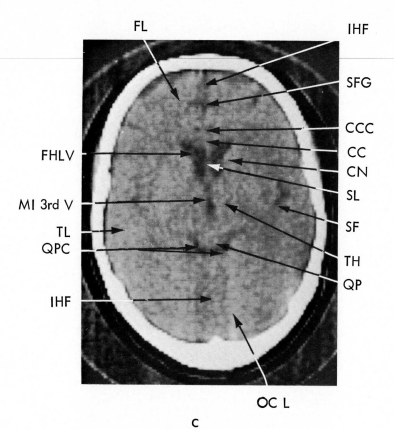

C

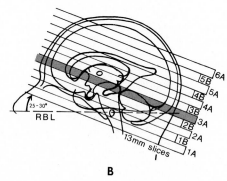

B

FIGURE A–20 *A*. Diagram of brain at the 3A level.
B. Miniature of Figure A–4 for orientation. *C*. Tomographic
cut at the 3A level.

FL	=	FRONTAL LOBE
FHLV	=	FRONTAL HORN, LAT. VENTRICLE
MI 3rd V	=	MASSA INTERMEDIA IN 3rd VENTRICLE
TL	=	TEMPORAL LOBE
QPC	=	QUADRIGEMINAL PLATE CISTERN
IHF	=	INTERHEMISPHERIC FISSURE
IHF	=	INTERHEMISPHERIC FISSURE
SFG	=	SUPERIOR FRONTAL GYRUS
CCC	=	CISTERNA CORPUS CALLOSI
CC	=	CORPUS CALLOSUM
CN	=	CAUDATE NUCLEUS
SL	=	SEPTUM LUCIDI
SF	=	SYLVIAN FISSURE
TH	=	THALAMUS
QP	=	QUADRIGEMINAL PLATE
OC L	=	OCCIPITAL LOBE
LN	=	LENTICULAR NUCLEUS
TV	=	THIRD VENTRICLE
A	=	ATRIUM

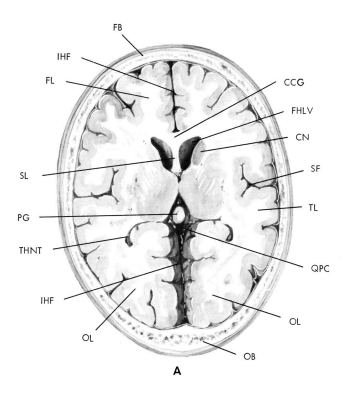

A

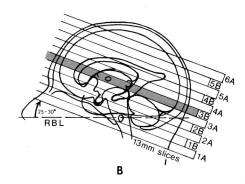

B

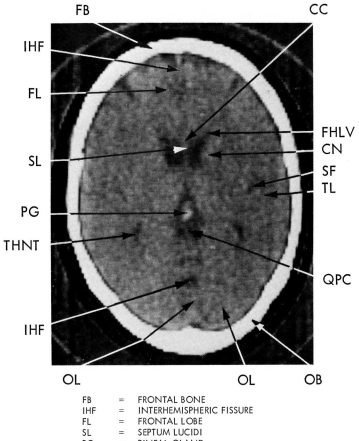

FB	=	FRONTAL BONE
IHF	=	INTERHEMISPHERIC FISSURE
FL	=	FRONTAL LOBE
SL	=	SEPTUM LUCIDI
PG	=	PINEAL GLAND
THNT	=	TEMPORAL HORN NEAR TRIGONE
IHF	=	INTERHEMISPHERIC FISSURE
OL	=	OCCIPITAL LOBE
CC	=	CORPUS CALLOSUM
FHLV	=	FRONTAL HORN, LAT. VENTRICLE
CN	=	CAUDATE NUCLEUS
SF	=	SYLVIAN FISSURE
TL	=	TEMPORAL LOBE (SUPERIORLY)
QPC	=	QUADRIGEMINAL PLATE CISTERN
OB	=	OCCIPITAL BONE

C

FIGURE A–21 *A*. Diagram of brain at the 3B level. *B*. Miniature of Figure A–4 for orientation. *C*. Tomographic cut at the 3B level.

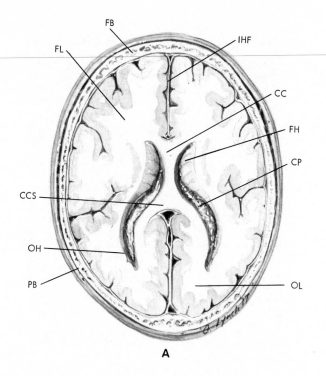

A

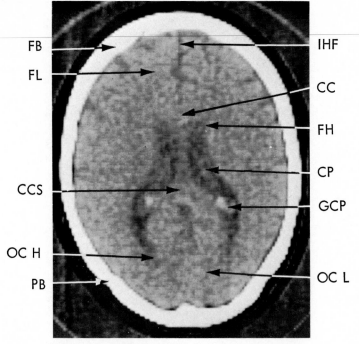

FB = FRONTAL BONE
FL = FRONTAL LOBE
CCS = CORPUS CALLOSUM SPLENIUM
OC H = OCCIPITAL HORN, LAT. VENT.
PB = PARIETAL BONE
IHF = INTERHEMISPHERIC FISSURE
CC = CORPUS CALLOSUM
FH = FRONTAL HORN, LAT. VENT.
CP = CHOROID PLEXUS, LAT. VENT.
GCP = GLOMUS (WITH CALCIUM),
CHOROID PLEXUS IN TRIGONE, LAT. VENT.
OC L = OCCIPITAL LOBE

C

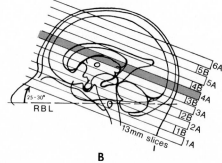

B

FIGURE A–22 *A*. Diagram of brain through at 4A level. *B*. Miniature of Figure A–4 for orientation. *C*. Tomographic slice at 4A level.

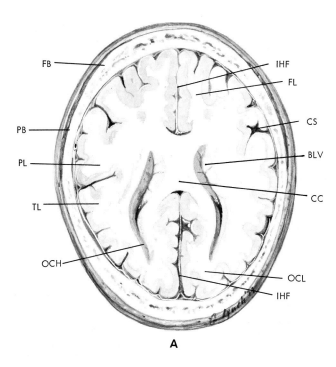

A

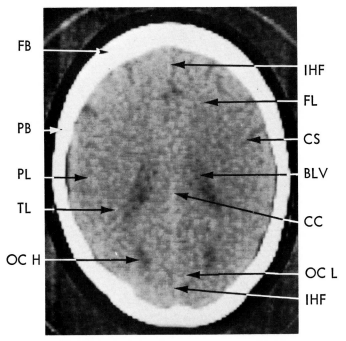

FB	=	FRONTAL BONE
PB	=	PARIETAL BONE
PL	=	PARIETAL LOBE
TL	=	TEMPORAL LOBE
OC H	=	OCCIPITAL HORN, LAT. VENT.
IHF	=	INTERHEMISPHERIC FISSURE
FL	=	FRONTAL LOBE
CS	=	CENTRAL SULCUS
BLV	=	BODY, LAT. VENTRICLE
CC	=	CORPUS CALLOSUM
OC L	=	OCCIPITAL LOBE
IHF	=	INTERHEMISPHERIC FISSURE

C

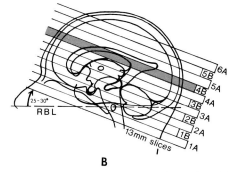

B

FIGURE A–23 *A*. Diagram of brain at the 4B level. *B*. Miniature of Figure A–4 for orientation. *C*. Tomographic slice at level 4B.

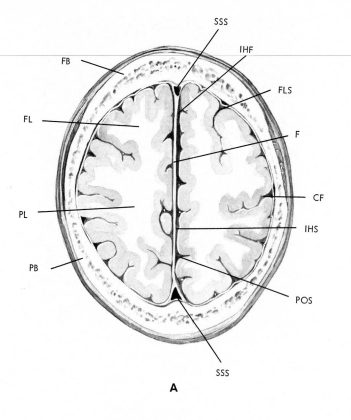

A

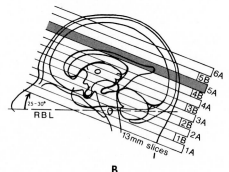

B

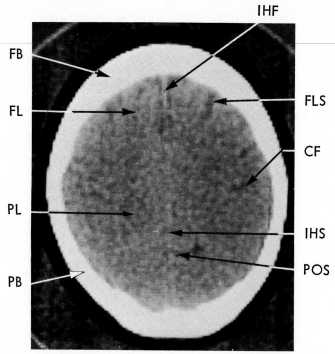

FB	=	FRONTAL BONE
FL	=	FRONTAL LOBE
PL	=	PARIETAL LOBE
PB	=	PARIETAL BONE
IHF	=	INTERHEMISPHERIC FISSURE
FLS	=	FRONTAL LOBE SULCUS
CF	=	CENTRAL FISSURE
IHS	=	INTERHEMISPHERIC SULCUS
POS	=	PARIETO-OCCIPITAL SULCUS
SSS	=	SUPERIOR SAGITTAL SINUS
F	=	FALX
SSS	=	SUPERIOR SAGITTAL SINUS

C

FIGURE A–24 *A*. Diagram of brain at the 5A level. *B*. Miniature of Figure A–4 for orientation. *C*. Tomographic slice at the 5A level.

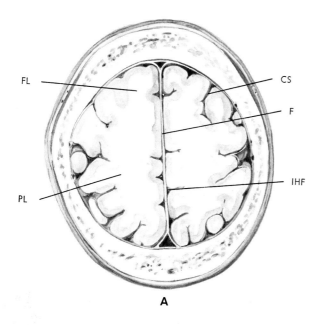

A

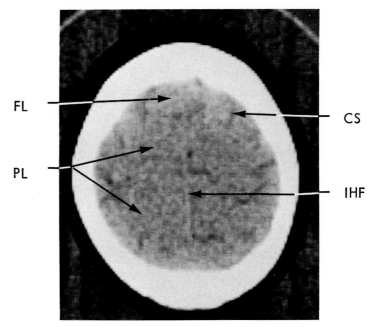

FL = FRONTAL LOBE
PL = PARIETAL LOBE
CS = CENTRAL SULCUS
IHF = INTERHEMISPHERIC (LONGITUDINAL) FISSURE
F = FALX

C

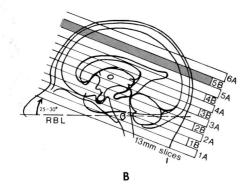

B

FIGURE A–25 *A*. Diagram of brain at the 5B level. *B*. Miniature of Figure A–4 for orientation. *C*. Tomographic slice at the 5B level.

ACA   MCA

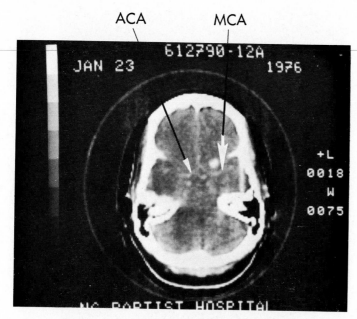

ACA - ANT. CEREBRAL ART.
MCA - MIDDLE CEREBRAL ART.

FIGURE A-26 Computed tomograph at the 2A level immediately following the infusion of 300 ml. of 25 per cent Reno-M-30-DIP (diatrizoate meglumine) for contrast enhancement of the blood vessels and other structures in the brain. Note the demonstration of the internal carotid artery in cross section as it divides into the anterior cerebral and middle cerebral arteries. The middle cerebral artery in its first portions is clearly shown.

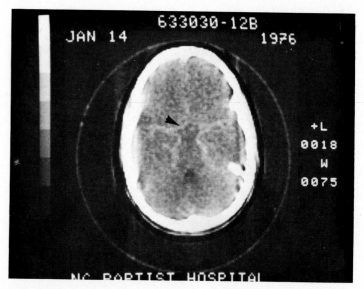

→ CIRCLE OF WILLIS WITH CONTRAST AGENT

FIGURE A-27 Computed tomograph at the 2B level with contrast infusion (enhancement) demonstrating the circle of Willis.

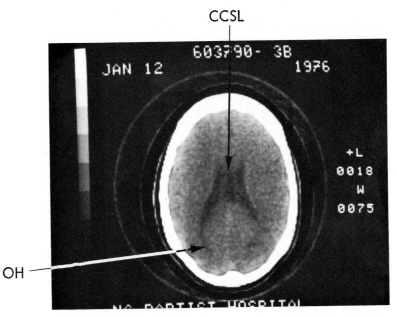

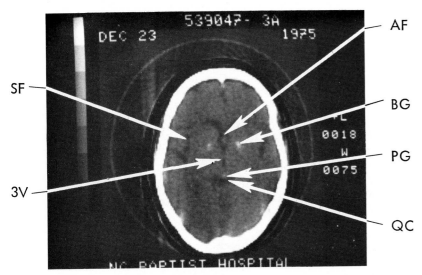

SF – SYLVIAN FISSURE
3V – THIRD VENTRICLE
AF – ANTERIOR FORNIX
BG – CALCIFIED BASAL GANGLIA
PG – PINEAL GLAND
QC – QUADRIGEMINAL CISTERN

FIGURE A–28 Computed tomograph at the 3A level, showing more clearly some of the structures that have been previously depicted. There is calcium deposit in the basal ganglia, structures much more frequently calcified by computed tomography than on conventional radiography.

CCSL – CISTERNA CAVUM SEPTUM LUCIDI
OH – OCCIPITAL HORN, LAT. VENTRICLE

FIGURE A–29 Computed tomograph at the 3B level, 25 to 30 degrees to Reid's base line, showing clearly the cisterna cavum septi pellucidi as well as the occipital horns of the lateral ventricle.

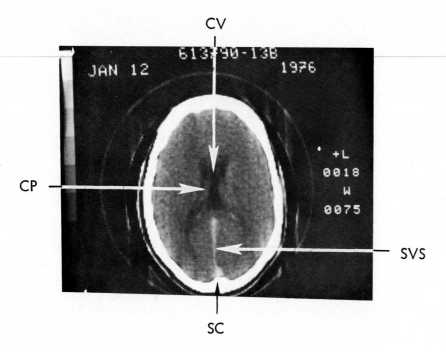

CV — CAVUM VERGI
CP — CHOROID PLEXUS, LAT. VENTRICLE
SC — SINUS CONFLUENS
SVS — STRAIGHT VENOUS SINUS

FIGURE A–30 Computed tomograph at the 3B level following contrast enhancement with infusion of contrast agent and showing such structures as the cavum vergi, the choroid plexuses of the lateral ventricles, the straight venous sinus, and the sinus confluens.

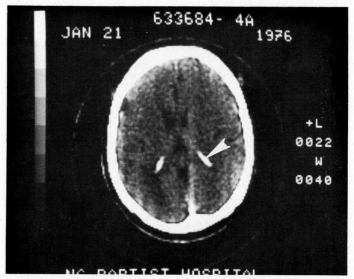

→ BILAT. CALCIFIED GLOMERA OF CHOROID PLEXUSES

FIGURE A–31 Computed tomograph at the 4A level, 25 to 30 degrees to Reid's base line. This shows bilateral calcified glomera of the choroid plexuses (arrow).

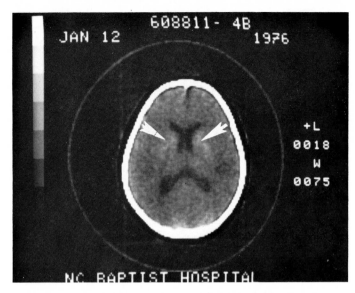

→ FAINTLY CALCIFIED BASAL GANGLIA

FIGURE A–32 Computed tomograph at the 4B level showing faintly calcified basal ganglia. The anterior and posterior limbs of the internal capsules separate the head of the caudate nucleus, partially calcified, from the putamen, also partially calcified. Even the thalamus can be separated.

Appendix B

Computed Whole Body Tomography

Isadore Meschan, M.A., M.D.

W. Martin Dinn, M.D.
Assistant Professor, Department of Radiology, State University of New York,
Upstate Medical Center, Syracuse, New York

with anatomical sketches by
George C. Lynch
Professor of Medical Illustration, Bowman Gray School of Wake Forest University,
Winston-Salem, North Carolina

INTRODUCTION

Computed head tomography was introduced in 1972 by Ambrose and Hounsfield (see discussion in Appendix A on computed tomography of brain and skull). In February 1974, the first ACTA total body scanner went into operation at Georgetown University Medical Center. Since then, a moderate number of whole body scanners made by different manufacturers have been installed in several institutions throughout the world.

Computed Tomographic Equipment

As shown in Appendix A, the basic computed tomographic (CT) equipment consists of the following: (1) a patient table; (2) an x-ray scanning unit that moves at 1- to 10-degree intervals through a 180- to 360-degree arc; (3) an x-ray control unit that energizes the x-ray tube (or x-ray tubes), resulting in the emission of highly collimated beams of x-rays; (4) receptor devices that receive the "remnant radiation" on the far side of the patient after it has passed through the patient; (5) a computer that summates the photons of energy transmitted through the patient in each pass; (6) a computer that reconstructs the summated photons of radiation into an image that can be viewed on a cathode ray tube; and (7) a photographic unit that records the image from the face of the cathode ray tube. To assist in these basic functions there are motor generators, high-voltage generators, cooling oil pumps, and a teletype apparatus to "instruct" the computer devices regarding scanning operations and image data manipulations. The scanning device, consisting of an x-ray tube (or x-ray tubes) on one side and scintillation or gas-filled detectors on the other, is spoken of as a "gantry."

With the early models that were designed to examine the head, the patient's head was introduced into a flexible water bag within an opening in the gantry. The water bag served to limit the dynamic range of radiation to which the detectors would be exposed. (It is electronically more difficult to maintain the calibration of the detectors over the very wide range required if the detectors are exposed to the raw x-ray beam as it scans beyond the edge of the patient's head.) The water bag also served as a reference medium for relative x-ray attenuation with respect to water.

In the newer CT systems the water bag has been abandoned; a hole through the gantry in a "doughnut" configuration permits any part of the patient's body to be introduced for CT examination. Although some units still surround the body part examined with unit density material, devices using such an approach are less than satisfactory, since they result in the loss of information-bearing photons before they reach the detectors and also result in unnecessary irradiation of the patient.

The scintillation or gas-filled detectors opposite the x-ray tube not only are more sensitive than x-ray film in discriminating fine differences in x-ray attenuation, but the collimators of these detectors also reduce the amount of scattered radiation, thus preventing further degradation of the image.

The Head Computed Tomographic Scanner (see also Appendix A)

The first scanner was developed by Emitronics Limited of England, which published a report of its products in 1972 at the Annual Congress of the British Institute of Radiology; this scanner, however, was specifically designed for brain scanning. By mid-1973 the first *head* CT scanner was being made in the United States. The first unit with whole body scanning capability—the ACTA scanner—now being manufactured by the Pfizer Medical Systems, was introduced early in 1974. Other companies soon announced production of similar devices. At this writing (May, 1977), over 15 companies world-wide have entered the computed tomography market.

Design of Scanning Apparatus. In the four years since the first commercial units were available, the time required to obtain a CT image has been reduced by many orders of magnitude. In 1977, scan times are quoted in terms of seconds, rather than minutes. The diminishing scan time is the consequence of two basic design improvements, which in turn result in more efficient data collection and less mechanical motion of the x-ray source and detectors. These two developments are the following:

1. The geometry of the x-ray beam has changed from the original

narrow beam of x-rays to a thin, fanlike beam. The fastest scanners available today employ a wide-angle fan beam and several hundred detectors in a rotational design.

2. The mechanical motion of the x-ray source and detectors has been diminished. The early CT scanners moved in 1-degree increments following the completion of each lateral translational scan until an arc of 180 degrees was completed. The most recently developed two-motion (translate-rotate) CT scanners are able to complete a scan in 2 to 20 seconds by utilizing the fan beam geometry and multiple detectors. Two-second CT scanners that are single motion (rotation) scanners are now available. This single motion scanning is accomplished by a bank of detectors as well as by a fan beam geometry, and the source and detectors rotate simultaneously around the patient. A no-motion CT scanner will probably be available in the not-too-distant future; in such a scanner, stationary fan beams will impinge on stationary arcs of hundreds of detectors. Such a design would permit one to "suspend" cardiac motion by the extremely rapid scan time. Electrocardiographic "gating" would also allow one to obtain an image of the heart in any selected phase of the cardiac cycle. For example, the heart could be scanned only during the peak of diastole, and by means of intravenous contrast enhancement, the chambers would be clearly visualized.

Computer Hardware and Software. Apart from the design changes in the scanning apparatus, there has been significant improvement in the computer hardware and software. Changes in the algorithms have resulted in the attainment of image reconstruction within seconds after scanning. Usually, with the two-motion body scanners now available, the minimum scanning time averages 16 seconds, whereas a complete image requires from 30 to 80 seconds. Minimum scanning time on a one-motion scanner ranges from 2 to 8 seconds; the total time needed to obtain an image averages about 1.4 minutes. The combination of all of these devices has made feasible extremely rapid scanning and rapid reconstruction.

The detail in the reconstructed image depends, in part, on the number and size of the squares used by the computer to reconstruct the image. Each square represents a finite area in the cross section of the patient's head or body, and the computer assigns a specific average density to each square, thereby reflecting the number of x-ray photons computed to have been absorbed by that volume of tissue. The entire cross section could be divided into only four boxes, with each box having one homogeneous density representing the average absorption of all the tissue in that area, but such an approach would offer no useful reconstruction of the actual structures within each box. It is thus apparent that the smaller and more numerous the computed boxes are, the more representative the reconstruction will be. Since each of these boxes represents not only an area of tissue but also a finite thickness of tissue, the term *voxel* (volume element) has been applied. When the voxel is displayed on a cathode ray tube, it is referred to as a *pixel* (picture element). The dimensions (given in voxels or pixels) of the reconstructed image represent the matrix size. The early CT scanners used a matrix of 80 × 80 voxels, resulting in an image composed of visible and, therefore, objectionable boxes. Currently, most CT systems use a matrix of 256 × 256 voxels or 320 × 320 voxels. This yields an image in which the voxels are not readily apparent.

There is a limit to how fine a matrix one can use in image reconstruction. As the voxel gets smaller and smaller, one starts to detect the random statistical fluctuation of x-ray photons passing through each tiny volume of tissue, rather than the linear attenuation coefficient of this tiny tissue volume. To avoid this problem of the very fine matrix (512 × 512 or finer), one must increase the number of photons passing through the patient—that is, one must increase the radiation dosage.

The tissue volume represented by each picture element in the display matrix has been significantly reduced in the new matrices; at present, element size ranges from 1 × 1 mm. to 2 × 2 mm. in cross section. Moreover, the scan slices, when such are employed, can now become collimated from 13 mm. to 3 mm. in width so that the tissue volume represented by each picture element ranges anywhere from 3 to 68 cu. mm. These changes have increased both image resolution and detection of smaller tumors or other abnormalities in the areas scanned.

Speed is particularly important, since respiratory and peristaltic motion seriously degrade the computed tomographic image. Moreover, while rotational fan-beam scanners can collect more readings in a shorter period of time, their detectors must be very carefully calibrated with respect to each other in order to obtain good images. Any mismatches will result in undesirable artifacts.

Radiation Exposure of Patient. Another important consideration is radiation exposure to the patient. With most of the current CT scanners, the radiation skin dose received by the patient during an abdominal examination is less than during the average barium enema. Nevertheless, one must strive to minimize the dose as much as possible, in particular, by confining the examination to the anatomic region of interest or suspicion. With one representative CT system, the Ohio Nuclear Delta-50 scanner, the skin dose on the side of x-ray entry is approximately 1.25 rads, and on the exit side the dose is 0.25 rads per CT "slice."

In the reconstructed image, the computer assigns each voxel a relative density number based on an arbitrary scale of -1000 to $+1000$. This scale is mathematically related to the linear attenuation coefficient of the tissue represented by that voxel. On this scale, air is assigned a density of -1000; water, a density of 0; and compact bone, $+1000$. Some CT systems use a more contracted scale of -500 to $+500$; in all likelihood, however, the larger scale will be universally adopted. Most CT systems provide an electronic device at the display console that permits the observer to sample any area of the image and receive a computer readout of the density number of the selected area.

Currently Available CT Scans of the Body

The ensuing pages present examples of currently available CT scans of the body. The images were selected at segmental levels below the calvaria. Computed tomography is a rapidly advancing field, and its full potential is yet to be realized. The examples included here, represent the current state of the art. Although computed tomography has made a dramatic appearance on the horizons of medical imaging, there still remains a need for the more familiar modalities previously described: angiography, pneumoencephalography, conventional radiography, ultrasonography, and radionuclide imaging. The various roles of these modalities is beyond the scope of this text.

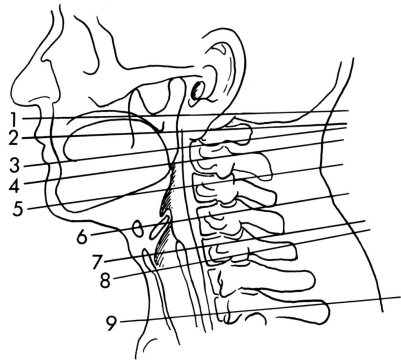

FIGURE B–1 Line diagram showing the position of the computed tomographic cuts of the lower face and neck.

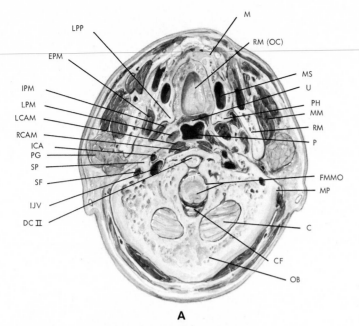

A

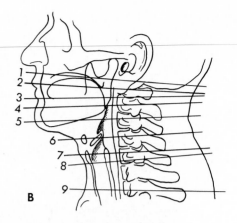

FIGURE B–2 *A.* Diagram of lower face at level No. 1, showing anatomic parts encountered in this slice. *B.* Miniature of Figure B–1 for orientation. *C.* Computed tomograph obtained.

B

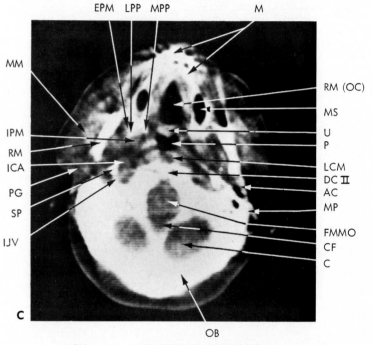

C

EPM	=	EXTERNAL PTERYGOID MUSCLE
LPP	=	LATERAL PTERYGOID PLATE
MPP	=	MEDIAL PTERYGOID PLATE
M	=	MAXILLA
MM	=	MASSETER MUSCLE
IPM	=	INTERNAL PTERYGOID MUSCLE
RM	=	RAMUS OF MANDIBLE
ICA	=	INT. CAROTID ARTERY
PG	=	PAROTID GLAND
SP	=	STYLOID PROCESS
IJV	=	INT. JUGULAR VEIN
RM (OC)	=	ROOF OF MOUTH (ORAL CAVITY)
MS	=	MAXILLARY SINUS
U	=	UVULA
P	=	PHARYNX
LCM	=	LONGUS CAPITIS ANTERIOR MUSCLE
DC II	=	DENS OF C II
AC	=	AUDITORY CANAL
MP	=	MASTOID PROCESS
FMMO	=	FORAMEN MAGNUM AND MEDULLA OBLONGATA
CF	=	CEREBROSPINAL FLUID
C	=	CEREBELLUM
OB	=	OCCIPITAL BONE

LPM	=	LEVATOR PALATINI MUSCLE
RCM	=	RECTUS CAPITIS ANTERIOR MUSCLE
SF	=	STYLOMASTOID FORAMEN
PH	=	PTERYGOID HAMULUS

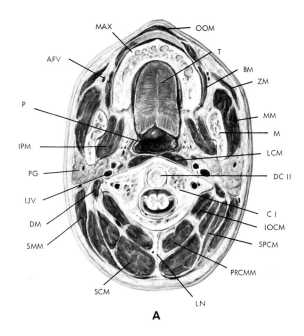

A

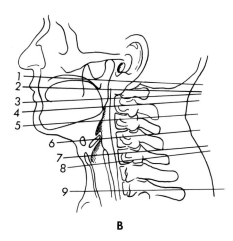

FIGURE B–3 *A*. Diagram of lower face at level No. 2, showing anatomic parts encountered in this slice. *B*. Miniature of Figure B–1 for orientation. *C*. Computed tomograph obtained.

B

MAX	=	MAXILLA
AFV	=	ANT. FACIAL VEIN
P	=	PHARYNX
IPM	=	INT. PTERYGOID MUSCLE
PG	=	PTERYGOID GLAND
IJV	=	INT. JUGULAR VEIN
DM	=	DIGASTRIC MUSCLE
SMM	=	STERNOCLEIDOMASTOID MUSCLE
SCM	=	SEMISPINALIS CAPITIS MUSCLE
OOM	=	ORBICULARIS ORIS MUSCLE
T	=	TONGUE
BM	=	BUCCINATOR MUSCLE
ZM	=	ZYGOMATIC MUSCLE
MM	=	MASSETER MUSCLE
M	=	MANDIBLE
LCM	=	LONGUS CAPITIS MUSCLE
DC II	=	DENS OF C II
CI	=	C I
IOCM	=	INF. OBLIQUE CAPITIS MUSCLE
SPCM	=	SPLENIUS CAPITIS MUSCLE
PRCMM	=	POST. RECTUS CAPITIS MUSCLE
LN	=	LIGAMENTUM NUCHAE

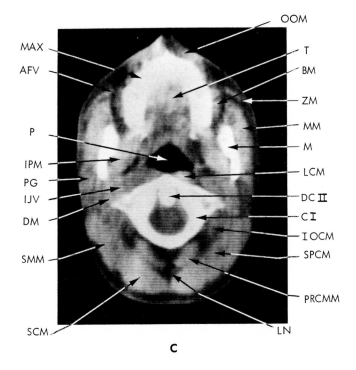

C

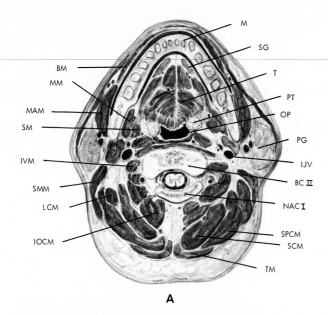

A

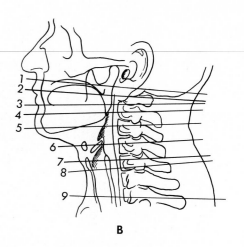

B

FIGURE B-4 *A.* Diagram of lower face at level No. 3, showing anatomic parts encountered in this slice. *B.* Miniature of Figure B-1 for orientation. *C.* Computed tomograph obtained.

BM	=	BUCCINATOR MUSCLE
MM	=	MYLOHYOIDEUS MUSCLE
MAM	=	MASSETER MUSCLE
SM	=	STYLOGLOSSUS MUSCLE
IVM	=	INTERTRANSVERSARIUS MUSCLE
LCM	=	LONGISSIMUS CAPITIS MUSCLE
IOCM	=	INF. OBLIQUE CAPITIS MUSCLE
M	=	MANDIBLE
T	=	TONGUE
PT	=	PALATINE TONSIL
OP	=	OROPHARYNX
IJV	=	INT. JUGULAR VEIN
BC II	=	BODY OF C II
SMM	=	STERNOCLEIDOMASTOID MUSCLE
NAC I	=	NEURAL ARCH C I
SPCM	=	SPLENIUS CAPITIS MUSCLE
SCM	=	SEMISPINALIS CAPITIS MUSCLE

C

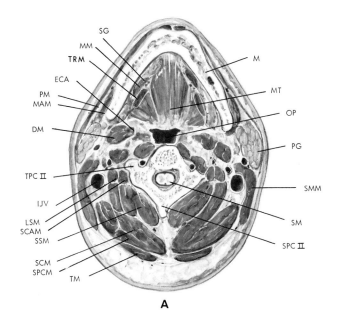

A

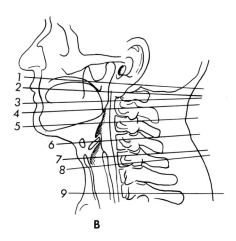

FIGURE B–5 *A*. Diagram of lower face at level No. 4, showing anatomic parts encountered in this slice. *B*. Miniature of Figure B–1 for orientation. *C*. Computed tomograph obtained.

B

SG	=	SUBLINGUAL GLAND
MM	=	MYLOHYOIDEUS MUSCLE
TRM	=	TRIANGULARIS MUSCLE
ECA	=	EXTERNAL CAROTID ARTERY
PM	=	PLATYSMA MUSCLE
MAM	=	MASSETER MUSCLE
DM	=	DIGASTRIC MUSCLE
PG	=	PAROTID GLAND
IJV	=	INTERNAL JUGULAR VEIN
SCAM	=	SCALENUS MEDIUS MUSCLE
LSM	=	LEVATOR SCAPULAE MUSCLE
TPC II	=	TRANSVERSE PROCESS C II
SSM	=	SEMISPINALIS CERVICIS MUSCLE
SPCM	=	SPLENIUS CAPITIS MUSCLE
SCM	=	SEMISPINALIS CAPITIS MUSCLE
TM	=	TRAPEZIUS MUSCLE
SPC II	=	SPINOUS PROCESS C II
M	=	MANDIBLE
MT	=	MUSCLE OF TONGUE
OP	=	OROPHARYNX
BC II	=	BODY OF C II
SMM	=	STERNOCLEIDOMASTOID MUSCLE
SM	=	SPINAL MEDULLA
SSM	=	SEMISPINALIS CERVICIS MUSCLE

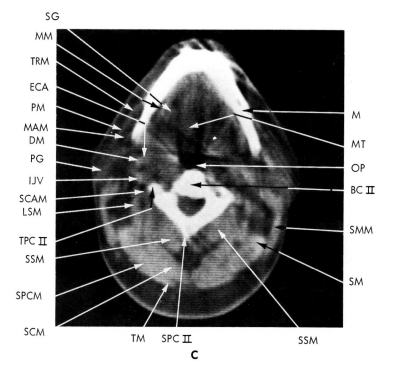

C

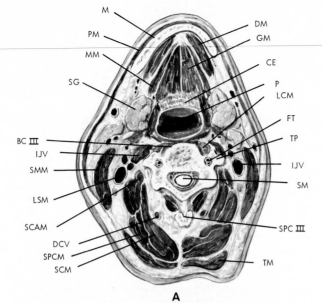

A

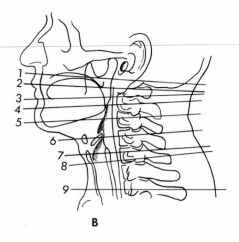

B

FIGURE B–6 *A.* Diagram of lower face at level No. 5, showing anatomic parts encountered in this slice. *B.* Miniature of Figure B–1 for orientation. *C.* Computed tomograph obtained.

PM	=	PLATYSMA MUSCLE
CE	=	CARTILAGE OF EPIGLOTTIS
MM	=	MYLOHYOIDEUS MUSCLE
P	=	PHARYNX
SG	=	SUBMAXILLARY GLAND
BC III	=	BODY OF C III
IJV	=	INTERNAL JUGULAR VEIN
LSM	=	LEVATOR SCAPULAE MUSCLE
SCAM	=	SCALENUS MEDIUS MUSCLE
SMM	=	STERNOCLEIDOMASTOID MUSCLE
DCV	=	DEEP CERVICAL VEIN
SPCM	=	SPLENIUS CAPITIS MUSCLE
SCM	=	SEMISPINALIS CAPITIS MUSCLE
TM	=	TRAPEZIUS MUSCLE
SSM	=	SEMISPINALIS CERVICIS MUSCLE
M	=	MANDIBLE
DM	=	DIGASTRIC MUSCLE
GM	=	GENIOHYOID MUSCLE
LCM	=	LONGUS COLLI MUSCLE
TP	=	TRANSVERSE PROCESS
FT	=	FORAMEN TRANSVERSARIUM
SM	=	SPINAL MEDULLA
SPC III	=	SPINOUS PROCESS C III

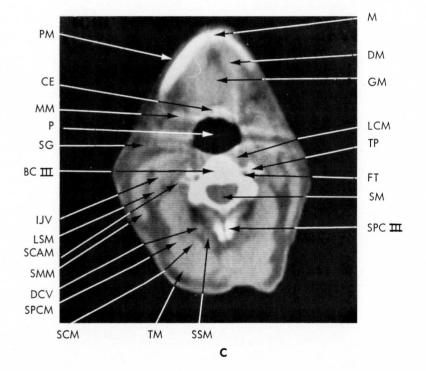

C

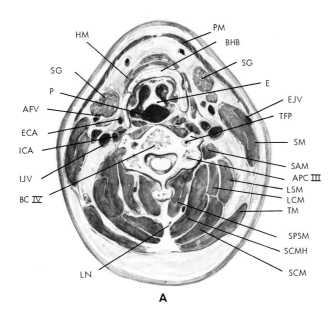

A

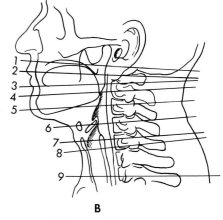

FIGURE B–7 *A*. Diagram of neck at level No. 6, showing anatomic parts encountered in this slice. *B*. Miniature of Figure B–1 for orientation. *C*. Computed tomograph obtained.

B

HM	=	HYOGLOSSUS MUSCLE
SG	=	SUBMAXILLARY GLAND
P	=	PHARYNX
AFV	=	ANT. FACIAL VEIN
ECA	=	EXTERNAL CAROTID ARTERY
IJV	=	INT. JUGULAR VEIN
ICA	=	INT. CAROTID ARTERY
BC IV	=	BODY OF C IV
BHB	=	BODY OF HYOID BONE
PM	=	PLATYSMA MUSCLE
E	=	EPIGLOTTIS
TFP	=	TRANSVERSE FORAMEN AND PROCESS
EJV	=	EXT. JUGULAR VEIN
SAM	=	SCALENUS ANTERIOR MUSCLE
SM	=	STERNOCLEIDOMASTOID MUSCLE
APC III	=	ANTERIOR PROCESS C III
SSM	=	SEMISPINALIS CERVICIS MUSCLE
LSM	=	LEVATOR SCAPULAE MUSCLE
LCM	=	LONGISSIMUS CAPITIS MUSCLE
TM	=	TRAPEZIUS MUSCLE
SCM	=	SEMISPINALIS CAPITIS MUSCLE
SPCM	=	SPLENIUS CAPITIS MUSCLE
LN	=	LIGAMENTUM NUCHAE

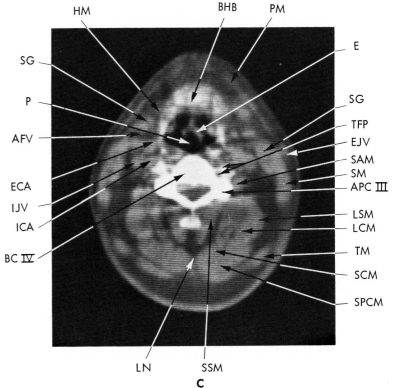

C

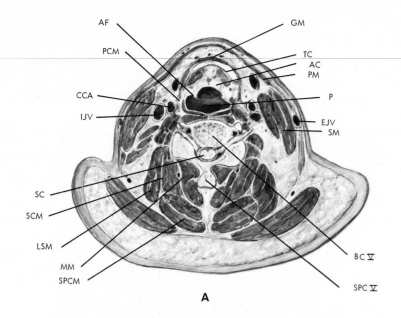

A

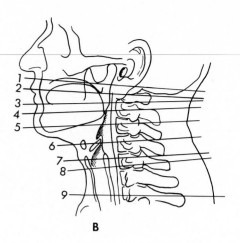

FIGURE B–8 *A*. Diagram of neck at level No. 7, showing anatomic parts encountered in this slice. *B*. Miniature of Figure B–1 for orientation. *C*. Computed tomograph obtained.

B

PCM	=	PHARYNGEAL CONSTRICTOR MUSCLE
AF	=	ARYEPIGLOTTIC FOLD
GM	=	GENIOHYOID MUSCLE
CCA	=	COMMON CAROTID ARTERY
IJV	=	INTERNAL JUGULAR VEIN
MM	=	MULTIFIDUS MUSCLE
SPCM	=	SPLENIUS CAPITIS MUSCLE
SPC Ⅴ	=	SPINOUS PROCESS C-Ⅴ
SC	=	SPINAL CORD
TC	=	THYROID CARTILAGE
AC	=	ARYTENOID CARTILAGE
PM	=	PLATYSMA MUSCLE
EJV	=	EXTERNAL JUGULAR VEIN
P	=	PHARYNX
SM	=	STERNOCLEIDOMASTOID MUSCLE
BC Ⅴ	=	BODY OF C Ⅴ
LSM	=	LEVATOR SCAPULAE MUSCLE
SCM	=	SEMISPINALIS CAPITIS MUSCLE
TM	=	TRAPEZIUM

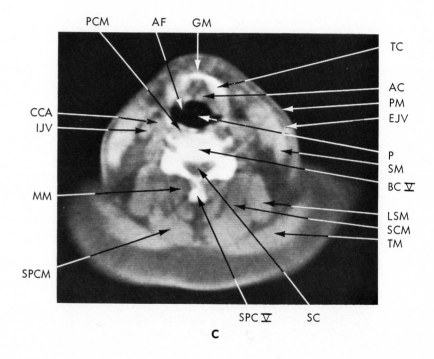

C

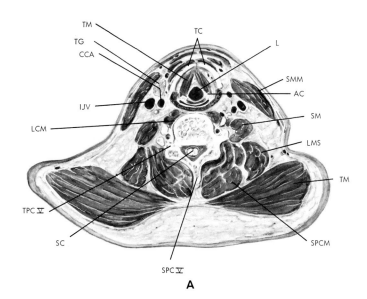

A

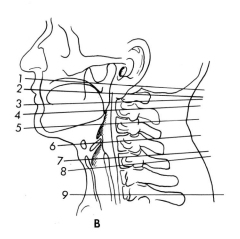

FIGURE B–9 *A.* Diagram of neck at level No. 8, showing anatomic parts encountered in this slice. *B.* Miniature of Figure B–1 for orientation. *C.* Computed tomograph obtained.

B

CCA	=	COMMON CAROTID ARTERY
TC	=	THYROID CARTILAGES
IJV	=	INT. JUGULAR VEIN
LCM	=	LONGUS COLLI MUSCLE
TPC V	=	TRANSVERSE PROCESS C V
SC	=	SPINAL CORD
SPC V	=	SPINOUS PROCESS C V
L	=	LARYNX
SMM	=	STERNOCLEIDOMASTOID MUSCLE
AC	=	ARYTENOID CARTILAGE
SM	=	SCALENUS MUSCLES
LMS	=	LEVATOR MUSCLE OF SCAPULA
BC V	=	BODY OF C V
TM	=	TRAPEZIUS MUSCLE
TG	=	THYROID GLAND
SPCM	=	SPLENIUS CAPITIS MUSCLE

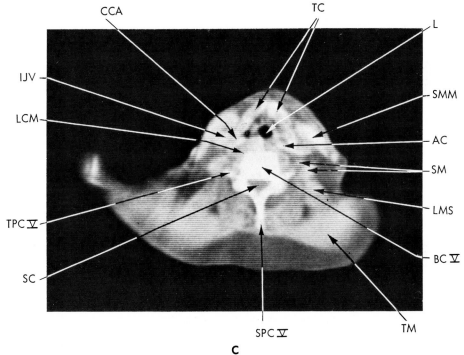

C

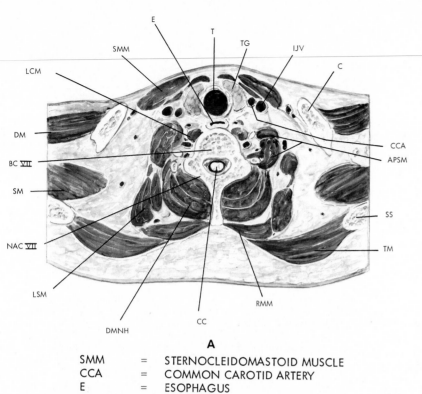

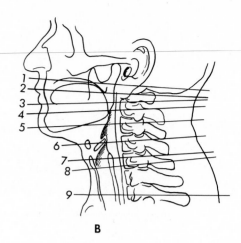

FIGURE B–10 *A.* Diagram of neck at level No. 9, showing anatomic parts encountered in this slice. *B.* Miniature of Figure B–1 for orientation. *C.* Computed tomograph obtained.

A

SMM	=	STERNOCLEIDOMASTOID MUSCLE
CCA	=	COMMON CAROTID ARTERY
E	=	ESOPHAGUS
T	=	TRACHEA
TG	=	THYROID GLAND
IJV	=	INT. JUGULAR VEIN
C	=	CLAVICLE
DM	=	DELTOID MUSCLE
BC VII	=	BODY OF C VII
SM	=	SUPRASPINATUS MUSCLE
NAC VII	=	NEURAL ARCH C-VII
LSM	=	LEVATOR SCAPULAE MUSCLE
DMNH	=	DEEP MUSCLES OF NECK & HEAD
CC	=	CERVICAL CORD
LCM	=	LONGUS COLLI MUSCLE
RMM	=	RHOMBOID MINOR MUSCLE
TM	=	TRAPEZIUS MUSCLE
PSM	=	POST. SCALENE MUSCLE
HH	=	HEAD OF HUMERUS
SS	=	SPINE OF SCAPULA
ASM	=	ANT. SCALENE MUSCLE

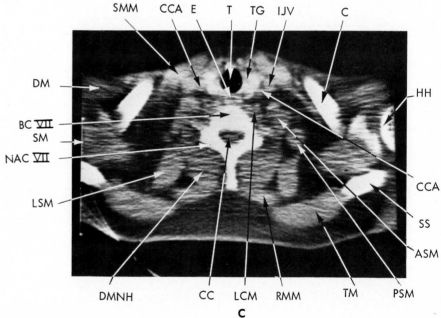

C

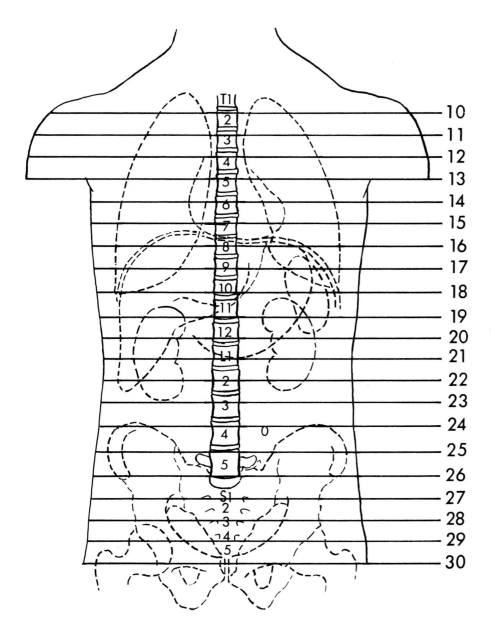

FIGURE B-11   Line drawing showing the position of the computed tomographic cuts of the thorax and abdomen.

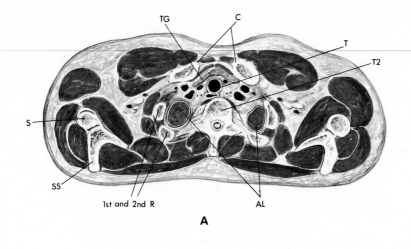

A

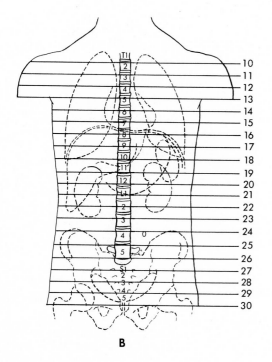

B

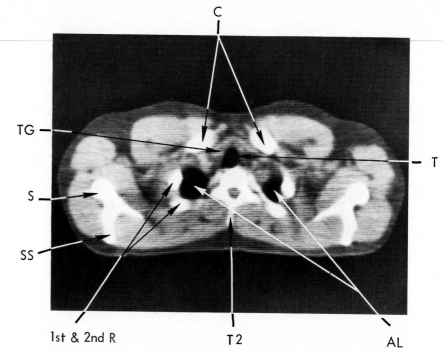

FIGURE B–12 *A.* Diagram at shoulder level (T2) at cut No. 10, showing anatomic parts encountered in this slice. *B.* Miniature of Figure B–11 for orientation. *C.* Computed tomograph obtained.

C	=	CLAVICLES
TG	=	RIGHT LOBE OF THYROID GLAND
S	=	SCAPULA
SS	=	SPINE OF SCAPULA
1st & 2nd R	=	1st AND 2nd RIBS
T 2	=	T 2 LEVEL
T	=	TRACHEA
AL	=	APICES OF LUNG

C

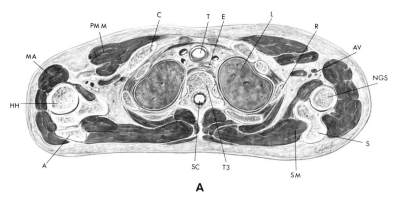

A

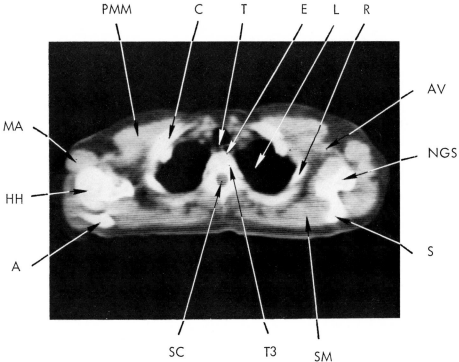

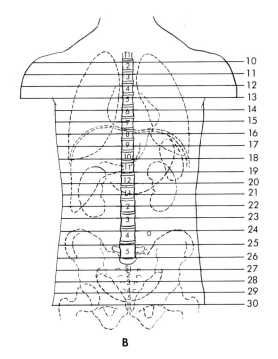

B

FIGURE B–13 *A.* Diagram at thoracic level (T3) at cut No. 11, showing anatomic parts encountered in this slice. *B.* Miniature of Figure B–11 for orientation. *C.* Computed tomograph obtained.

PMM	=	PECTORALIS MAJOR MUSCLE
C	=	CLAVICLE
T	=	TRACHEA
E	=	ESOPHAGUS
L	=	LUNG
R	=	RIB
MA	=	MUSCLES OF ARM
HH	=	HEAD OF HUMERUS
A	=	ACROMION
SC	=	SPINAL CORD
T3	=	T3 LEVEL
SM	=	SUPRASPINATUS MUSCLE
AV	=	AXILLARY VESSELS
NGS	=	NECK AND GLENOID OF SCAPULA
S	=	SCAPULA

C

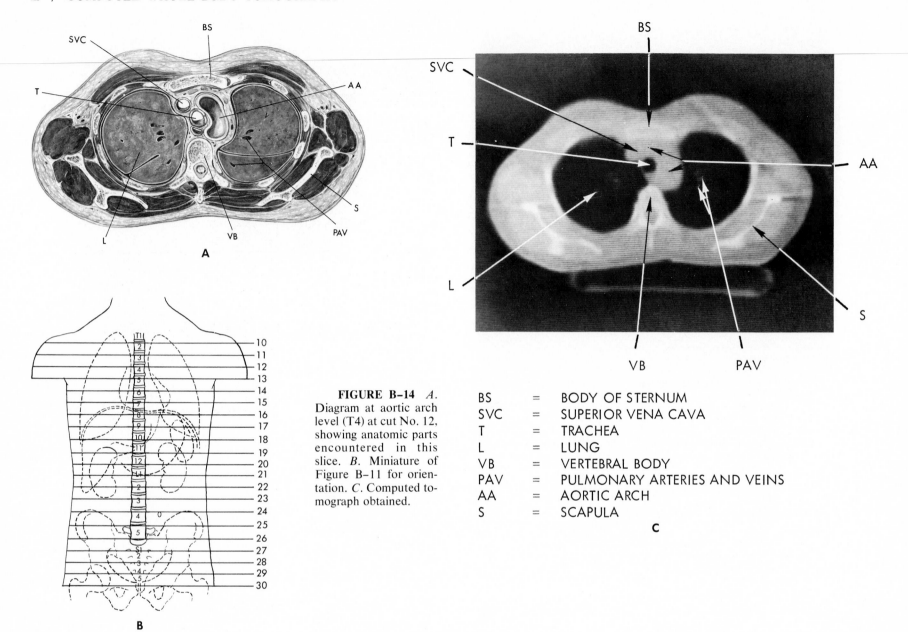

FIGURE B–14 *A.* Diagram at aortic arch level (T4) at cut No. 12, showing anatomic parts encountered in this slice. *B.* Miniature of Figure B–11 for orientation. *C.* Computed tomograph obtained.

BS	=	BODY OF STERNUM
SVC	=	SUPERIOR VENA CAVA
T	=	TRACHEA
L	=	LUNG
VB	=	VERTEBRAL BODY
PAV	=	PULMONARY ARTERIES AND VEINS
AA	=	AORTIC ARCH
S	=	SCAPULA

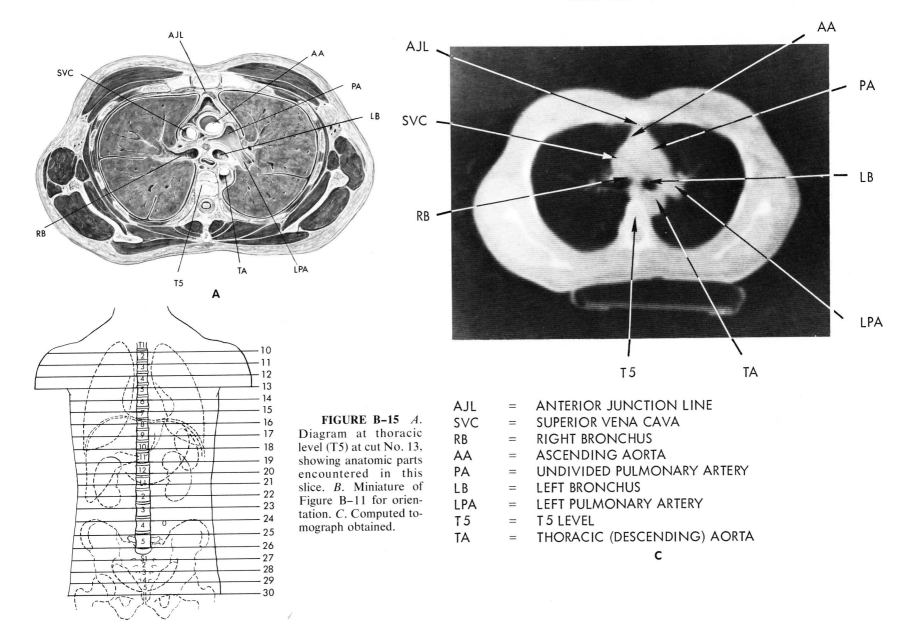

FIGURE B–15 *A.* Diagram at thoracic level (T5) at cut No. 13, showing anatomic parts encountered in this slice. *B.* Miniature of Figure B–11 for orientation. *C.* Computed tomograph obtained.

AJL	=	ANTERIOR JUNCTION LINE
SVC	=	SUPERIOR VENA CAVA
RB	=	RIGHT BRONCHUS
AA	=	ASCENDING AORTA
PA	=	UNDIVIDED PULMONARY ARTERY
LB	=	LEFT BRONCHUS
LPA	=	LEFT PULMONARY ARTERY
T 5	=	T 5 LEVEL
TA	=	THORACIC (DESCENDING) AORTA

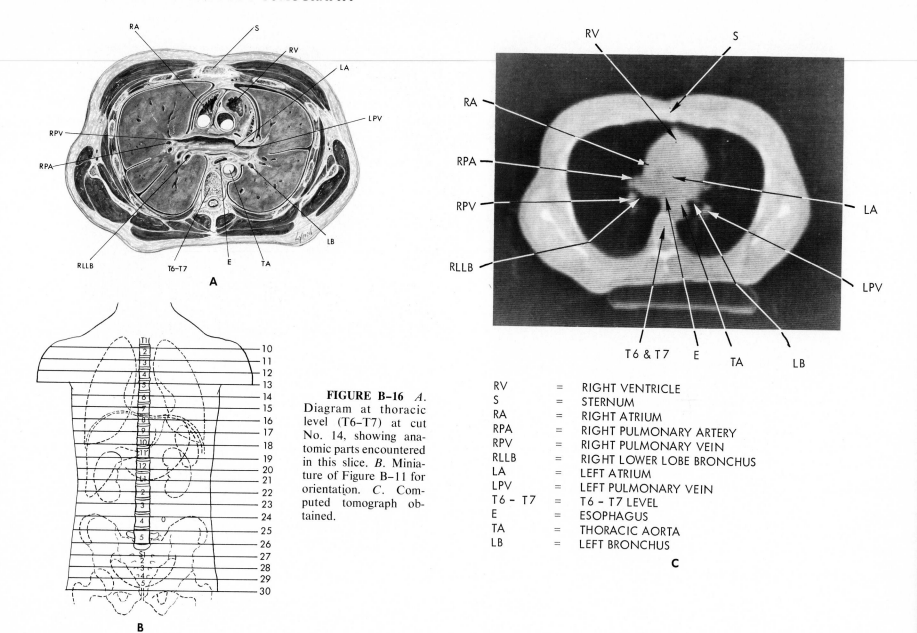

A

B

FIGURE B–16 *A.* Diagram at thoracic level (T6–T7) at cut No. 14, showing anatomic parts encountered in this slice. *B.* Miniature of Figure B–11 for orientation. *C.* Computed tomograph obtained.

C

RV	=	RIGHT VENTRICLE
S	=	STERNUM
RA	=	RIGHT ATRIUM
RPA	=	RIGHT PULMONARY ARTERY
RPV	=	RIGHT PULMONARY VEIN
RLLB	=	RIGHT LOWER LOBE BRONCHUS
LA	=	LEFT ATRIUM
LPV	=	LEFT PULMONARY VEIN
T6 – T7	=	T6 – T7 LEVEL
E	=	ESOPHAGUS
TA	=	THORACIC AORTA
LB	=	LEFT BRONCHUS

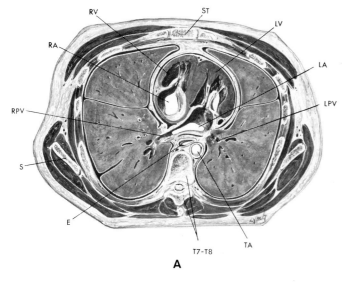

A

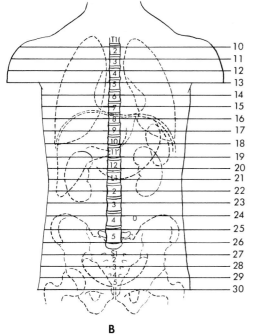

B

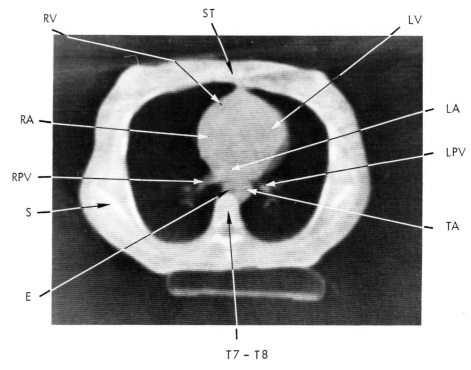

T7 - T8

C

FIGURE B–17 *A.* Diagram at thoracic level (T7–T8) at cut No. 15, showing anatomic parts encountered in this slice. *B.* Miniature of Figure B–11 for orientation. *C.* Computed tomograph obtained.

RV	=	RIGHT VENTRICLE
RA	=	RIGHT ATRIUM
RPV	=	RIGHT PULMONARY VEIN
S	=	SCAPULA
E	=	ESOPHAGUS
T7 – T8	=	T7 – T8 LEVEL
ST	=	STERNUM
LV	=	LEFT VENTRICLE
LA	=	LEFT ATRIUM
LPV	=	LEFT PULMONARY VEIN
TA	=	THORACIC AORTA

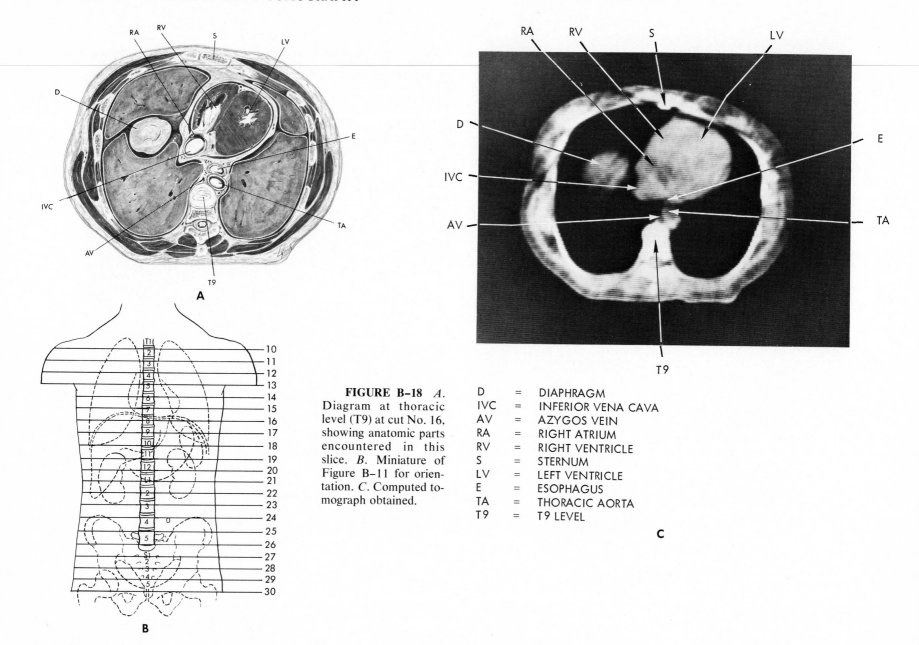

FIGURE B–18 *A*. Diagram at thoracic level (T9) at cut No. 16, showing anatomic parts encountered in this slice. *B*. Miniature of Figure B–11 for orientation. *C*. Computed tomograph obtained.

D	=	DIAPHRAGM
IVC	=	INFERIOR VENA CAVA
AV	=	AZYGOS VEIN
RA	=	RIGHT ATRIUM
RV	=	RIGHT VENTRICLE
S	=	STERNUM
LV	=	LEFT VENTRICLE
E	=	ESOPHAGUS
TA	=	THORACIC AORTA
T9	=	T9 LEVEL

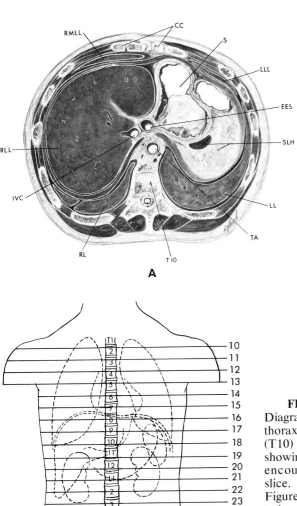

A

B

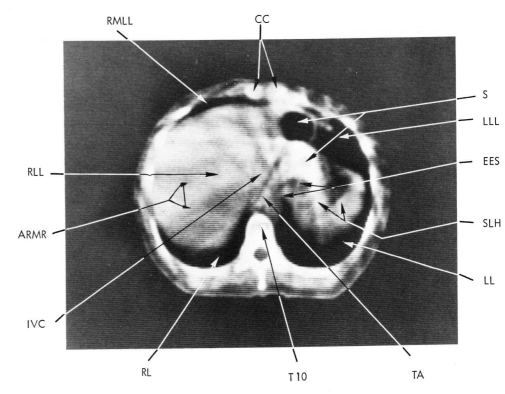

C

FIGURE B–19 *A.* Diagram at junction of thorax and abdomen (T10) at cut No. 17, showing anatomic parts encountered in this slice. *B.* Miniature of Figure B–11 for orientation. *C.* Computed tomograph obtained.

RLL	=	RIGHT LOBE, LIVER
ARMR	=	ARTIFACT FROM RESPIRATORY MOTION OF RIBS
IVC	=	INFERIOR VENA CAVA
RL	=	RIGHT LUNG (LOWER LOBE)
T10	=	T10 LEVEL
TA	=	THORACIC AORTA
RMLL	=	RIGHT MIDDLE LOBE OF LUNG
CC	=	COSTAL CARTILAGES
S	=	STOMACH
LLL	=	LINGULA LEFT LUNG
EES	=	ESOPHAGUS ENTRY TO STOMACH
SLH	=	SPLEEN AND LEFT HEMIDIAPHRAGM
LL	=	LEFT LUNG

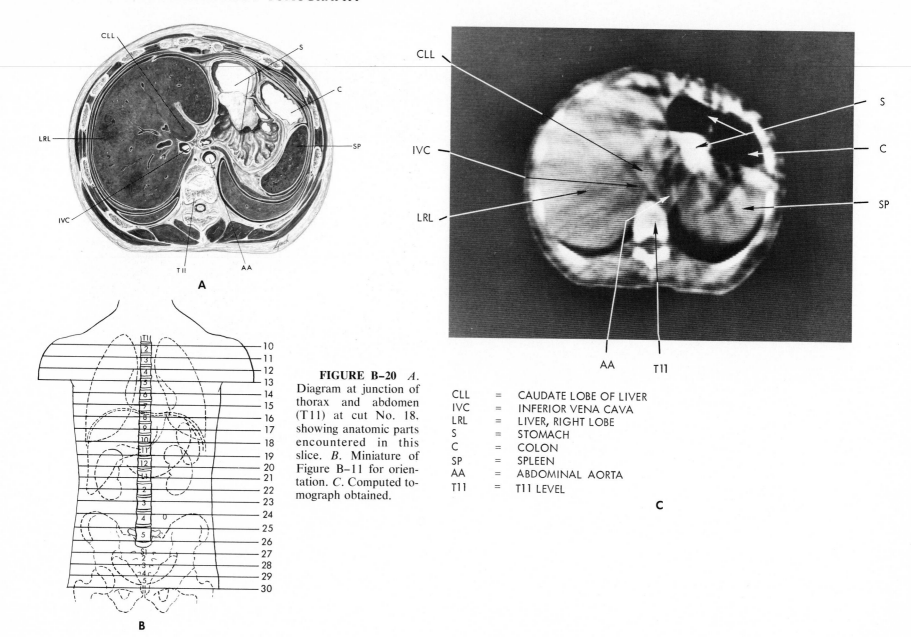

FIGURE B–20 *A*. Diagram at junction of thorax and abdomen (T11) at cut No. 18, showing anatomic parts encountered in this slice. *B*. Miniature of Figure B–11 for orientation. *C*. Computed tomograph obtained.

CLL	=	CAUDATE LOBE OF LIVER
IVC	=	INFERIOR VENA CAVA
LRL	=	LIVER, RIGHT LOBE
S	=	STOMACH
C	=	COLON
SP	=	SPLEEN
AA	=	ABDOMINAL AORTA
T11	=	T11 LEVEL

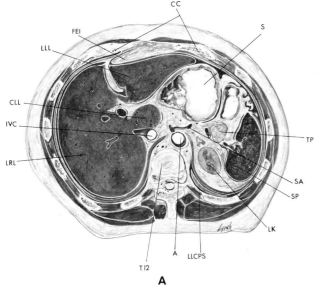

A

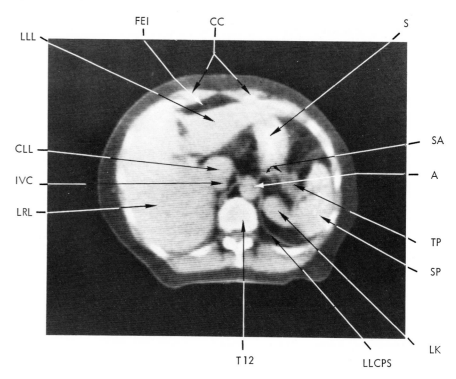

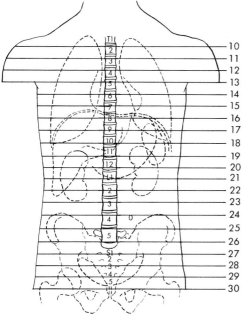

B

FIGURE B–21 *A.* Diagram at upper abdomen level (T12) at cut No. 19, showing anatomic parts encountered in this slice. *B.* Miniature of Figure B–11 for orientation. *C.* Computed tomograph obtained.

LLL	=	LIVER, LEFT LOBE
CLL	=	CAUDATE LOBE OF LIVER
IVC	=	INFERIOR VENA CAVA
LRL	=	LIVER, RIGHT LOBE
FEI	=	FAT, EXTRAPERITONEAL AND INTRAPERITONEAL
CC	=	COSTAL CARTILAGES
S	=	STOMACH
SA	=	SPLENIC ARTERY
A	=	AORTA
TP	=	TAIL OF PANCREAS
SP	=	SPLEEN
LK	=	UPPER POLE LEFT KIDNEY
LLCPS	=	LEFT LUNG IN COSTOPHRENIC SULCUS
T12	=	T12 LEVEL

C

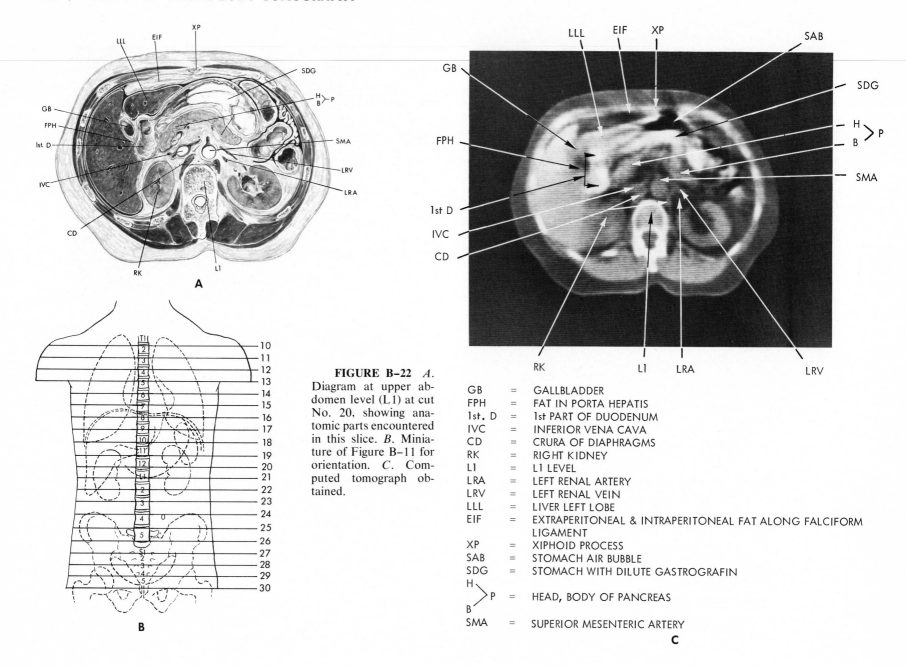

FIGURE B–22 *A.* Diagram at upper abdomen level (L1) at cut No. 20, showing anatomic parts encountered in this slice. *B.* Miniature of Figure B–11 for orientation. *C.* Computed tomograph obtained.

GB	=	GALLBLADDER
FPH	=	FAT IN PORTA HEPATIS
1st. D	=	1st PART OF DUODENUM
IVC	=	INFERIOR VENA CAVA
CD	=	CRURA OF DIAPHRAGMS
RK	=	RIGHT KIDNEY
L1	=	L1 LEVEL
LRA	=	LEFT RENAL ARTERY
LRV	=	LEFT RENAL VEIN
LLL	=	LIVER LEFT LOBE
EIF	=	EXTRAPERITONEAL & INTRAPERITONEAL FAT ALONG FALCIFORM LIGAMENT
XP	=	XIPHOID PROCESS
SAB	=	STOMACH AIR BUBBLE
SDG	=	STOMACH WITH DILUTE GASTROGRAFIN
H, B > P	=	HEAD, BODY OF PANCREAS
SMA	=	SUPERIOR MESENTERIC ARTERY

C

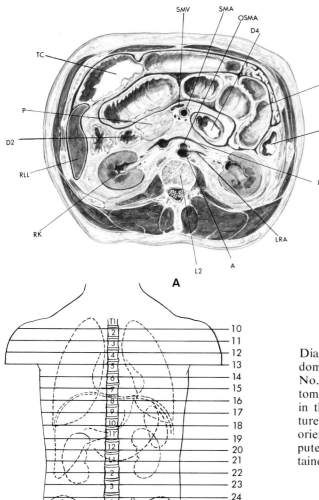

A

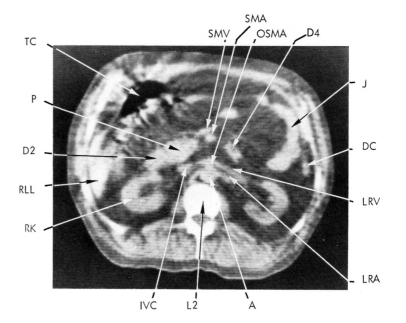

C

B

FIGURE B–23 *A.* Diagram at upper abdomen level (L2) at cut No. 21, showing anatomic parts encountered in this slice. *B.* Miniature of Figure B–11 for orientation. *C.* Computed tomograph obtained.

TC	=	TRANSVERSE COLON
P	=	HEAD OF PANCREAS
D2	=	2nd PORTION OF DUODENUM
RLL	=	RT. LOBE OF LIVER
RK	=	RT. KIDNEY
IVC	=	INFERIOR VENA CAVA
L2	=	L2 LEVEL
A	=	AORTA
SMV	=	SUPERIOR MESENTERIC VEIN
SMA	=	SUPERIOR MESENTERIC ARTERY (MORE DISTAL)
OSMA	=	ORIGIN OF SUPERIOR MESENTERIC ARTERY
D4	=	4th PORTION OF DUODENUM
J	=	JEJUNUM
DC	=	DESCENDING COLON
LRV	=	LT. RENAL VEIN
LRA	=	LT. RENAL ARTERY

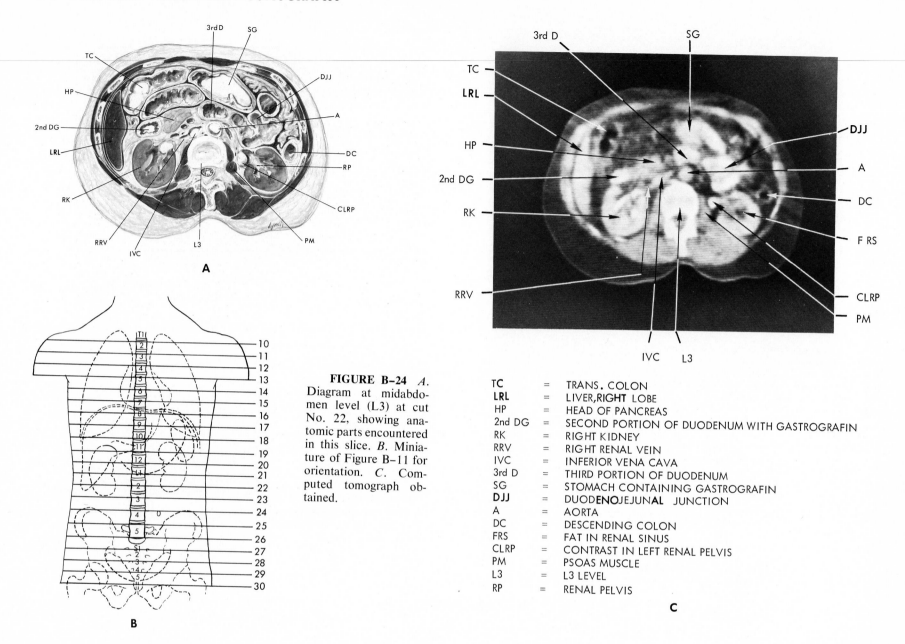

FIGURE B–24 *A.* Diagram at midabdomen level (L3) at cut No. 22, showing anatomic parts encountered in this slice. *B.* Miniature of Figure B–11 for orientation. *C.* Computed tomograph obtained.

TC	=	TRANS. COLON
LRL	=	LIVER, **RIGHT** LOBE
HP	=	HEAD OF PANCREAS
2nd DG	=	SECOND PORTION OF DUODENUM WITH GASTROGRAFIN
RK	=	RIGHT KIDNEY
RRV	=	RIGHT RENAL VEIN
IVC	=	INFERIOR VENA CAVA
3rd D	=	THIRD PORTION OF DUODENUM
SG	=	STOMACH CONTAINING GASTROGRAFIN
DJJ	=	DUOD**ENO**JEJUN**AL** JUNCTION
A	=	AORTA
DC	=	DESCENDING COLON
FRS	=	FAT IN RENAL SINUS
CLRP	=	CONTRAST IN LEFT RENAL PELVIS
PM	=	PSOAS MUSCLE
L3	=	L3 LEVEL
RP	=	RENAL PELVIS

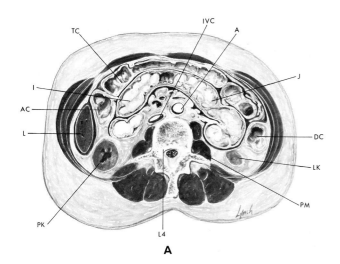

A

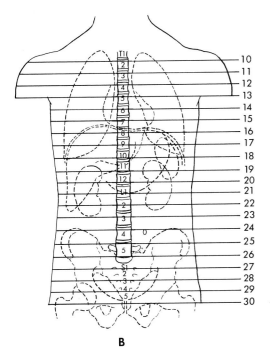

B

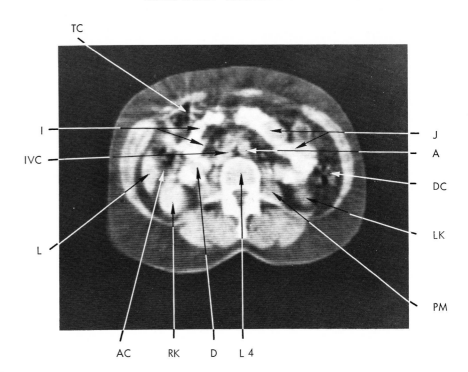

C

FIGURE B–25 *A*. Diagram at midabdomen level (L4) at cut No. 23, showing anatomic parts encountered in this slice. *B*. Miniature of Figure B–11 for orientation. *C*. Computed tomograph obtained.

TC	=	TRANS. COLON
I	=	ILEUM
IVC	=	INF. VENA CAVA
L	=	LIVER (RT. LOBE)
AC	=	ASCEND. COLON
RK	=	LOWER POLE RT. KIDNEY
D	=	JUNCTION OF 2nd AND 3rd PORTIONS OF DUODENUM.
L 4	=	L 4 LEVEL
J	=	JEJUNUM
A	=	AORTA
DC	=	DESCEND. COLON
LK	=	LEFT KIDNEY (LOWER POLE)
PM	=	PSOAS MUSCLE

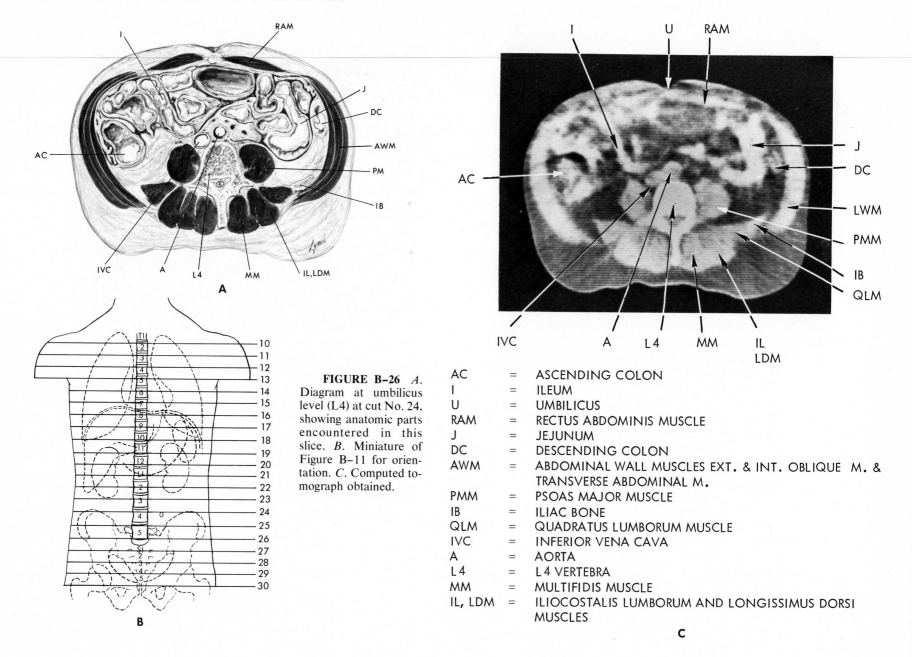

FIGURE B–26 *A.* Diagram at umbilicus level (L4) at cut No. 24, showing anatomic parts encountered in this slice. *B.* Miniature of Figure B–11 for orientation. *C.* Computed tomograph obtained.

AC	=	ASCENDING COLON
I	=	ILEUM
U	=	UMBILICUS
RAM	=	RECTUS ABDOMINIS MUSCLE
J	=	JEJUNUM
DC	=	DESCENDING COLON
AWM	=	ABDOMINAL WALL MUSCLES EXT. & INT. OBLIQUE M. & TRANSVERSE ABDOMINAL M.
PMM	=	PSOAS MAJOR MUSCLE
IB	=	ILIAC BONE
QLM	=	QUADRATUS LUMBORUM MUSCLE
IVC	=	INFERIOR VENA CAVA
A	=	AORTA
L 4	=	L 4 VERTEBRA
MM	=	MULTIFIDIS MUSCLE
IL, LDM	=	ILIOCOSTALIS LUMBORUM AND LONGISSIMUS DORSI MUSCLES

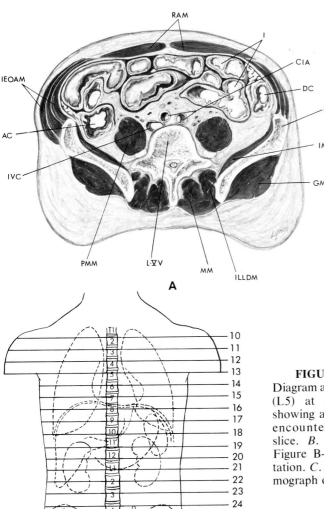

A

B

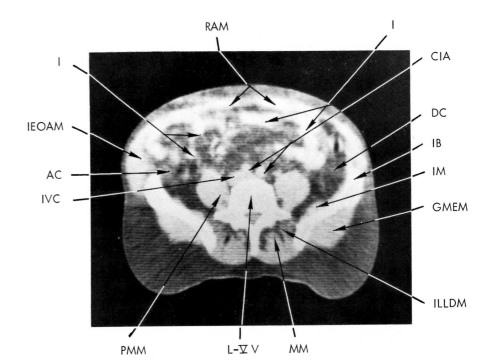

C

FIGURE B–27 *A.* Diagram at *lumbar* level (L5) at cut No. 25, showing anatomic parts encountered in this slice. *B.* Miniature of Figure B-11 for orientation. *C.* Computed tomograph obtained.

RAM	=	RECTUS ABDOMINIS MUSCLES
I	=	ILEUM
CIA	=	COMMON ILIAC ARTERIES
DC	=	DESCENDING COLON
IB	=	ILIAC BONE
IM	=	ILIACUS MUSCLE
GMEM	=	GLUTEUS MEDIUS MUSCLE
ILLDM	=	ILIOCOSTALIS LUMBORUM & LONGISSIMUS DORSI MUSCLES
MM	=	MULTIFIDIS MUSCLE
L-Ⅴ V	=	L-Ⅴ VERTEBRA
PMM	=	PSOAS MAJOR MUSCLE
IVC	=	INF. VENA CAVA
AC	=	ASCENDING COLON
IEOAM	=	INT. AND EXT. OBLIQUE ABD. MUSCLES

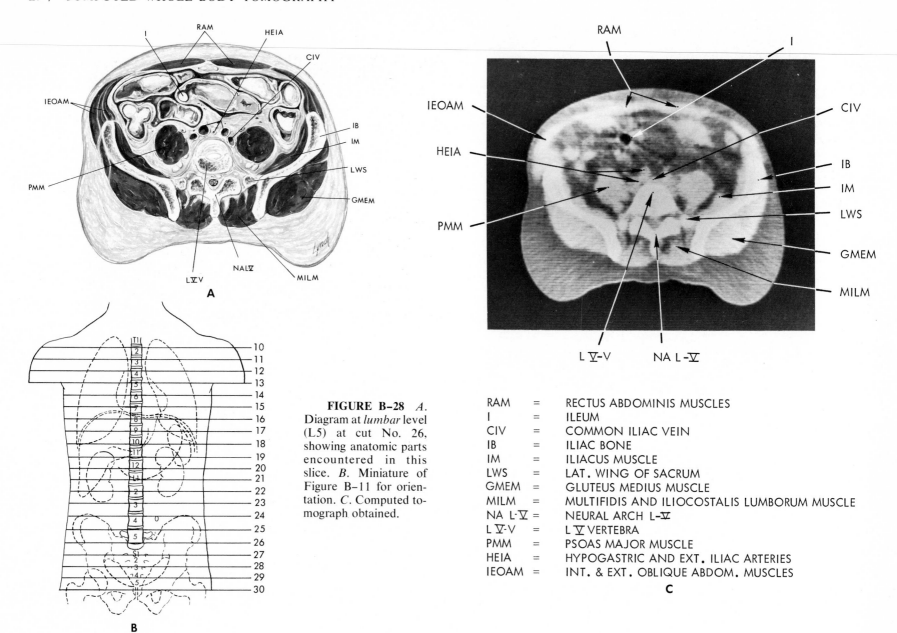

FIGURE B–28 *A.* Diagram at *lumbar* level (L5) at cut No. 26, showing anatomic parts encountered in this slice. *B.* Miniature of Figure B–11 for orientation. *C.* Computed tomograph obtained.

RAM	=	RECTUS ABDOMINIS MUSCLES
I	=	ILEUM
CIV	=	COMMON ILIAC VEIN
IB	=	ILIAC BONE
IM	=	ILIACUS MUSCLE
LWS	=	LAT. WING OF SACRUM
GMEM	=	GLUTEUS MEDIUS MUSCLE
MILM	=	MULTIFIDIS AND ILIOCOSTALIS LUMBORUM MUSCLE
NA L-Ⅴ	=	NEURAL ARCH L-Ⅴ
L Ⅴ-V	=	L Ⅴ VERTEBRA
PMM	=	PSOAS MAJOR MUSCLE
HEIA	=	HYPOGASTRIC AND EXT. ILIAC ARTERIES
IEOAM	=	INT. & EXT. OBLIQUE ABDOM. MUSCLES

C

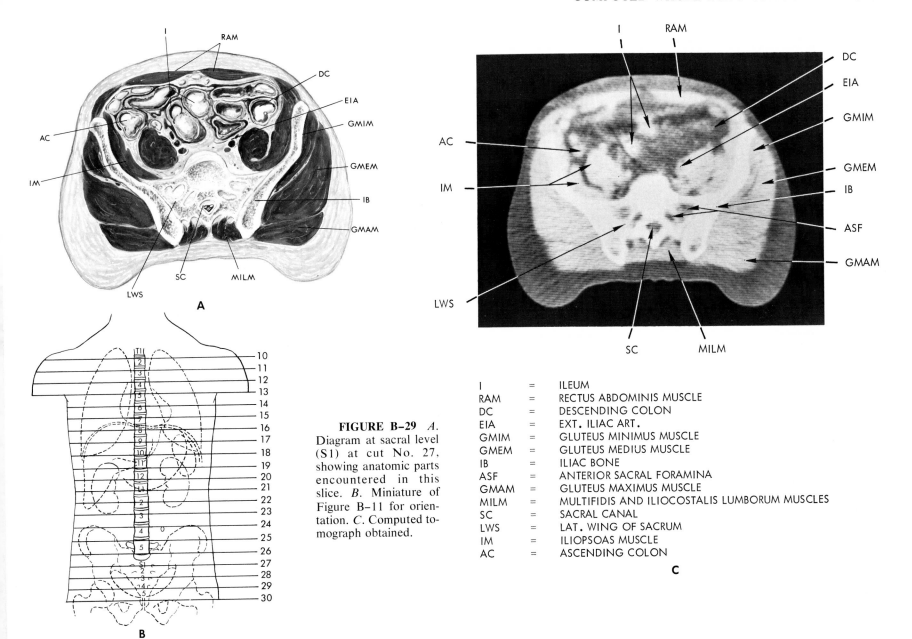

FIGURE B-29 *A*. Diagram at sacral level (S1) at cut No. 27, showing anatomic parts encountered in this slice. *B*. Miniature of Figure B-11 for orientation. *C*. Computed tomograph obtained.

I	=	ILEUM
RAM	=	RECTUS ABDOMINIS MUSCLE
DC	=	DESCENDING COLON
EIA	=	EXT. ILIAC ART.
GMIM	=	GLUTEUS MINIMUS MUSCLE
GMEM	=	GLUTEUS MEDIUS MUSCLE
IB	=	ILIAC BONE
ASF	=	ANTERIOR SACRAL FORAMINA
GMAM	=	GLUTEUS MAXIMUS MUSCLE
MILM	=	MULTIFIDIS AND ILIOCOSTALIS LUMBORUM MUSCLES
SC	=	SACRAL CANAL
LWS	=	LAT. WING OF SACRUM
IM	=	ILIOPSOAS MUSCLE
AC	=	ASCENDING COLON

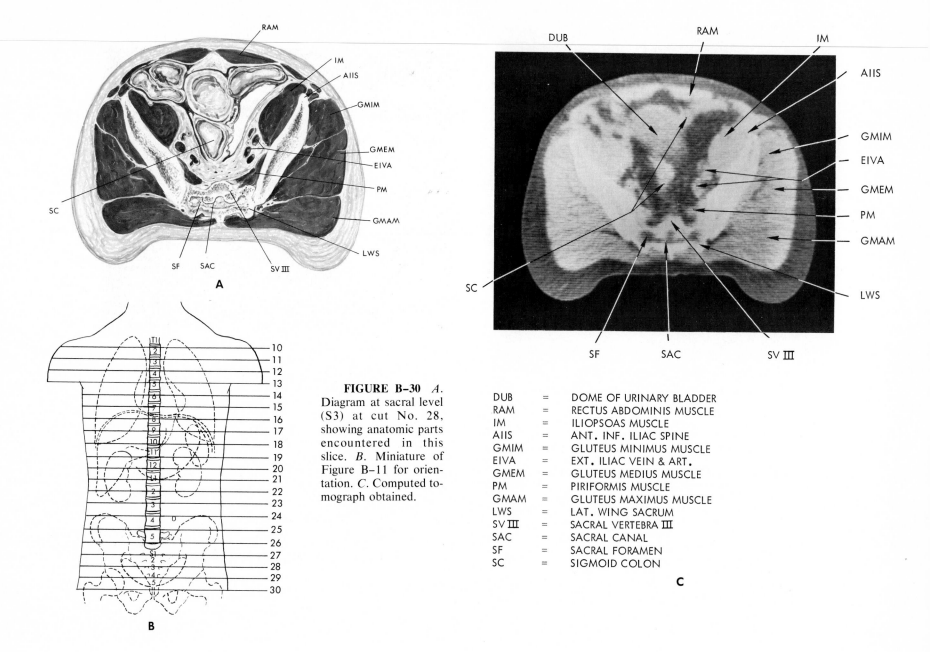

FIGURE B–30 *A.* Diagram at sacral level (S3) at cut No. 28, showing anatomic parts encountered in this slice. *B.* Miniature of Figure B–11 for orientation. *C.* Computed tomograph obtained.

DUB	=	DOME OF URINARY BLADDER
RAM	=	RECTUS ABDOMINIS MUSCLE
IM	=	ILIOPSOAS MUSCLE
AIIS	=	ANT. INF. ILIAC SPINE
GMIM	=	GLUTEUS MINIMUS MUSCLE
EIVA	=	EXT. ILIAC VEIN & ART.
GMEM	=	GLUTEUS MEDIUS MUSCLE
PM	=	PIRIFORMIS MUSCLE
GMAM	=	GLUTEUS MAXIMUS MUSCLE
LWS	=	LAT. WING SACRUM
SV III	=	SACRAL VERTEBRA III
SAC	=	SACRAL CANAL
SF	=	SACRAL FORAMEN
SC	=	SIGMOID COLON

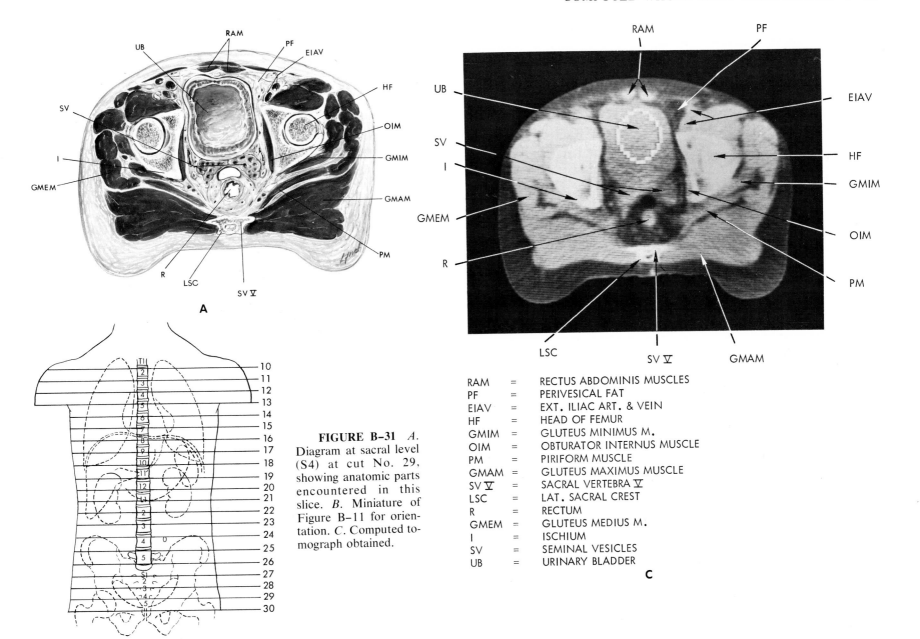

FIGURE B–31 *A.* Diagram at sacral level (S4) at cut No. 29, showing anatomic parts encountered in this slice. *B.* Miniature of Figure B–11 for orientation. *C.* Computed tomograph obtained.

RAM	=	RECTUS ABDOMINIS MUSCLES
PF	=	PERIVESICAL FAT
EIAV	=	EXT. ILIAC ART. & VEIN
HF	=	HEAD OF FEMUR
GMIM	=	GLUTEUS MINIMUS M.
OIM	=	OBTURATOR INTERNUS MUSCLE
PM	=	PIRIFORM MUSCLE
GMAM	=	GLUTEUS MAXIMUS MUSCLE
SV V	=	SACRAL VERTEBRA V
LSC	=	LAT. SACRAL CREST
R	=	RECTUM
GMEM	=	GLUTEUS MEDIUS M.
I	=	ISCHIUM
SV	=	SEMINAL VESICLES
UB	=	URINARY BLADDER

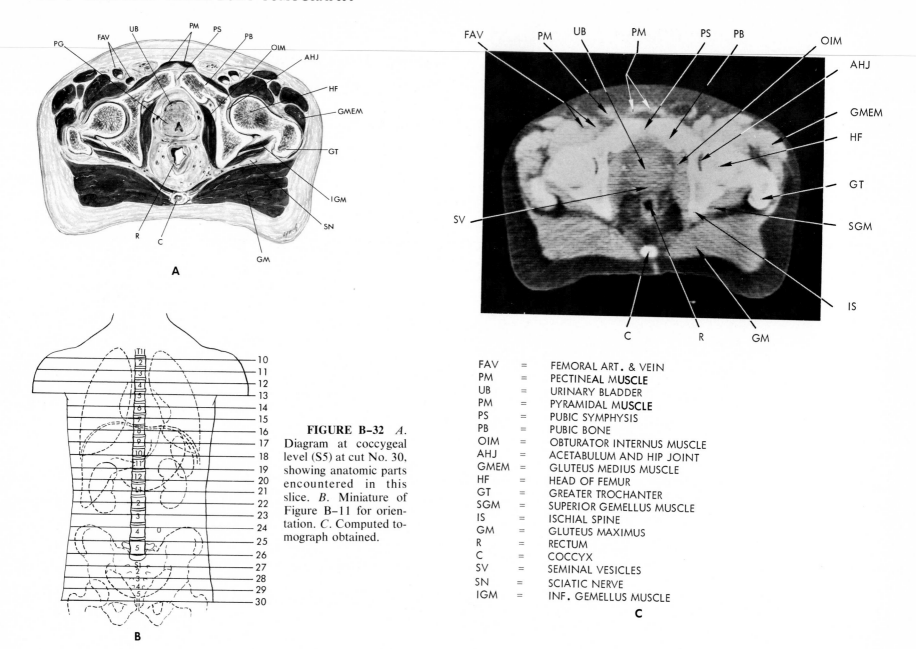

A

B

FIGURE B–32 *A.* Diagram at coccygeal level (S5) at cut No. 30, showing anatomic parts encountered in this slice. *B.* Miniature of Figure B–11 for orientation. *C.* Computed tomograph obtained.

FAV	=	FEMORAL ART. & VEIN
PM	=	PECTINEAL MUSCLE
UB	=	URINARY BLADDER
PM	=	PYRAMIDAL MUSCLE
PS	=	PUBIC SYMPHYSIS
PB	=	PUBIC BONE
OIM	=	OBTURATOR INTERNUS MUSCLE
AHJ	=	ACETABULUM AND HIP JOINT
GMEM	=	GLUTEUS MEDIUS MUSCLE
HF	=	HEAD OF FEMUR
GT	=	GREATER TROCHANTER
SGM	=	SUPERIOR GEMELLUS MUSCLE
IS	=	ISCHIAL SPINE
GM	=	GLUTEUS MAXIMUS
R	=	RECTUM
C	=	COCCYX
SV	=	SEMINAL VESICLES
SN	=	SCIATIC NERVE
IGM	=	INF. GEMELLUS MUSCLE

C

REFERENCES*

Ambrose, J.: Computerized X-ray scanning of the brain. J. Neurosurgery, *40*:679–695, 1974.

Ambrose, J., and Hounsfield, G.: Computerized transverse axial tomography. Br. J. Radiol., *46*:148–149, 1973.

Eycleshymer, A. C., and Schoemaker, D. M.: A Cross-Section Anatomy. New York, Appleton-Century-Crofts, 1970.

Gonzalez, C. F., Grossman, C. B., and Palacios, E.: Computed Brain and Orbital Tomography. Technique and Interpretation. New York, John Wiley & Sons, 1976.

J. Lloyd Johnson Associates: The effect of computed tomography on hospital practice. Northfield, Ill., J. Lloyd Johnson Associates, 1976.

Meyers, M. A.: Dynamic Radiology of the Abdomen: Normal and Pathologic Anatomy. New York, Springer-Verlag, 1976.

New, P. F. J., and Scott, W. R.: Computed Tomography of the Brain and Orbit. Baltimore, The Williams & Wilkins Co., 1975.

Ter-Pogossian, M. (ed.): Workshop on Reconstruction Tomography in Diagnostic Radiology and Nuclear Medicine: Proceedings. Baltimore, University Park Press, 1977.

Whalen, J. P.: Radiology of the Abdomen: Anatomic Basis. Philadelphia, Lea & Febiger, 1976.

*Only a few of the major references are listed here, since the student may find more extensive bibliographies within these major publications.

Index

to Computed Tomography of Brain and Whole Body